BIOCHEMICAL DISORDERS
IN HUMAN DISEASE

Biochemical Disorders in Human Disease

Edited by

R. H. S. THOMPSON

M.A., D.Sc., D.M., F.R.C.P., F.C.Path.

Courtauld Professor of Biochemistry, University of London
(Middlesex Hospital Medical School)

and

I. D. P. WOOTTON,

M.A., Ph.D., M.B., B.Chir., M.C.Path.

Professor of Chemical Pathology, University of London
(Royal Postgraduate Medical School)

THIRD EDITION

With 174 Illustrations

ACADEMIC PRESS · NEW YORK
1970

Academic Press, Inc.
111 Fifth Avenue
New York, New York 10003

Library of Congress Catalog Number 73—100993

Published simultaneously in
Great Britain by
J. & A. Churchill 104 Gloucester Place, London

Printed in Great Britain

CONTRIBUTORS

JAMES E. ASHMORE, M.S., Ph.D.
> Professor and Chairman of Pharmacology, Indiana University Medical Centre, Indianapolis.

P. M. F. BISHOP, D.M., F.R.C.P., F.R.C.O.G.
> Consultant Endocrinologist Emeritus to Guy's Hospital; Hon. Consultant Endocrinologist, Chelsea Hospital for Women.

THOMAS H. BOTHWELL, M.D.
> Tutorial Physician, University of the Witwatersrand, Johannesburg, South Africa.

G. S. BOYD, Ph.D., F.R.I.C.
> Reader, Department of Biochemistry, University of Edinburgh.

E. G. L. BYWATERS, M.B., B.S., F.R.C.P.
> Director of the Special Unit for Juvenile Rheumatism, Canadian Red Cross Memorial Hospital, Taplow, Bucks.; Consultant Physician (Rheumatism), Hammersmith Hospital; Senior Lecturer in Medicine, Royal Postgraduate Medical School, London, W.12.

I. CHANARIN, M.D., D.C.P., M.C.Path.
> Reader in Haematology, St. Mary's Hospital Medical School; Consultant Haematologist, St. Mary's Hospital, London, W.2.

R. W. CHARLTON, B.Sc., M.D., F.R.C.P.E.
> Professor of Experimental & Clinical Pharmacology, University of the Witwatersrand Medical School, Johannesburg; Senior Physician, Johannesburg Hospital.

S. COHEN, Ph.D., M.D., F.C.Path.,
> Professor of Chemical Pathology in the University of London at Guy's Hospital Medical School; Consultant Chemical Pathologist, Guy's Hospital, London, S.E.1.

J. N. CUMINGS, M.D., F.R.C.P., F.C.Path.
> Professor of Chemical Pathology in the University of London at the Institute of Neurology; Consultant Pathologist, The National Hospital for Nervous Diseases, London, W.C.1.

M. H. DRAPER, M.B., B.S., Ph.D.
> Senior Principal Scientific Officer, Agricultural Research Council Poultry Research Centre, Edinburgh; Honorary Senior Lecturer, Department of Physiology, University of Edinburgh.

RUSSELL FRASER, M.D., F.R.C.P., D.P.M.
> Professor of Clinical Endocrinology in the University of London at the Royal Postgraduate Medical School; Consultant Physician, Hammersmith Hospital, London, W.12.

vi CONTRIBUTORS

L. E. GLYNN, B.Sc., M.D., F.R.C.P., F.C.Path.
Director of the Department of Pathology, Canadian Red Cross Memorial Hospital, Taplow, Bucks.

A. H. GOWENLOCK, Ph.D., M.Sc., M.B., B.Ch., M.C.Path., F.R.I.C.
Reader in Chemical Pathology, University of Manchester; Consultant Chemical Pathologist, Manchester Royal Infirmary.

C. H. GRAY, M.D., D.Sc., F.R.C.P., F.R.I.C., F.C.Path.
Professor of Chemical Pathology in the University of London at King's College Hospital Medical School; Consultant Chemical Pathologist to the King's College Hospital Group, London, S.E.5.; Honorary Lecturer in Biochemistry, University College, London, W.C.1.

HENRY T. HOWAT, M.D., F.R.C.P.
Lecturer in Medicine, University of Manchester; Physician, Manchester Royal Infirmary.

A. E. KELLIE, D.Sc., F.R.I.C.
Professor of Steroid Biochemistry in the University of London at The Middlesex Hospital Medical School, London, W.1.

DONALD LONGSON, M.B., F.R.C.P.
Consultant Physician, Manchester Royal Infirmary, Manchester 13; Lecturer in Clinical Endocrinology, University of Manchester.

IAIN MACINTYRE, Ph.D., M.B., Ch.B., M.C.Path.
Professor of Endocrine Chemistry in the University of London at the Royal Postgraduate Medical School; Consultant in Chemical Pathology, Hammersmith Hospital, London, W.12.

NOEL F. MACLAGAN, D.Sc., M.D., F.R.C.P., F.R.I.C., F.C.Path.
Professor of Chemical Pathology in the University of London at the Westminster Medical School; Consultant Chemical Pathologist, Westminster Hospital, London, S.W.1.

R. MAHLER, B.Sc., M.B., Ch.B., F.R.C.P.
Professor of Metabolic Medicine, Welsh National School of Medicine; Honorary Consultant Physician, United Cardiff Hospitals.

W. J. MALAISSE, M.D.
Assistant Director, Laboratory of Experimental Medicine, The University, Brussels.

N. H. MARTIN, B.Sc., B.M., F.R.C.P., F.R.I.C., F.C.Path.
Professor of Chemical Pathology in the University of London at St. George's Hospital Medical School; Consultant Chemical Pathologist, St. George's Hospital, London, S.W.1.

M. D. MILNE, M.D., F.R.C.P.
Professor of Medicine in the University of London at Westminster Medical School; Consultant Physician, Westminster Hospital, London, S.W.1.

R. Passmore, M.A., D.M., F.R.S.E.
Reader in Clinical and Industrial Physiology, University of Edinburgh.

W. S. Peart, M.D., F.R.C.P., F.R.S.
Professor of Medicine in the University of London at St. Mary's Hospital Medical School; Consultant Physician, St. Mary's Hospital, London, W.2.

I. F. Sommerville, Ph.D., M.D.
Endocrinologist, Chelsea Hospital for Women; and Institute of Obstetrics and Gynaecology, London, S.W.3.

R. H. S. Thompson, M.A., D.Sc., D.M., F.R.C.P., F.C.Path.
Professor of Biochemistry in the University of London at The Middlesex Hospital Medical School; Consultant Biochemist, The Middlesex Hospital, London, W.1.

H. S. Wiggins, B.A., Ph.D.
M.R.C. Gastro-enterology Research Unit, Central Middlesex Hospital, Park Royal, N.W.10.

J. Wolff, M.D., Ph.D.
National Institute of Arthritis and Metabolic Diseases, National Institutes of Health, Department of Health, Education and Welfare, Bethesda, 14, Md.

Gunter Wolfram, M.D.
Research Assistant in Medicine, Medical Polyclinic, University of Munich.

I. D. P. Wootton, M.A., Ph.D., M.B., B.Chir., M.C.Path.
Professor of Chemical Pathology in the University of London at the Royal Postgraduate Medical School; Consultant Chemical Pathologist, Hammersmith Hospital, London, W.12.

Peter H. Wright, M.D.
Associate Professor of Pharmacology, Indiana University Medical Centre, Indianapolis.

O. M. Wrong, D.M., F.R.C.P.,
Professor of Medicine, University of Dundee; Consultant Physician, Dundee Royal Infirmary.

Kenneth L. Zierler, A.B., M.D.
Professor of Medicine, The Johns Hopkins University; Physician, The Johns Hopkins Hospital, Baltimore 5.

Nepomuk Zöllner, M.D.
Associate Professor of Internal Medicine; Leitender Oberarzt, Medical Polyclinic, University of Munich.

PREFACE TO THE THIRD EDITION

FIVE years have now elapsed since the publication of the second edition of this book, and the further advances that have taken place during this time in our knowledge of the biochemical abnormalities in disease, and the biochemical factors concerned in the newer methods of treatment, have continued unabated. It seemed therefore that the time was ripe for a further revision of this field of knowledge.

Although we have adhered to the general approach adopted in the earlier editions, individual authors have been invited to deal with their topics in such a way as to include recent developments without, if possible, unduly increasing the overall length of their contribution. It has therefore not been an easy task, and we are grateful to the authors not only for agreeing to revise their chapters, but also for their ready understanding of what was wanted from them. Our thanks are also due to those authors who have collaborated with us for the first time in this edition. Because of the recent striking advances in our knowledge of the genetic code and of the factors concerned in cell division, growth and development we have thought it desirable to include in this edition a chapter on the biochemistry of neoplastic disease.

We also wish to acknowledge with gratitude the help provided by Mr. W. Hill, Librarian, Guy's Hospital Medical School, who has again prepared the index to this book, and by Miss Rosemary Tilden who has surveyed the lists of references for each chapter, and for her help in reading the proofs. Lastly, we wish to mention the help and unfailing co-operation which we have received from our publishers, Messrs. J. & A. Churchill, Ltd., of London, and the Academic Press, Inc., of New York.

R. H. S. THOMPSON
I. D. P. WOOTTON

November 1969

CONTENTS

Chapter 1

THE CHEMICAL ANATOMY OF THE HUMAN BODY

by

R. PASSMORE and M. H. DRAPER

Physiology Department, Edinburgh University
and the Agricultural Research Council, Poultry Research Centre, Edinburgh

AMONGST other things, the human body is a chemical engine, continually converting the chemical energy obtained from the food into mechanical work and heat: it is also a storehouse containing reserves of fuel and of components necessary for replacing worn out parts of the engine. An inherent difficulty in studying disease processes arises because it is impossible for the chemist to separate accurately those parts of the body belonging to the engine from those that are stores. Thus muscle tissue is the main working component of the body, but it also contains important reserves of protein and of potassium (K). Adipose tissue is primarily a fuel depot, but it has an additional role as an insulator and conserver of heat, and also, as recent research has shown, in the conversion of one fuel, carbohydrate, into another, fat. Bone is primarily a supporting structure, but it is also a store of calcium (Ca) and sodium (Na). This distinction between a store and a reserve is useful. A store is a surplus of material, which can be utilized without in any way disturbing function (e.g. fat in adipose tissue). A reserve is material which may be lost in an emergency, but this loss is deleterious and must be replaced quickly if health is to be maintained (e.g. water in all tissues). However, this distinction is not always easy to make.

The chemical composition of the human body has been determined by analyses of cadavers (Widdowson, McCance & Spray, 1951; Widdowson & Dickerson, 1964). This is a cumbersome and messy procedure, and insufficient data have been collected to allow accurate statements of the range of variation of the material. However, in the last 20 years a variety of indirect methods have been used for measuring the amounts of the different chemical substances present in the living human body, particularly the use of radioisotope dilution methods (Moore, 1965). These have added greatly to our knowledge of the chemical anatomy of man, and are proving increasingly useful in clinical science.

Starvation and obesity are two well-known conditions in which the composition of the body is altered. Sixty years ago there was much public interest in professional fasting men. The effects of total deprivation of food for periods up to 30 days were studied in these men by physiologists. The results were collected together and admirably presented by Lusk (1928). The circumstances of the Second World War created an enormous interest in the more practical problem of partial starvation, as it presented in enemy-occupied countries and in prison camps. Today the interest appears to have changed and now lies in the starvation secondary to chronic gastro-intestinal disease, and to toxic starvation in patients with chronic sepsis not responding to antibiotics. It is not mere chance that the major modern textbook on the subject is by a distinguished American professor of surgery; Moore's book (1959) is certain to become a classic and is strongly recommended to all serious students and especially to those who aim at becoming surgeons.

With the increasing mechanization of industry and great improvements in transport, most of us are using our muscles less and less. This decreased expenditure of energy is not on the whole being met by a corresponding decrease in food intake; as a result, stores of fat are laid down. Obesity continues to increase in all prosperous industrialized countries and is a topic for much speculation. Little is known yet about the fundamental chemical pathology of this disequilibrium. There are also many other conditions in which there are important changes in the chemical anatomy of the body, for example the toxaemias of pregnancy.

The Chemical Composition of a Normal Man

Table 1.1 shows the chemical composition of a man, who would certainly be considered normal. The figures are rounded off and easy to remember.

TABLE 1.1

A normal chemical composition for a man weighing 65 kg.

	kg.	%
Protein	11·5	17·7
Fat	9·0	13·8
Carbohydrate	0·5	0·8
Water	40·0	61·6
Minerals	4·0	6·1

It would be impossible and unprofitable to describe an average man, giving a mean composition with all the usual statistical adjuvances. Physiologists have always needed a normal man and traditionally he has weighed 70 kg. This man appears to have been born in a physiological laboratory in Germany in the nineteenth century. He comes of large stock and has been well fed and is much bigger than the majority of the male citizens of the world. Our 65 kg. man is certainly more representative of his species. Table 1.1 would also describe a normal healthy woman, albeit a somewhat large and lean specimen. The differences in body composition of men and women will be discussed later.

Before going on to describe how the data in Table 1.1 have been obtained and to indicate some-

thing of the range of variations, we record how the total weight of the body might be distributed amongst the different organs. Table 1.2 shows a list of weights of organs, which can be considered normal, but, of course, there are considerable

TABLE 1.2

A normal size for the organs of a man weighing 65 kg.

	kg.	%
Skeletal muscle	30	46
Skeleton	10	15
Skin and subcutaneous adipose tissue	9	14
Blood	5·5	8·5
Gastro-intestinal tract	3·0	4·6
Liver	1·5	2·3
Brain	1·4	2·2
Lungs	1·0	1·5
Heart	0·35	0·54
Kidneys	0·30	0·46
Spleen	0·15	0·23
Bladder	0·15	0·23
Remainder	2·65	4·44
Total	65·0	100

variations. It is not always realized how much of the body is skeletal muscle. Skeletal muscle, the skeleton and skin and subcutaneous tissue may make up 75% of body weight.

Body Water

Reliable estimations of the total body water can be made using the dilution technique. This depends upon the fact that if a known quantity (Q) of a substance is dissolved in an unknown volume (V) of fluid, in which it is freely diffusible, and subsequently the concentration (C) of the substance in the solution determined, then the volume of the fluid can be calculated from the equation:

$$V = Q/C.$$

There are a number of substances, such as deuterium, urea and the drugs antipyrine and amino-antipyrine, which appear to diffuse evenly throughout all the water in the tissues of the body. These substances can be used to measure body water by the dilution technique. A known amount of the substance is given by mouth or intravenous injection. After an interval of time to allow for alimentary absorption and diffusion throughout the body, a sample of venous blood is taken and the concentration of the test substance in the serum estimated. Then the size of the "space" occupied by the substance in the body can be calculated. This "space" equals the total body water, provided the assumption that the substance is evenly distributed throughout all the body water is justified. Corrections to the amount of substance given have to be made to allow for losses in excretion and metabolism and, in the case of urea, for endogenous production. Practical details can be found in the following papers: for deuterium (Solomon, Edelman & Soloway, 1950), for urea (McCance & Widdowson, 1951), for antipyrine (Soberman, Brodie, Levy, Axelrod, Hollander & Steele, 1949), and for amino-antipyrine (Huckabee, 1956) and for tritium (Liebman, Gotch & Edelman, 1960).

If facilities for estimations are available, then deuterium is the simplest and most reliable substance to use. The urea, antipyrine and amino-antipyrine methods require only routine laboratory equipment. The urea method is perhaps the least reliable, because of the added complication of having to allow for endogenous production.

In our normal man (Table 1.1) the total body water is given as 40 l. or 61·5% of the body weight. The body water can vary from 50 to 70% of body weight in health depending on how fat the subject is. The former figure would be found in a well-covered person and the latter in a very thin one. This will be discussed further in the succeeding two sections.

Age and body water. The percentage of water in the body falls with age (McCance & Widdowson, 1951). The water content of the foetus is high and may be as much as 85%. In the full-term new-born infant the body water is usually between 75 and 80% of body weight. Muscle cells of the new-born contain 90% water, whereas at maturity they contain about 75% water (Widdowson & Dickerson, 1964). In early infancy there is a rapid fall and at the age of 6 months the child has reached or is rapidly approaching the adult figure of about 60%. There is a slight indication that this drying up of the tissues with age, which is a marked feature of foetal life and early infancy, may continue throughout a healthy life at a very slow rate. It is certainly unusual to meet anyone of 90 years or more who has not obviously shrivelled, as has been well described by Charles Dickens (1867): "Anyone may pass, any day, in the thronged thoroughfares of the metropolis, some meagre, wrinkled, yellow old man . . . This old man is always a little old man. If he were ever a big old man, he has shrunk into a little old man; if he were always a little old man, he has dwindled into a less old man." Plethoric people are reputed to be short lived. Perhaps the key to a long and happy life is the ability to dry up slowly and gracefully.

Body Fat

Density measurements. A fat man floats in water more easily than a thin one. If a man is weighed first in air and then under water, his density can be measured. A description of the necessary tank and equipment is given by Brožek, Henschel & Keys (1949). The procedure is simple and also pleasant for the subject (we write from personal experience) and it is surprising that the method has not been more used.

TABLE 1.3

Some values for the amount of fat present in the human body obtained by underwater weighing

City	Age	Fat as a percentage of body weight		Reference
		Mean	Range	
Men—				
Edinburgh . .	18–22	11	5–27	Macmillan *et al.* (1965)
Tokyo . .	22	12	6–22	Arimoto (1963)
Minnesota . .	25	14	...	Keys (1955)
Minnesota . .	55	26	...	Keys (1955)
Women—				
Edinburgh . .	18–22	26	18–35	Macmillan *et al.* (1965)
New York State .	16–30	29	20–38	Young *et al.* (1963)
Tokyo . .	21	23	13–33	Arimoto (1963)
Minnesota . .	24	25	...	Keys (1955)
New York State .	50–60	42	29–55	Young *et al.* (1963)
Minnesota . .	56	38	...	Keys (1955)

The calculation of the body fat depends on the following considerations. The density of samples of human fat has been accurately measured (Keys & Brožek, 1953) and ranges from 0·898 to 0·901, so there is little variation. The density of the fat-free human body cannot be measured and is usually assumed to be 1·10. The figure will vary according to the size and density of the bony skeleton and also to the proportion of water present. If the density of fat is taken as 0·90 and of the fat-free body as 1·10, it is easy to construct a table giving the proportion of fat in a body of known density. Normal values for the density of men and women are given in Table 1.3.

In calculating the density, it is necessary to allow for the buoyancy given by the residual air in the lungs when the subject is submerged. This is of the order of 1 to 2 l. and may vary greatly. The volume of this air must be measured by a washout procedure immediately the subject comes up from the water. The volume of gas present in the alimentary canal at any one time is normally small (less than 200 ml.) and may be neglected.

A more sophisticated method has been developed whereby the greater solubility of an isotope of krypton (^{85}Kr) in fat than water is utilized. In careful hands this has given satisfactory results (Hytten, Taylor & Taggart, 1966).

The normal fat content of the body. The citizens of Minneapolis were the first to be weighed underwater in sufficient numbers to allow calculations of the normal fat content of the body and Table 1.3 shows the results and those of later studies. A fat content of 14% is certainly normal for a healthy young male and on average young ladies are plumper than this. The increased fat content of the older men and women is a measure of their middle-age spread.

Measurements of subcutaneous fat. A simpler and more rapid method of assessing body fat than underwater weighing would obviously be useful. A variety of calipers have been constructed for measuring the thickness of subcutaneous tissues. Edwards, Hammond, Healy, Tanner & Whitehouse (1955) have designed suitable calipers which have been widely used in Britain. They describe their use and discuss their reliability. Brožek & Keys (1951), using calipers of a different design, have made simultaneous measurements of skin fold thickness and body density. They publish regression equations giving the relation of body density to skin-fold thickness at various sites. There is no doubt that in suitable hands calipers can give measurements which are a useful index of body fat. Their correct use needs great care, if consistent results are to be obtained.

Tables giving the percentage of fat in the whole body for a given skin fold thickness are available. (Durnin & Rahaman, 1967).

Lean Body Mass

If the total body fat has been determined by underwater weighing, then a calculation of the lean body mass can be made.

$$\text{Lean body mass} = \text{total body weight} - \text{total body fat.}$$

Lean body mass can also be calculated from a measurement of total body water. Analyses of human carcasses indicate that in health the fat-free human body contains between 69 and 74% of water (Keys & Brožek, 1953), which is the approximate water content of carcasses of animals from which all visible fat has been stripped (Pace & Rathbun, 1945). Then,

$$\text{lean body mass} = \text{total body water} \times \frac{100}{70}.$$

The accuracy of such assessments depends on the reliability of the figure 70 taken as the percentage of water. It is unlikely to be out by more than 5%.

Calculations of lean body mass based on simultaneous measurements of body density and total body water agree remarkably well (Osserman, Pitts, Welham & Behnke, 1950). As the methods are completely independent, this agreement gives confidence in both. Nevertheless the assumptions necessary (the arbitrary figures which must be chosen for the density and water content of the lean body mass) preclude either method from ever being very precise. In general these methods do not permit accurate analyses of the chemical nature of small changes in body weight, such as may occur over a period of a few days.

A new method for the indirect determination of the lean body mass and hence of the body fat is based on the fact that there is a natural isotope of potassium, ^{40}K, which is present in a fixed proportion (0·0118%) of all K found in the body. The total ^{40}K content of a living man can be measured (Forbes, Gallup & Kursh, 1961), though the large counting chamber necessary is very expensive. From the total ^{40}K content of the body, the total K can then be calculated. The lean body mass has a constant K content, about 68 m-equiv./kg. In this way measurements of ^{40}K provide a theoretically simple, but in practice expensive, means of determining lean body mass.

Extracellular Fluid

A number of substances, inulin, sucrose, mannitol, Na thiocyanate and the ions $SO_4^=$, ^{82}Br$^-$ and

^{24}Na$^+$, if injected into the body, occupy a "space" or volume of fluid which is of approximately the same size and much less than the deuterium "space" or total body water. It is known that these substances either do not cross the cell membranes and enter the cells, or only do so in small amounts. In consequence the "space" which they occupy is used as a measure of the extracellular fluids. In our normal man the extracellular fluid volume is 15 l. or 23% of body weight.

This percentage of the body weight, attributable to the extracellular fluid, is slightly higher than figures often given by American writers. Thus Moore (1959) states that normal values for extracellular fluid, as determined with thiocyanate or radioactive Na, fall between 15 and 20% of body weight. This difference from our man probably arises because Americans tend to have more fat. On p. 417 of his book, Moore gives the composition of a normal man aged 30 years and weighing 70 kg. The measured total body water is 39·8 l. and the measured extracellular fluid is 16·4 l. Thus, this healthy American citizen closely resembles our hypothetical normal man, except that he is heavier by 5 kg. of extra fat. At the present time, it is quite impossible to set accurate limits for the size of the extracellular fluid volume in health.

Whereas there is good agreement between the values obtained for total body water using the substances mentioned on p. 2, there is no similar agreement between the values obtained for the extracellular fluid volume by the different methods. Na thiocyanate and ^{24}Na$^+$ give consistently higher values in the same subjects than do inulin, sucrose and mannitol (Schwartz, Schachter & Freinkel, 1949). Values obtained with SO$_4$= and Br$^-$ are usually intermediate. Gamble, Robertson, Hannigan, Forster & Farr (1953) found that the Na space was consistently greater than the sucrose space by about 5 l. The low values with the carbohydrates are probably due to their inability to penetrate fully into the water in the connective tissues and especially into the tendons. Na ions are known to be able to penetrate into the cells to a small extent and hence the ^{24}Na$^+$ space may be expected to be a little larger than the true extracellular fluid volume. Thus it can be appreciated that no molecule has the ideal properties necessary for the accurate definition of a space, which can be accepted as representing truly the extracellular fluids. The thiocyanate space is easily determined (Lavietes, Bourdillon & Klinghoffer, 1936) and has perhaps been more used than any of the other measures.

The plasma volume. The extracellular fluid is composed of two parts, an intravascular portion, which is the blood plasma, and an extravascular portion which is the true interstitial fluid actually in contact with the cells. The plasma volume can be measured by the dilution technique using the dye Evans blue (Gregersen, 1944). This dye after intravenous injection is attached to the plasma albumin and so leaves the circulation slowly; its concentration in the plasma is easily determined, so that it is a convenient substance for measuring plasma volume. Serum albumin labelled with ^{131}I is also sometimes used for measuring plasma volume.

Some serum albumin is always slowly passing across the capillary walls and so the use of this substance, labelled either with Evans blue or with ^{131}I, may give a high value for the plasma volume. As the rate of diffusion of the label throughout the plasma is rapid, the venous sample for measurement of dye concentration can be taken within a few minutes of injection. In this time, in health, an insignificant proportion of the labelled albumin will have passed out of the circulation. However, if the capillary permeability is greatly increased, as may happen after burns, traumatic shock and in severe septic conditions, the labelled protein may leave the circulation so rapidly as to invalidate its use for measuring plasma volume. In such circumstances, if a measure of plasma volume is required, it is necessary to use the more complicated methods based on labelling the red cells with isotopic chromium, iron or phosphorus, and so determining their volume (Sterling & Gray, 1950); with this and the haematocrit value of the blood the plasma volume can be calculated.

A normal figure for the plasma volume is 3 l., leaving 12 l. as the value for the interstitial fluid.

Water in the alimentary canal. A normal intake of water with the fluids drunk and in the food is about 2·5 l./day. In addition water to the extent of about 8 l./day is passed into the alimentary canal in the secretions of the various digestive glands. This water is rapidly absorbed, and almost completely, for faecal water is usually less than 100 ml./day. There is no satisfactory method of estimating how much water is present in the alimentary canal of man at any one time. Gotch, Nadell & Edelman (1957) measured the water present in the alimentary tract in 13 subjects at post-mortem and found the average amount was 407 ml. (range 164–843). In health the amount is probably small, but in various gastro-intestinal diseases large quantities of water may be present in the gut and subsequently lost in the faeces or vomit. In this way the extracellular fluid can be severely depleted.

Transcellular water. The division of total body water into extracellular water and intracellular water is an over-simplification. In a healthy subject there is also the small quantity of cerebrospinal fluid, ocular fluid and fluid in joints and serous cavities. These have been formed from the extracellular fluid by passage across cells, and so they are sometimes known collectively as *transcellular water*. In disease large accumulations of transcellular water can appear, for example, in the peritoneal and pleural cavities. This water is removed from the extracellular fluid and is sometimes described as *sequestrated fluid*, because it is effectively lost to the body. In such cases it is important to realize that the extracellular fluid must be replenished by the amount of the sequestrated fluid.

Oedema. In oedema, either generalized or local, the extracellular fluid volume increases and oedema fluid may amount to many litres. With the water retention, there is also marked Na retention (see below). Pitting oedema in the legs does not occur until the amount of collected tissue fluid has increased the limb volume by 8% (Drury & Jones, 1927). This clinical sign is therefore an insensitive test for an increased extracellular fluid volume. Probably this must be increased by at least 2 l. before generalized oedema can be detected clinically.

Dehydration. A rapid reduction of body water by 2 l. will make the subject feel very thirsty and uncomfortable; the dehydration is usually obvious to an observer. With a loss of 4 l. the subject is seriously ill, and few survive a loss as great as 8 l. of body water. In mild dehydration the water lost is probably all extracellular; when it is severe, the cells will also give up some water.

The obligatory water loss from the body is about one litre a day, of which 400 ml. will be in the urine and 800 ml. from the skin and lungs, against which 200 ml. of metabolic water may be set. This minimum loss is reached only under the best possible conditions, for example at rest in a temperate climate on a diet low in protein and salt. It must be remembered that a seriously ill patient in a hospital must lose at least this amount of water daily. In the tropics, or if the patient has fever, the loss will be much greater. A man might be expected to survive 4 to 8 days without water, provided sweat losses were at a minimum. In a hot desert, the survival time would be much less, as is well known.

Man, like other animals, has no true store of water. The 4 to 8 l. which may be lost might be considered a reserve, which can be spared in an emergency, but only at the expense of much discomfort and loss of working ability. It was an old military fallacy that men could be trained to withstand a reduced water intake. This is not possible. The human body cannot adapt to a lowered water content, nor can the obligatory water losses be lowered. Training and discipline can, of course, teach men and women how to husband a limited water supply, but this is not a physiological problem.

Active Cell Mass

Active cell mass may be defined by the equation

cell mass = total body weight − body fat − extracellular fluid − skeletal minerals.

The first three factors on the right can be measured and for the fourth an intelligent guess must suffice. In our normal man

$$\text{cell mass} = 65 - 9 - 15 - 4$$
$$= 36 \text{ kg. or } 55 \cdot 4\% \text{ of body weight.}$$

Alternatively we may calculate the cell water

cell water = total body water − extracellular water.

In our man the cell water is 25 kg. Then, if it be assumed that the average water content of the cells is 70%,

$$\text{cell mass} = \text{cell water} \times \frac{100}{70}.$$

Calculated in this way, the cell mass of our man is 35·7 kg.

The figure of 70% for the water content of the cells can only be an approximation. It is not yet practicable to analyse human cells directly except the blood corpuscles. The composition of cells can only be calculated after first analysing whole tissue and also determining the extracellular fluid volume of the tissue. Knowing the amount and composition of a sample of tissue and also of the extracellular fluid within it, the composition of the cells can be obtained by subtraction.

About three quarters of the cell mass is made up of muscle cells. Muscle tissue has frequently been analysed, and in adult human muscle the water content has seldom been found to differ significantly from 80% (Widdowson & Dickerson, 1964). The chloride space of human muscle tissue is about 18%. Thus 18% of muscle weight can be attributed to extracellular fluid. This means that human muscle cells contain about 75% water. However, the cells of some other tissues contain less than 70% water. This is certainly true for red blood cells, probably true for connective tissue (Manery, 1954) and possibly for brain cells.

Accurate information about the water content of cells is needed and would be most useful.

Calculations of the active cell mass are frequently made by those engaged on research into metabolic disorders of man. They are seldom either practical or necessary for the physician or surgeon. Nevertheless, the concept is useful to the practising doctor.

Body composition and therapeutics. Body weight is often used as a measure of body size both in medicine and in physiology. With the introduction of many powerful new drugs, increased precision in dosage is necessary. It is becoming common to see the recommended dose for a new drug expressed in units/kg. of body weight. This is sound provided the patient has a normal body composition, but may lead to serious error in the very fat and the very thin or in the oedematous or dehydrated patient. The danger is especially real in the very young. Many anaesthetics and some sedatives are soluble in lipids and large doses may be needed for the obese; correspondingly the thin and wasted will need relatively less, even on a weight basis.

The weighing machine may thus give quite a false impression of the amount of protoplasmic material, which the doctor is trying to influence by treatment, because the active tissue may be diluted by such varying amounts of lipid and water. In practice, these considerations can nearly always be met by an intelligent clinical appraisal of body composition without resort to laboratory analyses. Daily measurements of body weight are most useful as an index of changes in body composition, especially when oedema is present.

Body composition and the basal metabolic rate. Traditionally this is expressed in units of surface area. This is because the metabolism of animals as diverse as the mouse, the rabbit, the dog, man and the horse proceeds at approximately the same rate when expressed per unit of surface area (Rubner's Law). Expressed per unit of body weight the smaller animals have a much higher metabolism, but with increasing size the ratio of surface to weight is much reduced. However, it is very doubtful if surface area is a valid means for expressing differences of metabolism within members of the same species. There is no doubt that the statement that women have a basal metabolic rate some 10% lower than men, which has been reported by many observers, is correct—provided the results are given in terms of surface area. This is not due to women having a metabolism more economical than man in some mysterious way, but to the simple fact that women, as a sex, are fatter (Table 1.3). If basal metabolism is expressed in

terms of active tissue, cell mass or lean body mass, the sex difference disappears. A good discussion of the relation of basal metabolism to body composition is given by Behnke (1953) and some detailed experimental observations by Wedgwood, Bass, Klimas, Kleeman & Quinn (1953) and by Macmillan, Reid, Shirling & Passmore (1965).

Electrolytes in the Body Fluids

Table 1.4 gives a list of concentrations of the principal electrolytes in the extracellular fluid and in the cell water. It is easy to obtain a sample of plasma for analysis, and for all practical purposes the concentration of the principal ions in the

TABLE 1.4

The distribution of ions in the intracellular water and in the extracellular fluid in a normal man (m-equiv./l.)

Cations	Intracellular	Extracellular
Na$^+$	10	145
K$^+$	150	5
Ca^{2+}	2	2
Mg^{2+}	15	2
	177	154
Anions		
Cl$^-$	10	100
PO$_4^{3-}$	90	2
HCO$_3^-$	10	27
SO$_4^{2-}$	15	1
Organic acid	—	5
Protein	52	19
	177	154

plasma is identical with their concentration in the rest of the extracellular fluid. (The greater concentration of protein in the plasma has a small effect on the ionic distribution.) A great deal is now known about the effect of metabolic disturbances on the plasma electrolytes and this knowledge is of increasing value in therapeutics.

The values given in Table 1.4 for the principal ions in plasma are reliable figures which might be expected in a normal man. There are some doubts as to the state of ionization of the Mg and Ca in the plasma (for Ca it is about 50%): there are further doubts about the state of ionization of the PO$_4$ and protein present. Indeed the figure for protein has been calculated so as to make up the balance sheet for a neutral solution.

As samples of cell water for analysis cannot be obtained, the electrolyte content of the cells can only be determined indirectly. The calculated cell concentrations given in Table 1.4 are thus much less reliable than the direct analyses of plasma, but they are certainly of the right order. Very little is known about the form of the Mg and Ca in the cells; the PO_4 content of cells may well vary considerably with their metabolic activity. The figures in Table 1.4 merely give some guidance as to the order of magnitude of the common ions in cells; unfortunately, at present our knowledge of intracellular ionic concentrations is too vague to be of clinical value.

Sodium. In the great majority of people in health the level of plasma Na lies between 140 and 150 m-equiv./l. A figure of 136 or lower is strongly suggestive of a disturbance of normal levels, which may be serious.

In a hot climate, where there can be large losses of Na in the sweat and where the dietary intake of salt may be low, a primary Na deficiency often gives rise to plasma levels of around 130. Similarly in Addison's disease there is excessive loss of Na. Here it is in the urine and arises from a failure of reabsorption in the renal tubules due to a lack of adequate aldosterone secretion; plasma levels may be around 130 and indicate an overall deficiency of Na.

In temperate climates, a low plasma Na is seldom so simply explained in this way. It is more likely to occur in a situation (e.g. the presence of cardiac oedema or ascites and liver cirrhosis), where the total amount of Na in the body is increased, but so also is the extracellular fluid volume: with a failure of osmotic control, the extracellular fluid may become diluted with a fall in plasma Na concentration. Thus, in practice the interpretation of a low serum Na is often difficult. Ideally we would want to know, in addition to the extracellular Na concentration, the intracellular Na concentration and the total amount of Na in the body. Fortunately, although little is known about intracellular Na concentrations in health and disease, it is possible to get a measure of the total available in the body.

From Tables 1.1 and 1.4 it can be calculated that the total Na content of the extracellular fluid and the cells is 2425 m-equiv. Using radioactive Na the total exchangeable Na in the body can be measured; Miller & Wilson (1953) found values ranging up to 3140 m-equiv. The total exchangeable Na is less than the total Na in the tissues because there is some Na bound without water in the mineral skeleton. Most of the Na in bone is in a form which does not exchange with the circulating ion, but about a quarter is exchangeable. This may amount to 1000 m-equiv.

This exchangeable Na in bone may be considered as a store which can be drawn on in an emergency. In relation to possible needs, it is not large: moderately severe sweating (6 l./day at 50 m-equiv./l.) could lead to daily losses of Na of over 300 m-equiv. A dietary intake of more than 150 m-equiv./day is unusual. The kidneys in health conserve the body's Na very effectively, and a urine which is almost Na-free can be formed. Nevertheless, the reserves in bone could only meet the losses incurred in severe sweating for a few days. As is well known, such circumstances rapidly lead to evidence of Na deficiency, unless salt is added to the diet.

Potassium. The cells contain 3500 m-equiv. or more of K, whereas the extracellular fluid contains less than 100. In health the plasma level usually lies between 4·0 and 5·0 m-equiv./l. There is no appreciable store in the bones. Muscle cells contain about four-fifths of all the K in the body.

As K is present in all cells, both vegetable and animal, all unprocessed foods contain the element and all ordinary diets provide ample amounts (50–150 m-equiv./day). A primary dietary deficiency of K never arises.

As sweat contains 5–10 m-equiv./l. of K, losses by this route are seldom significant.

Losses of K from the gastro-intestinal tract may be large. Diseases of the intestinal tract associated with diarrhoea or vomiting, whether acute or chronic, frequently lead to K deficiency. The gastro-intestinal secretions, especially saliva, gastric juice and intestinal juice, contain important amounts (Kruhøffer & Thaysen, 1960). The normal daily secretion into the intestinal canal is large and probably amounts to 8 l. of fluid. This will contain up to 100 m-equiv. of K. In health this is almost all reabsorbed; the daily output in the faeces is 10 m-equiv., or even less. However, as much as 200 m-equiv./day can be lost from the body in severe diarrhoea or vomiting. Diarrhoea and vomiting are always associated with partial or complete starvation: this leads to a breakdown of cell protein and increased renal excretion of nitrogen. With this breakdown there is also loss of K from the cells, which is excreted in the urine.

The chief clinical features of K deficiency are muscular weakness and mental apathy. These, of course, are not specific and may easily be overlooked in a patient with severe gastro-intestinal disease. The heart muscle is affected along with the other muscles and electrocardiographic changes may assist in the early diagnosis.

Reserves of K are small. Subjects on an artificial low-K diet lost initially 20 to 40 m-equiv./day in the urine (Moore, Boling, Ditmore, Sicular,

Teterick, Ellison, Hoye & Ball, 1955). When the total losses amounted to 200 to 300 m-equiv., evidence of K deficiency began to appear. This loss of some 6 to 10% of the total body K could occur in 1 to 2 days with acute intestinal disease. It is important to realize that normally the kidneys do not conserve K to a significant extent, and renal losses will be added to alimentary losses. However, after about a week on artificially low-K diets, renal adaptation may occur, and as little as 1 m-equiv./day may be lost in the urine. If vomiting is present, the loss of the Cl ions will cause a metabolic alkalosis. This reduces the effective reserve of K in the cells, and evidence of deficiency may arise after a loss of only 100 m-equiv. (Moore et al. 1955).

Chronic diarrhoea, caused either by disease or the misuse of purgatives, will also lead to K deficiency. Here, however, adaptive changes may occur. Renal losses will be low and the plasma level can fall to 2 m-equiv./l., which would be fatal in an acute condition, without serious consequences (Schwartz & Relman, 1953).

Wasting diseases of all types are associated with loss of K. If cell protein is being utilized as a source of energy, then the cells shrink and K is lost. Analyses of human muscle tissue showed that in 1 kg. there were 92·2 m-equiv. of K and 30·8 g. of N (Dickerson & Widdowson, 1960). The ratio of K/N is 3·0 m-equiv./g. Balance studies show that K and N are lost from the body in approximately this ratio when there is tissue wasting, e.g. in obese patients on a strict reducing regimen (Passmore, Strong & Ritchie, 1958), though there are wide individual variations. In tissue wasting associated with the metabolic response to injury, K losses may be high and a K/N ratio up to 10 has been found (Howard, 1955). When tissue is being laid down, as in convalescence, positive balances of K and N in a ratio of about 3·0 can be observed. In such circumstances, if the patient can eat a good mixed diet and can digest and absorb it, the extra K required by the tissues will be provided therein.

Plasma K levels do not necessarily reflect accurately the level of K in the cells and so are an uncertain diagnostic guide. Thus, in uncontrolled diabetes, the tissue wasting may cause large losses of cell K, yet the plasma level may be raised above the normal. The total amount of K in the extracellular fluids is only about $\frac{1}{40}$ of the amount in the cells. A sudden outpouring of less than 0·5% of the K in the cells could raise the concentration in the plasma by 20% (from 5 to 6 m-equiv./l.) in the absence of a rapid excretory response by the kidneys. Acidosis and other factors may com-

plicate the situation in diabetes. Thus a high plasma value may be present when the cells are seriously depleted. A low level in the plasma, 3·5 m-equiv. or less, is always indicative of an overall deficiency, but is not a good measure either of its extent or of the consequent danger to the patient.

Finally, K deficiency is particularly important in gastro-intestinal disease of infancy and early childhood; it is certainly a common contributory cause of death in kwashiorkor.

Calcium. The total content of Ca in the body is about 1·2 kg. or 60,000 m-equiv. Relative to Na, this is a very large amount, but the vast majority of it is incorporated in the skeleton. The quantity in the extracellular fluid is about 40 m-equiv., and the amount in the cells is probably not very much greater. The concentration in the plasma is 5 m-equiv./l., but about half of this is bound to the proteins and hence will not equilibrate with the extracellular fluid. Of the remainder, most is in the ionized form. Very little is known about the intracellular form of the Ca, and the great influence of the extracellular Ca depends on the concentration of the ionized form of the Ca and not the overall Ca concentration, which remains remarkably constant at 10 mg./100 ml. or 5 m-equiv./l. Ca metabolism is fully discussed in Chapter 22.

Magnesium. The body of an adult contains about 30 g. of this metal, most of which is found in the bones. The concentration in the plasma is 1·5 to 2 m-equiv./l., of which perhaps a third is bound to protein. The concentration in cells is much higher, about 15 m-equiv./l. Inside the cells, the metal appears to be concentrated within the mitochondria, and it is an essential part of many enzyme systems responsible for the transfer of energy.

The daily intake of Mg in the diet normally lies between 200 and 400 mg./day (17–34 m-equiv.) and a primary dietary deficiency seldom, if ever, occurs in man, though it is well known in cattle. In man, Mg deficiency arises when there are excessive losses from the gastro-intestinal tract, from chronic diarrhoea or an ileal fistula. Until recently the condition has been generally overlooked, largely because it is nearly always associated with symptoms of other deficiencies, e.g. of K and Ca. The principal clinical features have been described by Hanna, Harrison, MacIntyre & Frazer (1960), and are depression, muscular weakness, vertigo and liability to convulsions. If these are present in any patient who has had chronic diarrhoea, Mg deficiency may be suspected, and the suspicion is strengthened if the plasma level is below 1·5 m-equiv./l. and the electrocardiograph shows low voltages. The diagnosis can be confirmed if giving Mg intravenously (100–200 m-equiv. over 4 hours) produces a prompt clinical improvement. Mg deficiency has been shown to be present in many children with kwashiorkor (Montgomery, 1961).

With large-scale electrolyte replacements becoming increasingly important, especially with the growing use of the artificial kidney, maintaining the Mg levels in cells and plasma is becoming a practical problem. The new method of estimating Mg in micro quantities in biological materials using the atomic absorption spectrometer greatly facilitates the control of Mg levels in body fluids.

Anions. The chief anions in the extracellular fluid are Cl^- and HCO_3^-. The important role of these ions in the regulation of the acid-base balance of the body is well known. The chief anion in the cells is phosphate. Very little is known about variations in the concentration of this and other anions in the cells, either in health or disease. This is due largely to the difficulty of estimations of cell contents.

Dynamic Considerations

The cells of the various tissues of the body are seldom in direct contact with a capillary wall, as can easily be seen under the light microscope. The gap between the cells and the capillaries seen under the microscope is not an empty space, but in life is occupied by an extracellular fluid, which can flow freely around the cells. It is filled by a variety of intercellular substances, some of which are formed into well-defined fibres—the collagen, reticular and elastic fibres. These materials and a ground substance containing mucopolysaccharides provide a structure through which water, electrolytes and nutrients do not diffuse as freely and rapidly as in simple solution. Intercellular substances may bind water and electrolytes, and so modify their free movements. However, they do not prevent movement, for there are continuous rapid fluxes of water and ions across both the cell membranes and the capillary walls. With the aid of isotopic techniques, it has been possible to measure some of these fluxes in the whole animal and in isolated animal tissues. An idea of the speed of turnover of substances between the various water compartments of the body can be gained from the time taken for an injected quantity of isotope to reach equilibrium in the intact human. Thus ^{42}K, ^{24}Na and deuterium oxide reach equilibrium in about 30, 16 and 4 hours respectively (O'Meara,

Birkenfeld, Gotch & Edelman, 1957). It is likely that in a vascular tissue such as muscle equilibrium is reached in about one-third of the above times. So far, the fluxes of ions across the cell-membrane have been studied extensively only in the squid nerve and frog striated muscle (Hodgkin, 1957). In single frog muscle fibres the average influx and efflux of Na was found to be about 4×10^{-12} mole/cm.^{2}/sec., and the average K influx about 5×10^{-12} mole/cm.^{2}/sec. (Hodgkin & Horowicz, 1959). The significance of these figures becomes apparent when it is realized that if the K influx stopped, a typical muscle would lose about 25% of its K in four hours. In warm-blooded animals the fluxes are greater. In the rat diaphragm, for example, about 40% of the K is exchanged in 30 min. (Creese, Hashish & Scholes, 1958). So far it has been difficult to get consistent measurements of fluxes in warm-blooded animals. Thus, it is impossible to calculate, with precision, the extent of these fluxes in the human body as a whole. However, it would seem probable that hundreds of litres of water enter and leave the intercellular spaces each day and also several kilograms of salts. The intercellular spaces are certainly not static, but are filled with material which is being changed constantly and rapidly. The capillary walls and the cell membranes provide barriers, which some substances may cross readily and others may find insurmountable or can only pass infrequently.

The capillary wall. This is freely permeable to water and dissolved substances of low molecular weight. Large molecules (e.g. plasma albumin) do not pass across freely, but they are not completely retained within the capillaries, for small amounts of plasma proteins can always be found in lymph draining the tissues. Even large structures such as a white blood corpuscle can occasionally pass through the wall and in some circumstances (e.g. acute inflammation) they can pass in very large numbers.

Some of the forces which drive fluids across the capillary walls were first described over 70 years ago by Starling (1895). He postulated that fluid movements were determined by the balance between hydrostatic pressure within the vessel tending to drive fluid out and osmotic pressure, provided by the plasma proteins, tending to draw it in. This simple model still provides a useful first approximation as to how the capillary barrier works. Movements of fluid across the barrier are undoubtedly in part determined by considerations of hydrostatic and osmotic pressures. However, it does not provide a full explanation, for example the onset of the oedema in starvation (McCance,

1951) and in renal disease (Peters, Wakeman, Eisenman & Lee, 1929) is closely related but not precisely determined by the degree of reduction of the osmotic pressure, consequent upon the fall in level of the plasma albumin. Pappenheimer (1953) has discussed carefully the physical forces operating across the capillary wall, and has pointed out that at the dimensions of a capillary diffusion may play a dominant role in fluid exchanges.

The structure of the capillary walls has been extensively studied with the electron microscope. The old concept of junctions between the endothelial cells, which were reputed to be filled with a "cement" through which material could pass, has received little support. Vacuoles, 500–650 Å in diameter, can be seen in the cytoplasm of the cells and it is possible that these are formed at one surface of the cell, which they then cross, and are discharged at the other (pinocytosis). However, the importance of this process is not yet known. Florey (1962) gives an excellent summary, illustrated with many electron micrographs, of modern views on capillary structure.

Zweifach (1949) has emphasized that the arrangement of capillaries in a tissue is often complex and far from a simple channel from metarteriole to venule. In these situations local contractions or dilatations of the metarteriolar wall or precapillary spincter can markedly alter the balance of osmotic and hydrostatic forces in the area without any change in the systemic pressure.

The cell membranes. These present a barrier quite different from the capillary walls, for they are not only impermeable to large molecules such as proteins but they also provide an obstruction to the free passage of particles as small in radius as 3·4 Å, e.g. the hydrated Na ion. However, the smaller hydrated K and Cl ions, radius about 2·2 Å, are able to cross much more freely. Thus, as far as the cells are concerned, Na ions are osmotically effective in bringing about movements of water.

That cells maintain a high K content and yet the cell wall is freely permeable to K appears as a paradox. Certainly in nerve and muscle (Hodgkin, 1957; Ussing, 1960), and probably in all cells, portions of the cell membrane are able to combine chemically with K and Na ions. In some as yet unknown way, these ions can then be passed on from regions where the electro-chemical potential is low to regions where it is high. This involves work and the expenditure of chemical energy. Thus those Na ions, which in small numbers are continually entering the cell where they maintain an intracellular concentration of about 10mM, are

pumped uphill across the cell membrane to the extracellular fluid, where the concentration of the Na ions is about 145 mM. On the return stroke of the pump, K ions are drawn in from a region of low concentraton (4 mM) to a region of high concentration (145 mM). In this way the composition of the cells is kept constant, despite large fluxes across the membranes. When a muscle or nerve cell is active, there is a temporary and local breakdown of the membrane barrier to the passage of Na ions, which for a brief period pass freely into the cells. These ions are then actively pumped out during the recovery period. This movement of ions is responsible for the action potentials in all excitable tissues (Hodgkin, 1957).

The chemical nature of the Na pump is not yet established with certainty; but several theories have been put out (Ussing, 1960; Skou, 1965). ATP is certainly used as a source of energy for the pump, which also consumes O_2. In some tissues one molecule of O_2 has been shown to be associated with the extrusion of 4 Na ions (Conway, 1960).

O_2 is thus needed to maintain the dynamic state of chemical equilibrium between the cell fluids and the extracellular fluids. How much O_2 is needed for this purpose cannot be calculated with precision, but it is certainly a significant proportion of the total O_2 consumption of a man at rest.

Chemical Activity in the Various Organs of the Human Body

Regional blood flow. In the last 20 years techniques have become available for passing catheters into most of the large veins in a living man. In this way, samples of the venous blood draining the various organs have been withdrawn for analysis. If, in addition, samples of arterial blood are obtained, it is possible to calculate the blood flow through the organs using the Fick principle. Table 1.5 shows how a cardiac output of 5 l./min. might be distributed in a resting normal man. The references in the table each describe a study, in which measurements have been made on several healthy subjects.

The principal findings have all been confirmed in other laboratories, but the total information available does not justify the giving of averages with the appropriate ranges and standard deviations. The figures given in the Table have been selected from the authors' protocols and rounded off. There is no doubt that each represents a normal value, which might be found in a healthy man.

TABLE 1.5

Distribution of the blood flow to the principal organs in a resting normal man weighing 65 kg.

Organ	Weight (g.)	Blood flow ml./min./100 g.	Blood flow total ml./min.	Cardiac output %	Reference
Liver (including splanchnic area)	1500	100	1500	30	Myers (1947)
Brain	1400	50	700	14	Lassen (1959)
Kidneys	300	400	1200	24	Cargill (1949)
Heart	350	63	220	4·4	Bing *et al.* (1949)
Skeletal muscles	30,000	2	600	12	Mottram (1955)
Remainder (by difference)			780	15·6	Lassen *et al.* (1964)
			5000	100	

The partition of the resting metabolism. Catheterization of the large veins in man has also made possible calculations of the O_2 consumption of individual organs. If the blood flow through an organ is known and also the difference between the O_2 content of the arterial and venous blood, then the rate of O_2 utilization is easily obtained. Brožek & Grande (1955) were the first to use such data to partition the O_2 consumption of a resting adult man, and Table 1.6 is a modified version of their analysis.

The figures for the percentage distribution of the O_2 consumption in the different organs, which are given in the last column of the table, indicate the main sites of chemical activity in the body. It will be seen that the liver can justify its old reputation as "the chief chemical workshop of the body". However, the brain, resting skeletal muscle and the "remainder" are not far behind. Much of the O_2 consumption in the "remainder" is probably attributable to the chemical activities of adipose tissue, which is now known to be a metabolically active organ (see Chapter 2). The kidneys, although receiving about one-quarter of the cardiac output, utilize less than one-tenth of the total O_2. Most of this O_2 will be needed to bring about the ionic exchanges already discussed.

In a trained athlete, O_2 consumption may be increased 20 times, up to 5 l./min. Nearly all this extra O_2 is utilized by the skeletal muscles, where the metabolic rate may be increased 100-fold. There will also be a large increase in utilization by cardiac muscle. However, even when the body is at rest, the heart is working and, as Table 1.6 shows, its O_2 consumption is high. Such a high increase in O_2 consumption is only possible in the exception-

TABLE 1.6

Distribution of the oxygen utilization amongst the principal organs in a resting normal man weighing 65 kg.

Organ	Blood flow ml./min.	Arterial-venous O_2 difference ml./100 ml.	Oxygen used ml./min.	Resting metabolism %
Liver (including) splanchnic area)	1500	4·5	67	27
Brain	700	6·7	47	19
Kidneys	1200	1·4	17	7
Heart	220	12·0	26	10
Skeletal muscles	600	7·5	45	18
Remainder (by difference)			48	19
Total			250	100

(For references see Table 1.5)

ally fit. An elderly patient, or someone with a cardiac or pulmonary disability, will be able to get around and lead an ordinary quiet life, if they can raise their resting O_2 consumption four-fold. Walking at a modest pace involves O_2 expendi-

tures of around 1 l./min. This involves increases in the metabolic activity of skeletal muscles by about 15 times. Thus, in even a moderately active individual, skeletal muscle is the chief site of the body's chemical reactions.

References

ARIMOTO, K. (1963). Personal communication.

BEHNKE, A. R. (1953). *Ann. N.Y. Acad. Sci.*, **56**, 1095.

BING, R. J., HAMMOND, M. M., HANDELSMAN, J. C., POWERS, S. R., SPENCER, F. C., ECKENHOFF, J. E., GOODALE, W. T., HAFKENSCHIEL, J. H. & KETY, S. S. (1949). *Amer. Heart J.*, **38**, 1.

BROŽEK, J. & GRANDE, F. (1955). *Human Biol.*, **27**, 22.

BROŽEK, J., HENSCHEL, A. & KEYS, A. (1949). *J. appl. Physiol.*, **2**, 240.

BROŽEK, J. & KEYS, A. (1951). *Brit. J. Nutrit.*, **5**, 194.

CARGILL, W. H. (1949). *J. clin. Invest.*, **28**, 533.

CONWAY, E. J. (1960). Ciba Foundation Study Group No. 5, "Regulation of the Inorganic Ion Content of Cells". London, Churchill.

CREESE, R., HASHISH, S. E. E. & SCHOLES, N. W. (1958). *J. Physiol.*, **143**, 307.

DICKENS, C. (1867). "Little Dorrit", chapter 31. London, Chapman & Hall.

DICKERSON, J. W. T. & WIDDOWSON, E. M. (1960). *Biochem. J.*, **74**, 247.

DRURY, A. N. & JONES, N. W. (1927). *Heart*, **14**, 55.

DURNIN, J. V. G. A. & RAHARMAN, M. M. (1967). *Brit. J. Nutr.* **21**, 681.

EDWARDS, D. A. W., HAMMOND, W. H., HEALY, M. J. R., TANNER, J. M. & WHITEHOUSE, R. H. (1955). *Brit. J. Nutrit.*, **9**, 133.

FLOREY, H. W. (1962). "General Pathology", 3rd Ed., pp. 40–97. London, Lloyd-Luke.

FORBES, G. B., GALLUP, J. & HURSH, J. B. (1961). *Science*, **133**, 101.

GAMBLE, J. L., ROBERTSON, J. S., HANNIGAN, C. A., FORSTER, C. G. & FARR, L. E. (1953). *J. clin. Invest.*, **32**, 483.

GOTCH, F., NADELL, J. & EDELMAN, I. S. (1957). *J. clin. Invest.*, **36**, 289.

GREGERSEN, M. I. (1944). *J. Lab. clin. Med.*, **29**, 1266.

HANNA, S., HARRISON, M., MACINTYRE, I. & FRAZER, R. (1960). *Lancet*, **2**, 172.

HODGKIN, A. L. (1957). *Proc. roy. Soc. B.*, **148**, 1.

HODGKIN, A. L. & HOROWICZ, P. (1959). *J. Physiol.*, **145**, 405.

HOWARD, J. M. (1955). *Amer. J. clin. Nutrition*, 3, 456.

HUCKABEE, W. E. (1956). *J. appl. Physiol.*, **9**, 157.

HYTTEN, F. E., TAYLOR, K. & TAGGART, N. (1966). *Clin. Sci.* **31**, 111.

KEYS, A. (1955). "Weight Control". Ed. Eppright, E. S., Swanson, P. & Iverson, C. A. Iowa, State College Press.

KEYS, A. & BROŽEK, J. (1953). *Physiol. Rev.*, **33**, 245.

KRUHOFFER, P. & THAYSEN, J. H. (1960). *Handb. exper. Pharmakol.*, Berlin, **13**, 508.

LASSEN, N. A. (1959). *Physiol. Rev.*, **39**, 183.

LASSEN, N. A., LINDBJERG, J. & MUNCK, O. (1964). *Lancet*, **1**, 686.

LAVIETES, P. H., BOURDILLON, J. & KLINGHOFFER, K. A. (1936). *J. clin. Invest.*, **15**, 261.

LIEBMAN, J., GOTCH, F. A. & EDELMAN, I. S. (1960). *Circulation Res.*, **8**, 907.

LUSK, G. (1928). "The Science of Nutrition", 4th edition. Philadelphia, Saunders.

McCANCE, R. A. (1951). Spec. Rep. Ser. med. Res. Coun. (Lond.), No. 275.

McCANCE, R. A. & WIDDOWSON, E. M. (1951). *Proc. roy. Soc. B.*, **138**, 115.

McCANCE, R. A. & WIDDOWSON, E. M. (1961). *Brit. med. Bull.*, **17**, 132.

MACMILLAN, M. G., REID, C. M., SHIRLING, D. & PASSMORE, R. (1965). *Lancet*, **1**, 728.

MANERY, J. F. (1954). *Physiol. Rev.*, **34**, 334.

MILLER, H. & WILSON, G. M. (1953). *Clin. Sci.*, **12**, 97.

MONTGOMERY, R. D. (1961). *J. Pediatrics*, **59**, 119.

MOORE, F. D. (1959). "Metabolic Care of the Surgical Patient". Philadelphia & London, Saunders.

MOORE, F. D. (1965). "The body cell mass and its supporting environment, body composition in health and disease". Philadelphia: Saunders.

MOORE, F. D., BOLING, E. A., DITMORE, H. B., Jr., SICULAR, A., TETERICK, A. E., ELLISON, S. J., HOYE, S. J. & BALL, M. R. (1955). *Metabolism*, **4**, 379.

MOTTRAM, R. F. (1955). *J. Physiol.*, **128**, 268.

MYERS, J. D. (1947). *J. clin. Invest.*, **26**, 1130.

O'MEARA, M. P., BIRKENFELD, L. W., GOTCH, F. A. & EDELMAN, I. S. (1957). *J. clin. Invest.*, **36**, 784.

OSSERMAN, E. F., PITTS, G. C., WELHAM, W. C. & BEHNKE, A. R. (1950). *J. appl. Physiol.*, **2**, 633.

PACE, N. & RATHBUN, E. N. (1945). *J. biol. Chem.*, **158**, 685.

PAPPENHEIMER, J. R. (1953). *Physiol. Rev.*, **33**, 387.

PASSMORE, R., STRONG, J. A. & RITCHIE, F. J. (1958). *Brit. J. Nutr.*, **12**, 113.

PETERS, J. P., WAKEMAN, A. M., EISENMAN, A. J. & LEE, C. (1929). *J. clin. Invest.*, **6**, 577.

SCHWARTZ, W. B. & RELMAN, A. S. (1953). *J. clin. Invest.*, **32**, 258.

SCHWARTZ, I. L., SCHACHTER, D. & FREINKEL, D. (1949). *J. clin. Invest.*, **28**, 1117.

SKOU, J. C. (1965). *Physiol. Rev.*, **45**, 596.

SOBERMAN, R., BRODIE, B. B., LEVY, B. B., AXELROD, J., HOLLANDER, V. & STEELE, J. M. (1949). *J. biol. Chem.*, **179**, 31.

SOLOMON, A. K., EDELMAN, I. S. & SOLOWAY, S. (1950). *J. clin. Invest.*, **29**, 1311.

STARLING, E. H. (1895). *J. Physiol.*, **19**, 312.

STERLING, K. & GRAY, S. J. (1950). *J. clin. Invest.*, **29**, 1614.

USSING, H. H. (1960). *Handb. exper. Pharmakol.*, *Berlin*, **13**, 1.

WEDGWOOD, R. J., BASS, D. E., KLIMAS, J. A., KLEEMAN, C. R. & QUINN, M. (1953). *J. appl. Physiol.*, **6**, 317.

WIDDOWSON, E. M. & DICKERSON, J. W. T. (1964). In Mineral Metabolism, II, Part A." Ed. Comar & Bronner, pp. 1–247. New York & London, Academic Press.

WIDDOWSON, E. M., McCANCE, R. A. & SPRAY, C. M. (1951). *Clin. Sci.*, **10**, 113.

YOUNG, C. M., BLONDIN, J., TENSUAN, R. & FRYER, J. H. (1963). *Ann. N.Y. Acad. Sci.*, **110**, 589.

ZWEIFACH, B. W. (1949). Basic Mechanisms in Peripheral Vascular Homeostasis, Tr. 3rd Josiah Macy, Jr., Conf. on Factors Regulating Blood Pressure. New York, Macy.

Chapter 2

NUTRITIONAL DISORDERS

by

R. Passmore and M. H. Draper

Physiology Department, Edinburgh University,
and the Agricultural Research Council, Poultry Research Centre, Edinburgh

THERE are four disorders arising from dietary causes which are widespread in the world today. Protein-calorie malnutrition takes an enormous toll of the lives of young children amongst the poor in Asia, Africa, Latin America and the Caribbean. Obesity contributes to the degenerative diseases which are so prevalent amongst the prosperous people of middle age, especially in North America and Europe. Starvation is fortunately less common, but the threat of famine is very near to millions of people in Africa and Asia. Further, many diseases of the gastro-intestinal tract and chronic infections, not responding to chemotherapy and antibiotics, lead to secondary starvation, in which the clinical features and chemical pathology are indistinguishable from primary starvation arising from lack of food. The dietary iron supply is only marginally adequate to meet the needs of women during their reproductive life and in all countries many women suffer much ill health from anaemia due to iron deficiency.

The classical deficiency diseases, scurvy, rickets, beriberi, pellagra and keratomalacia, are now relatively rare and seldom arise in epidemic proportions. One or other is still found in large numbers in a few countries and in all countries isolated cases may be seen, occurring among the poorest families, and in the occasional dietary crank. Keratomalacia, which is closely associated with protein-calorie malnutrition, is the most important of these diseases, for every year as many as 20,000 young children may become permanently blind from this cause (McLaren, 1963). The prevention of this disease presents a challenge to the hearts and minds of the prosperous world, which has not yet been taken up.

Knowledge of the classical deficiency diseases has long been sufficient to allow adequate treatment and prevention. A description of these diseases is given by Davidson & Passmore (1966), together with references to the literature in chemical pathology. In this chapter we confine ourselves to an account of the chemical pathology of starvation (calorie deficiency), obesity (calorie excess), and protein-calorie malnutrition.

CALORIE DEFICIENCY

Calorie deficiency in the adult falls into two broad categories, namely starvation proper, where the dietary input of energy is insufficient to maintain life for more than a short period, and partial calorie deficiency, where the input, although limited, is sufficient to enable the person to survive indefinitely, but with a greatly changed body composition and a severely reduced ability to expend energy in physical activities. This latter state of adaptation to a limited calorie intake is the fate of many millions of people in the world today. Both complete and partial starvation have been extensively studied and there is growing knowledge of the way the body can adapt to periods of food deprivation. In man's long history famine has frequently been his lot and it is scarcely surprising that some protective mechanism against periods of food shortage are present. What is becoming all too apparent is that man is ill adapted to survive in an environment of persistent and enduring food surplus.

Stores of Energy

It is well known that a man may survive complete starvation for periods of 60 days or more. One of the longest fasts, which was well documented, was the ordeal of Terence MacSwiney, the mayor of Cork, Ireland, who died after 74 days on hunger strike. The classic work on the physiology of starvation is the monumental study "The biology of human starvation" by Keys, Brožek, Henschel, Mickelsen & Taylor (1950). An important recent review is that by Grande (1964).

As discussed in Chapter 1, a man can survive without water for only a few days. His reserves of electrolytes will only last for a similarly short time, in the face of the heavy losses that may arise from gastro-intestinal disease or from exposure to a hot, dry climate. Table 2.1 shows in contrast the large stores of energy which are available should there be any sudden reduction in his food supply, a failure to absorb nutrients due to gastro-intestinal disease or a failure to utilize nutrients due to generalized toxaemia.

Table 2.1 gives values for the stores of available energy which could be considered normal. An alternative version of this table, with slightly different interpretations has been given by Drabkin (1959). The exhaustion times are calculated on the assumption of a utilization rate corresponding to a daily expenditure of 1600 kcal. This is a little above the expenditure of a man in bed at approximately the basal rate, but allows for only a small amount of activity. If hard work had to be carried out, daily expenditure would be much greater and the stores would run out sooner. The size of the stores is very variable and so greatly affects the exhaustion time. This will now be briefly discussed.

Carbohydrate

The total available carbohydrate of the body is not high and probably seldom exceeds 0·5 kg. There is also a similar amount present as polysaccharides in connective tissue, but this is not available for general metabolic use. Glycogen is the principle form in which carbohydrate is stored for energy in cells and the greatest quantity is present in the muscle cells at a concentration between 0·8 and 2·5 % (Hildes, Sherlock & Walshe, 1949). The liver may contain glycogen up to at least 6 % but this only amounts to 90 g. in the whole organ. It is known that liver glycogen can fall to low levels early in starvation, but muscle glycogen levels fall much less rapidly unless work is done; cardiac muscle glycogen does not ever appear to decrease (Lawrence & McCance, 1931) and it is probable that the glycogen level is little changed in starvation. The suggested figure of 150 g. in Table 2.1 as available for emergency use is probably generous and as this represents only 600 kcal. or about 12 hours' supply of energy, it is clear that during fasting the bulk of the energy must come from fat and protein. This is borne out by the fact that the respiratory quotient falls to below 0·75 after only a few hours of starvation and the level of ketone bodies in the blood then begins to rise. During the second day of starvation there is usually a well marked ketonuria. The blood glucose after an initial fall of some 10 to

TABLE 2.1

Normal stores of available energy in a man weighing 65 kg.

	Total body content (g.)	Available store (g.)	Available store (kcal.)	Daily utilization* (g.)	Exhaustion time (days)
Carbohydrate	500	150	600	All used in 1–2 days	Less than 1
Protein	11,000	2,400	9,600	60	About 40
Fat	9,000	6,500	58,500	150	About 40

* Assuming an energy expenditure of about 1600 kcal./day

20 mg./100 ml., changes little during starvation (Keys *et al.* 1950). The total glucose in the extracellular fluid is of the order of 15 g., which is trivial in terms of the total daily energy needs, but it is important to note that despite the severe strains on metabolism during starvation the level of the extracellular glucose concentration is held remarkably constant.

Protein

It is difficult to estimate the total amount of protein in the body, and in particular, although there are some techniques for assessing cell mass and hence cell protein, there is at present no way of estimating the collagen content of the body. Collagen is believed to make up about a third of the total protein in man and this fraction is relatively inert metabolically (Harkness, 1961). Of the remaining protein the bulk is present in skeletal muscle. During starvation there is atrophy of muscle and also a reduction in the protein content of the muscle cells. The most striking reductions in mass are found in the liver and intestines, but as these make up only some 7% of the total body weight (Table 1.2, Chapter 1) the main protein loss must come from muscle cells.

has in effect shrunk about its extracellular fluid which has changed little. In all about 10·6 kg of cell mass was calculated to have disappeared; if this cell mass is about 20% protein, this loss corresponds to 2100 g. of protein which supports the estimate of total reserve of 2400 g. given in Table 2.1. Holmes, Jones & Stanier (1954) studied the nitrogen (N) balance and changes in body weight in malnourished Africans for long periods during rehabilitation on protein-rich diets. Although the men were in positive N balance, they gained little weight. One man, Gabriel, during 109 days retained N equivalent to 4960 g. of protein, but only gained 2100 g. in weight. As the cell proteins increase, there is loss of water which could be extracellular, intracellular or a combination of both. Thus the body composition was changing although the change in body weight was small. Presumably this protein was used to replenish the reserves, principally in muscle. The situation concerning protein retention and the change in the composition of lean body mass, when undernourished subjects are given a good diet, is fully discussed by Holmes, Darke, Greaves & Read (1962).

During starvation some protein is lost inevitably

TABLE 2.2

Body weight and body composition in the Minnesota experiment of Keys et al. *(1950)*

	Control	12 weeks of semi-starvation		24 weeks of semi-starvation	
	kg.	kg.	loss	kg.	Final loss
Total body weight	69·4	57·3	−12·1	52·6	−16·8
SCN space	17·1	17·3	+ 0·2	17·8	+ 0·7
Fat	9·6	5·0	− 4·6	2·7	− 6·9
Active tissue	39·9	32·2	− 7·7	29·3	−10·6
Bone mineral	2·8	2·8	0·0	2·8	0·0

In Table 2.1 the reserve is put at 2,400 g., i.e., 22% of the total body protein but 33% of the cell protein. Table 2.2 is derived from the classic studies carried out during the Second World War at the University of Minnesota on 32 healthy young men who lived for 24 weeks on a diet providing just under 1600 kcal/day and made up mostly of cereals and vegetables. Although the results are not derived from subjects deprived of all food, there is no reason to think that the qualitative results are any different from those that would be obtained in complete starvation in about a quarter of the time. The striking finding is the great reduction in the active cell mass. The body

by "wear and tear" since no matter how much energy is supplied in the form of carbohydrate, there is always some loss of N in the urine. It is difficult to know the lower limit of this endogenous N loss since much depends on the previous nutritional history of the subject, but in healthy young men it would seem to be equivalent to about 20 g. protein/day. The bulk of the protein is mobilized for energy including some converted to the glucose needed to maintain blood glucose levels near normal, presumably to maintain the metabolism of the brain. Protein losses have been found to vary greatly in different subjects on starvation regimes. Usually 15% of calorie expenditure comes from proteins and 85% from fat. The figure of 60 g./day for the utilization of protein in starvation given in Table 2.1 is based on this. At such a rate the normal protein reserve would last a man for 6 to 7 weeks, if there are no replenishments. Lower figures for protein loss during starvation have been recorded (Lusk, 1928; Grande, 1964) and in such instances survival might be longer. In disease, especially in septic febrile conditions, protein catabolism may be greatly increased and the stores run out correspondingly faster.

Fat

The store of fat varies greatly from person to person. Fat people survive starvation longer than thin people. In a thin man it is possible that the fat stores may run out before the protein reserves, but the few analyses of bodies of people who have died from starvation have always revealed the presence of some fat. It was believed that if fat stores were depleted in starvation, the breakdown of protein to supply all the energy requirements would produce a premortal rise in urinary N. However, recent work on animals and a careful analysis of the literature has produced no acceptable evidence of such a premortal rise in any animal species (Keys *et al.* 1950; Grande 1964). The actual cause of death in starvation is complex and it seems that when the stores of body protein and fat are nearing total depletion, the rate of supply of nutrient fuels (e.g. glucose, free fatty acids, and α-ketoacids), required for cell metabolism is too low to maintain the conditions necessary for life (Kleiber, 1961).

The figures in Table 2.1 are useful as a reminder of the enormous amount of food that may be needed to rehabilitate a patient, who for any reason has become severely undernourished. Some 70,000 kcal. above his daily requirements must be given and absorbed. This can only be accomplished over a period of many weeks. Protein synthesis is always inefficient and thus costly in energy. To rebuild protein in the body, large intakes of carbohydrates are needed to supply extra calories. It must also be remembered that after a period of starvation the alimentary canal and liver regress and so preliminary refeeding must be undertaken cautiously. The figures also show that when a healthy, well fed person is suddenly struck by a grave emergency such as acute failure of the liver or kidneys, the problem of supplying food is of secondary importance. In such patients the issue, either death or recovery, is usually settled within two weeks. The normal calorie stores can cover this period. Although it is always advisable to try to give some nourishment, it is not desirable to complicate treatment unnecessarily by trying to cover all the calorie needs during a brief emergency. If 100 g. of glucose/day are given, this prevents the development of ketosis, and also reduces endogenous nitrogen metabolism to a minimum.

The Physiology of Calorie Deficiency

Our understanding of the physiology of calorie deficiency has been greatly advanced by the increasing number of careful studies on human volunteers throughout the world. In the Minnesota experiment the diet of cereals and vegetables, providing just under 1600 kcal./day was designed to resemble that in many parts of occupied Europe, where there were severe shortages of food. It was thus possible to measure under laboratory conditions, the effects of a long period of partial starvation. The results amplify and extend field observations carried out at about the same time in Europe and in the Far East, made under appalling circumstances and often by the sufferers themselves. References to reports of these studies were given in the first edition of this book. These and subsequent studies (*vide* Grande 1964) together with many important researches carried out before the First World War make it possible to set out briefly and concisely the effects of prolonged partial starvation on the chemistry of the human body. Our deeper understanding of why these changes occur has been greatly facilitated by the recognition of the key position of adenosinetriphosphate (ATP) in the processes of biological energy transformation (Krebs 1954). In brief the chemical energy present in the foodstuffs must be stored in the pyrophosphate bonds of ATP before it can be utilized for mechanical, osmotic or other forms of work. All the complex foodstuffs are processed, as far as energy yield is concerned, to a few hexoses, glycerol, some 20 amino acids and a few fatty acids. These tissue fuels are then converted in the cells to three key molecules, viz., acetic acid in the form of acetyl coenzyme-A, α-ketoglutaric acid and oxaloacetic acid. These substances then enter the citric acid cycle and their energy becomes available to synthesize ATP. All the carbon atoms of the common fatty acids, two-thirds of the carbon of carbohydrate and glycerol and a little less than half of the carbon of proteins is processed to 2-carbon active acetate which then enters the citric acid cycle. Here lie two cardinal points, firstly, the citric acid cycle cannot function properly if 2-carbon fragments are the sole molecules presented and, secondly, glucose cannot be synthesized from a source of 2-carbon fragments. Some 3-, 4- or 5-carbon α-ketoacids must form the starting point for glucose synthesis (pyruvic acid, oxaloacetic acid or α-ketoglutaric acid). It now becomes clear that in starvation protein becomes in essence the great reserve of carbohydrate since about half the amino acids of body proteins are glucogenic. Krebs (1964) has a discussion of the metabolic fate of amino acids and the scheme in Fig. 2.1 illustrating the metabolic pathways of the glucogenic amino acids to glucose and hence to glycogen, is from this review.

Obligatory for ultimate survival:

synthesis of body protein, which has its order of priorities ranging first from haemoglobin and certain enzymes, then a wide variety of cell proteins and lastly extracellular structural proteins.

Energy storage in the form of:

(a) glycogen in liver and muscle;
(b) fat depots;
(c) reserve proteins in cells, especially in muscle cells.

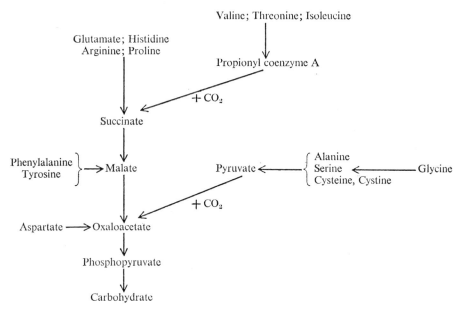

FIG. 2.1. Outline of metabolic pathways from amino acids to carbohydrate (Krebs, 1964).

Kinney (1962) has pointed out that the human body handles its energy sources on a priority basis which normal nutrition tends to mask and it is only when a significant degree of undernutrition exists that these priorities become apparent. Following Kinney the body's needs for foodstuffs can be listed in decreasing order of importance as follows:

Obligatory for immediate survival:

(a) 2-carbon active acetate fuel for the citric acid cycle to provide the essential ATP for cellular chemical energy;
(b) a continuous supply of 3- or more carbon α-ketoacids intermediates for this cycle;
(c) maintenance of blood glucose levels.

Looked at from the above viewpoint it can be seen that the essential ATP can only be generated by burning fat together with a quantity of carbohydrate intermediaries derived either from dietary carbohydrate or protein or, if there is no input of food, from tissue glycogen and protein. When after about 24 hours the reserve tissue glycogen is depleted, large quantities of cell proteins are broken down to supply both the essential carbohydrate intermediaries and to keep the cell glycogen "topped up" possibly as part of the mechanism which maintains blood glucose levels near normal in starvation.

If a group of previously well fed persons is forced to subsist on a daily diet of only 1600 kcal. their weight falls (Table 2.2). At first this fall is rapid but after a few weeks it slackens and when after 2–3 months about 25% of the initial body weight has been lost, no further losses may occur. The group may then continue to exist on such a diet for many months with no further loss of weight. Provided good medical and sanitary services are available, the death rate should be little higher than normal; but should the caloric content of the diet be lowered further, weight losses increase rapidly and deaths from starvation soon occur and become increasingly numerous. These are of course generalizations. The figure of 1600 kcal. is for adult men of weight about 65 kg. For women, children and persons of smaller build lower food intakes could be tolerated approximately in proportion to body weight in normal health. There are also many individual variations; some stand up to severe privations for longer times, others quickly succumb. Much depends on the degree of physical activity demanded of the group. If hard labour is forced upon them, then deterioration is more rapid and equilibrium is never reached.

Table 2.2 represents the results of semi-starvation over a period of many weeks. An idea of the adaptation of the body to this prolonged restrained energy input of 1600 kcal. per day can be obtained by calculating the energy represented by the lost tissues, taking active tissue to be 20% protein. During the first 12 weeks the average tissue mobilization for energy is 600 kcal./day, meaning that the overall average daily expenditure is some 2200 kcal./day. In the second period the tissue mobilization for energy has dropped to about 290 kcal./day, making the daily expenditure some 1890 kcal./day. Such average figures give an idea of the changes taking place; in fact by the end of the 24-week period the active cell mass of the body has shrunk so much that the body energy needs are almost in balance on the 1600 kcal./day of the diet.

Table 2.3 shows some results from experiments on young men subjected to two levels of drastic restriction of caloric input coupled with set exercises designed to maintain energy output at about 2600 kcal./day in each group. These results illustrate a number of important points; the weight loss in the first few days is greater than at any other period and much of this loss is water, not all of which can be accounted for in terms of active tissue loss. This water loss is a characteristic of the first week of starvation. Subsequently the calculated loss of tissue (protein x 5) and fat is greater than the actual weight loss; this indicates water retention which is initially not large and could be accounted for by a small increase in the extracellular space as indicated in Table 2.2. Alternatively it could be accounted for by the proteins leaving the cell and water moving into the cells, possibly accompanied by sodium ions. The next point is the clear demonstration of the protein-sparing action of carbohydrate; the group on the lower carbohydrate diet had to mobilize much more protein. This protein-sparing action of carbohydrate is a well known phenomenon (Munro 1951), but what is not well differentiated is the inevitable loss of "wear and tear" protein from that protein which must be mobilized to give the necessary carbohydrate intermediaries to keep the citric acid cycle generating ATP efficiently. In men doing hard work on a restricted food intake protein metabolism was found to contribute 10% of the total caloric deficit (Brožek et al. 1957). This means that 1 g. protein is metabolized for every 4 g. of fat. However, McCance & Strangeways (1954) found that adults during acute starvation without physical work needed twice this amount of protein. In Table 2.3 it can be seen that initially more protein is utilized per unit of fat than in the later stages. This could be explained by an initial loss of a true reserve

TABLE 2.3

Calculated losses of body substance during two regimens of low caloric diet
(After Brožek, Grande, Taylor, Anderson, Buskirk & Keys, 1957)

Dietary intake confined to carbohydrate (*a*) 1010 kcal./day (13 men)

(*b*) 580 kcal./day (6 men)

Days	Mean weight		Fat		Protein		H₂O	
	(*a*)	(*b*)	(*a*)	(*b*)	(*a*)	(*b*)	(*a*)	(*b*)
1– 3	800	733	200	198	40	66	560	469
4– 6	—	500	—	200	—	50	—	250
7–13	233	367	161	194	28	48	44	125
22–24	167	—	142	—	25	—	0	—

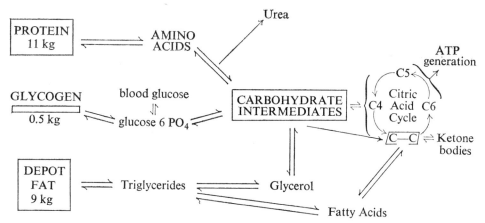

FIG. 2.2. Mobilization of body reserves for generation of ATP.

fraction of the sarcoplasmic protein in muscle cells. This protein can be sacrificed to keep the metabolism running with only minimal disturbances to overall metabolism. This state of affairs can only be maintained for a few days, when the metabolism adapts further to what may be called a siege economy. Here protein utilization is reduced to a minimum, and fat becomes the principal source of energy. This has some disadvantages in that ketone bodies begin to be produced in increased quantities. This results from a failure to metabolize completely the last stages of the degradation of triglycerides as well as the block to the proper metabolism of the ketogenic amino acids (leucine, lysine, methionine and tryptophan). Because of the greatly reduced glucose metabolism there is a greatly reduced activity of the hexose monophosphate shunt (Weber, 1959), which leads to a reduction in the amount of $NADPH_2$ which is crucial for the proper metabolism of those carbohydrate fragments which end up as acetone, acetoacetic acid and hydroxybutyric acid, the so-called ketone bodies. Figure 2.2 derived from Kinney (1962) summarizes the way in which the body reserves are mobilized to meet the needs for generating ATP and the maintenance of adequate carbohydrate levels.

An important aspect of the adaptation to caloric deficiency is reflected in the overall reduction in the basal metabolic rate. Table 2.4 shows the distribution of the energy expenditure during the control period and at the end of 6 months of semi-starvation in the Minnesota experiment. The conservation of energy due to the fall in the basal metabolism was 614 kcal./day. Evidence suggested that 65% of this saving was attributable to a reduction in the mass of actively

TABLE 2.4

Estimated partition of mean energy expenditure in kcal./day of 32 young men before and after 6 months semi-starvation (Taylor & Keys, 1950)

	Before	After
Basal metabolism	1576	962
Specific dynamic action	349	157
Cost of activity	1567	451
	3492	1570

metabolizing tissues, and a smaller part, 35%, to a decreased intensity of metabolism of the remaining tissue. A more marked saving was effected in the expenditure on muscular activities. This was not brought about by an increased efficiency of muscular action. Measurements on a treadmill showed that energy expenditure walking up a gradient was unchanged throughout the period of starvation, after correcting for the reduced work necessary to move the lighter body. The economy of movement is much more important. The semi-starved person thinks hard before he undertakes any action. No unnecessary movements are made. He always chooses the shortest possible route.

Water Metabolism—Famine Oedema

Changes in water metabolism are one of the characteristic features of starvation. The first week of starvation in healthy subjects results in a relatively large loss in weight most of which is water. Table 2.3 shows that despite the difference in caloric input the losses of water in the first few days are of the same order and are much greater than subsequent losses. In fact the net water loss diminishes with time, until a stage of water retention ensues which may in turn progress to oedema in prolonged severe calorie deficiency.

Famine oedema is the final stage in the sequence of pathological changes in water metabolism in severe starvation. McCance (1951) has collected a bibliography of over 500 references to the subject, and his review is an absorbing story of how famine oedema has fascinated and bewildered the medical profession for generations. The first symptom of the disturbed water balance is a nocturnal polyuria, which may arise soon after the onset of starvation and may seriously interfere with sleep. It often persists after oedema has appeared. The oedema disappears rapidly during rest in bed, only to reappear when the patient gets up. How rest in bed can cause an increased excretion of extracellular fluid is obscure; the nature of the cause of the oedema is not known with any certainty. Possibly several factors are involved.

(a) *A fall in the level of serum proteins.* Starling's postulate that the osmotic pressure of the plasma proteins plays a dominant role in determining the equilibrium between the plasma and tissue fluids has already been discussed in Chapter 1. This led to the view that famine oedema arises from a lowering of the level of plasma proteins, secondary to a deficient dietary intake of protein. Many observations made at the end of the First World War were consistent with this view, and it was postulated that a "critical level" of plasma protein was 5·5 g./100 ml., or of plasma albumin 2·3 g./100 ml., and that when levels fell below these values oedema developed. But observations have since been made showing beyond doubt that famine oedema can occur when levels of both total protein and albumin in the blood are normal. These cannot be critical factors in determining oedema, although they are certainly important. A brief discussion of other factors that may determine capillary permeability to water has been given in Chapter 1. How relevant these are to the causation of famine oedema is uncertain.

(b) *Impaired renal function.* A large number of investigators have shown that in famine oedema there is no gross disturbance of kidney function. Test doses of water and of Na salts are excreted in a manner similar to that in normal persons. McCance (1951) showed that a change from the recumbent to the erect position produced changes in the volume and composition of the urine and in the inulin and diodone clearances, which were similar in normal and undernourished persons when lying down.

(c) *A disturbed metabolism of antidiuretic hormone.* Gopalan (1950) found that Indian patients with famine oedema excreted in the urine a substance which had an antidiuretic effect on rats. He also found that the homogenized livers of starved rats were unable to destroy the antidiuretic action of posterior pituitary extracts at as fast a rate as the livers of normal rats. Others have claimed that rats fed on low-protein diets produce an excess of antidiuretic substance in the urine, as also do patients with cirrhosis of the liver (Ralli, Robson, Clarke & Hoagland, 1945). If a failure of the liver to destroy antidiuretic hormone produced by the posterior pituitary were a cause of famine oedema, it is difficult to see why persons with such oedema respond normally to test doses of water.

(d) *Abnormal secretion of adrenal cortical hormones.* The adrenal glands have often been reported to be enlarged in starvation, and Sinclair (1948) suggested that increased production of cortical hormones may increase reabsorption of water in the renal tubules and so promote the excess of extracellular fluid. There is, however, no evidence that there is overproduction of aldosterone or any other adrenal cortical hormone in starvation: the most that can be said for this hypothesis is that it is "not proven".

(e) *Vitamin deficiencies.* It is now well established that the full picture of calorie deficiency can arise with no gross deficiency of any vitamin. The oedema of wet beriberi has no relation to hunger oedema, and the latter is quite uninfluenced by thiamine therapy.

(f) *Reduction in tissue tensions.* The loss of fat and, to a lesser extent, of cell matter reduces the bulk of the body. The elasticity of the skin may not be sufficient to allow it to shrink sufficiently to fit the reduced body. Undernourished persons have typically a loose skin. Accurate measurements of tissue tension are difficult to make. Figures of between 2 and 4 cm. of water have been reported. A very small fall in the tension might result in water being drawn out of the cells into the tissue spaces. Youmans, Wells, Donley & Miller (1934) were the first to suggest that this may be an important factor in the production of oedema. It certainly explains two well-established clinical features. The marked effect of gravity on the distribution of the oedema becomes easily intelligible. It is also well known that famine oedema affects first and more severely men over 40 years of age. The loss of skin elasticity associated with ageing would readily account for the increased susceptibility of older persons. How it comes that men should be more prone to famine oedema than women is not clear.

(g) Fluid intake and output. Two other factors may affect water distribution in the underfed body. Starving persons often take much of their food in the form of thin soups. This may be because a little solid food appears more if it is suspended in a large volume of fluid. The bulk of fluid in the stomach may appease partially and for a brief time the sensation of hunger. To what extent the two appetites of hunger and thirst are dependent on each other is uncertain.

Famine oedema is usually associated with diarrhoea, even in the absence of intestinal infections. A simple famine diarrhoea was one of the most distressing and often fatal features of the Nazi concentration camps. The onset of oedema has frequently been reported to be associated with a bout of diarrhoea. It might be thought that the diarrhoea would reduce oedema by removing some of the excess fluid. This may be so, but protein and salts, especially K salts, are also lost in the bowel evacuations and this loss may aggravate the general starvation and so facilitate accumulation of extracellular fluid.

There can be no doubt that the origin of famine oedema is complicated. Indeed, it would be most surprising if any simple explanation of the mechanism of its production were forthcoming. An important characteristic is its variability from person to person and from day to day. For this reason, when there are reports in the literature of facts that appear to be conflicting, it is not necessary to assume that one set of observations is unreliable. In particular, the significance of negative data should not be overstressed. Oedema may well arise from a temporary or intermittent failure of several physiological functions.

Other changes. The weight changes and the disturbance of fluid balance leading to oedema are the main features of the chemical pathology of calorie deficiency. It is indeed remarkable how well the underfed body is able to carry on essential functions. In this respect the bone marrow provides an excellent example. In starving persons there is always some degree of anaemia: haemoglobin figures between 10 and 12 g./100 ml. are the rule; but severe anaemia never results and, if found, is indicative of other co-existent disease. The degree of anaemia found is compatible with atrophy of the bone marrow and shrinkage of the erythron (red cell population) on approximately the same scale as that of other cellular tissues.

The one definite change in the blood chemistry is a fall in the levels of the cholinesterases (Hutchinson, McCance & Widdowson, 1951). This fall occurs in the levels of both true and pseudo-cholinesterase. A similar fall has been reported by Waterlow (1950) in the liver and serum of malnourished infants. It is probable that the liver is the source of these enzymes and presumably this reflects a partial failure of liver function. The serum levels of other enzymes such as alkaline phosphatase are not lowered in subnutrition.

Surgical Starvation

Moore (1959, pp. 28–38) gives a very full account of changes in body composition as observed in surgical starvation. These resemble remarkably closely the changes already described in primary nutritional starvation. There are large losses of body fat and cell water and relatively large increases in extracellular water. The associated changes in electrolytes are important. Total exchangeable Na is little diminished from normal, and so is very high when expressed as a percentage of normal on observed weight. Total exchangeable K may be greatly reduced, and is a useful index of the loss of cell substance.

OBESITY

The number of obese people is probably increasing, both in Western Europe and in North America. The social, mechanical and metabolic disadvantages to health consequent upon carrying a large excess load of fat are well recognized. In the last decade there has been much interest in the problems of obesity, and new attempts have been made to understand the underlying chemical pathology.

Body fat can come only from the food consumed, so obesity is a sure and certain indication that the calories provided in the food have been in excess of the energy expended in maintaining the essential organs of the body and in physical activity. On this point there can be no doubt. Obesity arises from eating beyond one's needs. However, so much uncertainty surrounds all our present knowledge of the metabolic processes in human obesity, that there has been a natural tendency to discount the possibility of significant metabolic changes and to consider obesity as solely a psychological disorder. This, in fact, equates the disease with the sin of gluttony. This may be a true judgment on some fat people, but it seems very unlikely to apply to most. It would seem to us probable that in most obese people there is some disturbance in the chemical and other processes regulating energy intake and expenditure and so body composition and size.

Obese Tissue

The body does not lay down only excess fat: there is also some increase in body fluids and supporting tissue. Keys and Brožek (1953), as a result of measurements of body density on persons eating to excess, suggested that when the body either gains or loses weight "obese tissue" is either laid down or taken off: further this "obese tissue" is composed of 62% fat, 24% supporting cells and 14% extracellular fluid. It has a calorie value of 6·4 kcal./g. This conception has proved useful, but it is certain that the quantitative division of the gains or losses is not so precise as this. Indeed McCance & Widdowson (1951) found a distinct difference between fat men and fat women; the men usually showed a marked increase in non-fatty tissues, whereas in the women the excess weight was almost all fat.

Passmore, Strong & Ritchie (1958) made accurate measurements of the water balances and calorie balances of patients on a reducing regimen. From these they calculated the chemical composition of the tissue lost. In the first few days, much of the weight loss could be attributed to loss of water; subsequently little water was lost and on occasions, for periods of several days, some patients appeared to be gaining water. These observations have been repeated and extended by Ashley & Whyte (1961). There seems no doubt that fat people carry around a portion of body water, which may be as much as 2 to 4 litres, and which is very easily and quickly removed. It is the loss of this water in a few days which is responsible for the initial successes obtained by all the varied and much advertised "slimming cures". The mechanism behind this loss is unknown, but it is nearly always associated with a change over from a metabolic mixture, in which carbohydrate predominates, to one containing mostly fat. For a fuller discussion of this interesting point see Passmore (1961a). After this initial loss, fat people seem to retain their body water tenaciously, although losing fat and protein. It is as if their fundamental abnormality was a high body water, which cannot be reduced.

Thus the concept of "obese tissue", which we owe to Keys & Brožek, is certainly valuable, but it has not a fixed composition. Experience would indicate that the figures they gave (quoted above) represent an average, which would describe the nature of the tissue lost or gained over a period of a few weeks.

The Composition of Adipose Tissue

Chemical analyses and histological examinations of adipose tissue have been numerous (Hausberger & Hausberger, 1959; Bjurulf, 1959; Thomas, 1962). The fat content varies greatly but is usually of the order of 85%. The protein content is from 1 to 5%. Thomas (1962) and Hirsch & Goldnick (1964) have found that the N content and also the DNA content of samples of adipose tissue taken from obese subjects were only marginally less than in samples from lean subjects. In health the adipose tissue cells are already well loaded with lipid and there is little room for more when obesity develops. Some distension probably occurs, but even in people grossly overweight, the fat content is seldom over 90% and the protein content at least 2%. Hyperplasia of the tissue must occur with the formation of new cells. The following calculations show the importance of the fat-free components in adipose tissue. In a normal man there may be 7·5 kg. of adipose tissue; if the fat content is 85% there is over 1 kg. of fat-free cells and extracellular fluid and 200 g. of protein. In an obese patient with 50 kg. of adipose tissue, there may be 5 kg. of fat-free adipose tissue containing 1 kg. of protein. This corresponds to an organ which is more than three times larger than the normal liver. As *in vitro* studies indicate that it is metabolically active, adipose tissue may contribute a large part to the overall metabolism of an obese patient. To effect a cure of obesity, this new tissue must atrophy. How to bring this about is a therapeutic problem, which is not sufficiently discussed.

Reputed Causes of Obesity

There are a number of factors which have been reputed to be responsible for obesity for reasons which may appear sensible, but which have not been substantiated. As these are commonly quoted by patients and sometimes by their doctors, they merit brief considerations.

Endocrine factors. Although some diseases of the endocrine glands may give rise to obesity, in the great majority of obese patients endocrine functions appear normal; in particular, tests of thyroid function fall within the range found for persons of standard weight. If an endocrine factor is found in the future to be an important cause of obesity, then it is unlikely to be one of those well known today.

Psychological factors. Many obese people suffer from emotional disturbances, and the psychological factors that may be responsible are well described by Aldrich (1963). A few people become addicted to food, in a similar manner to that in which others get addicted to alcohol. Nevertheless many, perhaps most, obese people appear psychologically normal and to have mature personalities.

Excessive eating. Although gluttony inevitably leads to obesity, most obese people are obviously not gluttons. Whenever the food intake of a group of obese people has been accurately measured and compared with a group of controls (Swanson, Roberts, Willis, Pesek & Mairs, 1955; Johnson, Burke & Mayer, 1956; Stefanik, Heald & Mayer, 1959) they have been found to eat no more than normal.

Physical inactivity. In several studies (Dorris & Stunkard, 1957; Mayer, 1965; Bloom & Eidex, 1967) groups of obese subjects have been shown to be less physically active than controls. Bloom and Eidex have developed a device which records the time which a person spends upright. Whereas their lean subjects spent 35% of the 24 hours on their feet, obese subjects spent only 21%. It is also probable that large people in general eat less than would be expected for their size (Thomson, Billewicz & Passmore, 1961) and may be less active than small people. The probable cause of the increase in obesity which has occurred in all prosperous countries is reduced physical activity. There is nowadays much less need for either the worker in industry or the housewife in her home to use their muscles to do heavy muscular work. The great increase in the numbers of motor cars and television sets keeps people sedentary, when formerly they might have been physically active. Appetite, a control mechanism, which adjusts accurately food intake to food requirements in animals and men who are physically active, fails in many instances to reduce food intake in persons who lead sedentary lives. The sedentary life of most office workers is certainly unnatural in relation to man's evolutionary past.

Possible Metabolic Changes

Basal metabolism. Many years ago, it was reported that the basal metabolism of obese patients fell within the normal limits after correction for body size (Strang & Evans, 1929; Newburgh, 1944). There is no modern evidence to contradict this. Patients are not obese because they utilize less energy than normal either at rest or during physical activities. Indeed it is a common finding that the basal metabolism drops markedly early in the course of a reducing regime.

Luxus consumption. The German physician Grafe (Grafe & Graham, 1911; Grafe, 1933) postulated that there was a physiological mechanism, whereby food consumed in excess of requirements could be burnt off by increasing the rate of resting metabolism. Such a "Luxus consumption" mechanism, if it existed, would help to maintain normal weight and its absence might lead to obesity. The experimental evidence both in man and in animals on which Grafe based his theory lacks adequate controls and is unreliable. In studies on 16 individuals, some thin and some fat, who have been overfed under carefully controlled conditions in a metabolic ward, overfeeding led to no increase in the metabolic rates, other than a small rise attributable to the specific dynamic action of the extra protein consumed (Strong, Shirling & Passmore, 1967). There appears to be no mechanism whereby the body can dispose of excess dietary energy other than by storage in the tissues.

Alimentary absorption. It is conceivable that there might be a control mechanism in the intestinal tract enabling it to reject in the faeces a portion of any excess calories in the diet. Again a failure of such a mechanism could be a cause of obesity. Obese patients might have an exceptionally efficient mechanism for the digestion and absorption of food. However in the overfeeding experiments of Strong, Shirling and Passmore reported above, the proportion of the dietary calories lost in the faeces was the same when the subjects were overfeeding and when they were on diets which just met their energy needs. Losses of calories in the faeces are always small (in the absence of diarrhoea) and are not subject to any control.

Ketosis. It is an old observation of physicians that obese patients develop little or no ketosis when under dietary restrictions which might be expected to produce severe ketoacidosis. This has been confirmed in recent work. For instance, obese patients have been starved for periods ranging from 25 to 249 days (Thomson, Runcie & Miller, 1966); although some degree of ketonuria was noted in every patient, none of them had symptoms which could be associated with high levels of ketoacids in the urine. In a well controlled experiment on an artificial ketogenic diet Kekwick, Pawan & Chalmers (1959) showed that obese patients had much lower levels of ketoacids in their blood than normal subjects on the same regime. Although the varying circumstances that lead to ketonuria in man are well known and all are associated with an increase in the ratio of fat/carbohydrate oxidised (Passmore, 1961*b*), and the biochemical mechanisms in the liver that lead to the production of ketoacids are also well defined (Krebs, 1961), quantitative aspects of the metabolic changes in the liver have not been related to the levels of ketoacids appearing in the blood and urine.

Levels of free fatty acids (FFA) in the blood. Most workers find the FFA levels in the blood after an overnight fast higher in obese subjects than normal. Thus Opie & Walfish (1963) reported values of 482, 611 and 809 μ-equiv./l. in lean, moderately obese and grossly obese subjects respectively after a 13 hour fast. However after 21 hours fasting, the levels rose less in the obese and became 1040, 933 and 943 m-equiv./l. respectively. The levels may reflect a preference for fat rather carbohydrate metabolism in the obese.

Levels of triglyceride in the blood. These are often moderately raised in obesity. Albrink & Meigs (1965) found a positive correlation between the serum triglyceride level and skinfold thickness over the abdomen, provided the forearm skinfold thickness was low. Excess fat over the abdomen was interpreted as being an acquired characteristic arising from reactions to the environment, whereas fat on the arm was taken to be genetically determined. Thus, this change in serum lipids was not seen in subjects in whom genetic factors were considered to determine the obesity. Evans & Ostrander (1967) have also found a correlation between skinfold thickness and serum triglyceride level.

Carbohydrate metabolism. The glucose tolerance is frequently poor in obese subjects. This may be an early manifestation of the mild diabetic state that often arises after a prolonged period of obesity. However there appears to be no doubt that obese subjects handle a glucose load in a quantitatively different way from that of normal subjects. Gordon & Goldberg (1964) and Shreeve (1965) have each shown that after giving ^{14}C-glucose more ^{14}CO$_2$ appears in the expired air in normal than in obese subjects. Further after giving ^{3}H-glucose more ^{3}HOH is found in the body water in normal subjects. These facts are consistent with the view that in obesity carbohydrate metabolism is relatively reduced.

Metabolism of adipose tissue. The use of epididymal fat pads from the rat has revolutionised knowledge of lipid metabolism. Two large books (Renold & Cahill, 1965, and a symposium, New York Academy of Science, 1965) set out admirably much of this work. The enzymic mechanisms responsible for the synthesis and breakdown of triglycerides in the adipose tissue cell are now well described and also related to the ultrastructures of the cell. Adipose tissue is repeatedly changing from lipogenesis to lipolysis depending on whether the body is absorbing food or starving and drawing on the reserves of energy. The changeover is mediated by hormones, and insulin has a lipogenic action, whereas nor-

adrenaline, growth hormone and cortisol are lipolytic. The quantitative aspects of the hormonal control systems that determine the change from the one state to the other are not yet worked out.

There has also been a start in the study of the metabolism of human adipose tissue obtained either at surgical operations or by biopsy. Important papers are those by Carlson & Östman (1963), Hirsch & Goldnick (1964), Galton (1966), Bjorntorp & Martinsson (1967) and Galton & Bray (1967). From these two conclusions can be drawn. First the metabolism of human and rat adipose tissue are both qualitatively and quantitatively similar. Secondly any differences observed in the behaviour of adipose tissue obtained from thin and obese subjects are small, and those observed so far are of doubtful significance. The importance of standardizing the nutritional state of the subject from whom the biopsy is taken has only recently been appreciated, and accurate methods for determining levels of the various hormones in the blood at the time of the sampling are only now becoming available. Anaesthetics and other factors associated with surgery complicate the situation. Significant differences in the behaviour of adipose tissue from obese and lean subjects will be brought to light only by measurements of the enzymic activity in samples obtained under accurately controlled nutritional conditions and correlated with levels of blood hormones.

The Control System

The difference between static and developing obesity is important. Most obese patients are usually in the static state and the amount of triglyceride stored in the adipose tissue is accurately controlled, but the control is set at a higher level. If a patient gains 14 lbs. (6·3 kg.) in a year, the energy intake has been only of the order of 5% above requirement. When obesity develops insidiously over one or two decades, the misalignment of the weight control system is very small. Any change in either enzymic mechanisms or hormonal control is likely to be correspondingly small. It is also difficult, if not impossible, to tell whether any such differences that may be found are the cause or the effect of obesity.

In the decades 1940–60, there was much study of appetite and the mechanism of weight control. The existence of a satiety centre and feeding centre in the hypothalamus was established. The effects on the centres of such stimuli as the levels of blood glucose and FFA, environmental temperature and nervous impulses arising from the stomach were investigated. Mayer (1953) and

Brobeck (1960) were leaders in this field and their reviews are now classics. This work provides a reasonable account of the mechanisms that make a hungry animal or man seek food and consume it. However, as Yudkin (1965) had pointed out, hunger and appetite are not synonymous. Hunger is a primitive sensation, but in a prosperous society the presence of ample supplies of appetizing foods leads people to eat when they are not hungry. The difficult problem is the nature of the mechanism that stops people eating.

There is no doubt that the food intake is not accurately controlled to meet energy requirements on a day-to-day basis. Many studies have now been made in this country in which the food intake and energy expenditure of men and women leading their normal lives have been measured daily for 7 days (Durnin & Passmore, 1967). Over the period of a week, the two balance each other, often with remarkable precision; but on a daily basis food intake seldom provides precisely the energy requirements needed for activity (Durnin, 1961). In general our eating habits appear to vary more from day to day than does our physical activity. It is certain that we may run up either a credit or debit of up to 2000 kcal., the equivalent of two large meals, before making the necessary adjustments to the balance. In the overfeeding experiments of Strong, Shirling & Passmore (1967), the measurements of the RQ indicated that relatively little of the excess calories was laid down as fat in the first 4 days. Far more appeared to be stored as carbohydrate, and it would seem that the glycogen reserves may be increased by up to 1 kg. Discounting the liver which has a relatively small glycogen storage capacity, this means an increase in the glycogen content of skeletal muscle of about 3%. Saltin & Hermansen (1967) have shown that rises of this order occur in subjects in whom muscle biopsies have been done before and after a short period of feeding on a carbohydrate-rich diet.

Biological control mechanisms are concerned mostly with systems which either regulate the movement of muscle by nervous mechanisms or regulate the concentrations of substances in the blood by means which are predominantly hormonal. Comparatively simple feed-back models can be used to plan experimental studies of these controls. Obesity is a condition arising from the misalignment of a system which controls total quantities, not concentrations, on a time scale measured in days. Difficulties arise through ignorance of the nature of signals which transmit information about the size of the store and through the complexity of the factors that determine the motor control (feeding behaviour); these include social and psychological as well as physiological factors.

There are two lines of study which may be helpful in this respect, both of which have been almost completely neglected until recently. The first is the influence of the pattern of food intake, the number and size of meals eaten each day. The laboratory rat, if given free access to food, nibbles almost continuously throughout the night. However if access to food is restricted, adaptation to the new situation occurs quickly. This is accompanied by changes in the metabolism of adipose tissue. There is an increased RNA content of the tissue and an increase in the enzymic mechanism responsible for incorporation of carbohydrate and amino acids. In man those who eat 5 or more small meals a day tend to be less obese, to have a lower serum cholesterol and a better carbohydrate tolerance than those who eat 3 or fewer meals. These and other aspects of the effects of feeding patterns have been reviewed by Fábry & Braun (1967).

Secondly, the extent to which the taste influences food intake has not received the attention which it merits in a civilization served by a sophisticated food industry. Pangborn (1967) has written an admirable brief review on "some aspects of chemoreception in human nutrition" and provided a bibliography of over 3000 references on the sense of taste. Many of these papers are probably little known and might repay detailed study.

Conclusion

The only thing that can be said with certainty about the aetiology of obesity is that it arises when the intake of energy in the diet exceeds the output of energy in physical activities.

It can also be said that in contemporary prosperous countries attempts to prevent or treat the disease by dietary restrictions seldom meet with success, when the assessment is made after an interval of 6 months or more. In contrast, programmes to increase energy expenditure by active recreation either for a community or an individual patient are seldom advocated, and then usually in a half-hearted manner without professional advice. In our opinion, an obese person is more likely to be helped by a swimming instructor or a dancing mistress than by a dietician. The best chance is to consult all three.

PROTEIN–CALORIE MALNUTRITION

This term is now used to describe the clinical syndromes associated with a deficiency of calories and protein. Protein–calorie malnutrition is common in many parts of Asia, Africa, Latin America and the Caribbean. In many countries it is one of the main causes of death in children under 5 years of age and it is the most serious and widespread nutritional disorder in the world today.

Protein–calorie malnutrition has two characteristic extreme manifestations. At one end of the spectrum is calorie deficiency or marasmus. Characteristically it occurs in the first year of life or early in the second. A failure of lactation or death of the mother and repeated attacks of gastro-enteritis are common causes. It is becoming more common in the urban populations in the tropics, associated with a decline in traditional breast feeding and inadequate knowledge of sound methods of artificial feeding. The infant is seriously underweight with little or no subcutaneous fat and the muscles are wasted. The skin and hair are normally pigmented. Oedema is usually absent. The infant is miserable but responds to care and affection.

At the other end of the spectrum is protein deficiency or kwashiorkor. Characteristically it occurs in the second half of the second year of life or even later. The child has been weaned on to a diet of cereal paps or matoke bananas or cassava with no milk and little or no meat, eggs or fish. It is often precipitated by an attack of measles or some other acute infection. Oedema which may be severe is present. The subcutaneous fat may be present in normal amounts and the child may even be fat. This may mask the wasting of muscles, which is always present. The liver is enlarged and fatty. The skin and hair are underpigmented and a variety of dermatoses may be found. An associated vitamin A deficiency is common and may lead to keratomalacia. The child is miserable, but apathetic and generally antagonistic to attention.

Frequently a child cannot be classified into either of these two groups, but presents features of both, and may be said to be suffering from protein–calorie malnutrition. Among severe cases requiring admittance to hospital there is a high mortality despite the best treatment. In any area of the world where the disease is common for every child who is seriously ill with the disease, there will be many more whose health and development are impaired throughout the formative years of early life.

Protein–calorie malnutrition has an enormous literature. McLaren (1966) in a useful review discusses the prevalence, aetiology, diagnosis, prognosis and prevention. Brock (1966) has given an admirable account of the clinical features. Here we are concerned primarily with the chemical pathology. This is essentially the same in many respects in the marasmic child as in the adult suffering from the effects of chronic starvation; hence the following account is related mainly to kwashiorkor and the effects of protein deficiency. An admirable review of this aspect of the subject is that by Waterlow, Cravioto & Stephen (1960).

Body Composition

The total body water has been measured in children with kwashiorkor by Schnieden, Hendriekse & Haigh (1958) in Nigeria using deuterium, and by Smith (1960) in Jamaica using tritiated water. Both observers obtained values for several children, which were over 80% of body weight. This means that the body solids were less than 20% of body weight. Most of this will be protein and very little fat. A child with kwashiorkor aged 1 year may weigh only 5 kg., or half the weight of a normal child of that age. Table 2.5

TABLE 2.5

The chemical composition, which might be found in a normal child and in one with kwashiorkor, each aged 1 year

	Normal		Kwashiorkor	
	kg.	%	kg.	%
Body weight	10	100	5	100
Water	6·2	62	4·1	82
Protein	1·7	17	0·6	12
Fat	1·5	15	0·1	2
Minerals	0·6	6	0·2	4

shows the composition of such a child in comparison with that of a healthy child of the same age. The child with kwashiorkor may have laid down only one-third as much protein in the course of development as the normal child. He will also contain relatively much more water, and in this respect will resemble a foetus. The fat content may be as low as indicated in the table, but this is not a characteristic of all patients with kwashiorkor. If the child has received plenty of calories, fat may be present in normal amounts.

More recent studies (Hansen, Brinkman & Bowie, 1965; Garrow, Fletcher & Halliday, 1965) have confirmed the high water content of severely malnourished children. That this may rise to over 80% of the body weight is now well established. In such children the extracellular water is greatly increased, but not sufficiently to account for all the increase in total body water. Some overhydration of the cells must occur in these cases. However, in some children with kwashiorkor, treatment causes a reduction in the extracellular water which is greater than the reduction in total body water (Brinkman, Bowie, Friis-Hansen & Hansen, 1965). The treatment appears to cause a shift of some of the oedema water into the cells. This interesting observation indicates a difference between kwashiorkor and simple starvation.

Failure to Synthesize Serum Albumin

In severe kwashiorkor the serum albumin is always low. Dean & Schwartz (1953) found an average value of 1·51 g./100 ml. (range 0·76–2·17) which rose to a normal value of above 3·5 g./100 ml. on treatment. This rise is a useful measure for assessing the results of different methods of treatment. Using ^{131}I-albumin, it is possible to measure the albumin pool, which includes both extra- and intravascular protein. This may be reduced to 40% of normal (Gitlin, Cravioto, Frenk, Montano, Ramos-Galvan, Gomez & Janeway, 1958).

There is no doubt that this diminished serum albumin is an important cause of the oedema that is so frequently present. However, as in famine oedema, the relation between the clinical sign and the biochemical change is not precise, and other factors, as discussed on p. 22, may well be important. Dehydration may also be present and indeed it is not infrequent to find a child with obvious dehydration affecting the face and thorax and with gross oedema in the legs and around the hips. There is no simple explanation of this.

By contrast, the levels of serum globulin are usually well maintained. Indeed the gamma-globulin fraction is often higher than normal, probably due to the presence of infection (Rao, Swaminathan, Swarup & Patwardhan, 1959). Similarly, although some degree of anaemia is always found, the level of haemoglobin is not usually dangerously reduced and characteristically is between 7 and 10 g./100 ml. When amino acids are present in limited quantities, it would appear that the synthesis of globulins gets preference over that of albumins.

Failure to Synthesize Digestive Enzymes

The diarrhoea, which is so frequent and severe in advanced cases, is not usually caused by any infection. It is a result of a failure to digest the food consumed, following a diminished secretion of digestive enzymes. Thompson & Trowell (1952) aspirated the duodenal contents and determined the concentration of the pancreatic enzymes present. Soon after the patients were admitted, the mean value for amylase was one-tenth, for lipase one-quarter and for trypsin one-twelfth of the values obtained on the same patients after recovery had taken place. At post-mortem, atrophy of the acinous portion of the pancreas has been found (Davies, 1948), and calcification of the pancreas has been demonstrated radiologically in adults in areas where the disease is endemic (Zuidema, 1959; Shaper, 1960). Owing to this failure, there is an intolerance of many dietary substances, especially of fat and also frequently of starch and disaccharides. A vicious circle may be set up and patients become unable to utilize nutrients which they need. However, milk proteins are nearly always digested and absorbed. The diarrhoea causes losses of K, which may amount to 20–50 m-equiv./day (Hansen, 1956). Mg is also lost in large amounts in the stools (Montgomery, 1961). These cations are thus drained from the muscles and other tissues. Secondary deficiencies arising in this way contribute to the clinical picture and often appear to be the immediate cause of death.

Failure to Maintain the Normal Liver Structure

Protein is withdrawn from the liver cells, which are often distorted by droplets of fats, which may be large. The fat content of the organ may be as much as 40%. Senecal, Roullier, Camain & Dupin (1958), in an electron microscopic study of biopsy material, showed that the mitochondria were swollen and rarefied. After treatment these changes were reversed and granules of ribonucleic acid could be seen around the mitochondria, which suggested that they were participating in regeneration of cytoplasm.

Chemical analyses of biopsy material have been reported by Waterlow & Weisz (1956). Using the deoxyribonucleic acid (DNA) content of the liver as a basis for comparisons, they showed that the N present in the liver cells of malnourished infants rose after treatment from 49 to 83 mg.N/mg. DNA-P. This indicates that one-third of the cell protein had been lost. Despite this depletion, the usual tests show generally only slight impairment of liver function. Glycogen may be stored in normal amounts. Death is seldom attributable to liver failure.

With treatment the fat may be completely reabsorbed from the liver cells: in serial biopsies taken after a long follow-up period, the liver usually returned to a normal histological picture (Suckling & Campbell, 1957). Healing is generally complete and without fibrosis (Stein & Isaacson, 1960)—at least in Johannesburg where kwashiorkor is common, but not complicated by tropical infections. However, in Calcutta (Chandra, 1958) and elsewhere, it would appear that permanent liver damage with cirrhosis may follow.

These observations illustrate the immense reserves of function in the livers of young children and the great capacity of the organ for healing.

Failure to Maintain Muscle Substance

Skeletal muscle is the tissue quantitatively most depleted by protein lack. It is impossible at present to measure the mass of skeletal tissue in life and so there are no means of assessing accurately the severity of depletion of body protein. Estimations of body solids, derived from measurements of total body water, do not enable a distinction to be made between the protein, fat and minerals. Some indication of protein loss from muscles can be obtained by biopsy studies. Waterlow & Mendes (1957) obtained muscle biopsies before and after treatment in a series of children, and found that N rose from 237 to 343 mg./mg. DNA-P. The electrolyte content of muscle is also greatly changed. Montgomery (1961) in three biopsies found mean values for K, Mg and Na of 44, 8 and 71 m-equiv./kg. wet weight. These figures changed to 69, 11 and 69 respectively after 2 to 3 months treatment, but were still very different from values of 90, 20 and 50 reported in normal children's muscle. The total exchangeable K has also been shown to be markedly reduced: values of about 30 m-equiv./kg. of body weight, about 25 % below normal, were reported by Smith & Waterlow (1960). It is impossible to generalize about the relative deficiencies of N, K and Mg in muscle. Obviously the picture could not be expected to be the same in all patients. Looking at the published figures available, it would seem that the K/N ratio may often be markedly lowered in muscle in kwashiorkor. There is justification for emphasizing the importance of K deficiency in the tissues, when considering treatment, and also when discussing the possible ways in which the enzymic mechanisms in the cells may have failed. Too little is known as yet about the role of Mg deficiency in causing the various clinical and chemical disorders present in kwashiorkor. Our guess is that future work will emphasize the importance of this element in nutrition.

Collagen and Connective Tissue Metabolism

Despite the great reduction in the protein content of the body (Table 2.4), the collagen content is not reduced. Picou, Halliday & Garrow (1966) carried out carcass analyses on 10 malnourished Jamaican children. The total body protein con-

tent was reduced to 55–75 % of the amount expected for the child's height. Collagen protein was not reduced and formed 36 to 48 % of the total protein, whereas in adequately nourished children it forms 27 %.

That collagen metabolism is greatly reduced in the malnourished infant is indicated by the very low levels of urinary excretion of hydroxyproline (Picou, Alleyne & Seakins, 1965; Anasuya & Narasinga Rao, 1966). The urinary excretion of hydroxyproline in relation to creatinine has been used as an index of malnutrition and suggested as a means of screening large numbers of children (Whitehead 1965; Howells, Wharton & McCance, 1967). The use of such an index is still very much under trial.

Endocrine Changes

It is natural to attempt to explain the widespread metabolic disturbances that occur in protein–calorie malnutrition in terms of disorders of endocrine function. However, such attempts have been disappointing and in by far the majority of malnourished children endocrine function has appeared to be normal. It would seem that when the supply of protein is limited, it is reserved preferentially for the manufacture of the enzymes responsible for hormone synthesis.

The adrenal glands have been most extensively examined. In a recent study in Jamaica Alleyne & Young (1966) showed that in malnourished children plasma levels of 11-hydroxycorticosteroids were a little higher than normal and there was a good response to injected corticotropin. Increased adrenal cortical activity may indeed be partially responsible for the impaired glucose tolerance and the sodium retention characteristic of starvation and protein deficiency. Many other workers have found adrenal cortical function to be normal or slightly raised in the malnourished state.

Thyroid activity, as measured by the urinary excretion of ^{131}I, was found to be normal in most malnourished Jamaican children (Montgomery, 1962) although in a few it was just below the accepted range of normality. El-Gholmy, Ghaleb, Khalifa, Senna & El-Akkad (1967) report that in malnourished Egyptian children thyroid activity as judged by uptake of ^{131}I was often depressed, roughly proportional to the drop in the level of serum albumin. Yet there is no doubt that severe hypothyroidism is not a common feature of protein–calorie malnutrition. However, hypothermia is now well recognized as a serious complication occurring in some cases (Brenton, Brown & Wharton, 1967) and it is possible that in these a partial failure of thyroid function may be a contributory factor.

Glucose tolerance is often impaired. Baig & Edosien (1965) found that after an intravenous glucose load the level of blood insulin rose normally, but then soon fell. They suggest that the islet cells can respond effectively to a normal stimulus, but in the face of a massive challenge soon become exhausted because of a poor functional reserve, presumably due to diminished rate of protein synthesis.

There is no evidence of any failure of secretion of growth hormone by children with marasmus and kwashiorkor. In such children during dietary rehabilitation Hadden & Rutishauser (1967) found that injections of growth hormone did not affect absorption and retention of nitrogen or mobilization of free fatty acids. This was probably due to the fact that the dietary regimen had previously stimulated an adequate production of endogenous hormone. The plasma levels of growth hormone have also been reported to be high in kwashiorkor (Pimstone, Wittman, Hansen & Murray, 1966).

The Potassium Content of the Brain and Cerebral Function

Mental changes are characteristic of severe kwashiorkor. Using a whole body counter for the natural ^{40}K isotope of potassium, Garrow (1967) found that the head was more severely depleted than the rest of the body with kwashiorkor. The potassium loss is probably secondary to the metabolic effects caused by the dietary deficiency of protein. Whether potassium depletion of the brain is responsible for the mental changes seen in the acute stages of the disease is uncertain, but it is at least a reasonable hypothesis.

Much more speculative are the questions as to whether a period of severe malnutrition in early childhood or prolonged undernutrition in children and adolescence retards the normal process of mental development and leads to permanent intellectual failure. Brown (1965) has produced autopsy evidence that the weight of the brain in malnourished children in Uganda is less than normal, but the ratio brain weight/body weight is higher; this indicates that malnutrition impairs the growth of the brain less than the rest of the body. Stock & Smythe (1963) found that in an undernourished group of children in Cape Town both brain growth, as measured by head circumference, and I.Q. were significantly less than in normal controls; further, this gap was not closed during 7 years in which the children were followed up.

This difficult subject requires much more study before any firm conclusions can be made.

Possible Biochemical Lesions

The use of biopsy material and the development of analytical techniques applicable to samples of tissue of less than one milligram have made it possible to begin the study of the failure in disease of the enzymic processes responsible for protein synthesis. A paper by Waterlow (1961 a) on oxidative phosphorylation in the livers of normal and malnourished human infants would seem to point the line for much profitable work. He has shown that respiration is remarkably well maintained, even in livers which have been severely damaged and extensively infiltrated with fat; however, phosphorylation was usually slightly reduced and P uptake into phosphatidic acid generally greatly reduced. These results link together with the observations on the structural changes in the mitochondria of the liver cells described by Senecal and his colleagues (1958) and the finding of Vitale, Nakamura & Hegsted (1957) that in experimental Mg deficiency there is an impairment of oxidative phosphorylation in mitochondrial preparations. There are indications that protein synthesis in the tissues is thermodynamically not very efficient and the sources of the energy needed are obviously important. Clinically the child with kwashiorkor will recover quickly and grow well only if the diet provides him with ample calories as well as protein (Waterlow, 1961 b). At the mitochondrial level, energy-rich phosphate as well as amino acids are needed to make the cell proteins.

Some of the adaptive changes that occur in the livers of children on a low-protein diet have been described by Stephen & Waterlow (1968). The levels of amino acid activating enzymes were found to be high, whereas levels of argininosuccinase were low. Similar changes have been reported in rats on low-protein diets. The combined effect of these changes, it is suggested, is to increase the chance of an amino acid being incorporated into protein and a smaller chance of its conversion into urea.

The study of kwashiorkor is of immense practical importance; it can also be recommended as an academic exercise for biologists who are interested in the general problems of protein synthesis. For a proper understanding of this disease, the student has to range over fields as far apart as social psychology and molecular biology and to bring together a great diversity of knowledge.

References

ALBRINK, M. J. & MEIGS, J. W. (1965). *Ann. N.Y. Acad. Sci.*, **131**, 673.

ALDRICH, C. K. (1963). *Med. Clin. N. Amer.*, 77.

ALLEYNE, G. A. O. & YOUNG, V. H. (1966). *Lancet*, **1**, 911.

ANASUYA, A. & NARASINGA RAO, B. S. (1966). *Indian J. Med. Res.*, **54**, 849.

ASHLEY, B. C. E. & WHYTE, H. M. (1961). *Austral. Ann. Med.*, **10**, 92.

BAIG, H. A. & EDOZIEN, J. C. (1965). *Lancet*, **2**, 662.

BJORNTORP, P. & MARTINSSON, A. (1967). *Act. med. Scand.*, **181**, 359.

BJURUFF, P. (1959). *Act. med. Scand.*, **66**, Suppl. 349.

BLOOM, W. L. & EIDEX, M. F. (1967). *Metabolism*, **16**, 679.

BRENTON, D. P., BROWN, R. E. & WHARTON, B. A. (1967). *Lancet*, **1**, 410.

BRINKMAN, G. L., BOWIE, M. D., FRIIS-HANSEN, B. & HANSEN, J. D. L. (1965). *Pediatrics*, **36**, 94.

BROBECK, J. R. (1960). *Vitam. & Horm.*, **16**, 439.

BROCK, J. F. (1966). *Ann. Intern. Med.*, **65**, 877.

BROWN, R. E. (1965). *East African Med. J.*, **42**, 584.

BROŽEK, J. (1965). *Ann. N.Y. Acad. Sci.*, **131**, 1.

BROŽEK, J., GRANDE, F., TAYLOR, H. L., ANDERSON, J. T., BUSKIRK, E. R. & KEYS, A. (1957). *J. Appl. Physiol.*, **10**, 412.

BULLEN, B. A., REED, R. B. & MAYER, J. (1964). *Amer. J. Clin. Nutr.*, **14**, 211.

CARLSON, L. A. & ÖSTMAN, J. (1963). *Act. med. Scand.*, **174**, 215.

CHANDRA, N. K. (1958). *Brit. Med. J.*, **1**, 1263.

DAVIDSON, S. & PASSMORE, R. (1966). "Human Nutrition and Dietetics", Edinburgh and London, Livingstone.

DAVIES, J. N. P. (1948). *Lancet*, **1**, 317.

DEAN, R. F. A. & SCHWARTZ, R. (1953). *Brit. J. Nutr.*, **7**, 131.

DORRIS, R. J. & STUNKARD, A. J. (1957). *Amer. J. med. Sci.*, **223**, 622.

DRABKIN, D. L. (1959). *Perspect. in Biol. Med.*, **2**, 473.

DURNIN, J. V. G. A. (1961). *J. Physiol.*, **156**, 294.

DURNIN, J. V. G. A. & PASSMORE, R. (1967). "Energy, Work and Leisure", London, Heinemann.

EL-GHOLMY, A., GHALEB, H., KHALIFA, A. S., SENNA, A. & EL-AKKAD, S. (1967). *J. Trop. Med. Hyg.*, **70**, 74.

EVANS, J. G. & OSTRANDER, L. D. (1967). *Lancet*, **1**, 761.

FÁBRY, P. & BRAUN, T. (1967). *Proc. Nutr. Soc.*, **26**, 144.

GALTON, D. (1966). *Biochem. J.*, **101**, 164.

GALTON, D. J. & BRAY, G. A. (1967). *J. clin. Invest.* **46**, 621.

GARROW, J. S. (1967). *Lancet*, **2**, 643.

GARROW, J. S., FLETCHER, K. & HALLIDAY, D. (1965). *J. Clin. Invest.*, **44**, 417.

GITLIN, D., CRAVIOTO, J., FRENK, S., MONTANO, E. L., RAMOS-GALVAN, R., GOMEZ, F. & JANEWAY, C. A. (1958). *J. Clin. Invest.*, **37**, 682.

GOPALAN, C. (1950). *Lancet*, **1**, 304.

GORDON, E. S. & GOLDBERG, M. (1964). *Metabolism*, **13**, 775.

GRAFE, E. (1933). "Metabolic Diseases and their Treatment", Philadelphia, Lea & Febiger.

GRAFE, E. & GRAHAM, D. (1911). *Hoppe. Seyl. Z.*, **73**, 1.

GRANDE, F. (1964). In "Handbook of Physiology", Section 4, 911, Washington, U.S.A., American Physiological Society.

HADDEN, D. R. & RUTISHAUSER, I. H. E. (1967). *Arch. Dis. Childh.*, **42**, 29.

HANSEN, J. D. L. (1956). *South African J. Lab. clin. Med.*, **2**, 206.

HANSEN, J. D. L., BRINKMAN, G. L. & BOWIE, M. D. (1965). *South African Med. J.*, **39**, 491.

HARKNESS, R. D. (1961). *Biol. Rev.*, **36**, 399.

HAUSBERGER, F. X. & HAUSBERGER, B. C. (1959). *Anat. Rec.*, **65**, 135.

HILDES, J. A., SHERLOCK, S. & WALSHE, V. (1949). *Clin. Sci.*, **7**, 287.

HIRSCH, J. & GOLDNICK, R. B. (1964). *J. clin. Invest.*, **43**, 1776.

HOLMES, E. G., DARKE, S. J., GREAVES, J. P. & READ, W. W. C. (1962), *Quart. J. exper. Physiol.*, **47**, 15.

HOLMES, E. G., JONES, E. R. & STANIER, M. W. (1954). *Brit. J. Nutr.*, **8**, 173.

HOWELLS, G. R., WHARTON, B. A. & McCANCE, R. A. (1967). *Lancet*, **1**, 1082.

HUTCHINSON, A. O., McCANCE, R. A. & WIDDOWSON, E. M. (1951). *Spec. Rep. Ser. Med. Res. Coun. (Lond.)*, No. 275, 216.

JOHNSON, M. L., BURKE, B. S. & MAYER, J. (1956). *Amer. J. Clin. Nutr.*, **4**, 37.

KEKWICK, A., PAWAN, G. L. S. & CHALMERS, T. (1959). *Lancet*, **2**, 1157.

KEYS, A. & BROŽEK, J. (1953). *Physiol. Rev.*, **33**, 245.

KEYS, A., BROŽEK, J., HENSCHEL, A., MICHELSON, O. & TAYLOR, H. L. (1950). "The Biology of Human Starvation". Minneapolis, University of Minnesota Press.

KINNEY, J. M. (1962). In "Protein Metabolism". Ed. Gross, F., p. 275. Berlin, Springer Verlag.

KLEIBER, M. (1961). "The Fire of Life". New York, John Wiley.

KREBS, H. A. (1954). *Johns Hopkins Hosp. Bull.*, **95**, 34.

KREBS, H. A. (1961). *Biochem. J.*, **80**, 225.

KREBS, H. A. (1964). In "Mammalian Protein Metabolism". Eds. Munro, H. N. & Allison, J. B., p. 125. New York & London, Academic Press.

LAWRENCE, R. D. & McCANCE, R. A. (1931). *Biochem. J.*, **25**, 570.

LUSK, G. (1928). "The Science of Nutrition", 4th Edition, Philadelphia, Saunders.

McCANCE, R. A. (1951). *Spec. Rep. Ser. Med. Res. Coun.* (Lond.), No. 275, 21.

McCANCE, R. A. & STRANGEWAYS, W. M. B. (1954). *Brit. J. Nutr.*, **8**, 21.

McCANCE, R. A. & WIDDOWSON, E. M. (1951). *Proc. Roy. Soc. B.*, **138**, 115.

McLAREN, D. S. (1963). "Malnutrition and the Eye". New York, Academic Press.

McLaren, D. S. (1966). *Lancet*, **2**, 485.
Mayer, J. (1953). *Physiol. Rev.*, **33**, 472.
Mayer, J. (1965). *Ann. N.Y. Acad. Sci.*, **131**, 502.
Montgomery, R. D. (1961). *J. Pediat.*, **59**, 119.
Montgomery, R. D. (1962). *Arch. Dis. Child.*, **37**, 383.
Moore, F. D. (1959). "Metabolic Care of the Surgical Patient". Philadelphia and London, Saunders.
Munro, H. N. (1951). *Physiol. Rev.*, **31**, 449.
Newburgh, L. H. (1944). *Physiol. Rev.*, **24**, 18.
Opie, L. H. & Walfish, P. G. (1963). *New Eng. J. Med.*, **268**, 757.
Pangborn, R. M. (1967). In "The Chemical Senses and Nutrition". Ed. Kane, M. R. and Muller, O. Baltimore, Johns Hopkins Press.
Passmore, R. (1961 a). *Nutritio et Dieta*, **3**, 1.
Passmore, R. (1961 b). *Lancet*, **1**, 839.
Passmore, R., Strong, J. A. & Ritchie, F. J. (1958). *Brit. J. Nutr.*, **12**, 113.
Picou, D., Alleyne, G. A. O. & Seakins, A. (1965). *Clin. Sci.*, **29**, 517.
Picou, D., Halliday, D. & Garrow, J. S. (1966). *Clin. Sci.*, **30**, 345.
Pimstone, B. L., Wittman, W., Hansen, J. D. L. & Murray, P. (1966). *Lancet*, **2**, 779.
Ralli, E. P., Robson, J. S., Clarke, D. & Hoagland, C. L. (1945). *J. clin. Invest.*, **24**, 316.
Rao, K. S., Swaminathan, M. C., Swarup, S. & Patwardhan, V. N. (1959). *Bull. Wld. Hlth. Org.*, **20**, 603.
Renold, A. E. & Cahill, G. F. (1965). "Adipose Tissue", Washington, American Physiological Society.
Saltin, B. & Hermansen, L. (1967). In "Nutrition and Physical Activity". Ed. Blix, G. p. 32. Stockholm, Almquist & Wiksell.
Schnieden, H., Hendriekse, R. G. & Haigh, C. P. (1958). *Trans. Roy. Soc. trop. Med. Hyg.*, **52**, 169.
Senecal, J., Roullier, C., Camain, R. & Dupin, H. (1958). *Bull. Med. de l'A.O.F. Dakar*, **3**, 480.
Shaper, A. G. (1960). *Lancet*, **1**, 1223.
Shreeve, W. W. (1965). *Ann. N.Y. Acad. Sci.*, **131**, 464.
Sinclair, H. M. (1948). *Proc. Roy. Soc. Med.*, **41**, 541.
Smith, R. (1960). *Clin. Sci.*, **19**, 275.
Smith, R. & Waterlow, J. C. (1960). *Lancet*, **1**, 147.

Stefanik, P. A., Heald, F. P. & Mayer, J. (1959). *Amer. J. clin. Nutr.*, **7**, 55.
Stein, H. & Isaacson, C. (1960). *Med. Proc.*, **6**, 7.
Stephen, J. M. L. & Waterlow, J. C. (1968). *Lancet*, **1**, 118.
Stock, M. B. & Smythe, P. M. (1963). *Arch. Dis. Childh.*, **38**, 546.
Strang, J. M. & Evans, F. A. (1929). *J. clin. Invest.*, **6**, 277.
Strong, J. A., Shirling, D. & Passmore, R. (1967). *Brit. J. Nutr.*, **21**, 909.
Suckling, P. V. & Campbell, J. A. H. (1957). *J. Trop. Pediatrics*, **2**, 173.
Swanson, P., Roberts, H., Willis, E., Pesek, I. & Mairs, P. (1955). "Weight Control", p. 80. A symposium, ed. Eppright, E. S., Swanson P. & Iverson, C. A. Iowa, Iowa College Press.
Taylor, H. L. & Keys, A. (1950). *Science*, **112**, 215.
Thomas, L. W. (1962). *Quart. J. exper. Physiol.*, **47**, 179.
Thompson, M. D. & Trowell, H. C. (1952). *Lancet*, **1**, 1031.
Thomson, A. M., Billewicz, W. Z. & Passmore, R. (1961). *Lancet*, **1**, 1027.
Thomson, T. J., Runcie, J. & Miller, V. (1966). *Lancet*, **2**, 992.
Vitale, J. I., Nakamura, M. & Hegsted, D. M. (1957). *J. biol. Chem.*, **228**, 573.
Waterlow, J. (1950). *Lancet*, **1**, 908.
Waterlow, J. C. (1961 a). *Proc. Roy. Soc. B.*, **155**, 96.
Waterlow, J. C. (1961 b). *J. trop. Pediatrics*, **7**, 16.
Waterlow, J. C., Cravioto, J. & Stephen, J. M. L. (1960). *Adv. in Protein Chem.*, **15**, 131.
Waterlow, J. C. & Mendes, C. B. (1957). *Nature*, **180**, 1361.
Waterlow, J. C. & Weisz, J. (1956). *J. Clin. Invest.*, **35**, 346.
Weber, G. (1959). *Rev. Can. Biol.*, **18**, 245.
Whitehead, R. G. (1966). *Lancet*, **1**, 203.
Youmans, J. B., Wells, H. S., Donley, D. & Miller, D. G. (1934). *J. clin. Invest.*, **13**, 447.
Yudkin, J. (1965). *Lancet*, **1**, 1218.
Zuidema, P. J. (1959). *Trop. & Geograph. Med. Amsterdam*, **11**, 70.

P.S. In a Lecture given to the Royal College of Physicians (*Lancet*, 1968, **2**, 1091), Professor J. C. Waterlow has given an admirable account of modern views on the mechanism of adaptation to low protein intakes.

Chapter 3

DIABETES MELLITUS AND HYPOGLYCAEMIA

by

Peter H. Wright, James Ashmore and Willy J. Malaisse
Department of Pharmacology, University of Indiana, Indianapolis, Indiana, U.S.A., and
Laboratoire de Medecine Expérimentale, Université libre de Bruxelles, Belgium

THE history of the term "Diabetes Mellitus" is well known (Major, 1945). What is often forgotten is that it is descriptive of a syndrome, but gives no indication of aetiology. For almost half a century it has been known that the syndrome in man, which so closely resembles that produced first by von Mering & Minkowski (1889) after removal of the dog's pancreas, can be "cured" by the administration of insulin (Banting & Best, 1922). At that time it was considered that diabetes mellitus and insulin deficiency are synonymous, and for many years attention was concentrated on the restoration of this deficiency by administration of insulin and control of diet. In the clinical field, little else could be done for the diabetic patient, but it gradually became apparent that such treatment, whilst prolonging life, had a doubtful effect upon the appearance of lesions which now replace diabetic coma as the primary cause of death amongst diabetics.

In the experimental field, however, new techniques and an ever increasing volume of information concerning metabolic processes heralded a more basic approach to the problem of diabetes. In place of pancreatectomy, the administration of alloxan (see Lukens, 1948) and of guinea pig anti-insulin serum (Moloney & Coval, 1955) offered more convenient methods for the induction of insulin deficiency in experimental animals. It was shown that insulin promotes the entry of glucose into cells (Levine, Goldstein, Huddleston & Klein, 1950). The basic structure of insulin was determined (Brown, Sanger & Kitai, 1955), and methods devised for its bio- and immuno-assay at high dilution. Other hormones such as glucagon, growth hormone, adreno-corticotropic hormone and thyrotropic hormone were isolated and methods devised for their assay (Berson & Yalow, 1964a; Loraine & Bell, 1966). They, or crude extracts from the pituitary gland, were shown to have diabetogenic effects in experimental animals (see Young, 1951). The first real impact of these findings in the clinical field came when Bornstein & Lawrence (1951) showed that insulin does circulate in the blood of some, in fact most, human diabetics. In both the clinical and experimental fields it became possible to show that metabolism of carbohydrates, fats and proteins can be rapidly affected by adrenal, pituitary and thyroid hormones, and that these changes may play a part in the development of the diabetic syndrome. More quantitative estimates can now be made of the effects of physiological and pharmacological agents upon insulin secretion, and evidence is accumulating to show intimate relationships between the endocrine secretions of the body. As a result, we now have a better appreciation of the part played by insulin, or the lack of it, in the economy of both the normal and the diabetic subject. On balance, it also appears that insulin deficiency giving rise to the metabolic symptoms of the diabetic is due to secondary rather than primary failure of the insulin secretory mechanism.

As Wagener has pointed out (1945), "it is easy now to keep the average diabetic patient alive". He added, however, that "the main attention of the therapists should be devoted to the prevention of complications". Unfortunately, little or nothing of a basic nature is known about these "complications" which cause debilitating or even fatal forms of retinitis, nephropathy, neuropathy, and vascular occlusion. They may appear before or during the period of insulin deficiency, and are not dramatically improved or prevented by even the most stringent control of insulin deficiency. These "complications" still pose the greatest problem faced by the clinician, and no solution is likely to be found until the metabolic abnormality underlying their appearance has been identified.

The account which follows will deal with more recent developments in the experimental and clinical fields which appear to have a bearing on the problems associated with the nature and aetiology of diabetes. No attempt is made to recapitulate the wealth of information available in numerous textbooks concerning the treatment of diabetes. Attention will be focused on the metabolism of insulin; pertinent current knowledge and concepts of the metabolism of carbohydrates, fats and proteins; the clinical syndromes found in human diabetics and their diagnosis; and a discussion of the factors which may play parts in the aetiology of this disease. Finally, there is a short section dealing with hypoglycaemia. The object of this survey is to correlate, where possible, the main facts as they are now known, and to present the current problems in terms of questions which can only be answered in the future.

INSULIN

This hormone has been the subject of many reviews and symposia, but the most significant have been those published in the past decade (Stadie, 1954; Field, 1964; Levine & Mahler, 1964; Grodsky & Forsham, 1966). During this time, insulin has been successfully analysed and synthesized from its individual amino acids. Practical methods have been devised for its assay in small quantities, and these have been used to study the biosynthesis, secretion and transport of the hormone. Lastly, facts are emerging about the nature of insulin's biological activity and the part which it plays in the economy of the normal subject or animal.

Chemistry. In 1955, Brown *et al.* (1955) showed that insulin is a polypeptide composed of 51 amino acids arranged in two chains (the "A" and the "B" chains) joined to one another by two disulphide bridges; a third disulphide bridge joins two amino acids in the "A" chain. This basic structure, illustrated in Fig. 3.1, is common to molecules of insulin derived from the mammals, fishes and birds which have been investigated. In most cases, differences between molecules of insulin produced by different species are confined to the natures and sequences of amino acids in one or other of the chains. These differences are often minor (Table 3.1), but in insulins produced by the guinea pig and certain fishes they are pronounced (Smith, 1966). Dixon & Wardlaw (1960) were able to reconstitute the hormone from component chains and so produce hybrid molecules of insulin. Three groups of chemists in China, Germany and the United States now claim to have synthesized insulin from individual amino acids (Katsoyannis, Tometsko, Zalut & Fukuda, 1966; Du, Jiang & Tsou, 1965; Zahn, Gutte & Brinkhoff, 1965). The reported yields are low, and the biological activities of the products do not appear to be as great as those found for insulins of natural origins. These achievements should not, however, be under-rated, for they represent the first successful attempt to analyse and synthesize a protein.

Many questions about the insulin molecule

COMPOSITION OF HUMAN INSULIN

Position in Chain	"A" Chain	"B" Chain
	N-terminal	N-terminal
1	Glycine	Phenylalanine
2	Isoleucine	Valine
3	Valine	Asparagine
4	Glutamic Acid	Glutamine
5	Glutamine	Histidine
6	S--------- Cysteine	Leucine
7	Cysteine ------ S ----- S------ Cysteine	
8	Threonine	Glycine
9	Serine	Serine
10	Isoleucine	Histidine
11	S---------Cysteine	Leucine
12	Serine	Valine
13	Leucine	Glutamic Acid
14	Tyrosine	Alanine
15	Glutamine	Leucine
16	Leucine	Tyrosine
17	Glutamic Acid	Leucine
18	Asparagine	Valine
19	Tyrosine	S ------ Cysteine
20	Cysteine -------S	Glycine
21	Asparagine	Glutamic Acid
22		Arginine
23	C-terminal	Glycine
24		Phenylalanine
25		Phenylalanine
26		Tyrosine
27		Threonine
28		Proline
29		Lysine
30		Threonine
		C-terminal

FIG. 3.1. Basic structure of human insulin showing the natures and positions of individual amino acids in the "A" and "B" chains, and the N-terminal (NH_2) and C-terminal (COOH) ends of each chain.

still remain unanswered. For example, the sequence of amino acids in an insulin molecule can now be determined, but this does not appear to be the

TABLE 3.1

Sequences of amino acids in some mammalian insulin molecules

Species	"A" Chain			"B"
	8	9	10	30
Human	Threonine	Serine	Isoleucine	Threonine
Beef	Alanine	Serine	Valine	Alanine
Pork	Threonine	Serine	Isoleucine	Alanine
Sheep	Alanine	Glycine	Valine	Alanine
Whale	Threonine	Serine	Isoleucine	Alanine

only factor determining the properties of the molecule. Insulin molecules produced by the pig and sperm whale have identical sequences of amino acids in both chains (Table 3.1), but they have differing immunological properties (Berson & Yalow, 1961*a*). Moloney also suggests that after extraction from the pancreas insulin is not the same as the hormone formed in the pancreas during life and secreted into the blood (in Cameron & O'Connor, 1962). Until more is known of the molecule of insulin as it exists in the body, and of its physical nature in more than a single dimension, many present observations must remain unexplained.

Storage. Insulin is found in the islets of Langerhans, where it exists in the β-cells as granules which can be stained with aldehyde fuchsin or similar stains (Lazarus & Volk, 1962). Under the electron microscope, these granules take on different shapes in different species and appear to be enclosed in smooth membranous sacs (Lacy, 1957); Lazarus & Volk (1962) suggest that these sacs and not the granules take on the specific stains. Lazarus (1959) was the first to demonstrate glucose-6-phosphatase in the β-cell, and since then most of the enzymes required for glucose metabolism and protein synthesis have been demonstrated by similar histochemical methods (see Brolin, Hellman & Knutson, 1964).

For reasons which are understandable, little is known of the early stages of development of islets in man. Without the aid of specific stains, Pearce (1903) examined 21 human foetuses and concluded that structural maturity of the islets is achieved in the fourth month of intra-uterine life. Very recently, Steinke & Driscoll (1965) were able to extract insulin from the human pancreas between the twentieth and thirty-second week of foetal life; the content almost doubled between

then and birth, from 12·3 to 21·1 Units/g. More is known from experiments carried out in animals. After the seventeenth day of the 21 days of intra-uterine life, insulin can be extracted from the pancreas of the rat (Dixit, Lowe, Heggestad & Lazarow, 1964) but, as had been shown by Hard (1944), granules do not appear in the β-cells until the eighteenth day; granules do not appear in the α-cells until after birth. In the mouse, granules appear in the β-cells on the eighteenth day of the 20 days of intra-uterine life, but distinguishable α-cells are not seen until seven days after birth (Munger, 1958). In the rabbit, Bencosme (1955) was unable to demonstrate granules in the β-cells until about seven days after birth, complete differentiation of islet cells being achieved only after about three months of post-natal life. These widely varying rates of islet development require further investigation, especially with relation to pancreatic secretory activity; as does the much debated question of the origin of the islets themselves (Lazarus & Volk, 1962).

Measurement of insulin secretion. Specific confirmation of the role of glucose in the insulin secretory process has become possible with the introduction of highly sensitive and specific methods for the assay of insulin, and the development of suitable techniques for the study of islet tissue *in vitro*. For the quantitative estimation of insulin secretion, two principle methods are now employed:

(i) *Incubation and perfusion of pancreatic tissue in vitro.* By modification of a method originally described by Anderson & Long (1948), groups led by Grodsky and Sussman have studied insulin secretion into fluids perfusing the isolated rat pancreas (Grodsky, Batts, Bennett, Vcella, McWilliams & Smith, 1963; Sussman, Vaughan & Timmer, 1966*b*). The first extensive studies of pancreatic tissue incubated *in vitro* were reported by Coore & Randle (1964*b*), who used tissue from the rabbit. In both these methods, insulin accumulating in the perfusion or incubation medium was assayed by immuno-specific methods (see measurement of insulin in plasma), but the less specific methods of bio-assay have been used by others. To overcome the effect of a potent lytic substance released from incubated pieces of the rat's pancreas, Malaisse, Malaisse-Lagae & Wright (1967*f*) incorporated guinea-pig anti-insulin serum (GPAIS) in their incubation media, and calculated insulin secretion from the rate at which reactive antibodies to insulin disappeared from the medium. Finally, Lacy & Kostianowski (1967) have introduced a simple method for the isolation of individual islets from the mammalian pancreas. Collagenase is used to destroy the connective tissue of the gland, the islets then being separated from the acini by differential centrifugation in solutions of sucrose or, with less damage to the cells, by gravity in buffered solutions. Using groups of four to six of these islets, it has been possible to obtain reproducible estimates of secretion (Malaisse, Malaisse-Lagae, Lacy & Wright, 1967a). Though it is possible to obtain isolated islets from fishes (hagfish, toadfish, and members of the Cottus family) much more readily than from mammals, the insulins which they secrete do not react with the antibodies to mammalian insulins commonly used for immunoassays of insulin. For this reason, less is known of insulin secretion from the fish's than from mammalian pancreatic islets; but more is known of the metabolic processes involved in fish islets.

(ii) *Acute changes in the insulin content of the blood.* At best, these methods are quantitatively crude, but they were among the first to give important leads in the study of factors influencing insulin secretion. The first of these, and the only one which can be put to practical use in man, involves continuous study of the level of circulating insulin. Increased secretion of the hormone has been inferred from a rapid increase in the concentration of insulin after administration of a drug or metabolite. In experimental animals, similar studies have been reported, but attempts have also been made to collect blood issuing from the pancreas and so make a quantitative estimate of pancreatic insulin secretion; notable amongst these were the attempts of Metz (1960) and Seltzer (1962), both of whom used dogs. To circumvent the necessity for surgical interference and estimate all insulin secreted by the pancreas *in vivo*, Wright, Rivera-Calimlim & Malaisse (1966) injected known amounts of guinea pig anti-insulin serum intravenously into rats, and equated subsequent insulin secretion to the rate at which injected insulin antibodies were neutralized *in vivo*.

In addition to the evidence which has been obtained by these quantitative and semi-quantitative methods, morphological changes in the islets have been studied by both light and electron microscopy (Lazarus & Volk, 1962; Lacy, 1967). With the aid of these histological techniques, it has been shown that when the β-cell is stimulated, the granules within them migrate toward the periphery (margination of the granules). The sacs enclosing the granules fuse with the membrane of the cell, rupture and then release the granule into the interstitial space. This process, first observed in rat pancreas, has been termed "emiocytosis" (Lacy, 1961), and has been observed in other cells which contain granular secretory products. If

TABLE 3.2

Stimulants and inhibitors of insulin secretion in vivo or in vitro

Stimulants	Stimulant Activity	Inhibitors				
		Mannoheptulose Glucosamine	2-deoxy Glucose	α-adrenergic Agents*	Diazoxide	Atropine
1. Glucose	+++	+	+	+	+	−
2. Potassium	+					
3. 3′5′-adenosine monophosphate (Cyclic AMP)	+					
4. β-adrenergic agents**	±					
5. Glucagon	++			+	+	
6. ACTH	+					
7. TSH	+					
8. Theophylline, Caffeine	+++	+	+			
9. Gastro-intestinal factors	+					
10. Acetylcholine	+			+		+
11. Amino acids	+to++			−	−	
12. Sulphonylureas	+	−		+	±	

(*) Inhibition induced by α-adrenergic agents (adrenaline) is blocked by α-adrenergic blocking agents (phenoxybenzamine, phentolamine or ergotamine). (**) Isoproterenol stimulates *in vitro* when mixed with an α-adrenergic blocking agent (phenoxybenzamine) and is said to do so when given alone *in vivo*. Activities of stimulants are represented very crudely (+ to +++). Inhibitory effects have been agreed (+), not found (−), found by one observer but not by another (±), or have not been studied.

stimulation of the β-cells is continued, most of the granules disappear (degranulation) only to return when the stimulus is removed.

Physiological factors influencing insulin secretion. Under physiological conditions, insulin secretion is stimulated by glucose. Glucagon, certain amino acids, and a factor released from the gastro-intestinal tract may also play a part, but their exact physiological significances have yet to be determined. The only physiological inhibitor which has yet been found is adrenaline. Some of these factors are shown in Table 3.2.

concentration is less than about 100 mg./100 ml. but as the level is raised to 500–750 mg./100 ml. the rate of insulin secretion increases progressively to a maximum (Fig. 3.3).

The part played by glucose in the insulin secretory process has been studied with the experimental models described above. For reasons reported by Coore & Randle (1964*b*), it is assumed that the β-cell of the pancreas resembles the hepatic cell in being freely permeable to glucose. The cell itself contains many of the enzymes known to be necessary for the oxidation of glu-

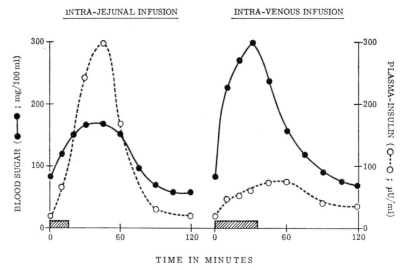

FIG. 3.2. Blood-sugar and plasma-insulin concentrations in normal human subjects following intrajejunal (15 min) and intravenous (35 min) infusion of the same amount of glucose (60g). (From McIntyre, Holdsworth & Turner, 1965.)

The administration of glucose (Fig. 3.2) causes a rapid increase in the level of circulating insulin in man, whether the hormone is assayed by biological or immunological methods (Vallance-Owen & Wright, 1960; Martin, Renold & Dagenais, 1958; Yalow & Berson, 1960). Glucose has also been shown to stimulate insulin secretion by perfused rat pancreas (Grodsky *et al.*, 1963; Sussman *et al.*, 1966*b*); by incubated pieces of rabbit (Coore & Randle, 1964*b*) and rat (Frerichs, Reich & Creutzfeldt, 1965; Malaisse *et al.*, 1967*f*) pancreas; and by isolated islets from rat pancreas (Lacy & Kostianowski, 1967). When the pancreatic tissue is exposed continuously to the same perfusion or incubation medium, insulin secretion occurs at a constant rate which increases with the glucose content of that medium. Thus Malaisse *et al.* (1967*f*) have shown that rat pancreas secretes small amounts of insulin *in vitro* when the glucose

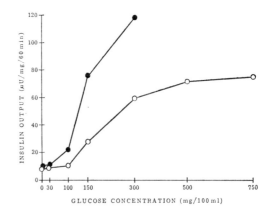

FIG. 3.3. Effects of glucose (open circles) and of glucose and theophylline (closed circles; 1.4 mM) during 60 minutes upon insulin output by pieces of incubated rat's pancreas (Malaisse, unpublished).

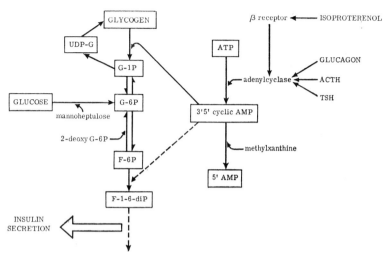

FIG. 3.4. Possible modes of action of substances stimulating or inhibiting insulin secretion *in vitro*. Those promoting the formation of 3'5'-cyclic AMP (β-adrenergic agents, glucagon, ACTH and TSH) or inhibiting its destruction (methylxanthines) promote insulin secretion by stimulating glycogenolysis or (possibly) phosphofructokinase. The sites of action of mannoheptulose and 2-deoxyglucose-6-phosphate, which inhibit glucose metabolism and the stimulant effect of glucose, are also shown. For further details, see text.

cose and the synthesis of proteins (see Field, 1964; Grodsky & Forsham, 1966), and of some importance may be the fact that it contains glucose-6-phosphatase (Lazarus, 1959). It has therefore been assumed that after entry into the β-cell, glucose can be metabolized by processes comparable to those found in other tissues.

There is now abundant evidence that glucose is only able to stimulate insulin secretion if it can be metabolized in the glycolytic pathway beyond the stage of fructose-6-phosphate (Fig. 3.4). Both *in vivo* (Wright *et al.*, 1966) and *in vitro* (Coore & Randle, 1964*b*), insulin secretion can be completely abolished by mannoheptulose which is known to inhibit the phosphorylation of glucose in the liver (Coore & Randle, 1964*a*). Glucosamine has a similar effect upon the phosphorylation of glucose and it too will inhibit insulin secretion *in vivo* and *in vitro* (Martin & Bambers, 1965). The isomerization of glucose-6-phosphate to fructose-6-phosphate can be competitively inhibited by 2-deoxyglucose-6-phosphate formed from 2-deoxyglucose; this is well known to occur in other tissues which are able to phosphorylate but not further metabolize 2-deoxyglucose (Wick, Drury, Nakoda & Wolfe, 1957). Such a process occurring in the β-cell would explain why 2-deoxyglucose also inhibits secretion of insulin by pieces of the rat's pancreas incubated in the presence of glucose (Malaisse *et al.*, 1967*f*); this

inhibitory effect is competitive. Further oxidation of fructose-6-phosphate appears to be necessary, for glucose will not stimulate insulin secretion *in vitro* either under anoxic conditions or under aerobic conditions when the media contain potassium cyanide or 2:4-dinitrophenol (Coore & Randle, 1964*b*; Malaisse *et al.*, 1967*f*). It is still not known at which point in the oxidative process glucose exerts its stimulant effect, and no metabolite of glucose along this pathway has yet been found which can exert a comparable stimulant action.

Other naturally occurring metabolites have been shown to influence insulin secretion *in vivo* or *in vitro*, but it is not clearly established in several instances whether these effects are produced independently or are mediated through modification of the metabolism of glucose. In the complete absence of glucose, only Grodsky's group have been able to stimulate insulin secretion with physiologically significant substances; with potassium they have produced such effects (Grodsky & Bennett, 1966). The significance of these observations is not known, but other observations suggest that modification of insulin secretion is more commonly associated with modification of effects produced by glucose. Amongst these are inhibitors (adrenaline) and stimulants (glucagon, adrenocorticotropin, thyrotropin, 3'5'-cyclic AMP, etc.).

(i) *Inhibitors*. Adrenaline has been shown to inhibit the effects of glucose upon insulin secretion both *in vivo* and *in vitro*. When adrenaline is infused into human subjects, it gradually raises the concentration of glucose in the blood, but the level of circulating insulin does not rise; infusion of glucose raises both. When the infusion is stopped, there is an immediate rise in the concentration of plasma-insulin and the blood-sugar concentration falls (Porte, Graber, Kuzuya & Williams, 1966). Insulin secretion by pieces of pancreatic tissue incubated with glucose is reduced when adrenaline is added to the medium (Coore & Randle, 1964*b*; Malaisse, Malaisse-Lagae, Wright & Ashmore, 1967*h*). The mechanism underlying this effect is not completely understood, but Malaisse *et al.* (1967*h*) have shown that it can be prevented by addition of an α-adrenergic blocking agent (phenoxybenzamine, phentolamine, etc.) to the medium in addition to the adrenergic agent.

(ii) *Stimulants*. When a predominantly β-adrenergic agent (isoproterenol) is added to the medium in which pancreatic tissue is incubated, it has a similar inhibitory effect, but this is converted to a stimulant action if an α-adrenergic blocking agent is also added (e.g. phenoxybenzamine). This stimulant action is weak, completely lacking when glucose is absent from the medium, and most marked at high glucose concentrations (Malaisse, Malaisse-Lagae & Mayhew, 1967*d*). The adenylcyclase system in the liver and other tissues (Robison, Butcher & Sutherland, 1967) is activated by β-adrenergic agents and other substances whose effects upon insulin secretion have been investigated. Stimulation of insulin secretion in man has been induced by injection of glucagon (Crockford, Porte, Wood & Williams, 1966; Samols, Marri & Marks, 1965; Karam, Grasso, Wegienka, Grodsky & Forsham, 1966) without any appreciable rise in the blood-sugar concentration. Glucagon will also stimulate insulin secretion by pancreatic tissue *in vitro* (Turner & McIntyre, 1966), but it only appears to do so when glucose is present in the medium (Malaisse *et al.*, 1967*d*). No secretion is induced by 3′5′-adenosine monophosphate (cyclic AMP) in normal pancreatic tissue unless glucose is present in the medium, and the same applies to theophylline and caffeine which inhibit breakdown of cyclic AMP in the liver. On the other hand, all these substances have maximal stimulant effects when glucose is present in the medium in high concentration (300 mg./100 ml.). The same was found to apply to adrenocorticotropic and thyrotropic hormones whose stimulant effects, however,

were much weaker than that of glucagon. From these observations, Malaisse *et al.* (1967*d*) concluded that the β-cell of the islet must contain an adenyl cyclase system similar to that found in adipose and hepatic tissue. They postulated, on the basis of the available evidence, that this system activates phosphorylase and (possibly) phosphofructokinase and that substances able to produce this effect are able to augment the effect of glucose upon insulin secretion (Fig. 3.4). Grodsky, Bennett, Smith & Schmid (1967) were able to stimulate secretion in the perfused rat's pancreas in the complete absence of glucose with both glucagon and theophylline, so the modes of action of these and related substances must still remain a matter of doubt.

Another possible physiological stimulant is a factor or factors released into the blood before or during the absorption of food from the gastro-intestinal tract. This hypothesis is based on the observation by Elrick, Stimmler, Hlad & Arai (1964) that oral administration of glucose gives rise to an elevation of the level of circulating insulin which precedes any appreciable rise in blood-glucose concentration, and is greater than that induced by infusion of glucose into a vein at a comparable rate (Fig. 3.2). This observation was confirmed by McIntyre, Holdsworth & Turner (1965) who considered that secretin might be the effective humoral agent. Unger, Ketterer, Eisentraut & Dupre (1966) found that both crude and purified preparations of secretin cause an almost immediate increase in the insulin content of pancreatico-duodenal venous blood in the dog without any appreciable increase in blood-glucose concentration. The purified preparation rapidly raises plasma-insulin concentration in man (Dupre, Rojas, White, Unger & Beck, 1966). An alternative suggestion by Samols *et al.* (1965) was that the humoral agent could be a form of glucagon released from the upper gastro-intestinal tract; they have since published evidence that the gut wall contains a substance with immunological properties similar to, but not always identical with, those of pancreatic glucagon (Samols, Tyler, Megyesi & Marks, 1966).

One other possible physiological stimulant is the parasympathetic system. Pancreatic tissue is supplied with nerves from both the sympathetic and parasympathetic systems, and it has been suggested that the parasympathetic fibres supply the cells of the islets (Richins, 1945). Vagal stimulation has been shown to stimulate insulin secretion in the dog (Kaneto, Kosaka & Nakao, 1967). It has also been shown that acetylcholine, in the presence of eserine and moderate concentrations of glucose (150 mg./100 ml.), will stimulate insulin secretion *in vitro*, an effect which is abolished by simultaneous addition of atropine (Malaisse *et al.*, 1967*h*).

Finally, mention must be made of the amino acids, several of which have been shown to stimulate insulin secretion. The best known is leucine which was first found to induce hypoglycaemia in certain cases of idiopathic hypoglycaemia of infancy (Cochrane, Payne, Simpkiss & Woolf, 1956). In normal adults, arginine, lysine, phenylalanine, and leucine have been shown to increase the level of circulating insulin (Floyd, Fajans, Conn, Knopf & Rull, 1966). Leucine and arginine are also effective in stimulating secretion from normal rat pancreas *in vitro*, and their effects are more potent than those of phenylalanine and tryptophan; lysine, histidine, valine and methionine appear to be inactive (Malaisse, unpublished).

The physiological significance of these observations has yet to be established, but certain conclusions do seem warranted. Schalch (1967) has recently shown that during acute stress and exercise, biochemical changes occur in man which are compatible with release of endogenous catecholamines, but which do not include any alteration in the level of circulating insulin. This finding, which is similar to that reported recently by Hertelendy, Machlin, Gordon, Horino & Kipnis (1966) following adrenaline injection into the pig, is consistent with the hypothesis that adrenaline plays a physiological role in the control of insulin secretion. The role of glucose itself is not certain except under the rare conditions in which marked hyperglycaemia exists. Under conditions approximating to normoglycaemia, it is possible that the "intestinal factor" may play a more dominant role in preventing the development of hyperglycaemia. An alternative possibility is that ingestion of food accompanied by the "gustatory reflex" could, by way of vagal stimulation, evoke the early secretion of insulin which follows. These and other possibilities have yet to be investigated, and explanations have to be found for altered responses to glucose which follow changes in the nutritional or endocrine status of an animal or man. Fasting or adrenalectomy reduces, and the administration of cortisone increases, sensitivity of the rat's secretory mechanisms to glucose (Malaisse, Malaisse-Lagae & Wright, 1967*g*; Malaisse, Malaisse-Lagae, McCraw & Wright, 1967*c*).

Pharmacological agents influencing insulin secretion. Reference has been made above to a number of agents which can affect insulin secretion, and which cannot be considered as physiological. Of more significance to the present topic, however, are two groups of compounds which have been used for therapeutic purposes in man—the sulphonylureas and the benzothiadiazines.

In a very exhaustive review of the literature available at that time, Duncan & Baird (1960) concluded that three facts had been established concerning the mode of action of the Sulphonylureas. These drugs induce hypoglycaemia only when endogenous or exogenous insulin is present *in vivo*; they stimulate release of insulin from the pancreas, at least initially, and reduce hepatic glucose release. They were constrained to admit, however, that the hypothesis attributing induced hypoglycaemia only to stimulation of insulin secretion was "not proven".

There is no doubt that these drugs do stimulate insulin secretion both *in vivo* and *in vitro*, but the mechanism is still debated (Levine & Mahler, 1964). Injection of sulphonylureas into rats or rabbits results in degranulation of the β-cells within a few hours (Lacy, 1961; Lazarus & Volk, 1962); emiocytosis similar to that seen after glucose administration is observed. When the isolated rat pancreas is perfused with the drug, an immediate increase in insulin concentration is observed in the perfusion fluid (Sussman *et al.*, 1966*b*). Variable responses have been observed during incubation of pancreatic tissue from the rat (Frerichs *et al.*, 1965; Malaisse, Malaisse-Lagae, Mayhew & Wright, 1967*e*) and rabbit (Coore & Randle, 1964*b*). When the secretory response was related to time of exposure of the tissue, glucose was found to exert a continuous effect for 2 hr., but the effect of tolbutamide was complete in 1 hr. and the tissue was then resistant to stimulation by both glucose and tolbutamide (Malaisse *et al.*, 1967*e*). Moreover, this stimulant effect was independent of the presence of glucose, and only adrenaline was able to inhibit it; mannoheptulose and diazoxide, though inhibiting the action of glucose, had no effect upon that of tolbutamide. Bellens observed (1961) that 1 hr. after administration of tolbutamide to the normal dog, a second dose of the drug did not induce the same response as the first; after the second dose the dog disposed of glucose at a slower rate than it did after the first. Our present knowledge of the actions of these drugs has not therefore advanced very much; they do appear to induce insulin secretion, but this effect is not sufficient to explain their hypoglycaemic action or their undoubted value in the treatment of certain diabetics.

The benzothiadiazines came into prominence as

potential inhibitors of insulin secretion when Goldner, Zarowitz & Akgun (1960) observed that chlorthiazide aggravates the signs of diabetes in a proportion of cases, but does not induce diabetes in normal human subjects. Diazoxide has since been used clinically to prevent onset of hypoglycaemia in human patients. Amongst its other effects, this drug has been shown to inhibit insulin secretion induced by glucose in slices of pancreatic tissue from the rabbit (Howell & Taylor, 1966), and in pieces of rat pancreas (Malaisse et al., 1967e). In rats the drug induces transient hyperglycaemia, but it fails to do so after either the pituitary or adrenal glands have been removed (Yabo, Viktora, Staquet & Wolff, 1965). This observation suggested that diazoxide may have two effects in vivo, both contributing to suppression of insulin secretion: a direct effect upon the islets, and an indirect one involving release of adrenaline from the adrenal glands. Subsequent observations in man have led to similar conclusions (Fajans, Floyd, Knopf, Rull, Guntsche & Conn, 1966; Graber, Porte & Williams, 1966).

Though it has not been used for therapeutic purposes, 2-deoxyglucose has been administered to man and has been found to elevate blood-sugar concentration without elevating the level of circulating insulin (Karam et al., 1966). In this case it does not appear that the sugar inhibits insulin secretion directly as it has been shown to do in vitro; it causes release of endogenous adrenaline which has the inhibitory effect (Laszlo, Harlan, Klein, Kirshner, Estes & Bogdonoff, 1961).

Biosynthesis. Present knowledge of the biosynthesis of insulin by the β-cell is mainly based on observations made with the islets of certain fishes; those of the goosefish and toadfish, for example, are easily obtained since they exist as nodules of tissue which are quite separate from the acinar pancreas. In such islets, as reviewed by Lazarow (in Leibel & Wrenshall, 1965), synthesis of insulin takes place on the ribosomes on an RNA template, each chain of amino acids (Fig. 3.1) being built up separately from the N-terminal to the C-terminal end (Humbel, 1965). There is evidence that the islets contain glutathione-insulin transhydrogenase (Kotoulas, Morrison & Recant, 1965) which can reversibly split all the disulphide bonds in the insulin molecule (Katzen, Tietze & Stetten, 1963), but there remains considerable doubt as to the way in which the two chains are joined together to give the complete insulin molecule (Humbel, 1966). From the microsomes, the newly synthesized insulin is transferred to the granules either directly or through transformation of the endoplasmic reticulum (see Brolin et al., 1964; Lacy, 1967). Since Lazarus's first histochemical demonstration of glucose-6-phosphatase in the β-cell (1959), many of the enzymes necessary for glucose oxidation and protein synthesis have been demonstrated in the β-cells of fishes or mammals either by histological or micro-chemical methods (see Field, 1964; Grodsky & Forsham, 1966). Further studies should therefore provide detailed information of the processes involved in biosynthesis of insulin in fishes.

Quantitative study of insulin biosynthesis in mammals is hindered by the fact that the islets of Langerhans are embedded in acinar tissue. Despite this fact, biosynthetically labelled insulin has been isolated from incubated pieces of rat, rabbit and ox pancreas (Mallory, Smith & Taylor, 1964). Like Humbel (1963), who used fish islets, Parry & Taylor (1966) were able to show that glucose and mannose stimulate the biosynthesis of insulin in mammalian islets, a process which is inhibited by mannoheptulose and dinitrophenol. Thus, those factors which stimulate insulin secretion may also stimulate biosynthesis of the hormone. Confirmation of this and other possibilities should be forthcoming as existing and new techniques are perfected. These include the isolation in large numbers of individual mammalian islets (Lacy & Kostianowski, 1967) and of individual insulin granules (Lindall, Bauer, Dixit & Lazarow, 1963); and the use of micro-methods for the study of enzymes in individual islets (Smith & Lacy, 1962; see Brolin et al., 1964).

Assay. Two broad groups of methods have been used to study insulin during its passage from the pancreas to the tissues which use it. These methods of assay have been reviewed (Vallance-Owen & Wright, 1960; Berson & Yalow, 1964a; Goetz, in Leibel & Wrenshall, 1965), so only brief mention need be made of their principles here.

(i) *Bio-assay.* Although Bornstein (1950) was the first to introduce a method capable of detecting small quantities of insulin, others failed to repeat his observations using adrenalectomized-hypophysectomized-alloxan-diabetic (ADHA) rats. Later investigators were able to show that plasma contains sufficient insulin to stimulate glucose uptake by the isolated rat diaphragm (Groen, Kamminga, Willebrands & Blickman, 1952; Randle, 1954; Vallance-Owen & Hurlock, 1954), or the production of radioactive carbon dioxide from ^{14}C-labelled glucose by the epididymal fat pad of the rat (Martin et al., 1958). Though these two methods are seldom used for routine purposes, they have provided useful if controversial information concerning the nature of insulin circulating in the blood and extracellular fluids.

(ii) *Immuno-assay*. These methods all depend upon the same basic reaction between mixtures of unlabelled and radio-iodinated (^{131}I- and ^{125}I-labelled) insulin on the one hand and antibodies to insulin produced by the guinea pig on the other. A fixed amount of the labelled hormone (usually porcine insulin for the assay of human plasma) is mixed with known amounts of unlabelled insulin

the ratio of "bound" to "free" insulin in the final reaction mixture will fall as the original amount of unlabelled hormone is raised. Individual methods differ only in the varying techniques used to separate "bound" from "free" insulin in the incubated mixtures (Fig. 3.5).

The original method for immuno-assay of insulin described by Yalow & Berson (1960) involved chromato-electrophoresis on filter paper. Whereas "free" insulin remained fixed to the

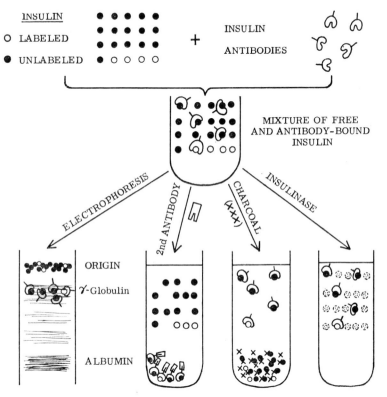

FIG. 3.5. Diagrammatic representation of the basic methods for immuno-assay of insulin showing separation of free from antibody-bound insulin by (1) chromato-electrophoresis on filter paper; (2) addition of a second precipitating antibody; (3) addition of charcoal or other substance capable of adsorbing free insulin; and (4) treatment with insulinase which degrades free insulin.

or the sample of plasma. When this mixture is exposed under standard conditions to a fixed amount of guinea-pig anti-insulin serum, some of the insulin reacts with the antibodies to become "bound", the excess remaining "free". It is assumed that the labelled hormone behaves toward the antibodies in the same way as the unlabelled insulin, so that as the amount of unlabelled insulin in the original mixture is raised, the proportion of "bound" labelled hormone in the final reaction mixture falls. Put another way,

paper at the point of application of the sample of incubated reaction mixture (the origin), "bound" insulin had an electrophoretic mobility comparable with the "inter γ-β" zone of the plasma-proteins. More routine use is now made of a second method based on original observations by Skom & Talmage (1958a). In this method (Morgan & Lazarow, 1963; Hales & Randle, 1963a), insulin "bound" by the antibodies is precipitated with the guinea-pig γ-globulins by serum from another animal (rabbit or goat) which contains antibodies to those globulins; the "free" insulin remains in solution. Various other methods have been used to achieve the separation of "free" from "bound" insulin in the final reaction mixture. Thus Grodsky & Forsham (1960) precipitated "bound" insulin with the globulins by means of sodium sulphite. Herbert, Lau, Gottlieb & Bleicher (1965) adsorbed the "free" insulin with charcoal coated with dextran, and Beck, Zaharko, Roberts, McNeil, King & Blankenbaker (1964) used "insulinase" to destroy it.

Transport. During almost two decades, a vast quantity of data has been published concerning insulin concentrations in the body's fluids, but there is still no unanimity concerning the form or

(Vallance-Owen & Wright, 1960), but it is generally considered to be more specific than the epididymal fat pad. The concentrations of insulin-like activity (ILA) obtained under similar conditions with the fat pad have ranged between about 50 and over 500 μU/ml. (Martin *et al.*, 1958; Froesch, Burgi, Ramseier, Bally & Labhart, 1963*a*).

In the case of the fat pad, it has been established that anti-insulin serum abolishes only part of the biological activity. In reviewing their work, Samaan, Frazer & Dempster (1963) support the contention that plasma contains two forms of insulin. The first they term "typical" since it resembles insulin extracted from the pancreas and

TABLE 3.3

Some properties of "Bound" and "Non-suppressible" insulin-like activity compared with those of "Free" and "Suppressible" insulin

	"Free" "Suppressible"	"Bound"	"Non-suppressible"
Molecular Weight	Less than 40,000	60,000 to 100,000	70,000 to 150,000
Electrophoretic Mobility	α_1-Globulin	from β to γ-Globulin	from α_2 to β-Globulin
Biological activity:			
(1) Muscle, *in vitro*	Active	Inactive	Active
(2) Adipose tissue, *in vitro*	Active	Active	Active
(3) *In vivo*	Active	Active	Active
Action of:			
(1) Anti-insulin serum	Inactivated	Not affected	Not affected
(2) Acid-ethanol	Extracted unchanged	Altered to "Free"	Extracted unchanged
(3) Performic acid	"A" and "B" Chains produced		No "A" or "B" Chains produced
(4) Reduced glutathione	Inactivated	Inactivated	Inactivated
(5) Alkali	Inactivated		Inactivated
(6) Heat (80°C)	Inactivated		Stable

(Results reported by Froesch, Muller, Burgi, Waldvogel & Labhart, 1966; Burgi, Muller, Humbel, Labhart & Froesch, 1966; Antoniades, Huber, Boshell, Saravis & Gershoff, 1965).

forms in which insulin is transported round the body. One side of the current argument is forcibly stated by Berson & Yalow (1965) who have studied sera by means of their immuno-assay method (Yalow & Berson, 1960). With this and similar methods, the normal resting level of circulating insulin in the fasting human subject is found to be less than 50 μU/ml. Using undiluted plasma, comparable but slightly higher levels are found with the isolated rat diaphragm (Vallance-Owen & Hurlock, 1954; Wright, 1957), and all this biological activity can be suppressed with guinea pig anti-insulin serum (Wardlaw & Moloney, 1961); much higher values are reported with the same methods when diluted plasma is assayed (Randle, 1954). This method is quantitatively inaccurate

can be inactivated with anti-insulin serum. The second was called "atypical" since it could not be inactivated with this serum; in their opinion it is a form of insulin derived from the "typical" form during passage through the liver. Froesch *et al.* (1963) also reported that only part of the insulin-like activity was "suppressible" with anti-insulin serum; the remainder was "non-suppressible" (Table 3.3). They differed in their conclusions as to the identity of "non-suppressible ILA" for they did not consider that this form could be converted to the "suppressible" form. Later, the same group extracted "non-suppressible" insulin-like substances from human serum and reported details of its physical and biological properties (Burgi, Muller, Humbel, Labhart & Froesch, 1966;

Froesch, Muller, Burgi, Waldvogel & Labhart, 1966). Like insulin, and as Samaan's group had previously claimed (Samaan *et al.*, 1963), it can be extracted with acid alcohol and its biological activity can be abolished by treatment with cysteine or glutathione. On the other hand it proved stable in solutions of high molarity and at high temperatures (80°C for 3 hr.), it had a much higher molecular weight (70,000 to 150,000), and did not yield detectable amounts of "A" or "B" chain when treated with performic acid. In a number of biological systems it exhibited activity which differed from that of insulin only in that it could not be suppressed with anti-insulin serum. They also observed that under a variety of circumstances, the level of "non-suppressible" insulin in plasma did not vary, a change which would not be expected if, as Samaan's group claimed, one form can be converted to the other.

In all the experiments reported by Samaan and Froesch, the fat pad was used exclusively for the assay of insulin-like activity. A second and more contentious theory has been put forward on the basis of experiments in which the fat pad and the rat's diaphragm have been used to study insulin-like activity in plasma. In this way, Antoniades and his group (Antoniades, Bougas, Camerini-Davalos & Pyle, 1964; Antoniades, Huber, Boshell, Saravis & Gershoff, 1965) have demonstrated a "free" and a "bound" form of circulating insulin. The "free" form resembles pancreatic insulin but the "bound" form differs from it in several respects (Table 3.3). It is absorbed by cation-exchange resins (e.g. Dowex-50), it has a molecular weight of more than 60,000, and moves with the β- and γ-globulins on electrophoresis; stimulates metabolism by the fat pad but not that of the rat's diaphragm, and may be converted to the "free" form with acid-alcohol or on treatment with an extract of adipose tissue (ATE). These essential properties have been confirmed by Shaw & Shuey (1963), but Meade, Stiglitz, & Kleist (1965), using an immuno-assay, were unable to reveal any increased activity in plasma after the various treatments suggested by Antoniades. According to Antoniades, circulating insulin exists mainly in the "bound" form, but, when glucose is administered, the concentration of "free" insulin rises steeply and that of the "bound" hormone falls, the "free" form returning rapidly to its original concentration. From this and other observations, Antoniades concludes that insulin is secreted from the pancreas in the "free" form and is converted into the "bound" form in the liver to act as a circulating depot upon which the tissues can call in time of need.

Heated discussion still continues concerning the validity and interpretations to be placed on these observations. However, it seems reasonable to conclude that all the immuno-assayable and part of the bio-assayable activity in blood-plasma is insulin. That portion of the bio-assayable insulin-like activity which cannot be detected by immuno-assay and which cannot be neutralized with anti-insulin serum does not, on the balance of present evidence, appear to be a form of insulin. More important than its identity is the question of its physiological significance. There is evidence that, unlike insulin, the majority of insulin-like substances in the blood do not leave the vascular space. They are present in much higher concentration in the plasma than in lymph and, unlike immuno-assayable insulin, do not increase in concentration in the lymph after administration of glucose (Rasio, Soeldner & Cahill, 1965). This suggests that the only cells likely to be influenced by the larger molecules which comprise the bulk of insulin-like substances in the blood are those which come into direct contact with the blood (e.g. hepatic cells). If it can be shown that the "non-suppressible" substance is actually a component of circulating blood, then its physiological significance can be assessed. Until then, however, the present rather unconstructive arguments are likely to continue.

Inhibitors. Much has been written about components and extracts of plasma which can interfere with the action of insulin *in vivo* or *in vitro* (see Berson & Yalow, 1964b) but only two will be considered here. In the present context they are important either as potential aetiological factors in diabetes ("synalbumin") or as insulin antagonists which can interfere with the effective treatment of diabetes (insulin antibodies). Only essential details of these two factors will be considered here (Table 3.4); their significance in diabetes will be discussed later.

TABLE 3.4

Some properties of insulin antibodies and synalbumin

	Antibodies	Synalbumin
Molecular Weight	ca 150,000	4,000
Electrophoretic Mobility	from β to γ Globulin	Albumin
Action of insulin on:		
(1) Muscle, *in vitro*	Inhibit	Inhibits
(2) Adipose tissue, *in vitro*	Inhibit	Does not inhibit
(3) *In vivo*	Inhibit	Unknown

(i) *The Vallance-Owen* (*"Synalbumin"*) *insulin antagonist.* This term was recently coined by Sherman (1966) to identify the material in an extract of plasma which, according to Vallance-Owen (see Leibel & Wrenshall, 1965), inhibits the effect of insulin upon glucose uptake by the isolated rat-diaphragm. As first reported by Vallance-Owen, Dennes & Campbell (1958), it occurs in extracts made from plasma with tri-chloroacetic acid and ethanol. These extracts consist predominantly of albumin but may be contaminated to a greater or lesser extent with α-globulins. It has been confirmed by some (Alp & Recant, 1964, 1965; Sherman, 1966) that this extract in a concentration of 5% (w/v) has no effect upon the basal rate of glucose uptake by the isolated rat diaphragm but inhibits the effect of added insulin (1 mU/ml.). If the extract is obtained from the plasma of diabetic patients, it continues to inhibit the effect of insulin when its concentration is reduced to 1·25%, but at this concentration, extracts from normal plasma have no inhibitory action. These observations have been flatly contradicted in reports by Keen (Cameron, Boyns, Jarrett & Keen, 1966a) who found that such extracts stimulate glucose uptake by the rat diaphragm and, with minor debatable exceptions, fail to inhibit the action of added insulin. This discrepancy remains unexplained, but Sherman (1966) has suggested that it could be due, in part at least, to minor but significant differences in the apparently identical techniques used for extraction of the plasma; Keen's extracts could have contained more α-globulin which is known to contain insulin. On the other hand, Keen used three samples of extract which had previously been examined by Ashton (1965) and, contrary to expectations, found no inhibitory effects in any of them; Ashton had reported two to be inhibitory.

When the epididymal fat pad is used instead of the rat diaphragm, metabolism is stimulated by the extract which does not inhibit the action of insulin (Alp & Recant, 1964; Cameron *et al.,* 1966a). There remains some doubt, however, as to the nature of the stimulant. Several of the stimulant actions resemble those of insulin but there are varying reports of the effects upon them of guinea pig anti-insulin serum. In some respects the stimulant is said to resemble "non-suppressible" insulin (Cameron, Boyns, Jarrett & Keen, 1966b).

In a recent report, Ensinck, Mahler & Vallance-Owen (1965) have suggested that the active component of their extract is not the albumin itself, but a small closely associated molecule which resembles the "B" chain of the insulin molecule.

This conclusion, and much of the experimental evidence upon which it is based, has been severely criticized by Berson & Yalow (1964b, 1965). Though merit is to be found in the arguments of both the proponents and opponents of the theory, there remains a basic question which has still to be answered. No matter what the nature of the substance which has been shown to have an inhibitory effect *in vitro,* it cannot yet be said that this same substance exists in the circulating blood of man. Only when it can be shown that this substance is a component of the circulating plasma will it be possible to assess its physiological significance and the part which it plays, if any, in the aetiology of diabetes.

(ii) *Insulin antibodies.* The antigenic potential of insulin had long been suspected, but real progress began with an observation by Banting, Franks & Gairns (1938). They found that the serum of an insulin-resistant, non-diabetic schizophrenic patient could protect mice from the convulsive effects of simultaneously injected insulin. Since then the existence of insulin antibodies has become universally recognized and the subject has been reviewed on several occasions (Prout, 1962; Berson & Yalow, 1964b, 1965; Wright, 1965; Pope, 1966).

Insulin antibodies in the serum of animals and man have been detected and assayed by three principal methods:

(a) *Neutralization of hormonal activity.* Neutralization of the effects of insulin in mice was used as a method of detection for many years, but is little used now (Davidson & Eddleman, 1950; Moloney & Coval, 1955). This technique is commonly used, however, for the identification of insulin; guinea pig anti-insulin serum inhibits the effects of insulin upon metabolism in the isolated rat diaphragm (Wright, 1959) and epididymal fat pad (Samaan *et al.,* 1963; Froesch *et al.,* 1963a).

(b) *Agglutination of insulin-coated erythrocytes.* Immune serum (i.e. serum containing antibodies to insulin) will agglutinate red cells which have been conjugated with insulin through bis-diazotized benzidine (Arquilla & Stavitsky, 1956a), or which have been tanned and then coated with the hormone (Yankelowitch, Massry & Gitter, 1956).

(c) *Combination with radio-iodinated insulin.* When immune serum is allowed to react with a mixture of unlabelled and a trace of radio-iodinated insulin, it binds the insulin in the "β-γ" fraction of the proteins. Radioactive material associated with "free" insulin can then be separated from the "bound" hormone by chromatography or chromato-electrophoresis on filter paper (Berson, Yalow, Bauman, Rothschild &

Newerly, 1956); chromatography on filter paper impregnated with ion-exchange resins (Kologlu, Wiesel, Positano & Anderson, 1963; Mitchell & Bradford, 1963); by precipitation with salts (Grodsky & Forsham, 1960), cold solutions of salt in ethanol (Gordis, 1960) or antibodies to the globulins in the immune serum (Skom & Talmage, 1958a); and with suspensions of cellulose (Wright & Malaisse, 1966) or charcoal coated with dextran (Herbert et al., 1965). Some of these methods, as outlined above, have been adapted for use in the immuno-assay of insulin in blood and other fluids (Fig. 3.5).

All animals appear to produce antibodies in response to repeated injections of insulin, but the guinea pig is unique in certain respects. The antibodies which it produces seem to react more strongly with insulin than do anti-insulin sera produced by other animals or by man. Guinea pig anti-insulin serum has, for example, a much more potent protective effect in mice and rats than sera from immunized human subjects, rabbits, sheep or horses (Moloney & Goldsmith, 1957; Wright, Kreisberg, Halpern & Dolkart, 1962). This property is also responsible for its use in the radio-immuno-assay of insulin (Yalow & Berson, 1960). Guinea pig anti-insulin serum is also unique in that it is the only anti-insulin serum which induces hyperglycaemia or, in sufficient dosage, frank diabetes in experimental animals (Moloney & Coval, 1955; Wright, in Leibel & Wrenshall, 1965). This immunological peculiarity of the guinea pig has yet to be explained, but this animal does produce an insulin molecule which differs markedly in structure from those of other mammals (Smith, 1966).

In other respects, the guinea pig responds to injections of insulin in a manner very similar to those of other mammals including man. Within a few weeks or months, antibodies to insulin can be detected in the plasma of human subjects by any of the more sensitive methods outlined above (Arquilla & Stavitsky, 1956b; Skom & Talmage, 1958b; Yalow & Berson, 1961). The presence of these antibodies, even in high concentration, is not accompanied in the normal animal or man by hyperglycaemia, and sera from such actively immunized subjects do not induce hyperglycaemia when injected into other animals. An exception was recently reported by Grodsky, Feldman, Toreson & Lee (1966) in two out of nine rabbits which, after only three injections of bovine insulin, became hyperlipaemic and frankly diabetic. When present in high concentrations, an exceptional finding in man, these insulin antibodies do give rise to resistance to the effects of injected insulin; this topic will be considered in more detail later.

By means of various technical methods it has been shown that the insulin antibodies produced by man, by rabbits and by guinea pigs are γ_1- or γ_2-globulins; insulin may also be bound by proteins in the β-globulins and these are thought to be responsible for allergic reactions to insulin (Prout, 1962). Studies of their reactions with insulin have shown that all three species produce heterogeneous antibodies. It has been suggested that man produces antibodies with two antigen-binding sites, insulin behaving as a monovalent antigen (Berson & Yalow, 1959a). Antibodies produced by the rabbit and guinea pig behave in a similar heterogeneous manner (Morse, 1960), antibodies produced by individual animals being directed toward different sites on the insulin molecule (Arquilla, Ooms & Finn, 1966). Arquilla's group also suggest that the types of antibody produced by guinea pigs may be genetically determined. For many years it was considered that insulin antibodies do not precipitate the antigen from solution but precipitating anti-insulin sera have been obtained from horses, guinea pigs and rabbits (Moloney & Aprile, 1959; Steigerwald, Spielmann, Fries & Grebe, 1960; Jones & Cunliffe, 1961; Birkinshaw, Randall & Risdall, 1962; Hirata & Blumenthal, 1963). By the less sensitive methods of bio-assay, little evidence of species-specificity has been found in anti-insulin sera from either experimental animals or man. However, Moloney & Aprile (1960) showed that the serum from horses treated with bovine insulin has little protective effect in mice against the cod's insulin; this insulin has a very different structure from that of bovine insulin (Smith, 1966). Using their more sensitive method, Berson & Yalow (1959b) were able to show that sera from patients treated with mixtures of bovine and porcine insulins react more strongly with bovine and sheep than with porcine and horse insulins. After treatment with porcine insulin, however, human patients' sera combined equally well with porcine, bovine, human and bovine deoxypeptide insulins until they were returned to treatment with the bovine hormone; their sera then showed ability to distinguish between the various insulins as described above (Berson & Yalow, 1963). Most human anti-insulin sera are not able to distinguish between insulins with the same amino acid sequences, but it has been reported that in a few instances such sera bind porcine insulin much more strongly than that of the sperm whale (Berson & Yalow, 1961a). Some human anti-insulin sera, but not all, are also able to distinguish between the homologous bo-

50 DIABETES MELLITUS AND HYPOGLYCAEMIA

vine hormone used for treatment and insulin from the tunny fish, which has a very different structure (Yalow & Berson, 1964).

From this and other evidence, it is apparent that much remains to be learned about the relationship between insulin's chemical and molecular structure on the one hand and the immunological response which this hormone evokes in man and in experimental animals. The problem is of some practical significance for it is encountered in a small group of diabetic patients who become resistant to insulin and have high levels of circulating antibodies.

METABOLIC ABNORMALITIES ASSOCIATED WITH DIABETES

Experimental Approach

According to classical concepts, diabetes mellitus is characterized by over-production and under-utilization of carbohydrate, but it has long been recognized that varying degrees of abnormal lipid and protein metabolism can co-exist. Much of our present knowledge of the metabolic defects associated with diabetes has been obtained with animals in various states of insulin deficiency. These have been induced by pancreatectomy, with alloxan, anti-insulin serum (A.I.S.), or manno-heptulose, which all have the effect of reducing the level of circulating insulin. It has also been found, however, that hyperglycaemic states can be induced with growth hormone and glucocorticoids, so that other hormonal factors are known to have diabetogenic effects. The principal hormone governing utilization of glucose is thought to be insulin, but growth hormone also appears to influence this process by inhibiting uptake of glucose in certain tissues. Over-production of glucose, or gluconeogenesis, is primarily regu-

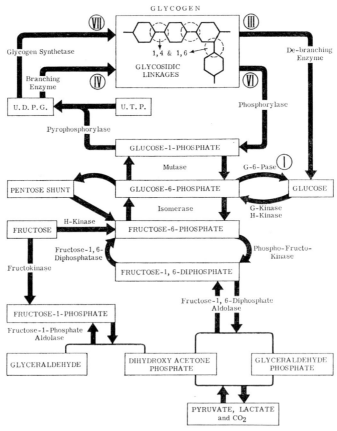

FIG. 3.6. Steps involved in the metabolism of glucose (G) and fructose (F) with emphasis upon intermediate metabolites (UTP = Uridine triphosphate; UDPG = Uridine diphosphoglucose) and enzymes (H = Hexo-). The roman numerals (I, III, IV, VI & VII) indicate the sites of impaired enzymic activity found in the corresponding types of glycogenoses discussed in the text. In hereditary fructose intolerance, hepatic activity of fructose-1-phosphate aldolase is reduced.

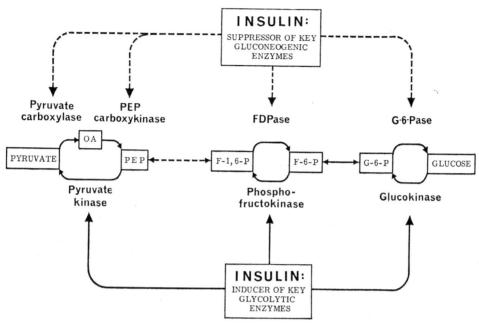

FIG. 3.7. The effects of insulin upon hepatic enzymes catalysing unidirectional reactions in the glycolytic pathway with suppression of the four principal gluconeogenic enzymes and induction of the glycolytic enzymes (From Weber, Singhal, Stamm, Lea & Fisher, 1966b).

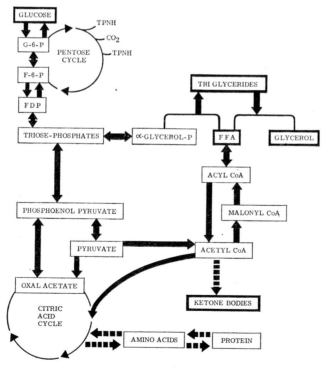

FIG. 3.8. Principal intermediate metabolites in pathways leading to the production of glucose, triglycerides, free fatty acids, glycerol and ketone bodies.

lated by the adrenal glucocorticoids, but glucagon may also play a part. In the following account each of these endocrine factors will be considered separately, attention being concentrated on their functions in the regulation of cellular metabolism and the inter-relationships between their actions. To facilitate understanding of the discussion, some of the processes involved in metabolism of carbohydrates, fats and proteins are shown in Figs. 3.6, 3.7 and 3.8.

Insulin

Lack of insulin is generally considered to be the major defect responsible for the clinical syndrome of diabetes mellitus. A growing body of evidence also indicates, however, that not all the metabolic abnormalities seen in the human diabetic can be attributed to insulin deficiency. It should be remembered, therefore, that the following discussion deals with metabolic effects which are mediated by insulin or observed in experimental states of insulin deficiency.

The primary action of insulin appears to be stimulation of entry of glucose into certain cells, principally muscle and adipose tissue. In addition, insulin is a potent anabolic agent which stimulates the synthesis of glycogen, protein and lipids. Whether these actions are inter-related is not yet established, but insulin probably plays a direct role in regulating a variety of biochemical systems. When intact animals are used, it is difficult to separate actions of insulin which are independent of its effects upon metabolism of glucose, but in several isolated tissues effects of insulin have been observed in the absence of glucose.

(i) *Glucose utilization.* Insulin stimulates utilization of glucose by intact animals *in vivo* and by isolated tissues *in vitro* (Renold, Ashmore & Hastings, 1956). It is thought to do so by facilitating the entry of glucose into individual cells, a phenomenon first described by Levine, Goldstein, Huddleston & Klein (1950). In their experiments with eviscerated nephrectomized hepatectomized dogs, Levine showed that intravenously injected non-metabolizable sugars distribute themselves in the extracellular water only. If insulin is injected, however, the volume of distribution is increased to that of the total body water. Subsequent work has shown that insulin stimulates specific transport systems for sugars in the isolated rat diaphragm (Kipnis & Cori, 1957), and that these systems are limited to muscle (Henderson, Morgan & Park, 1961) and adipose tissue (Renold, Crofford, Stauffacher & Jeanrenaud, 1965). Hepatic cells on the other hand are freely permeable to glucose (Cahill, Ashmore, Earle &

Zottu, 1958) and insulin has little if any effect upon utilization of glucose by the brain and other nervous tissue (Krahl, 1961).

The mechanism by which insulin stimulates entry of glucose into cells is largely unknown, but active transport does not appear to be involved; glucose moves from a relatively high concentration in the extracellular fluids to a low level within the cells. Randle & Smith (1958) postulated that energy is expended to keep glucose out of cells, and that insulin stimulates entry of glucose by diverting energy (in the form of ATP) to synthetic processes.

In conditions under which synthesis of ATP is reduced (anaerobiosis and certain poisons), for example, muscle cells become permeable to glucose. During exercise, which lowers levels of ATP, permeability of muscle cells is also increased (Helmreich & Cori, in Wolstenholme & O'Connor, 1956). How exercise increases permeability is not known, but utilization of glucose in severe exercise can reach a level, even in the insulin-deficient state, at which it induces fatal hypoglycaemia (Bewsher, Hillman & Ashmore, 1966).

Since adipose tissue contains a very high proportion of lipid (85%), the technical difficulties involved in demonstrating entry of glucose into the remaining small aqueous phase are legion. However, using tritiated water (^3H_2O) and ^{14}C-labelled sugars, Renold et al. (1965) were able to measure intracellular water by isotope dilution and could demonstrate competition between glucose and non-metabolized labelled sugars for entry into the cell. The kinetics of sugar transport in both muscle and adipose tissue were found to be consistent with a carrier mechanism.

In hepatic cells, which are freely permeable to glucose, the rate-limiting step in the metabolism of glucose appears to be its conversion to glucose-6-phosphate (G6P), a reaction which is catalysed by ATP and glucokinase and stimulated by insulin (Pietro & Weinhouse, 1960). Hepatic activity of glucokinase declines during starvation and on induction of experimental insulin deficiency (Sols, Salas & Vinuela, 1964). If administered *in vivo* several hours before sacrifice, insulin restores hepatic glucokinase activity to normal in the diabetic animal, but this effect can be blocked by administration of puromycin or other substances which inhibit synthesis of protein. On this basis, it has been suggested that insulin regulates the synthesis of hepatic glucokinase (Sharma, Manjeshwar & Weinhouse, 1964).

(ii) *Glycogen synthesis.* Increased amounts of glucose consumed by muscle in the presence of insulin are largely converted to glycogen (Larner, Villar-Palasi & Richman, 1959). Doses of insulin which do not induce hypoglycaemia are also able to increase deposition of hepatic glycogen *in vivo* (Bishop, Steele, Altszuler, Dunn, Bjerknes & de Bodo, 1965). These effects could be produced in three ways.

First, insulin can stimulate glycogen synthetase. Steiner, Randa & Williams (1961) have shown that hepatic activity of this enzyme is low in alloxan-diabetic rats and can be restored to normal by administration of insulin *in vivo*.

Secondly, insulin appears to catalyse the conversion of glycogen synthetase from the "D" to the "I" form. The "I" form of glycogen synthetase (Uridine-diphospho-glucose: α-glucan transglucosidase) is active in the absence of glucose-6-phosphate; but the "D" form requires glucose-6-phosphate as an essential co-factor for activity (Villar-Palasi & Larner, 1961). This transformation from the "D" to the "I" form requires ATP and appears to be analogous to the conversion of phosphorylase in the liver from the inactive to the active form (Sutherland & Rall, 1960).

A third mechanism could be through an action of insulin upon the adenyl cyclase system. Insulin, under the proper experimental conditions, will inhibit the activation of hepatic phosphorylase (Rosell-Perez & Larner, 1964). This could be due to a direct effect of the hormone upon the enzyme but it seems more likely that insulin would act indirectly by inhibiting the activation of adenyl cyclase, or in some other way reducing the levels of intracellular $3'5'$-cyclic AMP (Robison, Butcher & Sutherland, 1967).

(iii) *Glucose production.* One of the most controversial aspects of insulin is its action in the liver. Under certain circumstances insulin will inhibit hepatic production of glucose. Madison, Combes, Adams & Strickland (1961), by infusing insulin without inducing hypoglycaemia, were able to suppress hepatic output of glucose in dogs with porto-caval shunts. Using an isotope dilution technique, Dunn, Friedmann, Maass, Reichard & Weinhouse (1957) also observed acute effects of insulin upon hepatic production of glucose *in vivo*, but these were not confirmed in experiments in which hepatic production of glucose was measured by catheterization of the hepatic veins (Tarding & Schambye, 1958; Shoemaker, Mahler & Ashmore, 1959). It became apparent that effects of insulin could only be demonstrated in normal animals if the compensatory effects induced by hypoglycaemia could be avoided. Administered to the normal dog in appropriate dosage, insulin does inhibit hepatic output of glucose (Bishop

et al., 1965) and if insulin deficiency is induced with guinea pig anti-insulin serum, there is prompt increase in output which can be reversed as rapidly by administration of insulin (Franckson, Arnould, Malaisse & Conard, 1964). As in animals, insulin has an effect in man; as shown by catheterization of the hepatic vein, it decreases splanchnic production of glucose (Bearn, Billing & Sherlock, 1952). The role of insulin in the regulation of hepatic glucose production has been reviewed by Ashmore & Carr (in Litwack & Kritchevsky, 1964).

(iv) *Lipid metabolism.* Synthesis of fatty acids is markedly decreased in starvation and in various types of experimental diabetes. In the fabrication of long chain fatty acids, two biochemical steps are involved ; the carboxylation of acetyl-CoA to form malonyl-CoA, and the synthesis of the fatty acid from malonyl-CoA and TPNH. The conversion of acetyl- to malonyl-CoA is a rate-limiting enzymic reaction in the synthesis of fatty acids, and is inhibited by the fatty acids themselves and by their acyl-CoA esters (Numa, Matsuhashi & Lynen, 1961). Although insulin *per se* is not directly involved in either reaction, it may exert an indirect effect upon both. In the liver, for example, intracellular levels of fatty acids and acyl-CoA esters controlling synthesis depend in part upon the rate at which free fatty acids are mobilized from the extra-hepatic depots of adipose tissue. Insulin inhibits release of free fatty acids from these depots and could thus indirectly increase the synthesis of fatty acids in the liver by reducing the levels of free fatty acids and acyl-CoA esters in the hepatic cells.

Synthesis of fatty acids in partially purified fractions of liver cells may also be influenced by the rate at which fatty acids are esterified. Bortz, Abraham & Chaikoff (1963) showed that synthesis of fatty acids by "soluble fractions" of hepatic cells is increased when microsomal fractions are added. This stimulant effect appears to be due to the increased rate at which the added microsomes are able to esterify fatty acids. By reducing the levels of free fatty acids and acyl-CoA in the system, the microsomes would thereby remove their inhibitory effects upon acetyl-CoA carboxylase and so promote synthesis of fatty acids.

When added *in vitro*, insulin stimulates synthesis of fatty acids in isolated adipose tissue but only if glucose is also present (Jeanrenaud & Renold, 1960). Glucose is needed for the production of TPNH which is essential in the second (polymerization) stage of synthesis of the fatty acids; the reduced co-enzyme (TPNH) is produced during the oxidation of glucose by the pentose-pathway. Insulin stimulates metabolism of glucose through this pathway in adipose tissue, for C_1 in the glucose molecule is preferentially oxidized by this tissue *in vitro* when insulin is added to the medium (Ashmore, Cahill & Hastings, 1960). By stimulating metabolism of glucose through this pathway, therefore, insulin is able to stimulate production of TPNH, and so promote synthesis of fatty acids (Leboeuf & Cahill, 1960).

Release of fatty acids from adipose tissue depends upon the balance existing between two reactions—lipolysis and re-esterification. Lipolysis, the enzymic hydrolysis of triglycerides to give glycerol and fatty acids, is activated in adipose tissue by numerous hormones, including glucagon, TSH, ACTH, growth hormone and the glucocorticoids. Insulin has a direct effect on this process for, independent of any influence upon glucose metabolism, it prevents activation of the lipase which catalyses lipolysis (Ball & Jungas, 1964; Mahler, Stafford, Tarrant & Ashmore, 1963). Re-esterification, or the synthesis of triglycerides from fatty acids and α-glycerol phosphate in adipose tissue, is dependent upon metabolism of glucose for the production of α-glycerol phosphate; this tissue contains insufficient glycerol kinase to produce the α-glycerol phosphate needed for re-esterification. *In vivo*, therefore, insulin stimulates utilization of glucose with consequent increased production of α-glycerol phosphate, and so promotes re-esterification of free fatty acids in adipose tissue.

Randle, Garland, Hales & Newsholme (1963) have proposed that excessive mobilization of free fatty acids could inhibit utilization of glucose by a number of tissues, whether this is induced by growth hormone, catecholamines or insulin deficiency. Fatty acids can also increase production of glucose by the liver (Herrera, Kamm, Ruderman & Cahill, 1966; Struck, Ashmore & Wieland, 1966). Thus hyperglycaemia could result from any condition in which for any reason the levels of circulating free fatty acids are increased and, by regulating the release of these acids from adipose tissue, insulin could contribute indirectly to the regulation of carbohydrate utilization and gluconeogenesis in the body as a whole.

(v) *Protein metabolism.* Sinex, MacMullen & Hastings (1952) were the first to demonstrate an effect of insulin upon the synthesis of protein. Addition of the hormone to incubation media increased incorporation of ^{14}C-labelled amino acids into proteins of the isolated rat diaphragm. This has also been observed in isolated adipose tissue (Herrera & Renold, 1960). These effects appear to be independent of any action of insulin upon the metabolism of glucose, for incorporation of labelled amino acids into proteins is stimulated by insulin in the absence of glucose (Manchester & Krahl, 1959). There is some question as to whether this effect is related to the action of insulin upon transport of amino acids.

Manchester & Young (1959) have reported that in the isolated rat diaphragm, insulin increases the intracellular transport of only two amino acids—glycine and α-amino-isobutyric acid. If puromycin is added, however, insulin stimulates transport of many amino acids (Wool, in Karlson, 1965). From this it can be concluded that if the synthesis of proteins from amino acids is blocked, an effect of insulin upon transport of amino acids can be demonstrated. Manchester & Krahl (1959) have provided evidence that insulin can stimulate the synthesis of protein independently of its action upon amino acid transport. Thus, if the rat diaphragm is incubated with unlabelled amino acids and ^{14}C-labelled pyruvate, α-ketoglutarate or even with ^{14}C-bicarbonate, insulin will increase the incorporation of labelled carbon into protein; the degree of stimulation is the same as that observed when the labelled substrates are amino acids. Moreover, the presence of unlabelled amino acids, even in high concentration, does not reduce the rate of incorporation of ^{14}C from labelled pyruvate into tissue proteins. Actinomycin, which markedly inhibits synthesis of RNA in diaphragmatic muscle and somewhat reduces the incorporation of labelled amino acids into proteins, does not abolish the effect of insulin upon protein synthesis and is without effect upon insulin-activated transport of either glucose or α-amino-isobutyric acid (Wool, in Karlson, 1965).

The mode of action of insulin in promoting synthesis of proteins is still unknown, but Wool, Rampusad & Moyer (1966) have produced a provocative suggestion. Using ribosomes from the hearts of diabetic rats, they found reduced rates of protein synthesis, but if the animals were treated with insulin one hour before sacrifice, synthesis of proteins was restored to normal. Treatment with insulin *in vivo* also increased slightly the rate of protein synthesis from amino acids by ribosomes of normal rats. They suggested that insulin may produce configurational change in the ribosomes to alter their ability to bind either transfer RNA or messenger RNA, and so influence synthesis of proteins.

(vi) *Enzyme synthesis.* Besides affecting the actual conditions under which enzymes have to act in specific reactions, insulin influences the rates at which some enzymes are synthesized in the liver. Thus, when diabetes is induced in rats with alloxan, hepatic activities of three enzymes involved in glycolysis (glucokinase, phosphofructokinase and pyruvate kinase) decrease (Weber, Singhal, Stamm, Lea & Fisher, 1966b). If these diabetic animals are treated with insulin, hepatic activities of these three enzymes are restored to normal unless agents inhibiting synthesis of proteins (e.g. puromycin) are given simultaneously. At the same time that activities of the glycolytic enzymes decrease on induction of diabetes, those of four gluconeogenetic enzymes (glucose-6-phosphatase, fructose-1,6-diphosphatase, phospho-enol pyruvate carboxykinase and pyruvate carboxylase) increase and treatment of the diabetic animals with insulin suppresses their activity. These and other observations led Weber and his associates to suggest that insulin may act directly on DNA to modulate genetic information, and so stimulate or repress the synthesis of enzymes involved in the metabolism of glucose. Thus insulin appears to stimulate the synthesis of enzymes involved in glycolysis and suppress that of the gluconeogenetic enzymes, the latter effect (as outlined later) being opposed by the adrenal glucocorticoids (Weber, Singhal & Srivastava, 1965b). These effects are shown graphically in Fig. 3.7.

(vii) *Mucopolysaccharides and glycoproteins.* Widely distributed in the tissues of the body are a group of carbohydrates which consist of polymers of hexosamines, uronic acids and their sulphate esters. Bound to proteins, they comprise the mucopolysaccharides and glycoproteins which occur in plasma and connective tissue and are important components of "ground substance", blood-group polysaccharides, heparin and chondroitin sulphate. Although little is known of the regulation of their synthesis and metabolism, several hormones, including insulin, growth hormone and glucocorticoids, have been implicated in the regulation of their synthesis in skin and connective tissue (Asboe-Hansen, 1958).

In diabetes, increased levels of protein-bound glucosamine in the blood, and increased urinary excretion of hexosamines have been reported (Berkman, Rifkin & Ross, 1953). The significance of these abnormalities is still not known, but it has been suggested that abnormalities of metabolism of these substances are in some way connected with the incidence of diabetic "complications" in man (see below). Synthesis of protein-bound glucosamine in serum, kidney, lung, testis, liver and spleen from ^{14}C-labelled glucose is unimpaired in the alloxan-diabetic rat (Spiro, 1959), but in these same animals, as is well known, the synthesis of glycogen, another polysaccharide, is markedly reduced. Spiro (1963) therefore concluded that the synthesis of glucosamine from glucose, unlike that of glycogen, is not under the control of insulin, but it does appear that the primary site of synthesis of this amino-sugar is the liver (Spiro, 1959). There is no doubt that many of the lesions found in association with blood vessels in the retina, kidneys and elsewhere of human diabetics do contain large amounts of glycoprotein (Warren & Le-Compte, 1952; Bloodworth, 1963). The precise biochemical lesion which gives rise to them, however, has yet to be demonstrated.

TABLE 3.5

Metabolic effects of insulin

Affected process	Action of insulin — Mechanism	Responsive tissues
Glucose utilization	(1) Stimulation of glucose transport across membranes	Muscle and adipose tissue
	(2) Stimulation of glucokinase activity	Liver
Glycogen synthesis	(1) Activation of glycogen-synthetase	Muscle and adipose tissue
	(2) Induction of glycogen-synthetase activity	Liver
Protein metabolism	(1) Activation of systems for transport of amino-acids	Muscle, liver and adipose tissue
	(2) Stimulation of synthesis of proteins	Muscle, liver and adipose tissue
Lipid metabolism	(1) Indirect stimulation of fatty acid synthesis	Liver and adipose tissue
	(2) Inhibition of lipolysis	Adipose tissue

(viii) *Summary of effects produced by insulin.* A summary of the major effects of insulin upon isolated tissues is given in Table 3.5. Although this hormone may exert some effects in the brain, nervous tissue, leucocytes and elsewhere, its main actions are exerted in the liver, muscle and adipose tissue. Within these three tissues, sensitivity to the hormone varies widely. In muscle and adipose tissue, for example, acute effects of insulin are readily demonstrable, the hormone promoting entry of glucose into their cells and exerting a direct influence upon the synthesis of glycogen within them. In the liver, on the other hand, acute effects are not readily obtained. In time, insulin can exert effects upon hepatic utilization of glucose and synthesis of glycogen and fatty acids, but it is often difficult to tell whether these effects are due to direct or indirect actions of the hormone. At the moment it is the popular concensus of opinion that insulin has a direct effect upon hepatic phosphorylation of glucose (glucokinase) and upon glycogen synthesis (glycogen synthetase). On the other hand, synthesis of fatty acids in the liver appears to be secondarily influenced by changes in the hepatic levels of fatty acids and CoA-esters induced by effects of insulin in adipose tissue. In the adipose tissue, insulin may exert both a direct and an indirect effect. It directly inhibits lipolysis and indirectly stimulates re-esterification of fatty acids by promoting metabolism of glucose, both effects playing an important part in the synthesis of fatty acids and their release from adipose tissue.

Glucocorticoids

In the regulation of metabolism of carbohydrates, protein and lipids, the effects of insulin are opposed by those of the glucocorticoids (Ashmore, 1964). Thus diabetes can be induced with steroids (Ingle, 1941) and the symptoms and signs of diabetes ameliorated by adrenalectomy (Long & Lukens, 1936). At the cellular level, the stimulant effect of insulin upon utilization of glucose is opposed by a lesser inhibitory effect of the glucocorticoids. Insulin stimulates extrahepatic synthesis of protein and the steroids have an opposite effect, but in the liver both hormones stimulate protein synthesis. The glucocorticoids induce hepatic enzymes involved in gluconeogenesis. Mobilization of lipids is stimulated by glucocorticoids and inhibited by insulin. It can thus be seen that normal metabolism depends upon a balanced interplay between the actions of these two hormones, the glucocorticoids tending to exert diabetogenic effects.

(i) *Gluconeogenesis.* Glucocorticoids are primarily concerned with the breakdown of protein and the production of glucose. When administered to animals, the glucocorticoids increase the formation of glucose and glycogen in the liver, but this effect is preceded by increases in production of urea-nitrogen (Engel, 1950) and by hepatic uptake of amino acids (Christensen, in Wolstenholme & O'Connor, 1960a). What is not certain, therefore, is whether the effects seen in hepatic tissues are consequences of direct actions of glucocorticoids upon hepatic metabolism or secondary to extrahepatic catabolism of protein.

A direct effect of glucocorticoids has been demonstrated by Chambers, Georg & Bass (1965) who showed increased uptake of amino acids 60–120 min. after perfusion of the isolated rat liver with hydrocortisone. In liver slices, glucocorticoids have small but reproducible stimulant effects upon the incorporation of ^{14}C of labelled substrates into glucose (Haynes, 1962; Uete & Ashmore, 1963; Eisenstein, Berg, Goldenberg & Jensen, 1964), but in the isolated perfused liver no such uniform effect has been observed. Garcia, Williamson & Cahill (1966) and Struck *et al.* (1966) were unable to demonstrate any effect, but Exton & Park (1965) observed a reduced (net) rate of glucose production in perfused livers from adrenalectomized rats. Eisenstein, Spencer, Flatness & Brodsky (1966) have also demonstrated that dexamethazone, whether administered *in vivo* or added *in vitro*, stimulates conversion of alanine into glucose. Liver slices obtained from diabetic rats produce abnormally large amounts of glucose, but the rate can be reduced if the animals are first adrenalectomized (Ashmore, Hastings, Nesbett & Renold, 1956). Also, if cortisol or cortisone is administered to the adrenalectomized alloxandiabetic rat, there is a marked rise in blood-sugar concentration within 4–6 hr. at which time slices of liver are able to convert increased amounts of pyruvate to glucose.

(ii) *Glycogen deposition.* When glucocorticoids are injected into fasting rats, deposition of glycogen in the liver increases after a lapse of several hours (Hyde, 1957); this formed the basis of a standard method for bio-assay of glucocorticoids. This delay may provide the explanation for failure by many to demonstrate an effect of steroids upon hepatic metabolism *in vitro*. Evidence has been presented to suggest that glycogen deposited in the liver during stimulation with glucocorticoids is derived from glucose reaching the liver in the blood (Ashmore, Stricker, Love & Kilsheimer, 1961; Friedmann, Goodman & Weinhouse, 1965; Hornbrook, Burch & Lowry, 1965). It could be derived from lactate, but Hornbrook *et al.* (1965) have shown that although lactate will increase the levels of various glycolytic intermediates in the liver when administered *in vivo*, additional treatment with cortisol has no additive effect and cortisol given alone has no comparable effect. The only effects which cortisol did produce were decreases in the levels of glucose-6-phosphate and UDP glucose which appeared at the same time as the levels of glycogen were beginning to rise and suggested that activity of glycogen synthetase was increased.

(iii) *Glucose utilization.* It is difficult to demonstrate *in vivo* that glucocorticoids inhibit utilization of glucose (Long, Katzin & Fry, 1940; Munck & Koritz, 1962), but it has been shown with isolated tissues *in vitro*. In skin (Overell, Conden & Petrow, 1960), lymphoid (Jedeikin & White, 1958) and adipose tissue (Correa, Magalhaes & Krahl, 1960; Fain, Scow & Chernick, 1963), very marked inhibition of glucose uptake is produced by addition of adrenal steroids. Thus dexamethazone (1.5×10^{-8}M) has a strong inhibitory effect (-40%) upon utilization of glucose by mesenteric fat, but this effect is readily abolished by simultaneously added insulin (Leboeuf, Renold & Cahill, 1962).

In muscle, the entry of glucose into the cell is limited by insulin, but once inside its phosphorylation appears to be limited by growth hormone and glucocorticoids. Using perfused hearts from hypophysectomized alloxan-diabetic rats, Morgan, Henderson, Regen & Park (1959) were able to show that when given *in vivo*, both growth hormone and glucocorticoids would suppress phosphorylation by the isolated tissue exposed to insulin, maximum inhibition being obtained when both were present simultaneously.

(iv) *Protein and nucleic acid metabolism.* The catabolic effect of glucocorticoids upon protein was established by Long *et al.* (1940). They also cause the breakdown of lymphoid tissue and abolish immune responses in normal subjects (see Eisenstein, 1967). Depletion of tissue proteins is widespread, but glucocorticoids actually increase the total protein in liver, the gastro-intestinal tract, the urogenital organs and the plasma (albumin) (Silber & Porter, 1953). The changes which occur in the liver have been followed sequentially by Feigelson & Feigelson (1963).

Following a single injection of glucocorticoid, increased synthesis of protein can be detected in the liver in 4–10 hr. but other changes can be detected at a much earlier stage. One of the earliest is an increase in RNA nucleotidyl-transferase which appears within 30 min. and precedes a detectable increase of hepatic RNA at 90–180 min. (Lang & Sekeris, 1964). At the same time or slightly after, concentrations of RNA increase, the activities of certain hepatic enzymes rise (Table 3.6), and in two reports increased enzymic activity has been equated with increased synthesis of enzyme-protein (Greengard & Feigelson, 1962; Kenny, 1962). It has also been shown that substances capable of inhibiting synthesis of protein, are able to prevent the enzymic changes which corticoids induce (Weber *et al.*, 1966b). These observations therefore support the concept that hormones can activate synthesis of specific RNA which in turn catalyses the synthesis of enzymes.

(v) *Enzymic changes.* Not only do the glucocorticoids increase synthesis of enzymes in the liver, but they do so in a pattern consistent with their ability to increase glucose production. Thus in diabetic animals and in normal animals treated with glucocorticoids, hepatic activity of enzymes involved in gluconeogenesis is increased (Weber *et al.*, 1966b). Normal activities are restored if the diabetic animals are adrenalectomized or treated with insulin. These changes are summarized in Table 3.7 and have been mentioned (in part) above under the heading of insulin, but the interrelationship between insulin and the glucocorti-

TABLE 3.6

Effects of cortisol on hepatic enzyme activities and RNA synthesis in normal rats

Hours after Cortisol Injection	Hepatic RNA* (%)	Enzymic Activities (%)		
		Tryptophan Pyrrolase**	Tyrosine Transaminase**	Fructose-1,6-Diphosphatase*
0	100	100	100	100
4	124	280	240	140
8	250	700	340	145
12	140	880	700	160
24	100	400	250	200

All values are stated as percentages of those found in livers of normal rats (100%) and were obtained at stated intervals after a single injection of glucocorticoid. (After (*) Weber, Srivastava & Singhal, 1965b; and (**) Rosen & Nichol, 1964.)

TABLE 3.7

Hepatic enzyme activities in diabetic rats and normal rats treated with glucocorticoids and insulin

Enzyme	Diabetic	Corticoid-treated	Insulin-treated
Glycogen synthetase	Norm	Incr	Incr
Glucokinase	Decr	Norm	Incr
Pyruvate kinase	Decr	Norm	Incr
Phosphofructokinase	Decr		Incr
Glucose-6-phosphatase	Incr	Incr	Decr
Fructose-1, 6-diphosphatase	Incr	Incr	Decr
Phospho-enol pyruvate carboxykinase	Incr	Incr	Norm
Pyruvate carboxylase	Incr	Incr	Norm

Activities are stated as normal (Norm), increased (Incr) or decreased (Decr) in comparison with those observed in normal animals.

coids in controlling enzymic activities is best considered here.

In the diabetic animal or in the normal animal treated with glucocorticoids, hepatic activities of the "gluconeogenic" enzymes (glucose-6-phosphatase, fructose-1,6-diphosphatase, PEP-kinase and pyruvate carboxylase) are all increased. Those involved in glycolysis (glucokinase, phosphofructokinase and pyruvate kinase) show decreased activity in the liver. Increased synthesis of the "gluconeogenic" enzymes has been observed in experimental forms of insulin deficiency induced with alloxan, anti-insulin serum or mannoheptulose, and has been produced in normal animals treated with glucocorticoids. All these effects can be prevented by treatment with insulin and the levels of these enzymes in the liver are thought to be the result of stimulant and repressive effects of glucocorticoids and insulin, respectively, upon the synthesis of specific RNA. On the other hand, insulin promotes the synthesis of glucokinase and activates hepatic glycogen synthetase and pyruvate kinase, but it does not appear to increase the actual amounts of the latter two enzymes. As mentioned above, insulin appears to catalyse the conversion of glycogen synthetase from the "D" to the "I" form, and probably exerts an indirect effect upon the activity of pyruvate kinase by changing the levels of free fatty acids in the tissues (Weber, Hird-Convery, Lea & Stamm, 1966a).

It will be noticed that all the "gluconeogenic" enzymes which are induced by glucocorticoids and suppressed by insulin catalyse one-way reactions directed toward the production of glucose. Conversely those which are induced or activated by insulin and which also catalyse one-way reactions, promote reactions which lead to the storage of glycogen or the production of energy for synthetic purposes. The action of glucocorticoids on the first group of gluconeogenic enzymes seems clear, but it is not known how they act, if at all, upon the second.

(vi) *Lipid metabolism*. Synthesis of fatty acids is depressed in both the liver and adipose tissue of diabetic animals and is restored to normal in the liver (Brady, Lukens & Gurin, 1951), but not in adipose tissue (Jeanrenaud & Renold, 1960) by subsequent adrenalectomy. These findings are comparable with the idea, outlined above under the heading of insulin, that hepatic synthesis of fatty acids is largely regulated by intracellular levels of fatty acids and CoA esters, both of which rise in diabetes and are restored to normal levels after adrenalectomy. In adipose tissue, however, synthesis of fatty acids is dependent on simultaneous metabolism of glucose, which is depressed in diabetes and is not restored to normal levels after subsequent adrenalectomy. It therefore seems probable that the effects of corticoids upon hepatic synthesis of fatty acids are mediated through their influence upon the release of free fatty acids from adipose tissue. It is not known how the glucocorticoids influence such release, but Fain, Galton & Kouacev (1966) have demonstrated, as shown below, that both growth hormone and the glucocorticoids are needed to stimulate release of free fatty acids from adipose tissue, and they suggest that the effect is due to synthesis of a lipase.

When diabetic animals are adrenalectomized, concentrations of free fatty acids and glucose in the plasma fall. Ketoacidosis also disappears (Scow & Chernick, 1960), but production of ketone bodies by hepatic tissue can be rapidly increased again by administration of cortisol (Ashmore, 1964). Moreover, as Scow & Chernick (1960) have shown, diabetic acidosis does not develop if the rat is adrenalectomized or starved for six days before pancreatectomy. These observations suggest that development of ketoacidosis, like the suppression of fatty acid synthesis, is the result of excessive mobilization of peripheral fat and can be prevented by depletion of these depots (starvation) or inhibition of mobilization (adrenalectomy).

Glucagon

This hormone, produced by the α-cells of the pancreatic islets, is believed to exert its metabolic effects through stimulation of adenylcyclase and increased production of 3'5'-adenosine monophosphate (cyclic AMP). As an activator of adenylcyclase, glucagon appears to be more potent than adrenaline and several other hormones (Exton & Park, 1966). In the liver, glucagon initiates glycogenolysis (Sutherland & Rall, 1960), gluconeogenesis (Garcia et al., 1966) and ketogenesis (Struck, Ashmore & Wieland, 1965). In adipose tissue it stimulates lipolysis (Hagen, 1961) and in the pancreas, as shown above, it stimulates secretion of insulin.

(i) Glycogenolysis. The presence of glucagon in many preparations of insulin was first suspected because insulin was found to have a slight transient hyperglycaemic effect preceding the induction of hypoglycaemia; hence the name "hyperglycaemic factor" formerly given to glucagon. The effects of glucagon are often similar to those of adrenaline. They both activate adenylcyclase to produce more cyclic-AMP (Exton & Park, 1966), which in turn activates hepatic phosphorylase (Sutherland & Rall, 1960) and induces glycogenolysis. Though the final effects are comparable the initial sites of action of the two hormones probably differ. Thus the glycogenolytic effect of adrenaline, unlike that of glucagon, is readily inhibited by adrenergic blocking agents (Ashmore, Preston & Love, 1962). They also differ in their actions upon different tissues; both promote glycogenolysis in the liver but only adrenaline does so in muscle.

(ii) Gluconeogenesis. In addition to this marked effect upon glycogenolysis, glucagon has recently been shown to have other effects in the liver. Thus in the isolated perfused liver it increases production of urea nitrogen (Miller, 1965), and increases utilization of lactate and production of glucose (Schimassek & Mitzkat, 1963). It stimulates the conversion of lactate, pyruvate and alanine to glucose in the perfused liver (Garcia et al., 1966; Exton, Jefferson, Butcher & Park, 1966; Struck et al., 1966), the effect being proportional to the amount of hormone perfused (0·001 to 1·0 μg./ml.). These actions of glucagon are probably mediated by cyclic AMP, for the same effects can be obtained in the perfused liver with adrenaline (Exton & Park, 1966), theophylline, and cyclic AMP itself (Exton et al., 1966). From measurements of substrates in the liver before and after stimulation with glucagon, it has been concluded that the hormone promotes gluconeogenesis from lactate at some step during the conversion of pyruvate to phospho-enol pyruvate (Exton & Park, 1966; Williamson, 1967). This it could do by accelerating reactions involving pyruvate carboxylase or PEP-carboxykinase, or by inhibiting pyruvate kinase. Such effects may not be due to any direct

action of glucagon or cyclic AMP but could be the indirect result of actions of glucagon on lipid metabolism (see below).

(iii) Lipid metabolism. Production of ketone bodies by rat liver slices is slightly but sigificantly increased by glucagon (Haugaard & Haugaard, 1954), an effect which has been more clearly demonstrated in the isolated perfused liver (Struck et al., 1965). In adipose tissue, a number of hormones, including glucagon, are known to activate a lipase and increase release of glycerol and free fatty acids (Vaughan, Berger & Steinberg, 1964). It had been suggested that glucagon may act by the same mechanism in both tissues (Hagen, 1961) and evidence has now been furnished to show that the liver does in fact contain a lipase whose activity is increased by glucagon (Bewsher & Ashmore, 1966). Moreover, it appears that the effects of glucagon upon ketogenesis and gluconeogenesis may have a common basis through activation of cyclic AMP and of lipase.

It has been suggested that the ketogenic and gluconeogenic effects of glucagon could be due to hydrolysis of glycerides and concomitant increases in free fatty acids and acyl CoA esters (Struck et al., 1966). Added to perfusion media, fatty acids increase both gluconeogenesis and the production of ketone bodies by isolated rat livers (Struck et al., 1965). Fatty acids have also been shown to increase glucose production by kidney (Krebs, Speake & Hems, 1965) and liver (Haynes, 1965) slices. Conversion of alanine to glucose in the perfused liver is increased by linoleic (Herrera et al., 1966) and oleic (Williamson, Kreisberg & Felts, 1966a) acids. Hepatic production of glucose in vivo can also be increased by fatty acids (Friedmann, Goodman & Weinhouse, 1966). In each case, therefore, synthesis of carbohydrate is stimulated by fatty acids, but this does not imply that the synthesized glucose is derived from carbon atoms in the fatty acids. It appears that metabolites of the fatty acids and not the fatty acids themselves act as the stimulants.

Several modes of stimulation have been suggested. For example, CoA esters of fatty acids inhibit conversion of pyruvate to acetyl- CoA and could thus inhibit oxidation of pyruvate through the citric acid cycle. In fact, Herrera et al. (1966), have shown that the oxidation of ^{14}C-labelled alanine by the perfused liver is reduced by linoleic acid. Decreased oxidation of pyruvate and increased production of ketone bodies might also be due to inhibition of citrate synthetase by acyl-CoA esters (Wieland, Weiss & Eger-Neufeldt, 1964). Intracellular levels of acetyl CoA could play a role in the control of gluconeogenesis, for it is required in the carboxylation of pyruvate to form oxaloacetate, the first step in conversion of pyruvate to phospho-enol pyruvate (Utter, Keech & Scrutton, 1964). The relationship between ketogenesis and gluconeogenesis has recently been reviewed by Krebs (1966).

These observations are pertinent to changes in carbohydrate and fat metabolism which have been observed in acute insulin deficiency. Whether injected with anti-insulin serum or glucagon, rats rapidly develop signs of hepatic glycogenolysis, gluconeogenesis and ketogenesis (Wright, in Leibel & Wrenshall, 1965; Wagle & Ashmore, 1963; Exton et al., 1966). It is possible, therefore, that many of the signs of acute insulin deficiency such as those produced by anti-insulin serum could be due to actions of glucagon. The intracellular levels of glycolytic intermediates and metabolites of fatty acids produced by glucagon and by anti-insulin serum are consistent with one another and with the observed gluconeogenesis and keto-

genesis (Williamson, Wright, Malaisse & Ashmore, 1966b). Both sets of effects could be mediated through induced changes in hepatic levels of cyclic AMP which are known to be elevated in acute insulin deficiency. The inhibitory effect of insulin upon gluconeogenesis (Exton et al., 1966) may be related to the lower levels of cyclic AMP found in isolated tissues to which insulin has been added (Butcher & Sutherland, 1967).

(iv) *Amino acid and protein metabolism.* It has already been pointed out that glucagon increases urea production by the perfused liver (Miller, 1965). It also increases uptake of amino acids by hepatic cells (Chambers et al., 1965) and the levels of circulating amino acids in vivo (Foa, Galansino & Pozza, 1957). Glucagon inhibits the incorporation of labelled amino acids into proteins in slices of rat liver (Pryor & Berthet, 1960). It has rapid effects upon hepatic enzymes, increasing activities of PEP carboxykinase (Lardy, Foster, Shrago & Ray, 1964), tyrosine and phenylalanine transa-

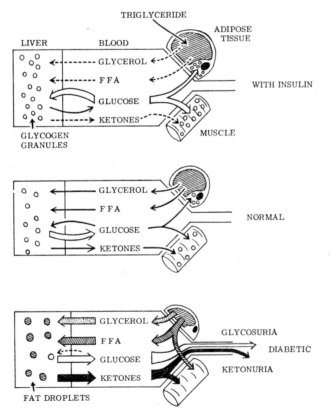

FIG. 3.9. Movements of glycerol, free fatty acids (FFA), glucose and ketones between the liver, muscle, and adipose tissue in the normal animal, the normal animal injected with insulin and the diabetic animal. Also shown are accumulations of glycogen and triglycerides.

minases (Greengard & Baker, 1966). Increased activity of these enzymes can be produced by increased levels of amino acids *per se*, so that the effect of glucagon could be indirect.

Growth Hormone

That the anterior pituitary gland plays a role in the regulation of carbohydrate metabolism was firmly established by Houssay (1936) and confirmed by many others (Young, 1953). This early work clearly showed that the gland produces a diabetogenic factor which was identified with its growth-promoting actions. Once it was recognized that growth hormone is species-specific, effects were demonstrated in primates (Knobil & Greep, 1959) and in man (Ikkos & Luft, in Wolstenholme & O'Connor, 1960*b*). Levine & Luft (1964) have analysed the various effects of this hormone which can be divided into two groups. First, it induces intolerance to carbohydrates, hyperglycaemia, ketonuria and glycosuria. Secondly, and not necessarily related to its diabetogenic effects, growth hormone causes retention of nitrogen, phosphorus and potassium, all of which are involved in growth. There is also evidence that growth hormone plays a part in the biosynthesis of collagen and chondroitin sulphate needed for the growth of bones (Daughaday & Kipnis, 1966).

The ketogenic and hyperglycaemic effects of growth hormone may be related to its effects upon mobilization of fatty acids from adipose tissue (Raben & Hollenberg, in Wolstenholme & O'Connor, 1960*b*). The hormone promotes lipolysis in adipose tissue and there is subsequent increased oxidation of fatty acids in the liver (Fain & Scow, 1965). For lipolysis *in vitro*, adrenal corticoids have to be present in the medium in addition to growth hormone, and then it is noted that lipolysis does not begin for several hours and can be prevented by adding actinomycin or puromycin to the medium at the beginning of incubation, or by injecting them *in vivo* before removal of the adipose tissue (Fain, Kouacev & Scow, 1965; Fain *et al.*, 1966). These results suggest that the lipolytic effect of growth hormone is not due to any direct action but involves some factor, possibly a lipase, whose synthesis is stimulated by the combined actions of growth hormone and glucocorticoids.

Apart from this, growth hormone has not been shown to have any effects upon reactions studied *in vitro*. Its actions *in vivo* could be due to the effects it has on the mobilization of free fatty acids. Thus the free fatty acids released from depots of fat could inhibit utilization of glucose by muscle (Randle, Garland, Hales & Newsholme, 1963)

and increase hepatic gluconeogenesis (Struck *et al.*, 1965). Possible inter-relationships between growth hormone and insulin in the control of carbohydrate and fat metabolism have been reviewed in detail by Randle, Garland, Hales, Newsholme, Denton & Pogson (1966).

Experimental Diabetes

By way of summary, the principal metabolic changes induced in the normal animal by injection of insulin and by removal of the endogenous source of insulin are illustrated in Fig. 3.9.

Insulin lowers the concentration of glucose in the blood as entry of glucose into muscle and adipose tissue is stimulated. In muscle the glucose is mainly deposited as glycogen. In adipose tissue some is deposited as glycogen and some provides α-glycerol phosphate which is esterified to augment deposits of triglyceride. Activation of the lipase in adipose tissue is depressed by the insulin so that lipolysis is reduced and the level of free fatty acids in the plasma falls. In the liver, deposition of glycogen is stimulated by insulin through its direct actions on synthetic enzymes (glucokinase and glycogen synthetase) and its indirect inhibitory effect upon glycogenolysis (phosphorylase). Activation of the hepatic enzymes involved in glycolysis provides the energy and substrates needed for increased synthesis of fatty acids and proteins.

When the normal animal is rendered diabetic by destruction or removal of its source of endogenous insulin, diabetes develops. Uptake of glucose by adipose tissue and muscle is suppressed and hepatic output of glucose rises; the latter effect could be due to glucagon. In adipose tissue, metabolism of glucose is reduced and insufficient α-glycerol phosphate is generated for the esterification of free fatty acids. In the absence of insulin, lipase activity increases and increased amounts of free fatty acids and glycerol are released into the blood. These are transported to the liver but during passage from the adipose tissue they further inhibit uptake of glucose by muscle which uses them as a source of energy. In the liver, the free fatty acids inhibit conversion of acetyl- to malonyl-CoA, and so inhibit synthesis of free fatty acids there. The intermediates involved in synthesis of free fatty acids are then degraded to aceto-acetic acid and β-hydroxybutyric acid which are released into the blood. Since the liver contains adequate amounts of α-glycerol phosphate, much of the free fatty acid reaching the liver is esterified and deposited as droplets of fat. Removal of insulin's suppressive effect upon synthesis of the gluconeogenic enzymes, leads to increased production of glucose from protein and increased excretion of nitrogen in the urine. In the end, therefore, the tissues of the body become adapted to catabolic as distinct from anabolic processes. These can be aggravated by additional secretion of endogenous glucocorticoids or ameliorated by hypophysectomy and adrenalectomy.

THE DIABETIC SYNDROMES

Though it had long been recognized that not all diabetics exhibit the same clinical syndromes, it was not until 1951 that any rational distinctions were made between them. Then Lawrence (1951) suggested that diabetics could be divided into those who were lipo-atrophic and those who were lipo-plethoric, or, as we know them today, the "juvenile-onset" and "maturity-onset" diabetics. In the same year, Bornstein & Lawrence (1951) also showed that "juvenile-onset", unlike "maturity-onset", diabetics have no detectable insulin in their blood. The two contrasting syndromes are summarized in Table 3.8.

Juvenile-onset diabetes. This group of patients, which comprises only a small fraction (5%) of the diabetic population, is so called because the first symptoms usually appear in youth at or about the age of puberty (White, 1956). When first seen by the doctor, the patient is often in a comatose or near comatose condition with a history of symptoms covering only a few days to a few weeks. These symptoms include the classical ones of polyuria, polydipsia, polyphagia and loss of body weight, with an increasing tendency toward weakness, lassitude and ultimately drowsiness. Evidence is found of wasting and dehydration associated with glycosuria and ketonuria. Depending upon the stage reached, there may be signs of coma, rapid deep but unobstructed respirations (Kussmaul), and signs of cardiovascular collapse. These patients seldom show evidence of cardiovascular disease, are normotensive, and sensitive to insulin. Following recovery from the initial attack of diabetic acidosis, they require little insulin for control during the first few months, but the required dose increases until they reach the age of about 21 years when they need 40 to 60 units of insulin per day. If insulin therapy is withdrawn for any reason, or if they undergo stress (infection, surgery, pregnancy, etc.), they become ketotic and, without adequate therapy, could die in coma.

Maturity-onset diabetes. The vast majority of diabetics fall into this category and in most cases develop their disease after the age of 40 years. The patient may be unaware of his or her condi-

TABLE 3.8

Comparison of juvenile- and adult-onset diabetic syndromes

	Juvenile-onset	Adult-onset
Proportional incidence (in diabetic population)	5% or less	80 to 90%
Age of onset	At puberty and usually less than 30 years	Usually over 35 years
Nature of onset	Acute—days to weeks	Insidious
Family History	Usually positive	Often positive
Symptoms	Polyuria, polydipsia and polyphagia	May be none (see text)
Signs	Wasted, dehydrated and sometimes comatose	Very commonly obese
Tendency to ketosis	Very prone	Little
Vascular changes:		
(1) Micro-angiopathy	Rare for first 5 years	Common
(2) Arteriosclerosis	Rare before 40 years	Common after 40 years
Insulin content of:		
(1) Pancreas	Very low or absent	Normal to low
(2) Plasma	Very low or absent	"Normal"
Response to intravenous:		
(1) Insulin	Sensitive	Commonly resistant
(2) Sulphonylureas	Absent after about 2 years	Sub-normal
Treatment with:		
(1) Diet	Ineffective without insulin	May be sufficient for control
(2) Insulin	Essential; commonly labile	Needed on some cases
(3) Sulphonylureas	Ineffective	May be effective

tion but, if questioned directly, commonly gives a history of loss of body weight, polydipsia, polyuria, pruritus or weakness. In about a quarter of the cases, however, no clear history of such symptoms can be elicited, the patient presenting with signs of cardiovascular disease (cardiac infarction, hypertension, renal disease, etc.) or neuropathies suggestive of diabetic "complications". These patients are often obese, commonly arteriosclerotic, and seldom show evidence of ketonuria. They tend to be resistant to treatment with insulin, and will usually survive on treatment with diet alone or in conjunction with insulin or one of the sulphonylureas. Although such patients are not usually prone to become ketotic, they may do so and develop diabetic coma when exposed to some severe stress (infection, surgery, etc.).

This division of diabetic patients into two groups is arbitrary and many patients may not fit completely into either category. An extreme example would be the rare syndrome of lipoatrophic diabetes of which only a few cases have been reported in the literature (Craig & Miller, in Williams, 1960; Marcus, 1966). These patients, as the name suggests, completely lack depots of subcutaneous or other fat; have intense hyperlipaemia; are extremely resistant to insulin in many cases; and show little tendency to become ketotic.

DIABETIC ACIDOSIS

No matter into which category he is placed, the diabetic may develop acidosis at any time, especially after exposure to stresses such as trauma, infection, surgery, etc. The clinical signs associated with impending and established diabetic coma have been mentioned briefly above. The sequences of clinical and metabolic events have only been studied once in man (Atchley, Loeb, Richards, Benedict & Driscoll, 1933), but they are very similar to those seen in pancreatectomized dogs (McArthur, Smart, MacLachlan, Terry, Harting, Gautier, Godley, Swallow, Simenone, Zygmuntowicz, Christo, Crepaux, Point & Benson, 1954), alloxanized rats (Knowles & Guest, 1954), and rats injected with guinea pig anti-insulin serum (Anderson, Kilbourn, Robinson & Wright, 1963). The developing syndrome can be attributed either directly or indirectly to insulin deficiency, and the signs are due to persistent hyperglycaemia or to the accumulation of keto-acids in the blood.

Accumulation of glucose in the blood, as explained above (Fig. 3.9), is due to reduced metabolism of glucose by the muscle and adipose tissues, to increased glycogenolysis in the liver, to

increased gluconeogenesis, and to increased intake of carbohydrate in the diet. When the concentration of glucose in the blood reaches about 180 mg./100 ml., osmotic diuresis commences (Brodsky, Rapaport & West, 1950) with increased urinary losses of sodium and chloride (Butler, 1950). Losses of extracellular water in the urine are made up by increased oral intake and by movements of water and potassium from the intracellular to the extracellular space. Provided renal function remains normal, the concentration of glucose in the blood seldom rises above about 500 mg./100 ml., and the concentrations of sodium, potassium, chloride and urea remain approximately normal. With the onset of renal failure, however, concentrations of glucose, potassium and urea tend to rise, and in advanced cases the heavy urinary losses may result in falls in the concentrations of sodium and chloride in the plasma.

With the development of insulin deficiency, lipolysis begins and induces hyperlipaemia and hyperketonaemia. The appearance of keto-acids in the blood leads to early reduction in the bicarbonate content of the plasma and the appearance of "ketone bodies" in the urine. Increased gluconeogenesis is reflected in increased urinary excretion of nitrogen. Whilst renal function remains normal, the kidneys are able to excrete keto-acids and nitrogenous products of metabolism, but once renal failure develops, a vicious cycle of events begins. Accumulating products of metabolism, especially the keto-acids and products of protein metabolism, reduce the bicarbonate content of the plasma to very low levels and ultimately reduce the pH of the blood. The developing acidosis augments losses of potassium, magnesium and phosphate from the cells. Thus in the advanced case, the patient suffers from metabolic acidosis and dehydration which together result in impaired cardiac function and developing coma. Coma and the hyperventilation seen in such patients have been attributed to the final fall in pH and reduced oxygenation of blood supplying the brain (Kety, Polis, Nadler & Schmidt, 1948).

The subject of diabetic acidosis has been reviewed many times (Guest, 1949; Butler, 1950; Daughaday, in Williams, 1960), and all are agreed that adequate treatment of the patient in diabetic coma depends upon an adequate assessment of the patient's condition on arrival at hospital. From their behaviour in balance studies during recovery it has been assessed that the average patient admitted in diabetic coma has lost (per Kg. body weight) 60 to 100 ml. water, 5–10 mEq sodium, 4–10 mEq chloride, 3–6 mEq potassium,

64 DIABETES MELLITUS AND HYPOGLYCAEMIA

and about 0·9 g. nitrogen (Danowski, Peters, Rathbun, Quashnock & Greenman, 1949; Butler; 1950; Nabarro, Spencer & Stowers, 1952; Martin, Smith & Wilson, 1958). In addition to being insulin-deficient, these patients are dehydrated, depleted of extra- and intra-cellular electrolytes, undernourished and in shock. Their treatment requires a well trained team of physicians, nurses, and laboratory technicians whose combined efforts should be directed toward correction of the insulin deficiency, replacement of fluid and electrolyte losses, and the prompt recognition and treatment of circulatory and other complications. Following these principles, covered in more detail by Daughaday (in Williams, 1960) and many others, the mortality rate in cases of diabetic acidosis has been reduced from 100% before the introduction of insulin to less than 5%.

ANATOMICAL LESIONS FOUND IN DIABETICS

Before the discovery of insulin almost half (48%) of the diabetics died in coma, but this figure has now dropped to 1·2% according to a recent study of a large number of patients (Root, in Williams, 1960). Most diabetic patients (76·5%) now die from what have been termed the "complications" of diabetes, the renal and vascular lesions found in most diabetics over the age of about 40 years. Future therapeutic measures, to be successful, must therefore be directed toward correcting or preventing these "diabetic complications". In addition to cardiovascular and other lesions to be found in non-diabetic members of the population, two groups have been attributed specifically to diabetes. There are the lesions responsible for or arising from reduced pancreatic islet function; and the specific "complications" to be found in or adjacent to blood vessels in the retina, kidneys, nervous system and elsewhere.

Pancreatic Lesions

The islets of Langerhans form only a small fraction (2% or less) of the total pancreatic tissue, but their growth is irregular (Ogilvie, 1937). In the first three years of life the total number of islets increases three-fold, but from then until the age of about 21 years the islets increase only in size. Relative to the rest of the body, the islet tissue increases more rapidly for the first three years, more slowly between the ages of 3 and 12 years, and at the same rate thereafter. Thus, according to Ogilvie (in Cameron & O'Connor, 1964), growth of islet tissue fails to keep pace with that of the rest of the body when the rate of

bodily growth is at its height and when, incidentally, diabetes occurs most frequently.

In established diabetes, little or no insulin can be extracted from the pancreatic tissue of juvenile diabetics, whilst that of the maturity-onset diabetic contains about half its normal complement (Wrenshall, Bogoch & Ritchie, 1952). In acute cases of juvenile diabetes dying within a few weeks or months of diagnosis, individual islets appear enlarged and contain cells with large discrete nuclei, abundant cytoplasm, some "hydropic" changes, but few or no granules (Maclean & Ogilvie, 1959; Gepts, 1965). This type of cell is seldom if ever found in young diabetics who have survived the initial acute attack of the disease. In such chronic cases, the islets are smaller and less numerous than normal and contain no identifiable β-cells; in fact, and contrary to many claims, the islets of the juvenile diabetic are never normal (Gepts, 1965). In the acute stage of the juvenile disease, the recognizable β-cells show marked evidence of synthetic activity, but with progress of the disease these cells disappear. In diabetics developing the disease later in life, the islets appear to be less numerous than normal and to contain fewer β-cells. Three other abnormalities may also be encountered:

(i) *Amyloid.* Originally described as "hyaline", amyloid deposits are most commonly seen in older patients (Ehrlich & Ratner, 1961). They appear in the interstitial spaces between the capillary walls and the islet cells and may completely replace the epithelial cells in the islets (Warren & Le Compte, 1952). In addition to comparable tinctorial properties, these deposits have the same fibrillar structure as amyloid produced experimentally and found in cases of primary amyloidosis in man (Lacy, 1967).

(ii) *Glycogen.* Originally described as examples of hydropic degeneration, deposits of glycogen may be found within the β-cells (Toreson, 1951). They appear following prolonged periods of hyperglycaemia and disappear when normoglycaemia is re-established (Lazarus & Volk, 1958). For this reason they are not thought to cause any permanent interference with islet function, though they could interfere with the function of a cell already embarrassed by the increased demands caused during persistent hyperglycaemia (Lacy, 1967).

(iii) *Fibrosis.* In juvenile diabetes in the chronic stage, marked fibrosis is usually seen, the β- and ultimately the α-cells being replaced (Gepts, 1965). In addition, evidence of fibrosis associated with the vascular system may be seen in older patients.

(iv) *"Insulitis."* This is a rare lesion confined to

children and young adults dying in the acute phase of the disease. It is characterized by infiltration of the islets by lymphocytes without any other obvious sign of inflammation or necrosis (Le-Compte, 1958). It has also been seen in cows (LeCompte, Steinke, Soeldner & Renold, 1966) and rabbits (Grodsky *et al.*, 1966) injected repeatedly with insulin in Freund's adjuvant.

(v) *Neonatal hyperplasia.* In new-born, usually stillborn, infants of diabetic mothers, the islets are larger and more numerous than normal (Cardell, 1953; Lazarus & Volk, 1962). They contain an abnormally high proportion of β-cells, and have high insulin contents (Rose, 1960; Steinke & Driscoll, 1965). Surrounding and sometimes infiltrating the islets are inflammatory cells of which the eosinophil predominates (Silverman, 1963). There may also be diffuse interstitial fibrosis which, in conjunction with the cellular infiltration, has been taken as presumptive evidence of a subacute form of interstitial pancreatitis (D'Agostino & Bahn, 1963). Some of these lesions have been produced experimentally. In the foetus of the normal rat, for example, insulin is present in the pancreas after 17 days of gestation, but if the mother is alloxan-diabetic the foetal pancreas before birth on the 22nd day contains less insulin although the islets are large, hyperplastic and hypertrophied (Kim, Runge, Wells & Lazarow, 1960; Dixit *et al.*, 1964). In the adult rat, an acute form of pancreatitis with haemorrhage, necrosis, oedema and infiltration of the acinar tissues with eosinophils, has been reported within 4–12 hr. of the injection of guinea pig anti-insulin serum (Lacy & Wright, 1966). The hyperplastic changes seen in foetal rats are very similar to those seen in the offspring of the diabetic mother, and may have the same aetiology. The acute allergic interstitial pancreatitis induced in rats with antibodies to insulin may represent an acute stage of the subacute lesion seen in man. Thus, it is known that antibodies to insulin can pass across the placenta from the maternal to the foetal circulation (Spellacy & Goetz, 1963a; Jorgensen, Deckert, Pedersen & Pedersen, 1966; Thorell, 1966). On the other hand, subacute pancreatitis is found in the offspring of mothers who have not received treatment with insulin, so it is far from certain that the lesions in man are produced by an immunological mechanism.

Micro-angiopathy

The renal lesions originally described by Kimmelstiel & Wilson (1936) and a unique form of retinopathy are the only two anatomical lesions which are generally accepted as typical of diabetes

mellitus in man. Both these lesions, however, have been attributed to a peculiar form of micro-angiopathy found not only in the retina and kidney but in other parts of the body (see Siperstein, Colwell & Meyer, 1964). Whether these vascular lesions are entirely responsible for all "diabetic complications" is still a matter for debate, but, for the purpose of the present discussion, this assumption is tentatively accepted.

One of the principal difficulties facing those who attempt to define the lesions specific to diabetes mellitus is the co-existence of degenerative lesions afflicting both diabetic and non-diabetic members of the population. In recent years, however, more attention has been paid to lesions in diabetic and non-diabetic subjects under the age of 40 years. Advantage has been taken of modern techniques to obtain objective as distinct from subjective assessments of accessible lesions and their progression with time. Such investigations will have to be carried out for many more years before these lesions are fully defined and their evolution explained, but a start has been made.

(i) *Retinopathy.* At about 20 years of age, only 5% of diabetics have diabetic retinopathy, but this figure rises to 84% at the age of 40 years (White, 1956). The prognosis for such patients is variable, in so far as visual acuity is concerned; it appears to be best in young patients and worst in those who have impaired vision when diabetes is first diagnosed (Caird & Garrett, 1963). According to one report (Lundbaek, 1953), about 3% go blind after 15 to 25 years. In fact, diabetic retinopathy, cataracts, and glaucoma pose a definite threat to the vision of the diabetic. The lesions which comprise diabetic retinopathy have been summarized by Wagener (1945), Becker 1952) and Ashton (1959). Venous engorgement, the first sign, is followed by the appearance of small saccular aneurysms at the venous ends of capillaries, mainly in the deep capillary plexuses of the posterior fundus. These aneurysms are associated specifically with capillaries, and may appear without simultaneous evidence of hypertension or arteriolar involvement. Hyaline material may be deposited within them and may completely obliterate the lumen of the vessel. Nearby, exudates and punctate haemorrhages are commonly found, and it can be shown that permeability of the capillaries is increased. The capillaries themselves are often grossly distorted and new ones may form in the later stages of the disease. "Of these features, the appearance of micro-aneurysms in an otherwise normal fundus is most characteristic of the diabetic state" (Ashton, 1959).

(ii) *Nephropathy.* Kimmelstiel & Wilson (1936)

were the first to describe nodular lesions in the glomeruli of diabetic patients, but in the next two decades the term "intercapillary glomerulosclerosis" came to mean "all things to all men" (Gellman, Pirani, Soothill, Muehrcke & Kark, 1959). Many have used the term "Kimmelstiel-Wilson syndrome" to describe the anasarcal condition sometimes seen in the terminal stages of diabetes, and have thereby implied that the lesions originally described by Kimmelstiel and Wilson are responsible. In fact, three lesions have been described (LeCompte, in Siperstein *et al.*, 1964).

(a) *Nodular glomerulosclerosis.* This is considered to be the most specific renal lesion associated with diabetes. In the early stages it consists of a spherical deposit of hyaline material which is stained deeply by the PAS (periodic acid-Schiff) method, and is seen at the periphery of the glomerular tuft in the inter-capillary tissues; one or more capillaries may be seen coursing over its surface. With increasing age, the number of affected glomeruli increases, and staining of the deposits becomes uneven; fat may appear in many of the nodules.

(b) *Diffuse glomerulosclerosis.* This lesion commences as a uniform thickening of the basement membrane of the glomerular capillaries and proceeds to involvement of the intercapillary tissues. These diffuse hyaline deposits can be stained by the PAS method, but, in the absence of nodular lesions, are difficult or impossible to differentiate from glomerulosclerotic lesions seen in non-diabetic subjects.

(c) *Exudates.* These, the least significant lesions, appear late in life and may be confused with the nodular lesions described above. They appear as crescents or caps either above the glomerular loop or on the inside of Bowman's capsule. They are strongly acidophilic and sometimes may be vacuolated.

Of these three lesions, the nodular one is specific but, in its absence, "most experienced pathologists do not diagnose the (more common diffuse) lesion with confidence, i.e. as a histologic entity" (LeCompte, in Siperstein *et al.*, 1964).

(iii) *Neuropathy.* The confusing literature dealing with neurological disorders associated with diabetes mellitus has recently been reviewed by Colby (1965). There is no specific disorder associated with this disease, symptoms and signs being found of various peripheral, autonomic, and central nervous disorders. Evidence of peripheral neuropathy, usually affecting the lower limb, is most common. From symptoms of distressing nocturnal pain and evidence of absent tendon reflexes, peripheral involvement can manifest

itself in the form of pareses and, in rare instances, a form of Charcot joint affecting the small bones of the foot. Spinal involvement may give rise to syndromes similar to those seen in tabes dorsalis and postero-lateral sclerosis. Gastro-intestinal disorders, including severe and distressing diarrhoea, may indicate an autonomic lesion. Involvement of the cranial nerves, especially the third and sixth, may give rise to pareses. In general, though the symptoms may be severe and the neurological signs very apparent, the pathological findings are not distinctive and are very variable.

These three pathological entities (retinopathy, nephropathy and neuropathy) have been considered under the heading of micro-angiopathy because there is increasing evidence that they are all manifestations of a common vascular lesion. The evidence for this comes both from clinical and pathological observations which were extensively discussed at a recent symposium (Siperstein *et al.*, 1964). In brief, the vascular lesions to be found in a diabetic are of two types (Colwell, 1965). First, there are the atheromatous and arteriosclerotic lesions of the larger blood vessels which probably develop more rapidly in diabetic than in non-diabetic subjects. Secondly, there are lesions which appear in the smaller arterioles, capillaries and venules, and are characterized by endothelial proliferation, thickening of the basement membranes and accumulations of hyaline deposits. According to one theory, these latter lesions, which are rarely found in patients who do not have diabetes, represent the result of abnormal glycoprotein metabolism; the hyaline deposits, like some glycoproteins, are deeply stained by the PAS method. Synthesis of glycoproteins is intimately related to the metabolism of glucose, but it is not dependent upon insulin (Spiro, 1963). According to many, therefore, abnormal metabolism of glucose should be a pre-requisite for the appearance of these lesions which should therefore be considered as "complications" of the disease and should be favourably influenced by good therapeutic control of diabetes. Others, on the other hand, point out that these disorders may appear long before any signs of insulin deficiency can be detected, and that they should not therefore be considered as "complications". They assert that the lesions "form part of the manifestation of a basic disorder, one of whose other manifestations is the metabolic disorder" (Colby, 1965), and they note that therapeutic control of the diabetes has a dubiously favourable effect upon their progression. Another distinct theory, originally suggested by Blumenthal, Berns, Owens & Hirata (1962), resulted from the observation that deposits of hyaline material in a wide variety of blood vessels in diabetic patients would react specifically with insulin conjugated to fluorescein isothiocyanate. This hypothesis, later formulated in greater detail (Blumenthal, Berns & Owens, 1963; Leibel & Wrenshall, 1965), implies that the lesions result from an auto-immune process, but this has still to be confirmed.

Further information will have to be obtained before any definite pronouncement can be made concerning either the basic natures or aetiologies of these lesions. A start has been made with the aid of modern techniques to follow the lesions which can now be recognized and are accessible in the living and otherwise healthy diabetic patient. Until more is known, however, it has to be confessed that we "still don't know why these lesions occur, how to prevent them or how to treat them" (Wagener, 1945).

DIAGNOSIS: TOLERANCE TESTS

The florid case of diabetes mellitus presents no great diagnostic problem to the clinician. In the case with a typical clinical history and prominent physical signs, little more is needed to establish the diagnosis than the finding of hyperglycaemia after an overnight fast or of glucose in the urine. Such a clinical picture, as will be emphasized below, represents a very late stage in the disease, and the real problem lies in the identification of mild cases and those who, though apparently normal at the time, could become diabetic in later life. On the assumption that florid diabetes is synonymous with insulin deficiency, tests have been devised to assess the ability of a patient's pancreas to secrete insulin in response to either a load of glucose (glucose tolerance tests) or a drug known to stimulate insulin secretion directly (tolbutamide test). A stress in the form of a small dose of glucocorticoid has been given to otherwise normal individuals to see whether this would reduce their responses to glucose or tolbutamide (steroid-glucose tolerance and steroid tolbutamide tests). Each of these tests is empirical and each has its uses, but none of them is perfect, and attempts are still being made to perfect their use (West, 1966). Before any of them can be applied it is essential that the subject should be well nourished; response to oral glucose, for example, is suppressed if a normal subject has lived on a low carbohydrate diet for only five days (Hales & Randle, 1963b). For this reason the subject is asked to take a high carbohydrate diet (300 to 400 g./day) for at least three days and to take no food for 8–12 hr. (overnight) immediately before the test is done. The test itself is started as early in the morning as is practicable with the subject still in the fasting state and at rest in bed.

(i) *Oral glucose tolerance test.* Glucose (100 g. or 1·75 g./kg. ideal body weight) is dissolved in flavoured water (ca. 400 ml.) and taken orally over a period of 5–10 min. The nausea and vomiting which this may sometimes cause can be avoided by using a carbonated flavoured solution of glucose (Glucola), which is said to be more palatable (Kent & Leonards, 1965). Venous or capillary blood is drawn before and at timed intervals (30, 60, 90 and 120 min.) after ingestion of the glucose for "true" sugar estimation.

(ii) *Intravenous glucose tolerance test.* In the test most commonly used now, glucose (25 g.) dissolved in water (50 ml.) is rapidly injected intravenously over a period of 2–4 min. Samples of blood are collected before and at 5 or 10 min. intervals up to 1 hr. after the midpoint of the infusion (Amatuzio, in Danowski, 1964).

(iii) *Intravenous Tolbutamide test.* A freshly prepared solution of sodium tolbutamide (1·0 g.) in distilled water (20 ml.) is injected intravenously at a constant rate over 2 min. Accurately timed samples of blood are withdrawn before, and 20 and 30 min. after the midpoint of the injection, the test being concluded after 30 min. with a glass of orange juice or with breakfast (Unger & Madison, in Danowski, 1964).

(iv) *Steroid tolerance tests.* The first of these was introduced by Fajans & Conn (1954), who administered cortisone in two doses 8½ and 2 hr. before ingestion of oral glucose; each dose consisted of 50 mg. cortisone acetate if the subject weighed less than 160 lbs. and 72·6 mg. for subjects weighing more. Long, Kilo & Recant (1964) gave a synthetic glucocorticoid (dexamethazone) at a constant dosage (3·0 mg.) and at the same times (8½ and 2 hr.) before intravenous injection of tolbutamide. These two tests are only used to study patients who have shown normal responses to either the oral glucose or intravenous tolbutamide tests.

In all of these tests, blood is collected into tubes containing fluoride, and some recommend that the plasma should be separated and used for subsequent sugar estimations (Zalme & Knowles, 1965). Concentrations of "true" sugar in these samples should be estimated using glucose oxidase, the Somogyi-Nelson method or with potassium ferricyanide in an automated method.

In each case the result of an individual test has to be compared with results obtained under the same conditions with normal subjects of comparable age and living under similar conditions.

After the age of about 40 years it is known, for instance, that the fasting level of blood-sugar rises (Silverstone, Brandfonbrener, Shock & Yiengst, 1957) and tolerance to either oral (West, Wulff, Reigel & Fitzgerald, 1964) or intravenous (Silverstone *et al.*, 1957) glucose decreases. In fact, if standards applicable to subjects under 40 years of age are applied to those over 60 years of age, the incidence of diabetes in old people would be more than 50%. It has also been shown that tolerance to glucose is much higher in East Pakistan and Malaya than it is in South America, the United States and Europe (West & Kalbfleisch, 1966). It is important to exclude diseases which could affect a subject's response. Abnormally rapid absorption of glucose from the intestines, such as may occur in thyrotoxicosis or after gastro-enterostomy, could raise the blood-sugar concentration rapidly after oral glucose. Slow absorption such as might occur in cases of pylorospasm, hypothyroidism or steatorrhoea, could cause delayed or minimal increases. In either of these cases an intravenous glucose tolerance test would be indicated. Organic disease of the liver, which plays an important role in homeostasis (Soskin, 1951), could also lead to incorrect interpretation of a response. These and other factors have to be considered before the result of any test can be correctly interpreted.

For diagnostic purposes, the oral glucose and intravenous tolbutamide tests are most commonly advocated. Conn & Fajans (1961) consider that the normal subject under 40 years of age should have a fasting blood-sugar concentration of less than 100 mg./100 ml. After an oral dose of glucose (1·75 g./kg. ideal body weight) the level should not rise above 160 mg./100 ml. after 1 hr., 140 mg./100 ml. after 90 min. and 120 mg./100 ml. after 2 hr. Others, such as Wilkerson (in Danowski, 1964), would accept somewhat higher upper levels of normality in the fasting state (110 mg./100 ml.) and 1 hr. after glucose (170 mg./100 ml.) but most are agreed on 120 mg./100 ml. as the upper limit of normality acceptable at 2 hr. It is possible for some patients to have levels below 120 mg./100 ml. at 2 hr. but above 160 mg./100 ml. at 1 hr. and above 140 mg./100 ml. at 90 min. (Conn & Fajans, 1961); such subjects are looked upon as "probable diabetics" and watched. Following the intravenous injection of tolbutamide, blood-sugar concentration normally falls rapidly in 20 min. to a value which is lower than 75% of the pre-injection level; after 30 min., virtually all normal subjects have levels which are less than 77% of the pre-injection level. By either of these tests the frankly diabetic subject is not difficult to identify, but especially when the fasting level of blood-sugar is within the normal range more false negative results are likely to be obtained with the tolbutamide test than after oral glucose (Unger & Madison, 1958).

As a diagnostic tool the intravenous tolerance test has limited applications; it has been used to study carbohydrate metabolism in pregnant women (Benjamin & Casper, 1966) and in cases of abnormal thyroid function (Elrick, Hlad & Arai, 1961) where gastro-intestinal absorption is abnormal. For research into carbohydrate metabolism in man it has proved valuable in getting quantitative estimates of glucose uptake by the tissues. Franckson, Ooms, Bellens, Conard & Bastenie (1962) have recently studied the changes induced by intravenously injected glucose and have emphasized that these must be taken into account before any "Glucose Assimilation Coefficient" can be interpreted correctly. For the first 15 min. the injected glucose redistributes itself in the extracellular space. Thereafter, and providing that sufficient glucose has been injected, it suppresses hepatic glucose output and the glucose content of the plasma falls exponentially. From about 15 to about 60 min. after injection, therefore, disappearance of glucose from the blood is due to uptake of that glucose by the tissues (liver muscle, adipose tissue and the brain). Under these conditions a Glucose Assimilation Coefficient (K) does reflect glucose uptake, but in diabetics hepatic glucose output is not suppressed by injected glucose and so "Increment Indices" (Amatuzio, in Danowski, 1964) in such cases should be interpreted with caution. Nonetheless it is true to say that injected glucose does disappear from the blood more slowly in diabetic (1·81 ± 0·51%/min.) than in normal (3·71 ± 0·40%/min.) subjects.

For the study of members of the population who could conceivably become diabetic, the two steroid tolerance tests have been used and will be considered later (see section on "The Natural History of Diabetes Mellitus"). Suffice it to say here that Fajans & Conn (in Leibel & Wrenshall, 1965) consider the first sign of insulin insufficiency to be present in a person who, after cortisone and an oral dose of glucose, has a blood-sugar concentration after 2 hr. of more than 140 mg./100 ml.; this is their definition of a "positive" response. After dexamethazone and intravenous tolbutamide, Long, Kilo & Recant (1964) found that abnormal responses were obtained more often with relatives of diabetics than with those having no family history of the disease; abnormal responses were found in six patients who subsequently developed diabetes.

The tests outlined above all have to be carried out under strictly standardized conditions, and are therefore not suitable for the study of large numbers of people in a community. Attempts are now being made to remedy this by using samples of blood drawn either one (Hayner, Kjelsberg, Epstein & Francis, 1965) or two (Kent & Leonards, 1965) hours after an oral dose of glucose. Others have investigated the possibility of using a standard meal of carbohydrate (75 g.) instead of the corresponding dose of glucose but this does not seem to induce sufficient hyperglycaemia (West et al., 1964). Those who appear to respond abnormally are being submitted to glucose tolerance tests and in this way it is hoped that the true incidence of diabetes in the population can be determined. Acceptable methods for the conduct of such surveys are still not agreed, since compromises have to be struck between practical and scientific considerations. For example, it is not agreed whether blood should be drawn 1 or 2 hr. after glucose is administered to subjects who have not fasted (Pratt, 1964). On the other hand a start has been made, and it is now obvious that amongst the older patients some new definition of diabetes is essential (Hayner et al., 1965).

DISTURBANCES OF ENDOCRINE FUNCTION ASSOCIATED WITH DIABETES

In most diabetics there is no overt or clearly defined evidence of deranged endocrine function, but there are certain endocrine conditions in which the patient may exhibit intolerance to

TABLE 3.9

Endocrine disorders associated with diabetes mellitus

Condition	Incidence	
	Diabetes in Condition	Condition in Diabetic Population
Acromegaly	15–25%	Less than 1%
Cushing's Syndrome	13%	Less than 1%
Thyrotoxicosis	Less than 6%	1–2·4%
Glucagon tumour	—	One case

(Information derived from sources given in text.)

glucose or frank diabetes. As shown in Table 3.9, these conditions are rarely responsible for diabetes in the general population. On the other hand, they have been and are being studied extensively since they demonstrate manifest

evidence that extra-pancreatic hormonal factors can induce diabetes and could in some less dramatic way play a part in evoking the "idiopathic" disease which is so much more common.

Growth Hormone

Though diabetes mellitus is found in 15 to 25% of acromegalics, acromegaly is seldom seen (1:500) in the diabetic population (Coggleshall & Root, 1940; McCullagh, 1956). In acromegalics, diabetes appears 10 to 15 years after the onset of acromegalic symptoms and signs; is more frequent in females than males; and is more common in the relatives of diabetic than non-diabetic subjects. The syndromes are comparable with the reversible (idiohypophyseal) and irreversible (metahypophyseal) diabetes induced in dogs with repeated injections of bovine growth hormone (Campbell, Chaikof & Davidson, 1954; Campbell & Rastogi, 1966a,b). Within a few days, injections of growth hormone (2 mg./kg. body weight/day) into normal dogs cause little change in blood-sugar concentration, but significant increases in the levels of circulating insulin and free fatty acids. At this stage, injected glucose evokes rapid and very marked secretion of endogenous insulin, but in spite of this the rate at which the injected glucose is removed from the circulation is reduced. After 9 to 11 days, resting concentrations of glucose and insulin in the blood may be markedly elevated, and, despite significantly increased mobilization of insulin, injected glucose is removed from the blood at a greatly reduced rate and the levels of free fatty acids do not fall to control levels. When injections of growth hormone are continued for 15 to 37 days, diabetes persists and insulin has to be administered after a further 44 to 150 days.

Similar changes can be induced with growth hormone in about four days in human patients with pan-hypopituitarism receiving thyroid extract, cortisone and androgens (Luft & Cerasi, 1964). By that time, there is hyperglycaemia accompanied by high levels of circulating insulin and free fatty acids, but, despite marked induced insulin secretion, these patients show a diabetic response to injected glucose. In acromegalics with normal or elevated resting levels of insulin and growth hormone in the blood, tolerance to glucose is often impaired even though large amounts of insulin may be secreted (Cerasi & Luft, 1964; Beck, Schalch, Parker, Kipnis & Daughaday, 1965). When insulin is injected (Landon, Greenwood, Stamp & Wynn, 1966; Roth, Glick, Yalow & Berson, 1963), concentrations of circulating growth hormone do tend to rise but the levels of free fatty acids in the blood either fail to fall or only do so to a slight extent.

Adrenal Hormones

The hormones secreted from the adrenal medulla (adrenaline) and cortex (cortisol, aldosterone) are all known or suspected to have diabetogenic effects in experimental animals or in man.

(i) *Adrenaline*. This hormone induces transient hyperglycaemia and elevation of the levels of free fatty acids in the blood. Induction of hyperglycaemia is probably due to (i) direct activation of hepatic phosphorylase; (ii) stimulation of release of glucagon from the α-cells of the pancreas and thence activation of the phosphorylase; and (iii) inhibition of insulin secretion from the pancreatic β-cells. It also activates lipase in depots of fat, thus stimulating release of free fatty acids into the blood. The rare phaeochromocytoma, a tumour of the adrenal medulla, induces paroxysmal or persistent hypertension in adults (Gifford, Kvale, Maher, Roth & Priestley, 1964) and in children (Stackpole, Melicow & Uson, 1963) who may also exhibit hyperglycaemia in the fasting state. A mistaken diagnosis of diabetes mellitus has been made in such cases, but the vascular and diabetic symptoms usually disappear with removal of the tumour.

(ii) *Glucocorticoids*. Cortisol stimulates gluconeogenesis, deposition of hepatic glycogen, uptake of amino acids and synthesis of RNA and protein in the liver, and, by mechanisms not yet fully understood, facilitates mobilization of fatty acids from adipose tissue (Ashmore & Morgan, in Eisenstein, 1967). These effects have been well demonstrated in adrenalectomized rats and in rats injected with adreno-cortical extracts (Long, Katzin & Fry, 1940).

In Addisons disease, as in the adrenalectomized animal, the blood-sugar concentration tends to be low and the patient is excessively sensitive to insulin (Fraser, Albright & Smith, 1941). Such adrenal insufficiency may be complicated by diabetes, the onset of which usually (63%) precedes that of Addison's disease. In this case, as after adrenalectomy of the pancreatectomized cat (Long & Lukens, 1936), sensitivity to insulin increases, ketonuria disappears, and the fasting level of blood-sugar falls (Crampton, Scudder & Davis, 1949). Treatment with insulin is often difficult, since these patients are very prone to develop signs of hypoglycaemia, and may do so at relatively high levels of blood-glucose. However, on judicious treatment with glucocorticoids, their insulin requirements are raised to values (*ca.*

50 U/day) found in comparable cases without adrenal insufficiency (Baird & Munro, 1954). Of the 113 cases reported in the literature up to 1965, only 16 were found to have tuberculous lesions in the adrenal glands, the remainder having unspecified (21) or atrophic (76) lesions (Solomon, Carpenter, Bennett & Harvey, 1965). In 28 of these cases (25%), there was also chronic lymphocytic thyroiditis and evidence in the blood of antibodies to both adrenal and thyroid tissues (Tzagournis & Hamwi, 1967). This condition, which is now being recognized more frequently, may therefore prove to be an example of a multiglandular auto-immune disease.

When glucocorticoids are administered for a prolonged period to man, as is sometimes necessary, they do not induce diabetes in subjects with no history of diabetes in the family but they may do so, even in therapeutic dosage, in the relatives of diabetics (Conn & Fajans, 1956). The effects of glucocorticoids in experimental animals have been reviewed by Levine & Mahler (1964) and, unlike those of growth hormone, are reversible even after prolonged administration. Hyperglycaemia, though present, is not necessarily prominent in animals treated with glucocorticoids but islet hypertrophy with degranulation of the β-cells is always seen in the pancreas and tolerance to glucose is frequently reduced. Cushing's syndrome in man, which is due to either an adrenocortical tumour or to adrenal hyperplasia, is predominantly but not entirely the result of excessive endogenous secretion of glucocorticoids (Liddle, in Eisenstein, 1967). The signs include marked wasting of muscular tissues and a centripetal redistribution of the depots of fat (Plotz, Knowlton & Regan, 1952; Soffer, Iannaconne & Gabrilove, 1961). Many of the patients have normal or almost normal fasting levels of blood-glucose, but about a quarter are glycosuric and about half of these are diabetic. Like normal subjects treated with a synthetic glucocorticoid (dexamethazone) for four days (Perley & Kipnis, 1966*a*), most patients with Cushing's syndrome (Klink & Estrich, 1964) secrete increased amounts of insulin in response to a load of glucose. On the other hand, despite the normal fasting levels, glucose tolerance is of the diabetic type in almost all cases of Cushing's syndrome. No cases of diabetic glomerulosclerosis have been reported but diabetic retinopathy has been observed. The prognosis for patients with Cushing's syndrome used to be poor, but many patients now survive after surgery, and tolerance to glucose is usually improved. At one stage it was thought that adrenalectomy might lead to improvement of retinopathy in diabetic patients, but this hope was not fulfilled (Malins, 1956).

(iii) *Aldosterone*. Conn (1965) has recently postulated that many cases of diabetes could be due to occult forms of aldosteronism. This postulate, which has yet to be confirmed, is based on the observation that approximately half of the patients from whom aldosterone-secreting tumours have been removed, have had impaired tolerance to glucose (Conn, Knopf & Nesbit, 1964). All these patients have hypertension and are thought to constitute about 15 % of the hypertensive population. Ostrander, Francis, Hayner, Kjelsberg & Epstein (1965) have also estimated that between 7 and 21 % of the hypertensive population have abnormalities of glucose metabolism. On this basis Conn considers that a high proportion of the population could be potentially diabetic due to a remediable lesion.

Thyroid

It is not known how the thyroid gland exerts its effects upon the metabolic processes of the body, but it probably influences a process which is fundamental and common to most tissues. In the present context it is sufficient to note that the thyroid accelerates oxidative processes and is necessary for normal synthesis of protein and for normal growth.

In experimental animals, the diabetogenic effect of the thyroid is much weaker than those of glucocorticoids and growth hormone. For example, meta-thyroid diabetes cannot be induced with thyroid extracts in the normal dog unless part of the pancreas has been removed (Houssay, 1944). On the other hand, extracts from the livers of rats treated with thyroxine will degrade insulin more rapidly than normal extracts or extracts from thyroidectomized rats (Elgee & Williams, 1955). In man, moderate doses of dessicated thyroid (25 mg./day) administered over nine weeks have little or no effect upon the response of the normal subject to either an oral dose of glucose or an intravenous injection of insulin (Danowski, Bonessi, Sarver & Moses, 1964). In established cases of thyrotoxicosis, however, the response to oral glucose is similar to that seen in some diabetics; insulin concentrations in the blood rise, but the glucose and free fatty acids in the blood remain elevated even after 3 hr. (Hales & Hyams, 1964.) After intravenously injected glucose, uptake of glucose by the tissues is either normal or slightly elevated in cases of hyperthyroidism but is reduced in the myxoedematous patient (Elrick et al., 1961; Lamberg, 1965). In hyperthyroidism it

is claimed that sensitivity of the tissues to insulin is either normal (Elrick et al., 1961) or, due to the presence of high concentrations of free fatty acids, reduced (Hales & Hyams, 1964). Glucagon also has a weaker hyperglycaemic effect (Lamberg, 1965). Several factors are said to play a part in producing these changes in subjects exposed to large amounts of endogenous or exogenous thyroid hormone (Abt, 1962). Reserves of hepatic glycogen become depleted, and increased gluconeogenesis with increased nitrogen excretion can occur, especially if intake of food does not keep pace with the increased rate of metabolism in the body. These, associated with the increased rate of destruction of endogenous insulin and the elevated levels of circulating free fatty acids, could lead to the diabetic response to glucose seen in hyperthyroidism. Evidence to suggest that the tissues themselves are less sensitive than normal to insulin is not convincing, but there is evidence to support the contention that the pancreas in hyperthyroidism is less sensitive than normal to glucose (Malaisse, Malaisse-Lagae & McCraw, 1967b).

In the diabetic population, the incidence of hyperthyroidism is of the order of 1 % (Pirart, 1965) to 2·4 % (Foster & Lowrie, 1938). Conversely, that of diabetes in cases of hyperthyroidism is higher in nodular-toxic (5·6 %) than in diffuse (1·7 %) goitre (Regan & Wilder, 1940). Myxoedema, most often seen in middle-aged obese women, occurs less frequently (0·4 %) in diabetes (Pirart, 1965). All are agreed that there is more than a fortuitous association between hyperthyroidism and diabetes. Most reports show that onset of hyperthyroidism precedes that of diabetes (Abt, 1962), but in Pirart's series this only occurred in about a third of the cases. Their coexistence is of clinical importance in that the thyrotoxic condition could precipitate severe diabetic complications such as ketosis, acidosis and coma, and the diabetic state could precipitate a thyroid crisis if not controlled (Abt, 1962). The association between diabetes and hypothyroidism may be of aetiological importance. It has already been pointed out that the rare co-existence of diabetes and hypo-adrenocorticism is also sometimes associated with hypothyroidism (Solomon et al., 1965), and that the adrenal and thyroid lesions may be the result of an auto-immune process. It seems possible, therefore, that diabetes could form part of some multiglandular auto-immune process in these particular cases. From the point of view of therapy, fluctuations in the state of thyroid activity have little effect upon diabetes, and do not influence a patient's insulin requirements (Pirart, 1965).

Pregnancy

The effects of diabetes upon the pregnant woman and those of the diabetic mother upon her unborn child have been well reviewed by Kyle (1963), and can be best considered under two headings.

(i) *The pregnant woman.* Normal pregnancy involves changes in hormonal balance, some of which are reflected in altered metabolism in the mother. During the first trimester the placenta forms rapidly increasing amounts of chorionic gonadotropin whose excretion in the urine reaches a peak after 80 to 90 days. Thereafter, and as the placenta takes over the functions of the corpus luteum, pregnanediol and oestriol excretion rise to reach a maximum at or just before delivery. Josimowich & MacLaren (1962) have also extracted from the placenta a further substance with lactogenic and growth-promoting activity. This substance, variously known as *growth hormone-prolactin* and *human placental lactogen* (*HPL*), has been localized in the syncytiotrophoblastic cells (Sciarra, Kaplan & Grumbach, 1963). Though immunologically similar to human growth hormone, it has been assayed by immunological methods (Beck, Parker & Daughaday, 1965; Kaplan & Grumbach, 1965a). After about eight weeks of pregnancy HPL can be detected in maternal plasma, and its concentration increases to a maximum during the second half of pregnancy. After delivery it entirely disappears from the mother's plasma within 60 min. Moreover, its concentration in the maternal plasma just before delivery is many times (x 600–1000) that of pituitary growth hormone. In the foetal circulation, on the other hand, growth hormone is present in high concentration and little or no HPL can be detected (Kaplan & Grumbach, 1965b; Beck et al., 1965). Thus, after the first trimester, maternal plasma contains relatively high concentrations of oestrogen, progesterone and placental lactogen. It is also said to contain cortisol in higher than normal concentrations but, for reasons which are still debated, the concentration of free and biologically active hormone is normal.

The effects of these hormonal changes in normal pregnancy are most apparent in the second and third trimesters. At term the concentrations of free fatty acids in the plasma are elevated, but they fall within a few days of delivery (Burt, 1960). If glucose is administered by mouth between the thirty-sixth week and term, glucose tolerance is usually normal but the moderate initial rise in plasma-sugar concentration is accompanied by a markedly greater rise in insulin concentration than is the case after delivery (Spellacy & Goetz,

1963b; Bleicher, O'Sullivan & Freinkel, 1964; Kalkhoff, Schalch, Walker, Beck, Kipnis & Daughaday, 1964). With this increased release of endogenous insulin, concentrations of free fatty acids fall in parallel with those found in the same test carried out after delivery. These changes in response to ingested glucose are now thought to be due to the circulating placental lactogen. This hormone in a purified form raises the level of free fatty acids in the plasma of hypopituitary dwarfs (Grumbach, Kaplan, Abrams, Bell & Conte, 1966), but has no growth-promoting activity (Schultz & Blizzard, 1966). Although much remains to be learned about the physiological functions of this hormone, its presence during the latter half of pregnancy does appear to be responsible for the observed alterations in response to glucose.

Detection of abnormal tolerance to an oral dose of glucose is made difficult by the changes which occur during pregnancy in gastro-intestinal function (Burt, 1962). When the results of oral and intravenous tolerance tests have been compared in small series of cases, they have often been found to conflict. In a recent large series (Benjamin & Casper, 1966) just over half the results (58%) were in agreement with one another, but most of the remainder suggested a normal response to intravenous and an abnormal one to oral glucose. This suggests that an abnormal response to oral glucose should be viewed with suspicion, but an abnormal one to intravenous glucose can be taken as more definite evidence of diabetes. Difficulty in establishing a diagnosis of diabetes during pregnancy is further compounded by the common finding (25%) of glycosuria even in the normal pregnant woman; and the appearance of lactosuria in many (51%) during the last six weeks of pregnancy. This glycosuria is due to increased glomerular filtration and a relatively smaller increase in tubular reabsorption.

Diabetes may commence at any stage of pregnancy, but it is most likely to do so during the second or third trimester; this is called "gestational diabetes". Such diabetics, and more especially those who acquire the disease before conception, are more than normally likely to develop metabolic complications of diabetes (acidosis, coma, etc.) which may be precipitated by infection, toxaemia or other obstetric complications. If the diabetes is well controlled, maternal mortality can be kept down to levels (0·3 to 0·7%) which are little above those found in a normal pregnancy (0·3 to 0·4%). Foetal mortality is adversely affected by diabetic complications, rapidly progressing hydramnios, toxaemia, and infections in the mother; it does not correlate well with the severity of the maternal diabetes as judged by the dosage of insulin needed for control. To prevent complications of the maternal diabetes, all are agreed that medical supervision of the patient from an early stage of pregnancy is essential. Granted good control, prognosis is poorest in those diabetics who develop the disease under the age of 10 years, have had it for more than 20 years and show marked evidence of diabetic micro-angiopathy (retinopathy, calcification of pelvic vessels, and chronic albuminuria). In this group, the worst of White's classification (in Joslin, Root, White & Marble, 1959), foetal wastage reaches 37 %. The incidence of toxaemia is hard to assess but it tends to appear at an earlier stage of pregnancy in the diabetic than in the non-diabetic patient, and when it occurs, foetal losses (23 %) tend to be higher than normal (10 %). Hydramnios occurs much more frequently (19 %) than it does in normal women (0·5 to 1·0 %), and gives rise to heavy foetal losses (39 %); its cause is unknown but foetal losses are mainly due to obstetric complications. Pyelonephritis occurs four times as frequently in diabetic as in normal pregnant women, and it too can lead to a high incidence of prematurity (24 %) or neonatal death (17 %). Even if these complications of pregnancy in the diabetic woman are satisfactorily anticipated and treated by a skilled team of physicians and obstetricians, there remains the danger of sudden intra-uterine death which occurs most frequently during the thirty-seventh to fortieth week.

It is agreed that survival of the foetus, other things being equal, is most likely after 36 weeks of gestation and that the risk of sudden intra-uterine death is the highest after 38 weeks. The exact time at which delivery should be induced is much debated, but methods are being used to assist in the making of this decision in individual cases. Thus it is known than in normal and diabetic pregnant women the rate of oestriol excretion in the urine rises after 20 weeks (Hobkirk, Blahey, Alfheim, Raeside & Joron, 1960). At term the rate usually exceeds 12 mg./day but if it falls for two days to 4 mg./day or less, foetal losses of 50 % may occur if the pregnancy is allowed to proceed (Kyle, Yalcin, Greese & Smith, in Leibel & Wrenshall, 1965). Delivery is therefore recommended either vaginally or, if circumstances warrant it, by Caesarean section after 36 weeks or when oestriol excretion falls to a low level.

(ii) *The foetus.* As judged by reports made of a number of series of diabetic pregnancies, foetal mortality has fallen from an average of 40 % between 1930 and 1940 to one of 15 % between 1950 and 1960. This has been largely due to close supervision of pregnancy itself, good timing of delivery and expert neonatal care. The lowest reported losses are of the order of 4 % for intra-uterine death and 9 to 17 % for the neonatal period (Gellis & Hsia, 1959). Having survived birth, the commonest cause of death in the neonatal period is acute respiratory distress due to atelectasis and hyaline membrane disease (Cornblath & Schwartz, 1966). This respiratory condition may account for 50 to 100 % of deaths occurring within the first 24 hr. of life, but in addition birth injuries (10 to 15 %) and congenital malformations may contribute. Many of the less severe anatomical malformations may not declare themselves until later in life, and their incidence (6 to 12 %), contrary to the conceptions of many, is not much greater than that found in normal children. Also, and contrary to common belief, the incidence of hydramnios does not correlate well with that of congenital abnormalities. In fact, the new-born child of the diabetic mother is really a premature infant, and is treated as such by the competent paediatrician.

The weight of such infants at birth is not a good criterion for judgement of prematurity. About a third of them weigh more than 4000 g., a weight achieved by only 0·5 % of normal new-born infants. The increased weight has been ascribed to retained water but there is indirect evidence that most is due to fat (Clapp, Butterfield & O'Brien, 1962). The state of bone development usually corresponds to the period of gestation, but the lengths of the bones may be greater than normal; if the mother has extensive vascular disease, the offspring may be small. In addition to these physical differences, the offspring of the diabetic mother has metabolic features which are similar to those of premature infants of normal mothers (Gellis & Hsia, 1959), but their most characteristic feature is an altered carbohydrate metabolism.

As already pointed out elsewhere, the pancreas of such an infant contains large hyperplastic islets of Langerhans (Cardell, 1953; Lazarus & Volk, 1962) with abnormally large amounts of stored insulin (Steinke & Driscoll, 1965). At birth the concentration of circulating insulin is high (Baird & Farquhar, 1962; Stimmler, Brazie & O'Brien, 1964; Chen, Adam, Laskowski, McCann & Schwarz, 1965) and that of glucose is somewhat lower than the maternal level. Within 30 min. the blood-sugar concentration falls to very low levels (ca. 30 mg./100 ml.) and may be slow to rise again. If infused with glucose, these infants dispose of it very rapidly (Baird & Farquhar, 1962), but they seldom die of hypoglycaemia, *per se*.

The prognosis for children of diabetic mothers cannot yet be fully assessed, but after the neo-natal period deaths occur most frequently in the first month of life and few occur after one year (Hagbard, Olow & Reinand, 1959). Nothing remarkable is noted in their development, either mental or physical, but no series of such children has been followed for a sufficient time to warrant more precise conclusions. In essence, therefore, these children appear to have good prospects for a full and normal life if they can survive life *in utero* and the transition from there to the outside world. Their prospects, in fact, depend very much upon the excellence of the medical and obstetric care lavished on their mothers during pregnancy, and the skill of the paediatrician who cares for them immediately after birth.

AETIOLOGY AND TREATMENT OF DIABETES MELLITUS

Payling-Wright (1950) emphasized that "pro-phylaxis and rational therapeutics in disease are both necessarily based on a knowledge of causes, and that when these are unknown, there is no adequate method of prevention, and treatment must remain empirical and symptomatic". In the case of diabetes mellitus, no fundamental cause is known and there are instances in which the disease is difficult to define and delimit from the normal. Some have even suggested that, like essential hypertension (Pickering, 1961), diabetes may

represent a quantitative rather than a qualitative deviation from the normal. Before considering aetiology, therefore, it is essential to define what we now mean by the words diabetes mellitus.

Natural History of Diabetes Mellitus

"It is incorrect to equate diabetes with hyper-glycaemia and glycosuria (Ellenberg, 1963)". "It is a genetically transmitted abnormality consisting of an elusive biochemical aberration which *may* eventually disclose its presence by evidence of diminished insulin activity (Conn & Fajans, 1961)." Quite apart from any consideration of its aetiology, many agree that the metabolic derange-ments constitute comparatively late manifesta-tions of the disease and are preceded in time by arbitrarily defined and less easily recognizable stages. In all, four stages were defined by Conn & Fajans (1961) and these are illustrated in Table 3.10.

(i) *Overt diabetes.* The overt or clinical (Fitz-gerald & Keen, 1964) diabetic has symptoms and physical signs directly referable to insulin defi-ciency. There is fasting hyperglycaemia and a glucose tolerance test is not needed for diagnosis. Evidence of diabetic angiopathy is usually present in older patients, but may be absent in newly diagnosed juvenile diabetics.

(ii) *Latent diabetes.* Latent, chemical (Camerini-Davalos, Caulfield, Rees, Lozano-Castaneda, Naldjian & Marble, 1963) or asymptomatic (Fitzgerald & Keen, 1964) diabetics have no symptoms directly referable to insulin deficiency,

TABLE 3.10

Natural History of Diabetes Mellitus in Man

	Prediabetes	Sub-clinical Diabetes	Latent Diabetes	Overt Diabetes
Symptoms of insulin deficiency	None	Suggestive History	Suggestive History	Present
Glucose Tolerance Test:				
(1) Fasting blood sugar	Normal	Normal	Above 110 mg./100 ml.	Above 110 mg./100 ml.
(2) 90 minutes after glucose	Normal	Normal	Above 140 mg./100 ml.	
(3) 2 hours after glucose	Normal	Normal	Above 120 mg./100 ml.	
Cortisone-Glucose Tolerance Test:				
(1) Result		"Positive"		
(2) 2 hours after glucose		Above 140 mg./100 ml.		
Synalbumin concentration	Increased	Increased	Increased	Increased
Vascular lesions	±	+	++	+++

Significant levels of blood-sugar concentrations (mg./100 ml.) determining category of the subject are taken from results published by Fajans & Conn (1954; in Liebel & Wrenshall, 1965) and by Conn & Fajans (1961).

but they may either be hyperglycaemic in the fasting state or respond abnormally to a load of glucose. Again, any degree of diabetic angiopathy may be found.

(iii) *Sub-clinical diabetes.* The sub-clinical, latent-chemical (Camerini-Davalos *et al.*, 1963) or latent (Fitzgerald & Keen, 1964) diabetic has no symptoms, a normal level of blood-sugar after fasting overnight and a normal response to a load of glucose. However, there may be a clinical history suggestive of a past diabetic episode (e.g. gestational diabetes), and the patient responds abnormally to glucose or tolbutamide after two doses of a glucocorticoid—the cortisone-glucose tolerance or steroid-intravenous tolbutamide tests. Evidence of diabetic angiopathy is usually but not always minimal or absent.

(iv) *Pre-diabetes.* The pre-diabetic or potential diabetic (Fitzgerald & Keen, 1964) is a person who shows no detectable evidence of insulin insufficiency, but does have "as yet undiscovered metabolic derangements which (*a*) lead eventually to insufficient insulin activity and (*b*) may give rise to the generalized angiopathy which characterizes the diabetic syndrome (Conn & Fajans, 1961)". If one accepts the thesis that diabetes has a genetic basis, then the pre-diabetic state exists "from conception to the demonstration of diminished insulin activity by whatever method is considered most sensitive at that time (Conn & Fajans, 1961)". A pre-diabetic state can be suspected in (*a*) non-diabetic subjects who are identical twins, parents or offsprings of overt diabetics; or (*b*) women who, though apparently normal at the time, have given birth to one or more large babies (Fajans & Conn, in Leibel & Wrenshall, 1965). In such subjects, who are now receiving increasing attention, it has been reported that after the intravenous injection of glucose, insulin and glucose levels in the blood run at a slightly higher but not always significantly different level from the normal; and that morphological changes can be seen in the conjunctival vessels, vessels of the ear lobe and in biopsy material from the kidneys (Camerini-Davalos, in Leibel & Wrenshall, 1965; Camerini-Davalos *et al.*, 1963; Rees, Camerini-Davalos, Caulfield, Lozano-Castaneda, Cervantes-Amezcus, Taton, Krauthammer & Marble, in Cameron & O'Connor, 1964).

Though Conn & Fajans define four stages in the development of overt diabetes, they do not consider that progression from the pre-diabetic to the overt diabetic state is relentless; it may never occur, may progress slowly or rapidly, and may be reversed at any stage. The reversible nature of this "dynamic state" may be illustrated by two examples. At one extreme are two cases, described by Harwood (1957) and by Peck, Kirtley & Peck (1958), who were admitted to a hospital in undeniable diabetic coma, were treated conventionally and were ultimately able to live normal or almost normal lives without any need for insulin or any overt signs of diabetes. The second and more common example is that of the woman who develops signs of diabetes during pregnancy, shows none after delivery and may live many more years without recurrence of diabetic symptoms (Kyle, 1963).

On this basis of classification, diabetes is only detected positively when some sign of insulin insufficiency becomes manifest. Yet it is well known that some of the "complications" of diabetes may appear before this stage is reached. Vallance-Owen (1966), on the other hand, claims that persons likely to develop the disease can be distinguished by the high concentrations of synalbumin present in their plasma. Since this insulin antagonist is dependent upon intact pituitary and adrenal glands, insulin deficiency is only likely to become apparent when adreno-cortical activity increases and may never develop at all.

Heredity and the Incidence of Diabetes

"Diabetes mellitus is in many respects a geneticist's nightmare. As a disease it presents almost every impediment to a proper genetic study which can be recognized (Neel, Fajans, Conn & Davidson, 1965)." In fact it seems as though we know little more about this aspect of the disease than Pavy (1885), when he said over 80 years ago that "there is no doubt that this disease runs in families".

Pincus & White (1933) were among the first to formulate a hypothesis on the basis of the higher incidence of diabetes in close relatives (parents and siblings) of diabetic as compared with normal subjects. They postulated that "the potentiality for developing diabetes is inherited as a simple Mendelian recessive". Then came the hypothesis that juvenile diabetes is due to the homozygous condition of a gene which in the heterozygous condition gives rise to maturity-onset diabetes (Harris, 1950; Lamy, Frezal & Rey, 1961). Simpson (1964) and Neel *et al.* (1965) consider it more likely that the disease is a condition subject to multifactorial inheritance. These conflicting hypotheses have been reviewed by Steinberg (in Leibel & Wrenshall, 1965) who, while rejecting the multifactorial theory, also considers that the other hypotheses either do not fit the facts or are not proven. He adds, as others have emphasized, that the main obstacle to successful genetic studies is the lack of knowledge of the basic nature of the disease; evidence of insulin insufficiency was used to identify persons covered by these studies.

Using synalbumin as a marker, Vallance-Owen (1966) now claims that the disease is inherited as an autosomal dominant characteristic, but that not all those affected will develop insulin insufficiency. Stimmler & Elliott (1964) claim to have found an insulin inhibitor whose inheritance is governed by a single autosomal gene. This inhibitor is considered to be an abnormal form of insulin by Elliott, O'Brien & Roy (1965). Whether any of these hypotheses are true or not remains to be seen, but it does seem obvious that little advance will be made until the basic lesion responsible for diabetes, if it exists, can be identified.

Environmental Factors Associated with Diabetes

Overt, but usually transient diabetes has been diagnosed soon after birth (Cornblath & Schwarz, 1966), but most cases occurring in youth have their onset at or about the age of puberty (White, 1956). In these cases both sexes are affected with equal frequency, but amongst the adult population curious and unexplained changes have occurred in this century. At the end of the last century, according to Pavy (1885), males (71%) predominated over females (29%) in the diabetic population. Malins, Fitzgerald & Wall (1965) have now reported that in Birmingham, England, the ratio of male to female diabetics fell during the first half of this century until 70% of diabetics were female in 1940. Now the ratio has reverted to that found by Pavy, with males once again predominating over females. The absolute incidence of diabetes is hard to assess, since the criteria for diagnosis have altered so much in the past 100 years and surveys of whole populations are only now becoming possible. However, one estimate (Augustine, 1964) suggests that 10% of the population of the United States either has or will develop the disease.

Hormonal factors play an obvious part in the production of some cases of diabetes mellitus. Thus, as already mentioned, acromegaly, Cushing's syndrome and thyrotoxicosis can all be associated with diabetes. It has also been reported that diabetes may be caused by a glucagon-secreting tumour (McGavran, Unger, Recant, Polk, Kilo & Levin, 1966). On the other hand these endocrine disorders are responsible for only a small fraction of the total number of diabetics seen in clinical practice (Table 3.9). The relationship between hormonal factors and the evolution of diabetes is best seen in pregnancy where, even in normal women, increased levels of free fatty acids and of insulin are found in the third trimester, and there is often evidence of increased resistance to the action of insulin. Here, the diabetogenic agent is thought to be *placental lactogen* (Kaplan & Grumbach, 1964). In non-pregnant women it now seems that the oral contraceptives may have a diabetogenic effect for they are said to reduce tolerance to glucose (Spellacy & Carlson, 1966; Buchler & Warren, 1966). Levels of circulating *growth hormone* are reported to be high in newly diagnosed mild cases of diabetes (Ehrlich & Randle, in Cameron & O'Connor, 1962; Pfeiffer, in Leibel & Wrenshall, 1965) but others have reported normal levels (Hunter, Clarke & Duncan, 1966). On the other hand the hypophysectomized juvenile diabetic is very sensitive to the effects of even small doses of growth hormone; within hours there is a dramatic worsening of the diabetic state with onset of severe acidosis (Luft, in Cameron & O'Connor, 1964). Hypophysectomized and non-hypophysectomized elderly diabetics on larger doses of growth hormone also develop glycosuria and hyperglycaemia but are less prone to become acidotic (Luft & Cerasi, 1964; Pfeiffer, in Leibel & Wrenshall, 1965). Removal of the pituitary gland may sometimes be followed by regression (Sprague, 1962) or even complete disappearance (Poulsen, 1953) of severe diabetic retinopathy. Increased *adreno-cortical* function has been clearly demonstrated in cases of Achard-Thiers syndrome, a rare condition characterized by onset of diabetes after the menopause in obese "bearded women" (Malaisse, Lauvaux, Franckson & Bastenie, 1965). In Pfeiffer's opinion (in Leibel & Wrenshall, 1965), the significant change in diabetes is not any absolute change in production of cortisol or ACTH but an inversion of the circadian rhythm of ACTH secretion. From these examples it can be concluded that there is rarely a clear association between the human diabetic syndromes and abnormalities of endocrine function other than that of the pancreatic islets. On the other hand, there is much indirect evidence that such abnormal endocrine function may precede the insulin deficiency.

A normal or mildly diabetic response to loading with glucose, accompanied by evidence of excessive release of endogenously secreted insulin, has been noted (Table 3.11) in late normal pregnancy (Kalkhof et al., 1964); in non-diabetic hypophysectomized patients treated with growth hormone (Luft & Cerasi, 1964); and in normal subjects treated for only a few days with a glucocorticoid

TABLE 3.11

Effects of hormones, pregnancy, obesity and mild diabetes upon the normal response to oral glucose

Condition	Fasting Plasma levels			After glucose	
	Glucose	FFA	Insulin	Glucose Tolerance	Insulin Response
Normal	N	N	N	N	N
Cortisol (Cushing)	N—Inc	Inc	N—Inc	N—Decr	Inc
Thyroxine (Thyrotoxic)	N—Inc	Inc	N	(Decr)	(N)
Growth hormone (Acromegaly)	N—Inc	Inc	Inc	N—Decr	Inc
Pregnancy	N	Inc	Inc	N—Decr	Inc
Obesity	N—Inc	Inc	Inc	N—Decr	Inc
Diabetes (mild)	N—Inc	Inc	N	Decr	N—Inc

Compared with the normal values (N), observations are increased (Inc), or decreased (Decr); in the case of thyrotoxicosis the change is dependant upon the method used for testing.

(Perley & Kipnis, 1966a). A similar response has been noted in non-diabetic subjects with two diabetic parents or an identical diabetic twin (Camerini-Davalos, in Leibel & Wrenshall, 1965). In mild cases of diabetes, administration of glucose is followed after 3–5 hr. by onset of hypoglycaemia with symptoms (Seltzer, Fajans & Conn, 1956). Levels of circulating insulin-like substances (fat pad) are also reported to be high in close non-diabetic relatives of diabetic patients (Steinke, Camerini-Davalos, Marble & Renold, 1961), and when glucose is given to some very mild cases of diabetes, the level of immuno-reactive insulin may rise to a high level (Yalow & Berson, 1965). Before or in the early stages of the disease, therefore, it is possible that increased function of the pituitary or adrenal glands or the placenta could place an extra strain upon the pancreatic islets which, if they are unable to adapt, might never recover their former function. In youth it is known that levels of circulating growth hormone are high and fluctuate over a wide range (Greenwood, Hunter & Marrian, 1964). The pancreatic islets are undergoing hypertrophic changes at a slower rate than is growth in the rest of the body (Ogilvie, 1937) and there is the coincidental sexual metamorphosis of puberty. Under such circumstances would not the added strain of infection or injury, so often seen before the onset of juvenile diabetes, be sufficient to overtax the pancreas of a susceptible individual? At the time of onset, if not later on, the pancreas of the diabetic can still secrete insulin in response to an injection of tolbutamide (Belle, Belmonte & Colle, 1967) and the islets contain β-cells which show marked synthetic activity (Gepts, 1965). In juveniles, therefore, it is possible that the endocrine system could play a role in the precipitation of diabetes, but in adults, except possibly the diabetic woman, the connection is less clear.

Diabetes which appears in adult life has several characteristics which differentiate it from the juvenile-onset syndrome. Amongst these is the fact that most of the adult diabetics are obese. In the non-diabetic obese subject the rate of cortisol production is greater than normal (Migeon, Green & Eckert, 1963; Copinschi, Cornil, Leclercq & Franckson, 1965) but not as great as the rate found in cases of Cushing's syndrome (Schteingart, Gregerman & Conn, 1963). When glucose is administered by mouth (Table 3.11), the response of the non-diabetic obese subject (by definition) is normal but the plasma-insulin level rises much more than it does in the non-obese person (Perley & Kipnis, 1966b). When glucose is rapidly infused intravenously, glucose uptake by the tissues, either in the presence or absence of injected exogenous insulin, is less than that found in non-obese non-diabetic controls (Franckson, Malaisse, Arnould, Rasio, Ooms, Balasse, Conard & Bastenie, 1966). Thus obesity, *per se*, induces the same type of changes as those caused by pregnancy, growth hormone and glucocorticoids; glucose uptake by the tissues is reduced despite an adequate supply of circulating insulin. With the development of diabetes, the pancreatic response to glucose may be slightly greater than that of the non-obese diabetic, but the response to tolbutamide is greater (Perley & Kipnis, 1966b). On the basis of similar observations it has been suggested that there may be two types of maturity-onset diabetes; that occurring in the obese subject which is due to peripheral insulin antagonism, and that due to pancreatic insulin deficiency (Karam, Grodsky, Pavlatos & Forsham, 1965).

The pancreas of the adult-onset diabetic does contain insulin, the amount being said to be about half the normal complement (Wrenshall *et al.*, 1952). In response to a single load of glucose (Table 3.11) it will secrete insulin after some delay and the level found in the blood may rise to much higher values than those seen in normal subjects (Yalow & Berson, 1960). However, if glucose is infused intravenously for seven days to keep the blood-sugar concentration up and so maintain a maximal stimulus to the pancreas, varying responses are obtained in diabetics (Seltzer & Harris, 1964). In the normal subject, the blood-sugar concentration does not rise and all of the infused glucose is retained but the plasma-insulin level is greatly increased throughout the infusion. Diabetics who can be controlled by diet alone and respond to tolbutamide also sustain high levels of circulating insulin, and are able to retain most of the infused glucose in spite of persistent hyperglycaemia. By contrast, however, elderly diabetics who do not respond to dietary treatment or tolbutamide excrete about half of the infused glucose and have more marked persistent hyperglycaemia; their plasma-insulin concentrations rise for only the first two days and then fall to almost zero. Thus, although the adult diabetic may have a reserve of pancreatic insulin, this is not inexhaustible, and any persistent strain, such as might be imposed by obesity, pregnancy or other stress, could be sufficient to precipitate insulin deficiency and the need for active treatment. Removal of such a strain could result in restoration of the reserves of insulin, reduction of tissue requirements by the tissues, and return to a normal metabolic economy. Such appears to be the explanation for disappearance of diabetic symptoms after delivery of the pregnant diabetic woman, and could be the reason for restoration of normal tolerance to glucose after weight reduction of the obese diabetic.

The Basic Lesion Responsible for Diabetes

In diabetes mellitus signs of insulin deficiency, either relative or absolute, co-exist with anatomical lesions which may or may not be causally related. To quote Payling-Wright (1950), "the nearer the causal chain approaches the final event, the more influential do individual factors become, until, with every abnormal state which constitutes a properly defined disease, and not a mere syndrome or symptom complex, it reaches the final link, the terminal and generally unique causal agent whose operation brings about the tissue disturbances that underlie and determine the distinctive 'clinical picture' of the disease". The ultimate causal agent of diabetes mellitus is not known, but attempts are being made to identify it.

In animals made diabetic by removal or destruction of the cells secreting insulin, vascular lesions such as those seen in the human diabetic have not been frequently reported; after eight years no strictly comparable lesions were found in pancreatectomized dogs (Ricketts, Test, Peterson, Lints, Tupikova & Steiner, 1959). In some rodents which develop diabetes spontaneously there is hope for better experimental models in the future. For example, in the Chinese hamsters (*Cricetulus griseus*) studied by Yerganian (in Leibel & Wrenshall, 1965) lesions have been regularly found which closely resemble the renal lesions seen in human diabetes (Meier & Yerganian, 1959). In the sand rat (*Psammomys obesus*), which normally lives a very frugal existence in the deserts of Egypt, diabetes can be induced by changing the diet from vegetables to a standard laboratory chow, and is characterized by an elevated level of circulating insulin (Hackel, Frohman, Mikat, Lebovitz, Schmidt-Nielson & Kinney, 1966). In a strain of mice (db) the disease is predictable, as it is inherited as a unit autosomal recessive, and is characterized by increased deposition of fat during early life (Hummel, Dickie & Coleman, 1966). These and other spontaneously appearing syndromes, discussed at a recent symposium (Renold & Dulin, 1967), present many of the features seen in the adult diabetic and should give valuable clues in the future to the aetiology of both the "complications" and the insulin-deficient states which characterize human diabetes.

In the meantime, and on the basis of observations made in man, theories are being put forward. Antoniades *et al.* (1964) suggest that the diabetic is unable to convert "bound" to "free" insulin. Vallance-Owen (in Leibel & Wrenshall, 1965) claims that they have abnormally high concentrations of circulating synalbumin, a characteristic which is inherited as an autosomal dominant (Vallance-Owen, 1966). Mainly on technical grounds, both these hypotheses have encountered severe criticism (Berson & Yalow, 1964b, 1965; Kipnis & Stein, in Cameron & O'Connor, 1964), but they could be used to explain one feature of diabetes. Diabetes has been called "the fatty acid syndrome" (Randle, Garland, Hales & Newsholme, 1963), and whilst "bound" insulin is only effective on adipose tissue, synalbumin will not inhibit the effect of insulin on that tissue (see above). Thus, either could be involved in the production of adiposity and the elevated levels of circulating free fatty acids, which, according to Randle's hypothesis (1966), can depress tolerance to glucose. A pancreatic as distinct from an extra-pancreatic lesion could be responsible for some cases of diabetes. Thus, "insulitis" seen in a few juvenile diabetics (Le Compte, 1958) is very similar to the lesion evoked in cows (Le Compte *et al.*, 1966) and rabbits (Grodsky *et al.*, 1966) by repeated injections of insulin. An auto-immune mechanism has also been postulated to explain the vascular lesions in older diabetics; the antigen is said to be an abnormal form of insulin secreted as a part of the normal process of ageing (Blumenthal, Goldberg & Berns, in Leibel & Wrenshall, 1965). Elliott *et al.* (1965) claim to have found an abnormal form of insulin in juvenile diabetics. The rare syndrome in which hypofunction is found simultaneously in the thyroid, adrenal and pancreatic insular tissues may also represent the result of a multiglandular auto-immune process (Solomon *et al.*, 1965). An additional factor which claims less attention than it did 10 years ago, is the possible part played by increased destruction of insulin in the diabetic (Mirsky, 1964). All these possibilities are being actively considered, but no single factor has yet been found to explain all the features of diabetes mellitus.

In view of this we are entitled to wonder whether diabetes mellitus is a disease or just a syndrome. Does the diabetic differ from the normal subject in a qualitative or in a quantitative respect; is the difference one of degree rather than kind? In the case of the young ketotic diabetic an abnormality exists; he makes and secretes no insulin with which he has to be provided if he is to survive. In many other cases, however, it is debatable whether the patient is the victim of a disease with a cause, or whether he stands at the fringe of the normal population from which he differs only in degree. What of the obese person, for example, who loses his diabetic stigmata after weight reduction; or the pregnant diabetic woman who is restored to normal after delivery? What of the old person whose only sign of diabetes is his "abnormal" tolerance to glucose? Some would claim that such persons are never entirely normal and that, at least in the first two instances, they have a hereditary trait. The nature of the trait and the lesions to which it gives rise and through which it is responsible for the appearance of diabetes are, however, still unknown.

Treatment of Diabetes Mellitus

Whatever the ultimate cause of the disease as a whole, insulin deficiency arises as the result of a severe acute or milder but chronic stress. The pancreas, after attempting or actually succeeding in adapting its activity to counteract this stress, ultimately fails completely, as in the juvenile diabetic, or is unable to meet all the demands of the tissues. Thus, treatment is directed toward either assisting the pancreas to meet the demands or substituting for its action with administration of exogenous insulin. Such treatment involves the use of insulin, diet, and general measures which have been described in detail in many textbooks, reviews and articles (see Williams, 1960; Joslin, Root, White & Marble, 1959) and will not be considered here. Instead, attention will be focused on two problems; the management of very early diabetes and of the insulin-resistant diabetic.

(i) *Early diabetes.* The greatest danger to the diabetic lies in the "complications" which he develops; any insulin deficiency is manageable by dietary or hormonal therapy. With the increasing realization of this fact, more and more patients are being found who have minor deficiencies of tolerance to glucose; they are either latent or subclinical diabetics according to the classification of Conn & Fajans (Table 3.10). As such they present few if any symptoms but are in a state where the syndrome could become overt and "complications" could arise. Under such conditions, the doctor is unable, at present, to rectify existing vascular lesions, but he can and should try to restore the equilibrium between pancreatic insulin supply and the demands of the tissues. If, as is often the case, the patient is obese, dietary restriction can be prescribed during weight reduction with an adequate maintenance diet thereafter. Conn (Conn & Fajans, 1961; and in Leibel & Wrenshall, 1965) has reported the effects of prolonged treatment with tolbutamide in nonobese asymptomatic diabetics who had not previously responded to dietary treatment alone. Among younger patients of less than 35 years of age, repeated glucose tolerance tests showed improvement in 19 out of 27 cases. In nine older subjects aged 37 to 49 years, only two showed any improvement over one to two years. This suggests, but does not prove, that prolonged treatment with the sulphonylureas may prevent ultimate failure of pancreatic function especially in younger patients. Provided the patient is of approximately normal weight and can be controlled by dietary measures or with small doses of insulin, prolonged use of the sulphonylureas also appears to be most successful for patients over 65 years of age (Powell & Howells, 1966). On the basis that even mild diabetes imposes a potential threat to the life of a patient, it does now seem worthwhile to seek out the early case and give treatment. Whether this will halt or delay onset of angiopathy is not known with any certainty, but available conventional methods of treatment might remove one of the potential causes of this complication.

(ii) *Insulin resistance*. Elevation of the level of circulating insulin is an early sign of diabetes and reflects resistance to the action of exogenous insulin. It may be due to overactivity of the pituitary or adrenal gland, or to factors associated with pregnancy or obesity. Where this is so, removal of the cause offers the best hope for cure of the insulin deficiency, but in a small proportion of cases resistance to exogenous insulin is due to antibodies to the insulin used for treatment. Up to 1961, at least 130 cases had been reported in which more than 200 units of insulin had to be given each day for control of the diabetic syndrome (Field, 1962). The highest dose which has ever had to be given is 177,500 units/day (Tucker, Klink, Goetz, Zalme & Knowles, 1964). In such cases where there is no other known cause for the resistance, high concentrations of antibodies to insulin have been found in the circulation. The level of circulatory antibodies cannot be correlated with the dose of insulin needed for clinical control, and Berson & Yalow (1961b) have suggested that a high rate of destruction of antibodies in the liver and elsewhere may be a determining influence. Steinke & Soeldner (1965), on the other hand, consider that resistance may be due to high concentrations of a strongly binding antibody or to failure of target tissues to respond even to free and biologically active insulin. Treatment of such cases has followed two main lines; first, adrenal steroids have been shown to reduce insulin requirements of the majority of 20 patients reported in the literature since 1948 (Shipp, Cunningham, Russell & Marble, 1965). In some patients the requirements drop within 2 to 5 days and may decrease further in following weeks. Those who appear to benefit most have had high doses of insulin for long periods, have unstable diabetic syndromes, a history of allergy to insulin, and frequent sterile abscesses at injection sites. Secondly, attempts have been made to use species of insulin which have a lower affinity for the circulating antibodies than the insulin (usually bovine and sometimes mixed with porcine) used previously for treatment. Some success has been achieved using porcine, dealanated porcine and even human insulin, but, probably due to the very

small differences in immunological properties of these insulins, their use has not always been successful (Akre, Kirtley & Galloway, 1964; Boshell, Barrett, Wilensky & Patton, 1964). Because of its very different immunological properties, Yalow & Berson (1964) have suggested the use of fish insulin at least in an emergency.

HYPOGLYCAEMIA

For about 40 years it has been recognized that when the concentration of glucose in the blood falls below 40 to 60 mg./100 ml., symptoms can arise which, in most instances, can be relieved by food or glucose. In recent reviews, authors have been careful to point out that hypoglycaemia which gives rise to these symptoms is not a disease but, like hyperglycaemia and glycosuria seen in diabetes, is a clinical sign (Conn & Seltzer, 1955; Marks & Rose, 1965; Yalow & Berson, 1965). The patient may complain of symptoms and exhibit signs suggestive of hypoglycaemia, but, unless it can be established that the blood-sugar concentration is low at the time, other causes could be responsible.

Not everyone agrees as to the basic causes of the symptoms which accompany hypoglycaemia, but they can be considered under two broad headings. First, there are symptoms and signs which resemble those produced by adrenaline; sweating, weakness, hunger, tachycardia, apprehension, etc. Secondly, there are the symptoms and signs referable to impaired neurological function; headache, confusion, listlessness, somnolence, coma, convulsions, defective memory, psychotic behaviour, mental deficiency, etc. The first group of signs and symptoms is commonly experienced by diabetic patients taking a slight overdose of insulin, but, if hypoglycaemia becomes profound and persists, the patient may become comatose, convulse and even die. Prolonged hypoglycaemia which may not involve loss of consciousness, and may be complicated by the appearance of angina, gives rise to the second group of symptoms and signs which, unlike the first, do not respond to glucose either as rapidly or as completely. In fact, if permanent damage has been done to the nervous system, recovery may be very slow if it occurs at all. Endogenous adrenaline is released when the blood-sugar concentration falls below a critical value, but signs comparable with those produced by adrenaline can be evoked in animals after the adrenal medulla has been removed. For this reason, some prefer to classify the symptoms associated with hypoglycaemia under the headings of acute, subacute and chronic neuroglycopenias on the assumption that they are all due to cerebral cellular dysfunction (Marks & Rose, 1965).

Hypoglycaemia may occur in a wide variety of diseases giving rise to symptoms and signs of greater or lesser clinical significance. The list of such diseases, if complete, would be lengthy and would include many in which hypoglycaemia is of minor clinical or academic importance. In the present account, therefore, attention will be concentrated on those conditions in which hypoglycaemia is a prominent feature and presents either urgent clinical problems or interesting academic features. Only passing mention will be made of treatment, which formed the subject of a recent

tissues other than the brain were to consume an inordinate proportion of the available glucose in the body. In other words, one could have hepatic and extra-hepatic lesions responsible for hypoglycaemia.

(i) *Hepatic disease.* Removal of an animal's liver results in hypoglycaemia and death unless glucose is continuously infused. Hepatic failure in man, however, is not usually characterized by hypoglycaemia which can occur with little evidence of hepatic damage, as judged by conventional tests. Hepatic disease is a common cause of hypoglycaemia only because hepatic disease is itself common, but spontaneous hypoglycaemia

TABLE 3.12

Clinical classification of the causes of symptomatic hypoglycaemia

Hypoglycaemia provoked by fasting	Hypoglycaemia provoked by other stimuli

1. Hepatic lesions
  Primary carcinoma
  Portal cirrhosis
  Malnutrition (Kwashiorkor)
  Glycogenoses (Types I, III,
    VI and VII)
	1. Iatrogenic hypoglycaemia
	  Insulin
	  Sulphonylureas
	  Alcohol
	  Other drugs and poisons

2. Pancreatic lesions
  Insulinomas
  Islet hyperplasia
	2. Hereditary fructose intolerance

3. Large extra-pancreatic tumours	3. Hereditary galactose intolerance

4. Endocrine diseases
  Hypopituitarism
  Adrenal insufficiency
	4. Essential reactive hypoglycaemia
	  Idiopathic
	  Diabetes mellitus
	  Post-gastrectomy

5. Idiopathic in infancy and childhood
  Transient neonatal
  Leucine sensitive
  Ketotic	

This list is not complete; for other causes consult reviews quoted in the text.

symposium (Boshell, 1966). The hypoglycaemic syndromes themselves will be considered under the two main headings shown in Table 3.12.

Hypoglycaemia Provoked by Fasting

The concentration of glucose in the blood falls when food is withdrawn but does not normally reach hypoglycaemic levels. The body reacts to conserve glucose for the brain by lowering the level of circulating insulin and raising that of growth hormone (Glick, Roth, Yalow & Berson, 1965). Fat is mobilized from the depots of adipose tissue for use by muscle and other energy-requiring tissues, and increased gluconeogenesis provides the glucose needed by the brain. During fasting, therefore, hypoglycaemia could develop if hepatic production of glucose were to fall or if

is seen in only a small proportion of such cases. It occurs, for example, only rarely in cases of infective hepatitis; as a late manifestation of portal cirrhosis; frequently in conditions of gross chronic malnutrition (Kwashiorkor); and very commonly in primary hepatic carcinoma. Much rarer, but of great academic interest, are the *glycogenoses* due to enzymic defects in the liver (Table 3.13).

The steps involved in the conversion of glucose into glycogen and those occurring during glycogenolysis are illustrated in Fig. 3.6. In the absence of one or (possibly) more of the enzymes involved in these reactions, a group of diseases can arise which is collectively termed glycogen storage disease, the glycogenoses or, after the man who first described one, von Gierke's disease (see

TABLE 3.13

Hepatic enzymatic defects in hereditary conditions causing hypoglycaemia

Name of Condition	Hepatic enzyme deficiency
Glycogenosis Type I	Glucose-6-phosphatase
Type III	Amylo-1, 6-glucosidase
Type VI	Phosphorylase
Type VII	Glycogen synthetase
Hereditary fructose intolerance	Fructose-1-phosphate aldolase (Fructose-1, 6-diphosphate aldolase)
Hereditary galactose intolerance	Galactose-1-phosphate uridyl transferase

Cornblath & Schwarz, 1966). In four of them (Types I, III, VI and VII), hypoglycaemia may arise and cause permanent mental deficiency. In the remainder, mentioned here only for the sake of completeness, hypoglycaemia either does not arise or is very mild.

In the first and commonest form (*Type I*), also called von Gierke's disease, there is little or no hepatic glucose-6-phosphatase. The child develops hepatomegaly in infancy; may become markedly hypoglycaemic on fasting; is stunted and may exhibit a variety of other lesions (Creveld, 1963).

After a brief fast (4–6 hr.), ketones appear in the urine and the concentrations of lactate, pyruvate, urate and free fatty acids rise as that of glucose falls in the plasma. At this stage, neither glucagon nor adrenaline can elevate the concentration of glucose in the blood in spite of the enormous amounts of hepatic glycogen; but they will elevate the level of circulating lactate. Presumptive evidence for a deficiency of glucose-6-phosphatase is based on a rise in circulating lactate without any increase in blood-glucose concentration following intravenous injection of fructose or galactose. For confirmation, absence of the enzyme from hepatic tissue has to be demonstrated. These children are highly susceptible to infection and, if they survive to adolescence, are likely to be mentally defective. One interesting point about them is that they may not develop cerebral manifestations of hypoglycaemia even though the blood-sugar concentration may be below 10 mg./100 ml. and evoking manifest evidence of endogenous adrenaline secretion.

When there is deficiency of the debranching enzyme (amylo-1,6-glucosidase), the clinical syndrome (*Type III*) is similar but less severe and the patient may well live to adulthood (Creveld & Huijing, 1964). Since the liver contains glucose-6-phosphatase, however, injected galactose and fructose will elevate blood-sugar concentration.

Glucagon and adrenaline are able to raise the blood-sugar concentration unless the short outer chains of the glycogen molecule (Illingworth, Cori & Cori, 1956) have already been mobilized by fasting for 12–14 hr. Absence of hepatic phosphorylase (*Type VI*), which hydrolyses about 90% of the normal glycogen molecule, may be a commoner defect than that of glucose-6-phosphatase (Hers, 1964) and may be difficult to distinguish from the syndrome due to deficiency of the debranching enzyme (*Type III*)'

Abnormal synthesis of glycogen occurs when there is deficiency of either the branching enzyme, amylo-1,4 → 1,6-transglucosidase (*Type IV*), or glycogen synthetase (UDPG-glycogen:glucosyl transferase; *Type VII*). In the absence of branching enzyme, an abnormal molecule of glycogen is produced, an amylopectin (Cori, 1953), and the patient develops progressive hepatic failure which proves fatal within about a year (Anderson, in Najjar, 1952). Only two cases have been described in which there were deficiencies of glycogen synthetase (Lewis, Spencer-Peet & Stewart, 1963). These children rapidly developed severe hypoglycaemia unless fed frequently; their livers contained little glycogen and after an overnight fast hyperglycaemia could not be induced with glucagon.

In the two remaining forms of glycogenoses (see Chapter 4), which are not represented in Fig. 3.6 or Table 3.13, hypoglycaemia is not a feature.

(ii) *Extra-hepatic lesions.* Uptake of glucose by extra-hepatic tissues may exceed the rate of hepatic production of glucose in cases of pancreatic insulinoma, some very large extra-pancreatic tumours, certain endocrine disorders, and in some rare but important conditions of infancy and early childhood. In all these conditions symptoms of hypoglycaemia can be precipitated by fasting alone but in some the liver may play a contributory part (Addison's disease) and in others, symptoms can be precipitated by other means (e.g. with leucine).

(a) *Pancreatic lesions.* Increased endogenous secretion of insulin has been associated with islet adenomas and carcinomas and, less definitely, with islet hyperplasia.

Adenomas of the islets of Langerhans giving rise to symptoms are most commonly diagnosed between the ages of 20 and 50 years but, as pointed out below, they may also occur in childhood. Usually benign and small (1–2 cm. diameter), they are composed largely of β-cells (Moss & Rhoads, in Howard & Jordan, 1960). Comparative absence of granules in the cells and the relatively low insulin contents of many of the tumours have led to the suggestion that they are unable to store insulin which they secrete continuously into the blood irrespective of the level of circulating glucose. Contrary to early reports (Lacy & Davies, 1959), insulin extracted from them appears to be normal (Taylor & Sheldon, 1964). The hypoglycaemia which they evoke is as much due to depression of hepatic glucose output as it is to stimulated peripheral uptake of glucose (Marks & Marrack, 1962). In response to an intravenous injection of tolbutamide or an oral dose of leucine, these tumours secrete large amounts of insulin (Samols & Marks, 1963; Floyd, Fajans, Knopf & Conn, 1964) and produce profound and prolonged hypoglycaemia (Fajans, Schneider, Schteingart & Conn, 1961). In the absence of such a stimulus, levels of circulating insulin may not be elevated and, if the tumour contains little insulin, tolbutamide may not induce a very marked effect. Use of these stimulants and coincidental measurement of circulating insulin do provide useful aids for the diagnosis of insulin secreting tumours, but reliance may have to be placed on clinical observations. The most useful of these is the triad of signs suggested by Whipple (1952) and comprising the observations of hypoglycaemic attacks during fasting or on exercise, a measured blood-sugar concentration of less than 50 mg./100 ml. after 12–24 hr. of fasting, and complete remission of symptoms on administration of glucose.

Hyperplasia of the islets of Langerhans, as already mentioned, is a prominent feature of the offspring of a diabetic mother. It also occurs occasionally in galactosaemia (Smetana & Olen, 1962) and in some cases of idiopathic hypoglycaemia of infancy (Haworth & Coodin, 1960). In these and other instances, the aetiological significances of the lesions are not known.

(b) *Extra-pancreatic tumours.* In over 60 reported cases, large mesenchymal tumours (770–20,000 g.) in the thoracic or abdominal cavities have been associated with symptomatic hypoglycaemia; most of these were low grade fibrosarcomas or spindle cell sarcomas (Silverstein, Wakim & Bahn, 1964). Primary hepatomas, virilizing adrenal tumours (Williams, Kellie, Wade, Williams & Chalmers, 1961) and a tumour causing signs of Cushing's syndrome (Eymontt, Gwinup, Kruger, Maynard & Hamwi, 1965) having the same effect are, along with other tumours, reviewed by Marks & Rose (1965). In each case, symptoms of hypoglycaemia disappeared with the removal of the tumour only to recur, in some instances, with renewed growth of

the neoplastic tissue. The cause of the hypoglycaemia is not known, but Samols (1963) suggests that it could be due to release from the tumour of insulin-like substances or of substances which sensitize the normal tissues to endogenously secreted insulin. Others, on the other hand, suggest that increased uptake of glucose by the large tumour itself could be responsible.

(c) *Endocrine disorders.* With the increasing use of hypophysectomy and adrenalectomy for the treatment of other diseases, hypofunction of the pituitary and adrenal glands becomes an important potential cause for hypoglycaemia. In hypothyroidism, mild hypoglycaemia may occur but is not prominent as a feature of the disease. There has been one recent and well documented case of a dwarfed child suffering hypoglycaemic attacks as a result of a specific deficiency of growth hormone (Wilder & Odell, 1965). Specific deficiencies of ACTH and adrenal tumours associated with synthesis of abnormal steroids have also been shown to cause hypoglycaemia, but in the vast majority of cases, either primary or secondary hypoadrenocorticism is responsible (Frawley, in Eisenstein, 1967).

In place of tuberculosis, atrophy is now the most common cause for Addison's disease, and circulating antibodies to adrenal tissue are being found in many patients (Blizzard & Kyle, 1963). If 90 to 95 % of the functional cortical tissue is destroyed, these patients are liable to develop hypoglycaemia during periods of anorexia or stress. Coma is rare but it has been described as a presenting feature (Gittleson, 1956). In hypopituitarism, however, coma, which is not entirely due to hypoglycaemia and is less likely to respond to intravenous injection of glucose, may well be the presenting sign (Sheehan & Summers, 1949). In both conditions, inability to react to hypoglycaemia is largely due to impaired gluconeogenesis aggravated in panhypopituitarism by the additional absence of growth hormone. In both conditions it is therefore dangerous to administer insulin, to even small doses of which (0·05 U/kg.) these patients are very sensitive (Fraser, Albright & Smith, 1941; Wajchenberg, Pereira, Pupo, Schnaeder, Cintra & Mattar, 1964).

(d) *Hypoglycaemia of infancy and childhood.* Hypoglycaemia occurring in the first six months of life is particularly important for if it is not treated effectively at that stage it can give rise to permanent cerebral damage and mental deficiency. In most cases the cause is not known but empirical methods have been devised for treatment.

(1) *Transient neonatal hypoglycaemia.* Some infants, more frequently male, with low birth

weights relative to their periods of gestation (less than 2,500 g.) may become transiently hypoglycaemic 24–72 hr. after birth. The majority, of whom 40 are reviewed by Cornblath & Schwarz (1966), then develop tremors, cyanosis, convulsions and irregularities of respiration which, though not indicative, are collectively very suggestive of hypoglycaemia. During these attacks, which respond to intravenous glucose, the blood-sugar concentration falls below 25 mg./100 ml. It is not yet possible to tell what permanent effect these attacks may have, for the syndrome was first recognized in 1959; but present evidence suggests that without adequate treatment the incidence of permanent cerebral damage may be high. The cause is also a matter of speculation.

(2) *Leucine-induced hypoglycaemia.* Since Cochrane *et al.* (1956) first reported a case, about 30 more have been described. Usually within six months of birth, the child develops hypoglycaemia either on fasting or on taking a feed containing large amounts of protein. Repeated attacks lead to stunting of growth and mental deterioration, but the condition appears to be self-limiting with disappearance of attacks after the age of 4 to 6 years (Cochrane, 1960). If leucine is administered, blood-sugar concentration falls and there is an increase in the level of circulating insulin (Yalow & Berson, 1960; Rosenthal, Metz & Pirani, 1964). To avoid attacks, a diet containing little protein is recommended (Roth & Segal, 1964) and diazoxide has been used successfully to suppress endogenous insulin secretion (Drash & Wolff, 1964).

(3) *Idiopathic hypoglycaemia of infancy.* Haworth & Coodin (1960) have reviewed 58 cases reported in the literature, and some of these would undoubtedly have proved sensitive to leucine. In most cases (60%), these infants are first affected before the age of 6 months and few respond to dietary treatment. Of the 21 cases showing subsequent evidence of mental retardation, 18 first developed symptoms within six months of birth. Most (17/24) responded to treatment with ACTH and some (15/25) benefited from pancreatectomy. The cause of this condition is not known and there is little evidence that it is familial, as McQuarrie (1954) had originally suggested.

(4) *Ketotic hypoglycaemia.* According to Colle & Ulstrom (1964), this may be the commonest form of hypoglycaemic syndrome to occur in early childhood. First observed between the ages of about 1 and 5 years, it subsides at 4 to 7 years without producing any permanent adverse effects. Individual attacks always start between 6 and 10 a.m. with symptoms ranging from listlessness and apathy to coma and convulsions. During attacks, which can be provoked by a ketogenic diet in 18–24 hr., the blood-sugar concentration falls below 40 mg./100 ml. and the urine contains acetone. If the patient is well nourished beforehand, attacks cannot be provoked by fasting alone, so they are thought to be due to chronic undernourishment associated with a defect in gluconeogenesis.

(5) *Other causes. Adenomas of the islets* are seldom found in children under the age of 4 years, a fact that is of great diagnostic importance (Boley, Lin & Schiffmann, 1960). These tumours are also rare, but as they cause a curable condition, it is important that they should be considered as a possible cause for hypoglycaemia. Hypoglycaemia, possibly due to insulin secreted from *hyperplastic islets*, may occur in the new-born infant of the diabetic mother but, though usually transient, it may give rise to severe symptoms. In some babies it is claimed that hypoglycaemia could be due to deficiencies of either glucagon or adrenaline but the evidence is not strong (see Cornblath & Schwarz, 1966).

Hypoglycaemia Provoked by Stimuli other than Fasting

Hypoglycaemia can be provoked by a number of substances which either inhibit gluconeogenesis or stimulate uptake of glucose by the tissues. It may arise in apparently normal human subjects after a meal containing a high proportion of glucose or easily assimilable carbohydrate (essential reactive hypoglycaemia.) The effect is better seen, in some cases, in the fasting subject, but does not occur unless the specific stimulus is also applied.

(i) *Iatrogenic hypoglycaemia.* In clinical practice, the commonest cause of hypoglycaemia is *insulin*, usually given for the treatment of diabetes, but also used in the past to induce "shock" in schizophrenic patients. It has been used to commit suicide (Blotner, 1954) and murder (Birkinshaw, Gurd, Randall, Curry, Price & Wright, 1958). Most diabetics are aware of the symptoms produced by a small overdose of insulin and which vary from patient to patient. Acute symptoms associated with a rapid fall in blood-sugar concentration are produced by soluble insulin and are seen most frequently in juvenile diabetics. Intermediate and long-acting insulin preparations give rise to symptoms such as drowsiness, lassitude, headaches, etc. in the early morning at the time of waking. In either case there is always the threat of coma which is better prevented than cured.

Hypoglycaemic symptoms following administration of the *sulphonylureas* are due to inappropriate dosage, impaired renal excretion of the drug, potentiation of their effects by other drugs, or their use in very elderly patients (see Galloway, in Boshell, 1966). Symptoms, not all of which may be due to hypoglycaemia, commence after 30–60 min., autonomic manifestations being less pronounced than those evoked by insulin. The drugs themselves are excreted in the urine unchanged (chlorpropamide) or as inactive derivatives (tolbutamide), but one (acetohexamide) is converted to derivatives which also have hypoglycaemic properties. Prolonged action is therefore likely to be due either to inadequate metabolism of the drug by the liver or to impaired excretion in the kidney.

The ingestion of *alcohol* may be followed by the onset of hypoglycaemia, an old observation which is now receiving close attention (Madison, 1966). Though it is most often seen in alcoholics, it can occur in persons with no evidence of hepatic disease or malnutrition. The fall in blood-sugar concentration is secondary to reduced output of glucose from the liver which in turn is due to reduced gluconeogenesis (Field, Williams & Mortimore, 1963; Freinkel, Arky, Singer, Cohen, Bleicher, Anderson, Silbert & Foster, 1965). It is now suggested that suppression of gluconeogenesis is secondary to the increased ratio of reduced to oxidized nicotinamide adenine dinucleotide ($NADH_2/NAD$) which is seen in the liver after administration of alcohol (Madison, Lochner & Wulff, 1967). In practice the patient is usually an alcoholic and he is most commonly seen first in coma.

Many other drugs are known to induce hypoglycaemia (see Marks & Rose, 1965); salicylates, monoamine oxidase inhibitors, thalidomide, metapyrone, some antihistaminic drugs and others could be mentioned.

(ii) *Hereditary fructose intolerance.* A small proportion of infants develop severe and protracted gastro-intestinal symptoms and hypoglycaemia after taking food containing fructose (sucrose, fruit juices, etc.). If fructose is withheld in time, complete recovery is assured, but if the diagnosis is not made, as is often the case with the first child in the family, repeated attacks are ultimately fatal. Administration of intravenous fructose causes prolonged hypoglucosaemia which is accompanied by a fall rather than any rise in the level of circulating insulin. The livers of these patients contain reduced amounts of fructose-1-

phosphate aldolase so that fructose-1-phosphate accumulates and the fructose content of the blood rises (Fig. 3.6; Table 3.13). It is now thought that the accumulating fructose-1-phosphate inhibits gluconeogenesis or the activation of phosphorylase or debranching enzyme, thus inducing hypoglycaemia by inhibiting release of glucose from the liver (Froesch, Wolf & Baitsch, 1963; Dubois, Loeb, Ooms, Gillet, Bartman & Champenois, 1961; Cornblath & Schwarz, 1966).

(iii) *Hereditary galactose intolerance.* In this condition, also rare, and due to a hepatic enzyme deficiency (Table 3.13), hypoglycaemia is not a prominent feature and when seen is probably the result of the chronic toxic effects of galactose upon the liver (Cornblath & Schwarz, 1966). Loeb (1962) has shown, however, that galactose will inhibit output of glucose from the livers of such patients. This ability appears to be shared by other sugars capable of inducing hypoglycaemia in man (Cahill, 1964).

(iv) *Essential reactive hypoglycaemia.* The commonest circumstance under which a patient will complain of symptoms suggestive of hypoglycaemia is 2–5 hr. after a meal. The symptoms include weakness, faintness, nervousness, palpitations, anxiety, irritability, hunger, headache, vertigo, etc., but seldom is there loss of consciousness which can be substantiated. Attacks are transient, more common in women than men, and first appear between the ages of 30 and 40 years in most instances. The patients are said to be "emotionally labile" or, according to Conn & Seltzer (1955), "intense, driving and intensely conscientious". For practical reasons it is frequently difficult to prove that these symptoms are associated with hypoglycaemia and in many cases they are ascribed to "psychological causes" (Marks & Rose, 1965). In some cases, however, the symptoms have been reproduced during prolonged glucose tolerance tests (5 hr.) and associations have been established with at least two organic diseases.

(a) *Diabetes mellitus.* Sussman, Stimmler & Birenboim (1966a) studied 14 normoglycaemic patients who had complained of such symptoms 3–5 hr. after meals. When given glucose by mouth they all became hypoglycaemic after 2–5 hr. with blood-sugar concentrations of less than 55 mg./100 ml. and all experienced symptoms which were relieved by glucose. According to their responses, these patients could be divided into three groups. Two groups showed no evidence of diabetes but their insulogenic responses were either normal or excessive; their levels of circulating insulin rose in 30–120 min. to either normal or excessively high levels. The third group, on the other hand, was frankly diabetic, the concentrations of both glucose and insulin rising to excessively high levels before the onset of hypoglycaemic symptoms. Many years previously, Seltzer, Fajans & Conn (1956) had made the same observations in a group of 110 mild diabetics with almost normal fasting blood-sugar concentrations, and had suggested that such a "reactive hypoglycaemia" could be the earliest manifestation of diabetes. Their observations amongst mild diabetics have been confirmed by others (Nydick, Samols, Kuzuya & Williams, 1964; Barnard, 1964; Yalow & Berson, 1965; Tittle & Kerr, 1966), some of whom have also demonstrated excessive release of insulin, often delayed, before the onset of hypoglycaemia.

(b) *Post-gastrectomy syndrome.* After gastrectomy it is not uncommon to find that the patient complains of extreme discomfort immediately following a meal. After $1\frac{1}{2} - 3$ hr., and in 15 to 50% of cases, the patient may complain of hypoglycaemic symptoms which can be severe (Conn & Seltzer, 1955; Yalow & Berson, 1965). Roth & Meade (1965) have now shown that these latter symptoms can be reproduced in normal subjects by administering an oral dose (100 g.) followed by an intravenous infusion (100 g.) of glucose over 1 hr. As in the gastrectomized patient given only the oral dose of glucose, the blood-sugar and plasma-insulin levels rise excessively in the first hour and are followed by hypoglycaemia with accompanying symptoms.

After gastrectomy there is little doubt that hypoglycaemia is secondary to the rapid intestinal absorption of glucose and the excessive stimulant effect of this upon insulin secretion. In the other cases, however, only speculation will be possible until more is known of the hormonal and other changes produced by ingested glucose or food.

References

Abt, A. F. (1962). *Metabolism,* **11,** 202.

Akre, P. R., Kirtley, W. R. & Galloway, J. A. (1964). *Diabetes,* **13,** 135.

Alp, H. & Recant, L. (1964). *Metabolism,* **13,** 609.

Alp, H. & Recant, L. (1965). *J. Clin. Invest.,* **44,** 870.

Anderson, J. W., Kilbourn, K. G., Robinson, J. & Wright, P. H. (1963). *Clin. Sci.,* **24,** 417.

Anderson, E. & Long, J. A. (1948). *Recent Progr. Hormone Res.,* **2,** 209.

Antoniades, H. N., Bougas, J. A., Camerini-Davalos, R. & Pyle, H. M. (1964). *Diabetes,* **13,** 230.

Antoniades, H. N., Huber, A. M., Boshell, B. R., Saravis, C. A. & Gershoff, S. N. (1965). *Endocrinology,* **76,** 709.

Arquilla, E. R. & Stavitsky, A. B. (1956a). *J. Clin. Invest.,* **35,** 458.

Arquilla, E. R. & Stavitsky, A. B. (1956b). *J. Clin. Invest.,* **35,** 467.

Arquilla, E. R., Ooms, H. & Finn, J. (1966). *Diabetologia,* **2,** 1.

Asboe-Hansen, G. (1958). *Physiol. Rev.,* **38,** 446.

Ashmore, J. (1964). *Diabetes,* **13,** 349.

Ashmore, J., Cahill, G. F. & Hastings, A. B. (1960). *Recent Progr. Hormone Res.,* **16,** 547.

Ashmore, J., Hastings, A. B., Nesbett, F. B. & Renold, A. E. (1956). *J. Biol. Chem.,* **218,** 77.

Ashmore, J., Preston, J. & Love, W. C. (1962). *Proc. Soc. Exp. Biol. Med.,* **109,** 291.

Ashmore, J., Stricker, F., Love, W. C. & Kilsheimer, G. (1961). *Endocrinology,* **68,** 599.

Ashton, N. (1959). *Lancet,* **2,** 625.

Ashton, W. L. (1965). *J. Endocr.,* **33,** 103.

Atchley, D. W., Loeb, R. F., Richards, D. W., Benedict, E. M. & Driscoll, M. E. (1933). *J. Clin. Invest.,* **12,** 297.

Augustine, J. (1964). "Diabetes Source Book". Publication No. 1168, U.S. Dept. Health, Education & Welfare, Washington, D.C.

Baird, J. D. & Farquhar, J. W. (1962). *Lancet,* **1,** 71.

Baird, I. M. & Munro, D. S. (1954). *Lancet,* **1,** 962.

Ball, E. G. & Jungas, R. L. (1964). *Recent Progr. Hormone Res.,* **20,** 183.

Banting, F. G. & Best, C. H. (1922). *J. Lab. Clin. Med.,* **7,** 251.

Banting, F. G., Franks, W. R. & Gairns, S. (1938). *Amer. J. Psychiat.,* **95,** 562.

Barnard, D. M. (1964). *J. Lancet,* **84,** 401.

Bearn, A. G., Billing, B. H. & Sherlock, S. (1952). *Clin. Sci.,* **11,** 151.

Beck, P., Parker, M. & Daughaday, W. H. (1965). *J. Clin. Endocr.,* **25,** 1457.

Beck, P., Schalch, D. S., Parker, M. L., Kipnis, D. & Daughaday, W. H. (1965). *J. Lab. Clin. Med.,* **66,** 366.

Beck, L. V., Zaharko, D. S., Roberts, N., McNeil, T., King, C. & Blankenbaker, R. (1964). *Life Sci.,* **5,** 545.

Becker, B. (1952). *Ann. Intern. Med.,* **37,** 273.

Belle, R. de, Bflmonte, M. M. & Colle, E. (1967). *Diabetes,* **16,** 215.

Bellens, R. (1961). *Acta Endocr.* (Kobenhavn), Suppl. **61,** 1.

Bencosme, S. A. (1955). *Amer. J. Anat.,* **96,** 104.

Benjamin, F. & Casper, D. J. (1966). *Amer. J. Obstet. Cynec.,* **94,** 566.

Berkman, J., Rifkin, H. & Ross, G. (1953). *J. Clin. Invest.,* **32,** 414.

Berson, S. A. & Yalow, R. S. (1959a). *J. Clin. Invest.,* **38,** 1996.

Berson, S. A. & Yalow, R. S. (1959b). *J. Clin. Invest.,* **38,** 2017.

Berson, S. A. & Yalow, R. S. (1961a). *Nature* (Lond.), **191,** 1392.

Berson, S. A. & Yalow, R. S. (1961b). *Amer. J. Med.,* **31,** 874.

BERSON, S. A. & YALOW, R. S. (1963). *Science*, **139**, 844.

BERSON, S. A. & YALOW, R. S. (1964a). In "The Hormones". (Eds. Pincus, J., Thimann, K. V. & Astwood, E. B.), Vol. IV, New York, Academic Press.

BERSON, S. A. & YALOW, R. S. (1964b). *Diabetes*, **13**, 247.

BERSON, S. A. & YALOW, R. S. (1965). *Diabetes*, **14**, 549.

BERSON, S. A., YALOW, R. S., BAUMAN, A., ROTHSCHILD, M. A. & NEWERLY, K. (1956). *J. Clin. Invest.*, **35**, 170.

BEWSHER, P. D. & ASHMORE, J. (1966). *Biochem. Biophys. Res. Comm.*, **24**, 431.

BEWSHER, P. D., HILLMAN, C. C. & ASHMORE, J. (1966). *Biochem. Pharmacol.*, **15**, 2079.

BIRKINSHAW, V. J., GURD, M. R., RANDALL, S. S., CURRY, A. S., PRICE, D. E. & WRIGHT, P. H. (1958). *Brit. Med. J.*, **2**, 463.

BIRKINSHAW, V. J., RANDALL, S. S. & RISDALL, P. C. (1962). *Nature* (Lond.), **193**, 1089.

BISHOP, J. S., STEELE, R., ALTSZULER, N., DUNN, A., BJERKNES, C. & DE BODO, R. C. (1965). *Amer. J. Physiol.*, **208**, 307.

BLEICHER, S. J., O'SULLIVAN, J. B. & FREINKEL, N. (1964). *N. Eng. J. Med.*, **271**, 866.

BLIZZARD, R. M. & KYLE, M. (1963). *J. Clin. Invest.*, **42**, 1653.

BLOODWORTH, J. M. B. (1963). *Diabetes*, **12**, 99.

BLOTNER, H. (1954). *Amer. J. Med. Sci.*, **227**, 387.

BLUMENTHAL, H. T., BERNS, A. W. & OWENS, C. T. (1963). *Lancet*, **2**, 783.

BLUMENTHAL, H. T., BERNS, A. W., OWENS, C. T. & HIRATA, Y. (1962). *Diabetes*, **11**, 296.

BOLEY, S. J., LIN, J. & SCHIFFMANN, A. (1960). *Surgery*, **48**, 592.

BORNSTEIN, J. (1950). *Aust. J. Exp. Biol. Med. Sci.*, **28**, 87.

BORNSTEIN, J. & LAWRENCE, R. D. (1951). *Brit. Med. J.*, **1**, 732.

BORTZ, W., ABRAHAM, S. & CHAIKOFF, I. L. (1963). *J. Biol. Chem.*, **238**, 1266.

BOSHELL, B. R. (1966). *Med. Treatm.*, **3**, 329.

BOSHELL, B. R., BARRETT, J. C., WILENSKY, A. S. & PATTON, T. B. (1964). *Diabetes*, **13**, 144.

BRADY, R. O., LUKENS, F. D. W. & GURIN, S. (1951). *J. Biol. Chem.*, **193**, 459.

BRODSKY, W. A., RAPAPORT, S. & WEST, C. D. (1950). *J. Clin. Invest.*, **29**, 1021.

BROLIN, S. E., HELLMAN, B. & KNUTSON, H. (Eds.) (1964). "The structure and metabolism of the pancreatic islets". New York, Pergamon Press.

BROWN, H., SANGER, F. & KITAI, R. (1955). *Biochem. J.*, **60**, 556.

BUCHLER, D. & WARREN, J. C. (1966). *Amer. J. Obstet. Gynec.*, **95**, 479.

BUKINAN, J., RIFKIN, H. & ROSS, G. (1953). *J. Clin. Invest.*, **32**, 414.

BURGI, H., MULLER, W. A., HUMBEL, R. E., LABHART, A. & FROESCH, E. R. (1966). *Biochim. Biophys. Acta.*, **121**, 349.

BURT, R. L. (1960). *Amer. J. Obstet. Gynec.*, **80**, 965.

BURT, R. L. (1962). *Diabetes*, **11**, 227.

BUTCHER, R. W. & SUTHERLAND, E. W. (1967). *Ann. N.Y. Acad. Sci.*, **139**, 849.

BUTLER, A. M. (1950). *New Eng. J. Med.*, **243**, 648.

CAHILL, G. F. (1964). *Advances in Enzym. Regulat.*, **2**, 137.

CAHILL, G. F., ASHMORE, J., EARLE, A. S. & ZOTTU, S. (1958). *Amer. J. Physiol.*, **192**, 491.

CAIRD, F. I. & GARRETT, C. J. (1963). *Diabetes*, **12**, 389.

CAMERINI-DAVALOS, R. A., CAULFIELD, J. B., REES, S. B., LOZANO-CASTANEDA, O., NALDJIAN, S. & MARBLE, A. (1963). *Diabetes*, **12**, 508.

CAMERON, J. S., BOYNS, D. R., JARRETT, R. J. & KEEN, H. (1966a). *Diabetologia*, **2**, 86.

CAMERON, J. S., BOYNS, D. R., JARRETT, R. J. & KEEN, H. (1966b). *Diabetologia*, **2**, 91.

CAMERON, M. P. & O'CONNOR, M. (Eds.) (1962). "Immuno-assay of Hormones". CIBA Foundation, Colloquia on Endocrinology. Vol. 14, London, Churchill.

CAMERON, M. P. & O'CONNOR, M. (Eds.) (1964). "The aetiology of Diabetes and its complications". CIBA Foundation, Colloquia on Endocrinology. Vol. 15, London, Churchill.

CAMPBELL, J., CHAIKOF, L. & DAVIDSON, I. W. F. (1954). *Endocrinology*, **54**, 48.

CAMPBELL, J. & RASTOGI, K. S. (1966a). *Diabetes*, **15**, 30.

CAMPBELL, J. & RASTOGI, K. S. (1966b). *Diabetes*, **15**, 749.

CARDELL, B. S. (1953). *J. Path. Bact.*, **66**, 335.

CERASI, E. & LUFT, R. (1964). *Lancet*, **2**, 769.

CHAMBERS, J. W., GEORG, R. H. & BASS, A. D. (1965). *Molec. Pharmacol.*, **1**, 66.

CHEN, C. H., ADAM, P. A. J., LASKOWSKI, D. E., MCCANN, M. L. & SCHWARZ, R. (1965). *Pediatrics*, **36**, 843.

CLAPP, W. M., BUTTERFIELD, L. J. & O'BRIEN, D. (1962). *Pediatrics*, **29**, 883.

COCHRANE, W. A. (1960). *Amer. J. Dis. Child.*, **99**, 476.

COCHRANE, W. A., PAYNE, W. W., SIMPKISS, M. J. & WOOLF, L. I. (1956). *J. Clin. Invest.*, **35**, 411.

COGGESHALL, C. & ROOT, H. F. (1940). *Endocrinology*, **26**, 1.

COLBY, A. O. (1965). *Diabetes*, **14**, 424 and 516.

COLLE, E. & ULSTROM, R. A. (1964). *J. Pediat.*, **64**, 632.

COLWELL, A. R. (1965). *Diabetes*, **14**, 110.

CONN, J. W. (1965). *New Eng. J. Med.*, **273**, 1135.

CONN, J. W. & FAJANS, S. S. (1956). *Metabolism*, **5**, 114.

CONN, J. W. & FAJANS, S. S. (1961). *Amer. J. Med.*, **31**, 839.

CONN, J. W., KNOPF, R. F. & NESBIT, R. M. (1964). *Amer. J. Surg.*, **107**, 159.

CONN, J. W. & SELTZER, H. S. (1955). *Amer. J. Med.*, **19**, 460.

COORE, H. G. & RANDLE, P. J. (1964a). *Biochem. J.*, **91**, 56.

COORE, H. G. & RANDLE, P. J. (1964b). *Biochem. J.*, **93**, 66.

COPINSCHI, G., CORNIL, A., LECLERCQ, R. & FRANCKSON, J. R. M. (1965). *Ann. Endocr.* (Paris), **26**, 170.

CORI, G. T. (1953). *Harvey Lect.*, **48**, 145.

CORNBLATH, M. & SCHWARTZ, R. (1966). "Disorders of carbohydrate metabolism in infancy". Philadelphia, Saunders.

CORREA, P. R., MAGALHAES, E. & KRAHL, M. E. (1960). *Proc. Soc. Exp. Biol. Med.*, **103**, 704.

CRAMPTON, J. H., SCUDDER, S. T. & DAVIS, C. D. (1949). *J. Clin. Endocr.*, **9**, 245.

CREVELD, S. VAN (1963). *Canad. Med. Ass. J.*, **88**, 1.

CREVELD, S. VAN & HUIJING, F. (1964). *Metabolism*, **13**, 191.

CROCKFORD, P. M., PORTE, D., WOOD, F. C. & WILLIAMS, R. H. (1966). *Metabolism*, **15**, 114.

D'AGOSTINO, A. N. & BAHN, R. C. (1963). *Diabetes*, **12**, 528.

DANOWSKI, T. S. (Ed.) (1964). "Diabetes mellitus, diagnosis and treatment". New York, American Diabetes Association.

DANOWSKI, T. S., BONESSI, J. V., SARVER, M. E. & MOSES, C. (1964). *Metabolism*, **13**, 739.

DANOWSKI, T. S., PETERS, J. H., RATHBUN, J. C., QUASHNOCK, J. M. & GREENMAN, L. (1949). *J. Clin. Invest.*, **28**, 1.

DAUGHADAY, W. H. & KIPNIS, D. M. (1966). *Recent Progr. Hormone Res.*, **22**, 49.

DAVIDSON, J. K. & EDDLEMAN, E. E. (1950). *Arch. Intern. Med.* (Chicago), **86**, 727.

DIXIT, P. K., LOWE, I. P., HEGGESTAD, C. B. & LAZAROW, A. (1964). *Diabetes*, **13**, 71.

DIXON, G. H. & WARDLAW, A. C. (1960). *Nature* (Lond.), **188**, 721.

DRASH, A. & WOLFF, F. (1964). *Metabolism*, **13**, 487.

DU, Y.-C., JIANG, R.-Q., & TSOU, C.-L. (1965). *Sci. Sinica*, **14**, 229.

DUBOIS, R., LOEB, H., OOMS, H. A., GILLET, P., BARTMAN, J. & CHAMPENOIS, A. (1961). *Helv. Paediat. Acta*, **16**, 90.

DUNCAN, L. J. P. & BAIRD, J. D. (1960). *Pharmacol. Rev.*, **12**, 91.

DUNN, D. F., FRIEDMANN, B., MAASS, A. R., REICHARD, G. A. & WEINHOUSE, S. (1957). *J. Biol. Chem.*, **225**, 225.

DUPRE, J., ROJAS, L., WHITE, J. J., UNGER, R. H. & BECK, J. C. (1966). *Lancet*, **2**, 26.

EHRLICH, J. C. & RATNER, I. M. (1961). *Amer. J. Path.*, **38**, 49.

EISENSTEIN, A. B. (Ed.) (1967). "The adrenal cortex". Boston, Little Brown.

EISENSTEIN, A. B., BERG, E., GOLDENBERG, D. & JENSEN, B. (1964). *Endocrinology*, **74**, 123.

EISENSTEIN, A. B., SPENCER, S., FLATNESS, S. & BRODSKY, A. (1966). *Endocrinology*, **79**, 182.

ELGEE, N. J. & WILLIAMS, R. H. (1955). *Amer. J. Physiol.*, **180**, 13.

ELLENBERG, M. (1963). *J. A. M. A.*, **183**, 926.

ELLIOTT, R. B., O'BRIEN, D. & ROY, C. C. (1965). *Diabetes*, **14**, 780.

ELRICK, H., HLAD, C. J. & ARAI, Y. (1961). *J. Clin. Endocr.*, **21**, 387.

ELRICK, H., STIMMLER, L., HLAD, C. J. & ARAI, Y. (1964). *J. Clin. Endocr.*, **24**, 1076.

ENGEL, F. L. (1950). *Recent Progr. Hormone Res.*, **6**, 277.

ENSINCK, J. W., MAHLER, R. J. & VALLANCE-OWEN, J. (1965). *Biochem. J.*, **94**, 150.

EXTON, J. H., JEFFERSON, L. S., BUTCHER, R. W. & PARK, C. R. (1966). *Amer. J. Med.*, **40**, 709.

EXTON, J. H. & PARK, C. R. (1965). *J. Biol. Chem.*, **240**, PC 955.

EXTON, J. H. & PARK, C. R. (1966). *Pharm. Rev.*, **18**, 181.

EYMONTT, M. J., GWINUP, G., KRUGER, F. A., MAYNARD, D. E. & HAMWI, G. J. (1965). *J. Clin. Endocr.*, **25**, 46.

FAIN, J. N., GALTON, D. J. & KOUACEV, V. P. (1966). *Molec. Pharmacol.*, **2**, 237.

FAIN, J. N., KOUACEV, V. P. & SCOW, R. O. (1965). *J. Biol. Chem.*, **240**, 3522.

FAIN, J. N. & SCOW, R. O. (1965). *Endocrinology*, **77**, 547.

FAIN, J. N., SCOW, R. O. & CHERNICK, S. S. (1963). *J. Biol. Chem.*, **238**, 54.

FAJANS, S. S. & CONN, J. W. (1954). *Diabetes*, **3**, 296.

FAJANS, S. S., FLOYD, J. C., KNOPF, R. F., RULL, J., GUNTSCHE, E. M. & CONN, J. W. (1966). *J. Clin. Invest.*, **45**, 481.

FAJANS, S. S., SCHNEIDER, J. M., SCHTEINGART, D. E. & CONN, J. W. (1961). *J. Clin. Endocr.*, **21**, 371.

FEIGELSON, P. & FEIGELSON, M. (1963). *J. Biol. Chem.*, **238**, 1073.

FIELD, J. B. (1962). *Ann. Rev. Med.*, **13**, 249.

FIELD, J. B. (1964). *Metabolism*, **13**, 407.

FIELD, J. B., WILLIAMS, H. E. & MORTIMORE, G. E. (1963). *J. Clin. Invest.*, **42**, 497.

FITZGERALD, M. G. & KEEN, H. (1964). *Lancet*, **1**, 1325.

FLOYD, J. C., FAJANS, S. S., CONN, J. W., KNOPF, R. F. & RULL, J. (1966). *J. Clin. Invest.*, **45**, 1487.

FLOYD, J. C., FAJANS, S. S., KNOPF, R. F. & CONN, J. W. (1964). *J. Clin. Endocr.*, **24**, 747.

FOA, P. P., GALANSINO, G. & POZZA, G. (1957). *Recent Progr. Hormone Res.*, **13**, 473.

FOSTER, D. P. & LOWRIE, W. L. (1938). *Endocrinology*, **23**, 681.

FRANCKSON, J. R. M., ARNOULD, Y., MALAISSE, W. & CONARD, V. (1964). *Diabetes*, **13**, 535.

FRANCKSON, J. R. M., MALAISSE, W., ARNOULD, Y., RASIO, E., OOMS, H. A., BALASSE, E., CONARD, V. & BASTENIE, P. A. (1966). *Diabetologia*, **2**, 96.

FRANCKSON, J. R. M., OOMS, H. A., BELLENS, R., CONARD, V. & BASTENIE, P. A. (1962). *Metabolism*, **11**, 482.

FRASER, R., ALBRIGHT, F. & SMITH, P. H. (1941). *J. Clin. Endocr.*, **1**, 297.

FREIDMANN, B., GOODMAN, E. H. & WEINHOUSE, S. (1965). *J. Biol. Chem.*, **240**, 3729.

FRIEDMANN, B., GOODMAN, E. H. & WEINHOUSE, S. (1966). *Fed. Proc.*, **25**, 347.

FREINKEL, N., ARKY, R. A., SINGER, D. L., COHEN, A. K., BLEICHER, S. J., ANDERSON, J. B., SILBERT, C. K. & FOSTER, A. E. (1965). *Diabetes*, **14**, 350.

FRERICHS, H., REICH, V. & CREUTZFELDT, W. (1965). *Klin. Wschr.*, **43**, 136.

FROESCH, E. R., BURGI, H., RAMSEIER, E. B., BALLY, P. & LABHART, A. (1963a). *J. Clin. Invest.*, **42**, 1816.

FROESCH, E. R., WOLF, H. P. & BAITSCH, H. (1963b). *Amer. J. Med.*, **34**, 151.

FROESCH, E. R., MULLER, W. A., BURGI, H., WALD-VOGEL, M. & LABHART, A. (1966). *Biochim. Biophys. Acta*, **121**, 360.

GARCIA, A., WILLIAMSON, J. R. & CAHILL, G. F. (1966). *Diabetes*, **15**, 188.

GELLIS, S. S. & HSIA, D. Y. (1959). *Amer. J. Dis. Child.*, **97**, 1.

GELLMAN, D. D., PIRANI, C. L., SOOTHILL, J. F., MUEHRCKE, R. C. & KARK, R. M. (1959). *Medicine*, **38**, 321.

GEPTS, W. (1965). *Diabetes*, **14**, 619.

GIFFORD, R. W., KVALE, W. F., MAHER, F. T., ROTH, G. M. & PRIESTLEY, J. T. (1964). *Mayo Clin. Proc.*, **39**, 281.

GITTLESON, N. L. (1956). *Brit. Med. J.*, **1**, 608.

GLICK, S. M., ROTH, J., YALOW, R. S. & BERSON, S. A. (1965). *Recent Progr. Hormone Res.*, **21**, 241.

GOLDNER, M. G., ZAROWITZ, H. & AKGUN, S. (1960). *New Eng. J. Med.*, **262**, 403.

GORDIS, E. (1960). *Proc. Soc. Exp. Biol. Med.*, **103**, 542.

GRABER, A. L., PORTE, D. & WILLIAMS, R. H. (1966). *Diabetes*, **15**, 143.

GREENGARD, O. & BAKER, G. T. (1966). *Science*, **154**, 1461.

GREENGARD, O. & FIEGELSON, P. (1962). *Biochem. J.*, **84**, 111 p.

GREENWOOD, F. C., HUNTER, W. M. & MARRIAN, V. J. (1964). *Brit. Med. J.*, **1**, 25.

GRODSKY, G. M., BATTS, A. A., BENNETT, L. L., VCELLA, C., McWILLIAMS, N. B. & SMITH, D. F. (1963). *Amer. J. Physiol.*, **205**, 639.

GRODSKY, G. M. & BENNETT, L. L. (1966). *Diabetes*, **15**, 910.

GRODSKY, G. M., BENNETT, L. L., SMITH, D. F. & SCHMID, F. G. (1967). *Metabolism*, **16**, 222.

GRODSKY, G. M., FELDMAN, R., TORESON, W. E. & LEE, J. C. (1966). *Diabetes*, **15**, 579.

GRODSKY, G. M. & FORSHAM, P. H. (1960). *J. Clin. Invest.*, **39**, 1070.

GRODSKY, G. M. & FORSHAM, P. H. (1966). *Ann. Rev. Physiol.*, **28**, 347.

GROEN, J., KAMMINGA, C. E., WILLEBRANDS, A. F. & BLICKMAN, J. R. (1952). *J. Clin. Invest.*, **31**, 97.

GRUMBACH, M. M., KAPLAN, S. L., ABRAMS, C. L., BELL, J. J. & CONTE, F. A. (1966). *J. Clin. Endocr.*, **26**, 478.

GUEST, G. M. (1949). *Amer. J. Med.*, **7**, 630.

HACKEL, D. B., FROHMAN, L., MIKAT, E., LEBOVITZ, H. E., SCHMIDT-NIELSEN, K. & KINNEY, T. D. (1966). *Diabetes*, **15**, 105.

HAGEN, J. H. (1961). *J. Biol. Chem.*, **236**, 1023.

HAGBARD, L., OLOW, I. & REINAND, T. (1959). *Acta Paediatr. Scand.*, **48**, 184.

HALES, C. N. & HYAMS, D. E. (1964). *Lancet*, **2**, 69.

HALES, C. N. & RANDLE, P. J. (1963a). *Biochem. J.*, **88**, 137.

HALES, C. N. & RANDLE, P. J. (1963b). *Lancet*, **1**, 790.

HARD, W. L. (1944). *Amer. J. Anat.*, **75**, 369.

HARRIS, H. (1950). *Ann. Eugen.* (Lond.), **15**, 95.

HARWOOD, R. (1957). *New Eng. J. Med.*, **257**, 257.

HAWORTH, J. C. & COODIN, F. J. (1960). *Pediatrics*, **25**, 748.

HAUGAARD, E. S. & HAUGAARD, N. J. (1954). *J. Biol. Chem.*, **206**, 641.

HAYNER, N. S., KJELSBERG, M. D., EPSTEIN, F. H. & FRANCIS, T. (1965). *Diabetes*, **14**, 413.

HAYNES, R. C. (1962). *Endocrinology*, **71**, 399.

HAYNES, R. C. (1965). *Advances Enzym. Regulat.*, **3**, 111.

HENDERSON, M. J., MORGAN, H. E. & PARK, C. R. (1961). *J. Biol. Chem.*, **236**, 273.

HERBERT, V., LAU, K. S., GOTTLIEB, C. W. & BLEICHER, S. J. (1965). *J. Clin. Endocr.*, **25**, 1375.

HERRERA, M. G., KAMM, D., RUDERMAN, N. & CAHILL, G. F. (1966). *Advances Enzym. Regulat.*, **4**, 225.

HERRERA, M. G. & RENOLD, A. E. (1960). *Biochem. Biophys. Acta*, **44**, 165.

HERS, H. G. (1964). *Advances Metab. Dis.*, **1**, 1.

HERTELENDY, F., MACHLIN, L. J., GORDON, R. S., HORINO, M. & KIPNIS, D. M. (1966). *Proc. Soc. Exp. Biol. Med.*, **121**, 675.

HIRATA, Y. & BLUMENTHAL, H. T. (1963). *J. Lab. Clin. Med.*, **62**, 683.

HOBKIRK, R., BLAHEY, P. R., ALFHEIM, A., RAESIDE, J. I. & JORON, G. E. (1960). *J. Clin. Endocr.*, **20**, 805.

HORNBROOK, K. R., BURCH, H. B. & LOWRY, O. H. (1965). *Biochem. Biophys. Res. Commun.*, **18**, 206.

HOUSSAY, B. A. (1936). *New Eng. J. Med.*, **214**, 961.

HOUSSAY, B. A. (1944). *Endocrinology*, **35**, 158.

HOWARD, J. M. & JORDAN, G. J. (Eds.) (1960). "Surgical diseases of the pancreas". Philadelphia, Lippincott.

HOWELL, S. L. & TAYLOR, K. W. (1966). *Lancet*, **1**, 128.

HUMBEL, R. E. (1963). *Biochim. Biophys. Acta*, **74**, 96.

HUMBEL, R. E. (1965). *Proc. Nat. Acad. Sci. USA*, **53**, 853.

HUMBEL, R. E. (1966). *Amer. J. Med.*, **40**, 672.

HUMMEL, K. P., DICKIE, M. M. & COLEMAN, D. L. (1966). *Science*, **153**, 1127.

HUNTER, W. M., CLARKE, B. F. & DUNCAN, L. J. P. (1966). *Metabolism*, **15**, 596.

HYDE, P. M. (1957). *Endocrinology*, **61**, 774.

ILLINGWORTH, B., CORI, G. T. & CORI, C. F. (1956). *J. Biol. Chem.*, **218**, 123.

INGLE, D. J. (1941). *Endocrinology*, **29**, 649.

JEANRENAUD, B. & RENOLD, A. E. (1960). *J. Biol. Chem.*, **235**, 2217.

JEDEIKIN, L. A. & WHITE, A. (1958). *Endocrinology*, **63**, 226.

JONES, V. E. & CUNLIFFE, A. C. (1961). *Nature* (Lond.), **192**, 136.

JORGENSEN, K. R., DECKERT, T., PEDERSEN, L. M. & PEDERSEN, J. (1966). *Acta Endocr.* (Kobenhavn), **52**, 154.

JOSIMOVICH, J. B. & MACLAREN, J. A. (1962). *Endocrinology*, **71**, 209.

JOSLIN, E. P., ROOT, H. F., WHITE, P. & MARBLE, A. (1959). "The treatment of diabetes mellitus". 10th Ed. Philadelphia, Lea & Febinger.

KALKHOFF, R., SCHALCH, D. S., WALKER, L., BECK, P., KIPNIS, D. M. & DAUGHADAY, W. H. (1964). *Trans. Ass. Amer. Physicians*, **77**, 270.

KANETO, A., KOSAKA, K. & NAKAO, K. (1967). *Endocrinology*, **80**, 530.

KAPLAN, S. L. & GRUMBACH, M. M. (1964). *J. Clin. Endocr.*, **24**, 80.

KAPLAN, S. L. & GRUMBACH, M. M. (1965a). *Science*, **147**, 751.

KAPLAN, S. L. & GRUMBACH, M. M. (1965b). *J. Clin. Endocr.*, **25**, 1370.

KARAM, J. H., GRASSO, S. G., WEGIENKA, L. C., GRODSKY, G. M. & FORSHAM, P. H. (1966). *Diabetes*, **15**, 571.

KARAM, J. H., GRODSKY, G. M., PAVOLATOS, F. C. & FORSHAM, P. H. (1965). *Lancet*, **1**, 286.

KARLSON, P. (Ed.) (1965). "Mechanisms of hormone action". London, Academic Press.

KATSOYANNIS, P. G., TOMETSKO, A. M., ZALUT, C. & FUKUDA, K. (1966). *J. Amer. Chem. Soc.*, **88**, 5625.

KATZEN, H. M., TIETZE, F. & STETTEN, DE W. (1963). *J. Biol. Chem.*, **238**, 1006.

KENNY, F. T. (1962). *J. Biol. Chem.*, **237**, 3495.

KENT, G. T. & LEONARDS, J. R. (1965). *Diabetes*, **14**, 295.

KETY, S. S., POLIS, B. D., NADLER, C. S. & SCHMIDT, C. F. (1948). *J. Clin. Invest.*, **27**, 500.

KIM, J. N., RUNGE, W., WELLS, L. J. & LAZAROW, A. (1960). *Diabetes*, **9**, 396.

KIMMELSTIEL, P. & WILSON, C. (1936). *Amer. J. Path.*, **12**, 83.

KIPNIS, D. M. & CORI, C. F. (1957). *J. Biol. Chem.*, **224**, 681.

KLINK, D. & ESTRICH, D. (1964). *Clin. Res.*, **12**, 354.

KNOBIL, E. & GREEP, R. O. (1959). *Recent Progr. Hormone Res.*, **15**, 1.

KNOWLES, H. C. & GUEST, G. M. (1954). *Diabetes*, **3**, 107.

KOLOGLU, Y., WIESEL, L. L., POSITANO, V. & ANDERSON, G. E. (1963). *Proc. Soc. Exp. Biol. Med.*, **112**, 518.

KOTOULAS, O. B., MORRISON, G. R. & RECANT, L. (1965). *Biochim. Biophys. Acta*, **97**, 350.

KRAHL, M. E. (1961). "The action of insulin on cells". New York, Academic Press.

KREBS, H. A. (1966). *Advances Enzym. Regulat.*, **4**, 339.

KREBS, H. A., SPEAKE, R. N. & HEMS, R. (1965). *Biochem. J.*, **94**, 712.

KYLE, C. K. (1963). *Ann. Intern. Med.*, Suppl. **3**, 1.

LACY, P. E. (1957). *Diabetes*, **6**, 498.

LACY, P. E. (1961). *Amer. J. Med.*, **31**, 851.

LACY, P. E. (1967). *New Eng. J. Med.*, **276**, 187.

LACY, P. E. & DAVIES, J. (1959). *Stain Techn.*, **34**, 85.

LACY, P. E. & KOSTIANOVSKY, M. (1967). *Diabetes*, **16**, 35.

LACY, P. E. & WRIGHT, P. H. (1966). *Diabetes*, **14**, 634.

LAMBERG, B. A. (1965). *Acta Med. Scand.*, **178**, 351.

LAMY, M., FREZAL, J. & REY, J. (1961). *Journees Ann. Diabet. Hotel Dieu*, 5.

LANDON, J., GREENWOOD, F. C., STAMP, T. C. B. & WYNN, V. (1966). *J. Clin. Invest.*, **45**, 437.

LANG, N. & SEKERIS, C. E. (1964). *Z. Physiol Chemie.*, **339**, 238.

LARDY, H. A., FOSTER, D. O., SHRAGO, E. & RAY, P. D. (1964). *Advances Enzym. Regulat.*, **2**, 39.

LARNER, J., VILLAR-PALASI, C. & RICHMAN, D. J. (1959). *Ann. N.Y. Acad. Sci.*, **82**, 345.

LASZLO, J., HARLAN, W. R., KLEIN, R. F., KIRSHNER, N., ESTES, H. & BOGDONOFF, M. D. (1961). *J. Clin. Invest.*, **40**, 171.

LAWRENCE, R. D. (1951). *Brit. Med. J.*, **1**, 373.

LAZARUS, S. S. (1959). *Proc. Soc. Exp. Biol. Med.*, **101**, 819.

LAZARUS, S. S. & VOLK, B. W. (1958). *Arch. Path.* (Chicago), **66**, 59.

LAZARUS, S. S. & VOLK, B. W. (1962). "The pancreas in human and experimental diabetes". New York, Grune & Stratton.

LEBOEUF, B. & CAHILL, G. F. (1960). *Fed. Proc.*, **19**, 226.

LEBOEUF, B., RENOLD, A. E. & CAHILL, G. F. (1962). *J. Biol. Chem.*, **237**, 988.

LE COMPTE, P. M. (1958). *Arch. Path.* (Chicago), **66**, 450.

LE COMPTE, P. M., STEINKE, J., SOELDNER, J. S. & RENOLD, A. E. (1966). *Diabetes*, **15**, 586.

LEIBEL, B. S. & WRENSHALL, G. A. (Eds.) (1965). "On the nature and treatment of diabetes". Amsterdam, Excerpta Medica Foundation.

LEVINE, R., GOLDSTEIN, M. S., HUDDLESTON, B. & KLEIN, S. P. (1950). *Amer. J. Physiol.*, **163**, 70.

LEVINE, R. & LUFT, R. (1964). *Diabetes*, **13**, 651.

LEVINE, R. & MAHLER, R. (1964). *Ann. Rev. Med.*, **15**, 413.

LEWIS, G. M., SPENCER-PEET, J. & STEWART, K. M. (1963). *Arch. Dis. Child.*, **38**, 40.

LINDALL, A. W., BAUER, G. E., DIXIT, P. K. & LAZAROW, A. (1963). *J. Cell. Biol.*, **19**, 317.

LITWACK, G. & KRITCHEVSKY, D. (Eds.) (1964). "Actions of hormones on molecular processes". New York, John Wiley.

LOEB, H. (1962). "Brussels Arscia", pp. 128.

LONG, C. N. H., KATZIN, B. & FRY, E. G. (1940). *Endocrinology*, **26**, 309.

LONG, C., KILO, C. & RECANT, L. (1964). *Diabetes*, **13**, 127.

LONG, C. N. H. & LUKENS, F. D. W. (1936). *J. Exp. Med.*, **63**, 465.

LORAINE, J. A. & BELL, E. T. (1966). "Hormone assays and their clinical application". 2nd Ed., Baltimore, Williams & Wilkins.

LUFT, R. & CERASI, E. (1964). *Lancet*, **2**, 124.
LUKENS, F. D. W. (1948). *Physiol. Rev.*, **28**, 304.
LUNDBAEK, K. (1953). *Acta Med. Scand.*, Suppl. 277, 143.
MCARTHUR, J. W., SMART, G. A., MACLACHLAN, E. A., TERRY, M. L., HARTING, D., GAUTIER, E., GODLEY, A., SWALLOW, K. A., SIMENONE, F. A., ZYGMUNTOWICZ, A., CHRISTO, E., CREPEAUX, J., POINT, W. W. & BENSON, J. A. (1954). *J. Clin. Invest.*, **33**, 420.
MCCULLAGH, E. P. (1956). *Diabetes*, **5**, 223.
MCGAVRAN, M. H., UNGER, R. H., RECANT, L., POLK, H. C., KILO, C. & LEVIN, M. E. (1966). *New Eng. J. Med.*, **274**, 1408.
MCINTYRE, N., HOLDSWORTH, C. D. & TURNER, D. S. (1965). *J. Clin. Endocr.*, **25**, 1317.
MACLEAN, N. & OGILVIE, R. F. (1959). *Diabetes*, **8**, 83.
MCQUARRIE, I. (1954). *Amer. J. Dis. Child.*, **87**, 399.
MADISON, L. L. (1966). *Advances Metab. Dis.*, **3**, in press.
MADISON, L. L., COMBES, B., ADAMS, R. & STRICKLAND, W. (1961). *J. Clin. Invest.*, **39**, 507.
MADISON, L. L., LOCHNER, A. & WOLFF, J. (1967). *Diabetes*, **16**, 252.
MAHLER, R., STAFFORD, W. S., TARRANT, M. E. & ASHMORE, J. (1963). *Diabetes*, **13**, 297.
MAJOR, R. H. (1945). "Classic descriptions of disease". 3rd Ed., Oxford, Blackwell.
MALAISSE, W., MALAISSE-LAGAE, F., LACY, P. E. & WRIGHT, P. H. (1967a). *Proc. Soc. Exp. Biol. Med.*, **124**, 497.
MALAISSE, W., MALAISSE-LAGAE, F. & MCCRAW, E. F. (1967b). *Diabetes*, **16**, 643.
MALAISSE, W., MALAISSE-LAGAE, F., MCCRAW, E. F. & WRIGHT, P. H. (1967c). *Proc. Soc. Exp. Biol. Med.*, **124**, 924.
MALAISSE, W., MALAISSE-LAGAE, F. & MAYHEW, D. A. (1967d). *J. Clin. Invest.*, **46**, 1724.
MALAISSE, W., MALAISSE-LAGAE, F., MAYHEW, D. A. & WRIGHT, P. H. (1967e). In "Tolbutamide after ten years". Amsterdam, Excerpta Medica Foundation. International Congress Series No. 149.
MALAISSE, W., MALAISSE-LAGAE, F. & WRIGHT, P. H. (1967f). *Endocrinology*, **80**, 99.
MALAISSE, W., MALAISSE-LAGAE, F. & WRIGHT, P. H. (1967g). *Amer. J. Physiol.*, **213**, 843.
MALAISSE, W., MALAISSE-LAGAE, F., WRIGHT, P. H. & ASHMORE, J. (1967h). *Endocrinology*, **80**, 975.
MALAISSE, W., LAUVAUX, J. P., FRANCKSON, J. R. M. & BASTENIE, P. A. (1965). *Diabetologia*, **1**, 155.
MALINS, J. M. (1956). *Lancet*, **1**, 530.
MALINS, J. M., FITZGERALD, M. G. & WALL, M. (1965). *Diabetologia*, **1**, 121.
MALLORY, A., SMITH, G. H. & TAYLOR, K. W. (1964). *Biochem. J.*, **91**, 484.
MANCHESTER, K. L. & KRAHL, M. E. (1959). *J. Biol. Chem.*, **234**, 2938.
MANCHESTER, K. L. & YOUNG, F. G. (1959). *Biochem. J.*, **72**, 136.
MARCUS, R. (1966). *Diabetes*, **15**, 351.
MARKS, V. & MARRACK, D. (1962). *Clin. Sci.*, **23**, 103.

MARKS, V. & ROSE, F. C. (1965). "Hypoglycaemia". Oxford. Blackwell.
MARTIN, J. M. & BAMBERS, G. (1965). *Amer. J. Physiol.*, **209**, 797.
MARTIN, D. B., RENOLD, A. E. & DAGENAIS, Y. M. (1958). *Lancet*, **2**, 76.
MARTIN, H. E., SMITH, K. & WILSON, M. L. (1958). *Amer. J. Med.*, **24**, 376.
MEADE, R. C., STIGLITZ, R. A. & KLEIST, T. J. (1965). *Diabetes*, **14**, 387.
MEIER, H. & YERGANIAN, G. A. (1959). *Proc. Soc. Exp. Biol. Med.*, **100**, 810.
MERING, J. VON & MINKOWSKI, O. (1889-90). *Arch. Exper. Path. u. Pharmakol.*, **26**, 371.
METZ, R. (1960). *Diabetes*, **9**, 89.
MIGEON, C. J., GREEN, O. C. & ECKERT, J. P. (1963). *Metabolism*, **12**, 718.
MILLER, L. L. (1965). *Fed. Proc.*, **24**, 737.
MIRSKY, I. A. (1964). *Diabetes*, **13**, 225.
MITCHELL, M. L. & BRADFORD, A. H. (1963). *Diabetes*, **12**, 257.
MOLONEY, P. J. & APRILE, M. A. (1959). *Canad. J. Biochem. Physiol.*, **37**, 793.
MOLONEY, P. J. & APRILE, M. A. (1960). *Canad. J. Biochem. Physiol.*, **38**, 1216.
MOLONEY, P. J. & COVAL, M. (1955). *Biochem. J.*, **59**, 179.
MOLONEY, P. J. & GOLDSMITH, L. (1957). *Canad. J. Biochem. Physiol.*, **35**, 79.
MORGAN, H. E., HENDERSON, M. J., REGEN, D. M. & PARK, C. R. (1959). *Ann. N.Y. Acad. Sci.*, **82**, 387.
MORGAN, C. R. & LAZAROW, A. (1963). *Diabetes*, **12**, 115.
MORSE, J. H. (1960). *Proc. Soc. Exp. Biol. Med.*, **103**, 494.
MUNCK, A. & KORITZ, S. B. (1962). *Biochim. Biophys. Acta*, **57**, 310.
MUNGER, B. L. (1958). *Amer. J. Anat.*, **103**, 275.
NABARRO, J. D. N., SPENCER, A. G. & STOWERS, J. M. (1952). *Quart. J. Med.*, **21**, 225.
NAJJAR, V. A. (1952). "Carbohydrate metabolism". Baltimore, Johns Hopkins Press.
NEEL, J. V., FAJANS, S. S., CONN, J. W. & DAVIDSON, R. T. (1965). In "Genetics and the epidemiology of chronic diseases". (Eds. Neel, J. V., Shaw, M. W. & Schull, W. J.) U.S. Public Health Service Publ. 1163.
NUMA, S., MATSUHASHI, M. & LYNEN, F. (1961). *Biochem. Z.*, **334**, 203.
NYDICK, M., SAMOLS, E., KUZUYA, T. & WILLIAMS, R. H. (1964). *Ann. Intern. Med.*, **61**, 1122.
OGILVIE, R. F. (1937). *Quart. J. Med.*, **6**, 287.
OSTRANDER, L. D., FRANCIS, T., HAYNER, N. S., KJELSBERG, M. O. & EPSTEIN, F. H. (1965). *Ann. Intern. Med.*, **62**, 1188.
OVERELL, B. G., CONDEN, S. E. & PETROW, V. (1960). *J. Pharm. and Pharmacol.*, **12**, 150.
PARRY, D. G. & TAYLOR, K. W. (1966). *Biochem. J.*, **100**, 2.
PAVY, F. W. (1885). *Lancet*, **2**, 1033 and 1085.

PAYLING-WRIGHT, G. (1950). "An introduction to pathology". 1st Ed., London, Longmans Green.

PEARCE, R. M. (1903). *Amer. J. Anat.*, **2**, 445.

PECK, F. B., KIRTLEY, W. R. & PECK, F. B. (1958). *Diabetes*, **7**, 93.

PERLEY, M. & KIPNIS, D. M. (1966a). *New Eng. J. Med.*, **274**, 1237.

PERLEY, M. & KIPNIS, D. M. (1966b). *Diabetes*, **15**, 867.

PICKERING, G. W. (1961). "The nature of essential hypertension". New York, Grune & Stratton.

PIETRO, D. L. DI & WEINHOUSE, S. (1960). *J. Biol. Chem.*, **235**, 2542.

PINCUS, G. & WHITE, P. (1933). *Amer. J. Med. Sci.*, **186**, 1.

PIRART, J. (1965). *Ann. Endocr.* (Paris), **26**, 27.

PLOTZ, C. M., KNOWLTON, A. I. & REGAN, C. (1952). *Amer. J. Med.*, **13**, 597.

POPE, C. G. (1966). In "Advances in Immunology". (Eds. Dixon, F. J. & Humphrey, J. H.). Vol. 5, New York, Academic Press.

PORTE, D., GRABER, A. L., KUZUYA, T. & WILLIAMS, R. H. (1966). *J. Clin. Invest.*, **45**, 228.

POULSEN, J. E. (1953). *Diabetes*, **2**, 7.

POWELL, T. & HOWELLS, L. (1966). *Diabetes*, **15**, 269.

PRATT, J. W. (Ed.) (1964). Conference on methodological approaches to population studies in diabetes. U.S. Public Health Service Publ. No. 1486.

PROUT, T. E. (1962). *J. Chronic Dis.*, **15**, 879.

PRYOR, J. & BERTHET, J. (1960). *Biochim. Biophys. Acto*, **43**, 556.

RANDLE, P. J. (1954). *Brit. Med. J.*, **1**, 1237.

RANDLE, P. J. (1966). *Diabetologia*, **2**, 237.

RANDLE, P. J., GARLAND, P. B., HALES, C. N. & NEWSHOLME, E. A. (1963). *Lancet*, **1**, 785.

RANDLE, P. J., GARLAND, P. B., HALES, C. N., NEWSHOLME, E. A., DENTON, R. M. & POGSON, C. I. (1966). *Recent Progr. Hormone Res.*, **22**, 1.

RANDLE, P. J. & SMITH, G. H. (1958). *Biochem. J.*, **70**, 501.

RASIO, E. A., SOELDNER, J. S. & CAHILL, G. F. (1965). *Diabetologia*, **1**, 125.

REGAN, J. F. & WILDER, R. M. (1940). *Arch. Intern. Med.*, **65**, 1116.

RENOLD, A. E., ASHMORE, J. & HASTINGS, A. B. (1956). "Vitamins Hormones" (N.Y.), **14**, 139.

RENOLD, A. E., CROFFORD, O. B., STAUFFACHER, W. & JEANRENAUD, B. (1965). *Diabetologia*, **1**, 4.

RENOLD, A. E. & DULIN, W. E. (Eds.) (1967). Brook Lodge Workshop on spontaneous diabetes in laboratory animals. *Diabetologia*, **3**, 63.

RICHINS, C. A. (1945). *J. Comp. Neurol.*, **83**, 223.

RICKETTS, H. T., TEST, C. E., PETERSEN, E. S., LINTS, H., TUPIKOVA, N. & STEINER, P. E. (1959). *Diabetes*, **8**, 298.

ROBISON, G. A., BUTCHER, R. W. & SUTHERLAND, E. W. (1967). *Ann. N.Y. Acad. Sci.*, **139**, 703.

ROSE, V. (1960). *Canad. Med. Ass. J.*, **82**, 306.

ROSELL-PEREZ, M. & LARNER, J. (1964). *Biochemistry* (Wash.), **3**, 81.

ROSEN, F. & NICHOL, C. (1964). *Advances Enzym. Regulat.*, **2**, 125.

ROSENTHAL, I. M., METZ, R. & PIRANI, C. (1964). *Amer. J. Dis. Child.*, **107**, 343.

ROTH, D. A. & MEADE, R. C. (1965). *Diabetes*, **14**, 526.

ROTH, J., GLICK, S. M., YALOW, R. S. & BERSON, S. A. (1963). *Metabolism*, **12**, 577.

ROTH, H. & SEGAL, S. (1964). *Pediatrics*, **34**, 831.

SAMAAN, N., FRASER, R. & DEMPSTER, W. J. (1963). *Diabetes*, **12**, 339.

SAMOLS, E. (1963). *Postgrad. Med. J.*, **39**, 634.

SAMOLS, E. & MARKS, V. (1963). *Brit. Med. J.*, **1**, 507.

SAMOLS, E., MARRI, G. & MARKS, V. (1965). *Lancet*, **2**, 415.

SAMOLS, E., TYLER, J., MEGYESI, C. & MARKS, V. (1966). *Lancet*, **2**, 727.

SCHALCH, D. S. (1967). *J. Lab. Clin. Med.*, **69**, 256.

SCHIMASSEK, H. & MITZKAT, H. J. (1963). *Biochem. Z.*, **337**, 510.

SCHTEINGART, D. E., GREGERMAN, R. I. & CONN, J. W. (1963). *Metabolism*, **12**, 484.

SCHULTZ, R. B. & BLIZZARD, R. M. (1966). *J. Clin. Endocr.*, **26**, 921.

SCIARRA, J. J., KAPLAN, S. L. & GRUMBACH, M. M. (1963). *Nature* (Lond.), **199**, 1006.

SCOW, R. O. & CHERNICK, S. S. (1960). *Recent Progr. Hormone Res.*, **16**, 497.

SELTZER, H. S. (1962). *J. Clin. Invest.*, **41**, 289.

SELTZER, H. S., FAJANS, S. S. & CONN, J. W. (1956). *Diabetes*, **5**, 437.

SELTZER, H. S. & HARRIS, V. L. (1964). *Diabetes*, **13**, 6.

SHARMA, C., MANJESHWAR, R. & WEINHOUSE, S. (1964). *Advances Enzym. Regulat.*, **2**, 189.

SHAW, W. N. & SHUEY, E. W. (1963). *Biochemistry* (Wash.), **2**, 286.

SHEEHAN, H. L. & SUMMERS, V. K. (1949). *Quart. J. Med.*, **18**, 319.

SHERMAN, L. (1966). *Diabetes*, **15**, 149.

SHIPP, J. C., CUNNINGHAM, R. W., RUSSELL, R. O. & MARBLE, A. (1965). *Medicine* (Balt.), **44**, 165.

SHOEMAKER, W. C., MAHLER, R. & ASHMORE, J. (1959). *Metabolism*, **8**, 494.

SILBER, R. H. & PORTER, C. C. (1953). *Endocrinology*, **52**, 518.

SILVERMAN, J. L. (1963). *Diabetes*, **12**, 327.

SILVERSTEIN, M. N., WAKIM, K. G. & BAHN, R. C. (1964). *Amer. J. Med.*, **36**, 415.

SILVERSTONE, F. A., BRANDFONBRENER, M., SHOCK, N. W. & YIENGST, M. J. (1957). *J. Clin. Invest.*, **36**, 504.

SIMPSON, N. E. (1964). *Diabetes*, **13**, 462.

SINEX, M., MacMULLEN, J. & HASTINGS, A. B. (1952). *J. Biol. Chem.*, **198**, 615.

SIPERSTEIN, M. D., COLWELL, A. R. & MEYER, K. (Eds.) (1964). "Small blood vessel involvement in diabetes mellitus". Washington, D.C., Amer. Inst. of Biological Sci.

SKOM, J. H. & TALMAGE, D. W. (1958a). *J. Clin. Invest.*, **37**, 783.

SKOM, J. H. & TALMAGE, D. W. (1958b). *J. Clin. Invest.*, **37**, 787.

SMETANA, H. F. & OLEN, E. (1962). *Amer. J. Clin. Path.*, **38**, 3.

SMITH, L. F. (1966). *Amer. J. Med.*, **40**, 662.

SMITH, C. H. & LACY, P. E. (1962). *Lab. Invest.*, **11**, 159.

SOFFER, L. J., IANNACONNE, A. & GABRILOVE, J. L. (1961). *Amer. J. Med.*, **30**, 129.

SOLOMON, N., CARPENTER, C. C. J., BENNETT, I. L. & HARVEY, A. M. (1965). *Diabetes*, **14**, 300.

SOLS, A., SALAS, M. & VINUELA, E. (1964). *Advances Enzym. Regulat.*, **2**, 177.

SOSKIN, S. (1951). *Postgrad. Med.*, **10**, 108.

SPELLACY, W. N. & CARLSON, K. L. (1966). *Amer. J. Obstet. Gynec.*, **95**, 474.

SPELLACY, W. N. & GOETZ, F. C. (1963a). *Lancet*, **2**, 222.

SPELLACY, W. N. & GOETZ, F. C. (1963b). *New Eng. J. Med.*, **268**, 988.

SPIRO, R. G. (1959). *Ann. N.Y. Acad. Sci.*, **82**, 366.

SPIRO, R. G. (1963). *New Eng. J. Med.*, **269**, 566 and 616.

SPRAGUE, R. G. (1962). *Diabetes*, **11**, 491.

STACKPOLE, R. H., MELICOW, M. M. & USON, A. C. (1963). *J. Pediat.*, **63**, 315.

STADIE, W. C. (1954). *Physiol. Rev.*, **34**, 52.

STEIGERWALD, H., SPIELMANN, W., FRIES, H. & GREBE, S. F. (1960). *Klin. Wschr.*, **38**, 973.

STEINER, D. F., RANDA, V. & WILLIAMS, R. H. (1961). *J. Biol. Chem.*, **236**, 299.

STEINKE, J., CAMERINI-DAVALOS, R., MARBLE, A. & RENOLD, A. E. (1961). *Metabolism*, **10**, 707.

STEINKE, J. & DRISCOLL, S. (1965). *Diabetes*, **14**, 573.

STEINKE, J. & SOELDNER, J. S. (1965). *Diabetes*, **14**, 432.

STIMMLER, L., BRAZIE, J. V. & O'BRIEN, D. (1964). *Lancet*, **1**, 137.

STIMMLER, L. & ELLIOTT, R. B. (1964). *Lancet*, **1**, 956.

STRUCK, E., ASHMORE, J. & WIELAND, O. (1965). *Biochem. Z.*, **343**, 107.

STRUCK, E., ASHMORE, J. & WIELAND, O. (1966). *Advances Enzym. Regulat.*, **4**, 219.

SUSSMAN, K. E., STIMMLER, L. & BIRENBOIM, H. (1966a). *Diabetes*, **15**, 1.

SUSSMAN, K. E., VAUGHAN, G. D. & TIMMER, R. F. (1966b). *Metabolism*, **15**, 466.

SUTHERLAND, E. W. & RALL, T. W. (1960). *Pharm. Rev.*, **12**, 265.

TARDING, F. & SCHAMBYE, P. (1958). *Endokrinologie*, **36**, 223.

TAYLOR, K. W. & SHELDON, J. (1964). *J. Endocr.*, **29**, 99.

THORELL, J. I. (1966). *Acta Endocr.* (Kobenhavn), **52**, 255.

TITTLE, C. R. & KERR, J. H. (1966). *Diabetes*, **15**, 212.

TORESON, W. E. (1951). *Amer. J. Path.*, **27**, 327.

TUCKER, W. R., KLINK, D., GOETZ, F., ZALME, E. & KNOWLES, H. C. (1964). *Diabetes*, **13**, 395.

TURNER, D. S. & McINTYRE, N. (1966). *Lancet*, **1**, 351.

TZAGOURNIS, M. & HAMWI, G. J. (1967). *Metabolism*, **16**, 213.

UETE, T. & ASHMORE, J. (1963). *J. Bio. Chem.*, **238**, 2906.

UNGER, R. H., KETTERER, H., EISENTRAUT, A. & DUPRE, J. (1966). *Lancet*, **2**, 24.

UNGER, R. H. & MADISON, L. L. (1958). *J. Clin. Invest.*, **37**, 627.

UTTER, M. F., KEECH, D. B. & SCRUTTON, M. C. (1964). *Advances Enzym. Regulat.*, **2**, 49.

VALLANCE-OWEN, J. (1966). *Diabetologia*, **2**, 248.

VALLANCE-OWEN, J., DENNES, E. & CAMPBELL, P. N. (1958). *Lancet*, **2**, 336.

VALLANCE-OWEN, J. & HURLOCK, B. (1954). *Lancet*, **1**, 68.

VALLANCE-OWEN, J. & WRIGHT, P. H. (1960). *Physiol. Rev.*, **40**, 219.

VAUGHAN, M., BERGER, J. E. & STEINBERG, D. (1964). *J. Biol. Chem.*, **239**, 401.

VILLAR-PALASI, C. & LARNER, J. (1961). *Arch. Biochem. Biophys.*, **94**, 436.

WAGENER, H. P. (1945). *Proc. Amer. Diab. Ass.*, **5**, 203.

WAGLE, S. R. & ASHMORE, J. (1963). *J. Biol. Chem.* **238**, 17.

WAJCHENBERG, B. L., PEREIRA, V. G., PUPO, A. A., SCHNAEDER, J., CINTRA, A. B. & MATTAR, E. (1964). *Diabetes*, **13**, 169.

WARDLAW, A. C. & MOLONEY, P. J. (1961). *Canad. J. Biochem. Physiol.*, **39**, 695.

WARREN, S. & LE COMPTE, P. M. (1952). "The pathology of diabetes mellitus". 3rd Ed., Philadelphia, Lea & Febinger.

WEBER, G., SINGHAL, R. L. & SRIVASTAVA, S. K. (1965a). *Proc. Nat. Acad. Sci.* (U.S.A.), **53**, 96.

WEBER, G., SRIVASTAVA, S. K. & SINGHAL, R. L. (1965b). *J. Biol. Chem.*, **240**, 750.

WEBER, G., HIRD-CONVERY, H. J., LEA, M. A. & STAMM, N. B. (1966a). *Science*, **154**, 1357.

WEBER, G., SINGHAL, R. L., STAMM, N. B., LEA, M. A. & FISHER, E. A. (1966b). *Advances Enzym. Regulat.*, **4**, 59.

WEST, K. M. (1966). *Arch. Intern. Med.*, **117**, 187.

WEST, K. M. & KALBFLEISCH, J. M. (1966). *Diabetes*, **15**, 9.

WEST, K. M., WULFF, J. A., REIGEL, D. G. & FITZGERALD, D. T. (1964). *Arch. Intern. Med.*, **113**, 641.

WHIPPLE, A. O. (1952). *Canad. Med. Ass. J.*, **66**, 334.

WHITE, P. (1956). *Diabetes*, **5**, 445.

WICK, A. N., DRURY, D. R., NAKADA, H. I. & WOLFE, J. B. (1957). *J. Biol. Chem.*, **224**, 963.

WIELAND, O., WEISS, L. & EGER-NEUFELDT, I. (1964). *Advances Enzym. Regulat.*, **2**, 85.

WILDER, J. F. & ODELL, W. D. (1965). *Metabolism*, **14**, 590.

WILLIAMS, R. H. (Ed.) (1960). "Diabetes". New York, Hoeber.

WILLIAMS, R., KELLIE, A. E., WADE, A. P., WILLIAMS, E. D. & CHALMERS, T. M. (1961). *Quart. J. Med.*, **30**, 269.

WILLIAMSON, J. R. (1967). *Advances Enzym. Regulat.*, **5**, 233.

WILLIAMSON, J. R., KREISBERG, R. A. & FELTS, W. P. (1966a). *Proc. Nat. Acad. Sci.* (U.S.A.), **56**, 247.

WILLIAMSON, J. R., WRIGHT, P. H., MALAISSE, W. & ASHMORE, J. (1966b). *Biochem. Biophys. Res. Commun.*, **24**, 765.

WOLSTENHOLME, G. E. W. & O'CONNOR, C. M. (Eds.) (1956). "Internal secretion of pancreas". CIBA Foundation, Colloquia on Endocrinology, Vol. 9, Boston, Little Brown.

WOLSTENHOLME, G. E. W. & O'CONNOR, M. (Eds.) (1960a). "Metabolic effects of adrenal hormones". CIBA Foundation, Group No. 6, London, Churchill.

WOLSTENHOLME, G. E. W. & O'CONNOR, M. (Eds.) (1960b). "Human pituitary hormones". CIBA Foundation, Colloquia on Endocrinology, Vol. 13, Boston, Little Brown.

WOOL, I. G., RAMPUSAD, O. R. & MOYER, A. N. (1966). *Amer. J. Med.*, **40**, 716.

WRENSHALL, G. A., BOGOCH, A. & RITCHIE, R. C. (1952). *Diabetes*, **1**, 87.

WRIGHT, P. H. (1957). *Lancet*, **2**, 621.

WRIGHT, P. H. (1959). *Biochem. J.*, **71**, 633.

WRIGHT, P. H. (1965). *Vitamins Hormones*, **23**, 61.

WRIGHT, P. H., KREISBERG, R. A., HALPERN, B. & DOLKART, R. E. (1962). *Diabetes*, **11**, 519.

WRIGHT, P. H. & MALAISSE, W. J. (1966). *Diabetologia*, **2**, 178.

WRIGHT, P. H., RIVERA-CALIMLIM, L. & MALAISSE, W. J. (1966). *Amer. J. Physiol.*, **211**, 1089.

YABO, R., VIKTORA, J., STAQUET, M. & WOLFF, F. (1965). *Diabetes*, **14**, 591.

YALOW, R. S. & BERSON, S. A. (1960). *J. Clin. Invest.*, **39**, 1157.

YALOW, R. S. & BERSON, S. A. (1961). *Amer. J. Med.*, **31**, 882.

YALOW, R. S. & BERSON, S. A. (1964). *New Eng. J. Med.*, **270**, 1171.

YALOW, R. S. & BERSON, S. A. (1965). *Diabetes*, **14**, 341.

YANKELOWITCH, T., MASSRY, S. & GITTER, S. (1956). *Diabetes*, **5**, 457.

YOUNG, F. G. (1951). *J. Clin. Endocr.*, **11**, 531.

YOUNG, F. G. (1953). *Recent Progr. Hormone Res.*, **8**, 471.

ZAHN, H., GUTTE, B. & BRINKHOFF, O. (1965). *Angew. Chem.*, **77**, 509.

ZALME, E. & KNOWLES, H. C. (1965). *Diabetes*, **14**, 165.

Chapter 4

GLYCOGEN STORAGE DISEASES AND GALACTOSAEMIA

by

R. MAHLER

Department of Metabolic Medicine, Welsh National School of Medicine, Cardiff

GLYCOGEN STORAGE DISEASES

IN 1857 Claude Bernard reported the isolation of glycogen from liver tissue. Since that time, glycogen has been an area of common interest to clinicians, chemists and biochemists; more recently, dating from the recognition of the glycogen storage diseases (Snapper & van Crefeld, 1928; von Gierke, 1929) it has also become an important field of study for geneticists.

When the glycogen diseases were first recognized, their metabolic basis was unknown and different forms were distinguished from one another primarily in accordance with the anatomical distribution of the major glycogen deposits. Two main types were recognized: a hepato-renal storage disease and a generalized disease with particular involvement of the heart (Pompe, 1932).

The discovery by Cori & Cori in 1952 of a specific enzyme defect in the hepato-renal type, the absence of glucose-6-phosphatase, was the break-through which led to the currently accepted classification of storage diseases into six different types (Table 4.1), each according to a specific enzyme defect, and each with its own unique clinical manifestations. In addition, well documented claims have been put forward in the last two or three years for the reality of yet other specific enzyme defects as possible primary causes of further types of glycogen storage diseases.

Claude Bernard also drew attention to the constancy of the "milieu intérieur". Its constancy depends upon the co-ordinated and self-regulating interaction of enzymes, metabolites and hormones, and because these interactions are so complex the study of homeostatic mechanisms in man is beset with great practical difficulties. It is also remarkable that the complete absence of an enzyme can be compatible with life, but, even under normal conditions, there are great variations in the activity of metabolic reactions, and the complete absence of an enzyme may be no more than an extreme example of

TABLE 4.1

Summary of the classified types of glycogen storage diseases

Type	Enzyme Defect	Tissues Affected	Clinical Features
I (von Gierke)	Glucose-6-phosphatase	Liver, kidney, gut	Hepatomegaly. Hypoglycaemia. Ketosis, acidosis
II (Pompe)	Acid maltase	Generalized, particularly heart, tongue, brain	Cardiomegaly. Heart failure, enlarged tongue, muscle weakness. Death in infancy
III (Limit dextrinosis)	"Debrancher"	Liver, heart, muscle, RBC, WBC	Hepatomegaly Moderate fasting hypoglycaemia. Muscle weakness and wasting.
IV (Amylopectinosis)	"Brancher"	Liver, spleen, heart, muscle, RBC	Cirrhosis. Hepatic failure
V (McArdle)	Muscle phosphorylase	Skeletal muscle only	Pain, stiffness, weakness on exercise only. Occasionally myoglobinuria
VI (Hers)	Liver phosphorylase	Liver, WBC	Hepatomegaly. Moderate fasting hypoglycaemia

individual variations of biochemical behaviour which are everywhere present in minor degree (Garrod, 1902). The glycogen storage diseases may be regarded as natural experiments, perhaps of evolution, and they present an opportunity for unravelling some of the interweaving complexities of biochemical control mechanism. They also present the clinician with the challenge to make use of the knowledge gained from such studies to arrive at an early diagnosis with the hope of relieving suffering and preventing permanent damage.

The story of the recognition of the various glycogen storage diseases illustrates how clinicians and biochemists depend upon one another to discover new facts and confirm the reality of their discoveries. It is the purpose of this article to correlate clinical, biochemical and genetic observations which have been made in the study of glycogen storage disease, and show how they have provided a better understanding of the normal metabolism of glycogen in man and of the defects that occur in these disorders.

Results of biochemical analysis of biopsy material and of functional tests are so dependent on technique, and vary so greatly from laboratory to laboratory, that it would be unwise in this article

to present absolute figures. Until methods are rigidly controlled, results between laboratories cannot easily be compared and investigations on abnormal tissues are only meaningful in the context of control studies performed in the same laboratory under the same conditions. Excellent reviews of practical methods have been published by Hers (1964a) for biopsy material, and by Cornblath & Schwartz (1966) for functional tests.

GLYCOGEN SYNTHESIS AND DEGRADATION

Glycogen Synthesis

In 1939, Cori, Schmidt & Cori accomplished the synthesis of glycogen *in vitro* from glucose-1-phosphate, using liver phosphorylase. Phosphorylase was known to be the enzyme responsible for the breakdown of glucose *in vivo*, and, although the conditions necessary to achieve the synthesis of glycogen *in vitro* are never likely to be present in the living cell, it came to be accepted that synthesis and degradation of glycogen occurred *in vivo* through the reversible action of this enzyme. But if it is accepted that this reaction can be reversible *in vivo*, then it is difficult to understand why activation of the enzyme, e.g. by adrenaline

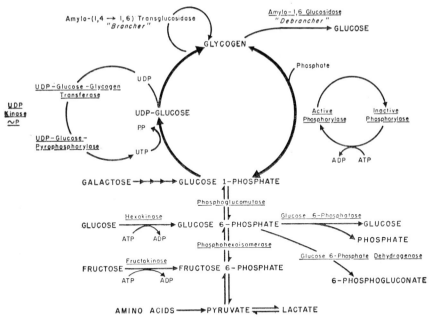

FIG. 4.1. Pathways of glycogen synthesis and glycolysis (from: Andersen, D. H., in "Biochemical Disorders in Human Disease", 2nd ed. p. 878).

or glucagon, invariably leads only to glycogen breakdown and never to the equilibrium between glycogenolysis and glycogenesis which would be expected from the usual considerations of enzyme kinetics. This difficulty was not resolved until 20 years later when two quite independent observations reinforced one another to emphasize the separateness of the synthetic and catabolic pathways and to confirm that each pathway was biologically important. In 1957, Leloir & Cardini described the role of a uridine diphosphate-requiring "glycogen synthetase" in the biosyn-

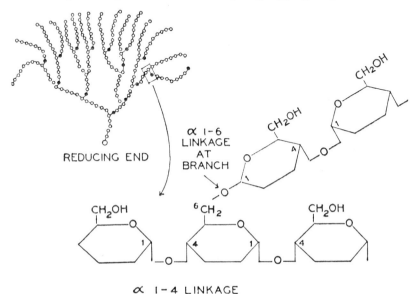

FIG. 4.2. Formation of a branch point in the glycogen molecule (from: Recant, L., *Amer. J. Med.*, 1955, **19**, 610).

thesis of glycogen and other polysaccharides, and in 1959, Schmid & Mahler, and Mommaerts *et al.* described a myopathy in which, although phosphorylase was absent, the muscles contained an excess of glycogen. These independent observations gave support to the view that in the living cell glycogen synthesis and degradation proceed by separate pathways, a view which was further strengthened by the observations of Grillo & Ozone (1962) that in chicken embryos, during growth, glycogen becomes detectable in the liver at the same time as glycogen synthetase, but before any phosphorylase activity is present.

The first step in glycogen synthesis is the reversible conversion of glucose-1-phosphate to uridine diphosphoglucose (UDPG) by a specific pyrophosphorylase (Fig. 4.1). The next step is the irreversible reaction of UDPG with "glycogen synthetase", in the presence of a few molecules of preformed glycogen acting as "primer", which lengthens the chain of glucose molecules by joining them to one another in an α-1,4-linkage. This reaction is stimulated by glucose-6-phosphate (Leloir, 1964) and by insulin (Larner *et al.*, 1964). When the chains have reached an average length of 6 to 11 glucose residues (Larner, 1964), "branching enzyme", (amylo-1,4 → 1,6-transglucosylase) transfers three or more units from the end of that chain to another chain (French, 1964), and forms a branch point by joining the transferred oligosaccharide in a 1,6 linkage to a glucose residue of the acceptor chain (Fig. 4.2). By the proper interaction in time and space of the two enzymes, glycogen synthetase and "branching enzyme", and in the presence of an adequate amount of substrate, a treelike molecule of glycogen is built up until it reaches a size when the peri-

phery becomes so densely packed that it is sterically impossible for regular branching to continue. The final molecule appears roughly spherical in shape under the electron microscope (Fig. 4.3), and contains about 122,000 glucose units with a total molecular weight of 2×10^6, and a volume of 200 Å^3, estimated by X-ray measurement (French, 1964). Larger units are also found because glycogen particles tend to aggregate. The tendency to aggregate is related to the nutritional state (Orrell *et al.*, 1964), and some types of glycogen storage disease may be recognized by the peculiar sedimentation pattern of their glycogen aggregates (Bueding *et al.*, 1964).

Glycogen Degradation

For the complete degradation of glycogen, at least two enzymes, phosphorylase and "debranching enzyme" (amylo-1,6-glucosidase) have to act in proper sequence. Through their action they yield a mixture of 93 % glucose-1-phosphate and 7 % glucose (Cori & Larner, 1951).

Phosphorylase attacks only the 1,4 glucosidic linkages of the outer chains of the glycogen molecule, with the formation of glucose-1-phosphate; the "debranching enzyme" acts on the 1,6 links with the production of free glucose. When phosphorylase acts on glycogen without "debranching enzyme" it produces a "limit dextrin". about whose precise structure there is still some disagreement, but it is clear that the action of the enzyme comes to an end before all the 1,4 linked glycosyl units have been removed (Walker & Whelan, 1960). The remaining glucose units on the chain, which are still covering a branch point, are removed by the enzyme, oligo-1,4 → 1,4-glucan transferase. This enzyme appears to be intimately associated with "debranching enzyme" (Brown & Illingworth, 1962), and transfers the few remaining oligosaccharides from one chain to another, thereby exposing the 1,6-linked branch point to the action of the "debranching enzyme".

Glucose-1-phosphate, which was formed by the action of phosphorylase, is subsequently converted to glucose-6-phosphate by phosphoglucomutase. In liver and kidney, glucose-6-phosphate can be converted to free glucose by glucose-6-phosphatase or may be converted to lactate by the glycolytic pathway, or may be oxidized through the pentose phosphate cycle, or re-used for glycogen synthesis.

The reactions described above are generally accepted to be the major pathways of glycogen degradation but other, non-phosphorolytic, pathways also exist whose importance in tissue meta-

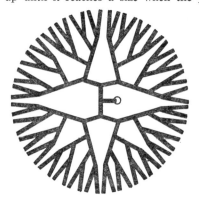

FIG. 4.3. A spherical aggregate of glycogen molecules (from: French, D., in "Control of Glycogen Metabolism" 1964, p. 11.)

bolism has only become apparent through a study of the glycogen storage diseases.

Hydrolytic enzymes capable of degrading most of the intracellular polymolecular compounds, including glycogen, are contained in the lysosomes, which play a role in the physiological and pathological autolysis of cells (de Duve, 1959). In the lysosome, glycogen is broken down by an acid maltase (Lejeune *et al.*, 1963) to form maltose and then glucose. Its importance in cell metabolism is shown by the fact that as long as the enzyme is present, there is only moderate accumulation of glycogen even in tissues in which phosphorylase or "debrancher enzyme" is absent, as in Types V, VI and III glycogenosis, but that in its absence, as in Type II glycogenosis (Hers, 1963), there is a huge accumulation of glycogen even though phosphorylase and "debrancher enzyme" remain active.

Other functionally distinct amylases and glucosidases have also been described, some in liver, others in muscle, through whose action oligosaccharides are formed with the subsequent liberation of glucose (Olavarria & Torres, 1962; Rutter & Brosemer, 1961; Rosenfeld, 1964). Their physiological role in glycogen metabolism is not yet established, but further studies on some of the as yet unidentified forms of glycogen storage diseases may clarify the situation.

The Cellular Control of Glycogen Synthesis and Breakdown

The amount of glycogen in a cell at any given moment represents the balance between the rate of glycogen synthesis and breakdown.

There is a close and complex inter-relationship between the activity of "glycogen synthetase" which controls synthesis and the activity of phosphorylase which determines the rate of glycogen breakdown. The activity of each enzyme is subject to intracellular and extracellular influences, such as hormones and metabolites, and the balance of the overall reaction is shifted by these factors in the direction appropriate to the metabolic needs of the body.

In the cell, both enzymes are closely associated with glycogen particles (Luck, 1961; Tata, 1964) and both enzymes exist in an active and an inactive form (Rosell-Perez *et al.*, 1962).

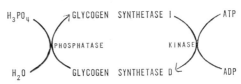

FIG. 4.4. The glucose-6-phosphate-dependent "D" form of glycogen synthetase is converted into the independent "I" form by the loss of a phosphate group and can be reconverted to the "D" form by phosphorylation.

The "inactive" form of glycogen synthetase becomes active in the presence of glucose-6-phosphate and has been named "D" form, because it is dependent for activity on glucose-6-phosphate. In these circumstances it may be almost as active as the glucose-6-phosphate independent "I" form (Fig. 4.4). In addition, the "D" form may be converted into the "I" form by removal of a phosphate group by a phosphatase and this reaction also requires the presence of glucose-6-phosphate. The "I" form can then be reconverted to "D" by a kinase, which phosphorylates the enzyme with the help of ATP. Thus the active "I" form is the dephosphorylated enzyme, while the inactive "D" form is in the phosphorylated state.

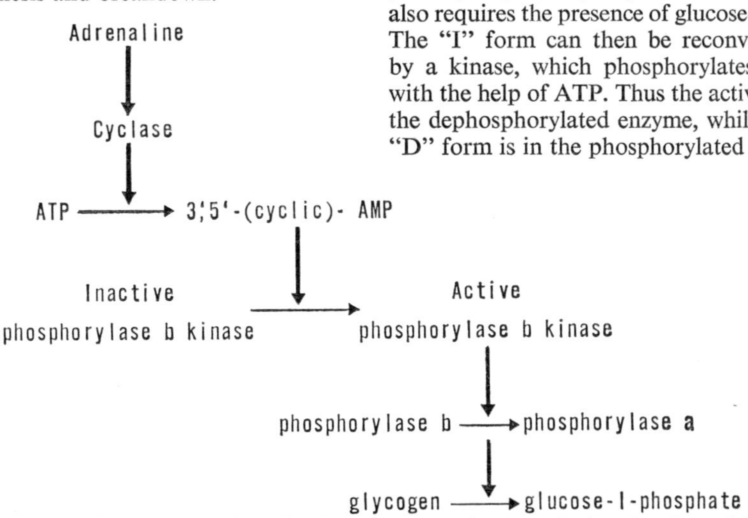

Adrenaline

↓

Cyclase

↓

ATP ⟶ 3',5'-(cyclic)- AMP

↓

Inactive ⟶ Active
phosphorylase b kinase   phosphorylase b kinase

↓

phosphorylase b ⟶ phosphorylase a

↓

glycogen ⟶ glucose-1-phosphate

FIG. 4.5. The cascade of enzyme reactions involved in the activation of phosphorylase which initiates the degradation of glycogen (from: Hales, N. C., in "Essays in Biochemistry" 1967, p. 97).

The rate of glycogen synthesis in muscle is also controlled by its own concentration of glycogen: when it is low, the active form of glycogen synthetase predominates and glycogen synthesis is increased (Danforth, 1965) and when it is high the inactive "D" form slows the rate of synthesis. In this way the cell protects itself against becoming overfilled with glycogen and this may explain how the glycogen concentration remains limited to 3 to 4% of fresh weight of muscle in those forms of glycogen storage disease in which glycogenolysis is blocked. Insulin also increases the proportion of "I" to "D" form (Larner et al., 1964) and this change correlates well with a greatly increased rate of glycogen synthesis in muscle after the administration of insulin.

The rate of glycogen breakdown is determined by the phosphorylase system. As in the case of glycogen synthetase, this system consists of an active and an inactive enzyme, and the rate at which glycogenolysis finally proceeds depends upon a cascade of enzyme reactions (Hales, 1967) which result in the activation of phosphorylase (Fig. 4.5).

The inactive form, phosphorylase b, is a dimer of molecular weight 250,000 and phosphorylase a is a tetramer of molecular weight 500,000 (Keller & Cori, 1955). An increase in phosphorylase activity can occur through two mechanisms analogous to those which increase glycogen synthetase activity (Fig. 4.6).

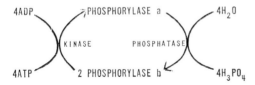

Fig. 4.6. The relationship between active and inactive phosphorylase.

The activity of "inactive" phosphorylase b can be increased by the presence of a high concentration of AMP and low concentrations of ATP and glucose-6-phosphate without being converted into the active a form. This mechanism probably accounts for the increased rate of glycogen breakdown in muscle under anaerobic conditions (Stadtman, 1966).

Alternatively, glycogenolysis in muscle increases when phosphorylase b is converted to phosphorylase a which occurs during muscle contraction or under the influence of adrenaline. The immediate mechanism of this conversion is the phosphorylation of two molecules of phosphorylase b with four molecules of ATP, catalysed by

phosphorylase kinase. This time, however, in contrast to glycogen synthetase "I", it is the phosphorylated enzyme which is the active form. The mechanism of activation of phosphorylase b under the influence of adrenaline is a complex reaction, because the kinase itself also exists in an active and inactive form. The conversion of the inactive into the active form of phosphorylase b kinase is accelerated by 3'5'-(cyclic)-AMP which in turn is formed by the action of a membrane-bound adenyl cyclase on ATP (Sutherland & Rall, 1960).

3'5'-(cyclic)-AMP occupies an important role in the activation of many different enzymes (Sutherland & Robison, 1966). In addition to its now well established effect on phosphorylase activation, it also influences the conversion of glycogen synthetase "I" to "D" (Huijing & Larner, 1966), so that adrenaline causes not only an increase in the rate of glycogenolysis, but also a decrease in the rate of glycogen synthesis.

It appears, therefore, that the amount of glycogen in a cell is controlled by complex and closely interwoven mechanisms, some of which are self-regulating and others which are subject to hormonal and nutritional influences in accordance with the metabolic needs of the organ or of the whole body.

The integrative action of intra- and extracellular processes in normal tissues makes it difficult to assess the biological importance of individual reactions, but the study of inborn errors of metabolism such as the glycogen storage diseases, often throws light on the control of the normal metabolic pathways, and much of what has been learnt about glycogen metabolism in general has been made possible through the detailed investigations of the glycogen storage diseases.

TYPE I GLYCOGENOSIS

Synonyms:

GLUCOSE-6-PHOSPHATASE DEFICIENCY, VON GIERKE'S DISEASE

This disease was the first of the glycogen storage diseases in which a specific enzyme defect was elucidated (Cori, 1954). It is due to the absence of glucose-6-phosphatase which is normally present only in liver, kidney and intestinal mucosa in significant amounts.

The clinical signs become obvious very early in life and can all be attributed directly and indirectly to severe and prolonged episodes of hypoglycaemia. Mortality is high, but if affected children survive the first four years, symptomatic improvement may occur through some adaptation of metabolic processes, although the enzyme defect remains permanent.

Biochemical Basis of Clinical Manifestations

In normal people the blood sugar level is maintained during fasting by the hepatic glucose output. In the liver, production of glucose depends upon glycogenolysis and gluconeogenesis, but all pathways ultimately converge upon one final common pathway, the hydrolysis of glucose-6-phosphate by the enzyme glucose-6-phosphatase with the liberation of glucose (Fig. 4.7).

phosphatase and distributed to the brain and other tissues by the blood stream.

In the absence of glucose-6-phosphatase, the normal steering of metabolic processes is distorted. Glucose is not produced from glucose-6-phosphate, but glycogen synthesis and lactate formation are both increased (Fig. 4.8). The enzymes concerned with glyconeogenesis from other sugars and from precursors such as amino acids may also be more active (Weber & Harpur, 1960), and the net result of these distortions is the accumulation of glycogen in liver cells.

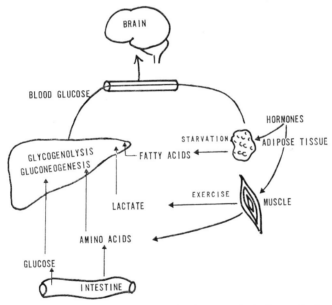

FIG. 4.7. During fasting the blood glucose level depends almost exclusively on the hepatic glucose output which is regulated by the activity of glucose-6-phosphatase.

The enzyme is therefore an important regulator in the maintenance of blood sugar level and in its absence hypoglycaemia in the fasting state is inevitable. Although glucose-6-phosphatase does not act directly on glycogen metabolism or on the glycolytic pathway, it exerts a widespread influence over the body's metabolism through its effect on the disposal of glucose-6-phosphate. This compound stands at one of the most important crossroads of carbohydrate metabolism: it serves not only as a substrate for glycogen synthesis, but also exerts a direct stimulating action on the activity of the uridine diphosphate-dependent glycogen synthetase (Leloir, 1964); it is also further metabolized to lactate through the glycolytic pathway and a portion of it passes through the pentose cycle; and it is hydrolysed to free glucose by glucose-6-

Abnormal deposits of glycogen also occur in kidney and intestinal mucosa, both of these being tissues in which glucose-6-phosphatase occurs normally but is absent in Type I glycogenosis (Williams *et al.*, 1963*a*; Öckerman, 1964).

Most of the clinical features of the disease appear early in the first year of life and are explicable as direct or indirect consequences of the enzymic defect. The liver contains more than 6% of its weight as glycogen and is greatly enlarged, causing a protuberant abdomen and often considerable abdominal discomfort because of its weight. In spite of its size, there are no signs of portal hypertension and all hepatic function tests, except those involving carbohydrate metabolism, show little, if any, abnormality.

The kidneys also contain more glycogen than

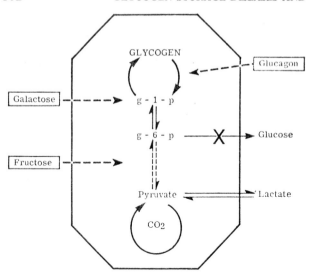

FIG. 4.8. Type I glycogen storage disease: there is no glucose-6-phosphatase activity in the liver.

normal and are usually radiologically, and often palpably, enlarged. But this enlargement has no recognizable direct effect on renal function, nor does the deposition of glycogen in the intestinal mucosa appear to cause any clinical manifestations.

Hypoglycaemia is responsible for most of the functional disturbances which are clinically apparent in Type I glycogenosis. Convulsions and mental retardation may be attributed to frequent episodes of prolonged and profound hypoglycaemia with blood glucose levels sometimes below 10 mg./100 ml. It is well recognized, however, that in this disease low glucose levels are not invariably associated with cerebral disturbances, and in these circumstances the brain may be using other available substrates, such as glycerol, or its glucose uptake may be facilitated by an increase in cerebral blood flow.

Prolonged hypoglycaemia causes secondary disturbances of lipid metabolism, including excessive mobilization of fat from adipose tissue depots, and synthesis of lipids in the liver. It is not clear, however, why some areas of the body, particularly the cheeks and buttocks, should remain well covered with fat, giving the child a "doll-like facies" (Cornblath et al., 1966) when fat is lost from other areas. Lipolysis in adipose tissue is increased when its supply of glucose is inadequate to provide glycerophosphate for re-esterification of fatty acids and is further stimulated and maintained through the action of adrenaline, growth hormone and perhaps cortisol, which are produced in response to hypoglycaemia and which also stimulate lipolysis (Steinberg, 1963). As a

result, glycerol and fatty acids are released into the circulation and carried to the liver, where they cause major quantitative changes in lipid metabolism. The usual fate of fatty acids in the liver is their degradation to acetyl-CoA, which then enters the Krebs cycle or is used for the synthesis of cholesterol; their re-esterification with glycerophosphate to form new triglycerides; and the synthesis of cholesterol and cholesterol ester which appear in the blood as lipoproteins. In glucose-6-phosphatase deficiency, the greatly increased flow of free fatty acids to the liver increases all these reactions. The amount of cholesterol in the blood increases and is deposited in the skin in the form of xanthomata. In some children these may appear as sudden eruptions of yellow papules, especially over the proximal parts of the upper and lower limbs. Although blood cholesterol is always above the normal level, the deposition of xanthomata, and particularly the waxing and waning of the eruptive phase, shows no clear relation to variations in the blood level. The triglyceride concentration is often high enough to give the plasma a creamy appearance and on ophthalmoscopy the retina appears as though a film of milk had been spread over it. Sometimes so much fat is stored in liver cells that it even exceeds their glycogen content.

A further consequence of the excessive flow of fatty acids to the liver is the appearance of keto-acids in the blood when the liver's capacity for oxidizing acetyl-CoA is exceeded. These acids contribute to the acidosis which is almost invariably present in children suffering from Type I glycogenosis.

Another cause of the metabolic acidosis is the high lactic acid concentration in the blood. Lactic acid, produced by muscle and other tissues, is usually removed from the circulation by the liver and metabolized via the Krebs cycle or converted to glucose and glycogen via gluconeogenetic pathways. In this disease, however, the liver itself produces so much lactic acid that it actually adds more acid to the blood, particularly when glycogenolysis is stimulated by hypoglycaemia or adrenaline. In addition to causing the usual features of acidosis, hyperlacticacidaemia is responsible for an unexpected metabolic complication, most commonly seen in those patients who survive into early adult life: lactic acid competes with uric acid for excretion by the kidney (Handler, 1960), and in the presence of a raised blood lactate level uric acid is retained in the blood and deposited as tophi in the large joints and in the skin. Thus the pain and discomfort of gout are added to these unfortunate patients' other symptoms (Kolb et al., 1955; Jeune et al., 1957; Howell et al., 1960; Holling, 1963; Powell et al., 1965). Renal excretion of uric acid is further diminished by the ketoacids which are frequently present in the blood of these patients (Goldfinger et al., 1965) and in addition there is some evidence that the biosynthesis of uric acid is also increased, possibly as the result of increased pentose cycle activity (Alepa et al., 1967).

Biochemical Diagnosis

(a) Glycogen content and structure. A normal liver may have a glycogen content of up to 5% of fresh weight, although in human liver obtained at operation the glycogen content rarely exceeds 3% of fresh weight. In Type I glycogenosis the glycogen content exceeds 5% but its fat content may be even greater. It is therefore preferable to refer glycogen content to a unit of nitrogen, protein or DNA, to avoid an underestimate of glycogen content due to "dilution" of the tissue with fat or other pathological material.

Glycogen from affected livers was isolated by Illingworth & Cori (1952) and shown to have a normal structure by complete degradation with phosphorylase and "debranching enzyme". More recently Manners (1964), using different enzymic and physical methods, has confirmed that the degree of branching and the length of outer chains of the glycogen from affected livers is the same as that present in normal livers.

Statistically, the glycogen content of muscle is not significantly greater than in normal muscle obtained under comparable conditions (Hers, 1964b). In individual cases, however, muscle

glycogen content may be moderately increased and this increase has been attributed to gluconeogenesis from lactate, induced by chronic hyperlacticacidaemia (Mahler, 1966a).

(b) Enzyme studies. In man, glucose-6-phosphatase activity is normally present in liver, kidney and intestinal mucosa (Williams et al., 1963a; Öckerman, 1964); it has been demonstrated histochemically in pancreatic islet cells (Lazarus, 1959), and is probably present in blood platelets (Linneweh et al., 1963a).

Glucose-6-phosphatase activity can be recognized in human embryonic liver as early as the tenth week of gestation (Villee, 1954). The influence of dietary variations and of hormones on its activity and its role in carbohydrate metabolism have been reviewed in detail by Ashmore & Weber (1959).

Enzyme activity in tissue homogenates is assayed by measuring the liberation of inorganic phosphate from glucose-6-phosphate at pH 6·5 (de Duve et al., 1949). The enzyme is easily destroyed if the tissue is not frozen quickly and partial loss of activity through inexpert handling may account for the wide variations observed in tissues obtained from normal human subjects. It is therefore very important to take a critical view of reports of "diminished" activity of this enzyme in glycogen storage diseases and to consider also the general problem of the mode of defining enzyme activity in pathological tissues, where "fresh weight" may contain a great deal of abnormal material such as glycogen or fat: "fresh weight" as a reference standard may therefore give an underestimate of enzyme activity. Moreover, because the liver of these patients is enlarged, it may well be that total glucose-6-phosphatase activity in the whole liver is normal or even greater than normal, even though "diminished activity" was found in the biopsy specimen. For these reasons, a diagnosis of Type I glycogen storage disease should only be based on the complete absence of glucose-6-phosphatase activity in tissue known to have been frozen immediately after taking the biopsy.

Although it is reasonable to infer that total absence of glucose-6-phosphatase activity implies that the enzyme protein itself is absent through a genetic defect of its synthesis, this has not yet been proven by immunochemical studies, as has been done in the case of other types of glycogenoses (Robbins, 1960; Layzer et al., 1967).

It is not entirely clear why the absence of glucose-6-phosphatase should result in an abnormal accumulation of glycogen. The enzyme is not directly concerned with glycogen synthesis or degradation, and there is no accumulation of glucose-6-phosphate in the affected liver (Hers, 1964a) which would cause an increase in activity of glycogen synthetase. Furthermore, there is no glucose-6-phosphatase activity in experimentally induced rat hepatomas, and yet their glycogen content is their very low (Ashmore & Weber, 1959). Further quantitative studies in the glycogen storage diseases on the inter-relationship of the various enzyme systems concerned with glycogen synthesis and degradation may eventually provide a better insight into the control of metabolic processes in normal conditions.

(c) *Functional tests.* Procedures which result in glycogenolysis or conversion of other hexoses to glucose normally produce a rise of the blood glucose level. In the absence of glucose-6-phosphatase, this response cannot take place but lactate is formed in excessive quantities (Table 4.2), which may sometimes be enough to aggravate a pre-existing acidaemia. It is therefore important to exercise care when carrying out these tests, particularly in very young children.

Adrenaline and Glucagon. Both hormones stimulate glycogenolysis through an action on phosphorylase. Glucagon is preferred for the test because it stimulates liver, but not skeletal muscle phosphorylase, and has none of the side effects of

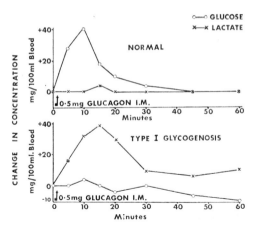

FIG. 4.9. In Type I glycogen storage disease, blood glucose does not rise after the injection of glucagon, but there is a sharp rise in blood lactate.

adrenaline. For the test, 0·5 mg. glucagon is given intramuscularly and serial blood samples obtained at 15 min. intervals over 2 hr. In glucose-6-phosphatase deficiency, there is usually no rise in blood glucose but there is always a significant rise in blood lactate during the first hour, and a concomitant fall in pH and plasma bicarbonate (Fig. 4.9). Occasionally a transitory

TABLE 4.2

Summary of the metabolic responses in the six types of glycogen storage disease

Type	I.V. Fructose or Galactose		Glucagon		Glycogen structure	Fat Metabolism	Blood lactate after ischaemic muscle exercise
I	Glucose Lactic acid	O ++	Glucose Lactic acid	O ++	Normal	All plasma lipids very high	Normal
II	Glucose Lactic acid	+ +	Glucose Lactic acid	+ +	Normal	Normal	Normal
III	Glucose	+	Glucose Fasting Post prandial	O +	Short outer chains	High fasting FFA	No rise
IV	Glucose	+	Glucose	±	Very long outer chains	Not reported	Not reported
V	Glucose Lactic acid	+ +	Glucose Lactic acid	+ +	Normal	High FFA uptake by muscle after exercise	No rise
VI	Glucose	+	Glucose	O	Normal	High cholesterol and neutral fats	Normal

O = No increase   ± = Poor increase
+ = Normal increase   ++ = Excessive increase

rise of the blood glucose level may be observed, particularly if the test is carried out within 1–2 hr. after a meal; it is probably due to glucose which has been liberated through the action of "de-branching enzyme" on newly synthesized outer branches of the glycogen molecule.

Conversion of Fructose and Galactose to Glucose

The fructose tolerance test (Hers & Malbrain, 1959) and the galactose tolerance test (Schwartz *et al.*, 1957) are probably the most useful functional tests for diagnosing the absence of glucose-6-phosphatase; no "false positives" have been reported with these two tests.

Fructose (0·5 g./kg. body weight) or galactose (1 g./kg. body weight) is rapidly given intravenously as a 25% solution. Blood samples are taken at 10 min. intervals for 1 hr. and glucose, lactate and the respective hexose estimated. In glucose-6-phosphatase deficiency there is no rise in blood glucose after the injection of either of these sugars, but blood lactate rises sharply (Fig. 4.10). The rise of the blood lactate level is greater

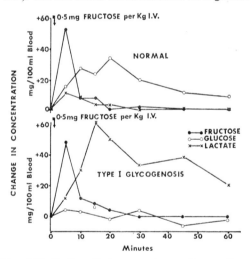

Fig. 4.10. In Type I glycogen storage disease, there is no rise in blood glucose after the infusion of fructose, but the lactate level rises considerably. Fructose disappearance from the blood is not delayed.

after fructose than after galactose and increases the risk of aggravating the existing acidosis; but the galactose test is more easily disturbed by other hepatic dysfunctions and may therefore sometimes give an apparently poor response. Impairment of hepatic function in that case will be evident from the peristence of a high blood galactose level.

Other Biochemical Studies

The glycogen content of erythrocytes (Sidbury *et al.*, 1961*a*) and of leucocytes (Williams & Field, 1963) is normal in patients suffering from glucose-6-phosphatase deficiency, but blood platelets, which normally exhibit some glucose-6-phosphatase activity, are said to have a raised glycogen content and loss of glucose-6-phosphatase activity (Linneweh *et al.*, 1963*b*).

Biochemical Genetics

The disease is transmitted as an autosomal recessive character. It is clearly not justifiable to investigate asymptomatic carriers of the trait by liver or kidney biopsy, but intestinal biopsy has come to be regarded as ethically acceptable and a significant decrease in intestinal glucose-6-phosphatase activity has been described in biopsies obtained from the parents of patients (Field *et al.*, 1965; Williams *et al.*, 1963*a*).

The claim by Hsia & Kot (1959) that heterozygous carriers could be detected by an increase in the glucose-6-phosphate content of erythrocytes could not be confirmed by Sokal *et al.* (1961) or by Oei (1962), but it has been reported (Linneweh *et al.*, 1963*b*) that heterozygotes have a higher than normal glucose-6-phosphate content in their blood platelets. The response of blood glucose to glucagon is too variable even in normal people to permit detection of a partial response which may occur in heterozygous carriers.

Course and Treatment

In general, the prognosis is poor in young children, but with careful management they may survive beyond their fourth year, and then the clinical manifestations of the disease tend to become milder (van Creveld, 1963). This may result from some adaptation of their metabolism to alternate pathways, although the primary biochemical lesion remains unaltered.

Prevention of hypoglycaemic episodes and maintenance of a normal blood glucose level may be attained by frequent feeding throughout the 24-hr. period, and it may be necessary to do this through the night as well as by day. The quantity and type of food must be geared to the child's requirements for growth and development, but an excess will inevitably result in deposition of more fat and glycogen. It is probably better to provide carbohydrate in the form of polymers of glucose, such starch, as or liquid glucose, than as milk and fruit which contain galactose and fructose, and are readily converted to glycogen and lactic acid.

Low urinary pH and ketonuria are a rough guide to the degree of acidosis, which, if necessary, may be corrected by adding sodium bicarbonate (0·2 to 0·4 g./kg./day) to the diet. Because the liver is already unable to metabolize lactate in the normal manner, lactate should never be given in an attempt to correct the acidosis.

Temporary benefit has been obtained from various forms of hormonal treatment. These have included glucagon, given several times per day, or a single injection of a long-acting zinc-glucagon, various steroids, and thyroxine. Although it is always worthwhile trying any of these methods in any particular patient, their beneficial action is unpredictable and inconsistent.

A paradoxical effect of alcohol, which may have therapeutic implications, was observed by Lowe & Mosovich (1965). In four patients infusions of alcohol resulted in a marked decrease in lacticacidaemia and in an increased responsiveness to glucagon, but to date there have been no further reports of this unexpected observation.

More recently an attempt has been made to by-pass the liver by anastomozing the portal vein to the vena cava to carry glucose absorbed from the intestine directly into the systemic circulation (Riddell & Davies, 1966). When examined 6 months after the operation, the child had grown 2 inches in height, was free of hypoglycaemic episodes on a normal diet and was able to attend an ordinary primary school.

In the not-too-distant future it may be possible to graft a liver from a normal donor (perhaps a pig) to provide a more "physiological hepatic glucose output" and to remove lactic acid from the circulation.

TYPE II GLYCOGENOSIS

Synonyms:

GENERALIZED GLYCOGENOSIS, POMPE'S DISEASE

In this disease, acid maltase is deficient and there is a great accumulation of glycogen in all the tissues of the body. Disturbances of carbohydrate or lipid metabolism are remarkable by their absence and the main symptoms are those of heart failure and muscular weakness, with death from heart failure at an early age.

Biochemical Basis of Clinical Manifestations

Perhaps the most remarkable aspect of this disease is the tremendous accumulation of glycogen in most of the tissues of the body with complete absence of any disturbance of carbohydrate metabolism. Its aetiology remained a mystery until 1963 when Hers reported that the lysosomes lacked their usual complement of α-1,4-glucosidase (Fig 4.11). The function of this enzyme in the removal of intracellular polysaccharides has been described on p. 99.

In most cases there is enlargement of the heart, and its glycogen content can become so great that it acts like a splint, preventing the myocardium from contracting efficiently, so causing heart failure. In some cases, the heart is less severely affected and the major affliction falls on skeletal muscle, causing mild to severe muscular weakness. One of the classical features of the disease is the grotesque enlargement of the tongue due to infiltration with glycogen.

α-1,4-glucosidase is not directly involved in glycolysis or gluconeogenesis and appears to play no role at all in glucose homeostasis. The body's

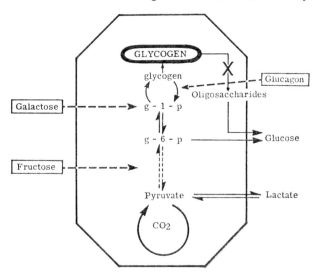

FIG. 4.11. Type II glycogen storage disease: there is no acid maltase in the lysomes. Glycogen is trapped in the lysosomes where it accumulates. Glycogen in the cytoplasm outside the lysosomes is accessible to the enzymes of the glycolytic pathway and there is no recognizable impairment of blood glucose metabolism.

metabolic requirements are met by glycogen which stays outside the lysosome and remains accessible to the enzymes of glycogenolysis.

Biochemical Diagnosis

(a) *Glycogen content and structure.* Glycogen accumulates in the lysosomes of most tissues and is separated from the cytoplasm by the lysosomal membrane. This prevents phosphorylase and other enzymes from degrading it so that glycogen accumulates in the lysosome until it becomes over-distended and ruptures; but before this happens, interference with the mechanical function of tissues may be sufficiently severe to cause the death of the patient.

The intravacuolar trapping of glycogen and the presence of free and metabolically available glycogen has been beautifully demonstrated by electron microscopy by Baudhuin *et al.* (1964).

The structure of the glycogen in Pompe's disease is normal (Hug, 1961). Progressive accumulation of glycogen was clearly demonstrated by Hug *et al.* (1966) who observed an increase of liver glycogen concentration from 6·6 to 10·6% over a period of 4 months.

(b) *Enzyme studies.* Hers (1963) described the properties of the enzyme after isolating it from lysosomes. Its action is that of a maltase, with a pH optimum of 4, which distinguishes it quite clearly from a neutral maltase found in the microsomal and soluble fraction of the cell. In human liver there is very little neutral maltase (Hers, 1964a) but its activity remains unchanged in the liver of patients with Type II glycogen storage disease (Hers, 1963).

The importance of acid maltase in preventing cells from becoming overdistended and damaged by glycogen is seen in glycogen storage diseases where other enzymes concerned with glycogenolysis are absent. In these diseases glycogen accumulation rarely exceeds 3 to 5% in muscle, in contrast to Pompe's disease, where failure of the lysosomal mechanism allows glycogen to accumulate to more than 10% of the weight of the muscle.

The enzyme must have some action in addition to the hydrolytic splitting of 1,4-linkages, because it can degrade the glycogen molecule completely which also contains 1,6 linkages at its branch points. But whether this action is carried out by the same enzyme or whether there is a 1,6-glucosidase associated with the α-1,4-glucosidase has not yet been resolved.

α-1,4-glucosidase activity in tissues from normal human subjects is greatest in the kidney, and is 5 to 10 times greater there than in liver, lung and

adrenals. Brain, heart, muscle, skin and adipose tissues have activities which are about 5 to 10% of that of liver. Normal leucocytes also contain α-1,4-glucosidase (Steinitz & Rutenberg, 1967). In three children with Pompe's disease studied by Steinitz &Rutenberg (1967), α-1,4-glucosidase activity was absent or very low in all tissues except the kidney but kidney glycogen content was normal. This may represent a special subtype of Type II glycogenosis, because kidney glycogen concentration was high in all other reported cases.

(c) *Functional tests.* There is no hypoglycaemia after fasting nor any other recognizable disturbance of carbohydrate metabolism.

Injections of glucagon and adrenaline, and galactose infusions all give a normal hyperglycaemic response, and there is a normal rise in blood lactate after ischaemic exercise (Mahler, 1966b).

Biochemical Genetics

Complete absence of α-1,4-glucosidase activity in leucocytes was reported in a patient at the age of 3 weeks by Huijing *et al.* (1963), before there had been sufficient time for much glycogen to accumulate in the tissues and this has also been found in other cases (Steinitz & Rutenberg, 1967). Examination of leucocyte α-1,4-glucosidase activity in both parents and one sibling of an affected child gave results which were intermediate between normal values and those obtained in patients with Pompe's disease; in another case the mother had normal leucocyte activity and the father an intermediate one. The disease is familial and as many as three affected siblings have been reported in a single family. It is probable that the disease is a genetically determined, autosomal recessive disorder.

Clinical Course

Death is usually due to heart failure or respiratory infection at an early age. However, a number of cases with a milder form of the disease have been described in which the heart was only slightly affected or not at all, and most of the clinical features were due to involvement of skeletal muscle. One child which died at the age of 4 years, had no cardiac enlargement, but had severe muscular hypotonia and was mentally retarded. There was no α-1,4-glucosidase in its tissues, but the muscle contained glycogen with abnormally short outer branches, which was attributed to the unusually high concentration of a neutral maltase in the muscles (Smith *et al.*, 1966).

There is no effective form of treatment, but

in one patient liver glycogen decreased after intramuscular injection of purified α-glucosidase (Baudhuin *et al.*, 1964).

TYPE III GLYCOGENOSIS

Synonyms:

DEBRANCHER DEFICIENCY,

AMYLO-1,6-GLUCOSIDASE DEFICIENCY,

LIMIT DEXTRINOSIS

In this disease the polysaccharide which accumulates in tissues through lack of debranching enzyme activity, has a structure that differs from normal glycogen and from the glycogen isolated from other forms of glycogenoses, in having short outer branches resembling a dextrin which is produced when the action of phosphorylase is allowed to continue until it reaches its limit: hence the name "limit dextrinosis" (Fig 4·12).

Biochemical Basis of Clinical Manifestations

In this disease the breakdown of the glycogen molecule is incomplete during fasting or with other glycogenolytic stimuli (adrenaline, glucagon). Thus glycogen accumulates because, as long as glucose is available, the chains of 1,4-linked glucose units elongate until they reach a critical length when a new 1,6-linked branch point is formed; the glycosyl chain proximal to this new branch point is then permanently trapped behind it.

Hepatic gluconeogenesis from hexoses and amino acids is not interfered with in any way and it is therefore not difficult to maintain the blood sugar at near normal levels even during fasting. There is consequently much less distur-

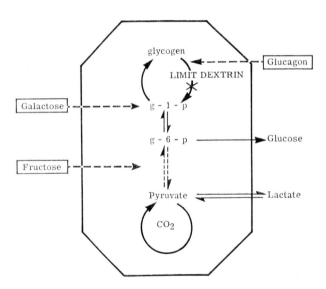

FIG. 4.12. Type III glycogen storage disease: debranching enzyme is deficient in liver and muscle. The glycogen molecule has short outer chains and resembles a dextrin.

The clinical manifestations of this disease are not as severe as those of Type I glycogenosis, but otherwise they are quite similar. Earlier descriptions of the hepatomegalic forms of glycogen storage disease did not distinguish "debrancher' from glucose-6-phosphatase deficiency. A few years ago van Creveld was able to re-examine two surviving patients whom he had described more than 30 years earlier and established that they were suffering from Type III glycogen storage disease (van Creveld, 1963; van Creveld & Huijing, 1964).

The usual clinical features of the disease are hepatomegaly and moderate hypoglycaemia on fasting, but a form presenting clinically as a myopathy has also been described (Oliner *et al.*, 1961).

bance of glucose homeostasis than in Type I glycogen storage disease and all other manifestations are less severe.

The liver is enlarged and contains a high percentage of limit dextrin, but its fat content is either normal or only moderately increased. The polysaccharide is also found in many other tissues, including erythrocytes and leucocytes, because the enzyme probably occurs in all tissues which are capable of forming glycogen. Lactic acidosis, which is often a serious complication of Type I glycogen storage disease, is not a feature of limit dextrinosis, probably because the amount of glycogenolysis is limited by the absence of "debranching enzyme".

Clinical manifestations of muscle involvement appear to be rare although a limit dextrin can be detected in the muscles of the majority of patients. The patient described by Oliner *et al.* (1961) showed many of the features of McArdle's disease (see p. 112), in particular, the absence of lactic acid production after ischaemic exercise. The myopathic type of limit dextrinosis may be one of the three forms postulated by Hers (1961), the other two being a pure hepatic and a hepatic-plus-muscular type, neither of which show clinical involvement of muscles (van Hoof & Hers, 1967). The severe myopathic form may be due to the absence of both amylo-1,6-glucosidase and transferase, the milder muscular forms being due to the absence of only one of the enzymes concerned with the debranching of glycogen.

Biochemical Diagnosis

(*a*) *Glycogen content and structure.* The amount of limit dextrin which accumulates in liver, muscle and myocardium (Illingworth, 1961) is quite considerable and often exceeds 10% of fresh weight. Erythrocytes (Sidbury *et al.*, 1961*b*) and leucocytes (Williams *et al.*, 1963*b*) also contain an excess of the abnormal glycogen. Hers (1964*a*) distinguishes at least two types of limit dextrinosis: in Type A, the content of limit dextrin is high in both liver and muscle and in Type B it is high in liver, but there is only a moderate amount in skeletal muscle. Type A occurs about three times as often as type B and all other subgroups together (van Hoof & Hers, 1967).

The abnormal structure of the glycogen was first described by Illingworth & Cori (1952) who subjected the polysaccharide, which they had isolated from affected tissues, to phosphorylase degradation. It yielded only a small amount (10 to 20%) of glucose-1-phosphate, which indicated that the outer chains consisted of short 1,4-linked glycosyl units. Normal human glycogen yields 28 to 34% of its glycogen as glucose-1-phosphate on degradation with phosphorylase. It was on the basis of this observation that Illingworth and Cori suggested that limit dextrinosis is caused by the absence of the "debranching enzyme".

(*b*) *Enzyme studies.* The development of a specific assay for the activity of amylo-1,6-glucosidase (Illingworth *et al.*, 1956) confirmed the suggestion that limit dextrinosis is due to the absence of "debranching enzyme".

The original assay technique was somewhat cumbersome, but recently Hers *et al.* (1967) described several elegant techniques depending upon incorporation of ^{14}C-glucose into the 1,6-links of glycogen, or on the release of ^{14}C glucose from labelled glycogen.

As indicated in the section on glycogen degradation, "debranching enzyme" appears to consist of two intimately associated enzymes, an amylo-1,6-glucosidase, the true debrancher, and a transferase (Brown & Illingworth, 1962). It may well be that there is a form of limit dextrinosis due only to transferase deficiency, but a separate assay for this enzyme would require the preparation of a polysaccharide with a very specific structure to act as substrate (Abdullah *et al.*, 1964), and this has not been accomplished yet.

Absence of "debranching enzyme" activity has been reported in liver, muscle, myocardium, erythrocytes and leucocytes of patients suffering from limit dextrinosis, but absence of the enzyme protein has not yet been demonstrated.

(*c*) *Functional tests.* Hypoglycaemia on fasting is usually the presenting symptom.

Glucagon. Stimulation of hepatic glycogenolysis with glucagon can be very helpful in diagnosis, as long as the result of the test is interpreted with care. In the fasting state, when the outer chains of the glycogen molecule are short, the blood sugar level does not rise in response to glucagon; but when the test is performed 2 or 3 hr. after a meal, when glycogen synthesis has lengthened the outer glycogen chains, there is a normal rise in blood sugar within 30 min. of the injection, because phosphorylase now has an adequate amount of 1,4-linked glycosyl units on which to act.

Conversion of Galactose and Fructose to Glucose

The intravenous injection of either of these hexoses results in a normal rise in blood sugar but without a rise in blood lactate. This indicates that conversion to glucose-6-phosphate is possible, and that there is normal hepatic glucose-6-phosphatase activity (Fig. 4.12).

Other Biochemical Tests

Polysaccharides react with iodine to give compounds which range in colour from red through various transitional colours to the deep blue of the starch-iodine complex, each with characteristic absorption spectrum (Krisman, 1962). Dextrins with very short outer chains (4 to 6 glucose units) have an absorption maximum at about 390 mμ, those with outer chains of normal length (8 to 12 units) give a red colour with an absorption peak at 460 mμ, while the long straight chains of starch have an absorption peak at 600 mμ. It is therefore possible to make a presumptive diagnosis of limit dextrinosis from a spectrophotometric analysis of the colour produced by staining the glycogen with iodine.

Biochemical Genetics

From an analysis of family histories it seems probable that the disease is inherited through a single recessive autosomal gene. In Hers' Type A, in which both liver and muscle are affected, the same gene probably controls the synthesis of "debranching enzyme" in both tissues, but the existence of Type B (only liver affected) complicates the situation and further studies are needed to determine whether the enzymes in the different tissues are under the same or separate genetic control.

It is possible to identify heterozygous carriers (parents of affected children) by the decrease in their leucocytes of amylo-1,6-glucosidase activity to about 50%, measured by a method which employs the incorporation of ^{14}C-glucose into glycogen (Chayoth et al., 1967). There is considerable variation of enzyme activity in leucocytes obtained from normal subjects and from heterozygous carriers, so that it is not possible to identify with absolute certainty any given individual heterozygote. The unaffected siblings of patients with Type III glycogenosis have also been studied and, statistically, the mean activity of amylo-1,6-glucosidase in their leucocytes falls between that of normals and that of heterozygous carriers, as would be expected on the basis that the siblings represent a mixture of normals and heterozygotes. Similar results have been reported by van Hoof (1967) for erythrocytes.

Course and Treatment

The chances of survival are good and some of van Creveld's own cases have lived for more than 30 years after the disease had first been diagnosed, albeit incorrectly (van Creveld, 1963); several cases have been discovered quite accidentally in their teens during investigations for some minor intercurrent illness. Growth and general development tend to be delayed in the first three or four years, but if the children are well cared for until then, most of their symptoms and signs disappear and mental development proceeds rapidly and becomes appropriate for their age. The liver diminishes in size, but usually remains palpable. In spite of the amelioration of the clinical features of the disease, the enzyme defect persists and was still present in fresh biopsies obtained in 1962 from van Creveld's early cases. The patient with severe myopathy described by Oliner et al. (1961) had no symptoms

until he was about 30 years old, but from then on his myopathy progressed slowly and relentlessly.

Maintenance of a normal blood sugar level is not too difficult, but feeding at 3 to 4 hourly intervals, including during the night, is often necessary in the first one or two years of life. Any excess carbohydrate is converted to glycogen in the liver, and the newly formed glycosyl units may then be trapped behind branch points. It may therefore be advisable to give injections of glucagon immediately after the main meals to prevent the outer chains of glycosyl units from lengthening sufficiently for a new branch point to be formed. Protein and amino acids in the diet are preferable to carbohydrate, because they can sustain the blood glucose level through gluconeogenesis although if given in excess, they too will be converted to glycogen. In a child with frequent and severe hypoglycaemic episodes, Starzl et al. (1965) anastomosed the portal vein to the inferior vena cava to by-pass the liver and distribute glucose absorbed from the intestine directly through the systemic circulation. They claimed an "encouraging result" for the operation in this patient.

TYPE IV GLYCOGENOSIS

Synonyms:

"BRANCHING ENZYME" DEFICIENCY
AMYLO-1,4→1,6-TRANSGLUCOSYLASE DEFICIENCY,
ANDERSEN'S DISEASE, AMYLOPECTINOSIS

In this disease a polysaccharide with an abnormal structure is deposited in tissues. It has long outer chains resembling a starch-like amylopectin and is probably formed through lack of the enzyme responsible for the formation of 1,6-linked branch points (Fig. 4.13). Hepatosplenomegaly, portal hypertension, ascites and jaundice are the clinical features of the disease and death occurs from hepatic failure at an early age.

Only two cases of this form of glycogen storage disease have been reported in the literature in detail (Anderson, 1952; Sidbury et al., 1962), and it is possible that the three patients described by Craig & Uzman (1958) as suffering from "a metabolic disorder with storage of an unusual polysaccharide complex" may also be cases of amylopectinosis.

Andersen's patient had been diagnosed during life as suffering from von Gierke's disease, and it was not until after the post-mortem examination when the liver glycogen was stained with iodine, that the structural abnormality of the glycogen was first suspected.

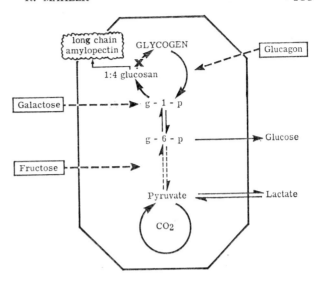

FIG. 4.13. Type IV glycogen storage disease: branching enzyme is absent. The glycogen molecule has abnormally long outer chains, but some degree of branching is present in the inner chains of the molecule.

Sidbury and his colleagues recognized the structural abnormality of glycogen isolated from the erthyrocytes four years before the child's death (Sidbury *et al.*, 1962), and attempted to delay the development of hepatic cirrhosis with steroid therapy.

Biochemical Basis of Clinical Manifestations

The clinical manifestations are those of hepatic cirrhosis. Fasting blood sugar levels are within normal limits, because there is no interference with gluconeogenesis.

Andersen suggested that the starch-like amylopectin in the liver may act as a foreign body which incites a fibrotic reaction, but if that were so it is surprising that a similar foreign body reaction is not observed in muscle, heart and other tissues where the same material is deposited. An alternative explanation offered by Sidbury *et al.* (1962) is that the cirrhosis is the result of liver cell malnutrition as in portal cirrhosis occurring in alcoholics.

Biochemical Diagnosis

(*a*) *Glycogen content and structure.* There is no excess of "glycogen" in the tissues, and, indeed, its concentration may be low. The abnormality resides rather in the structure of the glycogen, which is much less soluble in water than normal glycogen and has outer chains of 1,4-linked glycosyl units which are about twice as long as normal, as is shown by the fact that phosphorylase, acting alone, can degrade as much as

50% of the glycogen molecule (Illingworth & Cori, 1952).

Amylopectin accumulates not only in liver and red blood cells, but also in skeletal and smooth muscle, heart, renal tubules, reticulo-endothelial cells and spinal cord.

(*b*) *Enzyme studies.* Although the disease has been attributed to deficiency of the "branching enzyme", this was not confirmed by enzyme assay but only inferred from the structure of the deposited material. However, while it is true that the degree of branching of this polysaccharide is less than that of normal glycogen, the material does, nevertheless, exhibit a significant degree of branching overall and its abnormal structure is therefore probably not just due to the absence of branching enzyme.

In 1966, Brown referred to another patient, an 8-year old American Indian girl, in whom the diagnosis of "branching enzyme deficiency" was firmly established (Brown & Brown, 1966). Analysis of the liver glycogen showed that its outer chains were very long, resembling amylopectin, but that the inner chains were of approximately normal length, i.e. there were plenty of branch-points in the whole molecule. The enzyme was assayed directly by measuring the amount of glucose-1-phosphate polymerized. There was no measurable activity of the "branching enzyme" in liver or in leucocytes which confirmed the diagnosis, but the problem of the partial branching of the polysaccharide remains unsolved. There are probably two different branching enzymes, each having different specificities with regard to the length of the donor-chain, analogous to the "debranching enzyme" which also seems to consist of two functional and perhaps structural entities (Brown & Illingworth, 1966).

The activity of other enzymes in the liver has also been assayed and found to be decreased. But the results were referred to "fresh weight of tissue" and may therefore be misleading because of the presence of deposited material and fibrous tissue; in addition, the steroids which were used as therapy may also have had an influence on enzyme activities (Sidbury *et al.*, 1962).

(*c*) *Functional tests. Glucagon and adrenaline:* Intravenous injections of glucagon (100 μg./kg.) gave a poor response, but a somewhat better rise in blood sugar occurred after adrenaline. No completely satisfactory explanation can be offered for these results.

Other Biochemical Studies

Histochemical staining of the deposited material with iodine gives a characteristic lavender colour which can be identified spectrophotometrically by its peak absorption of light at 550 mμ, compared with that of a normal glycogen-iodine complex at 460 mμ (Illingworth & Cori, 1952).

The patients described by Craig & Uzman (1958), who may also have been cases of Type IV glycogenosis, had deposits of a material in their livers which was considered to be a mucopolysaccharide.

Oral and intravenous glucose tolerance showed no abnormality. All liver function tests were seriously impaired and serum transaminase levels were high. Blood lactate was not raised, there was no acidosis and the blood uric acid level was normal.

Biochemical Genetics

The brother of Andersen's patient died at the age of 7 months from an unspecified glycogen storage disease with clinical and histological features similar to those of his brother in whom the stored material had been characterized as amylopectin; two other pairs of siblings were referred to in Andersen's unpublished material (cited by Sidbury *et al.*, 1962). The patients described by Craig & Uzman (1958) were also related.

It may therefore be inferred that this is an inherited metabolic disorder, although its mode of inheritance cannot be determined on the information available. The red blood cells of the parents of these children have not been examined for the presence of amylopectin.

Course and Treatment

The two cases reported in detail died of progressive cirrhosis at the age of 17 and 42 months, but two of Andersen's patients reached the age of 11 and 12 years. Sidbury *et al.* (1962) attempted to delay the onset of portal fibrosis by treating the child with steroids to the point of inducing Cushingoid features, but it is impossible to decide whether the treatment had had any influence; it certainly did not prevent the eventual death from cirrhosis.

On theoretical grounds it should be possible to prevent excessive accumulation of glycogen by treatment with glucagon to prevent elongation of glycosyl chains.

It would also seem rational to attempt to prevent the development of portal cirrhosis with a porto-caval shunt. This diverts glucose from the liver and reduces the deposition of amylopectin and will also relieve portal pressure if that is already raised.

TYPE V GLYCOGENOSIS

Synonyms:

MUSCLE PHOSPHORYLASE DEFICIENCY,
MCARDLE'S DISEASE

This disease is due to the absence of phosphorylase in skeletal muscle, and glycogen accumulation is restricted to this tissue (Fig 4.14).

The first patient with this disease was described in 1951 by McArdle who made the important observation that glycogenolysis did not occur in the patient's forearm muscles after ischaemic exercise. In 1959 two further cases were reported independently by Schmid & Mahler, and by Mommaerts *et al.* and in both cases the metabolic lesion was shown to be due to the absence of muscle phosphorylase. The enzymic lesion was subsequently confirmed in McArdle's own patient (Mahler & McArdle, 1960), and since then more than 20 further cases have been reported in the literature.

McArdle's disease was the first example of a myopathy which could be clearly related to the absence of a single, specific enzyme. The elucidation of the enzyme defect came at a time when the biological importance of the newly-discovered pathway of glycogen synthesis via UDPG-glycogen synthetase had not yet been established in man, and provided a perfect model for illustrating in living tissues that glycogen synthesis and breakdown take place along different pathways. At the same time the knowledge of the existence of the phosphorylase-independent pathway of glycogen synthesis helped to explain how glycogen could accumulate in the patients' muscles in the absence of phosphorylase.

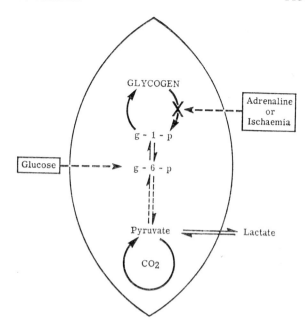

FIG. 4.14. Type V glycogen storage disease: phosphorylase is absent in muscle, but not in the liver.

Biochemical Basis of Clinical Manifestation

The main symptoms of McArdle's disease are pain and stiffness in muscles after moderately severe exercise. These symptoms are proportional to the severity and duration of the exercise and occur most commonly in the limb muscles, but other skeletal muscles such as the masseter may also become stiff and painful after arduous chewing. Steady, moderate exercise can be tolerated without trouble and even if some pain and stiffness do appear, they quite often disappear again as the exercise continues—a form of "second wind" (Pearson *et al.*, 1961).

McArdle observed localized swelling of muscles in his patient after ischaemic exercise and pressure on the muscle, and he noted that these swellings were electrically "silent", i.e. that the muscle at these sites was not actively contracting, but that true contracture of muscle fibres had taken place (McArdle, 1951). This observation, together with the failure of lactic acid production after ischaemia, suggested that glycolysis was blocked and that localized areas of ischaemic muscle might be in a state equivalent to "rigor mortis" (Bendall, 1960).

Energy for contraction is provided by a small store of creatine phosphate which is quickly exhausted, and also by a more sustained production of ATP (Szent-Györgyi, 1953), but ATP is also necessary for relaxation of muscle (Bendall, 1960). Most of the ATP is produced as a result of oxidation of fatty acids and glucose via the Krebs cycle, but in ischaemic conditions the only source of ATP is the metabolism of glycogen through the glycolytic pathway. As long as muscle blood flow, and hence oxygen supply, increases in proportion to the exercise, fatty acids are oxidized (Andres *et al.*, 1956), ATP can be produced and no physical difficulty will be encountered. In vigorous exercise, and especially on sustained contraction, blood flow becomes inadequate and muscle becomes relatively ischaemic. Glycogen, stored in the muscle fibres, now becomes the major and perhaps sole source for energy production by anaerobic glycolysis. In McArdle's disease, because of the absence of phosphorylase, the first step of glycogenolysis, the splitting of the 1,4 link between glucose units, cannot take place; no glucose-1-phosphate is produced; the glycolytic pathway is bereft of substrate and no ATP can be formed. The small store of creatine phosphate and ATP allows a few vigorous contractions to take place, but when this store is exhausted, the contracted muscle is unable to relax and remains in a rigor mortis-like contracture. Gradually, with the re-establishment of blood flow, relaxation occurs. The hyperaemia which follows ischaemic exercise in normal muscle, is usually attributed to the presence of intermediate metabolites of the glycolytic pathway. In McArdle's disease, muscle blood flow after ischaemic exercise is enormously increased – more than 5 times as much as in normal subjects (McArdle, 1951). It is clearly impossible to attribute this change to increased production of glycolytic metabolites in skeletal muscle, although the production of such metabolites in the smooth muscle of arterioles cannot be ruled out because it has been shown histochemically (Engel *et al.*, 1963) that this tissue does contain phosphorylase. Whatever the explanation, the greatly increased blood flow hastens recovery by bringing oxygen and fatty acids to the contracted muscle where they are extracted in large amounts (Mahler & McArdle, 1960) and oxidized to provide ATP for relaxation. The huge muscle blood flow after exercise may account in part for the severe dyspnoea which follows exercise (McArdle, 1951). Myocardial involvement has not been demonstrated by direct assay of myocardial phosphorylase, although in one patient suffering from McArdle's disease a conduction defect was displayed electrocardiographically (Ratinov *et al.*, 1965). It would be surprising if this were due directly to phosphorylase deficiency, because heart and muscle phosphorylase are immunologically distinct (Henion & Sutherland, 1957), and the production of the enzyme in each organ is therefore likely to be controlled by separate genes; for the same reason, liver phosphorylase is not affected in McArdle's disease.

Approximately a third of the reported cases have had episodes of myoglobinuria after severe exercise; but even in a given individual, this is not a constant feature and no satisfactory explanation has yet been found. It may be due to an abnormality of the muscle membrane and it is interesting in this context that the serum aldolase and creatine phosphokinase levels were grossly elevated in a patient after muscle biopsy (Mellick *et al.*, 1962).

Biochemical Diagnosis

(*a*) *Glycogen content and structure.* The glycogen content of muscle biopsies is usually about 3% of fresh weight, but in two patients it was within the normal range (about 1% of wet weight) (Mellick *et al.*, 1962; Engel *et al.*, 1963). The glycogen is structurally normal and is deposited in large amounts immediately below the sarcolemma and to a certain extent also between the myofibrils (Schmid & Mahler, 1959).

(*b*) *Enzyme studies.* Incubation of muscle homogenates with each of the glycolytic intermediates produced lactate, confirming that there was no block in the glycolytic pathway. Incubation without any addition or with the addition of purified glycogen did not produce lactate and direct assay for phosphorylase revealed that there was no enzyme activity in the muscle of these patients

(Schmid & Mahler, 1959; Mommaerts *et al.* 1959).

Absence of detectable phosphorylase activity may be due to a number of causes:

(1) Failure to convert inactive phosphorylase *b* to active phosphorylase *a* through lack of AMP or phosphorylase kinase. Assay for kinase activity in a patient's homogenate was normal, but the addition of AMP did not result in activation, suggesting that phosphorylase itself was absent.

(2) Activity affected by inhibitors: no inhibition was observed when pure crystalline phosphorylase was mixed with muscle homogenate.

(3) The enzyme protein may be absent because of a genetic failure: evidence from immunological studies using an antiphosphorylase serum confirmed that the enzyme protein was not present in muscle from a patient with McArdle's disease (Robbins, 1960).

These results are in keeping with the concept that McArdle's disease is a hereditary metabolic disorder. In fact, it is one of the few types of glycogen storage disease in which there is real evidence that the enzyme protein itself is absent and that the disease is not due to some factor inhibiting the action of the enzyme.

Phosphorylase activity in leucocytes is normal, and so is their glycogen content (Schmid & Mahler, 1959).

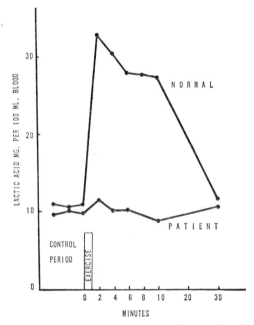

FIG. 4.15. Response to ischaemic exercise: in McArdle's disease there is no rise in blood lactate.

Other enzymes concerned with glycogen synthesis and degradation, including the "branching" and "debranching" enzymes, are all present and produce glycogen with a normal, branched structure and molecular aggregates which have a normal sedimentation coefficient (Bueding *et al.*, 1964).

(c) Functional tests. Ischaemic exercise. The test which led McArdle to postulate a block in the glycolytic pathway was the performance of ischaemic exercise in which there was no rise in the lactate concentration of venous blood coming from muscle (McArdle, 1951) (Fig. 4.15). This test is suggestive of phosphorylase deficiency but is not conclusive, as a block anywhere in the metabolic reactions which convert glycogen to lactate will give the same result. This has been described in a patient with Type III glycogenosis and also a patient whose muscles lacked phosphofructokinase (Oliner *et al.*, 1961; Layzer *et al.*, 1967).

Glucagon and adrenaline. Injections of glucagon and of adrenaline result in a normal blood glucose response, which confirms that hepatic phosphorylase activity is intact.

Other Biochemical Investigations

Incubation of whole blood produces a normal amount of lactic acid (McArdle, 1951). Myoglobinuria is inconstant, even in the same patient, after severe exercise.

Biochemical Genetics

Investigation of the family of the patient described by Schmid and Mahler revealed 3 affected cases among 13 siblings (Schmid & Hammaker, 1961). This and similar studies in other cases suggested that the disease is due to a single, recessive, autosomal gene. There is no simple test for detecting heterozygotes, because leucocyte phosphorylase is normal even in affected patients, and the lactate response to ischaemic exercise is too variable in normal subjects to permit identification of the heterozygous condition.

Course and Treatment

The disease may manifest itself early in life but usually the first symptoms begin during the second or third decade. In one family symptoms did not appear until both patients (brother and sister) were 49 years old (Engel *et al.*, 1963). Only a few patients have shown muscle wasting (Schmid & Mahler, 1959). Life expectancy is probably unimpaired, and McArdle's patient, who was first seen in 1949 when he was 30 years old, has now been observed for nearly 20 years without evidence of deterioration in muscle power beyond that expected from his age.

Temporary improvement of exercise tolerance can be achieved by giving glucose or fructose by mouth shortly before a strenuous bout of exercise, or by raising the blood sugar with an injection of glucagon (Schmid & Mahler, 1959). It has been suggested that fructose can be used directly by muscle (Pearson *et al.*, 1961; Mellick *et al.*, 1962), but Hers (1964*a*) believes that the improvement is more likely to be due to the rapid conversion in the liver of fructose to pyruvate which can then be used by the muscles.

Raising the plasma free fatty acid concentration also helps to provide the muscles with additional fuel for oxidation and formation of ATP. It is possible that the beneficial results from injections of glucagon and adrenaline are due as much to this effect as due to their hyperglycaemic effect. Ephedrine given orally, may also be effective (Mahler & McArdle, 1966).

TYPE VI GLYCOGENOSIS

Synonym:
HEPATIC PHOSPHORYLASE DEFICIENCY

This is a group of glycogen storage diseases rather than one specific and well-defined glycogenosis, in which liver glycogen concentration is high and liver phosphorylase activity low, but not absent (Hers, 1964*a*) (Fig. 4.16). Even this particular enzyme defect, which was first described by Hers in 1959, is not always present. In some clinically affected siblings of patients with phosphorylase deficiency, liver phosphorylase activity may be normal but one of the other enzymes of glycogen metabolism diminished. Hers (1964*a*) considers that approximately one third of all cases of glycogen storage disease seen by him belong to this rather ill-defined group.

Biochemical Basis of Clinical Manifestations

Hepatic glucose output in the fasting state depends upon the production of glucose from glycogen. Hypoglycaemia will ensue if phosphorylase activity is too low to allow adequate glycogenolysis to take place; it is unlikely, however, that hypoglycaemia from this cause alone would be severe, because the various pathways which permit gluconeogenesis from amino acids are not restricted. If hypoglycaemia is severe, it is probable that an associated enzyme defect is present. For instance, Sokal *et al.* (1961) and Illingworth & Brown (1964*a*) have described the association

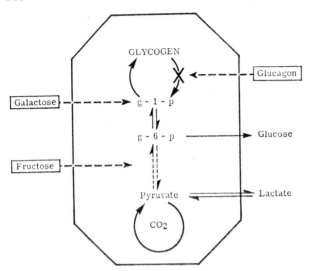

FIG. 4.16. Type VI glycogen storage disease: phosphorylase activity is diminished in the liver, but not in muscle.

of phosphorylase and glucose-6-phosphatase deficiency in children with severe hypoglycaemic episodes and other features of Type I glycogenosis.

Biochemical Diagnosis

(a) *Glycogen content and structure.* Increased liver glycogen concentration is perhaps one of the more consistent findings in this ill-defined group, but even this may not be the case when low liver phosphorylase activity is associated with some other enzyme defect, e.g. with glycogen synthetase deficiency (Parr *et al.*, 1965). To complicate the situation further, there is no clear division between normal and pathological concentrations of glycogen in the liver, and levels as high as 10% have been recorded after a meal in normal people (Young *et al.*, 1948). Muscle glycogen concentration remains normal in this group and erythrocyte and leucocyte glycogen is also normal. The structure of hepatic glycogen is normal.

(b) *Enzyme studies.* Phosphorylase activity in biopsy specimens of normal human liver is very variable and although in Hers' group of patients the mean phosphorylase activity was lower than normal, the difference was not significant. Nevertheless, in more than half the patients, liver phosphorylase activity was considerably less than normal. In view of the wide variations, a diagnosis of liver phosphorylase deficiency should not be made solely on the evidence of an enzyme assay, but clinical and genetic information must also be taken into account.

Liver phosphorylase exists in an active and an inactive form. The inactive form is converted to the active form by phosphorylase *b* kinase and a defect of the kinase system rather than of phosphorylase has recently been described in a child with progressive mental deterioration (Hug, 1967).

Leucocyte and liver phosphorylase have many properties in common and leucocyte phosphorylase activity is low in patients with a hereditary deficiency of liver phosphorylase (Hülsman *et al.*, 1961; Williams & Field, 1961). Although adrenal cortical phosphorylase also resembles liver phosphorylase (Riley & Haynes, 1963) no clinical manifestations of adrenal cortical dysfunction have been observed. Muscle phosphorylase is immunologically distinct from liver phosphorylase (Henion & Sutherland, 1957) and is therefore presumably under separate genetic control and its activity remains normal when liver phosphorylase activity is reduced.

(c) *Functional tests. Glucagon:* A poor hyperglycaemic response is usually obtained in patients in whom liver phosphorylase activity is low, but unfortunately this is not invariably the case in all patients of this group. Even in the same patient the response may sometimes be poor, and at other times normal.

Galactose infusion: A normal hyperglycaemic response is usually obtained unless an associated enzyme defect is present.

Biochemical Genetics

Low leucocyte phosphorylase activity has been found in the mother of each of 2 patients (Hülsmann *et al.*, 1961; Williams & Field, 1961), while the father's leucocytes had normal enzyme activity. This suggests a dominant form of inheritance and implies that not only the affected children, but also their clinically normal mothers were heterozygous for the abnormal gene. It is possible that the disease remained undetected during the mother's own childhood because of its mild and variable symptomatology.

Course and Treatment

No definite prognosis can be given in any one case but in general the disease is mild and there is no progressive deterioration. Heterozygous carriers for the gene can remain symptom-free and survive into adulthood and bear children. More severe symptoms and a poor prognosis are related to the simultaneous presence of other enzyme defects.

OTHER GLYCOGEN STORAGE DISEASES

Following the demonstration of a specific enzyme defect in McArdle's disease, the "index of suspicion" rose sharply and enzyme studies on muscle biopsies became much more frequent; and in a multi-enzyme system such as that concerned with glycogen metabolism, it was not surprising that within a short time several other enzyme defects were reported in myopathies in which storage of glycogen was also found.

Theoretically, a metabolic block anywhere in the glycolytic pathway between glycogen and pyruvate can lead to glycogen storage. To date, only two of the reported enzyme defects can be taken as proven; the others are less convincing and technical artefacts cannot be excluded.

PHOSPHOFRUCTOKINASE DEFICIENCY

There have been two detailed reports of patients in whom deficient phosphofructokinase activity in muscle appears to be the cause of a glycogen storage myopathy. One report (Tarui et al., 1965) deals with a Japanese family in which 3 siblings were shown to have almost complete lack of muscle phosphofructokinase, the other deals with one young American male (Layzer et al., 1967).

The clinical symptoms, which started in childhood, are similar to those of McArdle's disease, even to the extent of having occasional myoglobinuria after severe exercise. Cramp-like pain and stiffness in muscles after exercise are the cardinal features of the disease but at rest no abnormalities are detectable.

Biochemical Basis of Clinical Manifestations

The biochemical basis of the symptoms and signs in muscle phosphofructokinase deficiency is the same as in McArdle's disease, namely inadequate glycolysis when the muscle is relatively

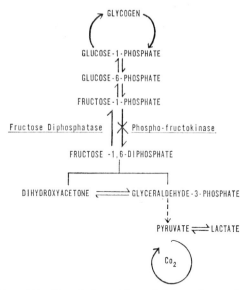

FIG. 4.17. Phosphofructokinase deficiency in muscle.

ischaemic and dependent for energy production solely on glycolysis (Fig. 4.17).

There are no clinical manifestations of carbohydrate intolerance or hypoglycaemia.

Biochemical Diagnosis

(a) *Glycogen content and structure.* Muscle contains more than twice the normal amount of glycogen. The structure of the glycogen is normal.

(b) *Enzyme assay.* Anaerobic glycolysis of muscle homogenate showed that lactate production from glycogen and hexose monophosphates was low, but that fructose-1,6-diphosphate was converted to lactate in quantities even greater than in normal controls.

When frozen muscle was analysed, it was observed that glycogen, glucose-1-phosphate and fructose-1-phosphate were present in excess, whereas fructose-1,6-diphosphate, the triose phosphates and pyruvate were present in amounts significantly less than in normal muscle. This suggested the presence of a block in the onward metabolism of fructose-1-phosphate and that the enzyme defect lay at the level of phosphofructokinase. Direct assay showed almost complete absence of phosphofructokinase activity (about 1% of normal).

In both studies, enzyme activity in the erythrocytes of affected patients was reported to be considerably less than normal (about 50%). The activity in leucocytes was normal (Layzer et al., 1967).

(c) *Functional tests*. The ischaemic exercise test as described by McArdle (1951) revealed a block in glycolysis by the absence of a rise in lactate concentration of blood coming from ischaemic muscles.

Biochemical Genetics

This is one of the few hereditary diseases in which absence of the muscle enzyme protein has been demonstrated by immunological techniques (Layzer *et al*., 1967).

Layzer and Rowland refer in their paper to immunological studies which suggest that human muscle, erythrocyte and brain phosphofructo-kinases are immunologically related, but are not identical. Erythrocyte enzyme activity was partly diminished but not blocked by muscle enzyme antibody, which suggests that the erythrocyte enzyme may be composed of "muscle" type as well as other subunits of the enzyme. Similarly, brain enzyme is likely to consist of "muscle" and other subunits and it is interesting to note that if the "muscle" subunit of the brain enzyme is deficient in these patients, it has no obvious metabolic or functional consequences.

Course and Treatment

All four cases were studied when they were in their late teens or older, but their symptoms had started in childhood. They showed no developmental abnormalities. No attempts at treatment have been reported. It would be interesting to observe the effect of fructose in these patients; if Hers' (1964a) view is correct that in McArdle's disease the improvement after fructose is indirectly due to its conversion to pyruvate in liver, then fructose could also be expected to help these patients. If, however, it is used directly by muscle, as suggested by Pearson & Rimer (1959) and by Mellick *et al*. (1962), then no benefit can be expected from its use in phosphofructokinase deficiency.

Measures designed to raise the plasma free fatty acid concentration should also be of some benefit.

PHOSPHOGLUCOMUTASE DEFICIENCY

A deficiency of this enzyme has been proposed as the possible cause of a glycogen storage disease in two patients (Thomson *et al*., 1963; Illingworth & Brown, 1964b). In Thomson's patient, the clinical manifestations were restricted to muscle, whereas the child described by Illingworth & Brown had marked hepatomegaly as well. Biochemical investigations and enzyme assays in the latter patient showed low phosphoglucomutase activity in liver and muscle, while glucose-6-phosphatase and muscle phosphorylase were normal. In Thomson's patient, the presence of other partial enzyme defects was inferred from incubation studies with various substrates, but only phosphorylase activity was assayed directly and found to be normal. If these observations are substantiated, it will be necessary to reconsider the pathway of the synthesis of glycogen from glucose when the conversion of glucose-6-phosphate to glucose-1-phosphate is throttled by the lack of the specific mutase (Fig. 4.1).

MULTIPLE ENZYME DEFICIENCIES ASSOCIATED WITH GLYCOGEN STORAGE

The familial occurrence of glycogen storage diseases and the demonstration of the absence of a specific enzyme protein is strong evidence that they are genetically determined. However, the demonstration of a single enzyme defect *in vitro* does not necessarily mean that it is the cause of the illness with which it is associated, nor does it preclude the presence of other biochemical abnormalities. It is therefore not entirely contrary to the "one gene, one enzyme" theory that several cases of glycogen storage disease have been reported in which there appear to be multiple enzyme defects. In none of these reports has the absence of the enzyme protein been proven, and in most cases enzyme activity was not completely absent, but only "diminished".

Enzymes work in a co-ordinated superstructure and not in isolated reactions and are kept in balance by a hierarchy of metabolic regulators such as hormones, co-enzymes and electrolytes. From the work of Jacob & Monod (1961) it is also probable that multi-enzyme systems develop in an integrated fashion, which is controlled by an "operon". The "operon" is thought to have overall control over the relative amounts in which all the enzymes concerned with glycogen catabolism are synthesized, and defects in its operation could account for multiple enzyme deficiencies.

Many enzymes exist in multiple molecular forms as isoenzymes, and the synthesis of each isoenzyme is probably under its own genetic control. It follows that the synthesis of a heterogeneous enzyme is controlled not by one single gene locus, but by several and that measurement of enzyme "activity" *in vitro* may not reflect the genetic abnormality. Cinader *et al*. (1966) have proposed a classification of various forms of protein polymorphism which is also applicable to hereditary enzyme defects:

(1) Proteins with similar functions may be present in all individuals of the species, but differ from one another in amino-acid sequences in limited regions of the molecule.

(2) A particular protein may be completely absent in different individuals.

(3) The quantity of the enzyme molecules may be severely diminished.

At present it is possible to demonstrate the defective action of an enzyme in the glycogen storage diseases, and in a few also the absence of the protein but not yet a defective structure. It is therefore not yet possible to express a definite view on the meaning of multiple enzyme defects in inborn errors of metabolism.

There are now several case reports of glycogen storage disease where two enzymes appear to be involved in the aetiology of the disease or where siblings do not always show the same enzyme defect (Lowe, et al., 1962; Calderbank, et al., 1960; Eberlein et al., 1962; Steinitz & Reisner, 1961; Abrahamov et al., 1961). There are many technical pitfalls in the biochemical analysis of tissue biopsies, particularly of pathological material, and it would be wise to be cautious before accepting in vitro evidence of deficient enzyme activity as equivalent to the genetically determined absence of that enzyme protein.

GLYCOGEN STORAGE DEFICIENCY DISEASE

Synonym:
GLYCOGEN SYNTHETASE DEFICIENCY

This disease was described and named in 1962 by Lewis et al. who found that liver glycogen synthetase activity was absent in a child with very low liver glycogen. A similar case, in which not only synthetase but also phosphorylase activity was absent in both liver and muscle, was reported more recently (Parr et al., 1965).

The clinical features of this disease are similar to those of Type I glycogenosis, with hypoglycaemia and secondary metabolic disturbances as the main features.

Biochemical Basis of Clinical Manifestations

In the absence of glycogen synthetase, glycogen cannot be stored in tissues and none is therefore available when it is needed to maintain hepatic glucose output during fasting. Nevertheless, it is not easy to explain the severity of the hypoglycaemia caused by fasting, because it should be possible to maintain a reasonable blood glucose level by gluconeogenesis (Fig. 4.7).

It was originally thought that poor gluconeogenesis might be caused by interference with steroid production in the adrenal cortex in which glycogen synthetase was also deficient. This suggestion, however, was not substantiated when it was found that fasting plasma cortisol levels were actually somewhat elevated (Spencer-Peet, 1964).

Mental deficiency is probably secondary to hypoglycaemia and was present in a pair of identical twins who had had frequent attacks of hypoglycaemia but is absent in their younger sister who has the same enzyme defect, but was protected against hypoglycaemia from birth by a careful dietary programme.

The other features, such as deposition of fat in the liver and ketosis, are evidence of disturbances of lipid metabolism secondary to hypoglycaemia.

Biochemical Diagnosis

(a) *Glycogen content.* The liver glycogen content in the first case was very low (0·45 g./100 g. wet weight) even though the blood sugar level had been maintained during the operation by an intravenous infusion of glucose. The lipid content of the liver was high (10%) (Lewis et al., 1963).

In the second case, liver and muscle glycogen were undetectable by chemical analysis and could not be demonstrated histochemically. No glycogen was found in kidney and adrenal gland when autopsy material was analysed, but marked "fatty metamorphosis" was seen in liver and kidney.

(b) *Enzyme studies.* Glycogen synthetase activity was not detectable in either case, even when assayed in the presence of glucose-6-phosphate which stimulates the synthetase.

In the first patient, liver phosphorylase and UDPG-pyrophosphorylase activities were within normal limits, but in the second patient there was an associated defect of both liver and muscle phosphorylase. Other enzymes concerned with glycogen synthesis were also reported to have low activities, but the extremely high fat content may have "diluted" these estimations.

Glucagon. Fasting caused a fall in blood glucose and in the fasting state there was no response to glucagon. In one of the children there was a normal response to glucagon after a meal (Spencer-Peet, 1964), which is difficult to explain, unless there had been some glycogen synthesis via phosphorylase in these circumstances. The child reported by Parr et al. (1965) did not have any injections of glucagon.

Biochemical Genetics

In the first family there were 3 affected children and one other child which became hypoglycaemic after fasting for 15 hr.; their father had glycosuria as a child and a "lag type" glucose tolerance curve.

In the second family, the disease was recognized only after death of one child which died aged 4 months and had three elder siblings who had died in early infancy with apnoea, coma and disturbances of the central nervous system. Fatty metamorphosis of the liver was present in these cases.

Course and Treatment

The first twins were not treated early enough to prevent repeated hypoglycaemic attacks and both now have permanent cerebral damage. Their younger sister, in whom hypoglycaemia was prevented from birth, has no evidence of mental defect.

Treatment rests on the prevention of hypoglycaemia by regular feeding at 6 hourly intervals by day and night.

GALACTOSAEMIA

Galactosaemia is a hereditary disorder due to an inborn error of metabolism which interferes with the conversion of galactose to glucose. The clinical consequences of the metabolic defect become apparent only when galactose is present in the diet, and are due to the intracellular accumulation of galactose-1-phosphate, an intermediate metabolite in the conversion of galactose to glucose. If the disorder is recognized early and a galactose-free diet instituted shortly after birth, no clinical manifestations develop, although the metabolic predisposition persists.

The first clear clinical description of the disease was given by von Reuss (1908), but Langstein & Steinitz (1906) had even earlier identified galactose as the sugar present in the urine of some breast-fed babies suffering from severe gastro-intestinal disorders. (It is also of interest, that the same investigators proved that lactase activity was normal in these children's intestinal fluid.)

Clinical Manifestations

At birth the infants appear quite normal, but within a few days or weeks of starting milk-feeds, irrespective of whether it is mother's or cow's milk, they become listless, begin to vomit and develop diarrhoea with all the clinical features of dehydration. If the disease is not recognized and milk is not withdrawn from the feeds, the liver and spleen become enlarged, jaundice develops, other signs of cirrhosis appear, and death may follow

quickly. In less severe cases, impaired growth and mental development become obvious by the second or third month, and cataracts may be detected in the eyes at an even earlier stage.

The course of the disease is often less severe and it may be some months before it is evident that the child is not thriving and developing at the proper pace, and the more striking features of the disease develop as the child continues to take milk-containing food.

The urine only contains galactose when there is galactose in the diet and during these episodes there is usually also some albumin and an excess of amino acids in the urine. But these renal abnormalities usually disappear when galactose is withdrawn from the diet.

Biochemical Basis of Clinical Manifestations

(a) *Normal galactose metabolism.* The metabolic pathway for galactose metabolism in microorganisms was established by Leloir and his associates (Caputto *et al.*, 1950) and its existence in man demonstrated by Kalckar *et al.* (1953).

In very young infants, the commonest source of galactose is lactose present in milk. The disaccharide lactose is split in the intestinal mucosa by the enzyme lactase to yield the monosacchrides glucose and galactose and both sugars are absorbed into the circulation.

In the cells the biologically important pathway of galactose utilization and its conversion to glucose occurs in four steps (Fig. 4.18). In galactosaemia, the enzymic failure is usually present at step 2, but recently a different type of galactosaemia has been described, which is due to a defect at the first metabolic step (Gitzelmann, 1965).

(1) Before galactose can take part in intracellular metabolic reactions, it must be phosphorylated by a galactokinase to yield galactose-1-phosphate.

(2) The next step is the transfer of the galactose moiety of galactose-1-phosphate to UDP-glucose with liberation of glucose-1-phosphate and formation of UDP-galactose. The reaction is catalyzed by the enzyme galactose-1-phosphate uridyl transferase.

(3) The galactose moiety combined with UDP in reaction 2 is then converted to UDP-glucose by a specific epimerase, UDP-galactose-4-epimerase, in the presence of NAD as co-enzyme. The enzyme derives its name from the fact that galactose is an epimer of glucose, differing in structure from glucose only at carbon-4.

(4) Finally, in a reaction which is not directly involved in the galactose-glucose interconversion,

UDP glucose is converted by a pyrophosphory-lase to glucose-1-phosphate which then enters the usual intracellular metabolic pathways.

Reaction 1 is irreversible *in vivo*, but the direction in which the other reactions may proceed depends on the metabolic state of the cell at any given time. Thus, in reaction 2, galactose-1-phosphate can be formed from glucose even when there is no galactose in the diet, and in reaction 3, UDP-galactose can be formed from UDP-glucose in similar circumstances. This makes it possible for galactose-containing compounds, such as the galactolipids of brain and structural galactose-containing polysaccharides such as chondroitin

and brain, but not in erythrocytes (Isselbacher, 1958; Ng *et al.*, 1964).

(ii) In erythrocytes, galactose-1-phosphate can be converted by phosphoglucomutase to galactose-6-phosphate (Posternak & Rosselet, 1954), which can then be oxidized to 6-phosphogalactonic acid by a hexose-6-phosphate dehydrogenase present in human erythrocytes (Inouye *et al.*, 1964) and in liver (Ohno *et al.*, 1966).

(iii) In liver cells, the enzyme galactose dehydrogenase can oxidize galactose to galactonic acid (Cuatrecasas & Segal, 1966), which is then converted to ketogalactonic acid and subsequently decarboxylated to xylulose.

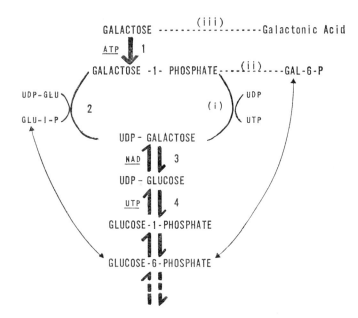

FIG. 4.18. Pathways of galactose metabolism. Steps 1, 2, 3, 4, are important in the conversion of galactose to glucose. Steps (i), (ii) and (iii) are alternate pathways which may be of some importance in galactosaemia.

sulphate to be synthesized from glucose in the complete absence of galactose from dietary sources. In reaction 4, UDP-glucose which is required in reactions 2 and 3, and also in the synthesis of glycogen and other polysaccharides, can be regenerated from glucose-1-phosphate.

(*b*) *Other pathways of galactose metabolism.* The following reactions are probably not very important in normal subjects, but may become important when the normal pathway of galactose metabolism is impaired.

(i) Galactose-1-phosphate may be incorporated into UDP-galactose by a specific UDP-galactose pyrophosphorylase which provides an alternate pathway to the transfer process of reaction 2 (Isselbacher, 1958). The enzyme occurs in liver

(*c*) *Galactose metabolism in galactosaemia.* An important clue to the metabolic lesion in galactosaemia came from the studies of Schwarz *et al.* (1956) on erythrocyte metabolism in galactosaemia. They observed that galactose-1-phosphate accumulated in red blood cells when galactosaemic infants were given a milk-containing diet and also that their red blood cells accumulated this compound when incubated *in vitro* in a medium containing galactose. These observations led them to postulate that the red blood cells of galactosaemic patients are unable to accomplish the transfer of galactose-1-phosphate to UDP (see reaction 2, Fig. 4.18). This was promptly confirmed by Isselbacher and his colleagues (1956) who showed that the enzyme galactose-1-phosphate uridyl transferase was deficient or absent in the patients' erythrocytes, although all the other enzymes involved in galactose utilization were present.

Galactose-1-phosphate uridyl transferase is normally present in red blood cells, and in liver (Anderson *et al.*, 1957), white blood cells (Weinberg, 1961) and fibroblasts (Krooth & Weinberg, 1961). In galactosaemic patients the activity of the enzyme in these cells is very low or unmeasurable. It has also been claimed that there is no transferase activity in the lens of galactosaemic subjects and that galactose-1-phosphate accumulates in this tissue when galactose is present in the diet (Lerman, 1959). Deficiency of transferase activity in red blood cells occurs not only in galactosaemic children who are actually suffering from the clinical manifestation of the disease, but has also been demonstrated in the cord blood of newly-born children before they have had any milk at all and also in nearly asymptomatic galactosaemic adults (Anderson *et. al.*, 1967*b*). Activity of the transferase enzyme in a liver biopsy specimen taken from a galactosaemic adult was very low when compared to that in the normal adult. These observations make it clear that this is a congenital disorder which persists into adult life. So far, of course, there has not been sufficient time since the discovery of the specific enzyme defect to prove that the defect persists in the same individual from an early age into adulthood.

A galactosaemic patient, who lacks the transfer enzyme, cannot utilize galactose adequately, so that galactose-1-phosphate accumulates in his cells and any galactose absorbed from the intestine persists in his extracellular fluid and plasma. The most striking demonstration of the failure to utilize galactose is seen in the test developed by Segal *et al.* (1962) in which $^{14}CO_2$ is measured in the expired air after an injection of radioactive galactose-1-^{14}C. In the majority of galactosaemic patients, virtually no radioactive CO_2 is produced. This test demonstrates the gross disturbance of galactose utilization in galactosaemia and underlines the biological importance of the transferase step in galactose metabolism.

A few galactosaemic patients do, however, produce almost normal amounts of radioactive CO_2 from galactose-1-^{14}C (Segal *et al.*, 1965). These patients were all negroes, and showed the usual clinical features of liver disease and failure to thrive and the development of cataracts, but they were able to metabolize galactose quantitatively like normal subjects. It would seem almost certain that in this variant of galactosaemia, galactose metabolism in the liver takes place by an alternate pathway, which may be via UDP-galactose pyrophosphorylase (see reaction (i), Fig. 4.18) or by oxidation by galactose dehydrogenase (reaction (iii), Fig. 4.18).

The significance of alternate pathways may also be seen clinically by the fact that galactosaemic children become more tolerant to galactose as they become older. They may be able to utilize galactose by conversion to galactose-6-phosphate, which can then be oxidized by glucose-6-phosphate dehydrogenase (see reaction (ii), Fig. 4.18). However, this possibility has not yet been demonstrated in a long term follow-up of any single individual.

Biochemical Basis of Toxic Effects

Galactose-1-phosphate has been implicated as the agent responsible for the toxic effects in liver, lens and brain. This belief was based on the observation that it accumulates in erythrocytes, but no direct measurement has been made to show that it also accumulates in other tissues. Absence of transferase activity has been observed in the lens of galactosaemic patients (Lerman, 1964), but it is not at all clear whether the lens does contain an excess of galactose-1-phosphate in galactosaemic patients. But this compound does accumulate in cataracts produced experimentally in animals by feeding diets high in galactose (Schwarz & Golberg, 1955).

In vitro, galactose-1-phosphate inhibits galactokinase, phosphoglucomutase, glucose-6-phosphatase and glucose-6-phosphate dehydrogenase, but it is not clear how this would explain the cellular damage (Sidbury 1961). Several of these enzymes are absent in other inborn errors of metabolism, e.g. in glycogen storage diseases, but cataract formation, aminoaciduria and cirrhosis of the liver do not occur in those diseases.

An alternative explanation for cataract formation has been proposed by Kinoshita (1965). He attributes it to hypertonicity and vacuole formation in lens fibres caused by the presence of dulcitol (van Heyningen, 1959), an alcohol formed from galactose by aldolase reductase which occurs in the lens. Although this mechanism may be the cause of cataract formation, it is unlikely to play an important part in damaging cells which are not as rigidly confined as those of the lens.

Another hypothesis for the toxic effects of galactose-1-phosphate is based on the observation of Pennington & Prankerd (1958) that the ATP content of galactosaemic red blood cells falls when galactose-1-phosphate accumulates and that normal glycolysis is disturbed in these cells. However, this observation could not be confirmed in a more recent study in which an adequate amount of glucose was provided in the incubation medium (Zipursky *et al.*, 1965) to allow glycolysis to proceed normally.

Important evidence against galactose-1-phosphate being the damaging agent comes from the discovery of a patient with cataracts and galactosuria but in whom the metabolic defect was due to the absence of galactokinase (Gitzelmann, 1965). If the enzyme defect extends to the lens, then galactose-1-phosphate cannot be formed and galactose itself would accumulate in the lens.

Though much is known at present about the biochemical aspects of galactose metabolism, there is still a lot of uncertainty about the consequences of the metabolic disturbances which express themselves clinically as interference with the function of many important organs.

Biochemical Diagnosis

The galactose tolerance test is now no longer used, because of its potential danger to the affected child, and because many other factors, quite unconnected with galactosaemia, can influence the disposition of injected galactose. In normal children, the intravenous injection of 0·5 g. galactose/Kg. results in a sharp peak and rapid disappearance of galactose from the blood and also a rapid rise in blood glucose as galactose is converted to glucose in the liver. In galactosaemic children the disappearance of galactose is very much slower and the glucose response correspondingly delayed (Cornblath & Schwartz, 1966) (Fig. 4.18). Occasionally, there may be a fall in blood sugar following galactose administration (Greenman, 1950), but this appears to be the case only in galactosaemic children in whom liver damage is present.

A valuable and safer investigation of galactose utilization can be carried out by injecting radioactive galactose-1-^{14}C and measuring the ^{14}CO$_2$ in expired air (Segal *et al.*, 1962). This test does not localize the metabolic defect, but gives valuable information concerning the overall utilization of galactose, which is virtually zero in the "classical" form of galactosaemia.

Hsia (1967) has reviewed the various methods available for examining specific enzyme activities in red blood cells and described how these can be used to distinguish a number of "variants" of galactosaemia.

Transferase activity is usually measured as originally described by Schwarz *et al.* (1956)

by estimating the amount of galactose-1-phosphate accumulating in erythrocytes incubated in the presence of galactose.

An *in vitro* test based on the conversion of galactose-1-^{14}C to ^{14}CO$_2$ by red blood cells has been used extensively by Isselbacher (1966), but like the *in vivo* test described by Segal, it can only give an indication of overall galactose metabolism in the red blood cell and does not localize the enzyme defect.

The remaining tests depend upon reaction 2 of the major metabolic pathway. The most extensively used test depends upon the rate of UDP-glucose disappearance, which is measured before and after incubation with galactose-1-phosphate, using a highly specific UDP-glucose dehydrogenase (Anderson *et al.*, 1957*b*), and has given good reproducibility when used for red blood cells.

Recently, Beutler & Baluda (1966) have developed a test which depends on the formation of glucose-1-phosphate and its onward metabolism via the hexose monophosphate shunt. In essence, the test depends upon the failure of NADPH formation in galactosaemic red blood cells because galactose-1-phosphate cannot be further metabolised in the absence of transferase activity. Using this test for screening purposes in over 2000 cases, Beutler, Baluda, Sturgeon & Day (1965) discovered a new genetic abnormality, the Duarte variant, in which transferase activity in erythrocytes of homozygotes is not completely absent as it is in the "classical" form, but is reduced to about 50% of that of normal subjects, while in heterozygtes the activity for the variant is 75% of normal. On electrophoresis, the homozygote for the Duarte variant shows a single band for transferase activity which differs in mobility from that of normal individuals, while the transferase of heterozygotes has two bands, one corresponding to the Duarte variant, the other to the normal band.

A further technique for measuring transferase activity involving reaction 2, (Fig. 4.18) depends on the rate of conversion of radioactive galactose-1-phosphate to UDP-galactose (Anderson *et al.*, 1957*b*). This method gives lower results than the UDP-glucose consumption tests, which may be due to the technique of the test or because the UDP-glucose consumption test is non-specific and measures changes other than those caused by transferase.

As a result of the various tests a number of variants of galactosaemia have been recognized with their own clinical and biochemical features. It is now no longer possible to regard galactosaemia as a single inborn error of metabolism, but rather as a group of diseases in which different metabolic disorders, produced by the presence of galactose in the diet, find rather similar clinical expression.

Biochemical Genetics

In the "classical" form of galactosaemia, transferase activity is undetectable in the homozygote, and is about 50% of normal in both of the heterozygous parents of affected homozygous children. This is consistent with an autosomal recessive mode of inheritance. Galactosaemia is a disorder with considerable clinical variability, and it has been suggested that some heterozygotes, although not showing the full clinical picture of galactosaemia, may suffer from varying degrees of milk intolerance (Hsia & Walker, 1961).

The availability of specific enzyme assays has made it possible to attempt an estimate of the incidence of galactosaemia in the population, but the figures vary greatly with the method used for enzyme assay. Schwarz et al. (1961) calculated the incidence of galactosaemia to be 1 in 70,000 births, but Hansen et al. (1964) have calculated an incidence of 1 in 18,000 births, while Beutler et al. (1967), on the basis of an estimated prevalence of heterozygotes in the population, expect a birth incidence of 1 in 25,000 to 30,000. The latest estimates by Beutler et al. (1967) have been corrected for the Duarte variant, in which the homozygote has transferase activity equal to that of the heterozygous carrier of "classical" galactosaemia and would have been counted in earlier surveys as a heterozygous carrier.

The genetic mechanisms involved in enzyme abnormalities are complex. Transferase activity in whole blood and in white blood cells of patients with Down's syndrome is 50% higher than normal (Brandt et al., 1963), which suggests that the locus for the enzyme may be situated on chromosome 21. It is particularly interesting that galactokinase activity of whole blood is also increased by 50% in these patients (Krone et al., 1964). It has been suggested that this is due to an alteration in the co-ordinated regulation of a multi-enzyme system, but other explanations, such as a change in some component of cirulating leucocytes in Down's syndrome, cannot be ruled out.

Course and Treatment

The clinical manifestations arise as a result of the ingestion of galactose. If the disease is not recognized, and milk feeds continue to be given, death usually occurs within a short time, but if all galactose-containing food is withheld, most of the clinical features usually improve, and even cataracts may clear up completely. Mental retardation is the only important feature which shows no improvement and for this reason early diagnosis remains essential.

Galactose-free diets are relatively simple to prepare for very young infants taking a formula diet, but later in life the temptation to eat food such as chocolate, bread, etc. which contain added lactose, is very great. Fortunately, tolerance to galactose seems to increase as the child gets older, but even then the patient should be encouraged as much as possible to avoid such foods.

It has also been suggested that during pregnancy a heterozygous mother, whose baby may be homozygous for the disease, should restrict the amount of galactose in her diet, because in some instances babies were born with cataracts and cirrhosis (Hsia & Walker, 1961).

References

Glycogen Storage Diseases

ABDULLAH, M., TAYLOR, P. M. & WHELAN, W. J. (1964). In "Control of Glycogen Metabolism", p. 123. Eds. Whelan, W. J. & Cameron, M. P. London., J. & A. Churchill.

ABRAHAMOV, A., MAGER, J. & SHAFRIR, E. (1961). Bull. Res. Coun. Israel, E., 9, 83.

ALEPA, F. P., HOWELL, R. R., KLINEBERG, J. R. & SEEGMILLER, J. E. (1967). Amer. J. Med., 42, 58.

ANDERSEN, D. H. (1952). In "Carbohydrate Metabolism". Ed. Najjar, V. A. Baltimore, Johns Hopkins Press.

ANDRES, R., CADER, G. & ZIERLER, K. L. (1956). J. clin. Invest., 35, 671.

ASHMORE, J. & WEBER, G. (1959). Vitamins and Hormones, 17, 91.

BAUDHUIN, P., HERS, H. G. & LOEB, H. (1964). Lab. Invest., 13, 1139.

BENDALL, J. R. (1960). In "Structure and Function of Muscle", p. 227. Ed. Bourne, G. H. New York, Academic Press.

BERNARD, C. (1857). C. R. Soc. Biol., 44, 578.

BROWN, B. I. & BROWN, D. H. (1966). Proc. Nat. Acad. Sci. U.S.A., 56, 725.

BROWN, D. H. & ILLINGWORTH, B. (1962). Proc. Nat. Acad. Sci. U.S.A., 48, 1783.

BROWN, D. H. & ILLINGWORTH, B. (1966). Biochem. J., 100, 8P.

BUEDING, E., ORRELL, S. A. Jnr. & SIDBURY, J. B. Jnr. (1964). In "Control of Glycogen Metabolism", p. 387. Eds. Whelan, W. J. & Cameron, M. P. London, J. & A. Churchill.

CALDERBANK, A., KENT, P. W., LORBER, J., MANNERS, D. J. & WRIGHT, A. (1960). *Biochem. J.*, **74**, 223.

CHAYOTH, R., MOSES, S.W. & STEINITZ, K. (1967) *Israel J. Med. Sci.* **3**, 422.

CINADER, B., DUBISHI, S. & WARDLAW, A. C. (1966). *Nature*, **210**, 1291.

CORI, G. T. (1954). *Harvey Lect.*, **48**, 145.

CORI, G. T. & CORI, C. F. (1952). *J. biol. Chem.*, **199**, 661.

CORI, G. T. & LARNER, J. (1951). *J. biol. Chem.*, **188**, 17.

CORI, C. F., SCHMIDT, G. & CORI, G. T. (1939). *Science*, **89**, 464.

CORNBLATH, M. & SCHWARTZ, R. (1966). "Disorders of Carbohydrate Metabolism in Infancy". p. 121. Philadelphia, W. B. Saunders Company.

CRAIG, J. M. & UZMAN, L. (1958). *Pediatrics*, **22**, 20.

CREVELD, VAN S. (1963). *Canad. Med. Assoc. J.* **88**, 1.

CREVELD, VAN S. & HUIJING, F. (1964). *Metabolism*, **13**, 191.

DANFORTH, W. H. (1965). *J. biol. Chem.*, **240**, 588.

Discussion (1964). In "Control of Glycogen Metabolism", p. 406. Eds. Whelan, W. J. & Cameron, M. P. London, J. & A. Churchill.

DUVE, DE C. (1959). In "Subcellular Particles", p. 128. Ed. Hayashi, T. New York, Ronald Press.

DUVE, DE C., BERTHET, J., HERS, H. G. & DUPRET, L. (1949). *Bull. Soc. Chim. Biol.*, **31**, 1242.

EBERLEIN, W. R., ILLINGWORTH, B. & SIDBURY, J. B., Jnr. (1962). *Amer. J. Med.*, **33**, 20.

ENGEL, W. K., EYERMAN, E. L. & WILLIAMS, H. E. (1963). *New Engl. J. Med.*, **268**, 135.

FIELD, J. B., EPSTEIN, S. & EGAN, T. (1965). *J. clin. Invest.*, **44**, 1240.

FIELD, R. A. (1966). In "The Metabolic Basis of Inherited Disease". 2nd ed., p. 163. Eds. Stanbury, J. B., Wyngaarden, J. B. & Fredrickson, D. S. New York, McGraw-Hill.

FRENCH, D. (1964). In "Control of Glycogen Metabolism", p. 7. Eds. Whelan, W. J. & Cameron M. P. London, J. & A. Churchill.

GARROD, A. E. (1902). *Lancet*, **2**, 1616.

GIERKE, VON E. (1929). *Beitr. path. Anat.*, **82**, 497.

GOLDFINGER, S., KLINENBERG, J. R. & SEEGMILLER, J. E. (1965). *New Engl. J. Med.*, **272**, 351.

GRILLO, T. A. I. & OZONE, K. (1962). *Nature* (Lond.), **195**, 902.

HALES, C. N. (1967). In "Essays in Biochemistry". **3**, 97. Eds. Campbell, P. N. & Greville, G. D. London, The Biochemical Society and Academic Press.

HANDLER, J. S. (1960). *J. clin. Invest.*, **39**, 1526.

HENION, W. F. & SUTHERLAND, E. W. (1957). *J. biol. Chem.*, **224**, 477.

HERS, H. G. (1959). *Rev. Intern. Hépatol.*, **9**, 35.

HERS, H. G. (1961). *Chemisch. Weekbl.*, **57**, 437.

HERS, H. G. (1963). *Biochem. J.*, **86**, 11.

HERS, H. G. (1964a). *Adv. in Metabolic Disorders*, **1**, 1.

HERS, H. G. (1964b). In "Control of Glycogen Synthesis". p. 151. Eds. Whelan, W. J. & Cameron, M. P. London, J. & A. Churchill.

HERS, H. G. & MALBRAIN, H. (1959). *Mod. Probl. Paediat.*, **4**, 203.

HERS, H. G., VERHUE, W. & HOOF, VAN F. (1967). *Europ. J. Biochem.*, **2**, 257.

HOLLING, H. E. (1963). *Ann. int. Med.*, **58**, 654.

HOOF, VAN F. (1967). *Europ. J. Biochem.*, **2**, 271.

HOOF, VAN F. & HERS, H. G. (1967). *Europ. J. Biochem.*, **2**, 265.

HOWELL, R. R., ASHTON, D. & WYNGAARDEN, J. B. (1960). *J. clin. Invest.*, **39**, 997.

HSIA, D. Y. & KOT, E. C. (1959). *Nature* (Lond.), **183**, 1331.

HUG, G. (1961). *Biochim. Biophys. Acta.*, **47**, 271.

HUG, G. (1967). *Amer. J. Med.*, **42**, 139.

HUG, G., GARANCIS, J. C., SCHUBERT, W. K. & KAPLAN, S. (1966). *Amer. J. Dis. Child.*, **111**, 457.

HUIJING, F., CREVELD, VAN S. & LOSEKOOT, G. (1963). *J. Pediat.*, **63**, 984.

HUIJING, F. & LARNER, J. (1966). *Proc. Nat. Acad. Sci.*, (U.S.A.), **56**, 647.

HÜLSMANN, W. C., OEI, T. L. & CREVELD, VAN S. (1961). *Lancet*, **2**, 581.

ILLINGWORTH, B. (1961). *Amer. J. Clin. Nutr.*, **9**, 683.

ILLINGWORTH, B. & BROWN, D. H. (1964a). In "Control of Glycogen Metabolism", p. 345. Eds. Whelan, W. J. & Cameron, M. P. London, J. & A. Churchill.

ILLINGWORTH, B. & BROWN, D. H. (1964b). In "Control of Glycogen Metabolism", p. 346. Eds. Whelan, W. J. & Cameron, M. P. London, J. & A. Churchill.

ILLINGWORTH, B. & CORI, G. T. (1952). *J. biol. Chem.*, **199**, 653.

ILLINGWORTH, B., CORI, G. T. & CORI, C. F. (1956). *J. biol. Chem.*, **218**, 123.

JACOB, F. & MONOD, J. (1961). *J. Mol. Biol.*, **3**, 318.

JEUNE, M., CHARRAT, A. & BERTRAND, J. (1957). *Arch. franç. pediat.*, **14**, 897.

KELLER, P. J. & CORI, G. T. (1955). *J. biol. Chem.*, **214**, 127.

KOLB, F. O., LALLA, DE J. W. & GOFMAN, J. W. (1955). *Metabolism*, **4**, 310.

KRISMAN, C. R. (1962). *Anal. Biochem.*, **4**, 17.

LARNER, J. (1964). In "Control of Glycogen Metabolism", p. 87. Eds. Whelan, W. J. & Cameron, & M. P. London, J. & A. Churchill.

LARNER, J., ROSELL-PEREZ, M., FRIEDMAN, D. L. & CRAIG, J. W. (1964). In "Control of Glycogen Metabolism", p. 273. Eds. Whelan, W. J. & Cameron, M. P. London, J. & A. Churchill.

LAYZER, R. B., ROWLAND, L. P. & RANNEY, H. M. (1967). *Arch. Neurol.*, **17**, 512.

LAZARUS, S. S. (1959). *Proc. Soc. Exptl. Biol. Med.*, **101**, 819.

LEJEUNE, N., THINÈS-SEMPOUX, D. & HERS, H. G. (1963). *Biochem. J.*, **86**, 16.

LELOIR, L. F. (1964). In "Control of Glycogen Metabolism", p. 71. Eds. Whelan, W. J. & Cameron, M. P. London, J. & A. Churchill.

LELOIR, L. F. & CARDINI, C. E. (1957). *J. Amer. chem. Soc.*, **79**, 6340.

LEWIS, G. M., STEWART, K. M. & SPENCER-PEET, J. (1962), *Biochem. J.*, **84**, 115P.

LEWIS, G. M., SPENCER-PEET, J. & STEWART, K. M. (1963). *Arch. Dis. Child.*, **38**, 40.

LINNEWEH, F., LÖHR, G. W., WALLER, H. D. & GROSS, R. (1963a). *Clin. Chim. Acta*, **8**, 343.

LINNEWEH, F., LÖHR, G. W., WALLER, H. D. & GROSS, R. (1963b). *Klin. Wschr.*, **41**, 352.

LOWE, C. U. & MOSOVICH, L. L. (1965). *Pediatrics*, **35**, 1005.

LOWE, C. U., SOKAL, J. E., MOSOVICH, L. L., SARCIONE, E. J. & DORAY, B. H. (1962). *Amer. J. Med.*, **33**, 4.

LUCK, D. J. L. (1961). *J. biophys. biochem. Cytol.*, **10**, 195.

MCARDLE, B. (1951). *Clin. Sci.*, **10**, 13.

MAHLER, R. (1966a). *Nature*, **209**, 616.

MAHLER, R. (1966b). Unpublished observations.

MAHLER, R. & MCARDLE, B. (1960). *Quart. J. Med.*, **29**, 638.

MAHLER, R. & MCARDLE, B. (1966). Unpublished observations.

MANNERS, D. J. (1964). In "Control of Glycogen Metabolism", p. 326. Eds. Whelan, W. J. & Cameron, M. P. London, J. & A. Churchill.

MELLICK, R. S., MAHLER, R. & HUGHES, B. P. (1962). *Lancet*, **1**, 1045.

MOMMAERTS, W. F. H. M., ILLINGWORTH, B., PEARSON, C. M., GUILLORY, R. J. & SERAYDARIAN, K. (1959). *Proc. Nat. Acad. Sci.* (U.S.A.), **45**, 791.

ÖCKERMAN, P. A. (1964). *Clin. Chim. Acta*, **9**, 151.

OEI, T. L. (1962). *Clin. Chim. Acta*, **7**, 193.

OLAVARRÌA, J. M. & TORRES, H. N. (1962). *J. biol. Chem.*, **237**, 1747.

OLINER, L., SCHULMAN, M. & LARNER, J. (1961). *Clin. Res.*, **9**, 243.

ORRELL, S. A., Jnr., BUEDING, E. & REISSIG, M. (1964). In "Control of Glycogen Metabolism", p. 38. Eds. Whelan, W. J. & Cameron, M. P. London, J. & A. Churchill.

PARR, J., TEREE, T. M. & LARNER, J. (1965). *Pediatrics*, **35**, 770.

PEARSON, C. M. & RIMER, D. G. (1959). *Proc. Soc. exp. Biol.* (N.Y.), **100**, 671.

PEARSON, C. M., RIMER, D. G. & MOMMAERTS, W. F. H. M. (1961). *Amer. J. Med.*, **30**, 502.

POMPE, J. C. (1932). *Nederl. Tijdschr. geneesk.*, **76**, 304.

POWELL, R. C., MAHLER, R. & DEISS, W. P., Jnr. (1965). *Clin. Res.*, **13**, 331.

RATINOV, G., BAKER, W. P. & SWAIMAN, K. F. (1965). *Ann. int. Med.*, **62**, 328.

RIDDELL, A. G. & DAVIES, R. P. (1966). *Proc. Roy. Soc. Med.*, **59**, 484.

RILEY, G. A. & HAYNES, R. C., Jnr. (1963). *J. biol. Chem.*, **238**, 1563.

ROBBINS, P. W. (1960). *Fed. Proc.*, **19**, 193.

ROSELL-PEREZ, M., VILLAR-PALASI, C. & LARNER, J. (1962). *Biochemistry*, **1**, 763.

ROSENFELD, E. L. (1964). In "Control of Glycogen Metabolism", p. 176. Eds. Whelan, W. J. & Cameron, M. P. London, J. & A. Churchill.

RUTTER, W. J. & BROSEMER, R. W. (1961). *J. biol. Chem.*, **236**, 1247.

SCHMID, R. & HAMMAKER, L. (1961). *New Engl. J. Med.*, **264**, 223.

SCHMID, R. & MAHLER, R. (1959). *J. clin. Invest.*, **38**, 2044.

SCHWARTZ, R., ASHMORE, J. & RENOLD, A. E. (1957). *Pediatrics*, **19**, 585.

SIDBURY, J. B., Jnr., CORNBLATH, M., FISHER, J. & HOUSE, E. (1961a). *Pediatrics*, **27**, 103.

SIDBURY, J. B., Jnr., GITZELMANN, R. & FISHER, M. J. (1961b). *Helv. paediat. acta*, **16**, 506.

SIDBURY, J. B., Jnr., MASON, J., BURNS, W. B., Jnr. & RUEBNER, B. H. (1962). *Bull. Johns Hopkins Hosp.*, **111**, 157.

SMITH, H. L., AMICK, L. D. & SIDBURY, J. B., Jnr. (1966). *Amer. J. Dis. Child.*, **111**, 475.

SNAPPER, I. & CREVELD, VAN S. (1928). *Bull. et mém. Soc. méd. hôp.* (Paris), **52**, 1315.

SOKAL, J. E., LOWE, C. U., SARCIONE, E. J., MOSOVICH, L. L. & DORAY, B. H. (1961). *J. clin. Invest.*, **40**, 364.

SOKAL, J. E., FLEISSNER, S., SARCIONE, E. J. & LOWE, C. U. (1961). *Nature*, **192**, 265.

SPENCER-PEET, J. (1964). In "Control of Glycogen Metabolism", p. 382. Eds. Whelan, W. J. & Cameron, M. P. London, J. & A. Churchill.

STADTMAN, E. R. (1966). *Adv. Enzymol.*, **28**, 41.

STARZL, T. E., MARCHIORO, T. L., SEXTON, A. W., ILLINGWORTH, B., WADDELL, W. R. & HERRMANN, T. J. (1965). *Surgery*, **57**, 687.

STEINBERG, D. (1963). In "The Control of Lipid Metabolism", p. 111. Ed. Grant, J. K. London, Academic Press.

STEINITZ, K. & REISNER, S. H. (1961). *Bull. Res. Coun. Israel, E.*, **9**, 84.

STEINITZ, K. & RUTENBERG, A. (1967). *Israel J. med. Sci.*, **3**, 411.

SUTHERLAND, E. W. & RALL, T. W. (1960). *Pharmacol. Rev.*, **12**, 265.

SUTHERLAND, E. W. & ROBISON, G. A. (1966). *Pharmacol. Rev.*, **18**, 145.

SZENT GYÖRGYI, A. (1953). "Chemical Physiology of Contraction in Body and Heart Muscle". New York, Academic Press.

TARUI, S., OKUNO, G., IKURA, Y., TANAKA, T., SUDA, M. & NISHIKAWA, M. (1965). *Biochem. biophys. Res. Comm.*, **19**, 517.

TATA, J. R. (1964). *Biochem. J.*, **90**, 284.

THOMSON, W. H. S., MACLAURIN, J. C. & PRINEAS, J. W. (1963). *J. Neurol. Neurosurg. Psychiat.*, **26**, 60.

VILLEE, C. A. (1954). *Cold Spring Harbor Symp. on Quant. Biol.*, **19**, 186.

WALKER, G. J. & WHELAN, W. J. (1960). *Biochem. J.*, **76**, 264.

WEBER, G. & HARPUR, E. R. (1960). *Metabolism*, **9**, 880.

WILLIAMS, H. E. & FIELD, J. B. (1961). *J. clin. Invest.*, **40**, 1841.

WILLIAMS, H. E. & FIELD, J. B. (1963). *Metabolism*, **12**, 464.

WILLIAMS, H. E., JOHNSTON, P. L., FENSTER, L. F., LASTER, L. & FIELD, J. B. (1963a). *Metabolism*, **12**, 235.

WILLIAMS, H. E., KENDIG, E. M. & FIELD, J. B. (1963b). *J. clin. Invest.*, **42**, 656.

YOUNG, N. F., ABELS, J. C. & HOMBURGER, F. (1948). *J. clin. Invest.*, **27**, 760.

Galactosaemia

ANDERSON, E. P., KALCKAR, H. M. & ISSELBACHER, K. J. (1957a). *Science*, **125**, 113.

ANDERSON, E. P., KALCKAR, H. M., KURAHASHI, K. & ISSELBACHER, K. J. (1957b). *J. Lab. Clin. Med.*, **50**, 469.

BEUTLER, E. & BALUDA, M. C. (1966). *J. Lab. Clin. Med.*, **68**, 137.

BEUTLER, E., BALUDA, M. C., STURGEON, P. & DAY, R. (1965). *Lancet*, **1**, 353.

BEUTLER, E., IRWIN, R., BLUMENFELD, C. M., GOLDENBURG, E. W. & DAY, R. W. (1967). *J. Amer. med. Ass.*, **199**, 501.

BRANDT, N. J., FORLAND, A., MIKKELSEN, M., NIELSEN, A. & TOLSTRUP, N. (1963). *Lancet*, **2**, 700.

CAPUTTO, R., LELOIR, L. F., CARDINI, C. E. & PALADINI, A. C. (1950). *J. biol. Chem.*, **184**, 333.

CORNBLATH, M. & SCHWARTZ, R. (1966). "Disorders of Carbohydrate Metabolism in Infancy". p. 165. Philadelphia, W. B. Saunders Company.

CUATRECASAS, P. & SEGAL, S. (1966). *Science*, **153**, 549.

GITZELMANN, R. (1965). *Lancet*, **2**, 670.

GREENMAN, L. (1950). *J. biol. Chem.*, **183**, 577.

HANSEN, R. G., BRETTHAUER, R. K., MAYES, J. & NORDIN, J. H. (1964). *Proc. Soc. Exper. Biol. Med.*, **115**, 560.

HEYNINGEN, VAN, R. (1959). *Nature*, **184**, 194.

HSIA, D. Y.-Y. (1967). *Metabolism*, **16**, 419.

HSIA, D. Y.-.Y. & WALKER, F. A. (1961). *J. Pediat.*, **123**, 635.

INOUYE, T., SCHNEIDER, J. A. & HSIA, D. Y.-Y. (1964). *Nature*, **204**, 1304.

ISSELBACHER, K. J. (1958). *J. biol. Chem.*, **232**, 429.

ISSELBACHER, K. J. (1966). In "The Metabolic Basis of Inherited Diseases". 2nd Ed. P. 183. Eds. Stanbury, J. B., Wyngaarden, J. B. & Fredrickson, D. S. New York, McGraw-Hill.

ISSELBACHER, K. J., ANDERSON, E. P., KURAHASHI, K. & KALCKAR, H. M. (1956). *Science*, **123**, 635.

KALCKAR, H. M., BRAGANÇA, B. & MUNCH-PETERSEN, A. (1953). *Nature*, **172**, 1038.

KINOSHITA, J. H. (1965). *Invest. Ophth.*, **4**, 786.

KRONE, W., WOLF, U., GOEDDE, H. W. & BAITSCH, H. (1964). *Lancet*, **2**, 590.

KROOTH, R. S. & WEINBERG, A. N. (1961). *J. Exp. Med.* **113**, 1155.

LANGSTEIN, L. & STEINITZ, F. (1906). *Beitr. chem. Physiol. Path.*, **7**, 575.

LERMAN, S. (1959). *Arch. Ophth.*, **61**, 88.

NG, W. G., BERGREN, W. R. & DONNELL, G. N. (1964). *Nature*, **203**, 845.

OHNO, S., PAYNE, H. W., MORRISON, M. & BEUTLER, E. (1966). *Science*, **153**, 1015.

PENNINGTON, J. S. & PRANKERD, T. A. J. (1958). *Clin. Sci.*, **17**, 385.

POSTERNAK, T. & ROSSELET, J. P. (1954). *Helv. chim. Acta*, **37**, 246.

REUSS, VON A. (1908). *Wien. med. Wschr.*, **58**, 799.

SEGAL, S., BLAIR, A. & TOPPER, Y. J. (1962). *Science*, **136**, 150.

SEGAL, S., BLAIR, A. & ROTH, H. (1965). *Amer. J. Med.*, **38**, 62.

SIDBURY, J. B. Jnr., (1961). "Molecular Genetics in Human Disease". Springfield, Ill, Charles C. Thomas.

SCHWARZ, V. & GOLBERG, L. (1955). *Biochem. et biophys. Acta*, **18**, 310.

SCHWARZ, V., GOLBERG, L. KOMROWER, G. M. & HOLZEL, A. (1956). *Biochem. J.*, **62**, 34.

SCHWARZ, V., WELLS, A. R., HOLZEL, A. & KOMROWER, G. M. (1961). *Ann. Human. Genet.*, **25**, 179.

WEINBERG, A. N. (1961). *Metabolism*, **10**, 728.

ZIPURSKY, A., ROWLAND, M., FORD, J. D., HAWORTH, J. C. & ISRAELS, L. G. (1965). *Pediatrics*, **35**, 126.

Chapter 5

DISEASES OF THE LIVER AND BILIARY TRACT

by

Noel F. Maclagan

Westminster Hospital Medical School, London

In view of the protean manifestations of liver disease it would be possible to discuss work in this field either from a functional or from a pathological viewpoint, since the two approaches are so intimately connected. In the present chapter a mixed approach has been employed and the subject will be considered under the headings indicated above.

BILE PIGMENT METABOLISM

Bilirubin has long been regarded as the chief pigment of bile and its metabolism has been the subject of extensive investigations since its isolation from gallstones by Staedeler in 1864. The normal pigment of stool, stercobilin, and the related urobilin of urine have been known since the work of Jaffé (1868) and have been regarded as originating entirely from the breakdown of haemoglobin. A re-orientation of our ideas on both these important points has taken place during the last decade.

The Structure and Origin of Bile Pigments

The constitution of bilirubin and of urobilin was established by Fischer and his colleagues (Fischer & Orth, 1937) during the period 1930–37.

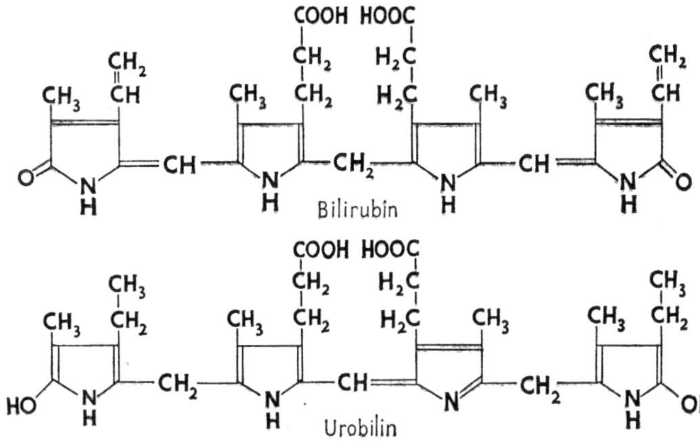

Fig. 5.1. Constitution of bile pigments.

Their structure is indicated in Fig. 5.1. Their obvious chemical relation to haem was, of course, anticipated in view of the large amount of experimental work which had been going on during the previous half century by Virchow (1847), Whipple (1922), Aschoff (1922), McNee (1923), and Mann (Mann, Sheard, Bollman & Baldes, 1926), which had shown clearly that the bile pigments could be formed in large amounts by the breakdown of haemoglobin. There was, however, some confusion as to the location of this process, which was originally thought to occur entirely in the liver. This conception arose from the well-known experiments of Minkowski & Naunyn (1886), which showed that even active haemolysis did not produce jaundice in the hepatectomized goose. It had been realized by McNee (1923) that the goose was a special case in this respect, as the liver contained nearly the whole of the available reticulo-endothelial cells in this species, and this obscurity was finally clarified when Mann and his colleagues (Mann *et al.* 1926) succeeded in performing hepatectomy in the dog. In this species jaundice regularly appeared in animals surviving the operation by more than 6 hr.

It is thus now generally accepted that the major portion of the circulating bilirubin is produced from haemoglobin breakdown in the reticulo-endothelial system, but the chemical pathway is still unsettled. Haematin was at one time considered as an intermediate in the process, but according to Lemberg & Legge (1949) a more likely possibility is choleglobin. This is a green iron-containing pigment retaining its connection with the original globin of the haemoglobin molecule; it can be converted to biliverdin and hence to bilirubin. Some support for this pathway has been given by Nakajima *et al.* (1963) who have isolated an enzyme "heme-α-methenyl oxygenase" which catalyses the conversion of the haemoglobin-haptoglobin complex to an iron-containing precursor of biliverdin. The relative importance of the different parts of the reticulo-endothelial system in this respect has also been investigated. In the hepatectomized dog the bone marrow is the principal site (Mann *et al.* 1926), but in human pathology the spleen is probably more important. More recently it has been recognized that some bilirubin is also produced by a direct *biosynthesis* in the liver and bone marrow (see "early" bilirubin below).

van den Bergh Reaction

The fact that bilirubin is altered by passage through the liver was recognized at an early date, and this subject is bound up with the well-known reaction of van den Bergh & Müller (1916). They revived an earlier reaction for bilirubin (Ehrlich, 1883) and showed that an acid diazotized solution of sulphanilic acid (the diazo reagent of Ehrlich) gave a red colour with bilirubin in *alcoholic* solution. This reaction, later known as the "indirect" reaction, was also obtained faintly with normal serum and more strongly with sera from cases of haemolytic jaundice. The accidental omission of alcohol from the mixture led to the observation that the reaction proceeded equally well in *aqueous* solution in the case of bile, and of sera from cases of obstructive jaundice (the "direct" reaction). These findings were rapidly confirmed and extended by McNee (1923) and by others.

The nature of the change in bilirubin produced by the liver has been the subject of great difference of opinion over the years. The obvious explanation of the facts noted above would be the existence of two separate substances, which was van den Bergh's original suggestion (van den Bergh & Müller, 1916). Others, however, sought to explain the different diazo reactions in terms of differences in protein attachment of bilirubin or in the presence of accelerating agents (Bollman, Sheard & Mann, 1927; Barron, 1931; Coolidge, 1940; Cantarow, 1944; Watson, 1946). The main

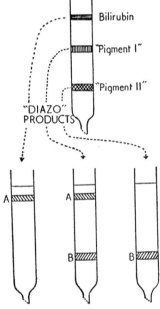

Fig. 5.2. Behaviour of plasma bile pigments and their "diazo" products on partition chromatograms (from Lathe, Biochemical Society Symposium, 1954).

obstacle to the acceptance of two distinct pigments was the failure to isolate them directly from jaundiced sera. The subject was reviewed by Gray (1953, 1961).

This long drawn-out controversy has now been settled by the work of Cole & Lathe (1953; Cole, Lathe & Billing, 1954), who employed a new method in the investigation of human jaundiced sera. Using reverse-phase partition chromatography on silicone-treated kieselguhr, they separated from jaundiced sera two direct pigments in addition to a less polar indirect-reacting substance which proved to be identical with bilirubin. These three substances when treated with the van den Bergh reagent give rise to two distinct diazo compounds as indicated in Figure 5.2. The formation of two diazo compounds by "pigment I" is in keeping with previous work on the chemistry of this reaction, which is thought to involve rupture of one of the C bridges in the tetra-pyrollic pigment with the formation of two di-pyrollic diazo compounds. Cole and Lathe considered that direct pigments I and II represented successive stages in the hepatic metabolism of bilirubin. They are both fairly unstable and readily converted to bilirubin by many of the processes, such as extraction by non-organic solvents, used by previous workers.

It seems likely that pigment I is the monoglucuronide of bilirubin and pigment II the diglucuronide (Billing & Lathe, 1956; Billing, Cole & Lathe, 1957; Schmid, 1957), but the possibility that pigment I represents an equimolecular complex of bilirubin and the diglucuronide has not been ruled out (Billing, 1965). This identification affords a complete explanation of the behaviour of bilirubin, pigment I and pigment II on diazotization referred to above. As shown in Fig. 5.3 during diazotization two products are formed from the monoglucuronide whereas only one is formed from the di-glucuronide. Methods for the quantitative estimation of pigments I and II are not entirely satisfactory but their relative proportions do not appear to have much clinical significance. However pigment II tends to predominate in the blood in post-hepatic jaundice while pigment I predominates in hepatic jaundice (Billing & Lathe, 1958; Hoffman, Whitcomb, Butt & Bollman, 1960). It should also be noted that other conjugates of bilirubin have been identified in blood and in bile, for example with taurine and with sulphate. These appear to form a small part of the total and have not yet assumed pathological importance in man (Billing, 1965). This work as a whole represents a major revolution in our views of the nature of circulating bilirubin.

The second revolution in this field concerns the origin of bile pigments. The earlier work of von Müller (1892), McMaster & Elman (1927), and others in animals with biliary fistulae had established that under the conditions of these experiments stercobilin and urobilin were only produced when bile entered the intestine. It therefore became accepted that they represented a further stage in the degradation of bilirubin brought about by intestinal bacterial action. Later work indicated the colon as the principal site of this change (Hollan, 1950). Since some urobilin was found in the bile it appeared likely that a fraction of the intestinal urobilin or urobilinogen was absorbed into the blood and re-excreted by the liver; the remainder reached the stool as stercobilin.

"Early" Bilirubin

This simple scheme appeared to provide a reasonable explanation of the well-known pathological alterations in urobilin and stercobilin excretion, and although more recent work indicated the existence of other related substances such as mesobilirubinogen and urobilin IXa (Gray, 1953), no other source of this group of pigments was suspected. It was therefore a surprise when the new isotope methods of investigation were applied to this problem and indicated unequivocally the presence of at least one alternative mode of production. This was done independently by three groups of workers in 1949 (Grinstein, Aldrich, Hawkinson & Watson, 1949; Gray, Neuberger & Sneath, 1950; London, West, Shemin & Rittenberg, 1950). The experiments were conducted by feeding glycine labelled with ^{15}N to normal subjects and also to patients with porphyria. It was well known from previous work that glycine is rapidly incorporated into the circulating haemoglobin so that degradation products arising by haemolysis should become labelled only after about 100 days, the normal life span of the erythrocyte. However, the stercobilin showed a marked peak in ^{15}N content during the second 4-day period as well as at the anticipated 100-day interval. This peak was much more marked in the individual with congenital porphyria, who excreted most of his labelled stercobilin before 20 days. Some typical results are shown in Fig. 5.4. It appears therefore that normally only about 70% of the stercobilin is formed from haemoglobin breakdown, about 20% by a rapid synthetic mechanism, and the remaining 10% by some slower undetermined method (Gray, 1953). Full confirmation of this concept has recently been available from observations on dogs with

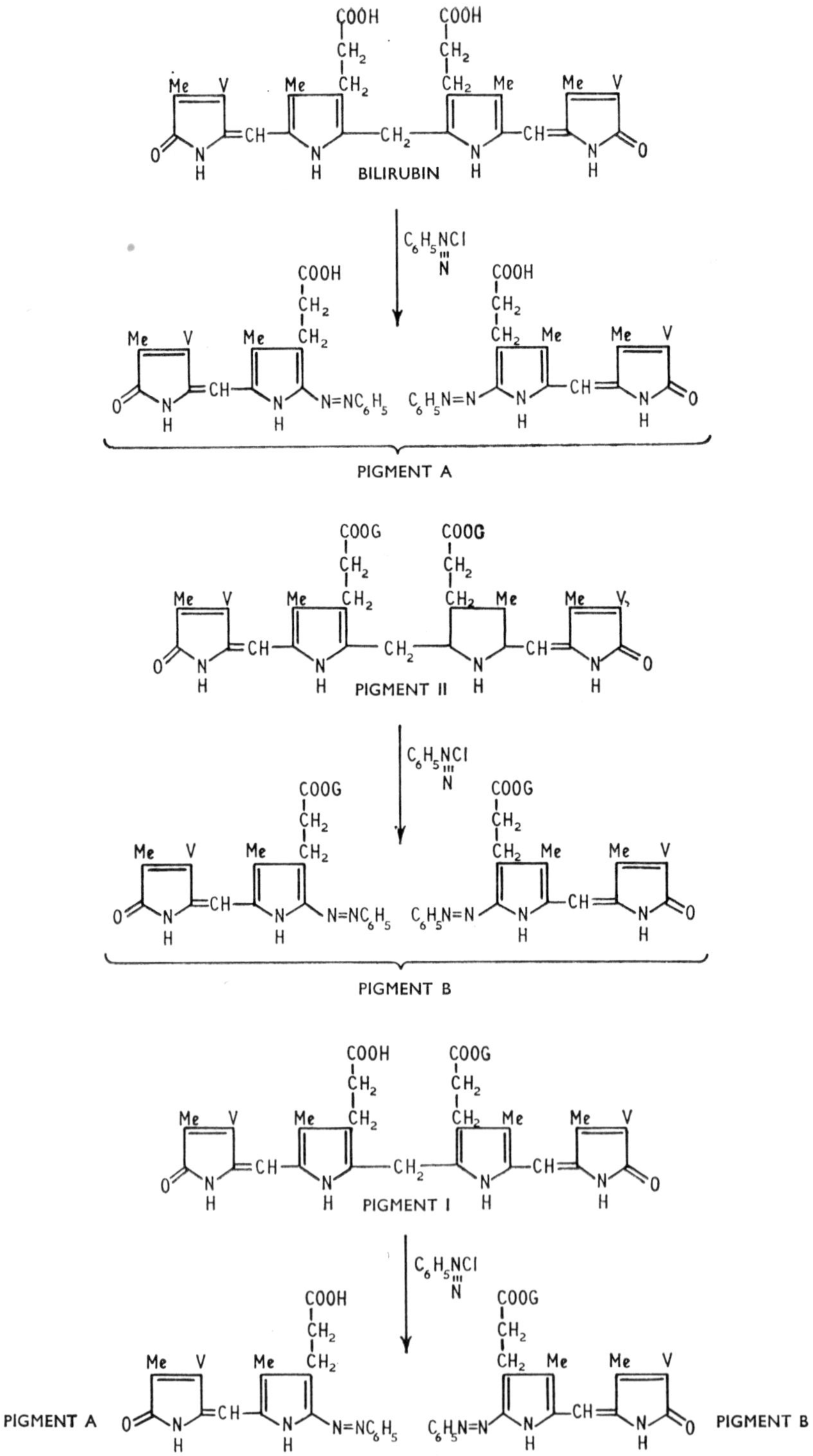

FIG. 5.3. The diazo reaction of bilirubin and its glucuronides (from Gray 1961).

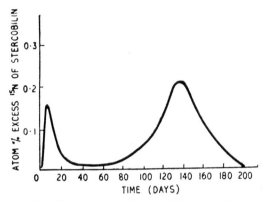

FIG. 5.4. ^{15}N contents of stercobilin hydrochloride samples obtained at various times after the administration to a normal subject of ^{15}N-labelled glycine (from Gray, "The Bile Pigments", Methuen, 1953).

biliary fistulae. When C^{14}-labelled glycine or δ-aminolaevulinic acid is administered a proportion of the label appears in the biliary *bilirubin* during the first five days. This "early bilirubin" appears in at least two fractions, the first at 24 hours being thought to represent a by-product of the synthesis of tissue haems, perhaps in the liver, while the second at 3–5 days is apparently associated with haemoglobin synthesis in the bone marrow (Israels, Yamamoto, Skanderberg & Zipursky, 1963).

JAUNDICE

Pathological Classification

The enormous literature on this subject reflects both the pathological and the biochemical difficulties which have been encountered in arriving at a satisfactory explanation of this common

and arresting symptom. The multiplicity of terms in use to describe the common forms is an indication that the classification has not yet reached finality. Most workers would, however, agree that there are three main pathological types of jaundice, as indicated in Table 5.1. It will be seen that the difference between the rival schemes is mainly one of terminology, except that Rich's (1930) classification differs more fundamentally as it does not make a primary distinction between mechanical biliary obstruction and intrahepatic causes; although this can be justified in terms of pigment metabolism it is confusing to clinicians, who are vitally interested in distinguishing between these two types and would prefer to avoid using the same name for both.

The other three proposals are substantially similar although the relative merits of the proposed terms can be argued at length. The virtue of McNee's "toxic and infective" group is that it at once suggests the two main types of agent responsible for the jaundice. On the other hand the word "obstructive" has unfortunately come to be used very loosely, e.g. to include "intra-hepatic obstruction" in hepatitis. With's classification is logical but the confusion of his "retention" jaundice with the earlier use of this term by Rich for a different condition is an obvious danger, and the word "lymphogenous" implies adherence to a theory of the mechanism of "obstructive" jaundice which is not universally accepted. On the whole, therefore, the writer prefers Lichtman's classification of *pre-hepatic*, *hepatic*, and *extra-hepatic*, although *post-hepatic* would appear a better term for the last variety. This is simple, unambiguous and easily understood, and expresses the main agreed differences between the three types without committing us to any assumptions

TABLE 5.1

Pathological classification of jaundice

Principal cause	Nomenclature according to			
	McNee (1923)	Rich (1930)	With (1944)	Lichtman (1942)
Excessive haemolysis	Haemolytic	Retention	Production	Pre-hepatic
Hepatocellular damage	Toxic and infective	Regurgitation	Retention	Hepatic
Mechanical obstruction of bile passages	Obstructive hepatic	Regurgitation	Lymphogenous	Extra-hepatic (post-hepatic)

as to the cause or the intimate mechanism of the jaundice. This is a useful negative advantage, since new causes are still being discovered and the finer details of the mechanism are in many cases incompletely understood. As with all classifications the terms are not necessarily mutually exclusive as more than one main cause may be operating in any particular case. Numerous examples of this dual aetiology will be found below.

During the last decade, the necessity for some extension of this simple nomenclature has been recognized. This arises because of the discovery of certain anomalous forms of jaundice which are discussed below, in which there is a complete dissociation of the different functions of the liver instead of a general failure. The best established of these is the group of conditions formerly referred to as "constitutional hyperbilirubinaemia" in which there is a selective failure to conjugate bilirubin with glucuronic acid due to lack of a specific liver enzyme or to transport failure. The functional disturbances in these are entirely different to those of general liver damage, and resemble in some degree those of pre-hepatic jaundice (see below).

combination of pathological findings which may result either from hepatic or from post-hepatic causes. These include accumulation of bile pigment in the liver cells, Kupfer cells and canaliculi with variable cellular infiltration in the portal zones. Electron microscopy reveals dilatation and swelling of the microvilli. The biochemical changes resemble those of post-hepatic jaundice but the serum alkaline phosphatase is not usually so high. It seems best to leave this condition in an equivocal position as shown since it does not represent a final diagnosis or classification. Although the differential diagnosis may be extremely difficult these cases will eventually prove to have a primary cause which is either in or outside the liver cell, and until the decision can be made the term cholestasis is the least objectionable in use; it is certainly preferable to "obstruction" since there is no evidence of mechanical obstruction in the hepatic examples of this condition.

Pre-hepatic, Haemolytic, or Retention Jaundice

As the various synonyms suggest, this variety is thought to be due mainly to over-production of bilirubin from excessive haemolysis. This may be

TABLE 5.2

Types of Jaundice

Type of Jaundice	Serum Bilirubin	Clinical Examples
Pre-hepatic	Unconjugated	Haemolytic conditions Neonatal jaundice.
Hepatic——pre-microsomal	Unconjugated	Gilbert's Crigler-Najjar.
hepatocellular	Conjugated	Hepatitis, Cirrhosis.
post-microsomal	Conjugated	Dubin-Johnson, Rotor, Drugs
cholestasis		Primary biliary cirrhosis.
Post-hepatic	Conjugated	Gall-stones, etc.

Table 5.2 represents an attempt by the author to bring this extra type of jaundice into relation to the others and incorporates proposals made by Nosslin (1960) and by Sherlock (1963) and Schiff (1963) and Billing (1963). The main new feature here is the concept that conjugation occurs in the microsomes for which good experimental evidence exists since the UDP glucuronyl transferase enzyme is mainly found in this site. The main difficulty is to fit in the term *"cholestasis"* which is becoming widely used to describe a

due either to abnormalities in the red cell, or to haemolysis of normal cells by abnormal antibodies or by extraneous haemolytic substances. It occurs typically in the congenital and acquired haemolytic anaemias, after transfusion of incompatible blood, and in malaria. It is also seen as a result of various poisons such as phenylhydrazine, snake venom, and occasionally sulphonamides. Haemolysis due to Rh-factor incompatibility is the main cause in haemolytic disease of the newborn, and bacterial or protozoal toxins and cold agglutinins may also be concerned in other cases (septicaemia, malaria, nocturnal and march haemoglobinurias). Further discussion of the causes of haemolysis will be found in haematological textbooks and special monographs (Wintrobe, 1967; Dacie, 1960).

In many of these conditions extensive haemolysis may occur without jaundice, as shown, e.g., by haemoglobinuria and/or excessive excretion of faecal stercobilin. For this reason it is generally assumed that a pure overload is insufficient to cause jaundice, but needs to be combined with some degree of liver cell damage, i.e. the jaundice is partly hepatic in origin. Such damage may either result directly from the toxic agent where present, or may be due to fatty infiltration of the liver associated with the anaemia which usually accompanies the other conditions. For this reason chronic extravascular haemolysis is more likely to produce jaundice than the acute intravascular variety.

The changes in pre-hepatic jaundice are fairly constant and include the following:

anaemia with reticulocytosis;
abnormal red cells or presence of haemolytic antibodies;
increased urinary excretion of urobilinogen and coproporphyrin;
increased excretion of faecal pigment, usually estimated as "faecal urobilinogen";
increase mainly in the unconjugated serum bilirubin fraction;
some bromsulphthalein retention;
other liver function tests mainly normal.

Particularly noteworthy for diagnosis are the haematological findings and the absence of bilirubin and bile salts from the urine, the nature of the serum bilirubin, and the normality of tests such as the serum alkaline phosphatase. In acute cases a sudden fall in the haemoglobin level or a failure of this level to respond to blood transfusion is an important sign, and in the newborn tests for maternal-foetal blood group incompatibility will be essential.

In the haemolytic anaemias the formation of pigment stones with possible post-hepatic jaundice is a complication which may cause difficulty in interpretation. Also, in cases with severe anaemia or severe toxic elements, some degree of overlap with hepatic types of jaundice may occur. Nevertheless the findings and clinical background are usually so typical that serious difficulties in diagnosis are rare.

A rare special variant of pre-hepatic jaundice is the "*shunt hyperbilirubinaemia*" of Israels, Suderman & Ritzman (1959). Here abnormal synthesis of early bilirubin occurs probably in the bone marrow, and signs of haemolysis are lacking. The mild jaundice of pernicious anaemia has similar features although here some haemolysis may also be present.

Hepatic Jaundice (1) *Pre-microsomal with Conjugation Failure*

It is remarkable that diseases such as infective hepatitis are not normally associated with conjugation failure, but this function can fail selectively in three conditions. Firstly in neonatal jaundice (see below) the virtual absence of conjugation during the first few days of life greatly increases jaundice due to physiological or to pathological haemolysis. Secondly there are two inborn errors of metabolism in which conjugation is defective. In the mild Gilbert's disease (1901), which is not uncommon, a transport defect in the liver cell is suspected. These individuals have a slight chronic jaundice with few symptoms and are usually discovered accidentally. A similar condition is seen in the Gunn strain of Wistar rats, which has been the subject of much investigation (Gunn, 1938; Schmid, 1965). The serum bilirubin is unconjugated and no obvious changes are seen in the urine or stool pigments. In the severe Crigler-Najjar (1952) syndrome, which is very rare, the hepatic UDP-glucuronyl transferase enzyme is completely absent from birth. The infants exhibit severe jaundice with unconjugated pigment and usually die early from kernicterus.

Hepatic Jaundice (2), *Toxic and Infective or Hepatocellular Jaundice*

Here all the functions of the liver are affected to some degree, although conjugation is usually normal. Infective hepatitis is the most familiar example of this variety, and although the liver is easily incriminated as the defective organ the detailed cause of the jaundice is still in dispute. Several different mechanisms have been suggested (Weinbren, 1952). The main pathological findings are those of centrilobular necrosis, but there may be sufficient swelling of the liver cells to cause blockage of the sinusoids or of the liver lymphatics. Alternatively, the whole architecture of the lobule may be destroyed in severe cases, or the infective process may single out the smaller bile capillaries in cholangiolytic hepatitis. These distinctions are interesting but to some extent academic, as they can rarely be demonstrated and may well co-exist. However, the pathological findings in "cholangiolytic" hepatitis are reasonably well defined as a necrosis confined to the peri-portal bile capillaries, and in this variety an abnormal permeability of these capillaries is the suggested cause of the jaundice. "Cholestasis" may be seen as in post-hepatic jaundice.

The causes of hepatic jaundice are numerous and will be partly discussed below (under acute hepatic necrosis). They include epidemic infective hepatitis, homologous serum jaundice, cholangio-lytic hepatitis, ascending cholangitis, cirrhosis and toxic hepatitis from drugs (chloroform, phosphorus, arsenic, trinitrotoluene, sulphonamides) and from bacterial toxins (septicaemia, peritonitis)

The biochemical findings in hepatic jaundice vary somewhat in the different varieties, but some or all of the following features are usually present:

> presence of bilirubin, urobilin, and bile salts in the urine;
> pale stool with low urobilinogen content;
> increase mainly in the conjugated bilirubin fraction;
> variable increase in total serum cholesterol, phospholipids, lipoproteins, iron, bile acids, alkaline phosphatase and transaminases;
> fall in serum albumin and/or rise in serum γ-globulin;
> fall in serum cholesterol/ester ratio and mucoprotein content;
> positive protein flocculation tests;
> bromsulphthalein retention;
> positive results with most other liver function tests, e.g. galactose tolerance, hippuric acid, etc.

Most of these changes are too well known to require detailed reference, but the statements concerning lipoproteins, iron, and mucoproteins depend upon contributions by Pierce, Kimmel & Burns, 1954; Ducci, Spoerer & Katz, 1952; Christian, 1954; and Greenspan, Tepper, Terry & Schoenbach, 1952). No special diagnostic advantage is at present claimed for the first of these procedures which is technically difficult, but the iron and mucoprotein estimations are further discussed below.

The extent to which these changes occur is variable from case to case depending upon the intensity, type and duration of the illness. In severe cases urobilin may disappear from stools and urine for periods of one or two weeks. Cases of purely toxic jaundice tend to show the least conspicuous changes, with abnormalities mainly in pigmentary tests, while in cholestasis the results may simulate to some extent those of post-hepatic jaundice (see below). The average case of

infective hepatitis, however, usually gives a typical and easily recognizable picture.

Hepatic Jaundice (3) *Post Microsomal, without Conjugation Failure*

Here conjugation proceeds normally but the conjugated pigment fails to reach the large bile ducts. Two varieties apparently due to inborn errors fall into this category. In the Dubin-Johnson (1954) syndrome the jaundice is of moderate severity and is accompanied by the deposition of a black pigment in the liver cells. In the Rotor (1948) syndrome the black pigment is missing but the condition is otherwise similar. Both these conditions are thought to represent failure of transport mechanisms within the liver cells.

Unfortunately jaundice due to certain drugs (see below) and a few cases of hepatitis present with very similar functional changes, usually with the histological appearances of cholestasis. These can be very difficult to distinguish from post-hepatic jaundice, even at laparotomy. A related condition is "recurrent intrahepatic cholestatic jaundice of pregnancy", which occurs during the last trimester and is thought to represent an unusual reaction to a steroid produced in pregnancy. The jaundice is accompanied by much pruritis and usually clears rapidly after the termination of pregnancy (Ljunggren, 1956; Sherlock, 1963).

Primary biliary cirrhosis (Hanot, 1876) (chronic intra-hepatic cholestasis, Sherlock, 1963) is another important example of this group. It occurs insidiously, usually in middle-aged women, and the symptomatology and biochemical changes resemble those of post-hepatic jaundice. The prognosis is bad, all patients dying after a few years. No mechanical obstruction is present. This disease is suspected of having an auto-immune basis, partly on account of the high levels of serum γ-globulin encountered.

Post-hepatic Jaundice

The factor of mechanical blockage is not in dispute here but the fine details are again undecided. As indicated by Rich's terminology there is evidence of regurgitation of bile into the blood stream, which may take place through the hepatic lymphatics or directly from the distended bile capillaries or possibly by both routes. In this respect the final mechanism is probably the same as in the milder cases of hepatitis. Since the failure to secrete bile is usually more complete and prolonged than in hepatitis, the degree of regurgitation tends to be greater, and in adults the most intense degrees of jaundice are seen most commonly in the post-hepatic variety. The qualitative changes in pigment metabolism are, however, virtually identical with those seen in hepatic jaundice. The suggestion has recently been made that the lack of distinction from hepatic jaundice may depend partly upon *deconjugation of bilirubin*, which has been shown to occur in the Gunn rat after ligation of bile ducts (Acocella, Tenconi, Armas-Merino, Raia & Billing, 1968).

Obstruction to the main bile passages may be caused by calculi, by strictures, and by a variety of malignant tumours originating in the bile ducts, pancreas, gall bladder, or by metastatic carcinoma in the portal fissure. Obstruction by plugs of mucus has been described, but is of doubtful validity.

The biochemical findings include:
bilirubin, urobilin and bile salts in the urine;
diminished or absent stool pigment;
increase mainly in the conjugated bilirubin fraction;
increase in total serum cholesterol, alkaline phosphatase, transaminases, phospholipids, bile salts, mucoprotein;
decrease in serum prothrombin and cholesterol/ ester ratio;
substantially normal results for serum proteins and protein flocculation tests;
variable impairment of bromsulphthalein retention, galactose tolerance, hippuric acid synthesis, etc.

The findings, particularly with the pigmentary tests, vary somewhat according to the completeness of the biliary obstruction, stool pigment, for example, being virtually absent in complete obstruction and usually present with an incomplete obstruction. Urobilinuria is thus confined to the incomplete variety. The duration of jaundice also has an important influence on tests such as galactose tolerance and hippuric acid, which may be normal in early cases but abnormal in late cases. It will be seen that the functional changes overlap to some extent with those of hepatic jaundice, but the biochemical picture is frequently distinctive enought to be of diagnostic help. The value of the various tests in the differential diagnosis of jaundice is discussed below.

While the above classification covers adequately the great majority of cases of jaundice in adults there is a residuum of conditions in which the pathology is either still in doubt or which possess some unique features requiring discussion. These include neonatal jaundice, and jaundice due to drugs.

Cholestasis. It will be seen from the above discussion that the condition labelled "cholestasis" is produced by a large number of hepatic and post-hepatic causes. The term implies a certain combination of clinical, histological, and biochemical features but is not a final diagnosis. The principal causes include mechanical obstruction of the bile passages, hepatitis, and many examples of jaundice due to drugs.

Neonatal Jaundice

Neonatal jaundice may be due to congenital obliteration of the bile ducts or to umbilical sepsis, but these conditions fall under the standard classification given above. The commoner types have, however, received much attention of recent years, and a considerable change of outlook has occurred as a result of the work of Mollison, Lathe and others. This reorientation is of interest not only for its own sake but for the analogies which it suggests in relation to the adult condition of constitutional hyperbilirubinaemia.

One important development has been the recognition of incompatibility of the Rh blood-group factors as the main cause of a particular type of haemolysis which may result in intra-uterine death or in a severe and dangerous neonatal jaundice (icterus gravis neonatorum, haemolytic disease of the newborn). More recently the existence of glucose-6-phosphate dehydrogenase deficiency has been recognized as a contributory cause, particularly in Greece (Doxiadis, Karaklis, Valaes & Stavrakakis, 1964). A full consideration of this question would be out of place here as it is fully dealt with in haematological and paediatric textbooks (Dacie, 1960; Gairdner, 1965).

Work on this subject has thrown much light on the milder types of neonatal jaundice, formerly regarded as physiological. In this condition the serum bilirubin is of the unconjugated variety and the earlier impression was of a pre-hepatic jaundice. This was thought to result from an accelerated destruction of red cells associated with the change from the neonatal haemoglobin level of about 20 g./100 ml. to the infantile value of 12 g./100 ml. This view was, however, challenged by Mollison (1948; Mollison & Cutbush, 1948) who showed that the degree of haemolysis at this time was not greatly excessive, and this has found general acceptance (Fashena, Bates & Reid, 1950; Arthurton, O'Brien & Mann, 1954). It appears, therefore, that we must regard this jaundice as partly hepatic in origin and due to the restricted ability of the liver in the newborn to excrete bilirubin in the bile. Thus it has been calculated that the neonatal liver can only excrete bilirubin in the bile at about 1–2% of the rate possible in the adult liver (Billing, Cole & Lathe, 1954). In these circumstances even a normal bilirubin production will result in jaundice. The pigment which accumulates is, however, unconjugated bilirubin since it has not been handled by the liver cell at all.

A recent development in this field is the sampling of amniotic fluid before birth. The bilirubin content of this fluid gives a good indication of the severity of the haemolytic process and may even constitute an indication for intra-uterine transfusion (Morris, Murray & Ruthven, 1967). The facility of conjugation rapidly increases during the first few days of life, but as would be expected it is inversely related to prematurity, so that premature infants become on the average more deeply jaundiced (Billing, Cole & Lathe, 1954). It should be added that these infants are not necessarily jaundiced at birth because of placental removal of bilirubin.

The accumulation of unconjugated bilirubin in the blood in haemolytic disease of the newborn may greatly exceed that seen in adult jaundice even when due to severe haemolysis, so that serum bilirubin values of 50 mg./100 ml. or more are not uncommon in cases due to Rh factor incompatibility. This accumulation frequently has important effects on the brain, where staining of the basal ganglia may occur with permanent structural damage (kernicterus). The serum bilirubin level is a useful guide as to the risk of this complication and modern treatment aims at avoiding levels above 20 mg./100 ml. by repeated exchange transfusions (Hsia, Allen, Diamond & Gellis, 1953). The increasing brain involvement associated with high values is clearly shown in Table 5.3. More recently Stern & Denton (1965) have shown that much lower levels of serum bilirubin, even below 10 mg./100 ml., may be associated with kernicterus in small premature infants with respiratory disease and acidosis. Exchange transfusion is naturally more difficult in these cases.

TABLE 5.3

Relation between maximum bilirubin concentration in the plasma and kernicterus (from Mollison & Cutbush, 1954)

Maximum bilirubin concentration (mg./100 ml.)	Total number of cases	Number with kernicterus
30–40	11	8
25–29	12	4
19–24	13	1
10–18	24	0

All this evidence appears to suggest that we should look upon bilirubin as a potentially toxic substance and its conjugation by the liver as a process of detoxication (Claireaux, Cole & Lathe, 1953).

At a slightly later period we have a new type of jaundice in breast-fed infants in which unusual quantities of progestational steroids are secreted into the breast milk. These steroids inhibit the glucuronyl transferase enzyme and hence lead to the perpetuation of neonatal jaundice with unconjugated hyperbilirubinaemia (Arias, Gartner, Seifter & Furman, 1964).

Jaundice Due to Drugs

Drugs may produce liver damage with or without jaundice by a variety of mechanisms (Sherlock, 1964). Firstly *pre-hepatic (haemolytic) jaundice* may be produced directly by phenylhydrazine or indirectly by drugs such as para-aminosalicylate, phenacetin or quinine which cause the formation of antibodies to the drug-erythrocyte complex. *Hepatic jaundice* may be of the following types:

(*a*) Generalized toxic action as with carbon tetrachloride or phosphorus.

(*b*) Hepatitis-like jaundice, as with iproniazid and its derivatives. This is a sensitivity reaction and is clinically and pathologically indistinguishable from infective hepatitis.

(*c*) Cholestatic type which may be a sensitivity reaction (chlorpromazine and derivatives) or dose-dependent as with C17- alkyl steroids such as methyl testosterone. Contraceptive pills contain progestogens of this type which, although rarely causing jaundice, have been accused of producing changes in liver function, particularly in older women (Borglin, 1965; Burton, Loudin, Wilson, 1967).

Other drugs may act by competition with conjugation or transport mechanisms (Novobiocin, Bunamiodyl). Rather unexpectedly the anaesthetic halothane, in spite of its chemical relationship to chloroform, is associated with a hepatitis-like picture. The complication is however so rare that doubt is still felt as to whether the halothane is the actual cause of the jaundice (National Halothane Study, 1966). Hepatotoxic substances may also occur in certain foodstuffs such as groundnuts and the role of alcohol is still debatable (see under cirrhosis).

Laboratory Distinction between Different Types of Jaundice

An enormous amount of work and much heartburning has gone into this subject, which is perhaps best considered on a historical basis.

Van den Bergh's discovery of the *direct reaction* given by certain sera with solutions of diazotized sulphanilic acid may be regarded as the pioneer observation. Although he did not make far-reaching claims for the test the impression soon gained ground that it was a valuable weapon in the differential diagnosis of jaundice and many of the textbooks of that time listed the three types of reaction—"prompt", "biphasic", and "delayed" —as though they were specific indications of post-hepatic, hepatic, and pre-hepatic jaundice respectively. There were, however, dissentient voices (Harrison, 1930), and it was eventually recognized that these three terms were difficult to define accurately by the visual methods then in use, and that in any case the overlap between the groups was considerable.

We were, however, left with the absence of a direct reaction and also of bilirubinuria as a valuable indication of pre-hepatic or haemolytic jaundice. The significance of urinary and faecal urobilinogen estimations was also very thoroughly explored, and the values and limitations of these tests were established (Watson, 1937, 1938, 1942). Once more their contribution was mainly in the direction of isolating haemolysis as a possible cause of jaundice, since the overlap between the hepatic and post-hepatic varieties was considerable. The virtual absence of faecal and urinary urobilin in *complete* biliary obstruction is, however, still a finding of some value.

The next phase was the exploration of a number of non-pigmentary tests which it was hoped would help in making the all-important distinction between hepatic and post-hepatic jaundice. This is obviously of the greatest clinical importance since the former requires medical treatment while surgery may be indicated in the latter. A considerable literature developed during the 1930–40 period on tests such as hippuric acid, galactose and laevulose tolerance, cincophen oxidation, the Takata-Ara reaction and the serum cholinesterase estimation (Jezler, 1930; Roe & Schwartzman, 1933; Quick, 1933, 1939; Stewart, Scarborough & Davidson, 1938; Maclagan, 1940; McArdle, 1940; Lichtman, 1942). All of these showed a statistical difference between the two types of jaundice, but no one of them proved reliable when extended to a large series of cases. During this period, however, the merits of serum alkaline phosphatase estimation were recognized, and the frequency of values over 30 units in post-hepatic jaundice was established (Roberts, 1933; King & Armstrong, 1934; Bodansky & Jaffé, 1934; Gutman, Olson, Gutman & Flood, 1940).

The next development, which is still proceeding, was the institution of the protein flocculation tests and of the electrophoretic technique to which they are linked, together with the idea of combining a number or "battery" of tests into a complete picture. The extensive literature on this subject was reviewed by Watson (1944), Maclagan (1948, 1955), Hoffbauer, Rames & Meinert (1949,) Popper, Bean, de la Huerga, Franklin, Tsumagari, Routh & Steigmann (1951) and Lichtman (1954) and recent work on the newer enzyme tests is discussed below. Table 5.4 presents the general trend of findings with those tests which show a reasonably significant and useful difference between the various types of jaundice.

This emphasizes the facts noted above that the pigmentary tests are useful and usually adequate for the diagnosis of pre-hepatic jaundice, but fail to discriminate between the two other varieties. The other tests listed are those most likely to distinguish hepatic from post-hepatic jaundice, but they all show some degree of overlap between the two types.

An all-important consideration in this connection is to know when the tests are sufficiently typical to permit diagnostic deductions and when they are not, and there is no doubt that failure to recognize the possibility of defeat has contributed much to the confusion in this subject. The writer's experience with 200 cases of jaundice studied with the thymol-phosphatase combination is summarized in Table 5.5.

It will be seen from this Table that 80% of the cases fell into areas which were homogeneous, so that, e.g., no cases of hepatic or pre-hepatic jaundice were found in the post-hepatic areas, and vice versa. The remaining 20% were, however, labelled "equivocal" as they occurred in a "no-man's land" common to all types of jaundice. When this scheme was advanced it was, of course, anticipated that occasional exceptions were to be expected and such cases have been reported by Coleman (1950). However, it appears otherwise to have met with fairly general acceptance (Maizels, 1946; Mawson, 1948; Hoffbauer et al. 1949; Ricketts, 1953; Wang, 1953), and probably represents the simplest useful combination of laboratory tests at present available for distinguishing post-hepatic from the other varieties of jaundice.

Other flocculation tests have also been used in combination with the serum alkaline phosphatase, and the merits of the prothrombin test have been particularly evident in the surgical jaundice group (Stein, 1944). Here the risk of haemorrhage is mainly due to low plasma prothrombin levels, which may arise either from liver damage or from

TABLE 5.4

Liver function tests of value in differential diagnosis of the common varieties of jaundice

	Types of jaundice		
Test	Pre-hepatic	Hepatic	Post-hepatic
Bilirubinuria	Usually absent	Present	Present
Urobilinuria	Frequently present	Usually present	Variable with degree of obstruction
Faecal urobilinogen	Increased	Usually diminished	Usually diminished
Serum bilirubin	Mainly unconjugated	Mainly conjugated	Mainly conjugated
Serum alkaline phosphatase	Normal	Normal or moderately raised	Much increased
5′-nucleotidase	Normal	Normal or moderately raised	Much increased
Serum aminotransferases (transaminases)	Normal	Very high in first week	Moderately raised
Protein flocculation tests	Normal or weakly positive	Usually positive	Negative except with much biliary infection
Serum proteins	Normal	Albumin low, γ-globulin high	α_2 globulin high
Prothrombin response to vitamin K	Not usually applicable	Impaired	Normal

TABLE 5.5

Thymol-phosphatase combination in 200 cases of jaundice
(after Maclagan, 1947)

No. of cases	Thymol flocculation test	Serum alkaline phosphatase (King-Armstrong units)	Diagnostic indication
38	0 or 1 +	Over 35 units	All post-hepatic
92	2 + or more	—	All hepatic or pre-hepatic
67	—	Under 15 units	All hepatic or pre-hepatic
40	0 or 1 +	15 to 35 units	All types—no differentiation

Note. In this table 1+ thymol flocculation indicates either incomplete flocculation, or complete flocculation with a turbidity of 4 units or less.

impaired absorption of vitamin K (due to lack of bile in the intestine). In the latter case a prompt return to normal is obtained with vitamin K therapy and failure of this return suggests either a hepatic type of jaundice or very severe secondary liver damage. In this event operation is either contra-indicated or carries a much increased risk. It should be noted that the prothrombin response to vitamin K is only available in patients whose prothrombin is initially below normal, which restricts the test to perhaps one third of all cases of jaundice (Stein, 1944).

The serum iron estimation has been suggested as a useful diagnostic agent, values above 300 μg./100 ml. favouring hepatitis as against obstructive jaundice (Ducci *et al.* 1952; Christian, 1954). A similar but inverse relationship also exists with the serum mucoprotein concentration, which is raised in post-hepatic jaundice, but lowered in hepatic jaundice (Greenspan *et al.* 1952). More recently the new enzyme tests described below have taken an important place in the diagnosis of acute hepatitis in which very high values, particularly for the transaminases, are usually seen during the first week of the disease. Unfortunately, these high values do not usually persist for more than a few days, so that the tests are not so useful in differential diagnosis after this time. The administration of cortisol is sometimes helpful, since this will usually reduce the intensity of jaundice due to hepatitis ("steroid white-wash") while it is without effect on post-hepatic jaundice (Sherlock, 1963).

Finally it must be admitted that most of the literature on the subject has been concerned with the presentation of data from typical cases of infective hepatitis and of post-hepatic jaundice and the differentiation is much more difficult in cases of long standing cholestasis. The functional changes in hepatic and in extra-hepatic cholestasis can be very similar and will not usually provide a firm basis for diagnosis after the first few weeks.

SERUM ENZYMES

During the last decade important new work has appeared on changes in the serum enzymes which occur in liver disease. This has consisted not only in the exploration of new enzymes but also in the further sub-division of those previously known, particularly by electrophoretic methods. The name "iso-enzymes" has been coined for these fractions with similar biochemical properties but different electrophoretic mobilities.

Alkaline Phosphatase

The status of the serum alkaline phosphatase (SAP) estimation in the hepatic field is too well known to require much elaboration. We may recall here that it is mainly raised in cases of post-hepatic jaundice, frequently to over 35 King-Armstrong units; moderate increases, usually below 35 units, occur in hepatitis and in other diseases of the liver such as abscess, amyloidosis, carcinomatosis, etc. The merits of combining alkaline phosphatase estimations with the thymol flocculation tests for the differential diagnosis of jaundice are discussed above.

The SAP is of course also raised in a variety of bone diseases, and here the use of electrophoresis to distinguish the two enzymes concerned may be useful. In Table 5.6 the main difference between the bone and liver enzyme is indicated, the latter having a faster mobility. It is true that in most cases the cause of a raised SAP is obvious on purely clinical grounds, but cases have been recorded where genuine doubt has arisen, and in which the iso-enzyme technique has been of value (Cooke & Zilva, 1961).

Aminotransferases (Transaminases)

The aminotransferases are enzymes of great importance in protein and amino acid metabolism, and they catalyse the exchange of the $=O$ for the $<^H_{NH_2}$ groups. The reactions concerned in the case of the aspartate and alanine aminotransferases (GOT and GPT) are illustrated in Fig. 5.5. The distributions of these two enzymes in various body tissues are shown in Table 5.7.

A variety of acceptable methods of estimation have been worked out depending upon colorimetric or spectrophotometric methods and the changes undergone by these two enzymes in liver disease have been extensively investigated. (See reviews by Wróblewski, 1958; and Wilkinson, 1961.)

The following account is based upon the results obtained in my department by Prof. J. H. Wilkinson and his colleagues, and is illustrated by Fig. 5.6. Broadly speaking, both aminotransferases are dramatically above normal for at least the first week of infective hepatitis. Moderate rises are also seen in the later stages of hepatitis and also in post-hepatic jaundice, in cirrhosis, and with hepatic carcinomatosis. In the case of aspartate aminotransferase values of above 150 Inter-

TABLE 5.6

Tissue of origin of serum iso-enzymes

Associated with serum globulin fraction	Alkaline phosphatase (1)	Lactic dehydrogenase (2)	Aspartate amino-transferase (3)
α_1	liver	heart	—
$\alpha_2(1a)$	bone	—	⎰ liver, heart
$\beta(1b)$	bone	—*	⎱
γ	—	liver	—

From data of (1a) Rosenberg (1959), (1b) Keiding (1959), (2) Vesell & Bearn (1957) and (3) Pryse-Davies & Wilkinson (1958).

* Other LDH iso-enzymes have been described but are not organ-specific.

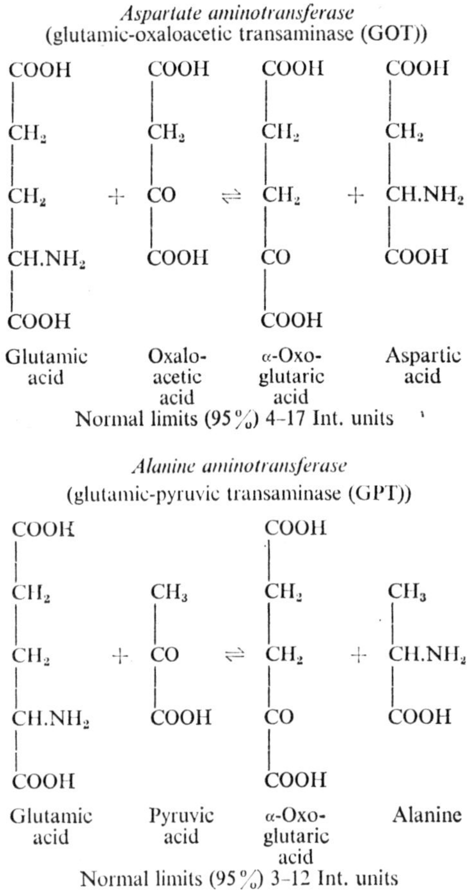

Aspartate aminotransferase
(glutamic-oxaloacetic transaminase (GOT))

COOH	COOH	COOH	COOH
CH$_2$	CH$_2$	CH$_2$	CH$_2$
CH$_2$ + CO	$\rightleftharpoons$ CH$_2$	+	CH.NH$_2$
CH.NH$_2$	COOH	CO	COOH
COOH		COOH	

Glutamic acid   Oxalo-acetic acid   α-Oxo-glutaric acid   Aspartic acid

Normal limits (95%) 4–17 Int. units

Alanine aminotransferase
(glutamic-pyruvic transaminase (GPT))

COOH		COOH	
CH$_2$	CH$_3$	CH$_2$	CH$_3$
CH$_2$ + CO	$\rightleftharpoons$ CH$_2$	+	CH.NH$_2$
CH.NH$_2$	COOH	CO	COOH
COOH		COOH	

Glutamic acid   Pyruvic acid   α-Oxo-glutaric acid   Alanine

Normal limits (95%) 3–12 Int. units

FIG. 5.5. Reactions catalysed by aminotransferases.

national units are almost confined to infective hepatitis, but are unfortunately usually only seen in the first week of the disease. Values up to this level may also occur in the other conditions mentioned and are not therefore so valuable in differential diagnosis. The alanine aminotransferase undergoes very similar changes in liver disease to those shown by aspartate aminotransferase, but it is much more specifically related to the liver (Table 5.7) and remains elevated rather longer in acute hepatitis.

Most workers have preferred to use aspartate aminotransferase for routine purposes since it is also useful in the cardiac cases, and clinical confusion between the two is unusual. If this should occur, the iso-enzyme technique is unfortunately not useful since the liver and heart enzymes have similar electrophoretic mobilities (Table 5.6).

Dehydrogenases

The lactic dehydrogenase (LDH) catalyses conversion of lactic to pyruvic acid and is widely distributed in the various body tissues. It is raised in the serum in a variety of conditions such as hepatitis, cardiac infarction, carcinomatosis, etc. (Wróblewski, 1959). Variations during the course of hepatitis are illustrated in Fig. 5.6, from which it can be seen that the rise is rather transient, occurring only during the first few days of the disease. The estimation does not therefore appear to be as useful as that of other enzymes in the investigation of patients with liver disease.

Recently the occurrence in serum of an enzyme acting on the next higher homologue of lactic acid—the α-hydroxybutyric dehydrogenase

TABLE 5.7

Comparison of enzyme activities in normal human tissue homogenates
(International units*/g. wet tissue)

Tissue	Glutamic[1] oxaloacetic transaminase	Glutamic[1] pyruvic transaminase	Lactic[2] dehydrogenase
Heart	75	3·4	79
Liver	68	21	123
Skeletal muscle	48	2·3	65
Kidney	44	9·1	—
Pancreas	13·4	1·0	—
Serum	0·01	0·008	0·12
Erythrocytes	5·1[3]	1·7[3]	29[3]

Figures calculated from data published by (1) Wroblewski & LaDue (1956), (2) Elliott & Wilkinson (1961), (3) B. A. Elliott (unpublished).

* μmoles substrate transformed per minute.

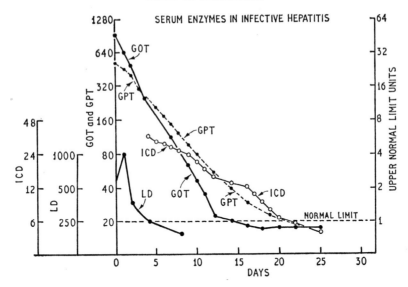

FIG. 5.6. Serum enzymes in infective hepatitis. Enzyme units on logarithmic scales with common upper normal limits. Drawn from data of Wilkinson (1961) and Sterkel, Spencer, Wolfson and Williams-Ashman (1958). Enzymes are given in International units (μmoles/min./l.).

(SHBD)—has been described by Elliott & Wilkinson (1961) and the use of this enzyme appears to be more promising in the liver field. The method of estimation is similar to that of LDH, but uses α-hydroxybutyric acid as substrate. High results occur both in acute hepatitis and in myocardial infarction, but the ratio SLD-SHBD appears to be a useful diagnostic feature, values over 1·5 being confined to cases of acute liver disease.

Variations in the isocitric dehydrogenases (ICD) have been investigated at length by Sterkel, Spencer, Wolfson & Williams-Ashman (1958) and changes of this enzyme in hepatitis appear to resemble fairly closely those of alanine aminotransferase, although they are quantitatively smaller (Fig. 5.6). The enzyme is said to be even more specifically related to the liver than alanine aminotransferase. Raised values are also seen in nutritional diseases of the liver such as kwashiorkor (Baron & Bell, 1960).

5'-nucleotidase

Adenosine-5'-phosphate is the substrate usually used to demonstrate this enzyme, and the level in serum varies normally between 1.6–17 International units per litre. As with SAP the highest values are found in post-hepatic jaundice, with moderate elevations in hepatic conditions; unlike the alkaline phosphatase no significant changes occur with bone disease (Wootton, 1964).

Other Serum Enzymes

The ornithine-carbamyl transferase is raised in many hepatic and intestinal diseases, and high values are said to indicate liver disease in cases where gross intestinal pathology is absent (Reichard, 1961). The β-glucuronidase is usually elevated in acute hepatitis and in cirrhosis, unless the disease is very severe, when values may fall *below* normal (Goldbarg, Pineda, Banks & Rutenburg, 1959).

The distribution of leucine aminopeptidase (LAP) appears to be similar to that of alkaline phosphatase, high values resulting from interference with biliary excretion from any cause. This enzyme has also a special relation to pancreatic disease where high values are very frequent, even in the absence of jaundice (Pineda, Goldbarg, Banks & Rutenburg, 1960). In jaundice values for LAP above 450 units suggest post-hepatic jaundice and it has been claimed that the findings are more consistent than those of SAP.

The use of many other enzymes and of various *enzyme ratios* has been advocated such as the aspartate aminotransferase/alanine aminotransferase and the aspartate aminotransferase/SAP ratio (Latner & Smith, 1958). The subject has been reviewed by de Ritis Giusti, Piccinino & Cacciatore (1965).

ACUTE HEPATIC NECROSIS

The recognition of the regional types of hepatic necrosis as a comparitvely common event has constituted a major development of liver pathology in recent years, and the exploration of the different types of necrosis and of the different agents and conditions which may cause them is still in progress. The following list, which is by no means exhaustive, represents the main varieties and/or agents at present recognized:

1. Virus infections,
   - (a) epidemic infective hepatitis
   - (b) homologous serum jaundice
   - (c) yellow fever
   - (d) infective mononucleosis
2. Bacterial infections,
   - (a) pneumonia
   - (b) septicaemia
   - (c) coli-typhoid infection
3. Protozoal infections — leptospirosis icterohaemorrhagica, malaria, syphilis
4. In major surgery — particularly when associated with anoxia, severe infection, extracorporeal circulation
5. Chemical poisons
   - (a) inorganic: arsenicals, phosphorus, gold, selenium
   - (b) organic: chloroform, CCl_4, trinitrotoluene, sulphonamides, atophan, cincophen, tannic acid.
   - (c) vegetable: "mushroom" poisoning
6. Experimental — poisons, low protein diets, cystine deficiency
7. Miscellaneous
   - (a) acute yellow atrophy
   - (b) cholangiolytic hepatitis

An important feature of most clinical varieties of this condition is the great variability in the intensity of the process, which may vary from a mild centrilobular necrosis with few symptoms to a massive necrosis involving one or more whole lobes of the liver with fulminating onset and rapid death. These fatal cases are fortunately rare. A further presumed common feature is the occasional sequel of chronic hepatitis and cirrhosis as a late complication. While this is well recognized in certain cases, e.g. infective hepatitis or cincophen poisoning, in others it has not been demonstrated with certainty; however, in view of the essential similarity of the pathological processes involved this possibility always merits consideration. The relation of these diseases to experimental hepatic necrosis is still the subject of dispute, but some valuable aetiological pointers have arisen from these studies. Certain aspects of each group which have been illuminated by recent work will now be considered individually.

Virus Infections

The commonest cause of icterus in temperate climates was generally known as "catarrhal jaundice" until just before the Second World War. This condition, which has now been re-named "infective hepatitis", had been described by Virchow (1847) under its former name because he considered that it was due to an acute inflammation in the duodenum causing blockage of the common bile duct by mucous exudate. Although Eppinger (1937) in the First World War gave a correct description of the disease, which was substantiated by liver function studies, accurate autopsy observations were necessarily few and the old name was perpetuated until the development of the punch-biopsy method by Roholm & Iversen (1939), which enabled histological observations to be made at all stages of the disease. These workers described a widespread centrilobular necrosis as a constant feature, and their results were confirmed and extended by Dible, McMichael & Sherlock (1943), and by Lucké (1944). Finally, the condition was transmitted to human volunteers by MacCallum & Bradley (1944), using bacteria-free blood, serum and faecal suspensions, thus indicating its virus nature. Although in some of these experiments the incubation period was very long, with inoculation by the naso-pharyngeal route the normal incubation period of about 30 days was seen. This disease may thus be said to have changed its name during the Second World War.

The same period saw the discovery of the important new disease now called "homologous serum jaundice", or simply "serum hepatitis". Although the condition must have existed previously (Hirsch, 1886), the first important outbreak in Great Britain was due to a batch of convalescent measles serum which caused cases of fatal jaundice among the children inoculated (McNalty, 1938). Once the long incubation period (about 3 months) had been recognized, the association with blood transfusion became apparent (Morgan & Williamson, 1943), and in 1944 MacCallum & Bauer produced jaundice in four out of eleven volunteer subjects inoculated with a pool of serum from a blood bank. Further examples of the disease include the large outbreak following prophylactic inoculation against yellow fever (human serum was added to the vaccine at that time) (Findlay, 1940), and numerous instances of syringe-transmitted hepatitis. The latter arose from the use of the same syringe for injecting a number of patients with, e.g., anti-syphilitic drugs, or even simply for the removal of blood, as in diabetic clinics.

It is evident, therefore, that the administration of even minute amounts of human blood or blood products from one subject to another is always a potentially dangerous procedure, and it is reasonably certain that homologous serum jaundice is due to a specific virus transmitted in this way. While some of the causes listed above can be eliminated by the proper sterilization of syringes, blood transfusion still carries this unavoidable risk, a risk which is naturally greater for pooled plasma than for whole blood which is not pooled (MacCallum *et al.* 1951). The overall attack-rate at the present time varies from 0·6–6·2 cases per 100 persons transfused with "average risk" material (Mosley & Dull, 1966).

Although the incubation period is so different, the signs and symptoms of the disease are indistinguishable from those of epidemic infective hepatitis, and liver biopsy studies have shown an identical histological picture. Changes in liver function may include all those listed under hepatic jaundice above. Demonstrable liver damage may sometimes be seen without jaundice, and even without a rise in the total serum bilirubin, although bilirubinuria will usually be found if sensitive tests are used (Pollock, 1945). While in most cases the functional impairment only lasts for a few weeks, it may last much longer (Kornberg, 1942) and may occasionally progress to cirrhosis.

In spite of these similarities the two viruses are immunologically distinct and one disease does not protect against the other (Neefe, Stokes & Gellis, 1945; Neefe, 1946). Further differences are the greater tendency to negative flocculation tests in serum jaundice (Maclagan, 1944b), and also the increased likelihood of serious interference with bile flow in this disease (Steigmann, Meyer & Popper, 1949). These two facts would suggest a significant association between serum jaundice and cholangiolytic hepatitis (see below). It may well be thought remarkable that the infective character of two such important diseases should have been recognized only during the last 20–30 years. The difficulties in establishing their nature appear to have been due mainly to the long incubation period in the case of serum jaundice, and to the rather sporadic incidence of infective hepatitis in settled populations, together with the technical difficulties of identifying the viruses concerned in the absence of any susceptible animal.

Yellow fever has been recognized as a virus infection causing jaundice for many years, but the hepatic lesion in glandular fever has only been studied more recently. Jaundice is only an occasional complication of this disease, and was at one time thought to be due to enlargement of lymphatic glands in the portal fissure causing biliary obstruction. However, recent work suggests that a true hepatitis similar to that of infective hepatitis is probably a constant feature, and liver function tests give abnormal results in a high proportion of cases. We must, therefore, remember the disease as a potential cause of liver damage.

Bacterial Infections

Liver involvement in severe bacterial infections is well recognized and may vary from the more usual cloudy swelling to an acute hepatic necrosis. The latter is a rather rare event, but is the probable cause of the mild jaundice which may accompany, for example, pneumonia. Under present conditions the more severe cases of jaundice are often associated with treatment by sulphonamides or other antibiotics which may perhaps contribute to the liver damage; such cases have been described by Irwin (1952). In these cases the liver function tests were those of a toxic rather than an infective jaundice, with normal alkaline phosphatase and protein flocculation tests.

Protozoal Infections

The principal new work here has concerned the fairly constant hepatitis which occurs in malaria and the nature of jaundice arising during antisyphilitic treatment. The latter is probably rarely due to syphilis, and appears to be of two unrelated types. It may occur within one or two weeks of the first injection, when probably it represents a true toxic reaction to arsenic. More usually, however, it appears at any time after the third month of treatment, and this variety is usually due to syringe transmission of the virus of homologous serum jaundice. This preventable condition has been discussed above.

The frequency of hepatic involvement in malaria has also been recognized; this work is considered below.

Chemical Poisons

These include industrial causes and those arising during therapy, e.g. sulphonamides, gold treatment of rheumatoid arthritis. In some cases the hepatic complications have been sufficiently severe to contra-indicate the use of the drug altogether (atophan, cincophen, tannic acid). Arsenic constitutes a special case which has been discussed above.

The case of selenium is of interest as it is of some importance in veterinary medicine and has been used to produce experimental liver necrosis. Animals fed with grain from seleniferous soils, or on a diet supplemented with selenium compounds, develop a massive necrosis very similar to that produced by cystine deficiency. It has been suggested that selenium may replace the sulphur in cystine causing an interference with its normal utlization in the body (Moxon & Rhian, 1943).

In this group of toxic hepatic necrosis as a whole, the liver function tests usually give rather different results from those seen in the infective types of hepatitis. The changes are mainly in the pigmentary tests, and in certain others such as cholinesterase, cholesterol/ester ratio, hippuric acid, etc., while the more reactive tests such as the serum alkaline phosphatase and protein flocculation tests are usually normal.

Experimental

Most recent work on experimental liver necrosis in animals has been carried out either with carbon tetrachloride or with various types of dietary deficiency. These two procedures give rise to very different liver lesions and much interest attaches to the possible clinical applications of the work (Stoner & Magee, 1957).

Carbon tetrachloride produces an acute centrilobular necrosis within a few hours of administration, affecting all the lobules simultaneously. After a single dose the animals either die rapidly or eventually recover completely, although a uniform fine cirrhosis can be produced by repeated sub-lethal doses (Cameron & Karunaratne, 1936). The similarity between this type of necrosis and that of infective hepatitis is fairly close, with the important exception that *massive* necrosis cannot apparently be produced by CCl_4 administration. This has been taken as evidence that massive necrosis is entirely distinct from zonal necrosis and is not just an extension of it (Hadfield, 1953). Some very interesting observations have been made by Rees & Sinha (1960) and by Rees, Sinha & Spector (1961) on the serum enzymes in experimental hepatic necrosis in rats

after CCl_4 and thioacetamide poisoning. Striking elevations of *iso*citric and glutamic dehydrogenases were demonstrated which could be almost prevented by the administration of the antihistamine drug "Phenergan", which has the effect of limiting cellular permeability; it was also successful in preventing the death of the animals. It will be interesting to see whether this observation can be exploited in the clinical field.

Protein deficiency on the other hand produces only a massive necrosis which occurs suddenly after a latent period of several weeks. This type of necrosis has been extensively studied, particularly by Himsworth & Glynn (1944) and by György (1944), and is thought to be due mainly to cystine deficiency. However, it can be prevented by a-tocopherol and also by a factor in casein which was shown to contain selenium (Factor 3 of Schwarz, 1951, 1960). It can also apparently be prevented by the simultaneous administration of antibiotics (Forbes, Leach & Williams, 1942), or by rearing the animals in a germ-free state (Luckey, Reyniers, György & Forbes, 1954). However, in the latter case the protection was shown to be due to a stimulation of appetite in the germ-free animals, for when they were restricted to a food consumption equal to that of the controls, hepatic necrosis appeared. Massive necrosis can also be produced experimentally by certain other poisons such as trinitrotoluene; these, however, require a latent period and associated protein deficiency for their action, and it has been suggested that they may act by combining with essential amino acids (Himsworth, 1947).

The morbid anatomy of experimental massive necrosis closely resembles that of acute yellow atrophy in man, and it is Himsworth's contention that the ultimate mechanism of both conditions depends upon a circulatory obstruction in the hepatic circulation consequent on swelling of the liver cells. This question is discussed more fully in the next section.

Acute Yellow Atrophy

A fatal form of massive liver necrosis involving the whole of one or more lobes has been recognized for many years, and has usually been described in association with pregnancy, with chemical poisons such as cincophen, nitrophenols, and trinitrotoluene, and with infective hepatitis both of the epidemic and serum varieties. It is generally regarded as simply an extreme form of hepatic necrosis of zonal type, in which the areas concerned have increased to involve the whole organ, but the recent work on experimental massive necrosis in animals referred to above has thrown doubt on this and has been interpreted by some workers as indicating an additional and fundamentally different mechanism.

The main arguments leading to this viewpoint are the striking resemblance between the condition of the liver in acute yellow atrophy and that seen in experimental massive necrosis produced by protein deficiency, and the difficulty of producing anything resembling a massive necrosis in mammals by the administration of poisons by themselves.

According to Himsworth & Glynn (1944), the additional factor which precipitates acute yellow atrophy in a patient with hepatic necrosis is a sudden swelling of the liver cells which obstructs the blood supply to one or more lobes of the liver. Such an event, which is, of course, not directly observable, they regard as also the probable cause of massive necrosis due to protein deficiency. It is therefore interesting to find a suggestive correlation between the severity of hepatic lesions and the previous nutrition of the patient. This is provided, e.g., by the comparative mortality rates in epidemics of infective hepatitis in well-nourished individuals as opposed to those suffering from various forms of malnutrition. Thus, in an epidemic of serum hepatitis in Brazil due to yellow fever vaccine, the mortality among the American troops was only 0·2% compared to a figure of 2·4% among the local population (Fox, Manso, Penna & Para, 1942). The association of acute yellow atrophy with pregnancy can also be plausibly attributed to a relative malnutrition due to vomiting and the extra demands of the foetus.

However, in other cases the disease may develop without any obvious background of this sort, for according to Lucké (1944) there was no observable difference in nutrition or in severity of early symptoms between his cases of infective hepatitis who died from massive necrosis and those who recovered. He did, however, mention persistent vomiting as an important prodromal symptom, and this could mean that the resulting nutritional disturbance was the actual precipitating factor. We may therefore reasonably conclude that some relationship with malnutrition has been established, although the mechanism by which this is made effective is at present a matter of speculation.

The recognition of this relationship has led to many attempts at treating cases of severe liver damage with high-protein diets and with cystine, methionine, and tocopherol (Latner, 1950; MacCallum, McFarlan, Miles, Pollock & Wilson, 1951). It is difficult to evaluate this form of treatment as control series were usually of necessity lacking, but encouraging results have been recorded in cirrhosis and in a few cases of severe acute necrosis. We might perhaps hope for more concrete effects in prophylaxis than in treatment of the established condition, but this possibility is hard to test.

Changes in liver function in acute yellow atrophy naturally tend to be well marked, and many or all of those listed above under "hepatic jaundice" can usually be demonstrated. In addition there may be others which are typical of the more severe degrees of liver failure such as gross amino-aciduria, with high blood amino acid levels, low values for blood urea, sugar, and fibrinogen, and elevated blood ammonia values. These are more fully discussed in a later section (Hepatic coma).

After Major Surgery

This is comparatively rare as a fatal complication, the overall incidence being about 1 per 10,000 operations. Most cases occur either as a result of blood transfusion (serum hepatitis) or in association with severe shock, infection or anoxia. Heart operations with extracorporeal circulation are particularly dangerous (22 cases per 10,000 ops.) and operations involving the liver or large vessels also show an increased incidence. Minor degrees of necrosis are probably much commoner and recovery may occur (for review see Maclagan, 1967).

HEPATIC CIRRHOSIS

In spite of the antiquity of this disease and of an immense amount of clinical, pathological, and experimental work, the actual pathogenesis of the condition remains either undecided or at best imperfectly explained. As in the case of massive necrosis the main problem at the present time is to reconcile the experimental and clinical findings, and no doubt one of the main difficulties here is in the considerable number of years needed to produce the final picture in man. This means that the initial stages are either never seen, or if seen cannot be correlated with the end-result. Nevertheless, the modern experimental approach has contributed many useful pointers and has suggested a number of possible relationships.

The definition of cirrhosis at once presents a difficulty as the word is often used to include the late results of cholangitis, syphilis, or chronic passive congestion. However, these forms will be excluded from the present account, which is concerned with that variety of coarse, hard fibrosis which is not due to any obvious inflammatory or circulatory cause and which involves a destruction of normal liver architecture. Livers of this type are not infrequently seen at autopsy in patients dying from unrelated complaints, indicating that the condition must be compatible with fair health for considerable periods. Patients dying of the disease, however, will have had some obvious symptoms and signs such as dyspepsia, ascites, oedema, or haematemesis.

The onset may be insidious without any apparent predisposing cause, but recognized aetiological factors are alcoholism, exposure to certain liver poisons such as atophan, cincophen, or trinitrotoluene, grossly deficient diets and previous attacks of virus hepatitis. The influence of deficient diets is seen particularly in the study by Gillman & Gillman (1945) of cirrhosis in South Africa; in this country the condition is common in the native population who live principally on maize meal, bean and fermented cows' milk. The traditional association with alcoholism is well accepted (Boles & Crew, 1940; Fagin & Thompson, 1944), but the degree of association appears to vary considerably in different countries. Thus Himsworth (1947), in Great Britain, appeared to find the association uncommon, while in the United States the majority of cases occur in heavy drinkers (Hall, Olsen & Davis, 1953). Although only some 8% of known heavy drinkers appear to develop cirrhosis (Kark, 1952) there is a definite relationship between the amount of alcohol consumed and the death-rate from cirrhosis (Klatskin, 1961).

It has always been very difficult to understand how such a variety of causes could produce a similar final condition, but the existence of two distinct types of cirrhosis provides a possible explanation and is strongly indicated by the results of recent experimental work. This dual theory of causation does not unfortunately mean that we can always guarantee to distinguish the two types of cirrhosis at autopsy, since the final results may be pathologically indistinguishable.

The distinction between these two types of *experimental* cirrhosis was extremely difficult owing to the apparent similarity of the types of diet which produced the two lesions and this aspect of the problem has been well reviewed by Himsworth (1947) and by Hadfield (1953). It will be sufficient here to recapitulate the main accepted features.

Diffuse hepatic fibrosis has usually been produced by diets deficient in the lipotropic factor choline, and is always preceded by a long period of extreme fatty infiltration. The nature of the lipotropic factors concerned in preventing fatty infiltration is considered elsewhere in this book, but it may be recalled here that the discovery was made by Best in 1932 as a result of studies of the fatty livers occurring in dogs after pancreatectomy. It was later found that methionine would also protect against this type of fatty liver, probably by serving as a methyl donor and thus contributing to choline production. This explains the deficiency produced by pancreatectomy, which interferes with protein hydrolysis and therefore with methionine absorption. A similar condition of diffuse hepatic fibrosis can also result from repeated sub-lethal doses of certain liver poisons such as CCl_4, which in single doses produces a recoverable centrilobular necrosis.

Post-necrotic scarring, however, is a sequel to massive necrosis of the liver in animals that recover from the condition. As we have seen, this is produced most readily by low-protein diets. While the essential protective factor here is cystine since methionine is a precursor of cystine it also protects against massive necrosis; this dual function of methionine goes far to explain many of the earlier obscurities of this subject. However, other factors such as tocopherol and antibiotics exert significant roles which have not yet been adequately explained.

In animals these two forms of liver lesion are said to be readily distinguishable, the diffuse type showing a fine uniform fibrosis with small nodules of fairly uniform size, while the post-necrotic type gives rise to a shrunken liver, with large irregular hyperplastic nodules. The suggestion, powerfully expressed by Himsworth (1947) in particular, is that the experimental diffuse fibrosis corresponds to multilobular cirrhosis in man while post-necrotic scarring is a sequel to a previous massive necrosis occurring during an attack of acute hepatitis.

There are many facts which support this conception. Firstly, the geographical distribution of cirrhosis referred to above fits in well with the deficiency of lipotropic factors in the diets in these areas, a deficiency which has been demonstrated by feeding such diets to rats (Gillman & Gillman, 1944). Secondly, the association with alcoholism is plausibly explained by the frequency of gross dietary deficiencies in this condition, due to anorexia and to economic factors. Some experiments of Best (Best, Hartoft, Lucas & Ridout, 1949) are of interest here, in which it was shown that fatty livers could be produced by diets in which calories were mainly supplied by sucrose, just as well as by diets in which alcohol served the same function. Thirdly, in the comparatively few cases of cirrhosis which can be traced back to an initial attack of acute hepatitis, the condition of the liver usually corresponds fairly closely to the post-necrotic scarring seen in animals. However workers in tropical countries are not agreed as to the relationship between the liver of protein deficiency (kwashiorkor) and cirrhosis (Waterlow & Bras, 1961) and tend to place more emphasis on the poisonous effects of certain herbs or moulds (see below). It may well be that in man fatty infiltration and cirrhosis are largely independent of each other.

To summarize this section therefore, we may conclude that although massive necrosis and fatty infiltration may both be causally related to hepatic cirrhosis, it is often impossible in the developed disease to decide which factor is the more important. These two factors may, of course, interact, so that errors of nutrition may adversely affect the victims of hepatitis, while hepatitis occurring in malnourished subjects is liable to be unusually severe.

Other Types of Cirrhosis

The discussion in the preceding section covers the common forms of cirrhosis, but somewhat similar degrees of hepatic fibrosis may occur in heart failure, cholangitis, hepatolenticular degeneration, haemochromatosis, syphilis, malaria and in Hanot's cirrhosis. Some of these are considered elsewhere in this book. An unusual type of cirrhosis occurring in Jamaica was described by Bras & Hill (1956) under the term *veno-occlusive disease* and apparently results from the consumption of senecio alkaloids consumed as "bush tea". The disease presents in childhood with ascites and an enlarged liver and is often fatal. The pathology appears to depend upon an occlusion of the small hepatic venules. Since this report from Jamaica, the disease has also been described in other parts of the world such as Indonesia. It is suspected that other "bush teas" may be factors in producing cirrhosis in Africa, and may even cause the high incidence of liver carcinoma in this country (Waterlow & Bras, 1961). Further natural hepatotoxins which may have similar relationships are the aflatoxins found in ground-nut meal contaminated with *Aspergillus flavus* (van der Zijden, Koelensmid, Boldingh, Barrett, Ord & Philp, 1962; Butler & Barnes, 1963). These produce various types of liver damage including fatty infiltration, cirrhosis and even hepatomas and such substances might well be consumed by native African populations in significant amounts (Lopez & Crawford, 1967).

Acute juvenile cirrhosis (Read, Sherlock & Harrison, 1963) occurs in young women and is associated with extreme hypergammaglobulinae-

mia. The possibility of an autoimmune basis for this disease is under discussion.

Functional Changes in Cirrhosis

It has already been mentioned that the symptomatology of hepatic cirrhosis is very variable, and the same may be said of the functional changes. Thus in certain latent or asymptomatic cases liver function may be almost normal (Ricketts, Kirsner, Palmer & Sterling, 1950), but in general obvious abnormalities are usually present. While any or all of the tests may be altered, the most constant and easily demonstrable changes are found in the serum proteins, the protein flocculation tests, the bromsulphthalein test and the urinary urobilinogen and coproporphyrin excretion. In latent cases the bromsulphthalein test appears to be the most sensitive of those tried (Cates, 1941; Mateer *et al.* 1947). Jaundice is frequently slight or absent, and the serum alkaline phosphatase may be either normal or raised. The flocculation tests are not uniformly positive in cirrhosis, but among the most sensitive of these is a modification of the old Takata-Ara reaction described by Maclagan, Bendandi & Cooke (1957). This mercuric chloride turbidity test, which employs a single tube under controlled conditions, was positive in 26 out of the 29 cases of hepatic cirrhosis studied.

The development of a collateral circulation in cirrhosis gives rise to the condition of portalsystemic encephalopathy discussed below under coma. Patients with cirrhosis exhibit an increased iron absorption which, when combined with a high iron intake, produced the haemosiderosis so commonly seen in the Bantu races in Africa (Bothwell, Abrahams, Bradlow & Charlton, 1965). This condition may be difficult to distinguish from idiopathic haemochromatosis (*q.v.*).

SECONDARY LIVER DAMAGE

The predominant role of the liver in detoxication processes is perhaps an explanation of the frequency with which the organ becomes secondarily involved in other diseases. Evidence for this involvement has been sought both by biochemical and by pathological methods, and the following list gives some of the conditions in which positive results have been obtained:

Burns, dermatitis, diabetes mellitus, heart failure, gastro-enteritis, glandular fever, malaria, sickle-cell anaemia, meningitis, obesity, peptic ulcer, pneumonia, pulmonary tuberculosis, surgical anaesthesia, rheumatoid arthritis, thyrotoxicosis, spinal cord injury, and after major surgery (see above).

In some of these conditions the liver damage is an incidental and perhaps unimportant finding, but in others it is intimately connected with the pathology of the disease and has implications in relation to treatment or prognosis. Some cases of interest are further discussed below.

In fatal cases of burns acute hepatic necrosis is a well-recognized post-mortem finding, and the excretion of toxic products by the liver is also suggested by the occasional presence of duodenal ulceration. In severe non-fatal cases many liver function tests give abnormal results, and a special study of the hippuric acid test was made by Boyce (1942). The writer has been impressed with the marked urobilinuria which is usually found, and with the progressive increase in excretion of this substance in fatal cases. In the pre-war period some at least of this liver damage in burns may have been due to tannic acid, a popular form of treatment which was subsequently shown to be definitely toxic to the liver (Wilson, MacGregor & Stewart, 1938; Clark & Rossiter, 1943). The situation would merit re-examination with cases treated by modern methods.

The enlarged fatty liver of diabetes mellitus is a significant complication, particularly in childhood and is presumably correlated to some extent with the lipaemia which is a constant feature in severe untreated cases. Milder degrees of fatty infiltration have also been demonstrated by liver biopsy studies (Zimmerman, MacMurray, Rappaport & Alpert, 1950), and positive results have been recorded with tests such as the serum colloidal gold reaction (Gray, Hook & Batty, 1946). In the latter study there was a significant correlation between the functional damage and inadequacy of diabetic control, but in the former the correlation was mainly with obesity, age and insensitivity to insulin. It is therefore suggested by Zimmerman et al. (1950) that pituitary over-activity may be responsible for the liver damage. A more recent review by Davidson (1954) regards the liver damage as resulting mainly from incomplete therapeutic control. A further complication here is the recent description of an hepatic form of diabetes occurring in cirrhosis and possibly due to an unusual inhibitor of insulin (Megyesi, Samols & Marks, 1967).

The existence of hepatic pathology in heart failure is obviously to be expected, and urobilinuria is a fairly constant finding. In addition a mild jaundice may be present, and positive flocculation tests and bromsulphthalein retention are commonly found (Bernstein, De Winn & Sinkins, 1942; Kissane, Fidler & Clark, 1947; Schalm & Hoogenboom, 1952). In one study the flocculation tests appeared to have some prognostic significance (Carter & Maclagan, 1946), but in general the functional change merely represents the degree of circulatory disturbance. The condition may progress to one of cardiac cirrhosis, a condition which has been extensively studied by Day & Armstrong (1940) and Kotin & Hall (1951). In general the liver changes in heart failure are of minor importance as compared with the condition of the heart itself, but they may well contribute to the production of the dyspeptic symptoms so common in this condition.

Gastro-enteritis might be expected to flood the portal circulation with toxic substances, and hepatic necrosis has been recorded in infantile acute gastro-enteritis by Schlesinger, Payne & Burnard (1949). Liver involvement was indicated by jaundice, hepatic enlargement and low plasma prothombin values. Five of their six cases recovered after treatment by protein supplements. More recently amino-aciduria in infantile diarrhoea has been ascribed to liver damage.

Although jaundice has long been known as an occasional complication of glandular fever, this was formerly thought to originate from pressure of enlarged glands in the portal fissure on the bile ducts. However, with the introduction of punch biopsy the reality of the hepatic pathology became recognized (Kilham & Steigman, 1942). The changes seen consist of a centrilobular necrosis very similar to that of infective hepatitis. A little later positive results with various liver function tests were reported in a high proportion of cases (Cohn & Lidman, 1946; Carter & Maclagan, 1946). This involvement is so constant that one feels that this condition should be seriously considered as a possible precursor of cirrhosis. In most cases, however, the hepatitis is mild and does not appear to complicate recovery, although positive flocculation tests may persist for some months (unpublished personal observation).

Nearly every liver function test which has been tried (except the serum alkaline phosphatase) appears to have given positive results in malaria, both in the natural and therapeutic varieties (Kopp & Solomon, 1943; Lippincott, Ellerbrook, Hesselbrock, Gordon, Gottlieb & Marble, 1945). It is thus no exaggeration to describe hepatitis as a feature of malaria rather than as a complication (McMahon, Kelsey & Drauf, 1954). The condition is a possible precursor of cirrhosis and the treatment of the hepatitis is an important part of the management of the disease.

The association of fatty infiltration of the liver with obesity has long been recognized, and a study by Zelman (1952) is of special interest as it related to 20 apparently healthy obese subjects. All of these had definite evidence of liver pathology as shown by needle biopsy and the bromsulphthalein test, and in addition many had positive results with other tests such as thymol turbidity and urine urobilinogen. The serum proteins were, however, normal. The somewhat similar findings in diabetes mellitus referred to above are of interest here.

The presence of metastatic carcinoma in the liver is a fairly frequent event and naturally affects liver function. The usual changes seen include urobilinuria with raised serum alkaline phosphatase levels; if the larger bile passages are involved the typical picture of post-hepatic jaundice is produced (Mendelsohn & Bodansky, 1952; Thomas & Zimmerman, 1952). Many other functions may be affected, but the serum proteins and at least some of the flocculation tests such as the thymol and zinc sulphate tests tend to be normal or only slightly altered. Of these the alkaline phosphatase is the most reliable indicator, and has found some application in the detection of such metastases (Shay & Siplet, 1954; Simons, 1954). It should be remembered, however, that some impairment of liver function is also found in cases of malignant disease without hepatic matastases (Abels, Rekers, Binkley, Pack & Rhoads, 1942). The significance of this finding is unknown, but it may well be partly related to malnutrition.

In sarcoidosis a raised plasma globulin may, of course, occur without actual hepatic lesions, but the disease frequently attacks the liver and in a case recently reported the hepatic changes were very prominent, producing jaundice and ascites as terminal symptoms (Branson & Park, 1954).

The condition of the liver in rheumatoid arthritis is difficult to define at the present time, principally on account of the inevitable scarcity of autopsy material. While needle biopsy studies have given mainly normal results (Movitt & Davis, 1953), a large number of different liver function tests have provided prima facie evidence of hepatic dysfunction (Rawls, Weiss & Collins, 1937; Carter & Maclagan, 1946; Swanson, 1949; Kalbak, 1951). The highest proportion of positive results has been recorded with the protein flocculation tests, which may merely reflect an autoimmune response, but others such as bromsulphthalein and urinary coproporphyrin have also given significantly abnormal findings. In a study in the writer's laboratory (Darby, 1954) a careful comparison was made between 50 cases of rheumatoid arthritis and 50 control patients with similar degrees of general restriction of activity, but not suffering from any disease known to affect the liver. The findings with flocculation tests, bromsulphthalein, and urinary coproporphyrin excretion were significantly more abnormal in the rheumatoid group. The suggestion is therefore that a mild functional liver impairment is frequently present in this disease and may represent a definite part of its pathology.

Considerable difference of opinion has also arisen as to the state of the liver in thyrotoxicosis. In fatal cases well-marked changes such as a fine cirrhosis and some fatty infiltration have been described, but in the milder examples work has been mainly confined to liver function tests, particularly the galactose tolerance, hippuric acid and bromsulphthalein tests.

The case of spinal injury is of some interest on account of the gross malnutrition and hypoproteinaemia which may be found in this condition. Definite evidence of liver damage was shown by Cooper, Rynearson & MacCarthy (1951) with the bromsulphthalein test, and such changes may well contribute to the metabolic problem. Hepatic damage following major surgery has been discussed above (under acute hepatic necrosis).

RELATION OF SYMPTOMS TO BIOCHEMICAL CHANGES

While many of the symptoms of liver disease are of somewhat obscure causation, a number of useful correlations have been established, and the present position in this respect is probably somewhat better than that obtaining in the case of uraemia.

Jaundice

The degree of jaundice is fairly accurately reflected by the serum bilirubin level, a value of 3 mg./100 ml. forming a rough dividing line between latent and manifest jaundice. This level, however, naturally varies with the type of light available, as jaundice is difficult to appreciate in artificial light. In addition to this there is a time lag between the rise of serum bilirubin and the staining of the skin so that the bilirubin estimation is particularly useful in the early stages of jaundice.

The greenish hue sometimes seen in cases of prolonged biliary obstruction is due to biliverdin, which can be estimated separately in the serum. Larson et al. (1947) have made a special study of this variety of jaundice, but it does not appear from their account that the biliverdin estimation is of any special diagnostic or prognostic value.

Pruritus

Although this symptom is generally ascribed to the accumulation of bile acids in the blood, no good correlation has been established with blood levels (Sherlock, 1963). Furthermore the pruritus seen in idiopathic jaundice of pregnancy is out of proportion to the degree of jaundice. However it seems likely that some biliary steroid is concerned since the itching is relieved by external biliary drainage and also by oral administration of the basic anion-exchange resin cholestyramine, which is thought to act by preventing re-absorption of bile acids (Datta & Sherlock, 1966).

Nausea and Vomiting

In view of the prominence of these symptoms in acute hepatitis it is perhaps surprising how little is known as to the mechanism involved. Reynell (1954) produced acute hepatic necrosis in rats by poisoning with carbon tetrachloride and followed gastro-intestinal movements by radiography. The barium meal was seen to remain in the stomach for periods of up to 72 hours in the poisoned animals. Ligation of the bile duct did not produce this effect, which was uninfluenced by vagotomy or by the administration of hexamethonium bromide. Rats are said not to vomit, but considerable anorexia was present. The results appear to throw some light on the subject but leave the actual mechanism still unexplained.

Oedema and Ascites

The relation between ascites and portal hypertension is well established, but in addition a correlation also exists with the level of plasma proteins. As in nephritis, formulae have been evolved relating these symptoms to colloid osmotic pressure and to particular functions of the albumin and globulin concentration. Thus, according to Iversen (1951) the best correlation is given by:

Colloid osmotic pressure (mm.Hg) = 3·5 × albumin + globulin (g/100 ml.).

The limiting value for the colloid osmotic pressure was 14·2, all patients with values below this figure having ascites. Other workers, however, have stressed the importance of an actual determination of the plasma osmotic pressure, which does not always agree with that given by the formula (Armstrong, Kark, Schoenberger, Shatkin & Sights, 1954). In spite of this no abnormal types of protein have actually been isolated in such cases.

A more recent formula for predicting ascites is that of Alkinson & Losowsky (1961), who found the following factor to be less than unity in all their cirrhotic patients with ascites:

$$\frac{10 \times \text{Serum albumin (g./100 ml.)} + 4}{\text{Intrasplenic pressure (cm. H}_2\text{O)}}.$$

Although theoretically sound this formula has the disadvantage of employing a pressure measurement which will not be available in all cases. The rate of turnover of ascitic protein has been studied with isotopically labelled (^{131}I) albumin and γ-globulin (Bauer, Blahd, Fields & Getchell, 1954). Rather unexpectedly these ascitic proteins had biological half-lives very similar to those of the plasma (16 days for albumin and from 10 to 13 days for γ-globulin).

The actual mechanism of fluid retention, as in many forms of chronic oedema, appears to depend upon the excessive secretion of aldosterone by the adrenal gland since very high values for urinary aldosterone excretion have been recorded in cirrhosis (Luetscher & Johnson, 1954). The antidiuretic hormone is not thought to be involved (Chaudhury, Chuttani & Ramalingaswami, 1961).

Coma

Although in severe liver failure coma may occasionally result from hypoglycaemia, the usual type seen is that described by Sherlock (1958) as "portal-systemic encephalopathy". This condition, which is accentuated by gastro-intestinal haemorrhage or protein feeding, is characterized by gross mental changes and "flapping tremor" as premonitory signs, followed by deep coma in severe cases.

The work of Sherlock and her colleagues has shown clearly that this type of coma is due to the absorption of some toxic nitrogenous compound or compounds from the intestine which by-pass the liver owing to the collateral circulation present. The exact nature of the toxins has not been determined with certainty, but there is a fair correlation between the depth of coma and the blood ammonium level, and the intestinal origin of this substance has been established (Sherlock, Summerskill, White & Phear, 1954). Normal values extend up to 3μg./ml., and while values up to double this level have been recorded in deep coma there was considerable overlap with the normal range. In view of this and of the technical difficulties of the estimation, it does not appear to have become a routine procedure.

The exact relationship between the raised blood ammonium and the coma is still undecided, since most of the theories previously advanced appear to have been disproved. One of these assumed the conversion of glutamate, known to be used in cerebral metabolism, to glutamine by combination with ammonium (Walshe, 1951), and this was supported by the finding of raised levels for glutamine concentration in the blood and cerebrospinal fluid (Walshe, 1953; Whitehead & Whittaker, 1955). Unfortunately, however, early reports on the favourable effects of glutamate administration were not confirmed. An alternative possibility was a deficiency of α-ketoglutarate, which might well combine with ammonium to produce glutamate (Weil-Malherbe, 1953). This again appears to have been disproved by the finding of *raised* blood levels of α-ketoglutarate in hepatic coma (Dawson, De Groote, Rosenthal & Sherlock, 1957). The subject is still under active investigation (Walshe, 1960; Sherlock, 1960). (Fenton, 1965).

CHOICE AND USES OF LIVER FUNCTION TESTS

There are some who find in the voluminous literature on this subject a confession of failure (Ivy & Roth, 1943; Himsworth, 1947), but it will be assumed that the reader of this book is convinced of the value of these tests and seeks guidance on the question of choice and interpretation. In this connection it is certainly important to have a clear idea as to exactly what clinical question is being asked of the tests employed, and to have a definite diagnosis in mind before they are undertaken. The motives for investigating cases of liver disease may be classified as follows:

(1) diagnosis
(2) to record the intensity of a pathological process
(3) prognosis.

Cases likely to be investigated may also be classified under one of the following headings:

(1) jaundice
(2) suspected liver damage in absence of jaundice
(3) hepatic enlargement
(4) suspected excessive haemolysis.

In the first group of cases the requirements may be either diagnostic or prognostic. Thus the cause of the jaundice may be unknown, or on the other hand the cause may be known but further information may be needed in cases of acute hepatitis, cirrhosis, or surgical jaundice, either as a record of progress or for prognosis. In the jaundiced group as a whole the pigmentary tests serve mainly to record the intensity of the jaundice and to suggest a haemolytic cause if present, while other types of test will usually be required for the other purposes outlined.

Suspected liver damage in the absence of jaundice covers a large number of possibilities. On the one hand we may be dealing with a case of pre- or post-icteric hepatitis or cirrhosis in which either confirmation of diagnosis is needed or prognostic information is sought. On the other hand we may be investigating a patient with heart failure, thyrotoxicosis, malaria, alcoholism or alimentary neoplasm with a view to estimating the degree of hepatic involvement. In this group as a whole there is little restriction on types of test, for any one may at times give useful information.

The differential diagnosis of hepatic enlargement overlaps to some extent with the last group, but in general we are concerned here in distinguishing a primary liver disease such as cirrhosis from secondary involvement of the liver as seen in, e.g., carcinomatosis or heart failure. Fortunately the biochemical changes in cirrhosis and in carcinomatosis are reasonably distinct from each other and are frequently of help in this type of case.

Although excessive haemolysis can occur without anaemia or jaundice, these two symptoms are likely to provide the main indications of severe chronic haemolysis. Haematological data are of primary importance here, but, when needed, confirmation can be obtained by the differential serum bilirubin determination and by the estimation of faecal urobilinogen. With the latter test we must now bear in mind the possibility of a non-haemolytic increase in faecal pigment, as noted above.

The first two motives listed above as reasons for undertaking liver function tests are too obvious to require much discussion, but the question of prognosis is less satisfactory. The difficulty of establishing significant correlation between the result of individual tests and long-term follow-up studies makes this field a rather speculative one, but a good case has been made out for the prognostic use of serum albumin estimations in hepatitis. Thus, Higgins, O'Brien, Stewart & Witts (1944) found that in their series, values below 3 g./100 ml. were associated with a duration exceeding 2 months and that values below 2 g./100 ml. were an indication of severe and usually irrecoverable liver damage. Similarly, low plasma fibrinogen and high amino acid values are only seen in severe liver failure. Failure of the plasma prothrombin to rise after vitamin K therapy is also a grave sign in surgical jaundice (Stein, 1944). In less severe cases of hepatitis the immediate prognosis is usefully correlated with serum bilirubin, bromsulphthalein retention and thymol turbidity (Kimmel, Burns, Harper, Dirstine & Higgins, 1954). Thymol turbidity sometimes remains positive for long periods after an attack of acute hepatitis, and in such cases may indicate an immunological response other than liver damage.

The scheme at present in use in the writer's laboratory is indicated below:

ROUTINE PROCEDURES

Tests	Methods
Serum bilirubin, conjugated and unconjugated, reading conjugated pigment at 10 min.	Malloy & Evelyn (1937)
Serum alkaline phosphatase.	King & Armstrong (1934)
Thymol turbidity and flocculation tests.	Maclagan (1944a, 1947)
Mercuric chloride turbidity test.	Maclagan, Bendandi & Cooke (1957)
Afternoon urine for urobilinogen, bilirubin, bile salts. Urobilinogen estimation may be corrected for urinary pH by the method of Bourke, Milne & Stokes (1965).	Watson, Schwartz, Sborov & Bertie (1944)
Bromsulphthalein test, 5 mg./kg. body weight (in non-jaundiced patients only).	Matteer, Baltz, Marion & MacMillan (1943)

SUPPLEMENTARY TESTS

Tests	Methods
Serum protein electrophoresis with scanning.	Kohn (1957)
Serum aspartate aminotransferase (SGOT).	Karmen, Wróblewski & LaDue (1955)
Serum alanine aminotransferase (SGPT).	Wróblewski & LaDue (1956)
Prothrombin response to vitamin K	Stein (1944)

The choice of suitable liver function tests is to some extent a matter of personal preference and this subject has given rise to considerable differences of opinion between workers in various centres. In so far as any consensus of opinion is discernible, there appears to be general agreement that no one test is suitable for all circumstances and that some combination or "battery" of tests is desirable. This viewpoint has been expressed particularly by Watson (1944) and by Lichtman (1954) who have at various times advocated the use of a formidable number of routine tests.

The element of personal choice enters strongly into this selection of tests and many workers might object to the omission of certain tests. The tests chosen are those which have been found by personal experience to be of greatest all-round value, most of them contributing in some degree both to diagnosis and prognosis. It is, however, impossible for any one worker to have really extensive experience of every proposed test, and it is not intended to express any criticism here of the different lists which have been proposed by other workers.

The routine tests listed above are best carried out during the afternoon on a day when ordinary meals have been taken. This proviso is particularly on account of the urobilinogen test, but also has the advantage of convenience for out-patient work, since the collection of specimens can be completed in about one hour and the patient need not fast. These routine tests will provide a record of the intensity of any jaundice which may be present, and will give a good indication of the probable type of jaundice on the lines indicated above. In the absence of clinical jaundice one or more of the tests may be sufficiently positive to provide supporting evidence for a diagnosis of, e.g., cirrhosis or non-icteric hepatitis.

If the results are negative or equivocal one or more supplementary tests may be needed, particularly in cases of suspected cirrhosis or in obscure jaundice. In the latter transaminase estimations are of particular value in cases seen reasonably early, whereas in cirrhosis either the bromsulphthalein test or the protein estimation are perhaps most likely to yield positive results, although it must be admitted that in latent or compensated cases all tests may sometimes be normal.

Serum electrophoresis is now a routine procedure and numerous semi-automatic scanning devices are now on the market which give quantitative results; some typical findings are given in Table 5.8. So far as liver disease is concerned the different results in hepatitis and cirrhosis on the one hand and in post-hepatic jaundice on the other are specially noteworthy. It may be mentioned here that the serum haptoglobins are reduced in many cases of liver damage. The

TABLE 5.8

Electrophoresis patterns in various hepatic diseases
(Modified from King & Wootton, 1959)

Condition	Albumin	α_1	α_2	β	γ
Normal	4·15	0·29	0·59	0·83	1·40
	± 0·35(S.D.)	± 0·07	± 0·07	± 0·10	± 0·19
Hepatitis	−	−			+
Cirrhosis	− −			+	+ +
Amyloidosis	−		+ +		
Carcinomatosis	−		+		
Post-hepatic Jaundice			+	+	
Myelomatosis ⎱ Macroglobulinaemia ⎰			"Paraprotein" in α_2-γ region		

$\left. \begin{array}{c} + \\ + + \end{array} \right\}$ = slight and large increases.

$\left. \begin{array}{c} - \\ - - \end{array} \right\}$ = slight and large reductions.

clinical value of this observation is in dispute (Owen, Podanyi & Smith, 1961; Williams, Speyer & Billing, 1961).

Finally the prothrombin response to vitamin K is not always carried out as a formal test, but the same information accrues in surgical cases from carrying out the estimation after vitamin K has been given as pre-operative preparation. A low prothrombin value at this time obviously implies a failure to respond, even though the initial value is missing and will usually indicate severe liver damage rather than biliary obstruction as a cause of the jaundice. In any case the risk of haemorrhage is considerable and the prognosis is poor.

References

ABELS, J. C., REKERS, P. E., BINKLEY, G. E., PACK, G. T. & RHOADS, C. P. (1942). *Ann. intern. Med.,* **16,** 221.

ACOCELLA, G., TENCONI, L. T., ARMAS-MERINO, R., RAIA, S. & BILLING, B. H. (1968). *Lancet,* **1,** 68.

ARIAS, I. M. (1960). Article in "Advances in clinical chemistry", Vol. 3. New York & London, Athlone Press.

ARIAS, I. M., GARTNER, L. M., SEIFTER, S. & FURMAN, M. (1964). *J. clin. Invest.,* **43,** 2037.

ARMSTRONG, A. R., KING, E. J. & HARRIS, R. I. (1934). *Canad. med. Ass. J.,* **31,** 14.

ARMSTRONG, S. H., KARK, R. M., SCHOENBERGER, J. A., SHATKIN, J. & SIGHTS, R. (1954). *J. clin. Invest.,* **33,** 297.

ARTHURTON, M., O'BRIEN, D. & MANN, T. (1954). *Arch. Dis. Childh.,* **29,** 38.

ASCHOFF, L. (1922). *Münch. med. Wschr.,* **69,** 1352.

ATKINSON, M. & LOSOWSKY, M. S. (1961). *Quart. J. Med.,* **30,** 153.

BARON, D. N. & BELL, J. L. (1960), *J. clin. Path.,* **12,** 385.

BARRON, E. S. G. (1931). *Medicine,* **10,** 77.

BAUER, F. K., BLAHD, W. H., FIELDS, M. & GETCHELL, G. (1954). *Metabolism,* **3,** 289.

BERGH, VAN DEN A. A. H. & MÜLLER, P. (1916). *Biochem. Z.,* **77,** 90.

BERNSTEIN, M., DE WINN, E. B. & SINKINS, S. (1942). *J. Lab. clin. Med.,* **28,** 1.

BEST, C. H., HARTOFT, W. S., LUCAS, C. C. & RIDOUT, J. H. (1949). *Brit. med. J.,* **2,** 1001.

BEST, C. H., HERSHEY, J. M. & HUNTSMAN, M. E. (1932), *J. Physiol.,* **75,** 56.

BILLING, B. H. (1963). *Postgrad. med. J.,* **39,** 176.

BILLING, B. H. (1965). "Progress in Liver Diseases", vol. 2. London, Heinemann.

BILLING, B. H., COLE, P. G. & LATHE, G. H. (1957). *Biochem. J.,* **65,** 774.

BILLING, B. H. COLE, P. G. & LATHE, (1954). *Brit. med. J,* **2,** 1263.

BILLING, B. H. & LATHE, G. H. (1956). *Biochem. J.,* **63,** 6P.

BILLING, B. H. & LATHE, G. H. (1958). *Amer. J. Med.,* **24,** 111.

BODANSKY, A. & JAFFÉ, H. L. (1934). *Proc. Soc. exp. Biol., N.Y.,* **31,** 107.

BOLES, R. S. & CREW, R. S. (1940). *Quart. J. Stud. Alcohol,* **1,** 464.

BOLLMAN, J. L., SHEARD, C. & MANN, F. C. (1927). *Amer. J. Physiol.,* **80,** 461.

BORGLIN, N. E. (1965). *Brit. med. J.,* **1,** 1289.

BOTHWELL, T. H., ABRAHAMS, C., BRADLOW, B. A. & CHARLTON, R. W. (1965). *Arch. Path.*, **79**, 163.

BOURKE, E., MILNE, M. D. & STOKES, G. S. (1965). *Brit. med. J.*, **2**, 1510.

BOYCE, F. F. (1942). *Arch. Surg.*, **44**, 789.

BRANSON, J. H. & PARK, J. H. (1954). *Ann. intern. Med.*, **40**, 11.

BRAS, G. & HILL, K. R. (1956). *Lancet*, **2**, 161.

BURTON, J. L., LOUDON, N. & WILSON, A. T. (1967). *Lancet*, **2**, 1326.

BUTLER, W. H. & BARNES, J. M. (1963). *Brit. J. Cancer*, **17**, 699.

CAMERON, G. R. & KARUNARATNE, W. A. E. (1936). *J. Path. Bact.*, **42**, 1.

CANTAROW, A. (1944). *Amer. J. digest. Dis.*, **11**, 144.

CARTER, A. B. & MACLAGAN, N. F. (1946). *Brit. med. J.*, **2**, 80.

CHAUDHURY, R. R., CHUTTANI, H. K. & RAMALINGA-SWAMI, V. (1961). *Clin. Sci.*, **21**, 199.

CHRISTIAN, E. R. (1954). *Arch. intern. Med.*, **94**, 22.

CLAIREAUX, A. E., COLE, P. G. & LATHE, G. H. (1953). *Lancet*, **2**, 1226.

CLARK, E. J. & ROSSITER, R. J. (1943). *Lancet*, **2**, 222.

COHN, C. & LIDMAN, B. I. (1946). *J. clin. Invest.*, **25**, 145.

COLE, P. G. & LATHE, G. H. (1953). *J. clin. Path.*, **6**, 99.

COLE, P. G., LATHE, G. H. & BILLING, B. H. (1954). *Biochem. J.*, **57**, 514.

COLEMAN, P. N. (1950). *Brit. med. J.*, **2**, 246.

COOKE, K. B. & ZILVA, J. F. (1961). *J. clin. Path.*, **14**, 500.

COOLIDGE, T. B. (1940). *J. biol. Chem.*, **132**, 119.

COOPER, I. S., RYNEARSON, E. H. & MACCARTHY, C. S. (1951). *J. Lab. clin. Med.*, **38**, 689.

CRIGLER, F. J. & NAJJAR, E. A. (1952). *Pediatrics*, **10**, 169.

DACIE, J. V. (1960). "The Haemolytic Anaemias", 2nd Ed. London, Churchill.

DARBY, P. W. (1954). Private Communication.

DATTA, D. V. & SHERLOCK, S. (1966). *Gastroenterology*, **50**, 323.

DAVIDSON, C. S. (1954). *Vitam. & Horm.*, **12**, 148.

DAWSON, A. M., DE GROOTE, J., ROSENTHAL, W. A. & SHERLOCK, S. (1957). *Lancet*, **1**, 392.

DAY, T. D. & ARMSTRONG, T. G. (1940). *J. Path. Bact.*, **50**, 221.

DE RITIS, F., GIUSTI, G., PICCININO, F. & CACCIATORE, L. (1965). *Bull. Wld. Hlth. Org.*, **32**, 59.

DIBLE, J. H., McMICHAEL, J. & SHERLOCK, S. (1943). *Lancet*, **2**, 402.

DOXIADIS, S. A., KARAKLIS, A., VALAES, T. & STAVRAKAKIS, D. (1964). *Lancet*, **2**, 1210.

DUBIN, I. N. & JOHNSON, F. B. (1954). *Medicine*, **33**, 155.

DUCCI, H., SPOERER, A. & KATZ, R. (1952). *Gastroenterology*, **22**, 52.

EHRLICH, P. (1883). *Z. anal. Chem.*, **22**, 301.

ELLIOTT, B. A. & WILKINSON, J. H. (1961). *Lancet*, **1**, 698.

EPPINGER, H. (1937). "Die Leberkrankheiten". Vienna, J. Springer.

FAGIN, I. D. & THOMPSON, F. M. (1944). *Ann. intern. Med.*, **21**, 285.

FASHENA, G. J., BATES, H. H. & REID, A. F. (1950). *Amer J. Dis. Child.*, **80**, 510.

FENTON, J. C. B. (1965). *J. clin. Path.*, **18**, 126.

FINDLAY, G. M. (1940). *J. R. Army med. Cps.*, **74**, 72.

FISCHER, H. & ORTH, H. (1937). "Die Chemie des Pyrrols". Leipzig, Akademische Verlagsgesellschaft.

FORBES, J. C., LEACH, B. E. & WILLIAMS, G. Z. (1942). *Proc. Soc. exp. Biol., N.Y.*, **51**, 47.

FOX, J. P., MANSO, C., PENNA, H. A. & PARA, M. (1942). *Amer. J. Hyg.*, **36**, 68.

GAIRDNER, D. (1965). "Recent Advances in Paediatrics", 3rd ed. London, Churchill.

GILBERT, A. & LEREBOULLET, P. (1901). *Sem. Medicale*, **21**, 241.

GILLMAN, T. & GILLMAN, J. (1944). *Nature Lond.*, **154**, 210.

GILLMAN, T. & GILLMAN, J. (1945). *J. Amer. med. Ass.*, **129**, 12.

GOLDBARG, J. A., PINEDA, E. P., BANKS, B. M. & RUTENBERG, A. M. (1959). *Gastroenterology*, **36**, 193.

GOLDBLATT, H. (1947). Report of pathologists on cirrhosis study. Josiah Macy Foundation 6th Conference on Liver Disease, p. 9.

GRAY, C. H. (1961). "Bile pigments in health and disease". Illinois, C. C. Thomas.

GRAY, C. H. (1953). "The bile pigments". London, Methuen.

GRAY, C. H., NEUBERGER, A. & SNEATH, P. H. A. (1950). *Biochem. J.*, **47**, 87.

GRAY, S. J., HOOK, W. & BATTY, J. L. (1946). *Ann. intern. Med.*, **24**, 72.

GREENSPAN, E. M., TEPPER, B., TERRY, L. L. & SCHOENBACH, E. B. (1952). *J. Lab. clin. Med.*, **39**, 44.

GRINSTEIN, M., ALDRICH, R. A., HAWKINSON, V. & WATSON, C. J. (1949). *J. biol. Chem.*, **179**, 983.

GUNN, C. K. (1938). *J. Heredity*, **29**, 137.

GUTMAN, A. B., OLSON, K. B., GUTMAN, E. B. & FLOOD, C. A. (1940). *J. clin. Invest.*, **19**, 129.

GYÖRGY, P. (1944). *Amer. J. clin. Path.*, **14**, 67.

HADFIELD, G. (1953). "Recent advances in pathology". Chapter X. The Liver. London, J. & A. Churchill.

HALL, E. M., OLSEN, A. Y. & DAVIS, F. E. (1953). *Amer. J. Path.*, **29**, 993.

HANOT, V. (1876). "Etude sur une Forme de Cirrhose Hypertrophique du Foie (Cirrhose Hypertrophique avec Ictère Chronique)". Paris, J. B. Bailliere.

HARRISON, G. A. (1930). "Chemical methods in clinical medicine". London, J. & A. Churchill.

HIGGINS, G., O'BRIEN, J. R. P., STEWART, A. & WITTS, L. J. (1944). *Brit. med. J.*, **1**, 211.

HIMSWORTH, H. P. (1947). Lectures on the liver and its diseases. Oxford, Blackwell Scientific Publications.

HIMSWORTH, H. P. & GLYNN, L. E. (1944). *Lancet*, **1**, 457.

HIRSCH, A. (1886). "Handbook of geographical and historical pathology". London.

HOFFBAUER, F. W., RAMES, E. D. & MEINERT, J. K. (1949). J. Lab. clin. Med., 34, 1259.

HOFFMAN, H. N., WHITCOMB, F. F., BUTT, H. R. & BOLLMAN, J. L. (1960). J. clin. Invest., 39, 132.

HOLLAN, O. R. (1950), Gastroenterology, 16, 418.

HSIA, D. Y. Y., ALLEN, F. H., JR., DIAMOND, L. K. & GELLIS, S. S. (1953). J. Pediat., 42, 277.

IRWIN, D. B. (1952). Brit. med. J., 1, 1379.

ISRAELS, L. G., YAMAMOTO, T., SKANDERBERG, J. & ZIPURSKY, A. (1963). Proc. 9th. Cong. Europ. Soc. Haemat., p. 891.

ISRAELS, L. G., SUDERMAN, H. J. & RITZMAN, S. E. (1959). Amer. J. Med., 27, 693.

IVERSEN, P. (1951). "Ciba Foundation Symposium on Liver Disease", p. 136. London, J. & A. Churchill.

IVY, A. C. & ROTH, J. A. (1943). Gastroenterology, 1, 655.

JAFFÉ, M. (1868). Cbl. med. Wiss., 6, 241.

JEZLER, A. (1930). Z. klin. Med., 114, 739.

KALBAK, K. (1951). Ann. rheum. Dis., 10, 182.

KARK, R. N. (1952). Nutrition in the practice of medicine, Nutrition Symposium Series No. 4, The National Vitamin Foundation, New York.

KARMEN, A., WRÓBLEWSKI, F. & LaDUE, J. S. (1955). J. clin. Invest., 34, 126.

KEIDING, N. R. (1959). Seand. J. Clin. Lab. Invest., 11, 106.

KILHAM, L. & STEIGMAN, A. J. (1942). Lancet, 2, 452.

KIMMEL, J. R., BURNS, T. W., HARPER, H. A., DIRSTINE, P. H. & HIGGINS, A. R. (1954). Gastroenterology, 26, 723.

KING, E. J. & WOOTTON, I. D. P. (1959). "Microanalysis in Medical Biochemistry", 3rd Ed. London, J. & A. Churchill Ltd.

KING, E. J. & ARMSTRONG, A. R. (1934). Canad. med. Ass. J., 31, 376.

KISSANE, R. W., FIDLER, R. S. & CLARKE, T. E. (1947). Amer. J. med. Sci., 213, 410.

KLATSKIN, G. (1961). Gastroenterology, 41, 443.

KOHN, J. (1957). Clin. Chem. Acta, 2, 297.

KOPP, I. & SOLOMON, H. C. (1943). Amer. J. med. Sci., 205, 90.

KORNBERG, A. (1942). J. clin. Invest., 21, 299.

KOTIN, P. & HALL, E. M. (1951). Amer. J. Path., 27, 561.

LARSON, E. A., EVANS, G. T. & WATSON, C. J. (1947). J. Lab. Clin. Med., 32, 481.

LATHE, G. H. (1954). Biochemical Society Symposia, No. 12, 34.

LATHE, G. H. & WALKER, M. (1958). Biochem. J., 70, 705.

LATNER, A. L. (1950). Brit. med. J., 2, 629.

LATNER, A. L. & SMITH, A. J. (1958). Lancet, 2, 915.

LEMBERG, R. & LEGGE, J. W. (1949). "Hematin compounds and bile pigments", Interscience Publishers Inc., New York, p. 453, Chemical mechanism of bile pigment formation and other irreversible alterations of haemoglobin.

LICHTMAN, S. S. (1942 & 1954). "Diseases of the liver, gall bladder and bile ducts", 1st and 3rd Ed. London, Kimpton.

LIPPINCOTT, S. W., ELLERBROOK, L. D., HESSELBROCK, W. B., GORDON, H. H., GOTTLIEB, L. & MARBLE, A. (1945). J. clin. Invest., 24, 616.

LJUNGGREN, G. (1956). Nord. Med., 55, 373.

LONDON, I. M., WEST, R., SHEMIN, D. & RITTENBERG, D. (1950). J. biol. Chem., 184, 351.

LOPEZ, A. & CRAWFORD, M. A. (1967). Lancet, 2, 1351.

LUCKÉ, B. (1944). Amer. J. Path., 20, 471.

LUCKEY, T. D., REYNIERS, J. A., GYÖRGY, P. & FORBES, M. (1954). Ann. N.Y. Acad. Sci., 57, 932.

LUETSCHER, J. A. & JOHNSON, B. B. (1954). J. clin. Invest., 33, 1441.

McARDLE, B. (1940). Quart. J. Med., 9, n.s., 107.

MacCALLUM, F. O. & BAUER, D. J. (1944). Lancet, 1, 622.

MacCALLUM, F. O. & BRADLEY, W. H. (1944). Lancet, 2, 228.

MacCALLUM, F. O., McFARLAN, A. M., MILES, J. A. R., POLLOCK, M. R. & WILSON, C. (1951). Infective hepatitis. Studies in East Anglia during the period 1943–47. Spec. Rep. Ser., Med. Res. Coun. Lond., No. 273.

MACLAGAN, N. F. (1944a). Brit. J. exp. Path., 25, 15.

MACLAGAN, N. F. (1944b). Brit. J. exp. Path., 25, 234.

MACLAGAN, N. F. (1944c). Proc. roy. Soc. Med., 37, 24.

MACLAGAN, N. F. (1947). Brit. med. J., 2, 197.

MACLAGAN, N. F. (1948). Brit. med., J., 2, 892.

MACLAGAN, N. F. (1955). Article in Schiff, L. Diseases of the liver. Philadelphia, J. B. Lippincott.

MACLAGAN, N. F. (1940). Quart. J. med., 9, 151.

MACLAGAN, N. F. (1967). Brit. J. Surg., Lister Centenary Number.

MACLAGAN, N. F., BENDANDI, A. & COOKE, K. B. (1957). Clin. Chim. Acta., 2, 49.

McMAHON, A. E., KELSEY, J. E. & DRAUF, D. E. (1954). Arch. intern. Med., 93, 379.

McMASTER, P. D. & ELMAN, R. (1927). Ann. intern. Med., 1, 68.

McNALTY, A. S. (1938). Annual Report of the Chief Medical Officer of the Ministry of Health, London, H.M. Stationery Office.

McNEE, J. W. (1923). Quart. J. Med., 16, 390.

MAIZELS, M. (1946). Lancet, 2, 451.

MALLOY, H. T. & EVELYN, K. A. (1937). J. biol. Chem., 119, 481.

MATEER, J. G., BALTZ, J. I., MARION, D. J. & MACMILLAN, J. M. (1943). J. Amer. med. Ass., 121, 723.

MAWSON, C. A. (1948), J. clin. Path., 1, 167.

MEGYESI, C., SAMOLS, E. & MARKS, V. (1967). Lancet, 2, 1051.

MENDELSOHN, M. L. & BODANSKY, O. (1952). Cancer, 5, 1.

MEULENGRACHT, E. (1939). Klin. Wschr., 18, 118.

MINISTRY OF HEALTH, MEDICAL RESEARCH COUNCIL AND DEPARTMENT OF HEALTH, SCOTLAND. *Lancet*, **1**, 1328.

MINKOWSKI, O. & NAUNYN, B. (1886). *Arch. exp. Path. Pharmak.*, **21**, 1.

MOLLISON, P. L. (1948). *Lancet*, **1**, 513.

MOLLISON, P. L. & CUTBUSH, M. (1948). *Lancet*, **2**, 522.

MOLLISON, P. L. & CUTBUSH, M. (1954) in GAIRDNER, D., "Recent advances in paediatrics", Chapter 5. Haemolytic diseases of the newborn, p. 110. London, J. & A. Churchill.

MORGAN, H. V. & WILLIAMSON, D. A. J. (1943). *Brit. med. J.*, **1**, 750.

MORRIS, E. D., MURRAY, J. & RUTHVEN, C. R. J. (1967). *Brit. med. J.*, **2**, 352.

MOSLEY, J. W. & DULL, H. B. (1966). *Anesthesiology*, **27**, 409.

MOVITT, E. R. & DAVIS, A. E. (1953). *Amer. J. med. Sci.*, **226**, 516.

MOXON, A. L. & RHIAN, M. (1943). *Physiol. Rev.*, **23**, 305.

VON MÜLLER, F. (1892). *Jber. schles. Ges. vaterl. Kult.*, *Med. Sekt.*, **70**, 1.

NAKAJIMA, H., TAKEMURA, T., NAKAJIMO, O. & YAMAOKA, K. (1963). *J. Biol. Chem.*, **238**, 3785, 3797.

NATIONAL HALOTHANE STUDY (1966). *J. Am. med. Ass.*, **197**, 725.

NEEFE, J. R. (1946). *Med. Clin. N. Amer.*, **30**, 1407.

NEEFE, J. R., STOKES, J. & GELLIS, S. S. (1945). *Amer. J. med. Sci.*, **210**, 561.

NOSSLIN, B. (1960). *Scand. J. Clin. Lab. Invest.*, **12**, Supplement 49.

OWEN, J. A., PODANYI, R. & SMITH, H. (1961). *Clin. Sci.*, **21**, 189.

PIERCE, F. T., KIMMEL, J. R. & BURNS, T. W. (1954). *Metabolism*, **3**, 228.

PINEDA, E. P., GOLDBARG, J. A., BANKS, B. M. & RUTENBERG, A. M. (1960). *Gastroenterology*, **38**, 698.

POLLOCK, M. R. (1945). *Lancet*, **2**, 626.

POPPER, H., BEAN, W. B., DE LA HUERGA, J., FRANKLIN, M., TSUMAGARI, Y., ROUTH, J. I. & STEIGMANN, F. (1951). *Gastroenterology*, **17**, 138.

PRYSE-DAVIES, J. & WILKINSON, J. H. (1958). *Lancet*, **1**, 1249.

QUICK, A. J. (1933). *Amer. J. med. Sci.*, **185**, 630.

QUICK, A. J. (1939). *Amer. J. digest. Dis.*, **6**, 716.

RAWLS, W. B., WEISS, S. & COLLINS, V. L. (1937). *Ann. intern. Med.*, **10**, 1021.

READ, A. E., SHERLOCK, S. & HARRISON, C. V. (1963). *Gut*, **4**, 378.

REES, K. R. & SINHA, K. (1960). *J. Path. Bact.*, **80**, 297.

REES, K. R., SINHA, K. P. & SPECTOR, W. G. (1961). *J. Path. Bact.*, **81**, 107.

REICHARD, H. J. (1961). *J. Lab. clin. Med.*, **57**, 78.

REYNELL, P. C. (1954). *Brit. J. exp. Path.*, **35**, 92.

RICH, A. R. (1930). *Bull. Johns Hopk. Hosp.*, **47**, 338.

RICKETTS, W. E. (1953). *Gastroenterology*, **23**, 391.

RICKETTS, W. E., KIRSNER, J. B., PALMER, W. L. & STERLING, K. (1950). *J. Lab. clin. Med.*, **35**, 403.

ROBERTS, W. M. (1933). *Brit. med. J.*, **1**, 734.

ROE, J. H. & SCHWARTZMAN, A. S. (1933). *Amer. J. med. Sci.*, **186**, 425.

ROHOLM, K. & IVERSEN, P. (1939). *Acta path. microbiol. scand.*, **16**, 427.

ROSENBERG, I. N. (1959). *J. clin. Invest.*, **38**, 630.

ROTOR, A. B., MANAHAN, I. & FLORENTIN, A. (1948). *Acra. med. Phillipine*, **5**, 37.

SCHALM, L. & HOOGENBOOM, W. A. H. (1952). *Amer. Heart J.*, **44**, 571.

SCHIFF, L. (1963). "Diseases of the Liver", 2nd Ed., p. 206. Montreal, Lippincott.

SCHLESINGER, B., PAYNE, W. W. & BURNARD, E. D. (1949). *Arch. Dis. Childh.*, **24**, 16.

SCHMID, R. (1957). *J. biol. Chem.*, **229**, 881.

SCHMID, R. (1965). "The Billiary System". Ed. Taylor, W., p. 205. Oxford, Blackwell.

SCHWARZ, K. (1951). *Proc. Soc. Exp. Biol. Med.*, **78**, 852.

SCHWARZ, K. (1960). *Nutr. Rev.*, **18**, 193.

SEEGMILLER, J. E., SCHWARTZ, R. & DAVIDSON, C. S. (1954). *J. clin. Invest.*, **33**, 984.

SHAY, H. & SIPLET, H. (1954). *J. Lab. clin. Med.*, **43**, 741.

SHERLOCK, S. (1958). "Diseases of the liver and biliary system". 2nd Ed. Oxford, Blackwell.

SHERLOCK, S. (1960). *Ann. Rev. Med.*, **11**, 47.

SHERLOCK, S. (1963). "Diseases of the liver and biliary system". 3rd Ed. Oxford, Blackwell.

SHERLOCK, S. (1964). *Proc. Roy. Soc. Med.*, **57**, 881.

SHERLOCK, S., SUMMERSKILL, W. H. J., WHITE, L. P. & PHEAR, E. A. (1954). *Lancet*, **2**, 453.

SIMONS, R. L. (1954). *Amer. J. med. Sci.*, **228**, 312.

STAEDELER, G. (1864). *Liebigs Ann.*, **132**, 323.

STEIGMANN, F., MEYER, K. A. & POPPER, H. (1949). *Arch. Surg.*, **59**, 101.

STEIN, H. B. (1944). *S. Afr. J. med. Sci.*, **9**, 111.

STERKEL, R. L., SPENCER, J. A., WOLFSON, S. K. & WILLIAMS-ASHMAN, H. G. (1958). *J. Lab. clin. Med.*, **52**, 176.

STERN, L. & DENTON, R. L. (1965), *Paediatrics*, **35**, 483.

STEWART, C. P., SCARBOROUGH, H. & DAVIDSON, J. N. (1938). *Quart. J. Med.*, **7** n.s., 229.

STONER, H. B. & MAGEE, P. N. (1957). *Brit. Med. Bull.*, **13**, 102.

SWANSON, J. N. (1949). *Ann. rheum. Dis.*, **8**, 232.

THOMAS, L. J. & ZIMMERMAN, H. J. (1952). *J. Lab. clin. Med.*, **39**, 882.

VAN DER ZIJDEN, A. S. M., BLANCHE KOELENSMID, W. A. A., BOLDINGH, J., BARRETT, C. B., ORD, W. O. & PHILP, J. (1962), *Nature* (Lond.), **195**, 1060.

VESELL, E. S. & BEARN, A. G. (1957). *Proc. Soc. exp. Biol. N.Y.*, **94**, 96.

VIRCHOW, R. (1847), *Virchows Arch.*, **1**, 379.

WALSHE, J. M. (1951). *Quart. J. Med.*, **20**, n.s., 421.

WALSHE, J. M. (1953). *Lancet*, **1**, 1075.

WALSHE, J. M. (1960). Article in Lectures on the Scientific Basis of Medicine. Vol. 8, p. 409. New York & London, Athlone Press.

WANG, I. (1953). *Brit. med. J.*, **2**, 971.

WATERLOW, J. C. & BRAS, G. (1961). "Modern Trends in Gastroenterology". Ed Card, W. I., 3, 158, London, Butterworths.

WATSON, C. J. (1938). "The pyrrole pigments", in Downey's Handbook of hematology. Vol. IV. London, Hamish Hamilton.

WATSON, C. J. (1942). *New Engl. J. Med.*, **227**, 665.

WATSON, C. J. (1944). *Amer. J. clin. Path.*, **14**, 129.

WATSON, C. J. (1946). *Blood*, **1**, 99.

WATSON, C. J., SCHWARTZ, S., SBOROV, V. & BERTIE, E. (1944). *Amer. J. clin. Path.*, **14**, 605.

WEIL-MALHERBE, H. (1953). *Lancet*, **2**, 623.

WEINBREN, K. (1952). *J. Path. Bact.*, **64**, 395.

WHIPPLE, G. H. (1922). *Physiol. Rev.*, **2**, 440.

WHITEHEAD, T. P. & WHITTAKER, S. R. F. (1955). *J. clin. Path.*, **8**, 81.

WILKINSON, J. H. (1961). Article in "Lectures on the Scientific Basis of Medicine". Vol. 9. London & New York, Athlone Press.

WILLIAMS, R., SPEYER, B. E. & BILLING, B. H. (1961). *Gut*, **2**, 297.

WILSON, W. C., MacGREGOR, A. R. & STEWART, C. P. (1938). *Brit . J. Surg.*, **25**, 826.

WINTROBE, M. M. (1961). "Clinical Haematology", 5th Ed. London, Kimpton.

WITH, T. K. (1944). *Acta med. scand.*, **119**, 214.

WOOTTON, I. D. P. (1964). "Micro-analysis in Medical Biochemistry", 4th ed. London, Churchill.

WRÓBLEWSKI, F. (1958). Article in "Advances in clinical chemistry", Vol. 1. New York & London, Academic Press.

WRÓBLEWSKI, F. (1959). *Ann. intern. Med.*, **50**, 62.

WRÓBLEWSKI, F. & LaDUE, J. S. (1956). *Pro. Soc. exp. Biol. N.Y.*, **91**, 569.

ZELMAN, S. (1952). *Arch. intern. Med.*, **90**, 141.

ZIMMERMAN, H. J., MACMURRAY, F. G., RAPPAPORT, H. & ALPERT, L. K. (1950). *J. Lab. clin. Med.*, **36**, 912 & 922.

Chapter 6

THE ANAEMIAS

by

I. CHANARIN

Experimental Haematology Research Unit, St. Mary's Hospital Medical School, London

THE ANAEMIA OF CHRONIC DISORDERS

ANAEMIA is common to a variety of disorders such as renal failure, rheumatoid arthritis, chronic infections and neoplastic disease. This anaemia has been termed the anaemia of infection, secondary anaemia as well as the anaemia of chronic disorders. The latter term used by Cartwright (1966) is perhaps the most acceptable. This is the commonest form of anaemia encountered in hospital practice and at the same time the most poorly understood.

Anaemia tends to develop during the first 6 to 8 weeks of the chronic disorder and thereafter to remain static unless there is marked deterioration in the clinical condition or unless it becomes complicated by iron deficiency or excessive red cell destruction (Cartwright & Wintrobe, 1952). It is difficult to obtain information about the frequency of anaemia amongst those at risk. However some anaemia was present in 42% of patients with chronic infections, 63% of patients with rheumatoid arthritis, 15% of patients with infective or neoplastic pulmonary diseases, and in over 70% of patients with malignant disease (Cartwright, 1966). In general the anaemia is moderate in degree, i.e. haemoglobin levels are often between 9 to 11 g./100 ml. but particularly in renal failure anaemia may be severe. Those with more active disease tend to be more anaemic and this is particularly true in rheumatoid arthritis (Jeffrey, 1953).

Changes in blood and marrow. The stained film of peripheral blood may not show any abnormalities, i.e. it is normocytic and normochromic, but in about one-third of patients the red cells appear hypochromic. Correspondingly the mean corpuscular haemoglobin concentration (MCHC) which is a valuable index of deficient haemoglobinization of the red cell, is reduced from the normal range of 32 to 36% to between 28 to 31%, and occasionally in renal failure the MCHC may be as low as 25 to 26%.

The marrow may appear to be normal morphologically but in a proportion of patients the erythroblasts show changes similar to those found in iron-deficiency anaemia, i.e. there are many late pyknotic normoblasts with irregular nuclei and ragged cytoplasm. These cells are similar to the micronormoblasts of iron deficiency. More important however is the disparity between the overall cellularity of the marrow fragments (as judged by the proportion of fat spaces to haemopoietic tissue in narrow fragments and by the cellularity of the trails of cells left by these fragments on the film as the marrow is spread) and the degree of anaemia. The cellularity of the marrow is either normal or occasionally somewhat hypocellular, and this suggests that the marrow has failed to become hyperplastic in response to the reduced haemoglobin level.

Changes in Iron Metabolism

Serum iron. The resemblance of the anaemia of chronic disorders to that of iron-deficiency is heightened by a reduction in the serum iron level in both conditions. This is usually reduced from a normal range of 60 to 200 μg/100 ml. to between 10 to 70 μg./100 ml. Because of the frequency with

which hypochromia and a reduced MCHC is present as well as a low serum iron concentration these cases are often regarded as being due to iron deficiency, and are given oral and parenteral iron therapy with no beneficial effect whatsoever. The fall in the serum iron level is very early in response to sepsis and may be observed within 24 hours of the onset of the disorder (Cartwright & Wintrobe, 1949).

Transferrin level. Characteristically the total iron-binding capacity of the serum is reduced in the anaemia of chronic disorders (Laurell, 1947). Values vary from 80 to 270 μg./100 ml. (Cartwright & Wintrobe, 1949) with a mean of about 200. By contrast the transferrin level is characteristically increased in iron-deficiency anaemia and this is valuable in distinguishing between these two anaemias. The reduction in transferrin levels is true of patients with acute infections, chronic infections such as tuberculosis and disorders such as rheumatoid arthritis (Bendstrup, 1953).

Iron stores. Decisive information is also obtained by staining spreads of the marrow aspirate by Perls' Prussian blue method. In contrast with iron-deficiency anaemia where stainable iron is absent, in the anaemia of chronic disorders the reticuloendothelial cells in the marrow fragments contain an abundance of stainable iron. Indeed often the amount of iron is increased. It is unnecessary to count the normoblasts containing stainable iron granules (sideroblasts), but when this is done the proportion of erythroblasts with iron granules is reduced from a normal range of 30–50% to less than 20% (Bainton & Finch, 1964). Perhaps it is as well to mention that the ringed-sideroblasts of the sideroblastic anaemias are not seen, since this anaemia also shares the morphological picture of hypochromia in blood films with abundant storage iron.

Iron absorption. The absorption of iron from the gut is decreased in patients with chronic disorders (Haurani, Green & Young, 1965), a not surprising observation in view of the more than adequate iron stores and the relatively normal or poor marrow cellularity.

	Normal subjects	Iron-deficiency anaemia	Anaemia of Chronic disorders
Blood film	Normochromic	Hypochromic	Normochromic or hypochromic
Serum iron	100 μg %	Low	Low
Transferrin	350 μg %	High	Low
Iron stores	normal	None	Normal or increased
Sideroblast count	30–50 %	Low	Low

Mechanism of the Anaemia

Impaired iron metabolism. Studies with radio-active iron have been carried out in patients with chronic infections, rheumatoid arthritis and carcinoma, and the results were reviewed by Cartwright (1966). Tracer doses of iron are cleared rapidly from the plasma, but the plasma iron turnover, and the incorporation of tracer iron into erythrocytes, is either normal or slightly above normal. Thus transferrin-bound iron is utilized adequately. When however radio-iron in the form of red cells is given the rate of reutilization is depressed (Freireich, Miller, Emerson & Ross, 1957) i.e. there is inadequate utilization of storage iron. This can also be inferred from the association of adequate iron stores, low serum iron levels and low sideroblast counts. Bothwell & Finch (1962) have suggested that the low transferrin level is due to adherence of transferrin to iron storage reticulum cells. The transfer of transferrin-bound iron from these cells to erythroblasts is normally accomplished by transient attachment of transferrin to the cell surfaces during which time iron is taken up and discharged.

Red cell survival. The considerable literature on mean cell life span in these disorders is reviewed by Cartwright (1966). In general there is a moderate shortening of mean life span. Survival of compatible donor cells given to patients with the anaemia of chronic disorders is generally moderately reduced with a mean cell life of 30 to 70 days. On the other hand there is no defect in the patient's own red cells as indicated by the normal survival of "patients" cells in a normal recipient (Hyman, Gellhorn & Harvey, 1956). Thus the modest shortening of the red cell life span is due to extracorpuscular factors. The nature of the factor or factors shortening the survival of the red cells is not known in the majority of patients where this occurs. In some cases with renal failure and disseminated carcinoma damage to red cells by passage through small irregular arterioles has been implicated (Brain, Dacie & Hourihane, 1962).

The modest diminution in red cell survival which has been demonstrated in these disorders is significant only because in the anaemia of chronic disorders the marrow is unable to show the normal response by an increased output, but remains normocellular or even hypocellular.

Associated complications. Particularly in rheumatoid arthritis true iron deficiency frequently complicates the picture. This is usually the result of long-term salicylate medication which produces gastro-intestinal blood loss. When this arises the anaemia responds to oral or parenteral iron therapy but the rise in haemoglobin concentration ceases at the level determined by the presence of the associated disorder.

Role of erythropoietin. Erythropoietin is a substance present in plasma and which stimulates erythropoiesis. It is possibly protein in nature and a possible site of production is the kidney. Cobalt administration on occasion produces a significant rise in haemoglobin concentration in the anaemia of chronic disorders, and Goldwasser, Jacobsen, Fried & Plzak (1957) showed an increased plasma erythropoietin activity following cobalt administration. Thus it has been speculated that the anaemia of chronic disorders is due to a failure to produce the erythropoiesis-stimulating factor, but evidence on this point is lacking.

Management. Only adequate control of the underlying disorder will correct the anaemia associated with these chronic disorders. When the anaemia is severe transfusion of red cells may be required.

INTRINSIC DISORDERS OF THE RED CELL

Inherited defects of the erythrocyte can involve the red cell membrane, the enzymic pathways which provide energy for the reactions which maintain the physical and biochemical *status quo* of the cell, or they can involve the haemoglobin moiety. Thus the disorders can be classified as

DEFECTS OF THE RED CELL MEMBRANE

(1) Hereditary spherocytosis

(2) Elliptocytosis

(3) Acanthocytosis

ENZYMIC DEFECTS

(1) *Hexokinase deficiency*

(2) *Defects of anaerobic glycolysis*
Pyruvate kinase deficiency
Triose phosphate isomerase deficiency
2, 3-diphosphoglycerate mutase deficiency

(3) *Defects of the hexose monophosphate shunt*
Glucose-6-phosphate dehydrogenase deficiency
Deficiency of erythrocyte glutathione
6-phosphogluconate dehydrogenase deficiency
Glutathione reductase deficiency

(4) *Hereditary methaemoglobinaemia*
DPNH-methaemoglobin reductase deficiency

HAEMOGLOBIN DEFECTS

(1) *Haem moiety*—erythropoietic porphyria
(2) *Globin moiety*
    Hb S, C, D and E
    Unstable haemoglobins—Zürich, Köln and others
    Hb M
    Thalassaemias

The Red Cell Membrane

A diagrammatic representation of the red cell membrane is shown in Fig. 6.1 (Weed & Reed, 1966). The structural components are lipids and proteins as well as ions and water. The phospholi-

choline and sphingomyelin (Weed & Reed, 1966).

Maddy & Malcolm (1965) have presented evidence that the protein in the red cell membrane is in the form of a coiled globular molecule. It contains sulphydryl groups and carbohydrate such as hexose, hexosamine and fucose as well as all the sialic acid present in the red cell membrane.

Many, if not all, of the enzymes of the glycolytic pathways are closely associated with the red cell membrane, and certainly glyceraldehyde phosphate dehydrogenase and phosphoglycerate kinase are firmly bound (Schrier, 1966). Cholinesterase too is part of the red cell membrane, as is adenosinetriphosphatase (ATPase).

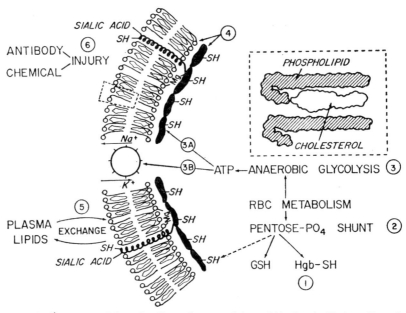

FIG. 6.1. Hypothetical structure of the red cell membrane and sites of biochemical lesions (1 to 6) (from Weed & Reed, 1966).

pids (phosphatidylcholine, phosphatidylserine, phosphatidylethanolamine and sphingomyelin) are arranged as a hydrophobic hydrocarbon tail and a surface polar group which is hydrophilic. Glycolipids and cholesterol are the other lipid constituents. All the lipid in the red cell can be recovered from the haemoglobin-free red cell ghost. *De novo* lipid synthesis does not occur in the mature erythrocyte, although inorganic phosphate is incorporated into phosphatidic acid at a very low rate through a phosphatase. There is, however, an exchange of various lipids with corresponding compounds in plasma, particularly of cholesterol which is exchanged completely in 12 hours and to a far less extent phosphatidyl-

The Enzymic Pathways

There are considerable differences between the metabolic capacity of reticulocyte-rich blood and blood having a normal reticulocyte complement. The reticulocyte still possesses some of the characteristics of the developing nucleated red cell, retaining both mitochondria and microsomes. The energy requirements of the reticulocyte depend on both aerobic pathways utilizing oxygen through mitochondrial phosphorylation and also on the anaerobic utilization of glucose. The reticulocyte can in fact utilize any of the intermediates that enter the tricarboxylic acid cycle, and is able to synthesize porphyrins and incorporate iron to form haem.

By contrast, the mature red cell is unable to synthesize protein and hence is unable to replenish its complement of enzymes. It is largely dependent for its energy requirements on anaerobic glycolysis. This energy is required for various activities that are essential for the viability of the red cell. These activities are the maintenance of the normal biconcavity despite the extreme buffeting and distortion of the red cell in its passage through capillaries, the pumping of sodium ions out of the red cell into plasma against the concentration gradient, and maintaining the levels of intracellular potassium and the maintenance of reducing conditions to keep haem iron in the ferrous form. The maintenance of a suitable oxidation-reduction potential depends not only on anaerobic glycolysis which forms DPNH but also on the hexose monophosphate shunt which regenerates TPNH. The latter pathway also maintains reduced gluthathione and impairment of this pathway as in glucose-6-phosphate dehydrogenase deficiency may be associated with a haemolytic process.

Defects of Red Cell Membrane
Hereditary spherocytosis

This disorder, which has been known for almost a century (Vanlair & Masius, 1871), is transmitted as an autosomal dominant characteristic. Generally a parent of a patient with this disorder will also show evidence of the disease and the exceptions have been attributed to a variation in penetrance of the gene leading to mild and not easily recognizable forms, but a mutation in the patient is also possible (Young, 1955). It is the commonest form of congenital haemolytic anaemia in people of North European origin.

Patients with this disorder come to clinical notice because of jaundice or splenomegaly, or because of some of the complications that may ensue viz. an aplastic crisis with severe anaemia, leg ulceration and occasionally gall stones. Many cases are found as a result of family studies initiated as a result of a case of hereditary spherocytosis being found in a member of the family.

Anaemia is not usually severe except at the height of an aplastic crisis and the haemoglobin concentration varies between 9 to 14 g./100 ml. The reticulocyte count is elevated from about 5% in the mildest cases to more than 30% in severe cases, and in the absence of splenectomy these high reticulocyte counts remain a permanent feature of the blood picture. A low reticulocyte count is an indication of an aplastic crisis, and on occasion may be the only evidence of such a crisis (Chanarin, Burman & Bennett, 1962).

The blood film shows spherocytosis i.e. many of the erythrocytes have lost their biconcavity, appear spheroidal with diminished diameter and stain in a more intense uniform manner. These changes may be mild or more severe. The older cells are more affected and the new polychromatic cells (reticulocytes) are evidently larger and tend to retain their biconcavity. Thus it would appear that the cells appear normal when delivered to the blood and become increasingly spherocytic with time.

Spherocytosis is not unique to hereditary spherocytosis. It is common to a variety of haemolytic anaemias, particularly those due to an autoimmune process and which are associated with a positive antiglobulin (or Coombs') reaction. Spherocytes are also frequent in haemolytic disease of the newborn due to ABO incompatibility. In this respect it is as well to note that more than half the newborn infants with hereditary spherocytosis become jaundiced (Stamey & Diamond, 1957) and may require exchange transfusion.

Apart from jaundice the almost constant clinical feature in hereditary spherocytosis is an enlarged firm spleen.

Laboratory studies. The striking abnormality in hereditary spherocytosis is that the red cells are unable to withstand the stress of incubation. In vivo this stress is brought about by sojourn in the spleen; in vitro this can be reproduced by incubating the red cells at 37°C. Splenectomy results in normal red cell survival. So much so, that in the rare cases where relapse occurs laparotomy will reveal residual or regenerated splenic tissue.

Characteristically the patient is jaundiced with a bilirubin level that rarely exceeds 5 mg. %. The direct van den Bergh reaction is negative, i.e. the bilirubin is not conjugated. Bile is absent from the urine, hence the term, acholuric jaundice for this disorder. However, urobilin is present in the urine and urobilinogen in large excess in the faeces. In a small number of mild cases the bilirubin level may be normal.

The osmotic fragility test on the red cells is abnormal. This test to some extent is a method of quantitating the degree of spherocytosis, and hence an abnormal result is found in all patients with spherocytosis irrespective of the cause. Nevertheless in the mild case where inspection of the blood film is indecisive the fragility test is useful. Unfortunately it is just in this type of case that changes may be relatively minor and call for a very careful and precise technique in the performance of the test. In some patients there are relatively small numbers of very fragile cells which are haemolysed between 0·75 to 0·55% of NaCl

solution; the result is also abnormal in 0·5%
saline, and thereafter the values are at the upper
limit of the normal range. These very fragile cells
provide a "tail" to the fragility curve. The majority
of patients however give more clearly abnormal
results.

The osmotic fragility test has also been used to
demonstrate the deleterious effects of incubation
upon the red cells in hereditary spherocytosis. The
effects of incubation can be tested in two ways.

Autohaemolysis. Sterile whole blood is incubated at 37°C for 48 hours. At the end of this time
less than 4·5% of normal cells have undergone
spontaneous haemolysis. In hereditary spherocytosis the amount of spontaneous haemolysis
exceeds this value often by a considerable amount.
This abnormality persists after splenectomy. The
range in 21 patients was 7·5 to 47·5%. The addition of glucose reduced the amount of haemolysis
both with normal blood and in hereditary spherocytosis (Selwyn & Dacie, 1954).

Osmotic fragility after incubation of blood. When
the blood has been incubated at 37°C for 24 hours
the increase in osmotic fragility is far greater in
hereditary spherocytosis than in controls.

The mean cell-life of red cells in hereditary
spherocytosis using the ^{51}Cr method may vary
from 18 to 27 days in very mild cases and less than
this in the majority of cases (Hughes-Jones &
Szur, 1957). The survival of the cells becomes
almost normal after splenectomy.

Complications. Gallstones may ultimately develop in about half the patients with hereditary
spherocytosis. They may be associated with the
usual symptoms of gallstone colic and sometimes
evidence of obstructive jaundice.

Intractable leg ulcers are an uncommon complication of a number of congenital haemolytic
anaemias. These are not associated with any
vascular abnormality and the reason for their
causation is obscure. In hereditary spherocytosis
they heal after splenectomy.

Temporary failure of marrow function, often
the result of trivial upper respiratory tract infections, is one of the serious complications of these
haemolytic anaemias. Often more than one member of the family may be affected, i.e. the so called
familial crisis. That these crises are due to transient marrow failure and not to increased red cell
destruction was indicated by Lyngar (1942) and
amply confirmed by others. The haemoglobin
declines rapidly to 2 to 3 g./100 ml. in severe cases
and the clue is given by the absence of reticulocytes if the case is seen early enough or by a
relatively low count where recovery has started.
As these cases are brought to clinical notice be-

cause of the anaemia it is unusual to see the patient
at an early stage. Thus recovery is generally under
way when the patient is seen, the phase of marrow
aplasia has already given way to recovery with
many early erythroblasts in the marrow and the
reticulocyte count is beginning to rise. Rapid
recovery ensues. The events initiating these dramatic changes remain obscure. The case reported by
Chanarin, Burman & Bennett (1962) excreted
large amounts of urocanic acid in the urine during
the period of observation which was the period of
marrow regeneration and this disappeared thereafter.

Treatment. This is splenectomy and results are
uniformly excellent.

Biochemical studies. The nature of the inborn
error of metabolism or structure in the red cell in
hereditary spherocytosis remains unknown.

The red cells in hereditary spherocytosis on incubation are unable to maintain their normal levels
of intracellular sodium (Jacob & Jandl, 1964).
Whereas normal red cells gain negligible quantities of sodium during the first 18 hours of incubation, the cells in hereditary spherocytosis accumulate sodium within 4 hours and this increases
steadily thereafter. Potassium loss is no different
from that in normal red cells. With this passage of
sodium into the cell water enters as well so that the
cell becomes spherocytic and liable to haemolyse.
The "sodium pump" which is concerned with the
expulsion of sodium from the cell is fully active in
hereditary spherocytosis and ^{24}Na is expelled
from the red cell in hereditary spherocytosis at a
greater rate than from a normal cell (Harris &
Prankerd, 1953; Jacob, 1966). Indeed it has been
calculated that both influx and egress of sodium
into the red cell is twice that of the normal cell.
This has suggested that there is an abnormal
permeability of the red cell membrane to this
cation. The expulsion of sodium requires energy,
and correspondingly the consumption of glucose
is about one-third greater than is the case with
normal cells (Mahler, 1965). It has been suggested
that the adverse effect of stasis or incubation upon
the red cells in hereditary spherocytosis is the
consequence of this hypermetabolic state which
exhausts the available supplies of glucose which
would normally be available from the plasma.
In vitro addition of glucose to the incubation
mixture diminishes lysis. The beneficial effect of
glucose is absent in some of the other congenital
haemolytic anaemias such as that due to pyruvate–
kinase deficiency and hence the autohaemolysis
test is of some value in the diagnosis of the doubtful case (Selwyn & Dacie, 1954). The energy for the
function of the sodium pump is provided via the

high-energy phosphate in ATP and the enzyme concerned, ATPase, is present in the red cell membrane and has been implicated in cation transport (Skou, 1965).

However persuasive this hypothesis is in rationalizing some of the events in hereditary spherocytosis, it is not likely to be the whole explanation. The spherocyte in hereditary spherocytosis is a much smaller cell than that produced by simple osmotic swelling in hypotonic solution of a normal red cell, i.e. the surface area is reduced in amount and the contents are more concentrated (Crosby, 1952). Hereditary spherocytosis is one of the few conditions where the mean corpuscular haemoglobin concentration (MCHC) is increased and values of 35 to 36% as opposed to a normal value of 32 to 33% are frequent. Indeed loss of surface area is as likely to be the explanation for spherocytosis as is osmotic swelling. Phospholipids constitute an important fraction of the red cell membrane although whether they function in cation transport is not known. There is evidence that the turnover of phospholipids is accelerated when there is increased sodium transport (Hokin & Hokin, 1963) and this applies equally to the red cell in hereditary spherocytosis (Jacob, 1966). Whittam (1964) has suggested that phospholipids may act as a binding material between other lipids and proteins in the red cell membrane and that increased sodium transport leads in turn to increased phospholipid turnover and loss of this material from the red cell membrane. That there is a marked loss of lipid on incubation of the red cells in hereditary spherocytosis has been reported by Prankerd (1960) and others. However the proportions of the different cholesterol and lipids fractions remain unchanged in the cell in hereditary spherocytosis i.e. there is no preferential loss of one or other constituent. This implies that small portions of the membrane are lost *in toto* and Weed & Reed (1965) have suggested on the basis of electron microscopy that there is actual loss of red cell fragments on incubation.

Elliptocytosis

Although oval red cells are not uncommonly encountered in routine haematological practice, elliptocytosis as part of a haemolytic anaemia is unusual. Like hereditary spherocytosis, inheritance follows a Mendelian dominant pattern.

A diminished red cell life span when present, may be fully compensated or the patient may show a varying degree of anaemia. Thus the reticulocyte count is elevated and the serum bilirubin may be slightly elevated. Oval densely staining elliptocytes reminiscent of the cells in hereditary spherocytosis may be present. The osmotic fragility test is normal in the elliptocytic trait and may be increased in some but not all cases with a haemolytic process. Autohaemolysis is normal.

It seems probable that the abnormality in shape is not the sole abnormality in the elliptocytic red cell when the mean cell-life is reduced. Dacie (1960) has suggested that the defect may be similar to that in hereditary spherocytosis, and cases with marked haemolysis are benefited by splenectomy.

Acanthocytosis

In this disorder which may be associated with a diminished red cell survival, the erythrocytes display large coarse irregular projections on their surface—hence the term acanthocyte or thorny red cell. The excuse for mentioning this disorder is that it is associated with a clear abnormality in the composition of the red cell membrane. Plasma lipids are markedly reduced and the normal ratio of plasma phosphatidylcholine to sphingomyelin (4 to 1) is reduced to either 3 to 2 or even to unity. The young erythrocytes are morphologically and chemically normal but in the circulation the ratio of phosphatidylcholine to sphingomyelin in the red cell membrane (normally 3 to 2) is reversed (Ways & Dong, 1965). Thus the lipid composition of the plasma influences the structure and composition of the red cell membrane and ultimately its survival in the circulation.

Enzymic Defects in the Red Cell

Selwyn & Dacie (1954) divided the patients with congenital haemolytic anaemia into two groups. The spherocytic group, i.e. hereditary spherocytosis, formed a well-knit clinical entity. There remained a group termed the nonspherocytic haemolytic anaemias which obviously comprised a number of disorders and which have only been partially unravelled in recent years.

Hexokinase deficiency. Valentine, Oski, Paglia, Baughan, Schneider & Naiman (1967) described a severe haemolytic anaemia in an infant. Investigation showed a decreased metabolism of glucose via the Embden-Meyerhof pathway but not via the pentose-phosphate shunt. Hexokinase was shown to decay with very marked rapidity in older erythrocytes but the enzyme was present in the patient's reticulocyte-rich blood. An autosomal recessive mode of inheritance was postulated.

Pyruvate-kinase deficiency. Following the original report by Valentine, Tanaka & Miwa (1961) of three patients with haemolytic anaemia due to a defect of pyruvate kinase more than 80 cases have been recorded (Keitt, 1966). It is transmitted as a

Mendelian recessive characteristic. The heterozygotes appear to be clinically normal, but there is a remarkable variation in the manifestations of the disease in homozygotes. It can be fully compensated with a normal haemoglobin level and a reticulocytosis that does not exceed 10% or the patient can be very anaemic with haemoglobin levels below 6 g./100 ml. (Bowman, McKusick & Dronamraju, 1965). All 12 patients studied by Grimes, Meisler & Dacie (1964) were anaemic and their reticulocyte counts ranged from 7 to 15% before splenectomy and from 20 to 78% in those who had undergone splenectomy.

The appearance of the red blood cells in stained films also reflects the variation in clinical severity of the disorder. The blood film may be unremarkable, with polychromasia and a tendency to macrocytosis, or there may be marked abnormalities in severely affected jaundiced infants, with macrocytosis, polychromasia, spherocytes and many irregularly contracted and "tailed" poikilocytes. These cases have many nucleated red cells in the peripheral blood (Oski & Diamond, 1963).

Splenectomy appears to benefit these cases to some extent. The obvious effect is in a sustained elevation of the post-splenectomy reticulocyte count suggesting that the spleen preferentially sequesters reticulocytes. Whether pyruvate-kinase-deficient reticulocytes are trapped more avidly than normal reticulocytes by the spleen is unknown, although this has been suggested by Bowman & Procopio (1963). Splenectomy is associated with an improved red cell survival. The autohaemolysis test may be normal or only marginally abnormal in half the cases. Haemolysis is not affected by the addition of glucose but is reduced by the addition of ATP (DeGruchy, Sanatamaria, Parsons & Crawford, 1960).

The metabolic defect. Pyruvate kinase catalyses the conversion of phosphoenolpyruvate to pyruvate and the red cells of patients with this

$$\text{phospho-} \underset{\text{enolpyruvate}}{} \underset{\overset{\text{ATP}}{\rightleftarrows}}{\overset{\text{ADP}}{}} \text{pyruvate} \underset{\overset{\text{DPN}}{\rightleftarrows}}{\overset{\text{DPNH}}{}} \text{lactate}$$

disorder have very low levels of this enzyme. Tanaka, Valentine & Miwa (1962) have described a method of assay which has proved to be readily reproducible. It is dependent on the conversion of phosphoenolpyruvate to pyruvate in the presence of ADP. Lactic dehydrogenase and DPNH are added so that pyruvate formed is converted to lactate with accompanying conversion of DPNH to DPN. The change in absorbance at 340mμ due to the oxidation of DPNH to DPN is measured. The normal range shows small variations in different hands and varies from 1·5 to 3·4 moles DPNH oxidized per minute by 10^{10} red cells. Values in heterozygotes are approximately one half that found in normal subjects, and the values in patients are well below the range in either of these groups. It is important that the red cell homogenate be relatively free of white blood cells since these too contain pyruvate kinase which is unaffected in patients lacking the red cell enzyme. However the white cell enzyme differs electrophoretically from that in the red cell and hence is presumably transmitted by a different genetic mechanism.

Why lack of pyruvate kinase should cause a haemolytic anaemia is not clear because pyruvate-kinase-deficient red cells are still able to utilize glucose at a rate that is often normal or only slightly abnormal (Grimes, Meisler & Dacie, 1964). They have suggested that the level of pyruvate kinase is adequate in young cells but declines rapidly with ageing and this results in a failure of glycolysis.

As expected, the red cells in pyruvate kinase deficiency show a low level of ATP and a high level of 2, 3-diphosphoglycerate. The low levels of ATP may result in difficulty in maintaining ionic balance, and there is some evidence that this leads to K loss from the cells which may also contribute to its final destruction.

Triosephosphate isomerase deficiency. Schneider, Valentine, Hattori & Heins (1965) described a haemolytic anaemia with splenomegaly, an undistinguished blood picture, and associated with a progressive neurological disorder producing spasticity. It appeared to have a recessive mode of inheritance, and in the families described by Valentine, Schneider, Bangham, Paglia & Heins (1966) consanguinity was present. Both red and white cells were affected and some patients had repeated episodes of intercurrent infections although the total white cell count was normal. There was generally only a moderate degree of anaemia except during episodes of infection when there was a rapid fall in haemoglobin level. Occasionally red cells resembling those seen in acanthocytosis were present. Autohaemolysis was abnormal in homozygotes and corrected by the addition of glucose, adenosine or ATP. Patients showed a marked reduction in activity of both erythrocyte and leucocyte triosephosphate isomerase. The activities of other enzymes were normal or elevated. An intermediate reduction of activity of the enzyme was found in both parents.

2, 3-diphosphoglycerate mutase deficiency. This rare defect too is the product of consanguinity in parents. A usually severe but sometimes mild haemolytic anaemia may be present in what is presumably a homozygous infant (Bowdler & Prankerd, 1964). A suitable assay method was described by Schröter (1965). The defect is a failure to convert 1, 3-diphosphoglycerate to 2, 3-diphosphoglycerate.

Deficiency of erythrocyte glutathione. A mild haemolytic anaemia due to lack of glutathione in red cells was described by Oort, Loos & Prins (1961). Normally erythrocytes are able to synthesize glutathione from glycine, cysteine and glutamic acid and this is controlled by an autosomal recessive gene. The red cells appeared normal, mild jaundice was present in some patients and Heinz bodies were readily produced by incubation with acetylphenylhydrazine. In this large Dutch family there were several consanguinous marriages, but parents of affected cases had normal GSH levels. The red cells in these patients are sensitive to drug-induced haemolysis.

Glutathione reductase deficiency. Löhr & Waller (1962) described a congenital nonspherocytic haemolytic anaemia due to deficiency of this enzyme. The activity of glutathione reductase was about 50% of that in normal red cells. These patients are also liable to drug-induced haemolytic episodes. Methods for assaying the level of glutathione reductase were described by Carson, Flanagan, Ickes & Alving (1956) and Beutler & Yeh (1963).

Glucose-6-phosphate dehydrogenase deficiency. Glucose is transported into the red cell by an active process and is then phosphorylated by the enzyme hexokinase which transfers phosphate from ATP to form glucose-6-phosphate. About 90% of the glucose-6-phosphate is utilized along the anaerobic glycolytic pathway to pyruvate and lactate (Fig. 6.2). About 10% of glucose is utilized by the hexose monophosphate or direct oxidative pathway. Here glucose is oxidized and decarboxylated. Whereas in the anaerobic pathway DPN is the principle coenzyme, in the hexosemonophosphate shunt it is TPN which is utilized and TPNH produced. This serves to convert oxidized glutathione (GSSG) to the reduced form (GSH). A supply of GSH is necessary for the normal survival of the red cell. Oxidation of GSH can result from direct reaction with a variety of drugs. If a supply of reduced GSH is not available oxidation can proceed to affect haemoglobin which becomes denatured to form Heinz bodies. A more physiological role for GSH in the red cell may lie in the disposal of hydrogen peroxide.

$$2\text{ GSH} + \text{H}_2\text{O}_2 \xrightarrow[\text{peroxidase}]{\text{GSH}} \text{GSSG} + 2\text{H}_2\text{O}$$

However red cells also contain catalases which are capable of destroying peroxides.

TPNH which arises via the hexose monophosphate pathway is also required for the reduction of methaemoglobin. One of the enzymes, though not the principle one concerned in methaemoglobin reduction is TPNH-dependent. A continuous supply of GSH and TPNH is achieved via the conversion of glucose-6-phosphate to 6-phosphogluconate. The enzyme catalysing the reaction is glucose-6-phosphate dehydrogenase (G-6-PD).

The earlier view was that an intact hexose monophosphate shunt was required only for overcoming the oxidative effects of exogenous agents. However, it is now known that G-6-PD deficient red cells may have a diminished survival in the circulation in the absence of any exogenous factors (Brewer, Tarlov & Kellermeyer, 1961), that G-6-PD deficiency may be the only defect found in some 30% patients with congenital nonspherocytic haemolytic anaemia (Newton & Bass, 1958), and that various illnesses may shorten the survival of these cells in the absence of any drug administration. Nevertheless the great importance of G-6-PD deficiency is that it renders such individuals susceptible to the action of a variety of haemolytic agents.

The locus for the enzyme G-6-PD is on the X-chromosome, i.e. it is a sex-linked characteristic and is transmitted by females to half their male offspring (Browne, 1957). Although most of the mothers show loss of G-6-PD deficiency of a less severe grade than do the patients, some females have normal levels of G-6-PD, and others levels as low as their affected male offspring. The explanation for this lies in the hypothesis put forward by Lyon (1961) which postulated that when two X-chromosomes are present in a cell one is inactivated and this inactivation can affect either the maternally derived or paternally derived chromosome in a random fashion. Thus the normal female, in fact, contains a mosaic of cells. In relation to G-6-PD the chromosome transmitting the defect may be suppressed in some erythroblasts but not in others. There is therefore a variable expression of the amount G-6-PD activity. The correctness of this hypothesis was demonstrated in relation to this enzyme by separation of the two types of red cells in heterozygous females (Sansone, Rasore-Quartino & Veneziano, 1963; Beutler & Baluda, 1964; Tönz & Rossi, 1964).

G-6-PD deficiency is the commonest of the enzyme defects affecting red cells. It has been estimated to affect more than 100 million people and to account for about 30% of cases of congeni-

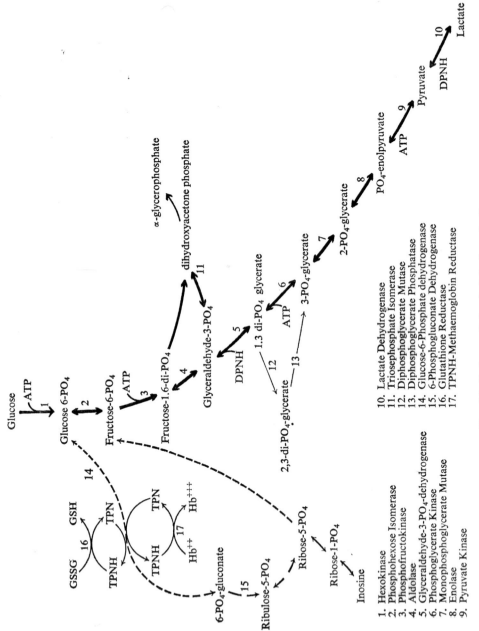

Fig. 6.2. Pathway of glycolysis in the red cell.

1. Hexokinase
2. Phosphohexose Isomerase
3. Phosphofructokinase
4. Aldolase
5. Glyceraldehyde-3-PO$_4$-dehydrogenase
6. Phosphoglycerate Kinase
7. Monophosphoglycerate Mutase
8. Enolase
9. Pyruvate Kinase
10. Lactate Dehydrogenase
11. Triosephosphate Isomerase
12. Diphosphoglycerate Mutase
13. Diphosphoglycerate Phosphatase
14. Glucose-6-Phosphate dehydrogenase
15. 6-Phosphogluconate Dehydrogenase
16. Glutathione Reductase
17. TPNH-Methaemoglobin Reductase

tal nonspherocytic haemolytic anaemia (Carson & Frischer, 1966). The deficiency was first detected in American negroes (Carson, Flanagan, Ickes & Alving, 1956) and has been found since in many parts of Africa, the Mediterranean countries, India, China and the Middle East. It has been suggested that G-6-PD deficiency, like the sickle cell trait, confers resistance to *Plasmodium falciparum* infestation.

Electrophoretic studies have indicated that there are a variety of genetically determined types of G-6-PD, and at least 22 types are listed by Carson & Frischer (1966).

Clinical presentation. Acute haemolytic episodes following ingestion of fava beans have been known to occur for centuries in the Mediterranean area and near East. The relationship of favism to G-6-PD deficiency only became apparent following studies with the anti-malarial drug primaquine in American soldiers. In a proportion of negro soldiers an acute haemolytic episode ensued. In the first two days after administration Heinz bodies were seen in the red cells, and thereafter the haemoglobin level declined reaching less than half its initial value in a severe case. A mild attack could pass unnoticed but a severe one was associated with pain, jaundice and a dark urine due to haemoglobinuria. Thereafter recovery with a reticulocytosis took place and recovery was not hindered by continued administration of the drug (Fig. 6.3).

In clinical practice the drugs which have been implicated in such attacks are shown in Table 6.1 taken from Beutler (1965).

Recovery from a haemolytic episode despite continued drug administration appears to be due to the fact that young red cells are relatively resistant to drug-induced haemolysis and that the older cells are preferentially destroyed (Beutler, Dern & Alving, 1954).

The biochemical sequence. When one of the drugs in Table 6.1 is given to G-6-PD-deficient subjects the following events occur: There is a disappearance of GSH from the red cells and a transitory increase in GSSG, methaemoglobin is formed followed by its denaturation to insoluble precipitates (Heinz bodies) which show up when stained in the wet with 0·5% methyl violet. All these events follow the failure of supply of TPNH almost all of which is provided by the hexose monophosphate pathway and which fails to function because aerobic glycolysis cannot be taken further than glucose-6-phosphate because of lack of G-6-PD.

The effects obtained depend on the dose of the drug, a larger dose being required to produce haemolysis in a female heterozygote with an intermediate degree of G-6-PD deficiency than is the case in a male. The effects also depend on the state of health of the individual and intercurrent illness greatly increases the susceptibility to drugs.

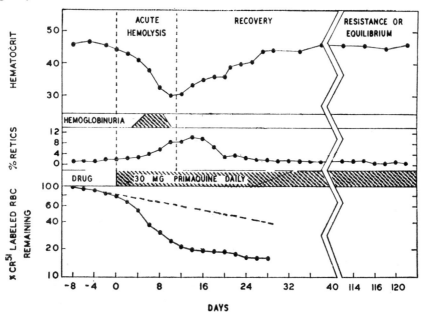

Fig. 6.3. The events of a drug-induced haemolytic episode in G-6-PD deficiency (from Carson & Frischer, 1966).

TABLE 6.1

Compounds known to have induced haemolysis of
G-6-PD-deficient red cells

(Beutler, 1965)

Analgesics
    Acetanilid
    Acetylsalicylic acid
    Acetophenetidin (phenacetin)
    Antipyrine
    Pyramidone

Sulphonamides and Sulphones
    Sulphanilamide
    Sulphapyridine
    N-Acetylsulphanilamide
    Sulphacetamide
    Sulphisoxazole (Gantrisin)
    Thiazolsulphone
    Salicylazosulphapyridine (Azulphadine)
    Sulphoxone
    Sulphamethoxypyridazine (Kynex)

Antimalarials
    Primaquine
    Pamaquine
    Pentaquine
    Quinacrine

Nonsulphonamide Antibacterial Agents
    Furazolidone
    Nitrofurantoin (Furadantin)
    Chloramphenicol
    Para-aminosalicylic acid

Miscellaneous
    Naphthalene
    Vitamin K (Water soluble analogues)
    Probenecid
    Trinitrotoluene
    Methylene blue
    Dimercaprol (BAL)
    Phenylhydrazine
    Quinine
    Quinidine

Diagnosis

(1) *Assay of G-6-PD*. A number of satisfactory assay procedures have been devised which depend on absorbency at 340 mμ due to reduction of TPN (Kornberg & Horecker, 1955). These provide a quantitative assay for G-6-PD.

(2) *Dye-linked techniques*. Methods which depend on decolorization of dyes such as methylene blue or brilliant cresyl blue have been widely used both as screening procedures and for large scale population studies (Bernstein, 1963; Tönz & Bethke, 1962).

(3) *Glutathione stability test*. Incubation of G-6-PD deficient blood with acetylphenylhydrazine causes a rapid decrease in the level of glutathione which can be measured (Beutler, 1957).

(4) *Methaemoglobin-reduction*. The reduction of methaemoglobin formed by the treatment of red cells with nitrite has also been used as a screening test for the deficiency (Brewer, Tarlov & Alving 1960).

Methaemoglobinaemia

About 1% of erythrocyte haemoglobin is in the form of methaemoglobin and as such cannot take part in oxygen transport. Methaemoglobin is constantly being formed, possibly at a rate of 3% of the total haemoglobin each day (Jaffe, 1966), and constantly being reduced to active haemoglobin. Accumulation of methaemoglobin can result from exposure to substances which increase the rate of oxidation or from an inability to reduce methaemoglobin formed at the usual rate. Systems in the red cell which remove potential oxidants are glutathione peroxidase and catalase, as well as ascorbic acid, glutathione and other sulphydryl compounds.

There are two forms of familial methaemoglobinaemia. One is transmitted by an autosomal recessive gene and affected patients are homozygotes. Their erythrocytes are markedly deficient in DPNH-methaemoglobin reductase activity (DPNH dehydrogenase). Intermediate levels of activity can be demonstrated in heterozygotes although there is no accumulation of methaemoglobin in these. The enzyme, DPNH-methaemoglobin reductase, has been isolated from normal red cells (Scott & McGraw, 1962). Subjects with hereditary methaemoglobinaemia have about 10% of normal activity of this enzyme.

Methylene blue given *in vivo* or in *in vitro* experiments is also able to convert haemoglobin iron from the ferric form to the ferrous form. Reduction of methaemoglobin in the presence of a dye requires TPNH regenerated in the hexose monophosphate pathway and an enzyme, TPNH methaemoglobin reductase, has been isolated from erythrocytes (Huennekens, Caffrey, Basford & Gabrio, 1957). In the absence of methylene blue this pathway operates slowly, and presumably the methaemoglobinaemia is due to deficiency of DPNH methaemoglobin reductase.

Reduced glutathione is also capable of a relatively slow reduction of methaemoglobin and it has been suggested that it is responsible for conversion of about 12 to 13% of methaemoglobin (Scott, Duncan & Ekstrand, 1965).

Seventy-one patients from 44 families with hereditary methaemoglobinaemia have been studied and shown to be deficient in DPNH-methaemoglobin reductase activity (Jaffe, 1966), and the total number of reported cases is about 250. The characteristic clinical picture is of a persistent state of grey cyanosis often present from birth without evidence of cardiac or pulmonary disease. The haemoglobin shows a characteristic absorption band at 632 mμ. Symptoms are few as concentrations of up to 25% methaemoglobin are well tolerated. Although these patients may have 20 to 50% methaemoglobin there is often a compensatory increase in the red cell count. Red cell survival is normal.

The other form of hereditary methaemoglobinaemia is associated with the presence of an abnormal haemoglobin involving amino acid substitutions in the globin portion. These haemoglobins, collectively termed haemoglobins M, have the amino acid substitution in the vicinity of the haem (See Fig. 6.4). This results in a functional anomaly wherein there is a reaction between the Fe^{++} of haemoglobin and an ionized side group of the new amino acid. Inheritance is via an autosomal dominant gene and heterozygotes are affected. The different varieties have been termed HbM Boston, HbM Milwaukee, HbM Saskatoon, HbM Iwate, HbM Hyde Park, etc. The proportion of abnormal haemoglobin is usually about 40% and apart from some cyanosis the patients are clinically well. HbM can be demonstrated on starch-gel electrophoresis.

HAEMOGLOBIN DEFECTS

Congenital Haemolytic Anaemia with Porphyria

This is a rare disorder appearing in early life wherein there is a defect in the biosynthesis of the haem portion of haemoglobin. Clinically there is skin photosensitivity which in time results in scarring of face and hands and red fluorescence of teeth under ultraviolet light. There is pigmentation of teeth and bones and splenomegaly. A haemolytic anaemia is present of varying severity. There is a large amount of porphyrin in the erythroblasts in the marrow and many normoblast nuclei fluoresce. The defect in haem synthesis is confined to the marrow. The urine contains large amounts of uroporphyrin I. Urinary protoporphyrin is not increased and excretion of delta-aminolaevulinic acid and porphobilinogen is normal. It has been suggested that there is a defect in the enzyme converting porphobilinogen to uroporphyrinogen.

Some patients are somewhat improved by splenectomy.

The Haemoglobinopathies

Haemoglobin consist of four polypeptide chains to each of which is attached an iron-containing haem portion. These chains interlock to form an ellipsoid with a M.W. of about 67,000. There are four different polypeptide chains in human haemoglobin and a fifth is found in young embryos. The four chains are called alpha, beta, gamma and delta.

There are three haemoglobins present in normal post-natal life. Haemoglobin A or adult haemoglobin constitutes about 97% of the total haemoglobin, haemoglobin A_2 is about 2·5% and foetal haemoglobin (haemoglobin F) is less than 1%. These haemoglobins differ in the composition of the polypeptide chains.

$$Hb\ A\ = \alpha_2\beta_2$$
$$Hb\ A_2 = \alpha_2\delta_2$$
$$Hb\ F\ = \alpha_2\gamma_2$$

All have a pair of alpha chains. Hb A has a pair of beta chains, Hb A_2 a pair of delta chains and Hb F a pair of gamma chains. Generally the production of alpha chains balances the combined production of other chains. The majority of abnormal haemoglobins involve an amino acid substitution in the beta chain. The alpha chains are affected in a form of thalassaemia termed alpha-thalassaemia where the rate of production is depressed. Depression of alpha chain synthesis results in the formation of abnormal tetramers, i.e. haemoglobins which contain four of the same polypeptide such as four β-chains (β_4 or Hb H) or four γ-chains (γ_4 or Hb Barts).

$$Hb\ H\ \ \ = \beta_4$$
$$Hb\ Barts = \gamma_4$$

Foetal haemoglobin is the principal haemoglobin in foetal blood. Its proportion decreases after about the fourteenth week and the proportion of Hb A increases. At birth Hb F is present in 70 to 80% concentration, and thereafter declines rapidly to reach adult levels after 5 to 6 months.

The formation of each polypeptide chain is genetically determined and transmitted as autosomal dominant characteristics. Each alpha chain contains 141 amino acid residues and each beta chain 146 (Fig. 6.4). There is a characteristic sequence of polar amino acids such as lysine and glutamic acid, dipolar such as tyrosine and glutamine, and nonpolar such as valine and leucine, so that when the chain is coiled the charged side groups are orientated towards the surface. Substitution of a single amino acid in the polypeptide chain can alter the surface charge of the haemoglobin molecule and thus lead to variation in electrophoretic mobility, an aspect utilized in the identification of the different haemoglobin types. To become a slow moving haemoglobin (Hb C, E or O) a negatively charged amino acid is replaced

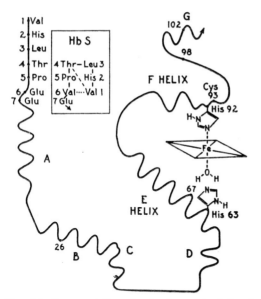

FIG. 6.4. Representation of a β-polypeptide chain of haemoglobin and the substitution in the globin chain in Hb S (from Heller, 1966).

by a positively charged one, for example, aspartic acid or glutamic acid is replaced by lysine or arginine. The opposite holds in a mutation resulting in a fast moving haemoglobin such as Hb I or Hb N.

Diagnostic methods

Blood picture. Generally the homozygous forms of the haemoglobin disorders are associated with a haemolytic anaemia which may be relatively mild, i.e. well compensated, but sometimes may be severe. Target cell formation in blood films is common and homozygous sickle cell disease is associated with sickle forms in the peripheral blood. When anaemia is severe as in homozygous form of thalassaemia the peripheral blood film may be bizarre in appearance. The blood picture is also modified by loss of splenic function either due to thrombosis of vessels and atrophy as in patients with sickle-cell disease, or surgically as is often the case in thalassaemia. This results in many normoblasts appearing in the blood and Howell-Jolly bodies which are nuclear remnants in the erythrocytes. In beta-thalassaemia the heterozygotes show target cell formation but heterozygotes in the case of other haemoglobinopathies appear haematologically normal.

Foetal haemoglobin. In general, investigations for an abnormal haemoglobin should be post-

poned until an infant is older than 6 months. The majority of haemoglobinopathies are mutations involving the β-chain. Only 20 to 30% of haemoglobin in the newborn is Hb A, i.e. containing β-chains and the rest is foetal haemoglobin ($a_2\gamma_2$). For this reason results may not be decisive until the proportion of adult haemoglobin has increased. In general foetal haemoglobin is more resistant to denaturation by extremes of pH. Thus red cells containing significant amounts of foetal haemoglobin can be recognized if adult haemoglobin is eluted from cells in a blood film by exposing them to a pH 3·2 buffer. Thereafter the slides are washed and counterstained with eosin or safranin. The remaining cells containing large amounts of foetal haemoglobin stain pink. This method is useful in studying admixtures of adult and foetal cells as in late pregnancy and after delivery.

Small quantities of foetal haemoglobin may be detected by the alkali denaturation method. Here the haemoglobin solution is exposed to sodium hydroxide for either one or two minutes and the reaction stopped by adding a saturated solution of ammonium sulphate. Details of this and other procedures are described by Lehmann & Huntsman (1966).

Sickle cells. Under low oxygen tension the solubility of sickle cell haemoglobin (Hb S) falls to 50 times less than that of normal Hb A and the Hb S molecules become crystalline. These crystalline structures align themselves to form long tactoids so that the red cell becomes distorted into a sickle shape. To test for this a small drop of blood is added to a large drop of freshly prepared 2% sodium metabisulphite solution on a slide. A cover slip is put on and the preparation examined after half and after one hour. In the trait (heterozygous condition) the red cell presents as a holly leaf shape (this must be distinguished from crenation) and in the homozygous state as long sickles.

Unstable haemoglobins (Hb H). A wet film examined under a cover slip after incubation with 0·5% brilliant cresyl blue as in a reticulocyte preparation will show up these fine inclusion bodies in the red cell. Indeed they may be spotted in the white cell counting chamber in doing a white cell count. Heinz bodies are also shown up by this method.

Electrophoresis. Excellent separation of the majority of abnormal haemoglobins as well as of Hb A_2 is achieved by electrophoresis using paper, cellulose acetate or starch, and elution of the haemoglobin permits quantitation of the proportion of different haemoglobins present. Excellent accounts of technique are available in a number of publications including that of Lehmann & Huntsman (1966).

Fingerprinting. The globin moiety of haemoglobin may be hydrolysed to peptides by trypsin and then subjected to 2-dimensional electrophoresis and chromatography. Any variation from the normal pattern can be determined and thus an amino acid substitution can be localized to a particular peptide.

Sickle-cell disease

Haemoglobin S has a wide distribution across tropical Africa as far south as the Zambesi River. It is also found along the Mediterranean coast of North Africa, Sicily, South Italy, Greece, Middle East, Arabian peninsula and India.

Heterozygotes, i.e. those with the sickle-cell trait (Hb AS), do not suffer from anaemia, their blood appears normal and the mean red cell life span is normal. Their red cells sickle under reduced oxygen tension and under special conditions producing anoxia. Thus rarely haematuria may be encountered, and symptoms may arise if the patients get severe pulmonary infection, under anaesthesia and in unpressurized aircraft.

The homozygotes, i.e. patients with sickle cell disease (Hb SS), tend to be tall. Leg ulceration is frequent. There may be slight jaundice and the liver may be enlarged. The spleen is generally not felt in adults and is often atrophic. The course of the disease is interrupted by "crises". These may be (1) Haemolytic in origin, i.e. there is increased red cell destruction usually associated with stasis in an infarcted area.

(2) Painful crises associated with infarcts. These are due to blocking of small vessels by sickle cells. In young children painful dactylitis occurs. Infarcts in the lung may present as acute chest pain and acute abdominal pain may simulate an acute abdominal catastrophe. Priapism and temporary or permanent blindness may occur.

(3) Megaloblastic crisis. Here there is aggravation of anaemia and the marrow shows severe megaloblastic haemopoiesis. This is invariably due to folate deficiency and responds specifically to folate therapy.

(4) Aplastic crisis. Less frequently developing anaemia may be the result of a temporary failure of haemopoiesis similar in type to that described in relation to hereditary spherocytosis. Pregnancy may carry considerable risk in these patients. Megaloblastic anaemia is frequent, and an aplastic crisis may be a fatal complication.

Anaemia is always present and the haemoglobin concentration varies from 5 to 10 g./100 ml. The blood film shows target cells and some partially sickled cells. The picture may be modified by splenic atrophy. The reticulocytes are raised and may vary from 10 to 40%. In a crisis there may be a leucocytosis of up to 30,000 cells/mm^3.

Diagnosis is made by demonstrating the presence of sickling, and electrophoresis will demonstrate that almost all the haemoglobin is Hb S with a small amount of Hb F.

The abnormality in the beta polypeptide chain consists of a replacement of a glutamic-acid residue by valine at the sixth position (Fig. 6.4). Hb S, and indeed all abnormal haemoglobins, seems to be made less efficiently and at a slower rate than Hb A. Thus the proportion of Hb S in patients with the trait is generally less than 45% and when folate deficiency supervenes with megaloblastic haemopoiesis the synthesis of Hb S may be almost completely suppressed (Heller, Yakulis, Epstein & Friedland, 1963). While megaloblastic the patient's red cells may fail to show adequate sickling, and electrophoresis may show only trace amounts of Hb S.

The extent to which the red cells in sickle-cell disease assume a sickle form in the circulation depends on the diminution of oxygen saturation in various organs. Deoxygenated sickle forms are thought to be incapable of passing through capillaries (Jandl, Simmons & Castle, 1961) and are probably removed by macrophages in spleen and liver.

Haemoglobin C, D and E disease

Homozygosity for these haemoglobins produces a relatively mild haemolytic anaemia with marked target cell formation in peripheral blood films. Haemoglobin C is found predominantly in West Africa, D in parts of India and E in Burma and other parts of the East. In the β polypeptide chains of Hb C the glutamic acid residue in position 6 is replaced by lysine, in Hb D amino acid 121 (normally glutamic acid) is replaced by glutamine and in Hb E the amino acid in position 26 (normally glutamic acid) is replaced by lysine.

Sickle-cell haemoglobin C disease

This is a common combination in West Africa. The anaemia is less severe than that found in SS disease although pregnancy may still prove a severe hazard due to megaloblastic anaemia and folate deficiency. These patients are also liable to infarcts. The retina may be involved and a characteristic syndrome is necrosis of the head of the humerus with painful abduction of the arm.

Sickle-cell thalassaemia

The diagnosis of sickle-cell thalassaemia depends on demonstrating a small amount of Hb A as one of the haemoglobin components. This is technically difficult. Clinically the disease is milder than SS disease.

The unstable haemoglobins

These patients have a haemolytic anaemia present from childhood and associated with an enlarged spleen, jaundice and dark urine. It is familial. Blood films show a small number of irregularly crenated red cells in some cases, and if the patient has undergone a splenectomy then the majority of red cells can be shown to have prominent Heinz bodies. In non-splenectomized patients Heinz bodies can be demonstrated by incubating a sterile blood sample at $37°C$ for 48 hours. Further, heating a haemolysate at $50°C$ for one hour causes a precipitate to form (heat stability test). Finally some cases are associated with a tendency to form methaemoglobin and a sensitivity to drugs, particularly sulphonamides. Hb Chesapeake is associated with polycythaemia since there is a failure to release oxygen from the haem.

These haemoglobins have been called Hb Zürich, Hb Köln, Hb St. Mary, Hb Seattle and a similar group of patients have been termed congenital Heinz body anaemia by Grimes, Meisler & Dacie (1964). In some the nature of the amino-acid substitution is known; in others the abnormality lies in the trypsin-resistant core of the chain and is therefore less accessible to analysis. In some cases an amino-acid deletion may be present (Hb Freiburg).

Electrophoresis shows an abnormal fraction comprising 10 to 14% of the haemoglobin migrating rather more slowly than Hb S. Nevertheless the proportion of abnormal haemoglobin may initially approximate to the amount generally present in heterozygotes, i.e. to just under half the total haemoglobin, and a considerable proportion of this is lost by precipitation and removal from the cell in the spleen.

The urinary pigment in these patients belongs to the group of bilifuscins. The presence of this dipyrrolic compound suggests that free haem is so rapidly released from the abnormal haemoglobin that not all is metabolized to bilirubin, and some follows other breakdown pathways. The abnormal release of haem has suggested that in these unstable haemoglobins the abnormality in the polypeptide chains lies in or near the helix in which haem is held. Haem is attached to histidyl residues at position 63 and 92 (Fig. 6.4). Hb

Zürich involves substitution of arginine in position 63, and Hb Köln a substitution of methionine at 98.

Haemoglobin associated with methaemoglobinaemia

These haemoglobinopathies are characterized by mutants which result in an accumulation of methaemoglobin. The patients are heterozygotes and the amino acid substitution has been determined in five of these mutants. Once again the substitution is in the vicinity of the haem and either the alpha or beta chain can be affected.

Haemoglobin	Designation of substitution
Hb M$_{Milwaukee}$	$\alpha_2\beta_2^{67\ Glu}$
Hb M$_{Boston}$	$\alpha_2^{58\ Tyr}\beta_2$
Hb M$_{Saskatoon}$ (Hb M$_{Chicago}$)	$\alpha_2\beta_2^{63\ Tyr}$
Hb M$_{Iwate}$ (Hb M$_{Kankakee}$)	$\alpha_2^{87\ Tyr}\beta_2$
Hb M$_{Hyde\ Park}$	$\alpha_2\beta_2^{92\ Tyr}$

Generally methaemoglobinaemia due to Hb M is not affected by methylene blue as the conversion to the ferric form is irreversible. The commonest form has so far proved to be Hb M$_{Boston}$.

Affected subjects are cyanotic but otherwise asymptomatic. The proportion of abnormal haemoglobin is generally about 40%.

Electrophoretic separation of Hb M from Hb A is best achieved if the entire sample is converted to methaemoglobin and separation on starch gel at pH 7·1 is used.

Thalassaemia

Unlike the other haemoglobinopathies no abnormalities of the polypeptide chains of the globin moiety have been detected in thalassaemia. Rather, current hypothesis favours the view that there is a failure to produce normal polypeptide chains in adequate amount.

Thalassaemia is the commonest abnormality of haemoglobin production with a high frequency in all the countries bordering the Mediterranean, and occurs in the Middle East, Arabia, India, China, Indonesia, the Philippines and New Guinea.

Thalassaemia is transmitted as an autosomal dominant characteristic. The clinical picture in the homozygote is of severe anaemia in infancy requiring repeated transfusion and proceeding to massive splenomegaly and iron-overload. Marrow hypertrophy causes bone changes, mongoloid facies, separation and thinning of the tables of the skull on X-ray with a "hair on end" appearance.

The haemoglobin level is between 3 to 7 g./100 ml. Reticulocytes are however only moderately elevated, often in the region of 10% and rarely exceed 15%, indicating a failure to produce enough red cells in response to anaemia.

The failure to make haemoglobin results in the production of red cells with a considerably reduced haemoglobin content. Thus these cells are "hypochromic" and the MCHC is low. In addition to severe hypochromia (but not iron deficiency) there are often many red cell fragments and normoblasts in the peripheral blood. The normoblast count can become very high after splenectomy.

Whereas the picture in the homozygote is uniformly severe, heterozygotes show a remarkable variation in the severity of the blood changes. Some patients show some target cell formation in blood films and virtually no other abnormality; others have moderate anaemia, splenomegaly, relatively high red cell counts, with some reduction of haemoglobin concentration; and others may have more severe degrees of anaemia.

It is of considerable importance to distinguish thalassaemia from iron-deficiency anaemia since simple blood examination will fail to differentiate the two. Often it is only when a course of iron therapy fails to produce a rise in haemoglobin that the possibility of thalassaemia comes to the fore. The serum iron and transferrin level is normal in thalassaemia, and marrow examination shows adequate iron stores when appropriate staining methods are used. However thalassaemia trait and iron-deficiency anaemia can co-exist.

Beta-thalassaemia major. This is the manifestation of the disease in homozygotes. There is a depression of beta-chain formation and hence of Hb A ($a_2\beta_2$). There is however no impediment to making Hb A$_2$ ($a_2\delta_2$) and Hb F ($a_2\gamma_2$). There is a marked elevation of the proportion of foetal haemoglobin which may comprise between 15 to 90% of the total. There may be some elevation of Hb A$_2$ and the rest is Hb A which comprises 20 to 80% of the total. Family studies will show that both parents are heterozygotes. The polyribosomes obtained from the erythroid cells of β-thalassaemic subjects have been shown to produce significantly fewer polypeptide chains than do the polyribosomes obtained from a series of control subjects. Thalassaemic ribosomes also incorporated considerably less labelled amino acids into

soluble haemoglobin than did preparations from patients with other haemoglobinopathies. Further, in β-thalassaemia the defect in the ribosome applies only to the synthesis of β-chains. Gamma chains were produced normally as judged by the capacity of the ribosomes to incorporate isoleucine into Hb F. This amino acid is absent from β-chains. The rate of Hb A synthesis per polyribosome in β-thalassaemia averaged about 10% of that found with ribosomes in control preparations (Burka & Marks, 1963; Marks & Burka, 1964). Bank & Marks (1966) suggested that the defect lay in some alteration in the messenger RNA and that the ribosomes themselves were capable of normal response to added synthetic messenger RNA.

Beta-thalassaemia minor. The diagnosis can be suspected from the blood picture and confirmation is sought by demonstrating an elevated level of Hb A$_2$ on starch gel electrophoresis. In these cases the range is between 2 to 5%. More than half the cases also have a raised level of foetal haemoglobin

Alpha-thalassaemia. The homozygous state is not compatible with life. Here one assumes that there is almost total suppression of a-chain formation, and thus the only chains that can be formed in any quantity are the tetramers such as Hb Barts (γ_4). If β-chain formation has commenced Hb H (β_4) will be present. This has been found in some still-born foetuses.

The heterozygous state for alpha-thalassaemia is so well compensated that the diagnosis may be impossible to make. Children in whom Hb Barts was known to be present in infancy, in later life show little abnormality other than some tendency to microcytosis. Hb Barts usually disappears 3 to 4 months after birth. On occasion the absence of an elevated Hb A$_2$ level in a patient suspected of having thalassaemia trait may lead to a suspicion that the patient has a-thalassaemia.

Haemoglobin H disease. Clinically these patients may have anaemia resembling an iron-deficiency anaemia and in these respects are similar to more severely affected patients with β-thalassaemia. The reticulocyte count is raised. Occasionally Hb H may appear in patients with acute leukaemia. Hb H denatures readily in the red cell and gives rise to Heinz bodies. On electrophoresis Hb H is easily recognized as it moves further than Hb A, i.e. it is one of the fast moving haemoglobins.

Other haemoglobinopathies

Persistance of foetal haemoglobin. The decline of gamma chain formation in the foetus and its replacement by β-chain formation is accompanied by a replacement of foetal haemoglobin

$(a_2\gamma_2)$ by Hb A $(a_2\beta_2)$. This change-over fails to occur in a benign disorder termed "Hereditary persistance of foetal haemoglobin". These patients are perfectly well and the blood picture is normal. However the heterozygotes have 15 to 20% foetal haemoglobin and homozygotes have all Hb F and no Hb A or Hb A_2.

Admixtures of abnormal haemoglobins

The diagnostic problem is often complicated because of combination of various abnormalities. Common combinations involve thalassaemia with haemoglobin S, C, D and E. Thus in sickle-cell-thalassaemia the predominant haemoglobin is Hb S. This is because the formation of structurally normal β-chain is depressed by the thalassaemia trait and there is overproduction of the β-chain bearing the substitution characteristic of Hb S. SC disease has been mentioned. The high F gene has been associated with both thalassaemia and Hb C and the blood picture in these is characterized by marked target cell formation.

THE AUTOIMMUNE HAEMOLYTIC ANAEMIAS

In this group of haemolytic anaemias the normal survival of the erythrocytes in the circulation is impaired by immunoglobulins on the red cell surface which bring about the rapid removal of these cells from the circulation. Dacie (1962) in an analysis of 175 cases seen over a period of 14 years grouped them as follows:

"*Idiopathic*" autiommune	108
"*Secondary*" autiommune	
Neoplastic—"Lymphomata"	20
Others	5
Virus pneumonia	11
Glandular fever	1
Other disorders	11
Disseminated lupus	6
Rheumatoid arthritis	3
Ulcerative colitis	2
Paroxysmal cold haemoglobinuria	8

In all, an antibody could be demonstrated either on the red cells by the direct antiglobulin test or in some cases in the serum particularly in those cases associated with "cold agglutinins".

There has been considerable interest in the mechanism whereby an immune reaction on the red cell surface leads to removal of the red cell from the circulation. Antibodies which bind complement are generally haemolytic. When a red cell has reacted with a specific antibody and is thereafter exposed to complement a hole with a clear rim is produced in the red cell membrane.

With human complement the average size of the hole on electron microscopy is 103 Å. The hole is similar with IgM and IgG immunoglobulins but varies with the source of complement (Rosse, Dourmashkin & Humphrey, 1966). This damage to the red cell membrane is followed by lysis. There is evidence that one completed complement sequence on the cell surface (i.e. C'1, C'4, C'2 and finally C'3 attached to the red cell-antibody complex) is sufficient to produce one hole and hence haemolysis (Mayer, 1961). Borsos, Dourmashkin & Humphrey (1964) suggested that C'2 was the limiting factor and that one hole in the red cell membrane resulted from each molecule of C'2 attached.

The other method by which red cells sensitized by antibody are removed from the circulation is by sequestration by the reticulo-endothelial system. The major sites of sequestration are the liver and spleen. Generally red cells damaged by agglutinating or complement-fixing antibodies are removed by the liver as are cells damaged by large doses of methaemoglobin-producing drugs or by prolonged heating (Mollison, 1962). Such injured cells may be removed from the circulation by a single passage through the organ, and since the liver receives a much greater volume of blood than the spleen it takes a greater part in the removal of such cells. Red cells coated with incomplete antibodies which do not fix complement are preferentially cleared from the circulation by the spleen. The amount of antibody on the red cell surface also influences the rate and site of sequestration. Red cells heavily coated with antibodies may be cleared by the liver and spleen. Mildly sensitized cells are cleared more slowly by the spleen (Crome & Mollison, 1964). Red cells sequestered in this manner are then thought to undergo erythrophagocytosis, and release of haemoglobin may result in haemoglobinaemia and disappearance of haptoglobins (Jandl, Richardson-Jones & Castle, 1957).

On the basis of the hypothesis put forward by Burnet (1959) the abnormal antibodies in autoimmune haemolytic anaemia arise from aberrations in the antibody-forming tissue, i.e. somatic mutation leads to the development of a clone of such antibody-forming cells. These antibodies are of two types: (1) *Warm antibodies*, generally incomplete and detected by the antiglobulin reaction, react best at 37°C. The red cells in some patients are agglutinated by an anti-γ-globulin serum; in others the red cells react with an anti-non-γ-globulin serum, i.e. the latter reaction is with complement on the red cell surface (2) *Cold antibodies*, which produce haemolysis, generally have both a high thermal amplitude, i.e. may be active at even 30°C, and are powerful agglutinins. About a third of the antibodies of warm type have some specificity within the Rh system, i.e on elution they may behave like anti-e, anti-c or anti-E, but generally non-specific activity is also present. Clinically patients may be very ill and jaundiced. Those with high titre cold agglutinins tend to show a Raynaud's phenomenon. Anaemia may be severe with reticulocytosis and the changes in red cell morphology depend on the severity of the process. There may be spherocytosis, auto-agglutination of red cells and in some cases marked poikilocytosis.

Treatment is with steroids, often in high dosage in the first instance. Transfusion should be avoided if possible as it is not feasible to attempt to maintain an adequate haemoglobin level by this means. Labelling the patient's own cells with ^{51}Cr and studying their rate of splenic sequestration by surface counting may be helpful in deciding whether splenectomy may help in cases not responding to steroids. Imuran has proved of some value in resistant patients (Hitzig & Massimo, 1966).

IRON DEFICIENCY

Many aspects of the physiology of iron in man are discussed in Chapter 7 by Charlton and Bothwell. Here the development, diagnosis and the consequences of iron deficiency are considered

Iron deficiency may be defined as a reduction of total body iron below levels which are normal (3 to 5 g.) for a particular subject.

Iron deficiency anaemia occurs when the total body iron becomes insufficient to maintain the normal haemoglobin mass (Conrad & Crosby, 1962) The sequence of changes that ensue in the development of iron deficiency has been studied by performing repeated venesections in volunteers.

The immediate consequence of regular and substantial blood loss is a fall in haemoglobin concentration. Until the iron reserves have been utilized there is an adequate increase in erythropoiesis, the amount of haemoglobin produced daily showing a three- to four-fold increase, and this is accompanied by a modest reticulocytosis which may reach 4% some 10 to 20 days after the commencement of blood loss. This phase is accompanied by an increase in red cell size (MCV) because reticulocytes tend to be larger than mature red cells.

Once iron reserves have been utilized and lack of iron becomes the limiting factor in erythropoiesis the serum iron level falls (normal range for the serum iron level is 60–200 μg./100 ml. with a mean of 125 μg./100 ml. in adult males and 110 μg./100 ml. in adult females). Generally the level does not fall below the normal range until about 500 mg. of iron has been lost and this fall is the earliest evidence of iron deficiency. This is followed by a rise in the transferrin level (normal adult range 300–340 μg./100 ml.). With continuation of blood loss there is a gradual reduction in red cell size which becomes evident some 90 to 120 days after commencement of venesection. Thus microcytosis with a reduced MCV is the first morphological evidence of iron deficiency anaemia. This is a commonplace clinical situation in normal pregnancy where the majority of women lack demonstrable marrow iron and many show microcytosis with moderately reduced haemoglobin levels. A decline in the proportion of haemoglobin in the red cell, i.e. a fall in the mean corpuscular haemoglobin concentration (MCHC) occurs subsequent to the decline in red cell size. Thus initially the haemoglobin concentration in the red cell is preserved at the expense of cell size but subsequently both decline. A reduced MCHC (normal range 32–36%) is a relatively late event in the development of iron deficiency anaemia.

Another early change consequent on depletion of iron stores is an alteration in the gastrointestinal absorption of iron. Normally only about 5–10% of oral iron is absorbed. Within a few days of the appearance of iron deficiency there is a change in the capacity of the gut to take up and retain food iron so that 20–40% of the available iron is absorbed (Hahn, Bale, Ross, Balfour & Whipple, 1943). Moderately iron-deficient red cells have a normal survival in the circulation but severely hypochromic ones (haemoglobin concentration less than 5 g./100 ml.) may only survive some 20–30 days.

Globin and haem are synthesized in the mitochondria of the developing erythroblasts and since iron is also attached to mitochondria, these structures are probably the site of haemoglobin formation. In iron deficiency protoporphyrin accumulates in the erythrocytes where it may be measured. Only in severe iron deficiency is there a failure to maintain iron-containing enzymes and with them epithelial surfaces. Such enzymes are cytochrome *c*, cytochrome oxidase and succinic dehydrogenase. Failure to maintain epithelial surfaces are seen in the characteristically spoon-shaped nails (koilonychia), the smooth sometimes painful tongue with angular stomatitis and in the symptom of dysphagia which may be accompanied by a pharyngeal web demonstrable on Ba swallow.

The relationship between iron deficiency and the gastric epithelium is of particular interest. Diminished HCl production has long been held to be a feature of chronic iron deficiency and atrophic changes on gastric biopsy are present in about three-quarters of patients (Coghill & Williams, 1958). About a quarter of patients with chronic iron deficiency anaemia develop antibodies against gastric parietal cells. There is some evidence that at least in younger subjects acid secretion may return following iron therapy (Jacobs, Lawrie, Entwistle & Campbell, 1966). Long term follow-up of patients with iron deficiency anaemia shows progression to gastric atrophy with pernicious anaemia appearing in some 5% of patients (Beveridge, Bannerman, Evanson & Witts, 1965).

Diagnosis. The diagnosis of iron deficiency in the absence of anaemia depends on the demonstration of diminished iron stores. This is readily accomplished by staining spreads of marrow from the sternum or other sites by Perls' prussian blue method. Particular attention is paid to marrow fragments which under low magnification normally show the blue-green colour of stained haemosiderin in reticulum cells. Their absence denotes diminished iron stores although examination under oil may still disclose iron granules in normoblasts (such cells are termed sideroblasts) or in storage reticulum cells. Marrow fragments as well as other material such as liver obtained by biopsy may be sectioned and stained for iron.

With the decline of iron stores the serum iron falls and is generally below 35 μg./100 ml. The transferrin level is generally between 350–500 μg./100 ml. so that the proportion of the total iron-binding protein carrying iron falls from about one-third to between 2–10%.

With iron-deficiency anaemia the haemoglobin level is reduced but it is difficult to recognize hypochromia with any degree of confidence in a stained peripheral blood film until the haemoglobin concentration falls below about 10·5 g./100 ml. On occasion microcytosis is a more obvious feature. Platelets are frequently abundant since chronic blood loss is a major cause of iron deficiency anaemia.

The MCHC is a reliable guide to established iron deficiency. Although 32% is the lower normal limit, in some laboratories 31% is accepted as normal.

Final proof of diagnosis rests with response to iron therapy although this should never be required as a diagnostic aid.

Ferrokinetics. A transferrin-bound dose of ^{59}Fe given intravenously in iron-deficiency anaemia is cleared from the plasma more rapidly than normal.

Almost all this iron is rapidly incorporated into red cells so that utilization is high. Iron turnover is generally reduced although results of such studies have been variable (Bothwell & Finch 1962).

Causes of iron deficiency. In order of importance a negative iron balance may result from

(a) Loss of iron from the body (blood loss).
(b) Increased requirement for iron (pregnancy).
(c) Inadequate absorption.
(d) Inadequate intake.

It should be only too evident that the cause of iron deficiency may be of greater importance than the anaemia itself, and that the important facet of the investigation of the iron deficiency lies not in establishing the presence of iron deficiency which is simple, but in establishing the cause, which may be a carcinoma of the stomach or caecum or uterus.

Blood loss is the only important route for the loss of significant quantities of iron from the body and the two major sites are the gastro-intestinal tract in both sexes and the uterus in women. Common lesions are nose bleeds, hiatus hernia, oesophageal varices, peptic ulcers, gastric carcinoma or polyps, salicylate erosions of the gastric mucosa, telangiectasia and angiomas of the gut, Meckel's diverticulum, Crohn's disease, ulcerative colitis, carcinoma of colon particularly caecum, and haemorrhoids. Bleeding disorders such as haemophilia may give iron deficiency particularly in children, and blood donors, especially women, are frequently iron-deficient. Hookworm infestation has a world-wide importance.

Menstrual blood loss though notoriously difficult to evaluate is the most significant cause of iron deficiency in women of childbearing age.

In general, blood loss becomes important when it exceeds some 6–8 ml. daily. This is equivalent to 3–4 mg. of iron and is the maximum amount that can be absorbed by iron-deficient subjects. Gastro-intestinal blood loss (and, with considerably more difficulty, menstrual blood loss) can be quantitated by labelling the patients' red cells with [51]Cr. The radioactivity in faeces is counted and by comparison with the radioactivity of whole blood, the blood lost into the gastro-intestinal tract is estimated. These tests in no way supplant the valuable methods which detect "occult blood" in faeces and these remain the standby for the detection of gastro-intestinal blood loss. Because of the notorious irregularity with which gastro-intestinal bleeds occur, it is necessary to be persistent in search for occult blood loss.

Increased iron requirement in pregnancy is due to an expansion of the maternal red cell mass, the provision of iron for the placenta and foetus and the loss of blood at delivery. There is increased requirement for some 450 mg of iron, three-quarters of which is taken up by the foetus and on a daily basis there is a need for 3–4 mg. during the second and third trimester. That this requirement often remains unfulfilled is shown in the study of Magee & Milligan (1951) where it was found that not only was the mean haemoglobin level in 2000 pregnant women less at the end of pregnancy than in the early weeks but that the mean haemoglobin level had still not been regained more than one year later. An increased requirement for iron is possible in polycythaemic patients and iron deficiency is usual in this group.

Inadequate absorption is evidently important in patients with disease of the upper gut such as gluten-sensitive enteropathy and is probably important in achlorhydric patients and after gastrectomy. The difficulties in assessing the absorption of iron are well illustrated by the varying views expressed concerning gastric acid and iron absorption, but recent studies agree that tracer doses are better absorbed when hydrochloric acid is present (Jacobs, Rhodes, Peters, Campbell & Eakins, 1966). There may well be one group of patients in whom the initial event is gastric atrophy with loss of acid and hence impaired iron absorption leading to iron deficiency. These may be the so-called "idiopathic hypochromic anaemia" group in whom repeated tests for occult blood are negative and in whom no other cause for iron deficiency is discernible. The other group may start with iron deficiency due to blood loss, and this in turn may produce atrophic gastritis and loss of acid secretion.

The third group in whom impaired iron absorption appears to be important is the post gastrectomy group. Post-war surgical enthusiasm has been such that some half-million people in the United Kingdom have undergone partial gastrectomies as have some 2–4% of the population of Sweden. After 5 years half the patients after partial gastrectomy have an iron-deficiency anaemia (Baird, Blackburn & Wilson, 1959). There is relatively poor absorption of food iron, and further, with the development of anaemia, the absorption of food iron tends to remain at the relatively low level found in non-anaemic subjects (Stevens, Pirzio Biroli, Harkins, Nyhus & Finch, 1959). The explanation is complex and reduction of acid secretion, by-pass of the duodenum and upper jejunum in the Polya operation, inadequate mixing of food, rapid gastric emptying and intestinal hurry may all contribute to the malabsorption of food iron.

It has been argued that reduction in the dietary intake of iron is never of sufficient importance to be the sole cause of an iron deficiency anaemia (Harris, 1963), and it is true that in practice an inadequate diet is frequently associated with menorrhagia, or a history of frequent pregnancies. It may well be a contributing factor in some patients.

Clinical aspects of iron deficiency anaemia. The onset of signs and symptoms are insidious and are those common to all anaemias. They are pallor, tiredness, weakness, palpitations, dyspnoea, oedema and even angina in severe cases. Nails tend to split easily and occasionally they may be spoon-shaped. The tongue is often smooth and sometimes painful. Occasionally the spleen may be enlarged. The anaemia is far more frequent in women particularly of childbearing age and in young children.

Treatment. Ferrous sulphate tablets containing 200 mg. of the salt and 60 mg. of elemental iron have the dual advantage of being the cheapest and the most efficacious form of therapy. Up to 6 tablets can be taken daily in treatment of iron deficiency, and treatment should be continued at a smaller dose level in an attempt to replenish iron stores.

THE MEGALOBLASTIC ANAEMIAS

These anaemias have in common a disordered mode of blood formation resulting in a reduced number of red cells which are larger than normal, in morphologically altered neutrophil polymorphs, which have an excessive number of lobes in the nucleus, and in diminished platelet formation. Although the most obvious effects of these disorders are upon blood-forming tissues, all dividing cells are affected and this affects most obviously the renewal of epithelial surfaces such as the skin and gastro-intestinal tract.

The biochemical lesion (or lesions) that is responsible for megaloblast formation is not known, but it affects biochemical pathways that come into play during the process of cell division. In its most severe form the cell is unable to replicate and dies *in situ*. In a less severe form a morphologically altered end-product appears, but appropriate treatment is able to alter the process and restore a more normal form of haemopoiesis in less severely affected cells. In the great majority of patients with a megaloblastic anaemia the cause lies in deficiency of folic acid or vitamin B_{12}. An identical anaemia may arise as a result of failure of nucleic acid synthesis in the rare disorder

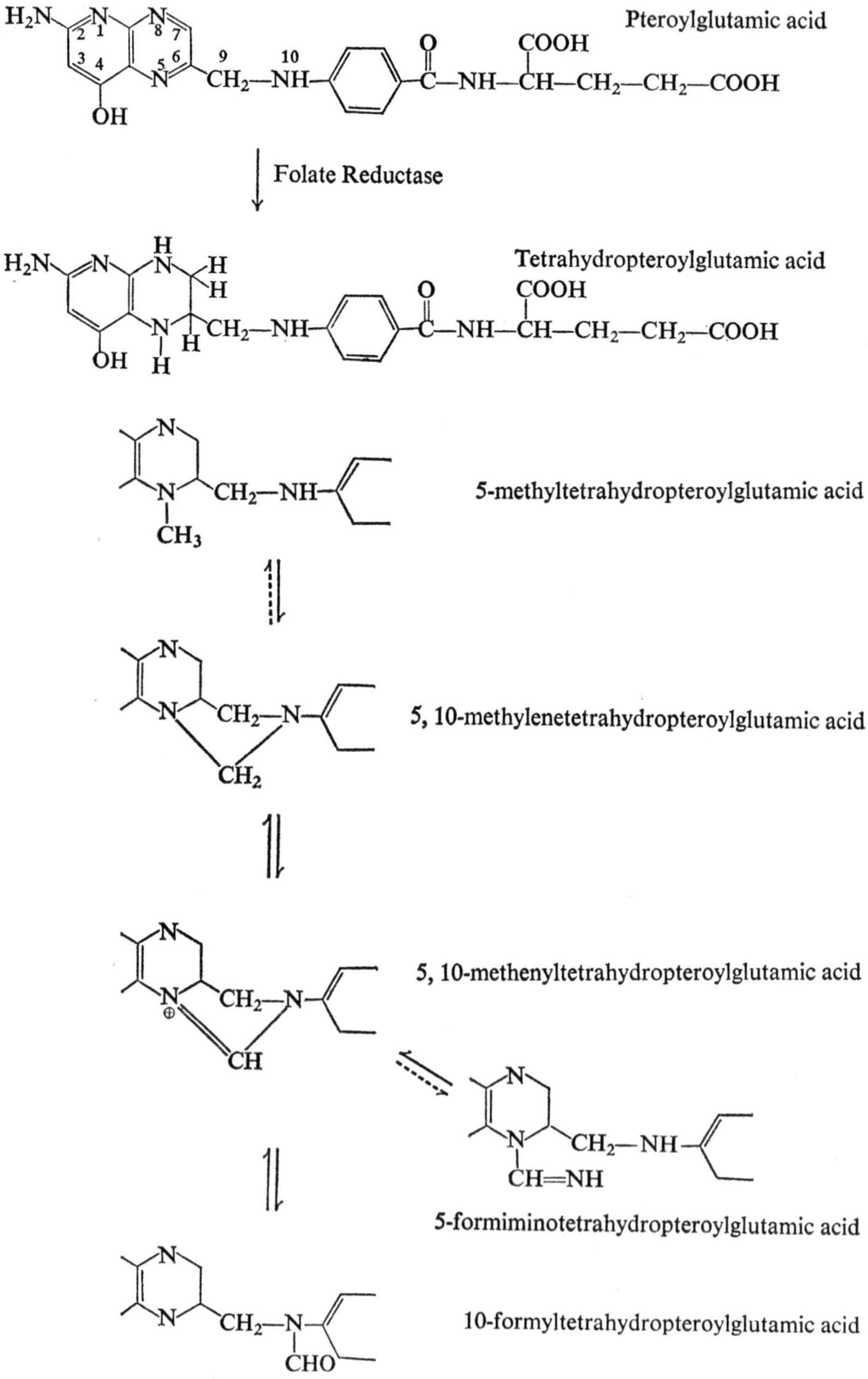

FIG. 6.5. Folic acid and the folate coenzymes.

termed hereditary orotic aciduria. Here there is failure to synthesize one of the basic components of nucleic acid, i.e. pyrimidine, because of an inability to convert orotic acid to uridine-5-phosphate. This severe megaloblastic anaemia does not respond to treatment with either folic acid or vitamin B_{12} but responds to therapy with oral uridine (Smith, Huguley & Bain, 1966). A morphologically identical picture emerges with administration of folate antagonists such as amethopterin, pyrimidine antagonists such as 2,4-diaminopyrimidine (Hamilton, Phillips, Sternberg, Clarke & Hitchings, 1954) and possibly purine antagonists such as 6-mercaptopurine.

Deficiency of vitamin B_{12} may also result in damage to nerve tissues, and since this effect may appear without any changes in the blood it must be presumed to take place through interference with biochemical pathways other than those concerned with cell replication. The nature of these pathways is obscure.

Chemistry of Folic Acid and Vitamin B_{12}
The folates

Pteroylglutamic acid (Fig. 6.5) consists of three portions: (1) a double ring structure called a pteridine or pterin, (2) p-aminobenzoic acid and (3) L-glutamic acid. The moiety composed of the pteridine and p-aminobenzoic acid is called pteroic acid. Organisms which require p-aminobenzoic acid utilize this substance for the biosynthesis of folic acid. Such organisms are sensitive to sulphonamides. Organisms which are resistant to sulphonamides are unable to utilize p-aminobenzoic acid and require a preformed form of folate.

The forms of folate which function as coenzymes are all derivatives of tetrahydropteroylglutamic acid (or tetrahydrofolate). This differs from pteroylglutamic acid in that it has become reduced, i.e. there are additional hydrogens in positions 5, 6, 7 and 8 of the pteridine ring (Fig. 6.5). This reduction is carried out by the enzyme, folate reductase. The usual substrate for this enzyme is a partially reduced form of folate, viz. dihydropteroylglutamic acid, which arises during the course of normal pyrimidine synthesis.

Folate reductase is the specific site of action of folate antagonists such as aminopterin, amethopterin (methotrexate) and dichloroamethopterin. These compounds bind irreversibly to folate reductase and so prevent regeneration of tetrahydrofolate from dihydrofolate. The overall effect is a pile up of dihydrofolate and shortage of tetrahydrofolate which is the form required for coenzyme function.

The development of resistance to folic acid antagonists is due to the development of high levels of folate reductase in the cells (Hakala, Zakrewski & Nichol, 1960). Further, the toxic effects of folate antagonists can be overcome by forms of folate which are already fully reduced. The only stable compound of this type is 5-formyltetrahydrofolate (folinic acid), which has a formyl or —CHO group in the 5 position.

The folate coenzymes function in the synthesis (and breakdown) of purines, pyrimidines, methionine and serine, and less directly in the synthesis of a variety of other important compounds. They do so by the transfer of a carbon unit usually derived from the breakdown of serine which is in turn converted to glycine. The single carbon unit is required at different states of reduction in different reactions. The most reduced form is the methyl form (—CH_3) required for the methylation of homocysteine to methionine. The folate coenzyme here is 5-methyltetrahydrofolate (Fig. 6.5).

5,10-methylenetetrahydrofolate (—CH_2—) is the coenzyme form of folate resulting from the transfer of a single carbon unit from serine. It is concerned with the transfer of a carbon to uridylate to form thymidylate. The enzyme 5,10-methylenetetrahydrofolate reductase converts this form of folate coenzyme to the 5-methyl form, a reaction that is largely irreversible.

5,10-methenyltetrahydrofolate (=CH—) has its single carbon unit in a still less reduced state, and this form is required in the earlier stages of purine synthesis, i.e. in adding a further carbon to glycine to form formylglycine, and so provide carbon 8 of the purine nucleus. This form of the folate coenzyme is formed from 5,10-methylenetetrahydrofolate by the enzyme 5,10-methylenetetrahydrofolate dehydrogenase.

The most oxidized form of carbon unit is formyl (—CHO) which arises from the 5,10-methenyl form via the enzyme 5,10-methenyltetrahydrofolate cyclohydrolase. It can also be formed by direct condensation of formate (HCOOH) with tetrahydrofolate via the enzyme formyltetrahydrofolate synthetase. This form of single carbon unit (—CHO) is required to complete purine synthesis, i.e. it provides carbon 2 of the purine nucleus. With the exception of 5-methylfolate these forms of folate coenzyme are interconvertible. The 5-methyl form is probably the main storage form of folate in the liver and other tissues. Tetrahydrofolate can be regenerated from the 5-methyl form only by the transfer of the methyl group to homocysteine to form methionine. Vitamin B_{12} is required for this reaction probably by acting as the acceptor of the methyl group to form methyl B_{12}.

Tetrahydrofolates are highly unstable, undergoing rapid oxidation under aerobic conditions.

The cobalamins

The cobalamin molecule consists of two major parts (Fig. 6.6) the corrin nucleus which consists of four reduced pyrrol rings (A, B, C and D) linked to a cobalt atom and a nucleotide set at right angles

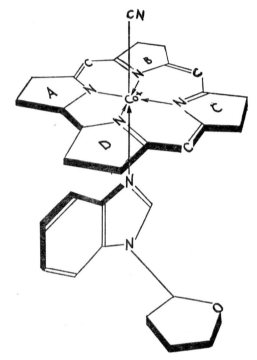

FIG. 6.6. Cobalamin nucleus.

to it. Following the addition of standard side chains to the corrin nucleus it is termed a "cobamide" as in vitamin B_{12}. The nucleotide in vitamin B_{12} contains 5,6-dimethylbenziminazole. It has a pentose sugar attached to it and this sugar is attached by a phosphate and carbon chain to pyrrole ring D of the cobamide nucleus. Four cobalamins are of importance in human physiology and pharmacology. These differ in the nature of the ligand attached to the cobalt atom.

Cyanocobalamin. Here a cyanide group is attached ionically to the cobalt atom. It is a stable compound although prolonged exposure to light results in a replacement of the —CN group by —OH.

Hydroxocobalamin. Here the ligand attached to

the cobalt atom is a hydroxo- (—OH) group. This compound is destroyed by ascorbic acid. It may function as a transient intermediary form in vitamin B_{12} metabolism. It is of therapeutic interest because it binds relatively strongly to plasma and hence after parenteral injection more of this form of vitamin B_{12} is retained than other forms. Thus it is preferred in the routine treatment of patients with pernicious anaemia and other forms of vitamin B_{12} deficiency.

Methylcobalamin. Here the ligand attached to the cobalt atom is the methyl group. It is one of the two forms functioning as a coenzyme in man. It has been identified in plasma and in the liver by Lindstrand (1964), and synthesized by Smith, Mervyn, Johnson & Shaw (1962). It is sensitive to light, which photolyses it to hydroxocobalamin.

Deoxyadenosylcobalamin. This is the other important coenzyme form of vitamin B_{12} and was first detected by Barker, Weissbach & Smyth (1958). The ligand attached to the cobalt atom is derived from adenosine. This appears to be the principal form of vitamin B_{12} in the liver and other tissues. It is extremely sensitive to light and an acidified solution (yellow) turns into a red solution due to formation of hydroxocobalamin within a few minutes of exposure.

Biochemical Reactions Involving Folate and Cobamide Coenzymes

(1) *Folate coenzymes* (Stokstad & Koch, 1967).
Serine-glycine interconversion. The overall reaction is catalysed by the enzyme *serine*

$$\underset{\text{serine}}{CH_2OH-\overset{\overset{\displaystyle NH_2}{|}}{CH}-COOH} \;\underset{\rightarrow}{\leftarrow}\; \underset{\substack{\text{glycine}\\ +\text{ "C"}}}{CH_2-COOH}$$

"carbon" unit

hydroxymethyltransferase (serine aldolase). Pyridoxal phosphate participates in the reaction and appears to be bound to the enzyme. It is assumed that serine is attached to pyridoxal phosphate and this results in freeing of the bond between the α and β atoms of serine. The β carbon then is transferred to tetrahydrofolate and glycine is released. Serine which may be synthesized from glucose is the main source of single carbon units.

Purine biosynthesis. Folate is concerned in two separate phases of purine synthesis. Glycinamideribonucleotide transformylase (GAR transformylase) is concerned with linking formate to glycine, the coenzyme being 5,10-methenyltetrahydrofolate.

Glycinamide ribonucleotide   formylglycinamide ribonucleotide

homocysteine   methionine

The closure of the purine ring is effected by 5-amino-4-imidazolecarboxamide ribonucleotide transformylase (AICAR transformylase) and the formyl donor is 10-formyltetrahydrofolate.

Pyrimidine biosynthesis. The conversion of uracil to thymine involves the addition of a methyl group to carbon 5.

Uracil   Thymine

The enzyme is *thymidylate synthetase* and, surprisingly, 5-methyltetrahydrofolate is quite ineffective as a methyl donor. The coenzyme form in fact is 5,10-methylenetetrahydrofolate and the substrate is deoxyuridine monophosphate. The transfer of this carbon unit is accompanied by its reduction to the methyl form and the hydrogen for this reduction is derived from the reduced pteridine moiety of tetrahydrofolate. As a result the coenzyme becomes oxidized to dihydrofolate. This in turn is regenerated to the tetrahydro form via folate reductase. The end product of the reaction is the formation of thymidine.

Methionine biosynthesis. The enzyme, which transfers the methyl group from 5-methyltetrahydrofolate to homocysteine, *5-methyltetrahydrofolate methyltransferase*, has vitamin B_{12} as a prosthetic group (Guest, Friedman, Woods & Smith, 1962). It has been postulated that the importance of this reaction lies not in the synthesis of methionine, which remains an essential amino acid, but in releasing tetrahydrofolate which would otherwise be trapped in the methyl-form (Buchanan, 1964). Because methyl B_{12} is the important prosthetic group in this reaction, in vitamin B_{12} deficiency methyl transfer from 5-methyltetrahydrofolate fails, there is trapping of

tetrahydrofolate in the methylfolate form and an overall failure of all reactions requiring the folate coenzymes (Herbert & Zalusky, 1962). In support of this hypothesis Waters & Mollin (1963) and others have found elevated levels of folate (probably methylfolate) in serum in untreated pernicious anaemia. On the other hand Chanarin & Perry (1968) have failed to demonstrate any defect in the handling of methylfolate in pernicious anaemia.

Histidine catabolism. Carbon 2 of the imidazole ring of histidine is transferred to tetrahydrofolate during normal histidine breakdown. This is not an important source of single carbon units, but this pathway has come into prominence because it is the basis for a biochemical test for folate deficiency in man viz. the urinary excretion of formiminoglutamic acid ("Figlu"). The breakdown of histidine is usually to urocanic acid, 4-imidazolone-5-propionic acid, formiminoglutamic acid and glutamic acid. In the last step (Fig. 6.7) tetrahydrofolate is the acceptor of the formimino-(—CH=NH) group, and the enzyme catalysing this transfer is *formiminoglutamate formimino-transferase*. 5-formiminotetrahydrofolate is converted to 5,10-methenyltetrahydrofolate by the enzyme *formiminotetrahydrofolate cyclodeaminase*.

(2) Vitamin B_{12} coenzymes

There are at least three types of reactions in which cobamide coenzymes are implicated. These are concerned with:

SINGLE CARBON-UNIT METABOLISM

(1) Methylation of homocysteine to methionine.
(2) Conversion of methanol and acetate to methane by methanobacteria.
(3) Formation of acetate from carbon dioxide by a clostridium.
(4) Methylation of soluble RNA in rats.

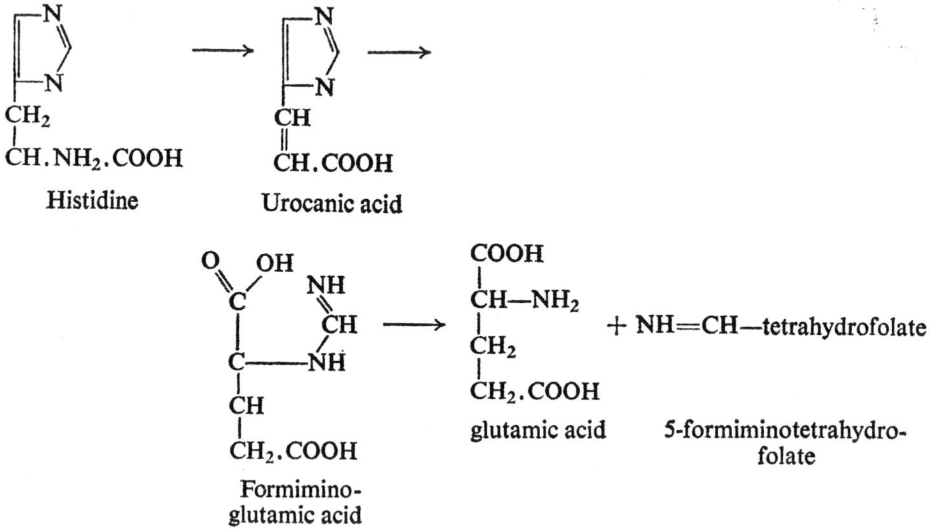

FIG. 6.7. Histidine catabolism.

ISOMERIZATION REACTIONS

    (5) Conversion of glutamic acid to methylaspartate in a clostridium.

    (6) Conversion of methylmalonyl coenzyme A to succinyl coenzyme A in both bacteria and mammals including man.

OXIDATION-REDUCTION REACTIONS

    (7) Conversion of a diol to an aldehyde in aerobacter.

    (8) Conversion of ribotides to deoxyribotides in *Lactobacilli*.

    (9) Lysine degradation by clostridia.

    (10) Ethanolamine degradation by clostridia.

Only three of these reactions, viz. (1), (4) and (6) have been demonstrated in mammals and these are discussed further.

Methionine synthesis. Woods, Foster & Guest (1965), suggested that there were two mechanisms whereby the methyl group of 5-methyltetrahydrofolate was transferred to homocysteine. One pathway required the triglutamate form of 5-methylfolate, i.e. 5-methyltetrahydropteroyltriglutamate, and here the methyl group was transferred directly to homocysteine. The alternative pathway with a monoglutamate, i.e. 5-methyltetrahydropteroylglutamic acid, required methyl B_{12} as an intermediary. The single carbon unit carried by the folate coenzyme is thus reduced to the methyl form, shunted to vitamin B_{12} and thence to homocysteine. Two other sub-

stances are required at catalytic levels, viz. S-adenosylmethionine and reduced flavinadenine dinucleotide.

Methylation of soluble RNA. Walerych, Venkataraman & Johnson (1966) in a brief report indicated that methylcobalamin could serve as a methyl donor for the direct methylation of s-RNA in rat liver.

L-*methylmalonyl-CoA mutase.* The last stage in the overall conversion of propionate to succinate, i.e. the conversion of L-methylmalonyl-CoA to succinyl-CoA, is brought about by the enzyme L-methylmalonyl-CoA-mutase, which has vitamin B_{12} coenzyme as a prosthetic group. The reaction in which there is internal rearrangement of the carbon chain is typical of a number of vitamin B_{12}-mediated reactions. The reaction is of special importance in ruminants such as sheep in which the fermentation of short chain fatty acids is the major source of energy. In these animals vitamin B_{12} is derived from synthesis by the bacteria in the rumen and subsequent absorption by the host. In sheep grazing on cobalt-deficient pastures lack of cobalt produces a failure of adequate vitamin B_{12} synthesis and these animals develop a disease known as pining, cured by vitamin B_{12} or by addition of cobalt to their diets (Marston, Allen & Smith, 1961). In vitamin B_{12} deficiency in both sheep and man, methylmalonic acid therefore appears in the urine.

$$
\begin{array}{c}
\mathrm{CH_3} \\
| \\
\mathrm{CH_2} \\
| \\
\mathrm{COOH}
\end{array}
\rightarrow
\begin{array}{c}
\mathrm{CH_3} \\
| \\
\mathrm{CH_2} \\
| \\
\mathrm{C{=}O} \\
\diagdown \mathrm{S{-}CoA}
\end{array}
\rightarrow
\begin{array}{c}
\mathrm{COOH} \\
| \\
\mathrm{H{-}C{-}CH_3} \\
| \\
\mathrm{C{=}O} \\
\diagdown \mathrm{S{-}CoA}
\end{array}
\rightarrow
\begin{array}{c}
\mathrm{COOH} \\
| \\
\mathrm{CH_2} \\
| \\
\mathrm{CH_2} \\
| \\
\mathrm{C{=}O} \\
\diagdown \mathrm{S{-}CoA}
\end{array}
$$

Propionic   Propionyl-   Methyl-   Succinyl-CoA
acid   CoA   malonyl-CoA

Nutritional Aspects of Folate and Vitamin B_{12} in Man

Folate. Folic acid is widely distributed throughout a variety of foodstuffs of both plant and animal origin. There are at least two forms of folate present in food:

(*a*) Forms available to microbiological assay organisms. *Streptococcus faecalis* is able to utilize monoglutamates other than 5-methylfolate. *Lactobacillus casei* is able to utilize both monoglutamates and triglutamates, i.e. having three glutamic acid residues linked by γ-glutamyl peptide bonds as well as 5-methylfolate.

(*b*) Forms not available to microbiological assay organisms. These may contain seven or more glutamic acid residues. Forms of folate having three or more glutamic acid residues are collectively termed polyglutamates or folic acid conjugates. Enzymes termed "conjugases" are present in tissues such as pancreas, kidney, and possibly intestinal juice which split off the glutamic acid chain and make the folates available to *Str. faecalis* and *L. casei* (Wright & Welch, 1943; Santini, Berger, Sheehy, Aviles & Davila, 1962).

The average daily cooked Western diet contains about 160 μg. of "free folate", i.e. as determined by direct assay with *L. casei* and about 500 μg. of conjugates, i.e. folate made available to *L. casei* by treatment with chick pancreas. Uncooked food, particularly if fresh, contains considerably more folate, but much of the folate is lost in the preparation of the food particularly if this is prepared by boiling in water. Canning of fruit, steaming of vegetables, and grilling meat results in loss of 70 to 95% of folate (Cheldelin, Woods & Williams, 1943).

A further difficulty stems from uncertainty as to whether the two forms of folate are equally available to man. It is likely that monoglutamates are easily absorbed since only about 20% of tritium-labelled pteroylglutamic acid is recovered from the faeces after small oral doses (Anderson, Belcher, Chanarin & Mollin, 1960); it is also likely that polyglutamates are less well absorbed and the most recent data suggest an absorption of some 25% of polyglutamates in a normal diet.

Vitamin B_{12}. Vitamin B_{12}, present in animal tissues and bacteria, is entirely absent from foods of plant origin, i.e. an exclusively vegetarian diet by man or animals leads to vitamin B_{12} deficiency. Nevertheless under normal conditions plant foods are likely to be contaminated by bacteria or by vitamin B_{12} from soil, water or by bacterial fermentation proceeding in the food and this provides trace amounts of vitamin B_{12}. There is relatively little loss of vitamin B_{12} in the preparation of food. Heat at alkaline pH might prove harmful. Only about 8% of vitamin B_{12} was lost in boiling liver, and meat broiled for 45 minutes lost 27% mostly in dripping from the meat (Heyssel, Bozian, Darby & Bell, 1966). Chung, Pearson, Darby, Miller & Goldsmith, (1961) found that a "high cost" American diet provided about 31·6 μg vitamin B_{12} daily, a "low cost" diet 16 μg and a poor diet only 2·7 μg vitamin B_{12} daily. The greater part of the vitamin B_{12} present in food appears to be available for absorption.

Requirement for vitamin B_{12} and folate. Various methods have been applied in determining folate requirements. These have varied from the determination of the daily dose of folate required to maintain serum folate levels while on a folate-free diet, following the change in folate status while on a folate-free diet (Herbert, 1962), and determining the minimum amount of folate required to produce a haematological response in folate-deficient megaloblastic anaemia. In general there is agreement that this amount is of the order of 100 to

200 μg. of folate daily. The total amount of folate in the body is about 15 mg. so that should intake cease, severe deficiency can arise in about 20 weeks

Daily loss of vitamin B_{12} from the body has been determined by loss of radioactivity in individuals receiving labelled vitamin B_{12}, by the time required for the development of vitamin B_{12} deficiency after total gastrectomy and by the amount of vitamin B_{12} required to produce an optimal haematological response in vitamin B_{12} deficient megaloblastic anaemia. By all these methods the daily vitamin B_{12} requirement is about 2 to 7 μg. daily. The total amount of vitamin B_{12} in the body is 3 to 6 mg. so that should intake cease deficiency will arise in about 5 years.

Physiological Considerations in Man

Little is known of the manner of absorption of folate by the gut. With large unphysiological doses of folate, rising blood levels are evident within the first 30 minutes after an oral dose. The site of absorption is no different from the bulk of other foodstuffs of similar chemical properties such as water-soluble vitamins, and the absorption of folate must not be regarded as primarily a function of the upper gut. Physiological doses of folate are transferred to the liver. Folate is normally present in large amounts in bile and undergoes an enterohepatic circulation (Baker, Kumar & Swaminathan, 1965).

The manner of absorption of vitamin B_{12} is unique. Normal gastric juice contains a mucoprotein, termed intrinsic factor by Castle (1929). This compound is a product of the parietal cell of the gastric mucosa in man and has a M.W. of about 60,000 as a monomer to 120,000 in the dimer form (Gräsbeck, Simons & Sinkkonen, 1966; Ellenbogen & Highley, 1967). Intrinsic factor is normally present in vast excess and only about 1% of the daily output is required for maximum absorption of a 1·0 μg dose of vitamin B_{12}. It can be assayed by a simple immunological method (Ardeman & Chanarin, 1963). Its secretion is stimulated by histamine and its analogues, by insulin, and by gastrin and its analogues, but not by cholinergic drugs such as carbachol.

Intrinsic factor binds vitamin B_{12} firmly and the intrinsic factor-vitamin B_{12} complex then enters the cells lining the villi of the distal gut, i.e. the ileum. Here there is a slow separation of vitamin B_{12} from intrinsic factor and peak blood levels of vitamin B_{12} after an oral dose are reached only some 10 hours after its administration (Booth & Mollin, 1956). The maximum amount of vitamin B_{12} that can be absorbed after a single oral dose

(or a single meal) is about 2·0 μg, but the delay in its transport across of the gut wall does not interfere with the uptake of a further dose of vitamin B_{12} given some 4 to 6 hours later (Heyssel, Bozian, Darby & Bell, 1966). When relatively large amounts of vitamin B_{12} are taken by mouth, e.g. 50 μg., and such amounts generally exceed the amount likely to be present in a single meal unless this contains large amounts of liver, some simple diffusion of vitamin B_{12} across the gut wall takes place with "early" elevation of serum levels.

Like folate, vitamin B_{12} is excreted in the bile and undergoes an enterohepatic circulation. Intrinsic factor is required for reabsorption of vitamin B_{12} secreted into the bile.

The Anaemia

The anaemia that arises as a result of deficiency of vitamin B_{12} is similar to that arising as a result of folate deficiency and there are no morphological features that characterize vitamin B_{12} deficiency as opposed to folate deficiency. However the morphological picture may be modified by accompanying iron deficiency and by loss of splenic function. Descriptions of the morphological changes in blood and marrow may be found in any standard haematological textbook. In general the degree of anaemia is variable, i.e. haemoglobin concentration may still be within the normal range or the anaemia may be severe. When little anaemia is present the stained peripheral blood film shows a macrocytosis with some slight variation in cell size. As the anaemia becomes more severe macrocytosis is more prominant and is accompanied by more marked variation in cell size. There is an increase in the number of neutrophils having five or more nuclear lobes; these do not normally exceed 3% of the total. With more severe anaemia there is leucopenia and a reduced platelet count.

The marrow shows that a megaloblastic form of erythropoiesis has replaced the normoblastic form, although in patients with little anaemia morphological changes are recognizable only in the haemoglobinized erythroblasts. Granulopoiesis is modified by the presence of a small number of obviously large metamyelocytes, i.e. giant metamyelocytes. It is debatable whether the presence of giant metamyelocytes alone, in the absence of recognizable change in the red cell precursors, should be regarded as adequate evidence of a megaloblastic process. It is the author's view that megaloblastic anaemia should not be diagnosed in the absence of megaloblast formation in red cell precursors irrespective of other findings

Accompanying iron deficiency may make these

changes more difficult to detect and may conceal them completely (Tasker, 1959). Under these circumstances the marrow examination should be repeated after adequate iron therapy. This situation is frequent in pregnancy and after partial gastrectomy.

The blood changes that characterize loss of splenic function (Howell-Jolly bodies, target cells, normoblasts, siderocytes in peripheral blood) are all exaggerated when there is an accompanying megaloblastic process. Their presence in the blood might suggest a post-gastrectomy-splenectomy picture or, in the absence of surgery, idiopathic steatorrhoea when the spleen tends to become atrophic.

Aids in Diagnosis

The diagnosis of megaloblastic anaemia. This depends entirely on the recognition of the morphological changes in peripheral blood and marrow. Although this recognition may be difficult in patients with little anaemia, the diagnosis should not be made unless these changes are clear cut. Ill-defined change should be ignored from the point of view of diagnosis although under some circumstances it may be desirable to measure the serum vitamin B_{12} level to exclude vitamin B_{12} deficiency. Such circumstances might be a neuropathy or a previous gastrectomy.

Biochemical findings common to all megaloblastic anaemias. Provided the anaemia is of sufficient severity a number of abnormal biochemical features are present. The serum bilirubin is often elevated although it is unlikely to exceed 2·5 mg./ 100 ml. unless there is hepatic damage. The bilirubin is conjugated. Urobilin excretion is increased

The serum iron is usually increased and the iron-binding capacity may be fully saturated. The earliest evidence of a response to specific therapy is a rapid fall in the serum iron level after 24 hours (Hawkins, 1955). There is a considerable increase in the serum lactate dehydrogenase activity and, to a lesser extent, β-hydroxybutyrate dehydrogenase activity in untreated megaloblastic anaemia (Hess & Gehm, 1955; Fleming & Elliott, 1964). The values for lactate dehydrogenase range from 1500 to 11,000 units/l. (Anderssen, 1964), i.e. they are far higher than in most other disorders. Nevertheless normal values are found in mildly anaemic patients. The origin of the enzyme is likely to be dead haemopoietic precursors in the marrow (Libnoch, Yakulis & Heller, 1966). Treatment of the anaemia is accompanied by a fall in lactate dehydrogenase activity in about 3 days followed by a slower return to normal levels after 2 weeks.

An aminoaciduria is common in untreated pernicious anaemia, and relatively high taurine excretion was noted by Weaver & Neill (1954). An increased excretion of hydroxyphenol compounds is present (Swendseid, Burton & Bethell, 1943). Although folic acid is able to bring about conversion of phenylalanine to tyrosine, pteridine compounds without the aromatic amine (i.e. lacking *p*-aminobenzoylglutamate) were more active (Kaufman, 1958), particularly pteridine methylated in the 6 and 7 positions.

Studies that Assess Vitamin B_{12} and Folate Status. Investigation procedures used in the study of patients with megaloblastic anaemia are listed in Table 6.2. It is fortunate that in such an investigation one is concerned with establishing deficiency of one of only two substances. It is rare for significant deficiency of both to be playing an aetiological role in a single patient. Thus confident exclusion of one of these substances immediately implicates the second substance as the deficient one. The desirable approach is to establish or to exclude vitamin B_{12} deficiency as the missing substance in the first instance. There are two reasons for doing

TABLE 6.2

Investigations useful in the diagnosis of the nature of the deficiency in a megaloblastic anaemia

Useful in vitamin B_{12} deficiency	Useful in folate deficiency
Serum vitamin B_{12} level	Red cell (and serum) folate level
Hepatic B_{12} level	Hepatic folate level
Methylmalonic acid excretion	Formiminoglutamic acid excretion
Absorption of vitamin B_{12}	Absorption of folate
Assay of intrinsic factor	Plasma clearance of i.v. folate
Antibodies to intrinsic factor	—
Haematological response to 2·0 μg parenteral B_{12} daily	Haematological response to 200 μg folate daily

so. Erroneous diagnosis and prolonged folate administration to a patient with vitamin B_{12} deficiency can precipitate subacute combined degeneration of the cord and this may prove only partially reversible on subseqent treatment with vitamin B_{12}. Secondly a more decisive outcome is likely with results of tests of vitamin B_{12} status than of folate status, i.e. when the serum vitamin B_{12} level or the absorption of vitamin B_{12} is normal then vitamin B_{12} deficiency can be excluded as the cause of the megaloblastic anaemia which can then be ascribed with every confidence to folate deficiency.

Tests of folate status give less decisive results. Because of the relatively short period of time that has to elapse before significant tissue depletion of folate arises this may be found in about one-third of unselected admissions to a general hospital (Leevy, Cardi, Frank, Gellone & Baker, 1965), and when special groups of patients are selected such as those with neoplasia the proportion of patients with abnormal results may approach 80%. These results are abnormal not because these tests are inadequate but because subclinical folate deficiency is so common in the general population

The serum vitamin B_{12} level. The normal range varies from 150 pg. to 900 pg./ml. and in vitamin B_{12} deficiency the level is considerably reduced from barely detectable levels to upwards of 100 pg./ml. (Mollin & Ross, 1957). Two techniques are available for determining the serum vitamin B_{12} concentration. The one is by microbiological assay using either *Euglena gracilis* or *Lactobacillus leichmannii* as test organisms, and the other an isotope method employing radioactive vitamin B_{12} (Anderson, 1964; Barakat & Ekins, 1961; Grossowicz, Sulitzeanu & Merzbach, 1962; Lau, Gottlieb, Wasserman & Herbert, 1965). With experience these methods are reasonably reproducible and reliable. A number of points of interpretation must be considered. The dividing line between normal and abnormal, as in all studies of this nature, is not as sharp as some publications would have us believe. A very small number of normal subjects may have vitamin B_{12} levels between 120 and 150 although investigation fails to reveal any abnormality. Further a small number of patients with pernicious anaemia may have levels as high as 170 pg./ml. (Ardeman, Chanarin, Krafchik & Singer, 1966). Reduced serum vitamin B_{12} levels occur in about 5% of normal pregnant women and these levels return to within the normal range after delivery. The serum vitamin B_{12} level may be low in megaloblastic anaemia due to folate deficiency and it rises to

within the normal range 2 to 3 weeks after the institution of folate therapy (Mollin, Waters & Harriss, 1961). This is particularly frequent in megaloblastic anaemia in pregnancy, due to anticonvulsant drugs and often in intestinal malabsorption syndrome. Thirdly the serum vitamin B_{12} level may be low in iron-deficiency and show a slow rise following many months of iron therapy (Cox, Meynell, Gaddie & Cooke, 1959). In all these conditions the absorption of vitamin B_{12} is normal and the low serum vitamin B_{12} level probably reflects an altered distribution of vitamin B_{12} in the body and not deficiency of the vitamin.

On the other hand a normal serum vitamin B_{12} level excludes vitamin B_{12} deficiency provided that normal values have been obtained with two independent serum samples. The necessity for this precaution arises from the ease with which trace amounts of vitamin B_{12} may contaminate bottles, syringes, etc. and it has been a common experience with paired samples that a low result may be obtained with one serum sample while the second from the same patient shows equivocal or clearly normal values. These dangers have been reduced by the use of disposable equipment. It is also as well to be aware that antibiotics may produce apparently very low values but often the clue is provided by the total absence of growth, i.e. the apparent result is less than that in the standard tube containing no added vitamin B_{12}.

Abnormally elevated vitamin B_{12} levels may be seen with blood samples taken within a few hours or days of a vitamin B_{12} injection, in chronic myeloid leukaemia, chronic myelofibrosis, polycythaemia vera and in liver disease associated with liver cell death such as hepatitis, cirrhosis and hepatic neoplasms.

Hepatic vitamin B_{12}. A piece of liver for assay of vitamin B_{12} is rarely available but where it is then it can provide valuable information. In vitamin B_{12} deficiency causing megaloblastic anaemia there is less than 0·2 μg. vitamin B_{12}/g. of wet liver. "Normal" liver has more than 0·2 μg./g. and the mean value is about 0.8 μg/g. (Anderson, 1965).

Methylmalonic acid excretion. The biochemical pathway concerned has been indicated. Normal subjects excrete less than 4·0 mg. of methylmalonic acid in the urine over 24 hours although some studies have reported values as high as 9 and 11 mg. (Cox & White, 1962; Gompertz, Jones & Knowles, 1967; Giorgio & Plaut, 1965). The majority of patients with untreated vitamin B_{12} deficiency due to pernicious anaemia excrete increased amounts in the urine. This may be only slightly more than in controls to quantities in excess of 500 mg. in 24 hours. Some patients after a partial gastrectomy and with pernicious anaemia and low serum vitamin B_{12} levels, however, may not have an increased excretion of methylmalonic acid (Holmberg, Jönemar, Norden, Ståhlberg & Tryding, 1966). Gompertz, Jones & Knowles (1967) have suggested that oral valine (5–10 g.) produced an appreciable increase in the urinary methylmalonic acid output in vitamin B_{12} deficiency.

At the moment the technique of estimation requires complex extraction procedures followed by gas chromatography or less satisfactory colorimetric or chromatographic techniques (Bashir, Hinterberger & Jones, 1966). When satisfactory techniques become available methylmalonic acid estimation is likely to be a useful aid in the diagnosis of vitamin B_{12} deficiency.

Absorption of vitamin B_{12}. The result of tests for the absorption of vitamin B_{12} is probably the most important single piece of information in the investigation of vitamin B_{12} deficiency. A low serum vitamin B_{12} level with malabsorption of vitamin B_{12} means vitamin B_{12} deficiency, but a low serum vitamin B_{12} level with normal absorption suggests that the low serum vitamin B_{12} may be due to any of the causes discussed above. The important exception here is found among vegetarians. In India many people for religious as well as for economic reasons eat basically polished rice, lentils, wheat, flour, boiled green vegetables and fruit, supplemented in some by milk and eggs. The mean serum vitamin B_{12} in a group of these subjects was 121 pg./ml. with more than half having levels of less than 100 pg./ml. (Mehta, Rege & Satoskar, 1964). In these subjects it may be presumed that the absorption of vitamin B_{12} is normal. With the important exception of dietary vitamin B_{12} deficiency lack of vitamin B_{12} arises only as a failure of its absorption.

Absorption tests are carried out with vitamin B_{12} labelled with one of the isotopes of Co. These are Co[56], half-life 77 days

    Co[57], half-life 270 days

    Co[58], half-life 71 days

    Co[60], half-life 5·27 years.

Their counting characteristics, emissions, liability to radiochemical decomposition as well as relative safety for use are discussed by Rosenblum (1962). For surface and whole body counting Co[58]-vitamin B_{12} is used, and for other work including the urinary excretion test Co[57]-vitamin B_{12} is the most desirable. The oral dose of vitamin B_{12} in absorption tests is generally either 0·5 μg. or 1·0 μg. and these generally have a specific activity of 0·5 to 1·0 μCi./μg. of vitamin B_{12}. Techniques

that are available for determining the absorption of this dose are:

Faecal excretion. The unabsorbed vitamin B_{12} is measured by collecting all the faeces until no more radioactivity is passed. This may take up to 8 days, although usually most is passed between days 2 to 4. Incomplete faecal collection is the bugbear of this method.

Urinary excretion method. Schilling (1953) found that if the oral labelled dose of vitamin B_{12} was accompanied or followed by an injection of about 1000 μg. of non-radioactive vitamin B_{12}, approximately one-third of the absorbed radioactive material was carried out into the urine with the non-radioactive vitamin B_{12} during the next 24 hours. This is the most convenient and the most widely used method of assessing the absorption of a dose of vitamin B_{12}.

Hepatic uptake method. Glass, Boyd & Stephanson (1954) noted that by placing a suitable scintillation counter over the subject's liver radioactivity due to vitamin B_{12} deposited in the liver could be counted. Counts should be done after a week when liver counts reach a peak and intestinal radioactivity has been largely eliminated. The principle advantage is that this method does not require the patient's cooperation in specimen collection.

Plasma radioactivity reaches a peak some 10 hours after the oral dose and may be counted (Booth & Mollin, 1956).

Whole body counting where available is a useful and quantitative means of assessing vitamin B_{12} absorption.

The results in control subjects are shown in Table 6.3. In vitamin B_{12} malabsorption the values are generally much lower. In intrinsic factor deficiency the absorption is improved significantly by repeating the test with normal gastric juice or an extract of dried hog pyloric mucosa. In anatomical abnormalities of the small gut such as blind loops or small intestinal diverticula the absorption is improved after a course of antibiotics. When the terminal ileum is diseased, resected or bypassed then absorption of radioactive vitamin B_{12} is not corrected by any of these measures.

Assay of intrinsic factor and antibodies to intrinsic factor. The commonest cause of vitamin B_{12} deficiency in many parts of the world is pernicious anaemia. Rapid diagnosis is possible by direct demonstration of the absence of intrinsic factor from the gastric juice. The presence of hydrochloric acid in the gastric juice excludes a diagnosis of pernicious anaemia but a histamine-fast achlorhydria may occur in the absence of

TABLE 6.3

The results of tests of vitamin B_{12} absorption in control subjects
(after Mollin, 1959)

	0·5 μg B_{12}		1·0 μg B_{12}	
	Range	Mean	Range	Mean
Faecal excretion (μg absorbed)	0·16–0·48	0·35	0·26–0·87	0·56
Urinary excretion (% oral dose in urine)	15·8–39·6	25·9	11·2–32·0	19·3
Plasma count—% $\left(\dfrac{\text{Plasma counts/litre}}{\text{counts of oral dose}} \times 100\right)$	1·01–2·58	1·51*	0·75–1·7	1·2**

* 12-hour plasma sample (Østergaard-Kristensen & Hald, 1962).
** 8-hour plasma sample (Armstrong & Woodliff, 1966).

pernicious anaemia. Antibody to intrinsic factor is present in the sera of 57% of patients with pernicious anaemia. Intrinsic factor that has reacted with its antibody is no longer able to bind labelled vitamin B_{12}. This observation forms the basis for a direct assay of intrinsic factor (Ardeman & Chanarin, 1963). The unit of intrinsic factor is that amount that binds 1·0 ng. of vitamin B_{12}. Normally 2000 units or more are excreted in the gastric juice in one hour after a histamine or gastrin stimulus. In pernicious anaemia 0 to 200 units may be excreted. Patients with gastric atrophy have intermediate values.

The presence of intrinsic factor antibody is also virtually restricted to pernicious anaemia and hence its demonstration is of great clinical value.

Red Cell Folate and Serum Folate values

Whereas a considerable measure of agreement is possible with results of vitamin B_{12} assays from different centres, the same cannot be said for the results of folate assays. Results of assays in some centres are three to four times higher than in others. The practical implications would be less if each centre determined their own normal range. Coupled with the frequency of abnormal results in the hospital population, the results should be treated as confirmatory and reliance placed on data that assess vitamin B_{12} status.

The range and mean of serum folate values from 18 reported series are:

	Serum folate ng./ml.	Mean
Lower limit	2·5– 8·0	4·8
Upper limit	7·4–45·0	16·0

In practice 5 ng./ml. may be taken as a lower normal limit with a range of 2 to 5 being indeterminate and values below 2 the expected finding in megaloblastic anaemia due to folate deficiency.

The red cells contain some 20 times more folate than does the serum and the result should be expressed in terms of packed red cells. Mollin & Hoffbrand (1965) find a normal range of 184 to 655 ng./ml. of packed red cells, and the author in 40 medical students a range of 116–410 ng. ml. A red cell folate of less than 100 ng./ml. is indicative of folate deficiency.

Hepatic folate. The normal hepatic folate content varies from 5·2 to 10·0 μg./g. of wet liver with a mean of 6·9. In folate deficiency the level is of the order of 1·0 μg./g. or less.

Formiminoglutamic acid excretion. Inability to metabolize this compound in folate deficiency forms the basis of a clinical test. Fifteen grams of L-histidine is given orally (10 times the normal daily intake) and all the urine passed in the next 8 hours is collected using a few ml. of N/HCl as preservative.

The presence of formiminoglutamic acid in the urine may be detected by paper or cellulose electrophoresis (Knowles, Prankard & Westall, 1960; Kohn, Mollin & Rosenbach, 1961) or by a quantitative enzymic assay (Luhby, Cooperman & Teller, 1959; Chanarin & Bennett, 1962a). In the qualitative methods the presence of any material is generally abnormal. With the quantitative assay normal subjects excrete 1 to 17 mg. of formiminoglutamic acid after a 15 g. loading dose of L-histidine (mean 9 mg.). In folate deficiency values between 20 to 1500 mg. may be found.

In liver disease, and in malnourished subjects there is a defect in the enzyme urocanase which converts urocanic acid to formiminoglutamic acid and thus there is a failure to metabolize histidine beyond the stage of urocanic acid. In these patients there is considerable urinary excretion of urocanate. On occasion however a feed-back inhibition of urocanase as a result of high formiminoglutamic acid levels may result in urocanic acid appearing with formiminoglutamic acid in the urine in patients with folate deficiency (Chanarin, 1963).

This test is of little value in the diagnosis of megaloblastic anaemia in pregnancy since changes in absorption of histidine in pregnancy, the lowered renal threshold for histidine, and passage of histidine across the placenta all tend to reduce urinary formiminoglutamic acid excretion (Chanarin, Rothman & Watson-Williams, 1963). Results are also unsatisfactory in folate deficiency due to anticonvulsant drugs (Reynolds, Milner, Matthews & Chanarin, 1966).

The absorption of folate. A folate absorption test provides useful evidence as to the cause of a folate deficiency state and the result parallels those obtained with faecal fat studies, urinary xylose excretion etc. The test may be performed by the comparison of the urinary excretion of an oral and parenteral 5 mg. dose of folate (Girdwood, 1956), by measuring the serum folate levels after an oral dose of 40 μg. folate/kg. body weight (Chanarin, Anderson & Mollin, 1958; Chanarin & Bennett, 1962 b) or by measuring the urinary or faecal excretion of tritium-labelled folate (Anderson, Belcher, Chanarin & Mollin, 1960). Following an oral dose of 40 μg. folate/kg. normal subjects have a peak serum folate value in the next 2 hours which exceeds 40 ng./ml. using *Str. faecalis* as the assay organism. In intestinal malabsorption the levels are much lower and may be zero.

Plasma clearance of intravenously injected folate (Chanarin, Mollin & Anderson, 1958). The rate of removal from the plasma of an intravenously injected dose of folate (15 μg./kg. of body weight) is a reliable guide of folate stores. The normal serum level 15 minutes after the injection as assayed with *Str. faecalis* is 21 to 80 ng./ml. (mean 40 ng.). In folate deficiency the 15 minute serum level is lower than 20 ng. and is often zero.

Haematological responses. The nature of a deficiency can be determined in a patient with a megaloblastic anaemia by demonstrating an optimal haematological response to either 2·0 μg. vitamin B_{12} parenterally daily for 10 days or 200 μg. folate daily either orally or by injection for the same length of time. An optimal response requires a peak reticulocyte response on day 5, 6 or 7, day 0 being the first day of treatment and the height of the reticulocyte response should be that expected from the degree of anaemia.

Initial red cell count /mm³	Expected approximate reticulocyte response %
1·0	40
1·5	30
2·0	20
2·5	15
3·0	10

The red cell count should exceed 3·0 million in 3 weeks

Causes of Folate Deficiency

Megaloblastic anaemia requiring therapy with folic acid may arise:

(1) When folate intake is inadequate either because of an inadequate diet or because of intestinal malabsorption. The causes of intestinal malabsorption include gluten-sensitive enteropathies in children and adults and tropical sprue.

(2) When requirement of folate is increased beyond that absorbed from dietary sources. The increased folate requirement is usually associated with an increased cell turnover. Here the most important cause is pregnancy and lactation but the principle is well illustrated by megaloblastic anaemia complicating a haemolytic anaemia or neoplasm such as a reticulosarcoma. The megaloblastic anaemia complicating chronic myelofibrosis may be of this type.

(3) When there is interference with the folate coenzymes; antifolate drugs are obvious examples, but the drugs used in the treatment of epilepsy such as primidone, phenytoin and barbiturates are of greater importance (Reynolds, Milner, Matthews & Chanarin, 1966; Reynolds, Chanarin, Milner & Matthews, 1966) as well as the antimalarial drug, pyrimethamine. Alcohol may have a direct effect on folate metabolism (Sullivan & Herbert, 1964).

Causes of Vitamin B_{12} Deficiency

Deficiency of vitamin B_{12} stems from a failure to absorb this substance.

(1) Dietary deficiency in strict vegetarians. There is no published case report of an adequate example of megaloblastic anaemia responding to oral doses of 2 to 5 μg. vitamin B_{12} daily.

(2) Failure of intrinsic factor secretion.
    Congenital failure to produce intrinsic factor.
    Pernicious anaemia.

Total gastrectomy.

Partial gastrectomy.

Caustic erosion of the stomach (one case).

(3) Disease of the small gut.

Gluten-sensitive enteropathy, tropical sprue, Crohn's disease, scleroderma, Whipple's disease.

Anatomical abnormalities of the small gut such as small intestinal diverticulosis, strictures, blind loops, anastomoses.

Congenital failure to absorb the intrinsic-factor vitamin B_{12} complex.

Fish tape worm (*Diphyllobothrium latum*— Finnish species only).

Many of the small gut lesions are associated with an abnormal intestinal bacterial flora which may be responsible for deviating vitamin B_{12} from the diet. These bacteria do not take up folic acid; in fact the organism may even excrete folate into the gut lumen which is then available for absorption. A similar mechanism may be operative in some patients after a Polya-type partial gastrectomy. In such patients temporary improvement in vitamin B_{12} absorption occurs after a course of antibiotics.

Clinical Syndromes

An exhaustive account of all the disorders associated with a megaloblastic anaemia is beyond the scope of this section. Instead the more important are surveyed.

Pernicious anaemia. This is the common cause of megaloblastic anaemia and vitamin B_{12} deficiency in people of European and in particular North European racial stock. It is rare below the age of 30 and the commonest age of diagnosis is the fifth and sixth decade. For every 10 men affected, some 17 women have the disease. Ten per cent. may have spinal cord involvement and 30% paraesthesiae.

The stomach shows gastric atrophy or severe atrophic gastritis. Every case has a histamine-fast achlorhydria with either absent or minimal intrinsic factor content in the gastric juice which is considerably reduced in volume. The absorption of vitamin B_{12} is always grossly impaired with less than 5% excretion of a $1\cdot0$ μg. oral dose of vitamin B_{12} in the Schilling test and always some correction when the test is repeated with a source of intrinsic factor (human gastric juice or hog gastric mucosal extract). However often the vitamin B_{12} absorption with intrinsic factor does not return to within the normal range, because many patients have intrinsic factor antibodies in the

gastric juice (Fisher, Rees & Taylor, 1966). The serum vitamin B_{12} level is low.

Parietal-cell antibodies are present in about 85% of patients, intrinsic factor antibodies in 57% and thyroid antibodies in about 30%.

There is a strong association between pernicious anaemia and other disorders showing autoimmune phenomena. These are thyroid disease, both Graves' disease, primary myxoedema and Hashimoto's thyroiditis, adrenal atrophy (Addison's disease) and hypoparathyroidism.

In addition pernicious anaemia shows a strong familial incidence, a family history of the disease being found in some 20% of patients and a high frequency of parietal cell and thyroid antibodies are present in healthy members of such families. It is likely that such families inherit an increased tendency to form organ-specific antibodies and to develop the diseases associated with these organs. The most extreme example is the group aptly termed "juvenile autoimmune pernicious anaemia" where in the second decade of life these children or teenagers develop pernicious anaemia, Addison's disease, hypoparathyroidism, monilia, dental abnormalities and sometimes other disorders (Sjöberg, 1966).

Finally 5–8% of patients with pernicious anaemia die of a carcinoma of the stomach.

Anaemia after gastrectomy. Total gastrectomy results in a cessation of vitamin B_{12} absorption. Megaloblastic anaemia is inevitable in those who survive. It is unlikely to appear in less than 2 years and most have manifested themselves after 5 years. These patients should be maintained on vitamin B_{12} once the operation has been performed.

Partial gastrectomy is followed by an iron deficiency anaemia in one-third to one-half of all patients. Anaemia is more frequent after the Polya operation than after a Billroth I gastrectomy, and is more frequent in women before the menopause. Low serum iron values are found in an even greater proportion of patients. Although iron deficiency is probably the result of poor absorption of food iron, the anaemia responds perfectly well to oral inorganic iron.

Megaloblastic anaemia does not appear before at least 5 years have elapsed after the operation, and can be expected in some 5–6% of all patients. In the majority it is due to vitamin B_{12} deficiency, but in perhaps 1 in 5 patients the cause is folate deficiency

There is a decline in the serum vitamin B_{12} with time after partial gastrectomy, and after 8 years about 20% of patients have low serum vitamin B_{12} levels. The frequency of vitamin B_{12} malabsorption has been found to be 30 % (Lous & Schwartz, 1959) but this value may be high because it is now known that the vitamin B_{12} absorption can be improved after partial gastrectomy when the test is accompanied by a stimulant to gastric secretion such as histamine (Turnbull, 1967) or by a meal.

In general the absorption of vitamin B_{12} after gastrectomy, when impaired, is improved by additional intrinsic factor. In 10 % of such cases it is not, and in these an abnormal bacterial flora in the blind loop of the Polya gastrectomy may be the explanation.

The diagnostic problem is often complicated because both iron deficiency and vitamin B_{12} deficiency may coexist. If the serum vitamin B_{12} level is normal then vitamin B_{12} deficiency can be dismissed. If it is low the situation should be reassessed following adequate iron therapy. A megaloblastic process may be revealed in the marrow following iron repletion; on the other hand an initially low serum vitamin B_{12} level may have risen to within the normal range following iron therapy. The combination of a low serum vitamin B_{12} level and impaired vitamin B_{12} absorption is of itself sufficient indication for institution of regular vitamin B_{12} therapy. A megaloblastic process in the presence of a normal serum vitamin B_{12} level or normal vitamin B_{12} absorption indicates that the cause is folate deficiency.

Abnormal small intestinal bacterial flora and megaloblastic anaemia. The small gut is normally sterile, being kept so by acid secretion from the stomach, absence of stasis and probably by immunoglobulins produced in the gut wall. The prime factor in the production of an abnormal resident gut flora is stasis of intestinal contents in diverticula, stagnant loops, behind strictures, or by interference with motility such as may occur in scleroderma, Whipple's disease, post-vagotomy, and with the use of ganglion-blocking agents. In general a bacterial flora which exceeds 10^5 organisms/ml. of intestinal fluid is significant of a resident flora. Coliform species are likely to be concerned with deviation of dietary vitamin B_{12} from the host. Bacteroides species which are obligatory anaerobes may be concerned with splitting of bile salts.

The effect of the abnormal flora is to produce vitamin B_{12} deficiency and even subacute combined degeneration of the cord; they may produce steatorrhoea because of deconjugation of bile salts; and urinary excretion of indican, because of the splitting of tryptophan to form indole, its hydroxylation in the gut and subsequent conjugation in the liver to indican which is excreted in the urine.

Four types of gut lesion may be encountered. Gut resection, often for Crohn's disease, forms one group; the other three are strictures (51 cases), anastomoses and fistulae (55 cases) and diverticulosis (76 cases), the numbers being the relative distribution among 182 patients taken from the literature. In general, symptoms referable to the abdomen tend to be more prominent than those due to anaemia. Dyspepsia, distension, nausea, vomiting, abdominal pain and prominent borborygmi may be present. Diarrhoea may be severe. Glossitis may be present and operation scars should be looked for. Malabsorption of vitamin B_{12} is almost the rule, and in all cases with a megaloblastic anaemia the serum vitamin B_{12} level is low. Only temporary improvement in vitamin B_{12} absorption follows the use of antibiotics, and where the lesion cannot be corrected surgically vitamin B_{12} therapy often with a low-fat, high-protein diet is called for.

Megaloblastic anaemia in childhood

Vitamin B_{12} deficiency. (a) Pernicious anaemia. An acquired deficiency of intrinsic factor with gastric atrophy and achlorhydria may appear in the second decade. It is associated with other endocrinopathies.

(b) Congenital intrinsic factor deficiency. Here there is a specific and isolated failure to elaborate intrinsic factor. The stomach is otherwise normal. These children present with a severe megaloblastic anaemia in the first two years of life. It is transmitted as a Mendelian recessive characteristic and other siblings are affected. This disorder does not bear any relationship to pernicious anaemia in adults (Miller, Bloom, Streiff, LoBuglio & Diamond, 1966). Trace amounts of intrinsic factor may be present and rarely may be sufficient to postpone the development of megaloblastic anaemia to the age of 8 (Reisner, Wolff, McKay & Doyle, 1951) and even later.

(c) Congenital vitamin B_{12} malabsorption. Here there is a failure of intestinal absorption of the vitamin B_{12}-intrinsic factor complex associated with an albuminuria (Imerslund, 1960; Gräsbeck, Gordin, Kantero & Kuhlbäck, 1960). It too is transmitted as a recessive characteristic and siblings are affected. It seems that there is a failure to take up a protein complex from the lumen of the gut and from the renal tubule into a lining epithelial cell.

Folate deficiency. The most important group of megaloblastic anaemias in infancy arise in association with protein malnutrition (Kwashiorkor) and with infection. This anaemia was present in 5·4 % of African children admitted to a hospital in Durban (Walt, Holman & Hendrickse, 1956), and was present in 6·3% of Jamaican paediatric admissions (MacIver & Back, 1960). The role of infection was difficult to evaluate and the mechanism of the anaemia is not understood.

Orotic aciduria. Failure in the pathway of normal pyrimidine synthesis resulted in a rare megaloblastic anaemia responding only to oral uridine. These children excrete large amounts of orotic acid in the urine, which may be in the form of crystals. There is also a failure of growth. There is a failure to convert orotic acid to orotidine-5′-phosphate and thence to uridine-5′-phosphate and enzyme activity responsible for these two steps was very low in leucocytes and red cells of patients with this disorder and their relatives (? heterozygotes) (Smith, Huguley & Bain, 1966).

Megaloblastic anaemia of pregnancy and lactation. A megaloblastic form of haemopoiesis may be suspected on careful examination of the blood in some 2% of pregnant women in Great Britain and unselected marrow examination shows megaloblastic haemopoiesis in 25%.

Normal pregnancy is associated with a progressive fall in vitamin B_{12}, red cell folate and serum folate levels. An oral supplement of 100 μg. of folate daily is required to prevent this fall in the red cell and serum folate levels.

The cause of the decline in folate stores in pregnancy is undoubtedly the demand for folate by the growing foetus. The frequency of megaloblastic anaemia is 10 times as high in twin pregnancy and the rate of folate clearance correlated well with the growth rate of the foetus (Chanarin, MacGibbon, O'Sullivan & Mollin, 1959).

Iron deficiency of greater or lesser degree is very common in pregnancy and Chanarin, Rothman & Berry (1965) produced evidence that folate deficiency was prevented by iron supplements, i.e. iron deficiency increased folate requirement. This view was supported by studies in combined iron and folate deficiency in hookworm infestation (Vitale, Seta & Hellerstein, 1965).

Prolonged lactation, the custom in some countries, may also place added burdens on the mother and give rise to a megaloblastic anaemia due to folate deficiency, possibly a combination of increased requirement and inadequate dietary intake (Shapiro, Alberts, Welch & Metz, 1965).

Megaloblastic anaemia due to anticonvulsant drugs. Although severe megaloblastic anaemia in epileptics taking anticonvulsant drugs is uncommon, minor degrees of megaloblastic change are common and were found by Reynolds, Milner, Matthews & Chanarin (1966) on marrow examination in 40% of treated epileptic patients. It is likely that the mode of action of these drugs is to interfere with folate coenzymes. Administration of folic acid, although improving their mental drive and alertness, generally had a deleterious effect on fit frequency suggesting that folate was neutralizing the action of the antiepileptic drug (Reynolds, 1967).

Intestinal malabsorption. Gluten-sensitive enteropathy usually involves the jejunum more severely than the ileum. Thus folate deficiency is usual, but vitamin B_{12} deficiency occurs in less than one-third of patients.

Tropical sprue has different manifestations in different parts of the world. As seen in South India it produces primarily vitamin B_{12} deficiency and vitamin B_{12} malabsorption. In Singapore it produces megaloblastic anaemia due to folate deficiency. Puerto Rican cases have combined deficiencies of both folate and vitamin B_{12}.

Nutritional folate deficiency. Although it seems probable that failure to eat enough folic acid in the diet is a likely cause of megaloblastic anaemia this is difficult to prove in practice. The diagnosis relies largely on exclusion of other known cases of folate deficiency and in this sense corresponds to an "idiopathic" category in diseases of other organs. Hurdle (1967) has found that old people with possible megaloblastic changes were taking only about 50 μg. of free folate in their diets which was less than a quarter of the folate intake of healthy control subjects. Such a diagnosis is likely in people eating only tea and toast, etc., over long periods (Gough, Read, McCarthy & Waters, 1963).

SIDEROBLASTIC ANAEMIAS

These anaemias, like those of thalassaemia and the anaemia of chronic infections are characterized by a failure to incorporate iron into haemoglobin. The disorder may appear in children, being transmitted as a sex-linked recessive characteristic in male siblings, or it may be acquired in adult life.

The diagnosis should be suspected from the peripheral blood film by the presence of a dimorphic blood picture, i.e. the simultaneous presence of hypochromic and normochromic red cells. Such an appearance in the blood usually results from iron therapy in an iron-deficiency anaemia or from transfusion of normochromic cells to an iron-deficient subject. Here this appears in the absence of these factors.

The marrow appearance is variable from an accumulation of basophilic erythroblasts on the one hand to the presence of late pyknotic normoblasts with irregular nuclei and "empty" or basophilic cytoplasm on the other. The clue is provided by the marrow stained by Perls' method for iron and this shows that the iron granules in normoblasts are arranged as a circle or semi-circle around the nucleus—this has been termed the "ringed sideroblast". The serum iron and the iron-binding capacity are generally normal. On occasion this anaemia may be associated with other evidence of iron overload including cirrhosis and skin pigmentation.

The anaemia is frequently associated with apparent deficiency of two other substances, viz. folic acid and pyridoxine. Folate deficiency may be suspected by a megaloblastic overlay in the marrow and this disappears with a variable haematological improvement on folate therapy. Pyridoxine "deficiency" is not necessarily accompanied here by abnormal results in the conventional tests for pyridoxine deficiency such as xanthurenic acid excretion, and only a therapeutic trial with large doses of pyridoxine (100 to 200 mg. daily) can decide whether any benefit appears. A significant proportion of younger patients achieve considerable haematological improvement with therapy but relapse on its withdrawal. Older patients tend to be resistant to therapy and may require transfusion. A similar form of anaemia may arise as a result of treatment with pyridoxine antagonists used in tuberculosis. These include cycloserine and pyrizinamide.

References

ANDERSON, B. (1964). *J. clin. Path.*, **17**, 14.

ANDERSON, B. (1965). *Ph.D. Thesis*, London.

ANDERSON, B., BELCHER, E. H., CHANARIN, I. & MOLLIN, D. L. (1960). *Brit. J. Haemat.*, **6**, 439.

ANDERSSEN, N. (1964). *Scand. J. Haemat.*, **1**, 212.

ARDEMAN, S. & CHANARIN, I. (1963). *Lancet*, **2**, 1350.

ARDEMAN, S., CHANARIN, I., KRAFCHIK, B. & SINGER, W. (1966). *Quart. J. Med.*, **35**, 421.

ARMSTRONG, B. K. & WOODLIFF, H. J. (1966). *Med. J. Aust.*, **1**, 709.

BAINTON, D. F. & FINCH, C. A. (1964). *Amer. J. Med.*, **37**, 62.

BAIRD, I. M., BLACKBURN, E. K. & WILSON, G. M. (1959). *Quart. J. Med.*, **28**, 21.

BAKER, S. J., KUMAR, S. & SWAMINATHAN, S. P. (1965). *Lancet*, **1**, 685.

BANK, A. & MARKS, P. (1966). *J. clin. Invest.*, **45**, 330.

BARAKAT, R. M. & EKINS, R. P. (1961). *Lancet*, **2**, 25.

BARKER, H. A., WEISSBACH, H. & SMYTH, R. D. (1958). *Proc. nat. Acad. Sci.*, Wash., **44**, 109.

BASHIR, H. V., HINTERBERGER, H. & JONES, B. P. (1966). *Brit. J. Haemat.*, **12**, 704.

BENDSTRUP, P. (1953). *Acta med. scand.*, **146**, 384.

BERNSTEIN, R. E. (1963). *Clin. chim. Acta.*, **8**, 158.

BEUTLER, E. (1957). *J. lab. clin. Med.*, **49**, 84.

BEUTLER, E. (1965). *Seminars in Hemat.*, **2**, 91.

BEUTLER, E. & BALUDA, M. C. (1964). *Lancet*, **1**, 189.

BEUTLER, E., DERN, R. J. & ALVING, A. S. (1954). *J. lab. clin. Med.*, **44**, 439.

BEUTLER, E. & YEH, M. K. Y. (1963). *Blood*, **21**, 573.

BEVERIDGE, B. R., BANNERMAN, R. M., EVANSON, J. M. & WITTS, L. J. (1965). *Quart. J. Med.*, **34**, 145.

BOOTH, C. C. & MOLLIN, D. L. (1956). *Brit. J. Haemat.*, **2**, 223.

BORSOS, T., DOURMASHKIN, R. & HUMPHREY, J. H. (1964). *Nature*, Lond., **202**, 251.

BOTHWELL, T. H. & FINCH, C. A. (1962). "Iron Metabolism", Churchill, London.

BOWDLER, A. J. & PRANKERD, T. A. J. (1964). *Acta haemat.*, Basel, **31**, 65.

BOWMAN, H. S., McKUSICK, V. A. & DRONAMRAJU, K. R. (1965). *Amer. J. hum. Genet.*, **17**, 1.

BOWMAN, H. S. & PROCOPIO, F. (1963). *Ann. intern. Med.*, **58**, 567.

BRAIN, M. C., DACIE, J. V. & HOURIHANE, D. O'B. (1962). *Brit. J. Haemat.*, **8**, 358.

BREWER, G. J., TARLOV, A. R. & ALVING, A. S. (1960). *Bull. Wld. Hlth. Org.*, **22**, 633.

BREWER, G. J., TARLOV, A. R. & KELLERMEYER, R. W. (1961). *J. lab. clin. Med.*, **58**, 217.

BROWNE, E. A. (1957). *Bull. Johns Hopk. Hosp.*, **101**, 115.

BUCHANAN, J. M. (1964). *Medicine*, Balt., **43**, 697.

BURKA, E. R. & MARKS, P. A. (1963). *Nature*, Lond., **199**, 706.

BURNET, M. (1959). *Brit. med. J.*, **2**, 645.

CARSON, P. E., FLANAGAN, C. L., ICKES, C. E. & ALVING, A. S. (1956). *Science*, **124**, 484.

CARSON, P. E. & FRISCHER, H. (1966). *Amer. J. Med.*, **41**, 744.

CARTWRIGHT, G. F. (1966). *Seminars in Hemat.*, **2**, 351.

CARTWRIGHT, G. E. & WINTROBE, M. M. (1949). *J. clin. Invest.*, **28**, 86.

CARTWRIGHT, G. E. & WINTROBE, M. M. (1952). In "Advances in Internal Medicine", **5**. Eds. Dock, W. & Snapper, I. The Year Book Publishers Inc. Chicago.

CASTLE, W. B. (1929). *Amer. J. med. Sci.*, **178**, 748.

CHANARIN, I. (1963). *Brit. J. Haemat.*, **9**, 141.

CHANARIN, I., ANDERSON, B. B. & MOLLIN, D. L. (1958). *Brit. J. Haemat.*, **4**, 156.

CHANARIN, I. & BENNETT, M. C. (1962a). *Brit. med. J.*, **1**, 27.

CHANARIN, I. & BENNETT, M. C. (1962b). *Brit. med. J.*, **1**, 985.

CHANARIN, I., BURMAN, D. & BENNETT, M. C. (1962). *Blood*, **20**, 33.

CHANARIN, I., MacGIBBON, B. M., O'SULLIVAN, W. J. & MOLLIN, D. L. (1959). *Lancet*, **1**, 634.

CHANARIN, I., MOLLIN, D. L. & ANDERSON, B. B. (1958). *Brit. J. Haemat.*, **4**, 435.

CHANARIN, I. and PERRY, J. (1968). *Brit. J. Haemat.*, **14**, 297.

CHANARIN, I., ROTHMAN, D. & BERRY, V. (1965). *Brit. med. J.*, **1**, 480.

CHANARIN, I., ROTHMAN, D. & WATSON-WILLIAMS, E. J. (1963). *Lancet*, **1**, 1068.

CHELDELIN, V. M., WOODS, A. M. & WILLIAMS, R. J. (1943). *J. Nutr.*, **26**, 477.

CHUNG, A. S. M., PEARSON, W. N., DARBY, W. J., MILLER, O. N. & GOLDSMITH, G. A. (1961). *Amer. J. clin. Nutr.*, **9**, 573.

COGHILL, N. F. & WILLIAMS, A. W. (1958). *Proc. roy. Soc. Med.*, **51**, 464.

CONRAD, M. E. & CROSBY, W. H. (1962). *Blood*, **20**, 173.

CONRAD, E. V., MEYNELL, M. J., GADDIE, R. & COOKE, W. T. (1959). *Lancet*, **2**, 998.

COX, E. V. & WHITE, A. V. (1962). *Lancet*, **2**, 853.

CROME, P. & MOLLISON, P. L. (1964). *Brit. J. Haemat.*, **10**, 137.

CROSBY, W. H. (1952). *Blood*, **7**, 261.

DACIE, J. V. (1960). "The haemolytic anaemias", part 1. The congenital anaemias, Churchill, London.

DACIE, J. V. (1962). "The haemolytic anaemias", part 2. The auto-immune anaemias, 2nd Ed. Churchill, London.

DEGRUCHY, G. C., SANTAMARIA, J. W., PARSONS, I. C. & CRAWFORD, H. (1960). *Blood*, **16**, 1371.

ELLENBOGEN, L. & HIGHLEY, D. R. (1967). *J. biol. Chem.*, **242**, 1004.

FISHER, J. M., REES, C. & TAYLOR, K. B. (1966). *Lancet*, **2**, 88.

FLEMING, A. F. & ELLIOTT, B. A. (1964). *Brit. med. J.*, **2**, 1108.

FREIREICH, E. J., MILLER, A., EMERSON, C. P. & ROSS, J. F. (1957). *Blood*, **12**, 972.

GIORGIO, A. J. & PLANT, G. W. E. (1965). *J. lab. clin. Med.*, **66**, 667.

GIRDWOOD, R. H. (1956). *Quart. J. Med.*, **25**, 87.

GLASS, G. B. J., BOYD, L. J. & STEPHANSON, L. (1954). *Science*, **120**, 74.

GOLDWASSER, E., JACOBSON, L. O., FRIED, W. & PLZAK, L. (1957). *Science*, **125**, 1085.

GOMPERTZ, D., JONES, J. H. & KNOWLES, J. P. (1967). *Lancet*, **1**, 424.

GOUGH, K. R., READ, A. E., McCARTHY, C. F. & WATERS, A. H. (1963). *Quart. J. Med.*, **32**, 243.

GRÄSBECK, R., GORDIN, R., KANTERO, I. & KUHLBÄCK, B. (1960). *Acta med. scand.*, **167**, 289.

GRÄSBECK, R., SIMONS, K. & SINKKONEN, I. (1966). *Biochim. biophys. Acta*, **127**, 47.

GRIMES, A. J., MEISLER, A. & DACIE, J. V. (1964). *Brit. J. Haemat.*, **10**, 281.

GRIMES, A. J., MEISLER, A. & DACIE, J. V. (1964). *Brit. J. Haemat.*, **10**, 403.

GUEST, J. R., FRIEDMAN, S., WOODS, D. D. & SMITH, E. L. (1962). *Nature*, **195**, 340.

GROSSOWICZ, N., SULITZEANU, D. & MERZBACH, D. (1962). *Proc. Soc. exp. Biol.*, N.Y., **109**, 604.

HAHN, P. F., BALE, W. F., ROSS, J. F., BALFOUR, W. M. & WHIPPLE, G. H. (1943). *J. exp. Med.*, **78**, 169.

HAKALA, M. T., ZAKREWSKI, S. F. & NICHOL, C. A. (1960). *Proc. amer. Ass. Cancer Res.*, **3**, 115.

HAMILTON, L., PHILLIPS, F. S., STERNBERG, S. S., CLARKE, D. D. & HITCHINGS, G. H. (1954). *Blood*, **9**, 1062.

HARRIS, E. J. & PRANKERD, T. A. J. (1953). *J. Physiol.*, Lond., **121**, 470.

HARRIS, J. W. (1963). "The Red Cell", Harvard Univ. Press, Mass.

HAURANI, F. I., GREEN, D. & YOUNG, K. (1965). *Amer. J. med. Sci.*, **249**, 537.

HAWKINS, C. F. (1955). *Brit. med. J.*, **1**, 383.

HELLER, P. (1966). *Amer. J. Med.*, **41**, 799.

HELLER, P., YAKULIS, V. J., EPSTEIN, R. B. & FRIEDLAND, S. (1963). *Blood*, **21**, 479.

HERBERT, V. (1962). *Trans. Ass. amer. Physicians*, **65**, 307.

HERBERT, V. & ZALUSKY, R. (1962). *J. clin. Invest.*, **41**, 1263.

HESS, B. & GEHM, B. (1955). *Klin. Wschr.*, **33**, 91.

HEYSSEL, R. M., BOZIAN, R. C., DARBY, W. J. & BELL, M. C. (1966). *Amer. J. clin. Nutr.*, **18**, 176.

HITZIG, W. H. & MASSIMO, L. (1966). *Blood*, **28**, 840.

HOKIN, L. E. & HOKIN, M. R. (1963). *Fed. Proc.*, **22**, 8.

HOLMBERG, C. G., JÖNEMAR, B., NORDEN, E. A., STÅHLBERG, K.-G., & TRYFING, N. (1966). *Scand. J. Haemat.*, **3**, 399.

HUENNEKENS, F. M., CAFFREY, R. W., BASFORD, R. E. & GABRIO, B. W. (1957). *J. biol. Chem.*, **227**, 261.

HUGHES-JONES, N. C. & SZUR, L. (1957). *Brit. J. Haemat.*, **3**, 320.

HURDLE, A. D. F. (1967). M.D. thesis, University of London.

HYMAN, G. A., GELLHORN, A. & HARVEY, J. L. (1956). *Blood*, **11**, 618.

IMERSLUND, O. (1960). *Acta paediat.*, Uppsala, **49**, Suppl. 119.

JACOB, H. S. (1966). *Amer. J. Med.*, **41**, 734.

JACOB, H. S. & JANDL, J. H. (1964). *J. clin. Invest.*, **43**, 1704.

JACOBS, A., LAWRIE, J. H., ENTWISTLE, C. C. & CAMPBELL, H. (1966). *Lancet*, **2**, 190.

JACOBS, A., RHODES, J., PETERS, D. K., CAMPBELL, H. & EAKINS, J. D. (1966). *Brit. J. Haemat.*, **12**, 728.

JAFFE, E. R. (1966). *Amer. J. Med.*, **41**, 786.

JANDL, J. H., RICHARDSON-JONES, A. & CASTLE, W. B. (1957). *J. clin. Invest.*, **36**, 1428.

JANDL, J. H., SIMMONS, R. L. & CASTLE, W. B. (1961). *Blood*, **18**, 133.

JEFFREY, M. R. (1953). *Blood*, **8**, 502.

KAUFMAN, S. (1958). *J. biol. Chem.*, **230**, 931.

KEITT, A. S. (1966). *Amer. J. Med.*, **41**, 762.

KNOWLES, J. P., PRANKARD, T. A. J. & WESTALL, R. G. (1960). *Lancet*, **2**, 347.

KOHN, J., MOLLIN, D. L. & ROSENBACH, L. M. (1961). *J. clin. Path.*, **14**, 345.

KORNBERG, A. & HORECKER, B. L. (1955). In "Methods in Enzymology", vol. 1, p. 323. Ed. Colowick, S. P. & Kaplan, N. O. Acad. Press, N.Y.

LAU, K.-S., GOTTLIEB, C., WASSERMAN, L. R. & HERBERT, V. (1965). *Blood*, **26**, 202.

LAURELL, C. B. (1947). *Acta. physiol. scand.*, **14**, Suppl. 46, 1.

LEEVY, C. M., CARDI, L., FRANK, O., GELLONE, R. & BAKER, H. (1965). *Amer. J. clin. Nutr.*, **17**, 259.

LEHMANN, H. & HUNTSMAN, R. G. (1966). "Man's Haemoglobins", North-Holland Publishing Co., Amsterdam.

LIBNOCH, J. A., YAKULIS, V. J. & HELLER, P. (1966). *Amer. J. clin. Path.*, **45**, 302.

LINDSTRAND, K. (1964). *Nature*, Lond., **204**, 188.

LÖHR, G. W. & WALLER, H. D. (1962). *Med. Klin.*, **57**, 1521.

LOUS, P. & SCHWARTZ, M. (1959). *Acta med. scand.*, **164**, 407.

LUHBY, A. L., COOPERMAN, J. M. & TELLER, D. N. (1959). *Proc. Soc. exp. Biol.*, N.Y., **101**, 350.

LYNGAR, E. (1962). *Nord. Med.*, **14**, 1246.

LYON, M. F. (1961). *Nature*, Lond., **190**, 372.

MACIVER, J. E. & BACK, E. H. (1960). *Arch. Dis. Childhd.*, **35**, 134.

MADDY, A. H. & MALCOLM, B. R. (1965). *Science*, **150**, 1616.

MAGEE, H. E. & MILLIGAN, E. H. M. (1951). *Brit. med. J.*, **2**, 1307.

MARKS, P. A. & BURKA, E. R. (1964). *Science*, **144**, 552.

MARSTON, H. R., ALLEN, S. H. & SMITH, R. M. (1961). *Nature*, Lond., **190**, 1085.

MAYER, M. M. (1961). "Experimental Immunochemistry". 2nd ed. Eds. Kabat, E. A. & Mayer, M. M. Charles C. Thomas, Springfield.

MEHTA, B. M., REGE, D. V. & SATOSKAR, R. S. (1964). *Amer. J. clin. Nutr.*, **15**, 77.

MILLER, D. R., BLOOM, G. E., STREIFF, R. R., LOBUGLIO, A. I. & DIAMOND, L. K. (1966). *New Engl. J. Med.*, **275**, 978.

MOHLER, D. N. (1965). *J. clin. Invest.*, **44**, 1417.

MOLLIN, D. L. (1959). *Brit. med. Bull.*, **15**, 8.

MOLLIN, D. L. & HOFFBRAND, A. V. (1965). In "Vitamin B$_{12}$ and Folic Acid". Ed. Bjorkman, S. E. p. 1. Munksgaard, Copenhagen.

MOLLIN, D. L. & ROSS, G. I. M. (1957). In "Vitamin B$_{12}$ und intrinsic Faktor". Ed. Heinrich, H. C. p. 413. F. Enke, Stuttgart.

MOLLIN, D. L., WATERS, A. H. & HARRISS, E. (1961). In "Vitamin B$_{12}$ und intrinsic Faktor". Ed. Heinrich, H. C. p. 737. F. Enke, Stuttgart.

MOLLISON, P. L. (1962). *Proc. roy. Soc. Med.*, **55**, 915.

NEWTON, W. A. & BASS, J. C. (1958). *Amer. J. Dis. Child.*, **96**, 501.

OORT, M., LOOS, J. A. & PRINS, H. K. (1961). *Vox Sang.*, **6**, 370.

OSKI, F. A. & DIAMOND, L. K. (1963). *New Engl. J. Med.*, **269**, 763.

ØSTERGAARD KRISTENSEN, H. P. & HALD, T. (1962). *Danish med. Bull.*, **9**, 167.

PRANKERD, T. A. J. (1960). *Quart. J. Med.*, **29**, 199.

REISNER, E. H., WOLFF, J. A., MCKAY, R. J. & DOYLE, E. F. (1951). *Pediatrics*, **8**, 88.

REYNOLDS, E. H. (1967). *Lancet*, **1**, 1086.

REYNOLDS, E. H., CHANARIN, I., MILNER, G. & MATTHEWS, D. M. (1966). *Epilepsia*, **7**, 261.

REYNOLDS, E. H., MILNER, G., MATTHEWS, D. M. & CHANARIN, I. (1966). *Quart. J. Med.*, **35**, 521.

ROSENBLUM, C. (1962). In "Vitamin B$_{12}$ und intrinsic Faktor". Ed. Heinrich, H. C. p. 306. F. Enke, Stuttgart.

ROSSE, W. F., DOURMASHKIN, R. & HUMPHREY, J. H. (1966). *J. exp. Med.*, **123**, 969.

SANSONE, G., ROSORE-QUARTINO, A. & VENEZIANO, G. (1963). *Pathologica*, **55**, 371.

SANTINI, R., BERGER, F. M., SHEEHY, T. W., AVILES,J. & DAVILA, I. (1962). *J. amer. diet. Ass.*, **14**, 562.

SCHEINDER, A. S., VALENTINE, W. N., HATTORI, M. & HEINS, H. L. (1965). *New Engl. J. Med.*, **272**, 229.

SCHILLING, R. F. (1953). *J. lab. clin. Med.*, **42**, 860.

SCHRIER, S. L. (1966). *Amer. J. Physiol.*, **210**, 139.

SCHRÖTER, W. (1965). *Klin. Wschr.*, **43**, 1147.

SCOTT, E. M., DUNCAN, I. W. & EKSTRAND, V. (1965). *J. biol. Chem.*, **240**, 481.

SCOTT, E. M. & MCGRAW, J. C. (1962). *J. biol. Chem.*, **237**, 249.

SELWYN, J. G. & DACIE, J. V. (1954). *Blood*, **9**, 414.

SHAPIRO, J., ALBERTS, H. W., WELCH, P. & METZ, J. (1965). *Brit. J. Haemat.*, **11**, 498.

SJÖBERG, K.-H. (1966). *Acta med. scand.*, **179**, 157.

SKOU, J. C. (1965). *Physiol. Rev.*, **45**, 596.

SMITH, E. L., MERVYN, L. JOHNSON, A. W. & SHAW, N. (1962). *Nature*, Lond., **94**,1175.

SMITH, L. H., HUGULEY, C. M. & BAIN, J. A. In "The metabolic basis of inherited disease". 2nd ed. Ed. Stanburg, J. B., Wyngaarden J. B. & Fredrickson, D. S. McGraw-Hill, New York.

STAMEY, C. C. & DIAMOND, L. K. (1957). *Amer.J. Dis. Child.*, **94**, 616.

STEVENS, A. R., PIRZIO-BIROLI, G., HARKINS, H. N., NYHUS, L. M. & FINCH, C. A. (1959). *Ann. Surg.*, **149**, 534.

STOKSTAD, E. L. R. & KOCH, J. (1967). *Physiol. Rev.*, **47**, 83.

SULLIVAN, L. W. & HERBERT, V. (1964). *J. clin. Invest.*, **43**, 1048.

SWENDSEID, M. E., BURTON, F. I. & BETHELL, F. H. (1943). *Proc. Soc. exp. Biol.*, N.Y., **52**, 202.

TANAKA, K. R., VALENTINE, W. N. & MIWA, S. (1962). *Blood*, **19**, 267.

TASKER, P. W. G. (1959). *Trans. roy. Soc. trop. Med. Hyg.*, **53**, 291.

TÖNZ, O. & BETKE, K. (1962). *Klin. Wschr.*, **40**, 649.

TÖNZ, O. & ROSSI, E. (1964). *Nature*, Lond., **202**, 606.

TURNBULL, A. L. (1967). *Brit. J. Haemat.*, **13**, 752.

VALENTINE, W. N., OSKI, F. A., PAGLIA, D. E., BANGHAN, M. A., SCHNEIDER, A. S. & NAIMAN, J. L. (1967). *New Engl. J. Med.*, **276**, 1.

VALENTINE, W. N., SCHNEIDER, A. S., BANGHAN, M. A., PAGLIA, D. E. & HEINS, H. L. (1966). *Amer. J. Med.*, **41**, 27.

VALENTINE, W. N., TANAKA, K. R. & MIWA, S. (1961). *Trans. Ass. amer. Physicians*, **74**, 100.

VANLAIR, C. & MASIUS (1871). *Bull. Acad. roy. Méd. Belg.*, **5**, 3rd series, 515.

VITALE, J. J., SETA, K. & HELLERSTEIN, E. E. (1965). *Fed. Proc.*, **24,** 718.

WALERYCH, W., VENKATARAMAN, S. & JOHNSON, C. B. (1966). *Fed. Proc.*, **25,** 785.

WALT, F., HOLMAN, S. & HENDRICKSE, R. G. (1956). *Brit. med. J.*, **1,** 119.

WATERS, A. H. & MOLLIN, D. L. (1963). *Brit. J. Haemat.*, **9,** 319.

WAYS, P. & DONG, D. (1965). *Clin. Res.*, **13,** 283.

WEAVER, J. A. & NEILL, D. W. (1954). *Lancet*, **1,** 1212.

WEED, R. I. & REED, C. F. (1965). *Blood*, **26,** 894.

WEED, R. I. & REED, C. F. (1966). *Amer. J. Med.*, **41,** 681.

WHITTAM, R. (1964). "Transport and Diffusion in Red Blood Cells". Williams & Wilkins, Baltimore.

WOODS, D. D., FOSTER, H. A. & GUEST, J. R. (1965). In "Transmethylation and methionine biosynthesis". Ed. Shapiro, S. K. & Schlenk, F. Univ. Chicago Press, Chicago.

WRIGHT, L. D. & WELCH, A. D. (1943). *Amer. J. med. Sci.*, **206,** 128.

YOUNG, L. E. (1955). *Trans. Ass. amer. Physicians.*, **68,** 141.

Chapter 7

IDIOPATHIC HAEMOCHROMATOSIS AND RELATED IRON STORAGE DISORDERS

by

ROBERT W. CHARLTON and THOMAS H. BOTHWELL*

C.S.I.R. Iron and Red Cell Metabolism Group, Department of Medicine, University of the Witwatersrand

THERE are normally between 3 and 4 g. of iron in the body of an adult (Granick, 1958). Two-thirds of this is *functional* iron, in the form of haemoglobin, myoglobin and tissue enzymes, while the surplus is deposited as *storage* iron in a number of organs. It is this fraction which is abnormally increased in the iron storage diseases.

The classical disease characterized by massive deposits of iron in the body is idiopathic haemochromatosis. In 1935 Sheldon analysed over 300 reported cases of this condition. He noted that the clinical disease usually manifested itself in middle age and that there were several characteristic features. Cirrhosis of the liver was invariable, while diabetes, skin pigmentation and endocrine changes were usually present.

Over the next 25 years much was learned about the exchange of iron between man and his environment. The limited capacity of the body to excrete the metal and the important role of the absorptive mechanism as a regulator of the body iron content were defined. Information of this type has led to the concept that idiopathic haemochromatosis is the end-result of a metabolic error in which iron balance is disturbed, with daily absorption slightly greater than excretion (Finch & Finch, 1955). At the same time it has become clear that iron overload can arise in other ways. It has been found to occur in subjects exposed over long periods to excessive quantities of dietary iron and it has been noted also in patients who have received many blood transfusions.

To understand the pathogenesis and significance of these different forms of iron overload it is first necessary to consider the normal pathways of iron exchange between man and his environment, and the factors which influence the distribution of iron within the body.

BODY IRON TURNOVER

Iron Excretion

It is essential to appreciate the limited loss of iron from the body. In the normal adult male the

* In receipt of grants from the National Institutes of Health, U.S.A. (AM04912-06) and from the Atomic Energy Board, South Africa.

total excretion amounts to between 0·5 and 1·0 mg. daily (Dubach, Moore & Callender, 1955; Moore, 1965). Most of this iron is lost in the faeces, where it is derived from the intracellular iron of exfoliated epithelial cells and from red blood cells. Small amounts of iron in desquamated cells from the genito-urinary tract and skin make up the total. The urinary iron loss is less than 0·1 mg. daily (Dagg, Smith & Goldberg, 1966), and desquamated epidermal epithelium contains approximately 0·2 mg. (Green, Charlton, Seftel, Bothwell, Mayet, Adams, Finch & Layrisse, 1968). It has been postulated that excessive sweating in the tropics may increase the daily iron loss from the skin to several mg. However, recent evidence suggests that the amount of iron lost by this route probably never exceeds 0·5 mg./day, even under the most extreme conditions (Moore, 1965; Green et al., 1966).

Menstruation and childbearing profoundly affect iron balance. The menstrual blood loss per period varies from 0·7 ml. to more than 500 ml., the median being about 25 to 30 ml. (Hallberg, Nilsson, Hogdahl & Rybo, 1965). In terms of daily iron balance this increases the mean excretion in normal women to approximately 1·3 mg., as compared with 0·6 mg. in males. Losses associated with pregnancy are also important. A quantity is donated to the foetus, blood is shed during parturition, and lactation represents a further loss. The total may amount to anything from 400 to 1000 mg. (Moore, 1965). This is balanced to a variable extent by amenorrhoea, and the net result can be an iron loss no greater than usual, or a loss as much as double the non-pregnant figure. Iron deficiency is therefore much commoner in females than it is in males and iron overload is much rarer. Iron deficiency in males with a reasonable dietary intake of iron is nearly always the result of pathological blood loss, and this is usually from the gastro-intestinal tract.

When the total body iron content is raised, iron excretion is somewhat increased. This is mainly due to the fact that each desquamated epithelial cell contains slightly more iron. However, there is some evidence that an additional mechanism for iron excretion exists in states of iron overload. Macrophages packed with iron are said to pass from the lamina propria of the intestine into the lumen (Thirayothin & Crosby, 1962; Astaldi, Meardi & Lisino, 1966). The maximum amount of iron which can be excreted when the body iron stores are increased is the subject of controversy at the present time. Some workers believe that it may be as much as 4 mg. per day (Crosby, Conrad & Wheby, 1963) while others have calculated it to be

not more than 2 mg. (Green et al., 1966). For the present purpose the quantity which can be lost is not important; the point which must be appreciated is that there are situations in which the excretory mechanisms of the body are inadequate to prevent the accumulation of massive iron deposits.

Since iron excretion is limited in the absence of blood loss, it follows that the iron content of the body is largely determined by the amounts absorbed from the gut.

Iron Absorption

Iron salts. Most of the information concerning the absorption of iron has been obtained from studies carried out with iron salts. Absorption takes place predominantly in the duodenum, and progressively diminishes down the small intestine (Brown & Justus, 1958). The amount absorbed is influenced both by factors acting within the lumen of the intestine and by the behaviour of the mucous membrane. Luminal factors affecting absorption include the amount and chemical form of the dietary iron, the gastric and pancreatic juices, and other dietary constituents such as phosphates, reducing substances and alcohol. Factors acting at the *mucosal* level include the amount of storage iron in the body and the rate of red blood cell production in the marrow.

Luminal factors. Although the intestinal mucous membrane exerts a considerable degree of control over the proportion of available iron taken up, absorption is nevertheless markedly affected by the amount of iron present in the lumen. Although the percentage absorption drops with increasing dosage, there is a progressive rise in the amounts retained (Bothwell, Pirzio-Biroli & Finch, 1958; Smith & Pannacciulli, 1958). The chemical form of the iron is also important. Iron in the ferrous state is absorbed about three times as well as ferric iron (Brise & Hallberg, 1962). While there is some evidence that ferric iron is converted to the ferrous state during its passage across the mucous membrane, the explanation for the greater absorption of ferrous iron may simply lie in its much greater solubility at the luminal pH. It has been shown *in vitro* that reducing the pH enhances the absorption of ferric iron (Jacobs, Bothwell & Charlton, 1966), which is considerably more soluble in acid than at a neutral or alkaline pH. This probably also explains the action of gastric hydrochloric acid in increasing the absorption of ferric iron, an effect which has been firmly established in several human studies (Jacobs, Bothwell & Charlton, 1964).

It seems probable that iron absorption is affected by the secretions of the pancreas as well as by the gastric hydrochloric acid. Several studies have demonstrated that many patients with chronic pancreatitis absorb iron excessively (Davis & Badenoch, 1962; Davis & Biggs, 1964; Deller, 1965). These clinical observations are supported by animal experiments in which pancreatectomy (Taylor, Stiven & Reid, 1931), ligation of the pancreatic duct (Taylor, Stiven & Reid, 1935), or ethionine-induced pancreatic damage (Kinney, Kaufman & Klavins, 1955) was followed by excessive absorption. The availability of the iron is presumably increased if the pancreatic secretions are reduced or abnormal. It is, however, uncertain that this organ plays a significant part in the physiological regulation of iron absorption.

In addition to digestive juices, other substances in the intestinal lumen may influence absorption. The overall effect of food is to diminish the uptake of iron (Sharpe, Peacock, Cooke & Harris, 1950), but certain dietary constituents may *enhance* absorption. These include reducing substances (Brise & Halberg, 1962) and alcohol (Charlton, Jacobs, Seftel & Bothwell, 1964). While the obvious explanation for the action of reducing substances such as ascorbic acid, cysteine and fructose, is the conversion of ferric iron to ferrous within the lumen, there is some evidence that they may also act within the cell to facilitate transport across the mucosa (Pollack, Kaufman & Crosby, 1964). Alcohol stimulates the secretion of gastric hydrochloric acid, and this probably accounts for its effect upon the absorption of ferric iron. These findings may have some relevance to the association between iron overload and the consumption of alcohol. Other substances in the diet *diminish* absorption by reducing the availability of the iron. Phosphates and phytates form insoluble complexes with iron. The eating of clay may be much commoner than is realized, and most clays profoundly depress iron absorption (Minnich, Okcuoglu, Tarcon, Arcasoy, Cin, Yorukoglu, Renda & Demirag, 1968). The association between clay-eating and iron deficiency is well established, and it has been suggested that the clay-eating (pica) is the cause of the iron deficiency.

Mucosal factors. The transport of iron across the mucous membrane into the portal circulation is an active metabolic process (Manis & Schachter, 1962; Jacobs *et al.*, 1966). The proportion of available luminal iron which the mucosal cells take up and transmit into the plasma is variable, and is influenced by factors such as the state of the body iron stores and the activity of the erythroid bone marrow. Absorption is enhanced if there is iron deficiency and depressed when the iron stores

are increased (Bothwell *et al.*,1958). Absorption is also closely linked to the rate of red blood cell production. Absorption is enhanced when erythropoietic activity is increased, and reduced when erythropoiesis is depressed (Bothwell *et al.*, 1958). The association between bone marrow activity and iron absorption is not surprising, since most of the absorbed iron is incorporated into haemoglobin in developing red cells.

While it is theoretically possible that these factors might modify absorption by changes in the secretions reaching the intestinal lumen, there is no convincing evidence that this occurs. The ability to absorb greater or smaller proportions of the available iron is a property of the mucous membrane itself (Manis & Schachter, 1966; Jacobs *et al.*, 1966). Several studies using experimental animals have revealed how the mucosal control of absorption may function. Normally only a proportion of the iron entering epithelial cells from the lumen is transported into the plasma (Conrad & Crosby, 1963; Crosby, 1963). The remainder is sequestered within mucosal cells in the form of ferritin (Charlton, Jacobs, Torrance & Bothwell, 1965). With the constant turnover of the duodenal epithelium, the cells progress towards the tips of the villi and exfoliate together with their trapped iron (Conrad & Crosby, 1963). In rats made avid for iron by venesection or some other manoeuvre, large quantities of iron rapidly cross the mucosa into the plasma, and little or none is sequestered as ferritin. When absorption is depressed, however, most of the iron taken up is held within the mucous membrane, and eventually discarded as the iron-containing cells are replaced from the intestinal crypts.

Dietary iron. Most of the dietary iron is tightly bound in organic molecules. These include haemoglobin, ferritin and haemosiderin from animal sources, plus phytoferritin (Hyde, Hodge, Kahn & Birnstiel, 1963) and a variety of poorly defined compounds in vegetables. Knowledge about the absorption of iron in these various forms is slowly accumulating, and it is apparent that there is considerable variation in availability. In general the iron in animal foodstuffs is more readily available than vegetable iron. The mean absorption of the iron in beef, chicken or fish muscle is about 10% in normal subjects and between 20 and 30% in iron deficiency (Moore & Dubach, 1951; Chodos, Ross, Apt, Pollycove & Halkett, 1957; Layrisse, 1966). The absorption of haemoglobin iron has been studied more fully. Normal individuals absorb about 10% and iron-deficient subjects 20% (Callender, Mallett & Smith, 1957; Turnbull, Cleton & Finch, 1962; Hussain, Walker,

Layrisse, Clark & Finch, 1965; Layrisse, 1966). There is evidence that haemoglobin iron is absorbed in a manner different from inorganic iron. In contrast to iron salts, the absorption of haemoglobin iron is not affected by substances such as reducing agents or phytates (Turnbull *et al.*, 1962).

With the exception of soya bean iron, the iron in vegetables is poorly absorbed. Less than 10% of the iron in wheat, corn, black beans and swiss chard is available even to iron-deficient subjects (Chodos *et al.*, 1957; Hussain *et al.*, 1965; Layrisse, 1966). The unavailability of most plant iron must be an important factor in the genesis of iron deficiency in areas of the world where the staple foodstuffs are of plant origin. Clearly the amount of iron which will be absorbed from a given diet cannot be predicted with any accuracy from the total iron content alone. It is necessary to consider also the chemical forms of iron present in the various constituents.

Normal Iron Balance

In order to maintain iron balance, an adult must absorb enough iron from the diet to make up the amount lost. In males a daily absorption of 0·5 to 1·0 mg. is sufficient, provided there is no blood loss (Moore, 1965). Gastro-intestinal bleeding for any reason, e.g. carcinoma or hookworm infestation, means that larger amounts must be absorbed. The physiological blood loss in females has the same consequence, the amount required depending on the menstrual flow. The daily figure is usually between 1·0 and 2·0 mg. Children need to absorb iron in excess of excretion to allow for growth. To provide a net gain of 0·5 mg. about 1·0 mg. must be absorbed daily. The average Western diet contains 10 to 15 mg. iron, but only a small proportion of this is available. Adult males and many females can absorb enough to stay in balance, but those females whose menstruation is excessive or who bear many children are often unable to replace their losses from the diet, and hence become iron-deficient. There is Swedish evidence that a menstrual blood loss of 60 ml. or more per month produces an iron requirement which cannot be supplied by the diet. As many as 18% of Swedish women fall into this category (Hallberg *et al.*, 1965). Diets in many other parts of the world contain less meat and fish, and consequently even smaller amounts of iron are available for absorption. A greater proportion of the population is therefore unable to maintain iron balance. In contrast, the diet consumed by the Bantu people in Southern Africa contains a large amount of inorganic iron (Walker & Arvidsson, 1953; Bothwell, Seftel, Jacobs, Torrance & Baumslag, 1964). As a consequence iron deficiency is uncommon in this group and iron stores are considerable in a high percentage of the adult population.

Internal Iron Transport and Storage

Iron transport. Iron in transit from one part of the body to another passes through the plasma bound to transferrin. This protein has a molecular weight of about 90,000, and is thought to consist of a single polypeptide chain with the ability to bind two atoms of ferric iron (Surgenor, Koechlin & Strong, 1949). It has the paper electrophoretic mobility of a β_1-globulin (Wallenius, 1952). More recent studies using starch-gel electrophoresis have revealed that there are 18 genetically determined variants, one of these being much commoner than the others (Giblett, 1966). By analogy with the haemoglobin variants, they probably differ from each other as a result of amino acid substitution, and it is possible that other substitutions which do not alter the electrical charge also occur. These transferrin variants do not appear to differ in their ability to bind and transport iron (Turnbull & Giblett, 1961).

The concentration of plasma iron is normally about 100 μg./100 ml., and the total iron-binding capacity slightly over 300 μg./100 ml. (Laurell, 1952). The protein is thus approximately one-third saturated with iron. About 30 mg. iron pass through the plasma each day (Huff, Hennessy, Austin, Garcia, Roberts & Lawrence, 1950; Bothwell, Callender, Mallett & Witts, 1956). Most of this iron is derived from the haemoglobin of red cells broken down in the reticulo-endothelial system and most of the iron leaving the plasma is delivered to the bone marrow. The major cycle of iron within the body thus involves the formation and breakdown of haemoglobin. Little exchange normally occurs between iron in the plasma and other tissues.

Storage iron. A variable amount of storage iron may be present in the body. The size of the stores can be assessed in several ways. During life the most accurate technique is to deplete the stores by repeated phlebotomies until anaemia develops (Finch, Haskins & Finch, 1950). The amount of storage iron can then be calculated from the volume of blood removed. Another method is to measure the urinary iron excretion after injecting a chelating agent such as desferrioxamine; individuals with large stores excrete more iron than normal (Bannerman, Callender & Williams, 1962;

Wohler, 1964; Fielding, 1965; Rosen & Tullis, 1966). The third technique is only applicable to necropsy studies. This is the chemical determination of the concentration of storage iron in the tissues (Mayet & Bothwell, 1964). Finally, a fair estimate can be offered by a trained observer from the histological examination of tissues stained for iron (Bothwell & Bradlow, 1960). However, care has to be exercised since this method has in the past given rise to some confusion (Charlton & Bothwell, 1966).

In general the iron stores in women are smaller than those in men. This reflects not only the greater losses via menstruation and childbearing but also the smaller quantities of food consumed. Individual differences result from variations in the diet and in the quantities lost. In addition to the individual variation, there are considerable differences between populations in different parts of the world. For example, the median hepatic concentration of storage iron in a group of male Indians from New Delhi was found to be 110 μg./ g. wet weight, compared with 831 μg./g. wet weight in male South African Bantu (Bothwell, 1966). Calculations from these figures indicate total body iron stores of approximately 300 to 400 mg. and 3·0 to 4·0 g. respectively. In Western countries the average adult male probably has between 1·0 and 1·5 g. of storage iron and females about half this amount. Iron overload in the haemochromatotic range is present if there is between 15 and 40 g. storage iron in the body (Sheldon, 1935).

The body stores of iron are located in the reticulo-endothelial system and in the parenchymal cells of the liver and skeletal muscles. Although the concentration of iron in the muscles is low, their large bulk makes them an important site for storage (Roth, Jasinski & von Bidder, 1951). There are approximately similar amounts of iron in the muscles, the liver and the bone marrow, with less in the spleen and small deposits in other organs.

Storage iron exists in two forms, *ferritin* and *haemosiderin*. Ferritin is soluble and not normally visible by conventional histological techniques. However, when a great deal is present in a cell a blue flush may appear after staining with potassium ferrocyanide (Cappell, Hutchison & Jowett, 1957). Ferritin is easily recognizable by electron microscopy, the molecules exhibiting a characteristic tetrad of electron-dense particles (Farrant, 1954). Chemically ferritin consists of a protein, apoferritin, and micelles of colloidal iron with the approximate composition $(Fe\ OOH)_8(FeOPO_3H_2)$ (Rothen, 1944; Michaelis, 1947). The molecular

weight of apoferritin is about 480,000 (Harrison, 1963). It is probably composed of 20 identical peptide chains arranged in spheres at the apices of a pentagonal dodecahedron (Harrison, 1963; Richter, 1963). The protein forms a shell around the iron micelles. There are probably six of these which are roughly spherical in shape (Muir, 1960). They are arranged at the vertices of a regular octahedron (Richter, 1963). Ferritin extracted from an organ such as the liver can be separated into fractions of differing iron content (Mazur, Litt & Shorr, 1950). On starch gel or polyacrylamide gel electrophoresis several fractions of different mobility can be demonstrated. These fractions appear functionally and serologically identical, but may differ in their iron contents (Kopp, Vogt & Maass, 1963) It has been shown that ascorbic acid and adenosine triphosphate are necessary for the incorporation of serum-bound iron into ferritin (Mazur, Carleton & Carlsen, 1961). The iron in ferritin exists in the ferric form and there is evidence that it can be removed *in vitro* by a number of reducing agents, leaving the apoferritin intact. It has been shown that the *in vivo* release of iron from ferritin can be effected by the enzyme xanthine oxidase (Mazur, Green, Saha & Carleton, 1958)

When intracellular iron is visible by light microscopy as golden clusters, or as blue granules after staining with potassium ferrocyanide, it is called *haemosiderin*. Haemosiderin is not a single substance. At least five forms have been distinguished (Richter & Bessis, 1965). One type is composed of aggregations of ferritin crystals, while another consists of collections of ferritin molecules without distinct crystalline arrangement. A third variety appears as closely-packed electron-dense particles within a single cytoplasmic membrane; many of the particles can be identified as the iron micelles of individual ferritin molecules. A fourth form is similar, but the iron particles are not ferritin micelles; this type is seen following the injection of parenteral iron preparations such as iron-dextran. Finally, there is a more complex variety of haemosiderin in which iron particles are mixed with lipid or other material. These bodies sometimes contain membranous complexes and have single or multiple unit membranes at their peripheries. It has been suggested that they are iron-loaded organelles.

From a functional as well as from a structural standpoint ferritin and haemosiderin are closely related (Shoden & Sturgeon, 1963). Their distribution is similar, and iron may be mobilized from each when needed (Shoden, Gabrio & Finch, 1953).

PATHOGENESIS OF IRON OVERLOAD

An absolute increase in the iron content of the body may arise in one of two ways. It is either due to excessive absorption from the gut or to the introduction of iron by a parenteral route (Bothwell & Finch, 1962). Absorption from the gut is greater than normal if large quantities of iron are present in the diet. In such circumstances the normal mechanisms for controlling absorption are presumably overwhelmed, and a positive iron balance results. Various sources of this extra iron have been recognized: these include home-brewed alcoholic beverages, wines, iron skillets, well-water and iron medicaments. An increase in the iron content of the body can also occur in conditions where the diet is normal, but in which the behaviour of the absorbing mechanism is deranged. The classical example of such a condition is the inherited metabolic disorder, idiopathic haemochromatosis. There is also recent evidence that inappropriately large amounts of iron may be absorbed from the gut in some subjects with chronic pancreatitis and in others with liver disease. In addition, it is known that iron absorption is increased in a number of so-called "iron-loading" anaemias. These include several chronic refractory anaemias in which there is intensive, but largely ineffective, proliferation of the erythroid marrow. Finally, iron overload can result from the repeated administration of iron given by a parenteral route. This occurs especially in patients with refractory anaemias who are kept alive by repeated blood transfusions. Since each half litre of blood contains approximately 250 mg. iron, such therapy leads to a steady build up in the iron content of the body.

While these different causes for iron overload are moderately clearcut, there is abundant evidence that more than one factor may be operative in certain situations. This is particularly true in the group of "iron-loading" anaemias. Although the inappropriate absorption of dietary iron is often a feature in patients with such disorders, they have usually been given large amounts of medicinal iron at some stage of the disease and have often required multiple blood transfusions. It is therefore clear that the pathogenesis of iron overload is often complex. In spite of this, it is helpful to consider the various types of iron overload under the following broad headings. Excessive amounts of iron may enter the body either *orally* or *parenterally*. *Oral* iron overload may result either from prolonged exposure to a high dietary intake of iron, or from the inappropriate absorption of iron present in normal amounts. *Parenteral* iron overload results either from multiple transfusions in the absence of blood loss, or from the injection of colloidal iron complexes.

Prolonged Exposure to a High Dietary Intake of Iron

In assessing the long-term effects of excessive dietary iron it is helpful to consider the iron overload which occurs in Southern Africa, since there is evidence that the majority of Bantu males are exposed to large quantities throughout their adult lives.

Iron overload in the South African Bantu

Tissue siderosis of varying degrees is very common in the adult Bantu of South Africa (Gillman & Gillman, 1951; Higginson, Gerritsen & Walker, 1953; Bothwell & Isaacson, 1962). The major source of the additional dietary iron is the iron containers used in the preparation of home-brewed alcoholic drinks, and it has been calculated that many Bantu derive between 50 and 100 mg. iron daily from this source alone (Walker & Arvidsson, 1953; Bothwell, Seftel, Jacobs, Torrance & Baumslag, 1964). Of lesser importance as a source of extra iron are the cooking pots which are still used in country areas. The iron in the drinks is inorganic and is absorbed to the same extent as simple ferric salts (Bothwell *et al.*, 1964). Although the proportion of iron absorbed from the daily intake decreases as the stores enlarge (Bothwell *et al.*, 1964), the controlling mechanisms are not able to prevent a net daily gain of about 2 to 4 mg. This is sufficient to account for the deposits found in middle age. In Johannesburg the incidence and severity of siderosis reflect the drinking habits of the Bantu population, so that marked iron overload is common in adult males, much less common in females, and does not occur in children. As many as 20% of Bantu males dying in hospital have hepatic iron concentrations in the range described in idiopathic haemochromatosis, i.e. more than 2% dry weight (Bothwell & Isaacson, 1962).

The distribution of iron in the majority of subjects is a characteristic one, with the major impact on the liver and reticulo-endothelial system (Higginson *et al.*, 1953; Bothwell & Bradlow, 1960). In the earliest phases, haemosiderin granules can be detected in the parenchymal cells of the liver and in Kupffer cells. As the concentration rises, increasing deposits are present in these sites, and haemosiderin is seen also in reticulo-endothelial cells throughout the body. The concentration of iron in the spleen is as high as or higher than that in the liver, and up to 10 g. iron may be stored in the reticulum cells of the bone marrow.

This pattern of distribution usually persists in even the severest grades of siderosis, and a striking feature is the absence of significant parenchymal deposits in organs other than the liver. The distribution is similar to that seen in experimental animals subjected to oral overload, and is quite different from that found in idiopathic haemochromatosis (Bothwell & Finch, 1962).

While a clear distinction can usually be drawn between the pathological findings in Bantu siderosis and in idiopathic haemochromatosis, this is not always so. A small proportion of siderotic Bantu develop portal cirrhosis, and in these subjects there is a redistribution of iron, with excessive deposits in the parenchymal cells of the pancreas, adrenals, thyroid, pituitary and heart (Bradlow, Dunn & Higginson, 1961; Isaacson, Seftel, Keeley & Bothwell, 1961). The reason for the altered distribution of iron in the siderotic Bantu with portal cirrhosis is not established. It may, however, relate to the high percentage saturation of plasma transferrin, since there is experimental evidence that iron is taken up more readily by tissues under such circumstances (Jandl, Inman, Simmons & Allen, 1959). Whatever the reason, there is no doubt that a small proportion of Bantu adults exhibit pathological findings very similar to those which occur in idiopathic haemochromatosis.

The clinical features in such individuals also bear some similarity to the idiopathic disease. For example, the results of one study showed that 20% of Bantu exhibiting siderosis and portal cirrhosis at necropsy were diabetic prior to death (Isaacson et al., 1961). In addition it has been found that between 5 and 10% of Bantu diabetics attending hospital have severe siderosis and portal cirrhosis (Seftel, Keeley, Isaacson & Bothwell, 1961). These patients differ from the majority of middle-aged Bantu diabetics in that they are underweight, and insulin is needed for control of the diabetes. However, clinical evidence of cardiac involvement, which is a distinctive feature in idiopathic haemochromatosis, has not been observed in the Bantu.

There are two other conditions which occur almost exclusively in Bantu adults with severe siderosis. The one is scurvy (Bothwell, Bradlow, Jacobs, Keeley, Kramer, Seftel & Zail, 1964), and the other is a form of marked osteoporosis which is found in middle-aged manual labourers (Grusin & Samuel, 1957). It has been suggested that the occurrence of scurvy in siderotic Bantu may be due to irreversible oxidation of available ascorbic acid by the iron deposits (Schulz & Swanepoel, 1962). Some support for this contention is provided by the fact that it is difficult to "saturate" such subjects with ascorbic acid. In addition, it has been shown that the administration of the vitamin to siderotic Bantu is followed by the urinary excretion of large quantities of oxalic acid, which is a major breakdown product of ascorbic acid (Seftel, Charlton, Jacobs & Bothwell, 1964). These findings may have some relevance to the collapse of lumbar vertebrae which occurs in middle-aged Bantu. Such subjects are not only heavily siderotic, but also often exhibit evidence of past or present scurvy (Seftel, Malkin, Schmaman, Abrahams, Lynch, Charlton & Bothwell, 1966)) It is known that ascorbic acid is necessary for the formation of bone matrix, and that guinea pigs maintained on a diet low in ascorbic acid develop osteoporosis (Hojer, 1923; Vilter, 1954). It is therefore possible that the irreversible oxidation of available ascorbic acid by heavy iron deposits may play a role in the causation of osteoporosis in the Bantu.

Other sources of excess dietary iron. It has been shown that most European and American wines contain several milligrams of iron per litre (MacDonald, 1963). In addition, there is evidence that alcohol itself potentiates the absorption of ferric iron by the gut (Charlton & Bothwell, 1966). On this basis, it might be expected that a form of dietary siderosis similar to that occurring in the Bantu, would be encountered in alcoholic subjects in other parts of the world. Indeed, it has been suggested that haemochromatosis in Western countries is always of this type (MacDonald, 1964). It should however, be noted that the mean iron content in most wines is approximately ten times *less* than that in the beverages consumed by the Bantu. This implies that very large quantities of wine would have to be consumed for severe siderosis to develop, and that the condition would therefore only occur in social derelicts. Direct chemical analysis of approximately 3000 necropsy specimens of liver from 15 countries has confirmed the rarity of severe siderosis in other population groups (Bothwell, 1967). Only three subjects had hepatic iron concentrations above 1% dry weight. In another study the chemical concentrations of hepatic iron were correlated with the previous drinking habits. Although the mean concentrations in heavy drinkers were somewhat raised, they were many times less than those found in siderotic Bantu (Powell, 1966). There is further evidence to indicate that *severe* dietary siderosis is rare outside South Africa. Since alcoholic drinks have been postulated as the major source of the extra dietary iron, it would be anticipated that significant iron overload would be common in alcoholic subjects with portal fibrosis or cirrhosis. The results of several studies indicate that this is not so (Kent & Popper, 1960; Zimmerman, Chomet, Kulesh & McWhorter, 1961; Block, Moore, Wasi & Haiby, 1965).

Other sources of excess dietary iron include well-water (Hiyeda, 1939), iron skillets (Moore, 1965) and medicaments (Turnberg, 1965). Severe siderosis has been described in Manchuria, and its incidence has been correlated with the high iron content of the local water (Hiyeda, 1939). The significance of the association is, however, not clear, and the condition includes certain bizarre features which seem to be unrelated to iron overload. Finally there are isolated well-documented examples of seemingly normal subjects who have developed iron overload after years of ill-advised iron medication (Turnberg, 1965).

Inappropriate Absorption from a Diet of Normal Iron Content

There are several conditions in which the absorbing mechanism for iron is disordered, so that increased amounts are absorbed from a normal diet. These include the disease idiopathic haemochromatosis, certain chronic refractory anaemias, chronic pancreatitis and both acute and chronic liver disease.

Idiopathic haemochromatosis. Idiopathic haemochromatosis is a rare hereditary disorder in which increased absorption of iron from the diet leads to excessive deposits of tissue iron (Finch & Finch, 1955; Bothwell & Finch, 1962). The disease is most often recognized clinically between the ages of 40 and 60 years, when the iron content of the body is usually between 15 and 40 g. These massive deposits can be adequately explained on a positive iron balance of 2 to 3 mg. daily occurring over many years. In the final clinical phase of the disorder cirrhosis of the liver is a feature, while diabetes, skin pigmentation and cardiac failure are often present (Sheldon, 1935; Finch & Finch, 1955).

Although it has been customary in the past to regard idiopathic haemochromatosis as a specific clinical and pathological entity, this concept has been broadened in the last few years. Since the disorder leads to disturbed iron balance, it is obvious that other factors which also affect iron balance may influence the expression of the disease in a given individual. Thus, more severe involvement would be expected if the dietary iron content were high, while only minor degrees of siderosis would occur if there were a small amount of iron in the diet. It is also apparent that the rate of iron loss from the body is of fundamental importance.

For example, the *clinical* manifestions of idiopathic haemochromatosis are uncommon in females. This can be explained by the fact that females tend to eat less than males and, in addition, they have greater physiological losses via menstruation and pregnancies. There is further evidence to show that other factors may also modify the course of the disorder. The most important of these is excessive consumption of alcohol. At least 30% of subjects with clinical manifestations give a history of having consumed excessive quantities of alcohol (Finch & Finch, 1955). There are several possible reasons for this association. It is known that many wines contain significant amounts of iron (MacDonald, 1963) and that alcohol itself may potentiate the absorption of iron (Charlton et al., 1964). In addition it seems probable that the deleterious effects of alcohol on the liver potentiate tissue damage, and so may precipitate liver failure in subjects who might otherwise have remained in an asymptomatic stage of the condition (Bothwell & Finch, 1962). These points are raised in order to underline the fact that subjects with clinical evidence of idiopathic haemochromatosis represent only a small proportion of affected individuals.

Genetic aspects. Evidence that idiopathic haemochromatosis is the result of an inborn error of metabolism has been obtained using a number of approaches (Crosby, 1966). Firstly, there are reports of more than one member of a family having suffered from the clinical disease (Bothwell & Finch, 1962). Secondly, increased iron stores have been demonstrated in affected relatives in several ways. These include the finding of elevated serum iron levels (Finch & Finch, 1955; Debre, Dreyfus, Frezal, Labie, Lamy, Maroteaux, Schapira & Schapira, 1958), varying degrees of excess storage iron found on liver biopsy (Bothwell, Cohen, Abrahams & Perold, 1959; Brick, 1961; Williams, Scheuer & Sherlock, 1962), and increased urinary excretion of iron after the administration of chelating agents (Powell, 1965). In addition, the degree of iron overload in some relatives has been assessed by subjecting them to repeated venesections (Perkins, McInnes, Blackburn & Beal, 1965; Balcerzak, Westerman, Lee & Doyle, 1966). Finally, increased absorption of iron has been demonstrated in a proportion of relatives of subjects with the disease (Williams, Pitcher, Parsonson & Williams, 1965; Balcerzak et al., 1966). The result of such studies suggest that the metabolic defect is inherited as an autosomal dominant (Balcerzak et al., 1966). However, the variation in the quantities of iron accumulated by affected members of families from the same household suggests that the expression of the gene is not uniform. The development of full-blown haemochromatosis by the age of 20 when neither parent exhibits more than minimal evidence of iron overload has been reported several times. These observations have led to the hypothesis that such individuals may be homozygotes. If this is correct, then the gene may perhaps be more accurately described as an intermediate rather than a dominant one (Williams *et al.*, 1962).

Nature of the metabolic defect. The nature of the metabolic defect in this condition has not yet been established. It has been suggested that the primary disorder lies in the pancreas. Pancreatic disease sometimes results in increased iron absorption, and the volume of pancreatic juice after secretin stimulation has been found to be abnormally increased in haemochromatosis (Marks & Banks, 1963; Perman & Bonera, 1964). However, this last abnormality may simply be a manifestation of cirrhosis. A second possibility is a defect in the mucosal apparatus for controlling iron absorption. It is easy to imagine how progressive iron overload could result from minor derangements in the mechanism whereby unwanted iron is sequestered in the form of ferritin within mucosal cells. Although there is as yet no definite evidence of such a derangement, it is of interest that small accumulations of ferritin are visible in the epithelial cells of the intestinal villi of normal humans on electron microscopy. It has been stated that these ferritin bodies are less frequently encountered in subjects with idiopathic haemochromatosis (Hartman, Conrad, Hartman, Joy & Crosby, 1963). A third possibility which has been investigated is that the plasma transferrin may be abnormal. No differences, however, have been detected on starch gel electrophoresis, salting out procedures and immunoprecipitin studies (Bothwell, Jacobs & Torrance, 1962). In addition, the *in vivo* clearance of iron bound to plasma from affected individuals is normal (Bothwell *et al.*, 1962; Wheby, Balcerzak, Anderson & Crosby, 1964). However, the uptake of iron *in vitro* has been reported to be more rapid (Ross, Kochwa & Wasserman, 1964). Finally, it is possible that the liver has an abnormal affinity for the metal in this disorder, and that the increased absorption from the gut is secondary to this. In this context there is some evidence that excessive amounts of plasma iron are taken up by the liver in subjects with the disease, even after energetic venesection therapy (Williams, Manenti, Williams & Pitcher 1966).

Possibly none of these suggested sites will eventually be established as the location of the metabolic error. It is also possible that more than one genetic abnormality has the same functional effect, and that there may be several types of idiopathic haemochromatosis.

Pathological findings. In the fully developed disease, widespread deposits of iron are visible as haemosiderin granules in the parenchymal cells of many organs. Several grams of iron are present in the liver, and concentrations are more than 10 times normal in the pancreas, thyroid, pituitary and heart. Lesser concentrations are present in the adrenal, spleen, kidney, testis, stomach and skin (Sheldon, 1935; Finch & Finch, 1955). In the liver the major deposits are in the parenchymal cells and lesser quantities are found in the Kupffer cells and in the portal tracts. The relatively low concentrations in the reticulo-endothelial cells of the liver, spleen and bone marrow are in striking contrast to the findings in Bantu with severe siderosis, since these subjects always show heavy reticulo-endothelial deposits (Bothwell, Abrahams, Bradlow & Charlton, 1965). In the pancreas most of the iron is found in the acini, and the major involvement in the adrenals is in the zona glomerulosa. In the heart, haemosiderin is deposited in the perinuclear regions of the muscle fibres. Associated pathological changes include portal cirrhosis and pancreatic fibrosis. Although the cirrhosis has been regarded as a constant pathological finding, there is recent evidence that hepatic involvement is sometimes less severe in young subjects succumbing to the cardiac complications of the disease (Charlton, Abrahams & Bothwell, 1967).

Clinical presentation. Clinical manifestations of idiopathic haemochromatosis occur 10 times more frequently in males than in females, and when the disease does manifest in females it tends to present at a somewhat later age (Finch & Finch, 1955). The clinical features in both sexes relate mainly to the liver, pancreas, heart and skin. The hepatic manifestations are the result of cirrhosis and its complications. It is, however, noteworthy that hepatic function is often excellent in those subjects not exposed to excessive alcohol (Bothwell & Finch, 1962). Although it is probable that the endocrine manifestations, such as loss of body hair, testicular atrophy, impotence and amenorrhoea, also reflect impaired hepatic function, this is not always so. In young, severely involved subjects the hypogonadism is striking, and yet liver function is usually good. The results of the few endocrine studies which have been done suggest that these manifestations are secondary to pituitary involvement (Bothwell & Finch, 1962). Diabetes is frequently present and is presumably the result of pancreatic damage. Insulin is usually needed for its control. Cardiac complications are common in the disease. The cardiopathy, which is characterized by various arrhythmias and progressive cardiac failure, is the usual cause of death in younger subjects with the disease (Bothwell & Alper, 1951). Skin pigmentation is present in more than 90% of patients. In about half iron deposits are demonstrable, while in the remainder it is the result of excessive melanin (Sheldon, 1935).

Laboratory diagnosis: There are a number of screening procedures of help in diagnosing haemochromatosis. Of these, the simplest is an estimation of the plasma iron level and of the percentage saturation of circulating transferrin. The plasma iron level is usually above 200 μg./100 ml. and the transferrin is completely or almost completely saturated (Bothwell & Finch, 1962). Although the raised plasma iron levels in the condition have been thought to be related to the increased stores, it is noteworthy that they have also been found to be high in some affected relatives at a time when stores were either normal or only moderately increased (Bothwell *et al.*, 1959). Another simple test which is of value is the examination of the urinary sediment for haemosiderin-containing cells, desquamated from the urinary tract (Rous, 1918). Recently more quantitative data have been obtained by measuring the amount of iron passed in the urine after the parenteral administration of desferrioxamine (Wohler, 1964; Ploem, De Wael, Verloop & Punt, 1966). When the screening procedures are positive, a more definite diagnosis can be made by examining a specimen of liver obtained by the puncture technique. It should show heavy parenchymal deposits of iron together with portal cirrhosis. Further confirmation of the diagnosis rests on the amount of excess iron present in the body. If subjects with idiopathic haemochromatosis are repeatedly venesected it is possible to remove more than 15 g. iron before significant anaemia develops (Bothwell & Finch, 1962). The response to venesection therapy therefore provides a useful way of distinguishing between massive iron overload and the lesser degrees which are sometimes present in subjects with alcoholic cirrhosis (Powell, 1965).

It must be appreciated that the various tests for disordered iron metabolism which are of help in diagnosis reflect only the degree of overload and are not specific for idiopathic haemochromatosis. It is therefore necessary to exclude the presence of sources of excessive dietary iron. Final proof of the presence of an inherited metabolic entity depends on the demonstration that a proportion of the patient's relatives exhibit evidence of disordered iron metabolism.

"Iron-Loading" Anaemias. Certain chronic refractory anaemias are sometimes complicated by the presence of severe iron overload. A feature common to them all has been intense, but largely ineffective, erythroid marrow activity (Kent & Popper, 1960). Examples include thalassaemia major, hereditary hypochromic anaemia, pyridoxine-responsive anaemia and refractory haemolytic anaemia associated with glucose-6-phosphate dehydrogenase deficiency. Excessive absorption of iron has been both directly demonstrated in these conditions (Price, Brown & Peters, 1959; Crosby & Sheehy, 1960; Erlandson, Walden, Stern, Hilgartner, Wehman & Smith, 1962; Weintraub, Conrad & Crosby, 1966) and inferred from the presence of considerable iron overload in the rare patient who has received neither medicinal iron nor transfusion (Ellis, Schulman & Smith, 1954; Byrd & Cooper, 1961; Horrigan & Harris, 1964; Canfield, Herman, Herman & Conrad, 1965; Weintraub *et al.*, 1966). In most of the published reports it is difficult to evaluate the relative importance of absorbed iron and of parenterally administered blood in the development of the iron overload. However, it is still possible to evaluate the contribution of orally derived iron in such anaemias if only those patients who were given less than 20 transfusions are considered. In fact, there are a number of reported cases in which little or nothing was given in the way of donor blood, and yet marked iron overload was present at necropsy (Wyatt, Mighton & Moragues, 1950; Bothwell, 1953; Kleckner, Baggenstoss & Weir, 1955; Wyatt, 1956). In an analysis of 22 reported cases who received 5 g. or less iron via transfusions, widespread siderosis was invariably present. Three showed increased portal fibrosis, 19 had portal cirrhosis and four had glycosuria (Bothwell & Finch, 1962). It is therefore apparent that clinical and pathological features very similar to those in idiopathic haemochromatosis are sometimes found in those refractory anaemias in which the overload is due to increased absorption from the gut.

Chronic pancreatitis and liver disease. Iron absorption from the gut is increased in some patients with chronic pancreatitis (Davis & Badenoch, 1962; Deller, 1965). In addition, it has been shown that the administration of pancreatic extract returns the enhanced absorption to normal. Some patients with liver disease also absorb excessively. These include both subjects with acute hepatitis (Turnberg, 1966) and a proportion of those with cirrhosis (Conrad, Berman & Crosby, 1962; Callender & Malpas, 1963; Davis & Biggs, 1964). It is possible that cirrhotic individuals absorb excessively because of associated pancreatic disease (Callender & Malpas, 1963). Folic acid deficiency may also play a part, since it sometimes leads to ineffective erythropoiesis and hence enhanced absorption (Herbert, Zalusky & Davidson, 1963). Although these findings are of interest there is no clear evidence as yet to indicate that any of these diseases leads to severe iron overload. This may relate to the degree of the absorptive defect and/or the length of time during which absorption is abnormal.

Parenteral Iron Overload

It is possible to achieve massive concentrations of iron in the bodies of experimental animals by administering iron complexes parenterally. Such studies have been carried out in a number of animal species using a variety of techniques (Brown, Dubach, Smith, Reynafarje & Moore, 1957). These complexes are taken up by the reticulo-endothelial system, and iron deposits are initially confined there. With the passage of time a certain amount of redistribution may occur, but this is a slow process and parenchymal deposits seldom reach significant proportions. A feature common to all these experimental investigations has been the absence of tissue damage.

In human subjects an analogous situation may arise when repeated transfusions are given over many years. Here, too, the initial impact is on the reticulo-endothelial system, but with the passage of time some redistribution into parenchymal cells occurs (Oliver, 1959; Bothwell & Finch, 1962). In order to gauge the significance of the condition it is helpful to consider only those subjects with aplastic anaemia, since absorption from the gut tends to be reduced when erythropoiesis is depressed (Bothwell *et al.*, 1958; Schiffer, Brann, Cronkite & Reizenstein, 1966). This means that all or almost all the iron eventually present must have been derived from donor blood. An analysis of 20 reported cases of this type who had received more than 100 transfusions revealed that cirrhosis was present in only one, although varying degrees of hepatic fibrosis were noted in 12 (Bothwell & Finch, 1962). These observations, together with those obtained in animal experiments, indicate that iron deposited in the reticulo-endothelial system is relatively innocuous.

RELATIONSHIP BETWEEN IRON OVERLOAD AND TISSUE DAMAGE

From the available evidence there is good reason to believe that iron overload of severe degree is potentially harmful to tissues. This relationship is, however, only a feature when the iron is present in parenchymal cells. A distribution of this type implies that the excessive iron has been derived from the plasma, and it is therefore most prominent in all those situations where absorption from the gut is increased. These include idiopathic haemochromatosis, Bantu siderosis and the "iron-loading" anaemias. Perhaps the best example is the disease idiopathic haemochromatosis, since a typical clinical and pathological picture eventually develops. Portal cirrhosis is the most constant of these manifestations, and there is abundant evidence from studies on relatives that severe hepatic siderosis *precedes* the development of the cirrhosis. This association has also been well demonstrated in siderotic Bantu. Several studies have shown a close relationship between the degree of overload and presence of portal fibrosis or cirrhosis. In one study a comparison was made between the histological findings and the chemical concentrations of iron present in the liver. It was found that moderately severe portal fibrosis or frank cirrhosis was present in the majority of livers in which the concentration of iron was more than 20 times normal (Bothwell & Isaacson, 1962). Although such changes were commoner in the older age groups, the cirrhosis could not be ascribed to this, since older male subjects without siderosis did not have more portal fibrosis than younger ones. The relationship between portal cirrhosis and siderosis was further clarified by another investigation in which measurements were made of iron concentrations in the livers of consecutive groups of Bantu subjects showing macroscopic and microscopic evidence of portal cirrhosis at necropsy (Isaacson *et al.*, 1961). It was found that severe siderosis was almost invariably present. In contrast, there appeared to be no correlation between the presence of post-necrotic cirrhosis and the degree of iron overload.

The incidence of insulin-dependent diabetes in idiopathic and Bantu haemochromatosis adds further weight to the concept that excessive iron deposits can lead to disordered function. While such associations are all suggestive, final proof of the noxious effects of severe siderosis must rest on the demonstration of increased survival rates in patients subjected to repeated venesections. Although there is a growing body of evidence suggesting that repeated phlebotomies ameliorate the course of the disease (Bothwell & Finch, 1962) absolute proof is still lacking. In this context, the cardiac manifestations of idiopathic haemochromatosis are of particular importance because of the uniformly bad prognosis in subjects exhibiting them. Recent isolated reports in which cardiac function has improved both subjectively and objectively after the removal of iron deposits are therefore of special interest (McAllen, Coghill & Lubran, 1957; Mirouze, 1964; Perkins *et al.*, 1965).

In spite of these various associations there are still unexplained discrepancies. For example, there is no doubt that a proportion of Bantu with massive hepatic deposits show little or no tissue damage (Bothwell & Isaacson, 1962). On available evidence it is therefore necessary to postulate that iron is only a low-grade fibrogenic agent, and

that other factors may influence the rate at which such changes develop. Of these the most important is certainly alcoholism, but other factors such as malnutrition, viral hepatitis and unknown toxins may also contribute. On this basis it might be expected that a subject with the metabolic defect associated with idiopathic haemochromatosis would be much more likely to develop clinical manifestations of the disorder if he took excessive alcohol. Such a concept is supported by the fact that siderotic experimental animals rapidly develop cirrhosis if exposed to hepatic toxins (Golberg & Smith, 1960).

References

ASTALDI, G., MEARDI, G. & LISINO, T. (1966). *Blood*, **28**, 70.

BALCERZAK, S. P., WESTERMAN, M. P., LEE, R. E. & DOYLE, A. P. (1966). *Amer. J. Med.*, **40**, 857.

BANNERMAN, R. M., CALLENDER, S. T. & WILLIAMS, D. L. (1962). *Brit. med. J.*, **2**, 1573.

BLOCK, M., MOORE, G., WASI, P. & HAIBY, G. (1965). *Amer. J. Path.*, **47**, 89.

BOTHWELL, T. H. (1953). *S. Afr. J. lab. clin. Med.*, **45**, 167.

BOTHWELL, T. H. (1966). *New Zealand Med. J.* Suppl. **65**, 880.

BOTHWELL, T. H. (1967). Unpublished observations.

BOTHWELL, T. H., ABRAHAMS, C., BRADLOW, B. A. & CHARLTON, R. W. (1965). *Arch Path.*, **79**, 163.

BOTHWELL, T. H. & ALPER, T. (1951). *S. Afr. J. clin. Sci.*, **2**, 226.

BOTHWELL, T. H. & BRADLOW, B. A. (1960). *Arch. Path.*, **70**, 279.

BOTHWELL, T. H., BRADLOW, B. A., JACOBS, P., KEELEY, K. J., KRAMER, S., SEFTEL, H. C. & ZAIL, S. (1964). *Brit. J. Haemat.*, **10**, 50.

BOTHWELL, T. H., CALLENDER, S., MALLETT, B. & WITTS, L. J. (1956). *Brit. J. Haemat.*, **2**, 1.

BOTHWELL, T. H., COHEN, I., ABRAHAMS, O. L. & PEROLD, S. M. (1959). *Amer. J. Med.*, **27**, 730.

BOTHWELL, T. H. & FINCH, C. A. (1962). "Iron Metabolism". Boston, Little Brown & Co.

BOTHWELL, T. H. & ISAACSON, C. (1962). *Brit. med. J.*, **1**, 522.

BOTHWELL, T. H., JACOBS, P. & TORRANCE, J. D. (1962). *S. Afr. J. med. Sci.*, **27**, 35.

BOTHWELL, T. H., PIRZIO-BIROLI, G. & FINCH, C. A. (1958). *J. lab. clin. Med.*, **51**, 24.

BOTHWELL, T. H., SEFTEL, H., JACOBS, P., TORRANCE, J. D. & BAUMSLAG, N. (1964). *Amer. J. clin. Nutr.*, **14**, 47.

BRADLOW, B. A., DUNN, J. A. & HIGGINSON, J. (1961). *Amer. J. Path.*, **39**, 221.

BRICK, I. B. (1961). *Gastroenterology*, **49**, 210.

BRISE, H. & HALLBERG, L. (1962). *Acta med. Scand.* **171** (Supp. 376).

BROWN, E. B., Jnr., DUBACH, R., SMITH, D. E., REYNAFARJE, C. & MOORE, C. V. (1957). *J. lab. clin. Med.*, **50**, 862.

BROWN, E. B., Jnr., & JUSTUS, B. W. (1958). *Amer. J. Physiol.*, **194**, 319.

BYRD, R. B. & COOPER, T. (1961). *Ann. int. Med.*, **55**, 103.

CALLENDER, S. T., MALLETT, B. J. & SMITH, M. D. (1957). *Brit. J. Haemat.*, **3**, 186.

CALLENDER, S. T. & MALPAS, J. S. (1963). *Brit. med. J.*, **2**, 1516.

CANFIELD, C. J., HERMAN, Y. F., HERMAN, R. H. & CONRAD, M. E. (1965). *J. lab. clin. Med.*, **66**, 96.

CAPPELL, D. F., HUTCHISON, H. E. & JOWETT, M. (1957). *J. Path. Bact.*, **74**, 245.

CHARLTON, R. W., ABRAHAMS, C. & BOTHWELL, T. H. (1967). *Arch. Path.*, **83**, 132.

CHARLTON, R. W. & BOTHWELL, T. H. (1966). "Progress in Haematology", Vol. 5, Grune & Stratton, New York.

CHARLTON, R. W., JACOBS, P., SEFTEL, H. & BOTHWELL, T. H. (1964). *Brit. med. J.*, **2**, 1427.

CHARLTON, R. W., JACOBS, P., TORRANCE, J. D. & BOTHWELL, T. H. (1965). *J. clin. Invest.*, **44**, 543.

CHODOS, R. B., ROSS, J. F., APT, L., POLLYCOVE, M. & HALKETT, J. A. E. (1957). *J. clin. Invest.*, **36**, 314.

CONRAD, M. E., Jnr., BERMAN, A. & CROSBY, W. H. (1962). *Gastroenterology*, **43**, 385.

CONRAD, M. E. & CROSBY, W. H. (1963). *Blood*, **22**, 406.

CROSBY, W. H. (1963). *Blood*, **22**, 441.

CROSBY, W. H. (1966). Heredity of Hemochromatosis. *In* "Controversy in Internal Medicine". W. B. Saunders & Co., Philadelphia.

CROSBY, W. H., CONRAD, M. E. & WHEBY, M. S. (1963). *Blood*, **22**, 429.

CROSBY, W. H. & SHEEHY, T. W. (1960). *Brit. J. Haemat.*, **6**, 56.

DAGG, J. H., SMITH, J. A. & GOLDBERG, A. (1966). *Clin. Sci.*, **30**, 495.

DAVIS, A. E. & BADENOCH, J. (1962). *Lancet*, **2**, 6.

DAVIS, A. E. & BIGGS, J. C. (1964). *Australas. Ann. Med.*, **13**, 201.

DEBRE, R., DREYFUS, J. C., FREZAL, J., LABIE, D., LAMY, M., MAROTEAUX, P. SCHAPIRA, F. & SCHAPIRA, G. (1958). *Ann. hum. Genet.*, **23**, 16.

DELLER, D. J. (1965). *Amer. J. dig. Dis.*, **10**, 249.

DUBACH, R., MOORE, C. V. & CALLENDER, S. T. (1955). *J. lab. clin. Med.*, **45**, 599.

ELLIS, J. T., SCHULMAN, I., & SMITH, C. H. (1954). *Amer. J. Path.*, **30**, 287.

ERLANDSON, M. E., WALDEN, B., STERN, G., HILGARTNER, M. W., WEHMAN, J. & SMITH, C. H. (1962). *Blood*, **19**, 359.

FARRANT, J. L. (1954). *Biochim. Biophys. Acta*, **13**, 569.

FIELDING, J. (1965). *J. clin. Path.*, **18**, 88.

FINCH, S. C. & FINCH, C. A. (1955). *Medicine*, **34**, 381.

FINCH, S. C., HASKINS, D. & FINCH, C. A. (1950). *J. clin. Invest.*, **29**, 1078.

GIBLETT, E. R. (1966). XIth Congress of the International Society of Haematology. Plenary Sessions. Sydney, Victor C. N. Blight, Government Printer.

GILLMAN, J. & GILLMAN, T. (1951). "Perspectives in Human Malnutrition". New York, Grune & Stratton.

GOLBERG, L. & SMITH, J. P. (1960). *Amer. J. Path.*, **36**, 125.

GRANICK, S. (1958). "Trace Elements". New York, Academic Press, Inc.

GREEN, R., CHARLTON, R., SEFTEL, H., BOTHWELL, T., MAYET, F., ADAMS B., FINCH, C. & LAYRISSE, M. (1968). *Amer. J. Med.*, **45**, 336.

GRUSIN, H. & SAMUEL E. (1957). *Amer. J. clin. Nutr.*, **2**, 323.

HALLBERG, L., NILSSON, L., HOGDAHL, A. M. & RYBO, G. (1965). *Act. Obstet. Gynec. Scand.*, **43**, Suppl. 7, 57.

HARRISON, P. M. (1963). *J. molecular Biol.*, **6**, 404.

HARTMAN, R. S., CONRAD, M. E., HARTMAN, R. E., JOY, R. J. T. & CROSBY, W. H. (1963). *Blood*, **22**, 397.

HERBERT, V., ZALUSKY, R. & DAVIDSON, C. S. (1963). *Ann. intern. Med.*, **58**, 977.

HIGGINSON, J., GERRITSEN, T. & WALKER, A. R. P. (1953). *Amer. J. Path.*, **29**, 779.

HIYEDA, K. (1939). *Jap. J. med. Sci.*, **4**, 91.

HOJER, J. A. (1923). *Acta Paediat.*, (Uppsala), **3**, Suppl. 48.

HORRIGAN, D. L. & HARRIS, J. W. (1964). *In* "Advances in Internal Medicine", Vol. XII. Chicago, Yearbook Medical Publishers Inc.

HUFF, R. L., HENNESSY, T. G., AUSTIN, R. E., GARCIA, J. F., ROBERTS, B. M. & LAWRENCE, J. H. (1950). *J. clin. Invest.*, **29**, 1041.

HUSSAIN, R., WALKER, R. B., LAYRISSE, M., CLARK, P. & FINCH, C. A. (1965). *Amer. J. Clin. Nutr.*, **16**, 464.

HYDE, B. B., HODGE, A. J., KAHN, A. & BIRNSTIEL, M. L. (1963). *J. ultrastruct. Res.*, **9**, 248.

ISAACSON, C., SEFTEL, H. C., KEELEY, K. J. & BOTHWELL, T. H. (1961). *J. lab. clin. Med.*, **58**, 845.

JACOBS, P., BOTHWELL, T. H. & CHARLTON, R. W. (1964). *J. appl. Physiol.*, **19**, 187.

JACOBS, P., BOTHWELL, T. H. & CHARLTON, R. W. (1966). *Amer. J. Physiol.*, **210**, 694.

JANDL, J. H., INMAN, J. K., SIMMONS, R. L. & ALLEN, D. W. (1959). *J. clin. Invest.*, **38**, 161.

KENT, G. & POPPER, H. (1960). *Arch. Path.*, **70**, 623.

KINNEY, T. D., KAUFMAN, N. & KLAVINS, J. (1955). *J. exp. Med.*, **102**, 151.

KLECKNER, M. S., BAGGENSTOSS, A. H. & WEIR, J. F. (1955). *Amer. J. Clin. Path.*, **25**, 915.

KOPP, R., VOGT, A. & MAASS, G. (1963). *Nature*, **198**, 892.

LAURELL, C.-B. (1952). *Pharmacol Rev.*, **4**, 371.

LAYRISSE, M. (1966). The XIth Congress of the International Society of Haematology. Plenary Sessions. Sydney, Victor C. N. Blight, Government Printer.

MACDONALD, R. A. (1963). *Arch. intern. Med.*, **112**, 184.

MACDONALD, R. A. (1964). "Hemochromatosis and Hemosiderosis". Charles C. Thomas, Springfield.

McALLEN, P. M., COGHILL, N. F. & LUBRAN, M. (1957). *Quart. J. Med.*, **26**, 251.

MANIS, J. G. & SCHACHTER, D. (1962). *Amer. J. Physiol.*, **203**, 73.

MANIS, J. & SCHACHTER, D. (1966). *Nature*, **209**, 1356.

MARKS, N. & BANKS, S. (1963). *S. Afr. Med. J.*, **37**, 1039.

MAYET, F. G. H. & BOTHWELL, T. H. (1964). *S. Afr. J. Med. Sci.*, **29**, 55.

MAZUR, A., CARLETON, A. & CARLSEN, A. (1961). *J. biol. Chem.*, **236**, 1109.

MAZUR, A., GREEN, S., SAHA, A. & CARLETON, A. (1958). *J. clin. Invest.*, **37**, 1809.

MAZUR, A., LITT, I. & SHORR, E. (1950). *J. biol. Chem.*, **187**, 473.

MICHAELIS, L. (1947). *In* "Advances in Protein Chemistry". Vol. III, New York, Academic Press.

MINNICH, V., OKCUOGLU, A., TARCON, Y., ARCASOY, A., CIN, S., YORUKOGLU, O., RENDA, F. & DEMIRAG, B. (1968). *Amer. J. clin. Nutrit.*, **21**, 78.

MIROUZE, J. (1964). *Sem. Hop. Paris.*, **43**, 2299.

MOORE, C. V. (1965). *Scand. J. Haemat. Series Haematologica*, **6**, 1.

MOORE, C. V. & DUBACH, R. (1951). *Trans. Ass. Amer. Phycns.*, **64**, 245.

MUIR, A. R. (1960). *Quart. J. exp. Physiol.*, **45**, 192.

OLIVER, R. A. M. (1959). *J. Path. Bact.*, **77**, 171.

PERKINS, K. W., McINNES, I. W. S., BLACKBURN, C. R. B. & BEAL, R. W. (1965). *Amer. J. Med.*, **39**, 118.

PERMAN, G. & BONERA, E. (1964). *Acta med. Scand.*, **175**, 787.

PLOEM, J. E., DE WAEL, J., VERLOOP, M. C. & PUNT, K. (1966). *Brit. J. Haemat.*, **12**, 396.

POLLACK, S., KAUFMAN, R. M. & CROSBY, W. H. (1964). *Blood*, **24**, 577.

POWELL, L. W. (1965). *Quart. J. Med.*, **34**, 427.

POWELL, L. W. (1966). *Australas. Ann. Med.*, **15**, 110.

PRICE, J. M., BROWN, R. R. & PETERS, H. A. (1959). *Neurology*, **9**, 456.

RICHTER, G. W. (1963). *Lab. Invest.*, **12**, 1026.

RICHTER, G. W. & BESSIS, M. C. (1965). *Blood*, **25**, 370.

ROSEN, B. J. & TULLIS, J. L. (1966). *J. Amer. med. Ass.*, **195**, 261.

ROSS, J., KOCHWA, S. & WASSERMAN, L. R. (1964). *Blood*, **24**, 850.

ROTH, O., JASINSKI, B. & VON BIDDER, H. (1951). *Helvet. Med. Acta*, **18**, 159.

ROTHEN, A. (1944). *J. biol. Chem.*, **152**, 679.

ROUS, P. (1918). *J. exp. Med.*, **28**, 645.

SCHIFFER, L. M., BRANN, I., CRONKITE, E. P. & REIZENSTEIN, P. (1966). *Acta Haemat.*, **35**, 80.

SCHULZ, E. J. & SWANEPOEL, H. (1962). *S. Afr. med. J.*, **36**, 367.

SEFTEL, H. C., CHARLTON, R. W., JACOBS, P. & BOTHWELL, T. H. (1964). *S. Afr. J. med. Sci.*, **29**, 97.

SEFTEL, H. C., KEELEY, K. J., ISAACSON, C. & BOTHWELL, T. H. (1961). *J. lab. clin. Med.*, **58**, 837.

SEFTEL, H. C., MALKIN, C., SCHMAMAN, A., ABRAHAMS, C., LYNCH, S. R., CHARLTON, R. W. & BOTHWELL, T. H. (1966). *Brit. med. J.*, **1**, 642.

SHARPE, L. M., PEACOCK, W. C., COOKE, R. & HARRIS, R. S. (1950). *J. Nutrit.*, **41**, 433.

SHELDON, J. H. (1935). "Haemochromatosis". London, Oxford Univ. Press.

SHODEN, A., GABRIO, B. W. & FINCH, C. A. (1953). *J. biol. Chem.*, **204**, 823.

SHODEN, A. & STURGEON, P. (1963). *Brit. J. Haemat.*, **9**, 513.

SMITH, M. D. & PANNACCIULLI, I. M. (1958). *Brit. J. Haemat.*, **4**, 428.

SURGENOR, D. M., KOECHLIN, B. A. & STRONG, L. E. (1949). *J. clin. Invest.*, **28**, 73.

TAYLOR, J., STIVEN, D. & REID, E. W. (1931). *J. Path. Bact.*, **34**, 793.

TAYLOR, J., STIVEN, D. & REID, E. W. (1935). *J. Path. Bact.*, **41**, 397.

THIRAYOTHIN, P. & CROSBY, W. H. (1962). *J. clin. Invest.*, **41**, 1206.

TURNBERG, L. A. (1965). *Brit. med. J.*, **1**, 1360.

TURNBERG, L. A. (1966). *Amer. J. dig. Dis.*, **11**, 20.

TURNBULL, A., CLETON, F. & FINCH, C. A. (1962). *J. clin. Invest.*, **41**, 1897.

TURNBULL, B. C. & GIBLETT, E. R. (1961). *J. lab. clin. Med.*, **57**, 450.

VILTER, R. W. (1954). In "The Vitamins". Eds. Sebrell, W. H. & Harris, R. S. Vol. 1. Academic Press, New York.

WALKER, A. R. P. & ARVIDSSON, U. B. (1953). *Trans. Roy. Soc. trop. Med. & Hyg.*, **47**, 536.

WALLENIUS, G. A. (1952). *Scandinav. J. clin. & lab. Invest.*, **4**, 24.

WEINBRAUB, L. R., CONRAD, M. E. & CROSBY, W. H. (1966). *New Engl. J. Med.*, **275**, 169.

WHEBY, M. S., BALCERZAK, S. P., ANDERSON, P. & CROSBY, W. H. (1964). *Blood*, **24**, 765.

WILLIAMS, R., MANENTI, F., WILLIAMS, H. S. & PITCHER, C. S. (1966). *Brit. med. J.*, **2**, 78.

WILLIAMS, R., PITCHER, C. S., PARSONSON, A. & WILLIAMS, H. S. (1965). *Lancet*, **1**, 1243.

WILLIAMS, R., SCHEUER, P. J. & SHERLOCK, S. (1962). *Quart. J. Med.*, **31**, 249.

WOHLER, F. (1964). *Acta Haemat.*, **32**, 321.

WYATT, J. P. (1956). *Arch. Path.*, **61**, 56.

WYATT, J. P., MIGHTON, H. K. & MORAGUES, V. (1950). *Amer. J. Path.*, **26**, 883.

ZIMMERMAN, H. J., CHOMET, B., KULESH, M. H. & McWHORTER, C. A. (1961). *Arch. int. Med.*, **107**, 494.

Chapter 8

PORPHYRIAS

by

C. H. GRAY

King's College Hospital Medical School, London

CLINICAL ASPECTS OF PORPHYRIA

THE porphyrias comprise a group of diseases associated with a primary abnormality of porphyrin synthesis. They were initially classified by Waldenström (1937) into acute porphyria and congenital porphyria and a third form—*porphyria cutanea tarda*.

In acute porphyria, inherited as an autosomal dominant, attacks of severe colicky abdominal pain and constipation are accompanied by lesions of the nervous system. These lesions may occur in the brain, brain stem, spinal cord, peripheral nerves or in the autonomic nervous system, and may present as a peripheral neuritis or as a paralysis sometimes ascending from the lower limbs and reaching the trunk, arms, neck and finally the respiratory centres in that order. Some cases may present with abdominal or neurological symptoms only, while in others the disease may be latent and then the biochemical abnormality is present without clinical symptoms. There has been said to be an abnormal mental state, but the mental features of the disease are often no different from the mental response of a normal individual to a frightening and painful illness (Ackner, Cooper, Gray, Kelly & Nicholson, 1961). Excellent accounts of the clinical aspects have been given by Vannotti (1954) and of the post mortem, morphological and biochemical findings by Perlroth, Tschudy, Marver, Berard, Zeigel, Rechcigl & Collins (1966).

In the single patient studied by Perlroth *et al.* excessive antidiuretic hormone activity before death could be correlated with lesions in the hypothalamus.

The attacks are frequently precipitated by the administration of barbiturates, sulphonamides or other drugs including oestrogens (Watson, Runge & Bossenmaier, 1962; Welland, Hellman, Gaddis, Collins, Hunter & Tschudy, 1964) and oral contraceptives (Rimington & de Matteis, 1965; Zimmerman, McMillin & Watson, 1966). Because the disease is essentially chronic in nature with acute exacerbations separated by periods of remission, Watson (1954) preferred the term "acute intermittent porphyria".

Congenital porphyria, a recessive disease, is characterized by a severe photosensitivity beginning at, or soon after, birth and persisting throughout life, and leading to very severe scarring and deformities. This form of the disease is not accompanied by abdominal or nervous system lesions. Large quantities of porphyrins are deposited in the bones, teeth and skin, which therefore become pigmented and present a characteristic red fluorescence in ultraviolet light (Borst & Koenigsdörffer, 1929). Episodes of haemolysis are common. In this form of the disease the abnormality of porphyrin synthesis almost certainly lies in the bone marrow, and for this reason Watson called this type "porphyria erythropoietica".

Porphyria cutanea tarda usually begins in early adulthood; photosensitivity is much less severe than in the congenital form and does not usually lead to scarring and deformities. The condition is now known to be heterogeneous and to consist of several distinct forms. Some present with mild abdominal colics in addition to the photosensitivity, and the condition is then often associated with alcoholism. In others the photosensitivity seems to be related to phases of hepatic dysfunction, when jaundice is also present (MacGregor, Nicholas & Rimington, 1952). This form was called *porphyria cutanea tarda hereditaria* or protoporphyria or coproporphyria since protoporphyrin and/or coproporphyrin are excreted in the faeces except during attacks of jaundice when the porphyrins accumulate in the blood and are excreted in the urine.

In some patients with protoporphyria or coproporphyria, the circulating red cells and their precursors in the bone marrow contain large quantities of free protoporphyrin (or less frequently coproporphyrin); this form of the disease, which is inherited as a dominant (Haeger-Aronsen, 1962; Redeker & Bryan, 1964) is therefore known as erythropoietic protoporphyria (Magnus, Jarrett, Prankerd & Rimington, 1961) or erythropoietic coproporphyria (Heilmeyer & Clotten, 1964). Unlike classical erythropoietic porphyria, haemolytic anaemia is uncommon in this disease, but the liver is usually enlarged and there is early cirrhosis with intrahepatic deposits of protoporphyrin (Porter, 1963; Porter & Lowe,

1963; Peterka, Fusaro, Runge, Jaffe & Watson, 1965; Cripps & Scheuer, 1965; Gray, unpublished observations). There is evidence that there is disturbance of porphyrin metabolism in the liver as well as in the bone marrow (Gray, Kulczycka, Nicholson, Magnus & Rimington, 1964) and this form of the disease might well be called "*porphyria erythropoietica et hepatica*". There is a recent suggestion, however, that in this condition much of the erythrocyte protoporphyrin may have been synthesised in the liver, carried in the plasma and absorbed by the erythrocytes (Nakao, Wada, Takahu, Sassa, Yano & Urata, 1967).

In an apparently benign form of coproporphyria, presumably not erythropoietic in origin, episodes of acute porphyria have followed barbiturates (Smart, Herbert, Whittaker & Barnes, 1965) or anticonvulsants or tranquilising drugs (Cowger & Labbe, 1965). There is also porphyria cutanea symptomatica, one group of which has been termed "cutaneous porphyria in the adult" by Bolgert, Canivet & Le Sourd (1953). On the other hand, a non-hereditary light-sensitive form occurs among the Bantu and seems to be associated with liver damage related to the ingestion of adulterated drinks and associated with alcoholism or excessive iron intake and dietary deficiencies.

In South Africa many white members of the population, all descendants of an early Dutch settler, suffer from a so-called "variegate" form in which a mild chronic photosensitivity may be

TABLE 8.1

Classification of porphyrias

1. Erythropoietic porphyria	(a) recessive (classical congenital porphyria)
	(b) dominant (*porphyria erythropoietica et hepatica* or erythropoietic protoporphyria or coproporphyria)
2. Acute intermittent porphyria	(a) manifest
	(b) latent
3. Hepatic cutaneous porphyria	
(a) hereditary	(i) *porphyria cutanea tarda* or protocoproporphyria (Waldenström, 1957)
	(ii) mixed porphyria (Watson, Pimenta de Mello, Schwartz, Hawkinson & Bossenmaier, 1951; Watson, 1954)
	(iii) variegate porphyria (Dean & Barnes, 1959; Dean, 1963)
(b) acquired	(i) symptomatic *porphyria cutanea tarda* (Waldenström, 1957)
	(ii) Bantu porphyria (Barnes, 1959)
	(iii) hexachlorobenzene porphyria (Cetingil & Ozen, 1960; Cam, 1957; Ockner & Schmid, 1961)
	(iv) griseofulvin porphyria (Rimington, Morgan, Nicholls, Everall & Davies, 1963)
	(v) porphyria of hepatic adenoma (Tio, Leijnse, Jarrett & Rimington, 1957)
4. Experimental porphyria	

associated with acute attacks of abdominal pain; often men are photosensitive with little or no colic, while their female relations with the disease have little photosensitivity and more abdominal symptoms (Dean & Barnes, 1959; Dean, 1963).

In Turkey between 1955 and 1960, the fungicide hexachlorobenzene caused an outbreak of a toxic form characterized by photosensitivity, pigmentation, hypertrichosis and evidence of hepatic damage; uroporphyrin and corproporphyrin were present in the urine (Cam, 1957; Ockner & Schmid, 1961; Peters, Johnson, Cam, Oral, Müftü & Ergene, 1966). Administration of the fungicide griseofulvin is also associated with disturbances of porphyrin metabolism (Rimington, Morgan, Nicholls, Everall & Davies, 1963).

The classification of the porphyrias is constantly being revised and Table 8.1 shows a useful classification that will be adopted in the present account; a detailed description of previous classifications has been given by Goldberg & Rimington (1962).

The porphyrias have hitherto been distinguished from the porphyrinurias in which there is an increased excretion of porphyrins in the urine and faeces, which does not seem obviously related to any abnormality of porphyrin biosynthesis, and which appears to be secondary to such diseases as haemolytic and pernicious anaemias (Watson, 1937), liver disease (Watson, Hawkinson, Capps & Rappaport, 1949), poliomyelitis (Watson, Schulze, Hawkinson & Baker, 1947) and lead poisoning (Watson, 1936). The quantities of porphyrins or of porphyrin derivatives excreted are usually much smaller in the porphyrinurias than in the porphyrias, but the colics and neuropathy of lead poisoning may simulate acute porphyria, especially when the excretion of urinary coproporphyrin (see below) is high, as it often is in lead poisoning. However, as will be seen later, the excretion of porphobilinogen in the urine is characteristic of acute intermittent porphyria and is never present in lead poisoning. It seems likely that more complete knowledge of the disturbances of metabolism in these diseases will reveal that differences between the porphyrias and the porphyrinurias are of degree only, and that all are essentially disturbances of porphyrin and haem biosynthesis.

CHEMISTRY OF THE PORPHYRINS

The porphyrins are red pigments with a cyclic tetrapyrrolic structure in which the four pyrrole rings are united through their α-carbon atoms by four methene ($=CH-$) bridges. The parent substance is porphin, in which the H atoms attached to the β-carbon atoms on the pyrrole nuclei are unsubstituted (Fig. 8.1). All the naturally occurring porphyrins may be regarded as derived from one or other of two uroporphyrins which are compounds with the eight hydrogen atoms of the

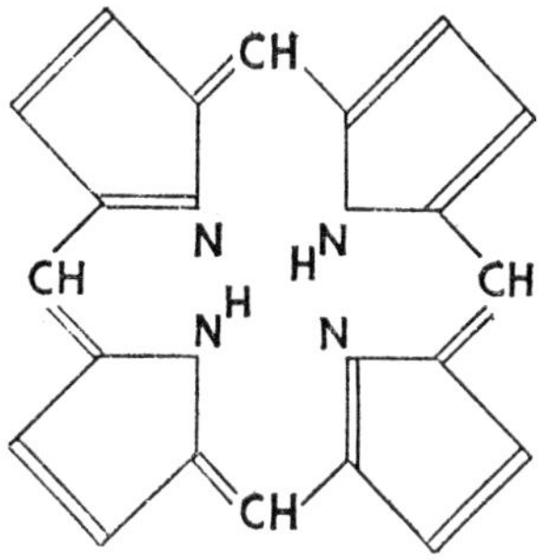

FIG. 8.1

β-carbon atoms of porphin replaced by four carboxy-methyl and four carboxy-ethyl groups. These substituents can be arranged around the porphin molecule in only four ways, so that four uroporphyrins—I, II, III and IV—are possible, corresponding to the analogous aetioporphyrins synthesized by Hans Fischer, and in which the β-constituents consist of four methyl and four ethyl groups (Fischer & Orth, 1937).

There is as yet no evidence that uroporphyrins II and IV, or porphyrins derived from them, occur in nature, all the naturally occurring porphyrins being theoretically derivable either from uroporphyrin I or uroporphyrin III. In the former, the carboxymethyl and carboxyethyl groups are attached alternately round the porphin ring, but in uroporphyrin III the positions of the groups attached to one pyrrole ring are reversed (Fig. 8.2). Oxidative decarboxylation of the four carboxymethyl groups can theoretically give rise to coproporphyrins I and III, each containing four methyl groups and four carboxyethyl groups (Fig. 8.3). Oxidative decarboxylation of two of the remaining carboxyethyl groups would form protoporphyrin IX, which therefore contains four methyl groups, two vinyl groups and two carboxyethyl groups attached to the β-carbon atoms in the pyrrole nuclei (Fig. 8.4). Fifteen arrangements of these substituents are possible, giving 15 isomers which were labelled by Hans Fischer as protoporphyrins I to XV (Fischer & Orth, 1937). Protoporphyrin IX, the structure formally derivable from coproporphyrin III in the above manner, is the only protoporphyrin so far found in nature, and its Fe complex is haem, the prosthetic group of haemo-

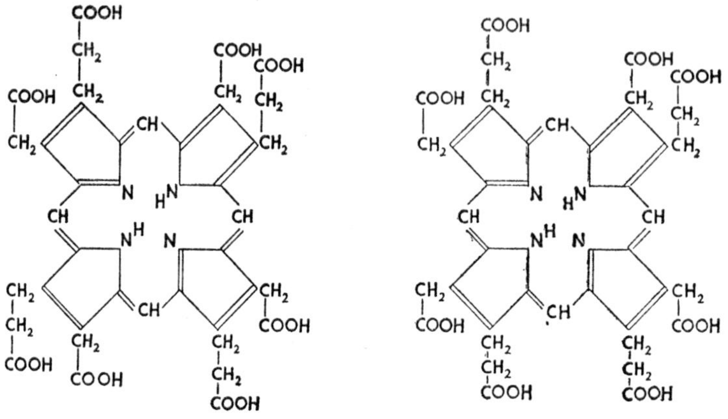

UROPORPHYRIN I   UROPORPHYRIN III

Fig. 8.2

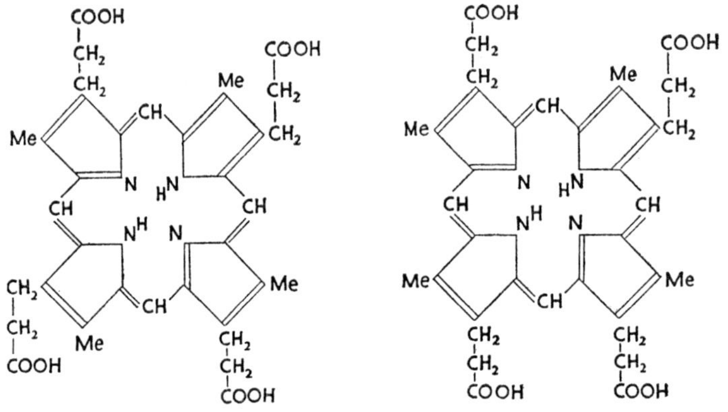

COPROPORPHYRIN I   COPROPORPHYRIN III

Fig. 8.3

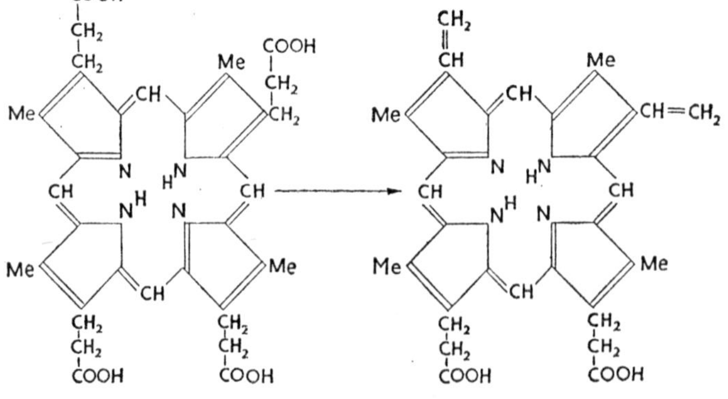

COPROPORPHYRIN III   PROTOPORPHYRIN IX

Fig. 8.4

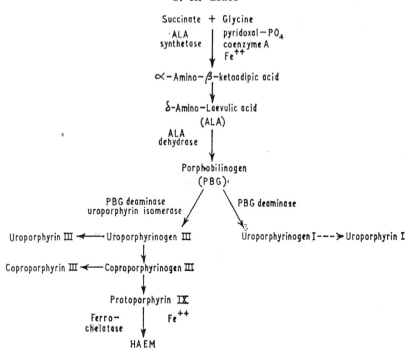

FIG. 8.5. The biosynthesis of haem.

globin, myoglobin, and many of the haem proteins. The prosthetic group of cytochrome *c* is protoporphyrin IX, in which the vinyl groups are linked with the cysteine groups of the apoprotein (Theorell, 1939), while the prosthetic group of chlorophyll is the Mg complex of a porphyrin derived from protoporphyrin IX (Granick & Gilder, 1947). As will be seen below, biosynthesis of protoporphyrin or haem takes place via the porphyrinogens in which the bridge carbon atoms linking the four pyrrole rings are methylene ($-CH_2-$) and not methene groups.

BIOSYNTHESIS OF PORPHYRINS

The main pathway of biosynthesis of porphyrins and of haem (Fig. 8.5) is now clearly established by the work of Shemin, Rittenberg, Neuberger and others. Succinyl coenzyme A, derived from acetate via the Krebs cycle and *a*-oxoglutarate*, is enzymically condensed (pyridoxal phosphate, coenzyme A and ferrous ions participating) with glycine (Fig. 8.6) to form

* Recent work suggests that in the porphyrias the excess succinyl coenzyme A required for synthesis of porphyrin precursors may be derived from some other source than the Krebs cycle; separate pools of succinyl coenzyme A may be concerned.

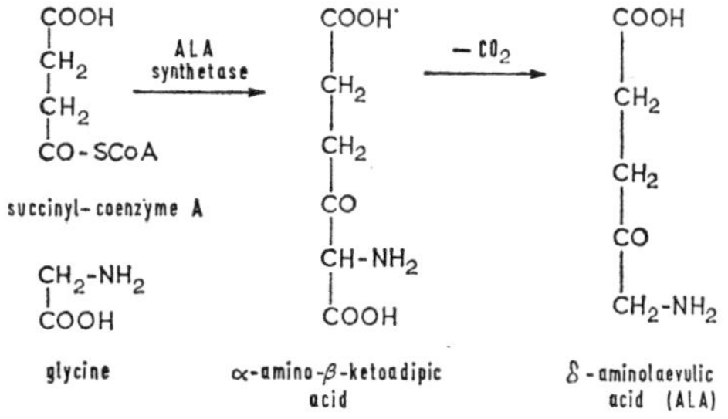

α-amino-β-ketoadipic acid, which rapidly loses CO_2 nonenzymically to form δ-aminolaevulic acid (ALA). Under the influence of the sulphydryl enzyme ALA dehydrase, two molecules of ALA then condense (Fig. 8.7) to form one molecule of the monopyrrole porphobilinogen (PBG), which was first observed in acute porphyria urine by Waldenström (1937), was isolated by Westall (1952), and was shown by Cookson & Rimington (1954) to have a structure of 2-aminomethyl-3-carboxymethyl-4-carboxyethylpyrrole (Fig. 8.7). Four molecules of the latter condense under a variety of conditions to give tetrapyrrolic compounds. In dilute acid solution uroporphyrin III is formed together with small quantities of other

FIG. 8.6. Formation of δ-aminolaevulic acid.

isomers. In the presence of red cell haemolysate, uroporphyrin III and the so-called pseudo-uroporphyrin are formed, unless the haemolysate is heated to 60° when uroporphyrin I is formed. The details of the condensation have been investigated by Bogorad (1958, 1960) using two enzyme preparations—porphobilinogen deaminase from

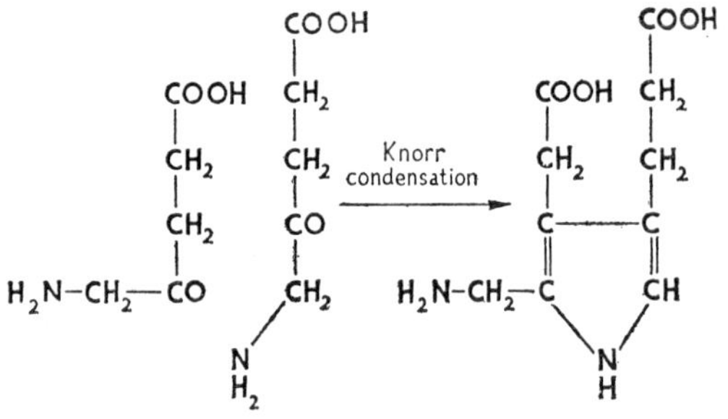

δ-NH$_2$-laevulic acid   porphobilinogen.

FIG. 8.7.

spinach leaves, and the other, uroporphyrinogen isomerase from wheat germ. The spinach preparation brings about the formation of uroporphyrinogen I while the isomerase, without activity by itself, causes uroporphyrinogen III formation in the presence of the deaminase. The corresponding porphyrins are readily formed in air by dehydrogenation.

A number of mechanisms have been proposed for the condensation of four molecules of PBG to form uroporphyrinogen III, in which the side groups are in the order AP . AP . AP . PA, where A is carboxymethyl and P is carboxyethyl (for review see Marks, 1962). Tripyrrylmethane and pentapyrrylmethane intermediaries have been proposed by Shemin, Russell & Abramsky (1955) and by Jackson & Macdonald (1957) respectively, in order to account for the inversion of the linkages of one of the pyrrole units, while Robinson (1955) has postulated migration of an aminomethyl group in a porphobilinogen molecule. These theories have been discussed by Rimington (1959), Bogorad (1960) and Gibson, Matthew, Neuberger & Tait (1961). A linear tetrapyrrolic compound may be formed by a series of successive electrophilic attacks by the $CH_2 . \overset{+}{N}H_3$ group of porphobilinogen molecules, firstly on a second porphobilinogen molecule and then in turn on the resulting dipyrryl and tripyrryl methanes. The order of the side chains will then be AP . AP . AP . AP. In the absence of the uroporphyrinogen isomerase there would be simple cyclization with the formation of uroporphyrinogen I. Matthewson & Corwen (1961) have suggested that three rings of

the tetrapyrrylmethane are in the pyrrolene, i.e. dihydropyrrole form, thus making the structure highly flexible. Under the influence of the isomerase the CH_2NH_3 group of the tetrapyrrylmethane is therefore able to attack, not the free α position of the other end pyrrole of the molecule, but the occupied α position of that pyrrole. The resulting cyclic structure then rearranges to form uroporphyrinogen III. Bullock (1965) has criticized this mechanism.

By whatever its mechanism of formation, uroporphyrinogen III is enzymically transformed into the tetracarboxylic coproporphyrinogen III, probably by stepwise decarboxylation with intermediate formation of hepta, hexa and pentacarboxylic porphyrinogens. Finally two of the four carboxyethyl groups of coproporphyrinogen III are oxidatively decarboxylated to form protoporphyrin by enzyme systems present in red cell systems and in the liver. The final incorporation of iron into the protoporphyrin molecules appears to be effected by an enzyme (ferrochelatase), and has been studied by Lockhead & Goldberg (1961).

CHEMICAL FINDINGS IN THE PORPHYRIAS

Acute Intermittent Porphyria

For many years it was believed that, while in acute intermittent porphyria the excreted porphyrins were of type III, in congenital porphyria the urine and faeces contained, respectively, mainly uroporphyrin I and coproporphyrin I. Isolation studies showed that the urine of acute porphyria contained increased amounts of coproporphyrin III, together with a porphyrin which was described as being uroporphyrin III (Waldenström, 1937). This worker also recognized that the porphyrin excreted in the urine in acute porphyria was partly excreted as a metal complex (often mistaken for haemoglobin) and partly in the form of the colourless precursor porphobilinogen. Porphobilinogen reacts with Ehrlich's aldehyde reagent (an acid solution of p-dimethylaminobenzaldehyde) to give a red pigment which differs, however, from that given by urobilinogen in having a 2-banded spectrum (Waldenström & Vahlquist, 1939) and in being insoluble in chloroform (Watson & Schwartz, 1941).

In acute intermittent porphyria, the essential abnormality of the urine is not the excretion of porphyrins but the excretion of the monopyrrolic porphyrin precursor, porphobilinogen, together with its metabolic precursor δ-aminolaevulic acid, as was shown by Granick & van den Schrieck

(1955); some patients with the full clinical features of the disease excrete urine normal in colour and containing no excess of preformed porphyrins. On standing, especially in acid solution, these urines darken owing to the formation of the porphyrins and a reddish-brown pigment, porphobilin (Brockman & Gray, 1953). The nature of the porphyrin formed from porphobilinogen depends upon experimental conditions. Indeed, Gibson & Harrison (1950) showed that preformed porphyrin in acute porphyria urines may be different from that obtained when porphobilinogen-containing urines are allowed to stand in light or are heated in acid. Cookson & Rimington (1954) and Mauzerall (1960a,b) have shown that the composition of the mixture of isomers formed from PBG is dependent on pH.

Congenital Erythropoietic Porphyria

In contrast to the porphyrins and precursors excreted in acute porphyria, the uroporphyrin I excreted in the urine in the congenital form of the disease is usually excreted in the free form. Urine from patients with congenital porphyria not only contains uroporphyrin I and coproporphyrin I, with 8 and 4 carboxyl groups respectively, but also small quantities of at least one other octacarboxylic porphyrin, perhaps uroporphyrin III, as well as porphyrins containing 7, 5 and 4 carboxyl groups (Rimington & Miles, 1951). The faeces contain large amounts of coproporphyrin I.

Erythropoietic Protoporphyria and Coproporphyria

In erythropoietic protoporphyria, the faeces contain a great excess of protoporphyrin—often 10 mg. or more per day (in coproporphyria the faecal porphyrin is coproporphyrin). The urine usually contains little or no excess of porphyrins or their precursors, but during periods of impaired hepatic function the concentration of protoporphyrin in the plasma increases as does the amount of porphyrin excreted in the urine. The most characteristic abnormality in this form of the disease is the greatly increased concentration of free protoporphyrin or coproporphyrin in the circulating erythrocytes. Protoporphyrin may be increased from the normal values of about 50 μg. to 2 mg. or more /100 ml. of red cells. In coproporphyria the erythrocyte coproporphyrin may be increased from the normal 2·5 μg. to 400 or 500 μg./100 ml. of red cells (Cripps, 1966).

Variegate Porphyria

Markedly increased amounts of copro- and protoporphyrin are consistently found in the faeces in both the acute and the remission phases in contrast to the slightly raised or normal amounts in acute intermittent porphyria. In the cutaneous phase, the excretion of ALA and PBG are normal or slightly raised, while during the acute attacks the excretion of these two porphyrin precursors is increased to values similar to those found in acute intermittent porphyria (Eales, Dowdle, Levey & Sweeney, 1966). Recently, Rimington & Lockwood (1965) have described some unusual hydrophilic peptide conjugates of a porphyrin, which Rimington, Lockwood & Belcher (1968) now believe to be characteristic of porphyria variegata.

Symptomatic Hepatic Cutaneous Porphyria

In symptomatic porphyria almost the only abnormalities are increases of urinary uroporphyrin and coproporphyrin. Apart from a questionable increase in faecal coproporphyrin, faecal and blood porphyrins are not raised.

Some porphyria urines contain in addition to, or instead of, porphobilinogen other porphyrin precursors which, in contrast to porphobilinogen itself, are extractable by organic solvents and do not react with Ehrlich's reagent (Raine, 1950; Watson, Pimenta de Mello, Schwartz, Hawkinson & Bossenmaier, 1951; Herbert, 1952). Sometimes this kind of porphyrin precursor may be a metal complex (Gray, 1951), but other precursors are often present and are converted into porphyrins by oxidation, e.g. by quinone or iodine. These precursors are usually present in the urine of patients with some forms of hepatic cutaneous porphyria; they are probably porphyrinogens.

Sano & Rimington (1963) have shown that in rabbits the porphyrinogens were more readily excreted in the urine than the corresponding porphyrins and that urinary excretion of the porphyrins diminished with decreasing carboxylation. Uroporphyrin and to a lesser extent coproporphyrin were excreted in the urine but protoporphyrin hardly at all. Excretion in the bile becomes more important when urinary excretion is low. Rimington (1963) has related these observations to the findings in human disease.

In all forms of porphyria except the erythropoietic forms, the serum iron or tissue iron stores, or both, together with the iron-binding capacity may be increased (Berlin & Brante, 1962).

EXPERIMENTAL PORPHYRIA

Schmid & Schwartz (1952) first showed that large quantities of porphobilinogen were excreted in the urine when sedormid was fed to rabbits. There was also a fall in the amount of liver catalase, and they thought that a block in the synthesis of this haem protein might lead to an accumulation within the body of porphyrin precursors including porphobilinogen, which because of its low renal threshold would be rapidly excreted. It seems more probable that, if there is indeed a deficiency in the synthesis of catalase, there must be a disturbance of the feed-back mechanism, whereby the availability of ALA and PBG for porphyrin formation is controlled by haem protein formation (see below); there would result an increased production of ALA and PBG. Goldberg (1954) has investigated the ability of a series of compounds related to sedormid to produce porphobilinogen in rats and rabbits, and has shown that the allylisopropyl acetamide (AIA) group is essential for this effect, and that allylisopropyl acetamide itself produces intense porphobilinogenuria in the rat and rabbit, without producing the narcosis produced by sedormid. However, the clinical features of rabbits with

porphyria induced by these compounds do not resemble those of human acute porphyria.

Hexachlorobenzene, the agent found by Ockner & Schmid (1961) to be responsible for the outbreak of toxic porphyria in Turkey, produces in rats a form of disease which seems closely related to that observed in the Turkish outbreak. These animals develop photosensitivity with tremor, ataxia, weakness and paralysis, and exhibit an excretion of PBG and ALA as well as of coproporphyrin and uroporphyrin. De Matteis, Prior & Rimington (1961) have studied the action of this compound in rabbits, guinea pigs, mice and rats and found some species differences in the response to this compound. The distribution of porphyrins in the carcasses suggested that the porphyria is of the hepatic type, with possible interference to the uroporphyrinogen-decarboxylating mechanisms.

The fungicide, griseofulvin, produces disturbances of porphyrin metabolism in mice very similar to those of *porphyria erythropoietica et hepatica* (erythropoietic protoporphyria) but the precise metabolic abnormalities responsible for the experimental condition have not yet been studied.

Table 8.2 summarizes the various forms of

TABLE 8.2

Porphyrinogenic Agent	Species	Metabolic Disturbances	References
Sedormid	rabbits	PBG and ALA excretion increased	Schmid & Schwartz (1952)
Sedormid and related compounds	rats	PBG and ALA increased	Goldberg (1954)
Allylisopropyl acetamide (AIA)	rabbits		Goldberg (1954)
Hexachlorobenzene	rats rabbits guinea pigs mice	PBG and ALA excretion increased coproporphyrin and uroporphyrin excretion increased	Ockner & Schmid (1961) de Matteis, Prior & Rimington (1961)
Dicarbethoxydihydro-cholidine (DDC)	guinea pigs	PBG and ALA increased	Granick & Urata (1963)
Griseofulvin	mice	urinary PBG and ALA increased faecal coproporphyrin and protoporphyrin increased hepatic and erythrocyte protoporphyrin greatly increased	De Matteis & Rimington (1963)
AIA, DDC, certain steroids	chick embryo liver cells	copro- and protoporphyrin increased liver copro- and protoporphyrin increased	Granick 1963; Granick & Kappas (1967); Kappas & Granick (1968)
Ethionine	rats		Palma-Carlos, Palma-Carlos, Gajdos-Török & Gajdos (1966)

experimental porphyria, together with the species in which they may be induced and the metabolic disturbances which result. Of these, those which have been most extensively studied are the conditions induced by AIA and dicarbethoxydihydrocholidine (DDC). Granick (1963) has found that tissue cultures of chick embryo liver cells provide a valuable *in vitro* test system for the investigation of porphyria-inducing drugs.

THE AETIOLOGY OF PORPHYRIA

Congenital Porphyria

In congenital porphyria it would appear that there is a genetically determined abnormality of the enzymic conversion of porphobilinogen to types I and III porphyrins in the bone marrow. This abnormality could be a deficiency or absence of uroporphyrin isomerase, although the enzyme from animal species has not yet been separated from the porphobilinogen deaminase. Normally there results a great predominance of type III porphyrins, which are used in the synthesis of haem-proteins together with a very small amount of type I porphyrins, the daily formation of which in normal man amounts to only a few hundred μg. which are readily eliminated. In congenital porphyria, however, the amount of type I porphyrins produced is very great and may amount to 100 mg. or more per day. These type I porphyrins are useless for prosthetic groups, and since they are not degraded to bile pigment they are excreted or deposited in the body, a well-recognized feature of the disease. The skin sensitivity in this condition is undoubtedly due to the photodynamic effects of the porphyrins, and Magnus, Porter, McCree, Moreland & Wright (1959) have found that the action spectrum as determined by the changes in skin sensitivity with wavelength corresponded to the spectral absorption of the porphyrins which have been shown to cause a release of histamine (Feldberg & Talesnik, 1953). More recently, Slater & Riley (1966) have shown that photosensitivity due to the chlorophyll degradation product, phylloerythrin, may be mediated by the release of lysosomal enzymes by the activity of free radicals; porphyrin-induced photosensitivity might result by a similar mechanism. Similarly, the uroporphyrin I demonstrated by Aldrich, Hawkinson, Grinstein & Watson (1951) in the red cells may lead to a photosensitized haemolysis of red cells. Haemolytic episodes are well recognized in congenital porphyria, and have been demonstrated both clinically (Guenther, 1925) and by isotope techniques (Gray, Muir & Neuberger, 1950). The increased rate of haemo-

lysis is compensated by increased haem synthesis, which aggravates the condition by causing increased production of type I porphyrins, which are by-products of that synthesis. Splenectomy is sometimes effective in reducing the rate of haemolysis, and therefore should ameliorate the condition. This was so in the case described by Aldrich *et al.* (1951), but not in the one described by Gray & Neuberger (1952). It is not possible, however, to explain the increased amount of stercobilin derived from the second metabolic source, i.e. that fraction rapidly labelled after administration of ^{15}N-glycine (Gray, Neuberger & Sneath, 1950). Equally difficult to explain are the high incorporation of ^{15}N into the haem and the enlarged pools of δ-aminolaevulic acid and porphobilinogen in this condition (Gray & Scott, 1960).

Acute Porphyria

There is no doubt that all the clinical features of acute intermittent porphyria are directly due to changes in the nervous system, although whether the lesions affect primarily the axon or the myelin sheath is still under discussion (Denny-Brown & Sciarra, 1945; Heirons, 1957; Goldberg, 1958, 1959; Cavanagh & Mellick, 1965; Annotation, Lancet, 1965; Gray, 1966). Goldberg, (1958) had earlier suggested that the abdominal pain and colics are caused by lesions in the pre-ganglionic motor fibres that innervate the viscera.

In this condition free porphyrins are present only in traces in the body and there is no photosensitivity.On the other hand, porphobilinogen and δ-aminolaevulic acid are excreted in large quantities. Berlin, Neuberger & Scott (1956) have found that ALA did not cause, despite the excretion of amounts of ALA and PBG comparable to those excreted by patients, clinical symptoms of acute porphyria in normal men, nor worsen those of patients with the disease. Neither PBG nor ALA is toxic (Goldberg, Paton & Thompson, 1954; Jarrett, Rimington & Willoughby, 1956) and the clinical condition is not directly related to the quantities of the two precursors excreted (Ackner *et al.*, 1961). The metabolic abnormality must always be present although its clinical effects do not usually become manifest until early adult life, and even then only when some additional factor precipitates a crisis. It therefore seems probable that the excretion of the two metabolites and the nervous system changes are separate manifestations of a metabolic event or series of events. There is evidence that an acute attack is precipitated by the administration of barbiturates (Goldberg, 1959), but known porphyric subjects may pass into an acute crisis without having had such drugs, so that other factors must also be concerned.

The condition is a genetically determined disease, and could be due to an enzyme deficiency, either causing a block in the conversion of porphobilinogen to porphyrins and haem in the liver, or associated with an excessive production of δ-aminolaevulic acid and of porphobilinogen in the body. In experimental porphyria in rabbits induced by administration of sedormid, Schmid & Schwartz (1952) have shown that there is a fall in the liver catalase, and it seems likely that this block in the formation of haem protein may be responsible for the accumulation of porphobilinogen in the body, leading to the excretion of the substance characteristic of this form of experimental disease. In human porphyria, however, there is no fall in liver catalase (Gray, 1950; Schmid & Schwartz, 1955), and it seems likely that porphobilinogen and δ-aminolaevulic acid are available in amounts in excess of what is required for normal haem synthesis. The fundamental lesion in acute porphyria must, therefore, be an abnormality of metabolism at or before the stage of ALA synthesis, and the determination of pool sizes and turnover rates of ALA and PBG (Gray & Scott, 1960) is now of academic interest only.

The disorder must be an excessive production of ALA, due either to a block in the catabolism of one of its precursors via an alternative pathway not leading to porphobilinogen and porphyrin formation, or to a block in the metabolism of ALA itself. The production of ALA and its disposal by PBG formation and by the other pathway is so regulated that normally little or no ALA and PBG are wasted. In acute porphyria this carefully balanced mechanism must be disturbed, so that quantities of ALA up to several hundred mg. in excess of that required by the body become available for disposal.

Richards & Scott (1961) have shown that the plasma glycine is not elevated in acute porphyria; it is therefore unlikely that any major pathway of glycine metabolism is blocked, although quantitatively minor but qualitatively important pathways may be affected. In the cycle proposed by Shemin (1956), ALA is deaminated to give α-oxoglutaraldehyde, which is then believed to be broken down to succinic acid and a one-carbon atom fragment at the oxidation level of formaldehyde. Richards & Scott (1961) attempted to assess the availability of these one-carbon atom fragments by determining the ability of the body to convert glycine to serine, a process requiring a one-carbon fragment. In three of six patients with acute porphyria the conversion of glycine to serine was abnormally low. This could mean either that the essential lesion in acute porphyria is not a defect in the utilization of ALA by pathways other than PBG formation, or else that the acute attack had ended in the three patients giving negative results in their tests.

The condensing enzyme responsible for the condensation of succinyl coenzyme A with glycine to form ALA can also bring about the condensation of acetyl coenzyme A with glycine to form amino-acetone. If for some reason the rate of production of acetyl coenzyme A were limited, the resulting deficiency of acetylcholine could interfere with transmission of the nerve impulse, and larger quantities of succinyl coenzyme A might react with glycine to form ALA. Sulphonamide drugs require acetylation, and their administration would make demands upon an already diminished production of acetyl coenzyme A and lead to an acute crisis. Such a theory would suggest that amino-acetone is a normal metabolite in the human subject and that amino-acetone would be absent from the urine of patients with acute porphyria. However, Tschudy, Welland, Collins & Hunter (1963) and Druyan & Haeger-Aronsen (1964) found no difference between the amino-acetone excretion of patients with acute porphyria and that of normal subjects. Moreover, Urata & Granick (1963) have shown that two distinct enzymes are responsible for the synthesis of amino-acetone and ALA respectively.

De Matteis & Rimington (1962) have pointed out that the synthesis of acetylcholine might be defective either on account of an interference with the acetylating mechanism or of a deficiency of the supply of coenzyme A, or of acetyl coenzyme A from pyruvate, or of NAD^+ or of available energy from adenosine triphosphate. Many of the features of acute porphyria could thus be attributed to interference at one or other of these points. Talman, Labbe, Aldrich & Sears (1959) have shown that sedormid interferes with purine synthesis, and that porphyrin production by chick embryos treated with sedormid is reduced when adenine (a constituent of AMP, ATP, NAD^+ and $NADP^+$) is also administered. The effect of barbiturates on porphyria could be due to their effect on oxidative phosphorylation which would decrease the availability of ATP for the synthesis of acetyl coenzyme A. This would provide a basis for the apparent benefit of adenosine monophosphate treatment of acute porphyria (see below).

Granick & Urata (1963) have shown that in experimental porphyria induced by AIA or DDC (see Table 8.2) in the guinea pig and in the chick embryo there is induction of a greatly increased synthesis of ALA synthetase (the rate-limiting enzyme in porphyrin biosynthesis) and the increased synthesis is inhibited by actinomycin D (Granick, 1963, 1966) and by puromycin (Marver, Tschudy, Perlroth & Collins, 1965). These observations suggest that these agents antagonize a repressor gene controlling the synthesis of ALA synthetase. Although these experimental porphyrias resemble acute intermittent porphyria in humans in their excessive excretion of ALA and PBG, they simulate none of the clinical features of the human disease. Nevertheless, hepatic ALA synthetase is also greatly increased in human patients (Perlroth, Tschudy, Marver, Collins, Hunter & Rechcigl, 1965; Perlroth et al., 1966) and in both human and experimental porphyria the excretions of ALA and PBG are reciprocally related to the dietary intake of carbohydrate and/or protein (Rose, Hellman & Tschudy, 1961; Welland et al., 1964). The AIA-induced increase of ALA synthetase in rats was reduced by carbohydrate feeding (Tschudy, Welland, Collins & Hunter, 1964). The evidence thus seems that in both experimental and human porphyria the essential lesion is the induction of ALA synthetase (see Rimington, 1966). Perlroth et al. (1966) have discussed the possible mechanism. The induction of ALA synthetase may be secondary to a genetic defect outside the pathway of porphyrin biosynthesis and which is responsible for the nervous system involvement. This would be supported by the excretion of porphyrin precursors which can occur in some patients during complete clinical remission. Alternatively since ALA synthetase is repressed by haem in Rhodopseudomonas spheroides and probably also in higher organisms, decreased amounts of a specific repressor haem in the liver might be responsible for the increased synthesis of ALA synthetase. Although the rate of haem synthesis in experimental porphyria is not low the structure of the haems concerned has not been fully characterized and the rate of production of a specific repressor haem might be diminished while leaving the total haem production within normal limits. On the other hand, if the neurological lesions are causally related to the increased rates of ALA and PBG formation, an abnormality of the control of ALA synthetase by the appropriate gene may be postulated, although it would not explain the failure of the neurological lesions to be correlated with the excretion of ALA and PBG. According to current ideas of the control of protein synthesis (Jacob & Monod, 1961) there is a genetic abnormality in the repressor-operon system controlling ALA synthetase synthesis. Perlroth et al. (1966) point out that if an abnormality of the repressor gene was responsible, synthesis of repressor would only be absent in a homozygote and acute intermittent porphyria would then be inherited as a recessive characteristic. Since the condition is dominant, there must be a mutation at an operator site so that the repressor can no longer inhibit the operon site controlling the structural gene transcribing the m-RNA responsible for the ribosomal synthesis of ALA synthetase. Such an operator-constitutive mutation, as previously suggested by Watson, Runge, Taddeini, Bossenmaier & Cardinal (1964), would account for the biochemical and genetic findings. However, the detailed mode of control of ALA and PBG excretion by drugs, by oestrogens and by carbohydrate content of the diet still requires elucidation.*

Granick & Kappas (1967) have recently shown that certain saturated steroid hormones or their precursors, especially pregnanolone (in the free but not in their conjugated forms) are highly potent in inducing porphyrin synthesis in cultures of chick embryo liver cells. Kappas & Granick (1968) have suggested that the exacerbations of human porphyria associated with puberty, the menstrual cycle, pregnancy or oral contraceptives might be related to endogenous production of similar compounds or to the exogenous administration of steroid hormones. These workers have also suggested that the effect of carbohydrate in reducing the excretion of ALA and PBG in porphyria may be due to the utilization of glucose for additional glucuronide synthesis, thus rendering the steroids inactive.

Until still more is known of the enzymic abnormalities in the human disease and the precipitating factors identified, the reason for the great variation in the clinical picture of the disease, and for the variations in the threshold of ALA production at which different individuals show clinical symptoms, cannot be understood. In some patients the motor nervous system is affected, and they are paralysed. In others, the autonomic nervous system is mainly affected and there is abdominal pain. The paralyses and central nervous system abnormalities develop with devastating suddenness, reaching their maximum within a few hours. The patient may then be left with residual lesions of the nervous system, despite recovery from the metabolic disturbance responsible.

There is urgent need to investigate the disturbances of carbohydrate, protein and fat metabolism which presumably must result in brain, liver and other tissues from the greatly increased pro-

* See Addendum p. 232.

duction of ALA. The observation of Smith & Taylor (1954) that the α-oxoglutarate concentration is increased in the blood of patients with acute porphyria has not been confirmed by others, although Joubert, McKechnie & Deppe (1963) have found decreased rates of pyruvate clearance and accumulation of α-oxoglutarate in the blood after pyruvate infusion in Bantu patients with porphyria. However, many other abnormalities of metabolism are associated with experimental porphyria. Liver lipid phosphorus and total lipid are increased in sedormid porphyria (Schwartz, 1955), as is fatty acid synthesis in the liver of AIA-treated rats. Taddeini, Nordstrom & Watson (1964) have found a marked elevation in cholesterol, total lipids and phospholipids after AIA and DDC treatment in rabbits. Gray & Waterfield (1965) have also shown that these agents profoundly disturb the incorporation of ^{14}C from [U-^{14}C]-glucose into protein and glycogen. De Matteis (1966), however, believes that the association of these changes with increased formation of ALA should be regarded as coincidental.

Symptomatic Hepatic Cutaneous Porphyria

Rimington (1963) has suggested that in some forms of hepatic cutaneous porphyria there may be an abnormality of the oxidation-reduction systems in the liver normally responsible for the oxidation of porphyrinogens to the protoporphyrin of haem. Uroporphyrinogens, the intermediate porphyrinogens in the biosynthetic pathway to protoporphyrin, may be oxidized in this condition to the corresponding porphyrins which cannot return to the biosynthetic pathway, and so accumulate in the tissues and are excreted. The oxidation to porphyrin might be due to a disturbance in the redox potential within the parenchymal cells. The ratios of $NAD^+/NADH$ and $NADP^+/NADPH$ in the liver might reflect this disturbance, and the ratios have been shown to be changed in the livers of rats with experimental porphyria (Slater & Ziegler, 1966).

Keen, Saunders & Eales (1966) have found that tissue cultures of chick embryo liver produce increased amounts of porphyrin when infected with *Aspergillus fungatus* and suggest that Bantu porphyria in South Africa might be due to fungal contamination of food or of intoxicating liquors.

Erythropoietic Protoporphyria

Little is known concerning the exact biochemical disturbance in erythropoietic protoporphyria. Gray *et al.* (1964) found that the incorporation of ^{15}N-glycine into the porphyrins of the erythro-

cytes, the plasma and faeces suggested that there was disturbance of porphyrin biosynthesis in both the liver and erythropoietic tissues. Granick (1966) has suggested that ALA synthetase is controlled by at least three operons, each with its own operator, structural gene and repressor. These three operons would be responsible for the control of ALA synthetase formation in the liver parenchymal cells, in the erythropoietic tissues and other tissues respectively, and abnormality of the first two could account for the features of erythropoietic porphyria as well as for the hepatic or erythropoietic manifestation of some forms of porphyria.

TREATMENT OF THE PORPHYRIAS

In the present state of knowledge, treatment of all forms of porphyria can only be symptomatic. Barrier creams, avoiding sunlight, and antibiotics for infected lesions are all that can be offered to the patient with congenital porphyria or with hepatic cutaneous porphyria, although the latter subjects should be advised to avoid alcohol. In congenital porphyria splenectomy may perhaps be considered if there is any evidence of considerably increased haemolysis.

The assessment of the efficacy of the different forms of treatment of acute porphyria is difficult because of the spontaneous remissions which occur in the disease, and also by the failure of clinicians to appreciate the explosive nature of the acute episode which is often quickly over, leaving neurological symptoms as sequelae which may take some months to improve, even though the responsible metabolic episode may have cleared up very quickly. Older forms of treatment included alkalis, various vitamin preparations, especially of the B complex, calcium, cortisone, ACTH and more recently BAL, but all have almost certainly been useless in the condition. Whether adenosine monophosphate found by Gajdos & Gajdos-Török (1961) to be effective in both the human disease and the hexachlorobenzene-induced experimental form of the disease will prove more efficacious than previous remedies remains to be seen. Peters (1960) has treated acute intermittent porphyria with chelating agents such as BAL or EDTA on the basis of an alleged increased body content of zinc which was supposed to interfere with enzyme activity. However, Olsson & Ticktin (1962) were unable to confirm any beneficial effect with EDTA nor could they demonstrate any abnormality of zinc metabolism in the disease. The synthesis of ALA is pyridoxine-dependent and it would seem logical to attempt to diminish ALA production by pyridoxine antagonists. Elder & Mengel (1966) found that deoxypyridoxine decreased the excretion of ALA and PBG during an asymptomatic phase in a patient with acute porphyria. On the other hand, Gray & Anderson (unpublished observation) found no clinical or biochemical improvement when a patient with some neurological symptoms was given the pyridoxine antagonist penicillamine. Subjects with acute porphyria must not take any sulphonamide or barbiturate drugs and should avoid oestrogens and oral contraceptives. Anticonvulsant and tranquillizing drugs have been reported to precipitate acute attacks in otherwise benign coproporphyria, but a tranquilliser such as chlorpromazine and others may do much to allay the patient's alarm, and re-establishment of proper feeding often reduces ALA and PBG excretion, with great improvement in the clinical condition. In the acute attack, and during the stages of recovery, pethidine and other morphine substitutes may be needed to alleviate severe pain and orthopaedic treatment necessary to minimize the effect of the paralyses. The poor nutrition and vomiting, which may sometimes accompany the acute attacks, may lead to Na and even K deficiency, and such patients may require strict control of the fluid, electrolyte and nutritional intake.

Chloroquine has been reported to have beneficial effects in cutaneous forms of porphyria (see Eales, 1961) but its effect in producing liver dysfunction argues against its use in this condition (Sweeney, Saunders, Dowdle & Eales, 1965).

The resin cholestyramine which has been found to bind uroporphyrin and coproporphyrin has been used successfully in the treatment of three patients with hepatic cutaneous porphyria presumably by interfering with the entero-hepatic circulation of the porphyrins (Stathers, 1966). Erythropoietic protoporphyria has been successfully treated with inosine according to Gajdos, Gajdos-Török, Mantz & Schirardin (1965).

In symptomatic porphyria the clinical features are said to be alleviated by repeated venesection (Epstein & Redeker, 1965).

CHEMICAL INVESTIGATIONS IN PORPHYRIA

Diagnostic Investigations

In most cases in which the clinical picture is typical, detailed quantitative and qualitative tests are unnecessary for clinical purposes, although they may be of the greatest importance in research. Methods which have been developed for the separation, purification and characterization of the constituents of these complex mixtures include adsorption chromatography (Nicholas, 1951), paper partition chromatography of the porphyrins (Nicholas & Rimington, 1949) and of their esters (Falk & Benson, 1954), and X-ray diffraction (Kennard & Rimington, 1953). Falk (1954) has produced an excellent review of this subject (see also Chu & Chu, 1966). More recently French & Thonger (1966) have used counter-current analysis for the identification of porphyrins.

Congenital porphyria. The diagnosis of congenital porphyria is readily confirmed by the pink or red colour of the urine, which on spectroscopic examination reveals the typical 4-banded spectrum of a free porphyrin, usually mainly the ether-insoluble uroporphyrin I with maxima at 612, 560, 539 and 504 mμ. In ultraviolet light, the urine fluoresces bright red.

Acute porphyria. In many patients the diagnosis of acute porphyria is first suggested by the voiding of urine of a colour varying from pale pink to deep mahogany, or which had become dark on standing. Porphobilinogen itself is a colourless chromogen, and the freshly voided urine is often of a normal colour even during the acute attacks. Preformed porphyrins are often present in the urine in the form of a metal complex, which gives a 2-banded spectrum at approximately 580 and 500 mμ, superficially resembling that of haemoglobin. The spectrum of the metal complex, unlike haemoglobin, is unaffected by reducing agents such as sodium hydrosulphite. The porphobilinogen is readily detected by the reaction with *p*-dimethylaminobenzaldehyde. During acute exacerbation of the disease this test may be positive even after the urine is diluted by as much as 1 in 10 or 1 in 20.

The urine (5 ml.) is treated with an equal volume of Ehrlich's reagent (2% *p*-dimethylaminobenzaldehyde in 6N-HCl). A red colour indicates the presence of porphobilinogen or of a urobilinoid. If urobilinoids are present, the Schlesinger reaction with zinc acetate after preliminary oxidation with iodine is positive; this reaction is negative if the Ehrlich reaction is due to porphobilinogen. The red solution obtained from porphobilinogen shows a 2-banded spectrum; that obtained from urobilinoids gives a one-banded spectrum in the green.

In the special test of Watson & Schwartz (1941) it is necessary to use a different reagent containing 0·7 g. *p*-dimethylaminobenzaldehyde, 150 ml. conc. HCl and 100 ml. water. An equal volume of the urine is treated with this reagent and then about three or four volumes of saturated sodium acetate are added. A red colour which cannot be extracted from the solution by chloroform indicates the presence of porphobilinogen, the red compound formed from a urobilinoid readily passing into the chloroform layer.

PBG and ALA may be estimated quantitatively by the method of Mauzerall & Granick (1956) which depends on the separation of PBG from ALA on ion-exchange columns, followed by estimations of the former with Ehrlich's reagent and the latter with the same reagent after condensation to a mono-pyrrolic compound with acetyl acetone. Haeger (1958) has found the normal daily excretion of PBG and ALA to be 0 to 1·5 mg. and 0·7 to 3·2 mg. respectively. Between the acute crises of acute porphyria there is a rough correlation between severity of symptoms and mean excretion of PBG and ALA, but considerable fluctuations in the excretion of these compounds occur, with no correlation between peaks of excretion and symptoms (Ackner et al., 1961). Some patients excrete considerable quantities of ALA and PBG although remaining symptomless, while others with no increased excretion have symptoms. In these last patients an hysterical overlay may cause the patient to believe he is suffering from an acute attack of porphyria whenever he experiences pain, whether this is due to the disease or not. At times of acute crisis, several hundred mg. of PBG and of ALA may be excreted.

In acute porphyria vomiting is frequently present and may lead to a salt-deficiency state, which has suggested to some workers that acute porphyria might be accompanied by adrenal insufficiency (Abrahams, Gavey & Maclagan, 1947). The blood urea is frequently raised, perhaps in part due to the salt deficiency, and perhaps also to some direct effect of the disease on the blood pressure which is raised during the acute exacerbation of the disease. In a high proportion of cases the serum K is low, even in patients in whom vomiting and dietary deficiency are insufficient to account for this. There is need for further investigation to elucidate the mechanism.

Hepatic cutaneous porphyria. The differential diagnosis of the various forms of hepatic cutaneous porphyria is more difficult. Qualitative examination of urine, faeces, blood, plasma and erythrocytes (Cripps, 1966) may frequently suffice, but in doubtful cases quantitative measurements may also be necessary. However, the excretion of coproporphyrin (but not uroporphyrin) is dependent upon urinary pH and none of the published figures have taken this into account (Bourke, Copeman, Milne & Stokes, 1966).

Qualitative Analysis
Urine. The urine (25 ml.) is acidified with 2 ml.

glacial acetic acid and extracted with an equal volume of ether. The ether solution is washed with water and then extracted with successive small volumes of 0·6N-HCl, until examination under ultraviolet light reveals that no red fluorescing porphyrin is being extracted. Simultaneous examination of normal urine may reveal that the urine under investigation contains large quantities of coproporphyrin. The methods for estimating urinary porphyrins have been evaluated by Fernandez, Henry & Goldenberg (1966).

Faeces. The faeces may similarly be examined by extracting with ethyl acetate after a preliminary extraction of fatty material with acetone. About 1 g. of the faeces should be used and an ethyl acetate extract obtained amounting to about 20 ml. Extraction of this extract with 0·15N-HCl will yield a coproporphyrin fraction, and on further extraction with 3N-HCl a protoporphyrin fraction will be obtained. Often the coproporphyrin and/or protoporphyrin fractions will fluoresce red in ultraviolet light to a much greater extent than the corresponding fraction from normal faeces studied simultaneously. The protoporphyrin fraction may often fluoresce red in subjects with gastro-intestinal haemorrhage (Barnes & Dean, 1959), and in normal individuals because of the presence of faecal protoporphyrin derived from the meat in the diet. This difficulty, as well as the interference by chlorophyll derivatives, which cause red fluorescence in the ethyl acetate extract, may be avoided by keeping the patient on a diet free from red meat and green vegetables. Although the quantity of the porphyrin in the urine or in the faeces is often much greater than is encountered normally, in hepatic cutaneous porphyria as well as in acute porphyria, during a remission phase, the quantity of the porphyrins may sometimes not be greatly in excess of normal. A quantitative determination is then necessary.

Plasma. If excess porphyrin is present the plasma will fluoresce pink or red in ultraviolet light.

Erythrocytes. The erythrocytes are best examined by ultraviolet microscopy using an iodine tungsten ultraviolet lamp (Cripps, Hawgood & Magnus, 1966), but in erythropoietic protoporphyria or coproporphyria a specimen of whole blood may be seen to fluoresce bright red in ultraviolet light.

Quantitative Analysis
Faecal and urinary porphyrins may be determined by the method of Rimington (1961) and erythrocyte and plasma porphyrins by that of Rimington et al. (1963) or as described by Gray

TABLE 8.3

	Urine				Stools			Erythrocytes			Plasma
	CP	UR	PBG	ALA	CP	PP	UR	CP	PP	UR	PORPHYRIN
Erythropoietic porphyria (Guenther's disease)	increased[1]	large[1] amounts	normal	normal	greatly[1] increased	normal	present[1]	greatly increased	often increased	greatly increased	present
Acute intermittent porphyria	slightly[1] increased	normal[2] or increased	greatly increased	greatly increased	slightly increased	normal	present	normal	normal	normal	absent
Porphyria variegata acute phase	increased	increased[3]	greatly increased	greatly increased	slightly increased	increased	absent	normal	normal	normal	present
chronic phase	variable	variable[3]	normal	normal	slightly increased	increased	present[3]	normal	normal	normal	absent
Erythropoietic protoporphyria	normal	normal[2]	normal	normal	variable	increased	absent	increased	greatly increased	normal	present
Erythropoietic coproporphyria	normal	normal[2]	normal	normal	increased	normal	absent	increased	normal	normal	present
Symptomatic hepatic cutaneous porphyria	slightly increased	greatly increased	normal	normal	increased	slightly increased or normal	absent	normal	normal	normal	present during hepatic dysfunction
Bantu porphyria[4]	increased	normal[2]	normal	normal	normal	normal	absent	—	—	—	
Hexachlorobenzene porphyria	increased	greatly increased	increased	increased	increased	increased	absent	increased	increased	normal	
Griseofulvin porphyria[5]	normal	normal[2]	normal	normal	increased	increased	absent				present

CP = Coproporphyrin; PP = Protoporphyrin; UR = Uroporphyrin; PBG = Porphobilinogen; ALA = δ-aminolaevulic acid.

[1] Type I porphyrins; [2] normal urine contains less than 30 μg. uroporphyrin/day, this amount may be detected only by special methods; [3] In porphyria variegata the ether-insoluble porphyrin appears to be an unstable hydrophilic porphyrin-peptide conjugate not a uroporphyrin; [4] Bantu porphyria is probably the same condition as symptomatic hepatic cutaneous porphyria; [5] Griseofulvin has also been said to precipitate acute attacks of acute intermittent porphyria (Redeker, Sterling & Bronow, 1964).

et al. (1964). ALA and PBG may be measured by the method of Mauzerall & Granick (1956).

In certain forms of hepatic cutaneous porphyria, hepatic dysfunction is frequently present, and tests of liver function may then be of value. In many of these cases it will be found that during remission the urine is practically free from porphyrin, the faeces containing large amounts, and fluorescing when examined in ultraviolet light. During attacks impairment of liver function

results in a diversion of the excretion of porphyrins from the hepatic route to the renal route. The porphyrins in the faeces become greatly diminished and considerable quantities appear in the urine. In these circumstances the blood itself may contain much porphyrin and fluoresce red in ultraviolet light (Gray, Rimington & Thomson, 1948; Macgregor *et al.* 1952).

Table 8.3 shows the results to be expected in the different forms of porphyria.

References

ABRAHAMS, A., GAVEY, C. J. & MACLAGAN, N. F. (1947). *Brit. med. J.*, **2**, 327.

ACKNER, B. G. C., COOPER, J. E., GRAY, C. H., KELLY, M. & NICHOLSON, D. C. (1961). *Lancet*, **1**, 1256.

ALDRICH, R. A., HAWKINSON, V., GRINSTEIN, M. & WATSON, C. J. (1951). *Blood*, **6**, 685.

ANNOTATION (1965). *Lancet*, **2**, 1336.

BARNES, H. D. (1959). *S. Afr. med. J.*, **33**, 274.

BARNES, H. D. & DEAN, G. (1959). *Brit. med. J.*, **2**, 365.

BERLIN, N. I., NEUBERGER, A. & SCOTT, J. J. (1956). *Biochem. J.*, **64**, 80, 90.

BERLIN, S. O. & BRANTE, G. (1962). *Lancet*, **2**, 729.

BOGORAD, L. (1958). *J. biol. Chem.*, **233**, 501, 510 & 516.

BOGORAD, L. (1960). In "Comparative Biochemistry of Photoreactive Systems". Ed. Allen, M. B. New York, Academic Press Inc., p. 227.

BOLGERT, M., CANIVET, J. & LE SOURD, M. (1953). *Sem. Hôp.*, Paris, **29**, 1587.

BORST, M. & KOENIGSDÖRFFER, H. (1929). "Untersuchungen über Porphyrine". Leipzig, Hirsch.

BOURKE, E., COPEMAN, P. W. M., MILNE, M. D. & STOKES, G. S. (1966). *Lancet*, **1**, 1394.

BROCKMAN, P. E. & GRAY, C. H. (1953). *Biochem. J.*, **54**, 22.

BULLOCK, E. (1965). *Nature*, **205**, 70.

CAM, C. (1957). *Nester.*, **1**, 2.

CAVANAGH, J. B. & MELLICK, R. S. (1965). *J. Neurol. Neurosurg. Psychiat.*, **28**, 320.

CETINGIL, A. I. & OZEN, M. A. (1960). *Blood*, **16**, 1002.

CHU, T. C. & CHU, E. J.-H. (1966). *Clin. Chem.*, **12**, 647.

COOKSON, G. H. & RIMINGTON, C. (1954). *Biochem. J.*, **57**, 476.

COWGER, M. L. & LABBE, R. F. (1965). *Lancet*, **1**, 88.

CRIPPS, D. J. (1966). *Trans. St. John's Hosp. Derm. Soc.*, **52**, 51.

CRIPPS, D. J., HAWGOOD, R. S. & MAGNUS, I. A. (1966). *Arch. Derm.*, **93**, 129.

CRIPPS, D. J. & SCHEUER, P. J. (1965). *Arch. Path.*, **80**, 500.

DEAN, G. (1963). "The Porphyrias. A Story of Inheritance and Environment". London, Pitman Medical.

DEAN, G. & BARNES, H. D. (1959). *S. Afr. med. J.*, **33**, 246.

DE MATTEIS, F. (1966). *Biochem. J.*, **98**, 23c.

DE MATTEIS, F., PRIOR, B. E. & RIMINGTON, C. (1961). *Nature*, **191**, 363.

DE MATTEIS, F. & RIMINGTON, C. (1962). *Lancet*, **1**, 332.

DE MATTEIS, F. & RIMINGTON, C. (1963). *Brit. J. Derm.*, **75**, 91.

DENNY-BROWN, D. & SCIARRA, D. (1945). *Brain*, **68**, 1.

DRUYAN, R. & HAEGER-ARONSEN, B. (1964). *Scand. J. clin. lab. Invest.*, **16**, 498.

EALES, L. (1961). *Ann. Rev. Med.*, **12**, 251.

EALES, L., DOWDLE, E. B., LEVEY, M. J. & SWEENEY, G. D. (1966). *S. Afr. med. J.*, **40**, 380.

ELDER, T. D. & MENGEL, C. E. (1966). *Am. J. Med.*, **41**, 369.

EPSTEIN, J. H. & REDEKER, A. G. (1965). *Arch. Derm.* **91**, 483.

FALK, J. E. (1954). *Brit. med. Bull.*, **10**, 211.

FALK, J. E. & BENSON, A. (1954). *Arch. Biochem.*, **51**, 528.

FELDBERG, W. & TALESNIK, J. (1953). *J. Physiol.*, **120**, 550.

FERNANDEZ, A. A., HENRY, R. J. & GOLDENBERG, H. (1966). *Clin. Chem.*, **12**, 463.

FISCHER, H. & ORTH, H. (1937). "Die Chemie des Pyrrols". Band II. Leipzig. Academische Verlagsgesellschaft M.B.H.

FRENCH, J. M. & THONGER, E. (1966). *Clin. Sci.*, **31**, 337.

GAJDOS, A. & GAJDOS-TÖRÖK, M. (1961). *Lancet*, **2**, 175.

GAJDOS, A., GAJDOS-TÔRÖK, M., MANTZ, I. M. & SCHIRARDIN, H. (1965). *Presse Med.*, **73**, 119.

GIBSON, K. D., MATTHEW, M., NEUBERGER, A. & TAIT, G. H. (1961). *Nature*, **192**, 204.

GIBSON, Q. H. & HARRISON, D. C. (1950). *Biochem. J.*, **46**, 154.

GOLDBERG, A. (1954). *Biochem. J.*, **57**, 55.

GOLDBERG, A. (1958). *Quart. J. Med.*, **28**, 183.

GOLDBERG, A. (1959). *Quart. J. Med.*, **28**, 196.

GOLDBERG, A., MOORE, M. R., BEATTIE, A. D., HALL, P. E., McCALLUM, J. & GRANT, J. K. (1969). *Lancet*, **1**, 115.

GOLDBERG, A., PATON, W. D. M. & THOMPSON, J. W. (1954). *Brit. J. Pharm.*, **9**, 91.

GOLDBERG, A. & RIMINGTON, C. (1962). "Diseases of Porphyrin Metabolism". Springfield, Illinois, Charles C. Thomas.

GRANICK, S. (1963). *J. biol. Chem.*, **238**, 2247.

GRANICK, S. (1966). *J. biol. Chem.*, **241**, 1359.

GRANICK, S. & GILDER, H. (1947). *Adv. Enzymology*, **7**, 305.

GRANICK, S. & KAPPAS, A. (1967). *J. biol. Chem.* **242**, 4587.

GRANICK, S. & URATA, G. (1963). *J. biol. Chem.*, **238**, 821.

GRANICK, S. & VAN DEN SCHRIECK, H. G. (1955). *Proc. Soc. exp. Biol. N.Y.*, **88**, 270.

GRAY, C. H. (1950). *Arch. intern. Med.*, **85**, 459.

GRAY, C. H. (1951). *Biochem. J.*, **48**, liv.

GRAY, C. H. (1966). *Acta med. Scand. Suppl.*, **445**, 41.

GRAY, C. H., KULCZYCKA, A., NICHOLSON, D. C., MAGNUS, I. A. & RIMINGTON, C. (1964). *Clin. Sci.*, **26**, 7.

GRAY, C. H., MUIR, H. M. & NEUBERGER, A. (1950). *Biochem. J.*, **47**, 542.

GRAY, C. H. & NEUBERGER, A. (1952). *Lancet*, **1**, 851.

GRAY, C. H., NEUBERGER, A. & SNEATH, P. H. A. (1950). *Biochem. J.*, **47**, 87.

GRAY, C. H., RIMINGTON, C. & THOMSON, S. (1948). *Quart. J. Med.*, **17**, 123.

GRAY, C. H. & SCOTT, J. J. (1960). In "2ème Colloque International de Biologie de Saclay". Paris, Presses Universitaires de France.

GRAY, C. H. & WATERFIELD, M. D. (1965). Proc. Int. Symposium on the Normal and Pathologic Metabolism of Porphyrins, St. Vincent, Italy. Panminerva Medica, p. 47.

GUENTHER, H. (1925). "Handbuch der Krankheiten des Blutes und der Blutbildenden Organe". Berlin, Vol. II.

HAEGER, B. (1958). *Lancet*, **2**, 606.

HAEGER-ARONSEN, B. (1962). *Lancet*, **1**, 1073.

HEILMEYER, L. & CLOTTEN, R. (1964). *Dtsch. med. Wschr.*, **89**, 649.

HEIRONS, R. (1957). *Brain*, **80**, 176.

HERBERT, F. K. (1952). *Biochem. J.*, **52**, xii.

JACKSON, A. H. & MacDONALD, S. F. (1957). *Canad. J. Chem.*, **35**, 715.

JACOB, F. & MONOD, J. (1961). *J. molec. Biol.*, **3**, 318.

JARRETT, A., RIMINGTON, C. & WILLOUGHBY, D. A. (1956). *Lancet*, **1**, 125.

JOUBERT, S. M., McKECHNIE, J. K. & DEPPE, W. M. (1963). *S. Afr. J. lab. clin. Med.*, **9**, 227.

KAPPAS, A. & GRANICK, S. (1968). *J. biol. Chem.*, **243**, 346.

KEEN, G. A., SAUNDERS, S. J. & EALES, L. (1966). *Lancet*, **1**, 798.

KENNARD, O. & RIMINGTON, C. (1953). *Biochem. J.*, **55**, 105.

LOCKHEAD, A. C. & GOLDBERG, A. (1961). *Biochem. J.*, **78**, 146.

MACGREGOR, A. G., NICHOLAS, R. E. H. & RIMINGTON, C. (1952). *Arch. intern. Med.*, **90**, 483.

MAGNUS, I. A., JARRETT, A., PRANKERD, T. A. J. & RIMINGTON, C. (1961). *Lancet*, **2**, 448.

MAGNUS, I. A., PORTER, A. D., McCREE, K. J., MORELAND, J. D. & WRIGHT, W. D. (1959). *Brit. J. Derm.*, **71**, 261.

MARKS, G. S. (1962). *Ann. Reps.*, **59**, 385.

MARVER, H. S., TSCHUDY, D. P., PERLROTH, M. G. & COLLINS, A. (1965). *Clin. res.*, **13**, 278.

MATTHEWSON, J. H. & CORWEN, A. H. (1961). *J. Amer. Chem. Soc.*, **83**, 135.

MAUZERALL, D. (1960a). *J. Amer. Chem. Soc.*, **82**, 2601.

MAUZERALL, D. (1960b). *J. Amer. Chem. Soc.*, **82**, 2605.

MAUZERALL, D. & GRANICK, S. (1956). *J. biol. Chem.*, **219**, 435.

NAKAO, K., WADA, O., TAKAHU, F., SASSA, S., YANO, Y. & URATA, G. (1967). *J. Lab. clin. Med.* **70**, 923.

NICHOLAS, R. E. H. (1951). *Biochem. J.*, **48**, 309.

NICHOLAS, R. E. H. & RIMINGTON, C. (1949). *Scand. J. clin. Lab. Invest.*, **1**, 12.

OCKNER, R. K. & SCHMID, R. (1961). *Nature*, **189**, 499.

OLSSON, R. A. & TICKTIN, H. E. (1962). *J. lab. clin. Med.*, **60**, 48.

PALMA-CARLOS, A., PALMA-CARLOS, M. L., GAJDOS-TÖRÖK, M. & GAJDOS, A. (1966). *Rev. Franc. Etudes Clin. et Biol.*, **XI**, 284.

PERLROTH, M. G., TSCHUDY, D. P., MARVER, H. S., BERARD, C. W., ZEIGEL, R. F., RECHCIGL, M. & COLLINS, A. (1966). *Amer. J. Med.*, **41**, 149.

PERLROTH, M. G., TSCHUDY, D. P., MARVER, H. S., COLLINS, A., HUNTER, G. W. & RECHCIGL, M. (1965). *J. clin. Invest.*, **44**, 1085.

PETERKA, E. S., FUSARO, R. M., RUNGE, W. J., JAFFE, M. O. & WATSON, C. J. (1965). *J. Amer. med. Assoc.*, **193**, 1036.

PETERS, H. A. (1960). In "Metal Binding in Medicine". Eds. Seven, M. S. & Johnson, L. A. Philadelphia, J. B. Lippincott Co. p. 190.

PETERS, H. A., JOHNSON, S. A. M., CAM, S., ORAL, S., MÜFTÜ, Y. & ERGENE, T. (1966). *Amer. J. Med. Sci.*, **251**, 314.

PORTER, F. S. (1963). *Blood*, **22**, 532.

PORTER, F. S. & LOWE, B. A. (1963). *Blood*, **22**, 521.

RAINE, D. (1950). *Biochem. J.*, **47**, xiv.

REDEKER, A. G. & BRYAN, H. G. (1964). *Lancet*, **1**, 1449.

REDEKER, A. G., STERLING, R. E. & BRONOW, R. S. (1964). *J. Amer. Med. Soc.*, **188**, 466.

RICHARDS, F. F. & SCOTT, J. J. (1961). *Clin. Sci.*, **20**, 387.

RIMINGTON, C. (1958). Assoc. of Clin. Pathologists Broadsheet, No. 21 (New Series).

RIMINGTON, C. (1959). *Brit. med. Bull.*, **15**, 19.

RIMINGTON, C. (1961). Assoc. of Clin. Pathologists Broadsheet, No. 36 (New Series).

RIMINGTON, C. (1963). *Ann. N.Y. Acad. Sci.*, **104**, 658.

RIMINGTON, C. (1966). *Acta med. Scand. Suppl.*, **445**, 11.

RIMINGTON, C. & DE MATTEIS, F. (1965). *Lancet*, **1**, 270.

RIMINGTON, C. & LOCKWOOD, W. H. (1965). Proc. Int. Symposium on the Normal and Pathologic Metabolism of Porphyrins, St. Vincent, Italy. Panminerva Medica, p. 60.

RIMINGTON, C., LOCKWOOD, W. H. & BELCHER, R. (1968). *Clin. Sci.*, **35**, 211.

RIMINGTON, C. & MILES, P. A. (1951). *Biochem. J.*, **50**, 202.

RIMINGTON, C., MORGAN, P. N., NICHOLLS, K., EVERALL, J. D. & DAVIES, R. R. (1963). *Lancet*, **2**, 318.

ROBINSON, R. (1955). "The Structural Relations of Natural Products". London, Oxford University Press, p. 25.

ROSE, J. A., HELLMAN, E. S. & TSCHUDY, D. P. (1961). *Metabolism*, **10**, 514.

SANO, S. & RIMINGTON, C. (1963). *Biochem. J.*, **86**, 203.

SCHMID, R. & SCHWARTZ, S. (1952). *J. lab. clin. Med.*, **40**, 939.

SCHMID, R. & SCHWARTZ, S. (1955). Personal Communication.

SCHWARTZ, S. (1955). *Fed. Proc.*, **14**, 717.

SHEMIN, D. (1956). "Currents in Biochemical Research". Ed. Green, D. E. New York and London, Interscience Publishers. p. 518.

SHEMIN, D., RUSSELL, C. S. & ABRAMSKY, T. (1955). *J. biol. Chem.*, **215**, 613.

SLATER, T. F. & RILEY, P. A. (1966). *Nature*, **209**, 151.

SLATER, T. F. & ZIEGLER, G. (1966). *Biochem. Pharm.*, **15**, 1279.

SMART, G. A., HERBERT, F. K., WHITTAKER, N. & BARNES, H. D. (1965). *Lancet*, **1**, 318.

SMITH, M. J. H. & TAYLOR, K. W. (1954). Unpublished observations.

STATHERS, G. M. (1966). *Lancet*, **2**, 780.

SWEENEY, G. D., SAUNDERS, S. J., DOWDLE, E. B. & EALES, L. (1965). *Brit. med. J.*, **1**, 1281.

TADDEINI, L., NORDSTROM, K. L. & WATSON, C. J. (1964). *Metabolism*, **13**, 691.

TALMAN, E. L., LABBE, R. F., ALDRICH, R. A. & SEARS, D. (1959). *Arch. Biochem. Biophys.*, **80**, 446.

THEORELL, H. (1939). *Biochem. Z.*, **301**, 201.

TIO, T. H., LEIJNSE, B., JARRETT, A. & RIMINGTON, C. (1957). *Clin. Sci.*, **16**, 517.

TSCHUDY, D. P., WELLAND, F. H., COLLINS, A. & HUNTER, G. W. (1963). *Lancet*, **2**, 660.

TSCHUDY, D. P., WELLAND, F. H., COLLINS, A. & HUNTER, G. W. (1964). *Metabolism*, **13**, 396.

URATA, G. & GRANICK, S. (1963). *J. biol. Chem.*, **238**, 811.

VANNOTTI, A. (1954). "Porphyrins". Translated by C. Rimington. London, Hilger & Watts.

WALDENSTRÖM, J. (1937). *Acta med. Scand. Suppl.* 82.

WALDENSTRÖM, J. (1957). *Amer. J. Med.*, **22**, 758.

WALDENSTRÖM, J. & VAHLQUIST, B. (1939). *Hoppe Seyl. Z.*, **260**, 189.

WATSON, C. J. (1936). *J. clin. Invest.*, **15**, 327.

WATSON, C. J. (1937). *J. clin. Invest.*, **16**, 383.

WATSON, C. J. (1954). "Advances in Internal Medicine", Vol. VI. Chicago, Year Book Publishers.

WATSON, C. J., HAWKINSON, V., CAPPS, R. B. & RAPPAPORT, E. M. (1949). *J. clin. Invest.*, **28**, 621.

WATSON, C. J., PIMENTA DE MELLO, R., SCHWARTZ, S., HAWKINSON, V. & BOSSENMAIER, I. (1951). *J. lab. clin. Med.*, **37**, 831.

WATSON, C. J., RUNGE, W. & BOSSENMAIER, I. (1962). *Metabolism*, **11**, 1129.

WATSON, C. J., RUNGE, W., TADDEINI, I., BOSSENMAIER, I. & CARDINAL, R. (1964). *Proc. nat. Acad. Sci.* (U.S.A.), **52**, 478.

WATSON, C. J., SCHULZE, W., HAWKINSON, V. & BAKER, A. B. (1947). *Proc. Soc. exp. Biol.*, (N.Y.), **64**, 73.

WATSON, C. J. & SCHWARTZ, S. (1941). *Proc. Soc. exp. Biol.*, (N.Y.), **47**, 393.

WELLAND, F. H., HELLMAN, E. S., GADDIS, E. M., COLLINS, A., HUNTER, G. W. & TSCHUDY, D. P. (1964). *Metabolism*, **13**, 232.

WESTALL, R. G. (1952). *Nature*, **170**, 614.

ZIMMERMAN, T. S., McMILLIN, J. M. & WATSON, C. J. (1966). *Arch. intern. Med.*, **118**, 229.

ADDENDUM

Goldberg and his colleagues (1969) have shown significant elevations of aetiocholanolone glucuronide, dehydroepiandrosterone glucuronide and sulphate or epiandrosterone sulphate in certain patients with acute intermittent porphyria and have shown that free dehydropeiandrosterone or its sulphate significantly elevated hepatic ALA synthetase in rats. They suggest that this abnormality of steroid metabolism in some patients with acute porphyria may explain certain clinical associations, such as the age of onset after puberty and the occurrence of attacks not attributable to exogenous factors.

Chapter 9

HYPERTENSION

by

W. S. Peart

St. Mary's Hospital Medical School, London

THE biochemical disturbances in any form of hypertension are considerable, and it is not always clear whether they are in any way causally related to the hypertension or whether they are some secondary happening (Peart, 1959*a*). In some cases this can be readily decided when a cure of the hypertension is possible by removing a gland or other organ thought to be concerned, and occasionally by reduction of the blood pressure using non-specific means, when some of the bio-chemical features revert to normal and are probably due to some consequence of the high blood pressure itself. A good example of the former state is the low plasma volume sometimes found in patients with phaeochromocytoma (Brunjes, Johns & Crane, 1960), probably due to the action of noradrenaline which increases filtration pressure in the capillaries (Folkow, Johansson & Mellander, 1961). This state is rapidly reversed on removing the tumour. An example of the latter state is the increased sodium-losing tendency of patients with hypertension (Brodsky & Graubarth, 1953; Cottier, Weller & Hoobler, 1958), and this can be blocked if the blood pressure is lowered by a variety of drugs, suggesting that the high arterial pressure itself is the main operative factor. It is not always easy to separate cause and effect, but this distinction must be kept in mind in the subsequent discussion on biochemical disturbances. Another important aspect hinges on homeostatic mechanisms into which the more modern but not more meaningful terms of positive and negative feed-back systems have been introduced. This simply means the tendency of the body to resist change in its normal functions and to return such a changed function to its normal state by variation in controlling mechanisms. In the cardiovascular field this is shown by return of an elevated blood pressure to normal by the action of baroreceptor reflexes, but not all homeostatic mechanisms are as rapid in action as this and the adjustments made, for example, to increases in blood volume which in turn have an action on venous pressure, cardiac output and urinary excretion, are of importance in relation to blood pressure (Borst & Borst-De Geus, 1963).

In systems with many variables acting upon them, the difficulty of deciding whether a normal value or function measured at a particular time necessarily means that this function might not have been deranged initially, is a considerable problem. In such a system, however, one of the controlling variables must necessarily become or remain abnormal, otherwise the state, for example, of hypertension could not exist. In assessing a situation this carries the implication, however, that all the variables playing a part are known if the part of the system which is thrown out of balance is to be readily discerned. It does not mean that the part of the system which is behaving differently is the cause of the imbalanced system, since it may represent purely the result of the homeostatic readjustments.

At the present time there are three main known systematic disturbances which may play a biochemical role in high arterial pressure.

I ELECTROLYTE CHANGES

Primary changes, due to Diseases of the Adrenal Cortex

Conn's syndrome. This in many ways is the classic example of such disease since the hypertension is usually readily reverted to normal by removal of the responsible cortical adenoma

(Conn, 1955). While the symptoms and signs vary, it is striking that they are usually much greater in the female than in the male, and characteristically include the following: weakness; cramps; paraesthesiae, especially in hands and feet; thirst; polyuria; paralysis and tetany; hypertension of variable degrees from very mild to the malignant phase. The biochemical features have been a subject of great controversy since they range from the easily diagnosed condition with hypokalaemic alkalosis and quite commonly elevated plasma sodium, to situations where the plasma electrolytes in themselves may be within normal limits (Cohen, Rovner, Conn & Blough, 1964; Conn, Cohen, Rovner & Nesbit, 1965). Typical figures

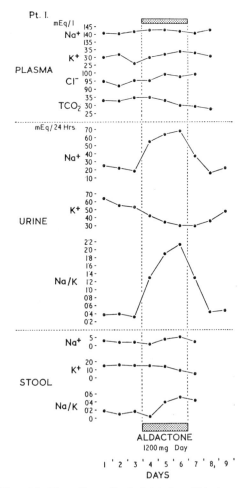

FIG. 9.1. The effect of administering Aldactone-A to a patient with Conn's tumour showing the immediate blocking effect of the action of aldosterone.

for a patient of the first type would be sodium 144 mEq./l., potassium 2 mEq./l. and bicarbonate 32 mMole/l., and the urine would remain alkaline. In this type of patient it seems likely that the biochemical disturbance as shown by the plasma figures is due to the action of aldosterone which usually reduces total body potassium and causes an inappropriately high potassium excretion relative to the plasma potassium level. A difficulty in looking at this situation is the widely variable figures of aldosterone secretion as measured by the technique of Kliman & Peterson (1960), and it has raised the suspicion that other steroids may be implicated that are currently being missed. However, there is no direct evidence for this as yet. The great characteristic of these patients where the sodium: potassium ratio in the saliva and more reliably in the stool is reduced, is their response to spironolactone (Aldactone-A), which, as shown in Fig. 9.1, readily blocks the action of aldosterone and returns the sodium:potassium ratio in saliva, urine and stool to normal (Brown, Davies, Lever, Peart & Robertson, 1965). The plasma potassium also quickly rises long before there is any correction of the external potassium balance, thereby suggesting that a change of intracellular to extracellular distribution has occurred. It cannot be claimed that this type of response proves the presence of a tumour since patients with secondary aldosteronism may show a similar response and secondary aldosteronism is not uncommon in cases of severe hypertension (Genest, Boucher, Nowaczynski, Koiw, de Champlain, Biron, Chrétien & Marc-Aurèle, 1964; Laragh, Ulick, Januszewicz, Deming, Kelly & Lieberman, 1960).

A greater problem arises in the second group of patients that Conn has recently claimed are not uncommon, who are normokalaemic throughout their observed course and may have quite low secretion rates of aldosterone and yet who harbour cortical adenomata, the removal of which is followed by a fall in blood pressure (Conn, *et al.*, 1965). They estimate that perhaps 20% of a hypertensive population may carry such tumours, and needless to say this view has aroused both surprise and opposition, and it is necessary to examine the main criteria on which this claim is based since there seems no doubt that patients with a normal blood potassium and no other evidence of the classical condition may have their blood pressure lowered by removal of such tumours. The question is how common the condition is in reality. Everything revolves around the assay of renin activity in the plasma and this will be discussed in full in a separate section. Since probably about 20% of a population of patients with high arterial pressure have a low or lower than normal plasma renin level (Brown, Davies, Lever & Robertson, 1964a) it is in this group that Conn believes this type of patient with adenoma is to be found. A criterion used in diagnosis is the finding of a low plasma renin which does not rise with exercise or sodium depletion. This carries the implication that aldosterone secretion is always raised in these patients; this is difficult to prove in many of them, and only time and the accumulation of more patients with post-operative follow-up will decide this issue. For decades pathologists have been pointing out adrenal cortical adenomata, sometimes especially marked in patients with hypertension. They have often been regarded as incidental or secondary to the hypertension, but now the position is open. Whether some of them may produce other steroids which are more hypertensive in their effects than aldosterone, remains to be seen. It is of interest that a large number of patients with hypertension treated randomly with big doses of spironolactone have their blood pressure lowered to normal levels, but whether this is due to the action of spironolactone independent of its aldosterone blocking action is not yet known (Peart—unpublished observations). A further point which arises is that many patients with Conn's syndrome of the hypokalaemic variety have a diabetic type of glucose tolerance curve. Initially it was thought that this was related to the hypokalaemia, and certainly restoration of potassium led to a return of the curve to normal (Conn, 1965). In the normokalaemic group an abnormality of glucose tolerance may also occur and it is now becoming common to find such abnormal glucose tolerance curves in a large number of subjects with hypertension and atheromatous vascular disease (Hood, Falkheden, Aurell, Olanders & Björk, 1967). This relation is of very uncertain meaning, and the argument must not be pushed too far in terms either of diabetes or of cortical adenomata.

It seems quite likely that a low plasma renin will be found in patients without a Conn's tumour since there are many factors which bear upon the level of plasma renin. Further, there is a not inconsiderable group of patients who have renal disease with signs of hyperaldosteronism. One of these with a renal artery stenosis and hypokalaemic alkalosis has been reported where correction of the renal artery stenosis had no effect on either the biochemical disturbances or the blood pressure, yet spironolactone reduced the blood pressure to normal, where it has remained for years, and the hypokalaemia was similarly

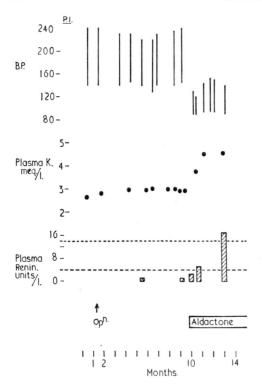

FIG. 9.2. The effect of Aldactone-A on the blood pressure, plasma potassium and renin in a patient with corrected renal artery stenosis (Opn.) where the operation failed to lower the blood pressure or alter any of the other values. This suggests the presence of a Conn's tumour. (From Brown, Davies, Lever & Robertson, 1964a).

reverted to normal (Peart, 1965a) (Fig. 9.2). Whether in fact the association which was thought at one time to be very marked between pyelonephritis, hypokalaemia and a Conn's tumour is a real one, or whether under some circumstances persistent stimulation of the adrenal cortex in the presence of renal disease leads to an autonomous cortex with adenomata, is still an open question, and some of the biochemical difficulties in differential diagnosis have been well brought out by Gowenlock & Wrong (1962). Although aldosterone is a poor pressor agent in the experimental animal, it may not be in man, in addition to which the duration of the disease in man has to be considered. Considerations of this sort led Conn et al. (1965) to wonder whether a long period wherein hypertension existed due to aldosterone preceded the development of frank hypokalaemia, and to postulate the normokalaemic association

of hypertension and adenoma. The most likely change that aldosterone produces is one involving transfer of sodium and potassium across smooth muscle cell membranes.

The response of blood pressure to surgery in established cases of tumour may be very rapid (days) or in some cases slow (weeks). The latter course may depend on the presence of vascular damage, as has been shown by the presence of fibrinoid necroses in renal arterioles (Brown, Davies, Lever, Peart & Robertson, 1964). Further, it may be expected that there will be some patients in whom vascular damage has proceeded so far that removal of a cortical adenoma will not be attended by a substantial fall in blood pressure. This is akin to the situation in unilateral renal disease where the opposite renal damage may maintain the hypertension (Wilson & Byrom, 1941). The circulation in patients with Conn's syndrome has been studied, and the presence of an increased plasma volume and its effects in altering ordinary circulatory reflex responses defined (Biglieri & McIlroy, 1966). The aldosterone secretion rate of a wide range of hypertensive subjects has been studied by Laragh and his colleagues (Laragh, 1961). They cannot find such a large number with increased aldosterone as Conn predicts, but again it might be best to reserve discussion for the association of cortical adenomata with hypertension and the effect on blood pressure following their removal, since, as has been stated before, aldosterone may not be the only hormone involved.

Cushing's syndrome. While it might be thought that the hypertension in Cushing's syndrome would be like that in Conn's syndrome, this is not proven. Most patients with this disorder do not have an increased secretion of aldosterone but do have a greater secretion rate of hydrocortisone, corticosterone and gonadal hormones. Hypertension of all grades up to the malignant phase is seen in well established cases, and because severe hypertension is uncommon in patients treated with cortisone-like steroids for varying disorders over long periods of time (Peart, 1959 b), the possibility is raised that some other steroid might be liberated with particular pressor effects that has so far escaped notice. This possibility should always be kept in mind, even though there is no direct evidence for it at present. Very few studies have been made but it seems likely that some electrolyte distribution change as in Conn's syndrome provides the basis of the hypertension. While the emphasis in Cushing's syndrome is usually on cortisol and its metabolites there are some patients who show mainly the androgenic aspects, and a patient seen recently at St. Mary's Hospital with hypertension and a large adrenal tumour, was secreting mainly corticosterone, a hormone which has been relatively neglected in this and other fields.

Adreno-genital syndrome. Attention was first directed to this in a series of children studied by Wilkins, Crigler, Silverman, Gardner & Migeon (1952) who were basically females although appearing to be male in their general body configuration, and who were found to have a high excretion of 17-ketosteroids. The blood pressure was reduced to normal by administration of cortisone, which decreased the excretion of 17-ketosteroids. The suggestion is that these subjects have a 21-hydroxylase defect which leads to the production of large amounts of androgen, presumably of a sort which does not depress ACTH. Administration of cortisol, in which they are deficient, suppresses the pituitary and reduces the drive to the suprarenals, thus lessening the androgenic metabolites. Because of the finding of tetrahydro-deoxycorticosterone in the urine of some patients with this condition, Eberlein & Bongiovanni (1956) suggested that the cause of the high blood pressure might be the production of DOCA. This also involves the lack of a second enzyme, 11-hydroxylase. More recently Biglieri (1965) has studied a patient with a distinct increase of deoxycorticosterone and his findings cast some doubt on the hypothesis that DOCA causes the hypertension, since despite a profound hypokalaemic alkalosis, the blood pressure was not elevated. The effect of DOCA could be blocked by spironolactone. In this particular case the very low blood volume might have been responsible for the postural hypotension noted.

The type of circulatory disorder which exists in any of these cases of hormonal hypertension is not clear. Conn's syndrome has been best studied, and the finding of an increased plasma volume may be relevant to the development of hypertension and therefore may contrast with the low plasma volume in the patient with excess of DOCA noted above, since it may be essential to have both the electrolyte effects of the mineralocorticoids plus the increased blood volume before hypertension can be brought about. DOCA itself is indeed a distinctly pressor agent, as was shown by the initial experiences in the treatment of patients with Addison's disease, where malignant hypertension occurred inadvertently in some patients given DOCA. Dosage may be very important here (Loeb, Atchley, Ferrebee & Ragan, 1939; McCullagh & Ryan, 1940; Thorn & Firor, 1940).

Secondary Changes

One of the striking features in some patients with hypertension is the development of low plasma sodium and potassium levels (Dollery, Shackman & Shillingford, 1959). When the plasma sodium is low, it is almost invariably accompanied by a low plasma potassium, but the converse is not true. In considering these changes the first thing to be excluded is whether the patients are receiving diuretics, since, while in hypertension the action of the commonly used diuretics of thiazide or frusemide type is to cause hypokalaemia, in some patients the plasma sodium is also lowered. The administration of potassium in conjunction is not enough in many patients to prevent hypokalaemia, and further, the administration of these diuretics may reveal an underlying deficiency of potassium and precipitate symptoms and signs sometimes of a dangerous kind such as paralysis. This is particularly so when they are administered to patients with Conn's syndrome.

Hyponatraemia. There is a small group of patients with severe hypertension, often of acute onset, who present with thirst, polyuria, weakness and malignant hypertensive changes in their fundi (De Camp & Birchall, 1958; Deming, 1954; Dollery, et al., 1959; Margolin, Merrill & Harrison, 1957; Øster, 1947). On investigation, the plasma sodium may be as low as 125–130 mEq./l., the potassium in the range 2·0–3·0 mEq./l., and the plasma bicarbonate between 30 and 35 mMole/l. These patients will often be found to have unilateral renal disease, sudden thrombosis in the renal artery, and embolus or rapid development of a stricture indicating perhaps thrombosis at an established stenosis. They offer a good prospect of cure of the hypertension by either nephrectomy or restoration of normal blood flow through surgery, and the mechanism of the hyponatraemia is obscure. It may be that because of the rapid elevation of pressure, the medullary blood flow rises very high and the concentration gradient of the kidney is grossly interfered with, allowing sodium to run out freely in the urine. Many of these patients are, in fact, excreting excessive amounts of sodium yet occasional patients are recorded who do not (Fitzgerald, Fourman, James & Scarborough, 1957). The fact that the potassium is also low suggests the influence of aldosterone, and while the effects in these patients are largely unrecorded, they would be expected to be very resistant to the usual sodium-retaining effects or, alternatively, under these circumstances aldosterone might be facilitating the excretion of sodium. Too few studies have been performed to draw any conclusion.

Hypokalaemia. This is very common in the studies of patients with moderate to severe hypertension, and while a low plasma potassium calls attention to the possibility of a Conn's syndrome, many patients will restore their potassium level to normal when the blood pressure is reduced by ordinary hypotensive drugs (Hilden & Krogsgaard, 1958). While it is usual to think of this as implying increased aldosterone secretion, this is by no means certain. In extensive studies, it has been shown that only those patients with severe hypertension have a high aldosterone secretion rate (Laragh, *et al.*, 1960). It has been previously claimed by Genest, Nowaczynski, Koiw, Sandor & Biron (1960) that all types of hypertensive patient have increased aldosterone secretion, but that those with the milder types have a more sporadic increase. The present weight of evidence suggests that it is only in the severe grades of hypertension that increased secretion rate is found. In view of the difficulty in diagnosing Conn's syndrome, the question of primary and secondary aldosteronism has to be examined. As noted before, in primary aldosteronism the plasma renin is low, so that hypokalaemia with an elevated plasma renin would be very much in favour of a secondary form of hyperaldosteronism and is an important point of differentiation. Whether the renin-angiotensin system is implicated in this hypokalaemia of hypertension is not certain since the correlation of plasma renin and plasma potassium is not so clear as with plasma sodium (Barraclough, Bacchus, Brown, Davies, Lever & Robertson, 1965).

Relation to Diuretic Treatment of Hypertension and Chronic Dialysis

Since one of the most strongly held beliefs about hypertension involves sodium retention in some way (Dahl, 1960), the effect of diuretics on hypertension deserves consideration. In general it may be said that while occasionally thiazides reduce the blood pressure considerably, this is rare, and a mild reduction in pressure is the rule, so that if the case was that the final path whereby hypertension is produced involves sodium content of the body as a whole, then this could not be supported. However, there is no strong evidence about sodium distribution and it could be argued that thiazides do not affect this important aspect of the action of sodium ion. This is brought out by the effects of spironolactone in the treatment of hypertension where it is apparent that, using fairly large doses, a much larger number of patients will show a considerable fall in blood pressure (Peart—personal observations). While it might be that

these patients harbour a Conn's tumour, the percentage that show a good response is surprisingly high. Since spironolactone is known to alter plasma potassium very rapidly without respect to the overall balance initially, this question of distribution may be important. The effects of chronic haemodialysis on the treatment of hypertension are also of real importance since they illustrate what may be done in the presence of abnormal kidneys. Scribner, Fergus & Boen (1965) first showed that intensive haemodialysis with removal of water and salt in large amounts led to a control of severe hypertension in most of their patients, whatever the underlying nature of the renal disease had been. Shaldon (1966) further showed that while these patients initially had the characteristic hypersensitivity to salt and water infusions, whereby the pressure would rise sharply even with relatively small infusions, after haemodialysis had been carried out intensively for many months and the blood pressure had become stable, this sensitivity was lost. His patients then behaved much as normal subjects. Whether this means that a prolonged de-salting process leads to marked haemodynamic alterations and, if so, how, cannot be answered at present. It does give food for thought in considering the haemodynamic situation in chronic renal failure and whether any of the factors implicated there, in terms of this increased sensitivity to blood volume changes, may play a part in other forms of hypertension in renal disease. It is not the only answer, however, since removal of diseased kidneys without change in fluid and electrolyte may bring about very quick change in blood pressure (Peart—personal observation).

II SYMPATHO-ADRENAL SYSTEM

The hypothalamo-sympathetic and adrenomedullary system may be considered as a whole, although most attention has been devoted to the function of sympathetic nerve endings, and the adrenal medulla is not considered of great importance in control of the circulation under ordinary circumstances except when a tumour appears there.

Functioning of the Sympathetic System

Knowledge has accrued mostly about the sympathetic efferent pathway, and relatively little is known about the central hypothalamic regions except that here are located the major stores of noradrenaline, 5-hydroxytryptamine and substance P. The fact that depletion of these stores by drugs such as reserpine is still compatible with adequate functioning of the sympathetic system, suggests that most of the stores of these sub-stances are not completely essential to a central function. The same also applies to sympathetic nerve-endings wherein lie most of the stores of noradrenaline. This suggests that only a few per cent of noradrenaline is needed for effective trans-mission of the nervous impulse, and the other stores are there for an as yet unknown purpose (for references see Proceedings of Second Cate-cholamine Symposium held in Milan, July 1965). One of the earliest ideas concerning hypertension was that excessive activity of the sympathetic nervous system might be responsible in some cases, and, while the evidence for this is tenuous (Pickering, 1936), the position has to be examined fairly carefully since the question asked is "How can a particular degree of sympathetic nervous activity be measured in the intact animal or man?" This falls into the following groups:

Physiological. In certain parts of the body it is possible to remove the effects of sympathetic tone by either nerve block or body warming (Lewis & Pickering, 1931; Pickering & Hess, 1933). This has been shown clearly in the hand where the effect of blocking the nerves with local anaesthetic has exactly the same effect on blood flow through the fingers as does body warming. The difference in flow produced by this procedure would then represent the degree of activity of the sympathetic nervous system under the prevailing conditions. It was by use of this sort of approach that Picker-ing (1936) was able to show that the increase in peripheral resistance in the hand in a wide variety of patients with hypertension was increased by some factor other than increased sympathetic tone. In present circumstances this sort of approach probably still offers the best measure of sympathetic activity but it has not been applied in other vascular territories.

Biochemical. When a nervous impulse passes down a sympathetic nerve to release noradrena-line, a fraction of the released hormone enters the blood stream and then is either re-stored in nerve endings, metabolized in various organs such as the liver, or excreted in the urine, together with its metabolic products. A further large fraction undergoes metabolic change within or close to the nerve ending due to the presence of the enzymes monoamine oxidase and catechol-O-methyl-trans-ferase. This results in production of various other metabolites, and the main final products which reach the urine include vanillylmandelic acid, metanephrine, normetanephrine, free amine and ethereal sulphate conjugates (for references see Proceedings of Second Catecholamine Sym-posium, 1965). If under ordinary circumstances

increased sympathetic activity led to the release of noradrenaline, which is metabolized in a predict-able way ultimately to reach the urine, then it might be possible to draw a quantitative relation between the metabolites appearing in the urine and the degree of sympathetic activity prevailing over a certain period of time. Similar arguments might be made about measurements of blood levels of noradrenaline and, in relation to the adrenal medulla, also of adrenaline. There are, however, some missing pieces of knowledge which are necessary if full use is to be made of this sort of approach. There is no particular correlation between known degrees of sympathetic activity and the amount of noradrenaline and adrenaline and their metabolites appearing in the urine. There are reports, however, which suggest that this line of reasoning may be quantitatively pos-sible. The original data of Luft & von Euler (1953) on patients with postural hypotension, probably due to decreased sympathetic efferent impulses, show a marked decrease in urinary noradrenaline. It seems very likely that this did reflect changed production in these patients, but what is not clear is whether, with an intact sympathetic system, there is any quantitative relation between change in activity and the amount of metabolite appear-ing in the urine. This is because we do not know quantitatively the fate of noradrenaline released in response to a sympathetic stimulus and, further, the precise distribution in quantitative terms between these various metabolic and humoral pathways. The presence of these large stores of noradrenaline which are not necessary for sympathetic activity is the major factor, and renders interpretation difficult. However, other studies and attempts at correlation with psycho-logical stress of different sorts have been made. In the field of hypertension, perhaps the most striking feature is the lack of difference between groups of normals and those with hypertension in respect of the amount of noradrenaline and adre-naline and their metabolites, whether studied by ordinary or isotopic methods (Crout, Pisano & Sjoerdsma, 1961; Gitlow, Mendlowitz, Kruk & Khassis, 1960). It might be thought easier to study blood levels and here the main problem has been one of methods, since the amounts of noradrenaline and adrenaline in the circulation are very small, and the methods of identification not as specific as could be wished. Despite this, there is support for the idea that further work on blood content may still yield results of value; as, for example, the demonstra-tion by Munro & Robinson (1958) of varying levels of amines in the blood of patients with transection of the cord at different levels, which would be expected to reduce the efferent sympathetic pathway by different amounts. With the exception of patients with phaeochromocytoma, no figures are available for patients with hypertension that enable firm conclusions to be drawn.

Pharmacological. Since many of the drugs used in the treatment of hypertension involve interference with the release, the stores in the nerve endings and the final effect on the smooth muscle cell of the arteriolar wall (e.g. reserpine, guanethidine, dibenyline), it was initially thought that they might throw light on the influence of the sympathetic nervous system. It is one of the remarkable things about hypertension that few very complete studies of the action of any of these commonly used drugs have been carried out, and certainly not in a way which answers this question. There is no doubt that sympathetic blockade must play quite a big part in the fall of blood pressure brought about by such drugs as guanethidine, which not only decreases stores of noradrenaline at nerve endings but also blocks the sympathetic impulse. This is not, however, to be taken as a measure of the degree of sympathetic activity in a particular patient, since removal of normal sympathetic tone at a time of increased vasoconstriction due to some other factor could well produce a very considerable effect which would be less apparent under normal circumstances.

So far none of these methods have yielded all the information it might be hoped, and the position about degrees of activity of the sympathetic nervous system still has to be left open.

Phaeochromocytoma

In this condition there is the clearest evidence of a circulating hormone capable of directly raising the blood pressure. The tumours most commonly occur in the suprarenal medulla, and more rarely in the retroperitoneal tissues between the kidneys (MacKeith, 1944). The chromaffin cells comprising these tumours receive their name because of the brown colour induced by treatment with chrome salts. This colour is characteristic of catecholamines, and these tumours were found to contain adrenaline-like substances by Labbé, Azérad & Violle (1929) and by Rabin (1929). The fact that the content of noradrenaline is often greater than that of adrenaline was first pointed out by Holton (1949). The content of these pressor amines is very high and may be up to 10 mg. amine/g. wet weight of tumour (von Euler, 1951; Goldenberg, Aranow, Smith & Faber, 1950; Hamilton, Litchfield, Peart & Sowry, 1953; Holton, 1949).

Patients with these tumours present commonly in two ways: (1) with paroxysms of hypertension; (2) with persistent hypertension. As we have seen, patients of the first type have attacks which can be reproduced by intravenous infusions of adrenaline and noradrenaline, and since the first demonstration by Beer, King & Prinzmetal (1937) of an adrenaline-like substance circulating in the blood during the attacks, further evidence has accrued. Engel & von Euler (1950) showed that the urinary excretion of adrenaline and noradrenaline was greatly increased in patients with phaeochromocytoma, and this has been confirmed by subsequent workers (Burn, 1953; Goldenberg & Rapport, 1951; Hamilton, et al., 1953). Following the paroxysms of hypertension associated usually with a cold, pale, sweating skin and forceful beating of the heart, the rate of urinary excretion of these pressor amines may rise up to 10 times the rate before the attack (Hamilton, et al., 1953). The total quantity of adrenaline and noradrenaline which is released into the circulation in these patients is often very great. Since only 0·3 to 0·4 % of infusions of these amines normally appears in the urine (von Euler & Luft, 1951; Goldenberg, 1951), and as some patients may excrete as much as 5 mg. of the free amines in 24 hours (Hamilton, et al., 1953), more than 100 mg. of the amines may have been released into the circulation in that time. This carries the possible implication that these patients are less sensitive to the pressor effects of the amines than normal. The means by which these large amounts of noradrenaline and adrenaline are removed from the body, are now much better known due largely to the discovery by Armstrong, McMillan & Shaw (1957) of 3-methoxy-4-hydroxymandelic acid, which is a main urinary metabolite of adrenaline and noradrenaline. Various other pathways have now been filled in (see Axelrod, Whitby, Hertting & Koping, 1960, for references).

The removal of the tumour in patients with paroxysmal attacks is curative, and the secretion of the pressor amines returns to within normal limits (Hamilton, et al. 1953).

Patients in the second category, with persistent hypertension, may be impossible to diagnose correctly on clinical grounds. For example, a female patient aged 36, seen at St. Mary's Hospital (under the care of Dr. J. W. Litchfield), had been hypertensive for 3 years, with symptoms only of an occasional throbbing headache. Her blood pressure under observation in bed remained steady at about 180/120 mm. Hg., and she had the retinal changes of malignant hypertension. There were no obvious renal abnormalities and no family history suggestive of hypertension. Her urinary excretion of free pressor amines expressed as (—)-noradrenaline/24 hours was 2400 and 900 μg. on successive days; while the highest figure obtained in 142 patients with "essential hypertension" was 100 μg./24 hours (Hamilton, *et al.*, 1953). A phaeochromocytoma was subsequently removed from the right suprarenal. The signs of malignant hypertension rapidly regressed. The exact role of the pressor amines in this type of hypertension is not well defined. Goldenberg & Aranow (1950) were the first to suggest that an additional mechanism was responsible for maintaining the blood pressure on the grounds that piperoxane, which will reverse the pressor effect of adrenaline, failed to lower the blood pressure on intravenous injection in some patients with a phaeochromocytoma. This reason may not be correct, since Prunty & Swan (1950) showed that piperoxane was relatively ineffective against circulating noradrenaline in man. There is some evidence that a further mechanism may exist, however, since the blood pressure of some patients does not fall after removal of the tumour, even when it is reasonably certain that no other tumour exists, as shown by a normal urinary excretion (Hamilton, *et al.*, 1953; Peart, 1954). It is quite likely that marked vascular or renal changes may be responsible for this maintained hypertension.

The actions of noradrenaline and adrenaline on the circulation largely explain the observed phenomena in these patients, but since the doses injected into the circulation are often very large, some unexpected observations have been made. In general the skin is pale due to the local action; sweating is often profuse, almost certainly due to a central action since neither of these amines cause sweating on local injection in man; headache and vomiting are severe due to the sharp rise in blood pressure, and a tachycardia is produced due either to the direct action of adrenaline in particular or a marked excess of noradrenaline, although in some cases a bradycardia is produced by reflex action through the vagus. This latter situation is only produced by infusions of noradrenaline. Occasionally blurring of vision, perhaps by direct action on the iris, and marked trembling, perhaps by action at neuromuscular junctions, is seen. When the latter is associated with a tachycardia, sweating and a raised metabolic rate, the diagnosis of thyrotoxicosis is often made, and if in addition glycosuria and an abnormal glucose tolerance curve are added to the findings, then the chance of misdiagnosis in terms of diabetes is added. Most of these effects are best reproduced by adrenaline and these manifestations are reversed by removal of the tumour. The swelling of the thyroid seen in attacks is due to the action of noradrenaline almost certainly on the vessels of the thyroid (Mowbray & Peart, 1960), since it can be reproduced by infusions only of noradrenaline and not of adrenaline. It seems likely that venoconstriction with increased blood flow due to the raised pressure operate to produce vascular swelling and oedema. However, many patients are seen who present with flushing and even hypotension (Leather, Shaw, Cates & Milnes Walker, 1962). The precise stage of an attack needs to be known since when prolonged infusions of these amines are stopped, a bright red flush is usual in normal subjects. Whether the hypotension which may then result is due to the release of a vasodilator that also causes the flush, is unknown (Lever, Mowbray & Peart, 1961). The occurrence of low blood volume in some of these patients is also striking (Brunjes, *et al.*, 1960) and may be due to the fact that noradrenaline, by virtue of its venoconstrictor action, increases the capillary venous pressure (Folkow, *et al.*, 1961), thus reducing plasma volume. This again may account for the high venous haematocrit seen in some of these patients.

The diagnosis of phaeochromocytoma can be supported in the laboratory using two methods: (1) biological and (2) chemical. The first depends on the excretion of the free amines, which are usually assayed by their ability to raise the blood pressure of a test animal (Engel & von Euler, 1950; Hamilton *et al.*, 1953), and the second used to depend on the detection of either the free amines or their catechol derivatives (von Euler & Floding, 1955; Goldenberg, Serlin, Edwards & Rapport, 1954). This latter method has now been superseded by those based on the detection of vanillylmandelic acid (VMA) (Gitlow *et al.*, 1960). There is as yet no simple quick method. With the biological methods, it is possible for the amine excretion to fall within normal limits if only slight attacks of hypertension occur (Litchfield & Peart, 1956), and it is important to differentiate adenaline from noradrenaline in the assay, since usually there is less of the former excreted and, even if the total excretion is within normal limits, an increased adrenaline excretion may point to a tumour. There are no reports of false negatives with the methods based on VMA excretion, but they can be confidently expected.

It is of great interest that in an organ which normally contains 80 to 90% adrenaline and 10 to 20% noradrenaline (von Euler, Franksson & Hellström, 1954), tumours arise in which noradrenaline is often greatly in excess of adrenaline.

The commonly postulated view of catechol metabolism is that noradrenaline is first formed and is then converted to adrenaline by methylation (Blaschko, 1942). The evidence is still incomplete, and the question arises as to whether within tumour cells methylation is defective, or whether different cells normally produce each amine separately. The latter possibility receives support from the finding that, in the foetus, the para-aortic glands (organs of Zückerkandl) contain cells which only produce noradrenaline (West, Shepherd, Hunter & MacGregor, 1953). As in many tumours with long metabolic pathways in the cells, the neoplastic process seems to interfere with the latter steps so that precursors of the final product appear in the blood and urine. Tumours, for example, which produce mainly hydroxytyramine have been reported (see von Euler, 1956, for references) as well as dopamine (Robinson, Smith & Whittaker, 1964).

III. RENAL FACTORS

Electrolyte and Water Balance

This has already been touched upon earlier and attention has to be drawn to the marked pressor sensitivity of patients deprived of their kidneys to relatively small intravenous infusions. Whether this is always due to a sharp increase in cardiac output or whether there is some alteration in peripheral resistance in addition, is not certain. The kidney in patients with hypertension handles salt and water in an abnormal fashion (Brodsky & Graubarth, 1953; Cottier, et al., 1958; Farnsworth & Barker, 1943). A salt and water load is excreted faster than normal, and the urine produced contains relatively more water than sodium. Conversely, the response of the "hypertensive" kidney to infusions of angiotensin is the reverse of normal in that instead of an antidiuresis and an antinatriuresis, a profuse diuresis and natriuresis may be produced (Brown & Peart, 1962). That this is purely a consequence of hypertension is shown by the return to a normal pattern on reducing the blood pressure by a variety of surgical procedures or drugs (Brown & Peart, 1962; Hollander, Chobanian & Burrows, 1956–57; Thompson, Silva, Kinsey & Smithwick, 1954). The nature of the alteration in the renal circulation that causes this unusual response, and which may be akin to the emotional diuresis and natriuresis readily produced in hypertensive subjects (Miles & de Wardener, 1953), is not known, but it points to the participation of the ion which many have regarded as of paramount importance in many forms of hypertension and which is being influenced purely

by the level of blood pressure and its effect on the kidney. In most forms of hypertension, save those related to over-activity of the adrenal cortex, there is no consistent relationship between blood pressure and measurements of total exchangeable sodium or potassium (Hollander, et al., 1956–57; Moore, Edelman, Olney, James, Brooks & Wilson, 1954; Ross, 1956). These measurements themselves, of course, are very much influenced by the relation between muscle mass, fat and extracellular fluid volume, so that a wide scatter may be expected in a normal population.

Adrenal Relationships

The initial relation of the adrenal to the kidney in hypertension was perhaps the observation of many pathologists that there seemed to be more cortical adenomata present in patients with hypertension with and without renal disease, than in other post-mortem cases. A more substantial quantitative relation was the observation of Goldblatt (1937) that removal of the suprarenals in dogs with renal clip hypertension led to a fall in blood pressure. This does not, of course, prove a particular causal relation since the same thing happens in a normal subject, and adrenalectomy in patients with malignant hypertension had a short vogue since the results were on the whole poor (Jeffers, Zintel, Hafkenschiel, Hills, Sellers & Wolferth, 1953; Thorn, Harrison, Merrill, Criscitiello, Frawley & Finkenstaedt, 1952). This did not apply to all cases, however, and at the time these studies were carried out it may well be that some small cortical adenomata of the type described by Conn were removed with curative results. Gross and his colleagues (Gross, 1960) first emphasized the close link between the kidney and adrenal in respect of renal clip hypertension in the rat and the intensive investigations of Davis and his colleagues (Davis, 1963) led to knowledge that the major stimulus to aldosterone secretion in the dog which had been bled heavily, resided in the kidneys. The demonstration by Genest et al. (1960) and Laragh, Angers, Kelly & Lieberman (1960) that angiotensin stimulated the production of aldosterone led naturally to the association of the renin-angiotensin system and the adrenal.

Renin–Angiotensin System

Renin. The enzyme renin was first extracted from the kidney by Tigerstedt & Bergman in1898. It was subsequently shown to be a protein with a molecular weight of about 40,000 (Peart, 1965b), and it has been obtained in a high state of purity from pig kidney (Peart, Lloyd, Thatcher, Lever, Payne & Stone, 1966). While very stable in crude preparation when it will withstand a pH range of 2 to 10, the purified preparations are unstable at room temperature, even on freeze-drying. In its enzymic properties, most studies have been made with either impure substrate or with a small synthetic substrate (Skeggs, Lentz, Kahn & Shumway, 1958; Skeggs, Lentz, Hochstrasser & Kahn, 1963), so that only limited statements can be made about its properties. However, the initial velocity

not only from plasma but also from kidney (Sen, Smeby & Bumpus, 1967), is a most interesting advance. Not only does it offer a tool to use in blocking the renin-angiotensin system *in vitro*, but also possibly *in vivo*. It remains to be shown whether it exists to a significant degree in the circulation, physiologically or pathologically.

Substrate. There is probably one major substrate in the α_2-globulin group, although others

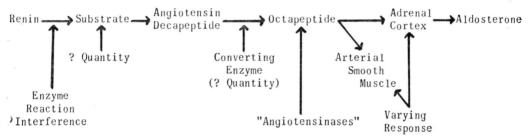

FIG. 9.3. The steps in the renin-angiotensin reaction with factors bearing on the rate of production and destruction of octapeptide and its ultimate action in the tissues.

of its reaction with a pure substrate follows zero order kinetics and the rate of reaction is fast. The optimum pH of reaction with plasma substrate is about 5·7, but there is a broad pH optimum so that the reaction still occurs at plasma pH. The bond specificity of the enzyme is not fully known, but Skeggs *et al.* (1963) showed that it would break the leucyl-leucine bond in a synthetic tetradecapeptide, the first 10 members of which form angiotensin decapeptide. The main steps in the reaction

have been claimed (Skeggs *et al.*, 1963), and the smallest peptide obtained by tryptic digestion of this group of proteins was the tetradecapeptide shown in Fig. 9.4 and which was subsequently synthesized (Skeggs, Kahn, Lentz & Shumway, 1957; Skeggs *et al.*, 1958).

Converting enzyme. Hitherto this enzymic activity was known to exist in the plasma and to be responsible for removing the terminal his-leu dipeptide from the decapeptide, producing the

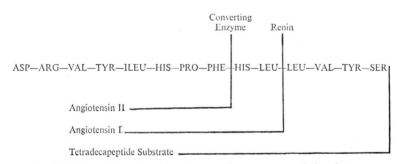

FIG. 9.4. The action of renin and converting enzyme on their substrates.

of renin with its plasma substrate are shown in Fig. 9.3, and it can be seen readily that there are many potential points of interference with the reaction before the final product angiotensin octapeptide appears, to produce most of the biological effects observed.

The recent description of a renin inhibitor of a mainly phospholipid composition, extractable

octapeptide (Skeggs, Kahn & Shumway, 1956). The activity was removed if plasma was made chloride-deficient, and further work has shown that the activity is metal-dependent, being removed by chelating agents such as EDTA and restored by metals, especially cobalt, zinc and calcium (Fitz, Boyd & Peart, in preparation). In plasma it is difficult to separate angiotensinase activity from converting enzyme activity and the recent work of Ng & Vane (1967) strongly supports the concept that conversion in the circulation principally occurs during the transit of angiotensin I through the lungs. Whether this is the only site of conversion in the circulation remains to be seen, but it certainly seems to be the major site in the anaesthetized dog since conversion in blood itself is very slow.

Angiotensin. The chemical structures of the angiotensin peptides initially isolated (Elliott & Peart, 1956 & 1957; Peart, 1955 & 1956; Skeggs, Marsh, Kahn & Shumway, 1955; Skeggs, Lentz, Kahn, Shumway & Woods, 1956) are shown in Fig. 9.5.

increased production of aldosterone by a direct action on the suprarenal cortex (Genest *et al.*, 1960; Laragh, *et al.*, 1960), and under certain circumstances, certainly in man, it seems to be the major controlling hormone for this production. It seems to act very early in the chain of aldosterone production yet it does not, in doses which stimulate aldosterone, increase production of cortisol or corticosterone (Blair-West, Coghlan, Denton, Goding, Munro, Peterson & Wintour, 1962). Of less certain nature is its action on the kidney where, while most of the actions seem explicable by a vascular effect (Peart, 1960), for example the antidiuretic antinatriuretic effect in normal man, it has been suggested that the diure-

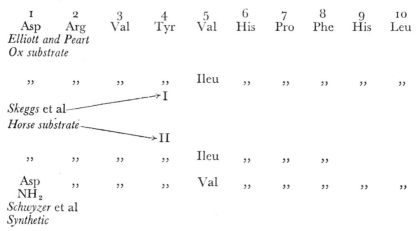

FIG. 9.5. Some natural and synthetic angiotensin peptides.

Pharmacological properties. The main action of angiotensin is as a pressor and vasoconstrictor substance as well as a stimulator of aldosterone production by the adrenal cortex. It seems to act as a universal vasoconstrictor with its main effects on the renal and splanchnic beds (Bock & Krecke, 1958; de Bono, Lee, Mottram, Pickering, Brown, Keen, Peart & Sanderson, 1963). There is evidence that it may act in part reflexly through the brain and the sympathetic outflow, as to the hand (Scroop & Whelan, 1966), and in some cases it may act by enhancing the final sympathetic nerve action without necessarily having to release increased amounts of noradrenaline from the vessel wall (McCubbin & Page, 1963*a* & *b*). It does, however, particularly in some animals, release adrenaline from the adrenal medulla by direct action after intra-arterial injection (Feldberg & Lewis, 1964). In ordinary physiological doses it seems to have little direct action on cardiac performance (Peart, 1965*b*). Its other major action is to cause

tic and natriuretic effect seen in some animals indicate a direct tubular effect on sodium reabsorption. That this might indicate an intrarenal role affecting sodium excretion has received much attention, but the evidence is not convincing.

Angiotensinases. Many enzymes will destroy angiotensin; while many are contained within various organs, some are both free and bound in blood and only fully revealed when blood is taken, and they may then readily destroy large amounts of angiotensin. Whether this activity exists freely in the circulation is at least open to some doubt due to their ready production *in vitro*.

Measurement of renin and angiotensin

Hitherto this has been performed by biological methods involving the final assay of angiotensin, usually on the blood pressure response of the anaesthetized rat or on an isolated smooth muscle preparation (see Renal Hypertertension,

1968, for references). The amount of angiotensin in the circulation in physiological or pathological situations is usually so low that the extraction, purification and subsequent assay have proved particularly difficult although some results have been achieved in this way (Scornik & Paladini, 1961; Boucher, Veyrat, de Champlain & Genest, 1964; Massani, Finkielman, Worcel, Agrest & Paladini, 1966). Most effort therefore was devoted to measurements of renin activity in plasma. This has involved a number of methods in which the plasma has been incubated alone with an effort made to inhibit angiotensinase activity. These methods are known collectively as "renin activity" methods. In some methods substrate is added to plasma to increase the amount of angiotensin formed per unit time, while in others the renin activity is extracted from the plasma and incubated with a prepared natural substrate (see Renal Hypertension, 1968, for references). The final product in most of these methods was probably angiotensin I or a partial mixture with angiotensin II, depending on whether the plasma converting enzyme was interfered with in the method. This probably led to

differences in the assay results since the biological test system might give a varying response to angiotensin I and II. A new approach to this problem has been gained through the development of radio-immunoassay of both angiotensin I and II (Boyd, Landon & Peart, 1967, 1968; Catt, Cain & Coghlan, 1967; Vallotton, Page & Haber, 1967). Such is the sensitivity of these methods that it is possible to measure normal levels of angiotensin II in the plasma, and since conversion of angiotensin I to II can be prevented, use can be made of simple incubation of the plasma in which the renin activity present produces angiotensin I which is measured by radio-immunoassay (Boyd, Adamson, Fitz & Peart, 1969). The antibodies raised to angiotensin I and II have a high degree of specificity so that these too may be assayed separately, even in the same mixture. It is not certain yet whether these methodological advances will produce radical change of view on the renin-angiotensin system, but the animals immunized to angiotensin already provide an interesting approach to the physiological and pathological role of this substrate, since the circulation in

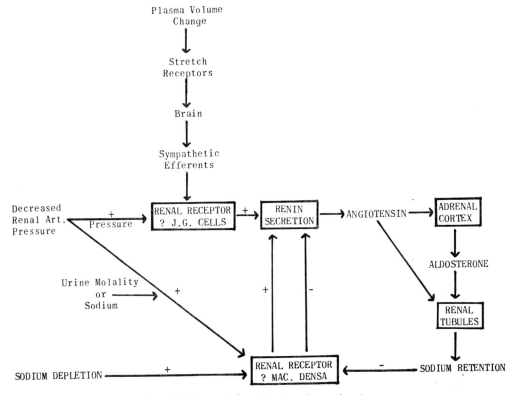

FIG. 9.6. Factors influencing the release of renin.

these animals contains amounts of antibody capable of blocking the angiotensin produced.

Plasma Levels of Renin and Angiotensin in Various Clinical States

These are under the control of various factors shown in Fig. 9.6. Reduction of pressure in the afferent arteriolar wall at the level of the juxtaglomerular apparatus seems to be of great importance in the acute release of renin in

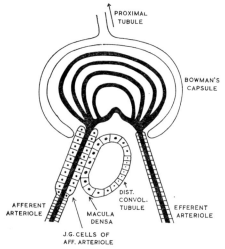

PROXIMAL TUBULE

BOWMAN'S CAPSULE

DIST. CONVOL. TUBULE

AFFERENT ARTERIOLE

MACULA DENSA

EFFERENT ARTERIOLE

J.G. CELLS OF AFF. ARTERIOLE

FIG. 9.7. The close anatomical relation between the macula densa of the distal convoluted tuble and the afferent arteriole.

response to changes in perfusion pressure (Corcoran & Page, 1942; Lever & Peart, 1962; Skinner, McCubbin & Page, 1963; Tobian, 1960). The fact that changes in the latter also cause changes in the composition of the urine draws attention to the possibility of the macula densa as another sensing

organ controlling renin release and seeming to be ideally situated anatomically (Fig. 9.7) by its contiguity with the afferent arteriolar wall (Thurau, 1964). This may explain some of the effects of injection of diuretics and solutions of different osmolality into the renal artery, although the precise sensing area of the kidney for these procedures is not known (Vander & Miller, 1964). Acute changes in plasma volume also produce their effect, and in particular decrease leads to increased output of renin, and the sympathetic nerves to the kidney seem to be very important as one part of the reflex arc involved in this response (Hodge, Lowe & Vane, 1966). The termination of the sympathetic nerves in different species seems to be rather different, however, and while some are close to the juxtaglomerular apparatus, this is not so in all (Barajas & Latta, 1963), and this aspect of renin release clearly needs more definition in different species. Finally, there is a close relation between the content of renin in the kidney and the action of adrenocortical hormones, particularly aldosterone (Gross, Loustalot & Sulser, 1956; Gross, Regoli & Schaechtelin, 1963). The administration of DOCA reduces the renal renin content to very low levels and, of course, high secretion rates of aldosterone produced by tumours depress plasma levels of renin (Brown, Davies, Lever, Peart & Robertson, 1964; Conn, Cohen & Rovner, 1964). This therefore gives in the normal situation a number of factors which may be operating to influence plasma renin and angiotensin levels. Those which increase and decrease the level under normal situations are shown in Table 9.1. Most of the data refer to renin levels, but it seems likely that angiotensin behaves similarly. It is found that the levels may be increased by alteration of posture so that the renin level rises on standing (Brown, Davies, Lever, McPherson & Robertson, 1966; Cohen

TABLE 9.1

Conditions which affect the plasma level of renin, renin activity or angiotensin

INCREASE	DECREASE
(a) *Physiological alterations*	(a) *Physiological alterations*
Reduction of blood volume	Increase of plasma volume
Reduction of sodium intake	Increase of sodium intake
Reduction of arterial pressure	Increase of plasma sodium
Reduction of renal arterial pressure	
Reduction of plasma sodium	
(b) *Clinical state*	(b) *Clinical state*
Cirrhosis of the liver with ascites	Conn's syndrome
Addison's disease	Cushing's syndrome
Pregnancy	Some cases of hypertension
Some cases of hypertension	Administration of DOCA and aldosterone
Administration of diuretics	

et al. 1964). Standing leads to a reduction in blood volume but whether this is the proper stimulus is not known. There is a diurnal swing in measurements of renin activity (Brown, Davies, Lever & Robertson, 1966a; Gordon, Wolfe, Island & Liddle, 1966), and over a longer term in the female there are changes related to the menstrual cycle (Brown, Davies, Lever & Robertson, 1964b). There does not seem to be any particular relation to age. There are fewer physiological alterations which lead to decrease, except in the negative sense by performing the opposite action to those which cause an increase. The precise figures for renin or angiotensin as normal values are not meaningful in the case of renin, since only laboratory standard units of differing size have been used, but in the case of angiotensin it is possible to be more precise in terms of synthetic asparaginyl[1] val[5] octapeptide (Peart, 1954) which has been used as a standard. Massani, Finkielman, Worcel, Agrest & Paladini (1966) found a mean level of about 100 ng./litre in a normal population, although there were some who had a much lower level than this, and this compares reasonably with a level of about 80 ng./litre found by Genest et al. (1964). Using an extraction method for measuring renin in plasma (Brown,

NORMALS

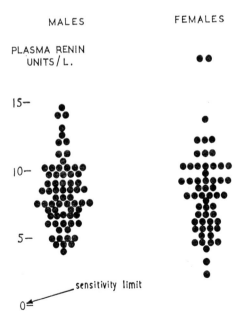

FIG. 9.8. The range of normal plasma renin values (St. Mary's Hospital units) showing that they are well above the sensitivity limit of the assay (From Brown, Davis, Lever, Robertson & Peart, 1964).

Davies, Lever, Robertson & Tree, 1964), the range of normal values is shown in Fig. 9.8, and this gives a basis for comparison with pathological states. The scatter noted in these figures may be related to posture or diet at the time that the blood was taken, since this was not standardized. In most of the clinical states to be considered, it is easy to see variations in some of the controlling factors already discussed (see Brown, Davies, Lever & Robertson, 1966b and Peart, 1965b, for references).

The radio-immunoassay of angiotensin II has allowed a re-examination of the quantitative aspect. In normal subjects on an ordinary diet and in a recumbent position for one hour before blood sampling, the plasma level of venous blood is of the order of 10 picograms/ml, while that of arterial blood is about twice as high. This is in line with previous work which suggests that angiotensin II is cleared from the blood in transit across most organs, except the lung, and that this is responsible for most of its disappearance after injection rather than by angiotensinase destruction in blood. So far the levels of angiotensin II in hypertension have shown an equal scatter with values of renin activity, being high in some cases of renal artery stenosis and malignant hypertension, and low in others with Conn's syndrome or of unknown origin (Boyd, Landon & Peart, 1967). The important fact gained by comparing plasma angiotensin levels during infusion of known amounts of angiotensin II with those found in some cases of hypertension is that there are some patients with levels high enough to cause a rise in blood pressure of a normal subject during intravenous infusion. Similarly in cases with secondary hyperaldosteronism, such as cirrhosis with ascites, pregnancy, and nephrosis, the plasma levels may be equally high, even though the blood pressure is normal. This immediately raises the question of sensitivity to infusions of angiotensin and whether this group is particularly insensitive or whether some subjects with hypertension are particularly sensitive to the prevailing levels of the hormone. So far no large discrepancies have been noted between levels of renin activity using the production rate of angiotensin I as determined by radio-immunoassay, and the prevailing levels of angiotensin II in the same patient. These might be expected if there is an alteration in renin activity introduced due to the methods of taking and incubating the blood: a failure of conversion of angiotensin I to II in the body; or an alteration in the metabolic clearance rate of angiotensin I and II.

Cirrhosis of the liver with ascites. In this situation plasma volume is low. There is also secondary aldosteronism and some of the highest aldosterone secretion rates are observed in this condition. Since the plasma renin level is also high, the question is whether this is because of the low plasma volume which stimulates renin production and then aldosterone, or whether some other factor is entering.

Addison's disease. The renin level here is high and the plasma volume and sodium are low. Since it has been shown that the plasma renin can be decreased by administration of cortisone and 9-α-fluorohydrocortisone with salt (Brown, Davies, Lever & Robertson, 1964*a*), the changes in plasma sodium and volume are probably important. Whether changes in plasma sodium alone are as important as alterations in plasma volume is uncertain, but in one case of dilutional hyponatraemia due to inappropriate secretion of antidiuretic hormone in a patient with carcinoma of the bronchus the plasma renin was not elevated. This suggests that plasma sodium is not always important (Brown, Davies, Lever & Robertson, 1965*a*).

Pregnancy. In this condition the plasma renin rises early in pregnancy and remains elevated only a short time after delivery (Brown, Davies, Doak, Lever & Robertson, 1963). The plasma volume here is elevated in contrast to the two previous conditions and the aldosterone secretion rate is again elevated from the early part of pregnancy (Sims, Meeker, Gray, Watanabe & Solomon, 1964). It is not known whether the renin-angiotensin system is responsible for this increase and it is a good example of a situation where one of the factors, namely a high plasma volume, which might theoretically lead to a lower plasma renin, may be overcome by another more strongly acting stimulus. Again since the source of the renin-like activity in pregnancy plasma is not certain [cf. amniotic fluid renin-like activity (Brown, Davies, Doak, Lever, Robertson & Tree, 1964)], this may be under different control from the ordinary physiological state.

Administration of diuretics. It is of some interest that the results in man of the administration of a potent diuretic like frusemide, which raises plasma renin and aldosterone levels concurrently (Fraser, James, Brown, Isaac, Lever & Robertson, 1965), contrast with those in the anaesthetized dog where osmotic diuretics were given into the renal artery (Vander & Miller, 1964). This latter procedure led to a fall in renin output by the kidney. The difference here may be that the total effect in man on plasma volume and sodium content be-

came the major factor in contrast to the local intra-renal effect of the diuretic. Nevertheless it points to the importance of knowing about the administration of diuretics in states where renin levels are being measured, and in particular congestive cardiac failure is a good example since big variations in plasma renin levels can readily be produced in this way (Brown, Davies, Lever & Robertson, 1964*a*).

Hypertension. Since hypertension is a syndrome containing many aetiological factors, it would not be expected that there would be any consistent relation between the level of plasma renin or angiotensin and the blood pressure itself; therefore it is not surprising that this is what is found. Even here, however, certain correlations of high significance have been established for both plasma renin and angiotensin. In the experimental animal in which hypertension has been mainly produced by renal artery clip, the relation is also becoming clearer. Whatever the underlying cause of hypertension, the plasma renin tends to be high if malignant hypertension is present, as shown by haemorrhages, exudates and papilloedema in the retinae (Brown, Davies, Lever & Robertson, 1965*b*), and conversely it is low in the presence of a Conn's tumour of the suprarenal cortex secreting an excess of aldosterone (Fig. 9.9) (Brown, Davies, Lever, Peart & Robertson, 1964; Conn *et al.*, 1964).

Turning to the wider group of patients with hypertension, those with proven renal artery stenosis have a variable level of renin, again linked to the presence of malignant hypertension but more convincingly to the level of plasma sodium, since the best correlation has been found between low levels of plasma renin and high levels of plasma sodium, and conversely (Fig. 9.10) (Brown, Davies, Lever & Robertson, 1965*c*). In those patients with hypertension of unknown origin, the same relation to plasma sodium is found, and it will be noted that quite a proportion, up to about one-third, have plasma renin levels at the lower level or below the normal level (Fig. 9.11). Conn (1964) has suggested that it is within this group that a large number will be found to have a tumour of the suprarenal cortex, even without the presence of a low plasma potassium which is usually used to indicate the presence of such a tumour (Conn *et al.*, 1965). In established cases of Conn's syndrome, the plasma renin may be elevated by the administration of spironolactone, which blocks the action of aldosterone (Fig. 9.9), and indicates that it is the final effect of this hormone, perhaps on electrolyte balance across cell membranes, which is res-

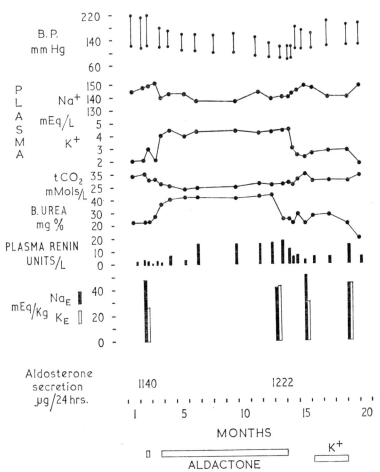

FIG. 9.9. The data on a patient with Conn's syndrome in whom a cure was subsequently brought about surgically. This shows that the administration of Aldactone-A brought the blood pressure to normal, reduced the plasma sodium, elevated the plasma potassium, decreased the plasma bicarbonate, increased the plasma urea, brought the plasma renin from its subnormal level (1–2 units/litre) up to normal (10–20 units/litre) and returned the exchangeable sodium and potassium pools in the body to normal, while having no effect on the markedly raised aldosterone secretion rate (From Brown, Davies, Lever, Peart & Robertson, 1965).

ponsible for lowering the plasma renin (Brown, Davies, Lever, Peart & Robertson, 1964). In experimental hypertension due mainly to renal artery clip, similar findings have been obtained with respect to renin as to angiotensin. In the few days following application of the clip the plasma renin level rises (Lever & Robertson, 1964) and then, as the pressure often rises higher still, so the plasma renin and angiotensin fall (Scornik & Paladini, 1961). The development of acute renal artery stenosis in a patient is shown in Fig. 9.12 and was associated with a very high plasma renin and aldosterone secretion rate

with a low plasma sodium and potassium. Many factors were probably operating here to give a high plasma renin. There is usually, however, no particular relation between a high level and a particular level of blood pressure, and it is quite possible to have hypertension with a normal level of renin and angiotensin. This leads to the conclusion that either the changes in renin and angiotensin are not in any way causally related to hypertension or else (since they often rise in the early phase of experimental hypertension) that a temporary rise induces some secondary change which maintains the high blood pressure after the

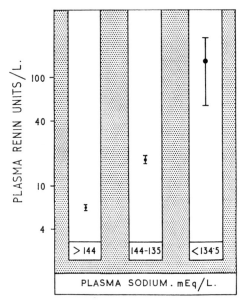

FIG. 9.10. The inverse relation between plasma renin and sodium levels in large groups of hyptertensive patients. (From Peart, 1966).

HYPERTENSION

renal artery stenosis   others

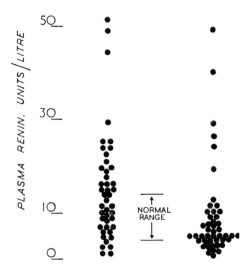

FIG. 9.11. Plasma renin levels in groups of patients with proven renal artery stenosis and those with hypertension of unknown origin. (From Brown, Davies, Lever & Robertson, 1964a).

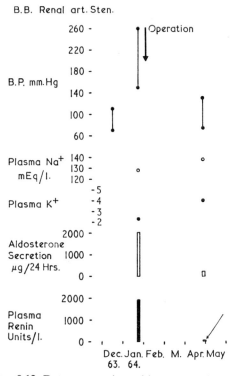

FIG. 9.12. Data on a patient with acute renal artery stenosis and malignant hypertension showing the low plasma sodium and potassium with grossly elevated aldosterone secretion rate and plasma renin level (normal 5–15 units/litre). Correction of the stenosis led to a return of all values to normal. (From Peart, 1965a).

renin and angiotensin levels have returned to normal. One way of looking at this situation is to consider the possibility of increased sensitivity to the action of angiotensin which has been touched on earlier. If some factors in hypertension led to increased sensitivity, then it would be possible to have this maintained by normal levels of renin and angiotensin as long as those factors continued to operate. While there is considerable variation and, in some patients with hypertension, marked sensitivity to the action of angiotensin (Kaplan & Silah, 1964), the case remains to be clearly demonstrated.

Intra-Renal Function

Because in many animals there are relatively large stores of renin in the juxtaglomerular apparatus and because it has also been demonstrated in lymph which drains the extracellular fluid of the kidney, it was natural to wonder about a possible intra-renal role since angiotensin has such potent effects on vessels, and even possibly directly on tubules (Lever & Peart, 1962; Peart, 1960; Thurau, 1964). There is not much direct evidence for this and certainly renin introduced directly into the renal artery in the conscious rabbit does not have an effect on renal function until it produces a pressor effect by systemic action (Boyd & Peart—in preparation). It is still possible that renin might enter the extra-cellular fluid in the kidney without passing through the blood stream, so that an intrarenal role could still be possible, and equally it may have a function within the cells of the juxta-glomerular apparatus which has not yet been defined. Another point to be made is that renin with a molecular weight of 40,000 is readily filtered at the glomerulus and that its failure to appear in the urine in any large quantities seems to be due to reabsorption in the proximal tubule of the kidney (Rappelli & Peart, 1968). While this probably has no physiological function, it means that factors interfering with the proximal tubule could influence the amount of renin escaping from the circulation.

The renin–angiotensin system has therefore emerged as of great importance in relation to aldosterone secretion and to changes in blood volume and of sodium balance, but its precise role in control of the circulation and of renal function, however, is still not clear.

Medullary Hypotensive Substances

Numerous extracts of kidney have in the past been claimed to have hypotensive effects on injection or even oral administration to various animals (Hamilton & Grollman, 1958). This field has become very much clearer since the initial demonstration of depressor materials (Hickler, Sarovis, Mowbray, Lauler, Vagnucci & Thorn, 1963; Milliez, Lagrue & Meyer, 1963; Muirhead, Brooks, Kosinski, Daniels & Hinman, 1966), and subsequently of the presence of prostaglandins in medullary extracts by different groups of workers. One of these extracts has been given the name Medullin and its activity claimed to be due to the presence of a particular prostaglandin (Lee, Covino, Takman & Smith, 1965). Another group of workers (Muirhead, 1967) claim that most of the activity in the renal medulla is due to another type of prostaglandin. These substances, which are widely distributed in the body and were first described in semen, have been shown to be extremely potent vasodepressor and vasodilator agents (Bergström, Duner, von Euler, Pernow & Sjövall, 1959). Whether they play either an intra-renal role or, by release in the blood stream, an extra-renal role involving control of the circulation, is not known, but their precise chemical definition leads to the belief that it will be possible readily to demonstrate them if they are indeed released from the kidney under different circumstances. Since one hypothesis of renal hypertension was that renal disease led to a lack of renal vasodepressor substances which were normally responsible for providing the balance to pressor mechanisms in the body (Grollman, Williams & Harrison, 1940), the discovery of these substances will enable this hypothesis to be adequately tested. So far Muirhead, Daniels, Pike & Hinman (1967) have claimed that administration of these substances to the animal which has become hypertensive after being deprived of its kidneys, will lower the blood pressure, but this does not, of course, mean that the blood pressure was raised because of their absence.

The main advances in our knowledge of high blood pressure have closely involved considera-tion of electrolytes, water, the suprarenal cortex and the renin-angiotensin system. Since many of the factors are completely interdependent, it is difficult to define the prime mover, and sometimes it would seem almost impossible to unravel the most important single factor in a clinical situation. However, in the experimental hypertension resulting from a renal artery clip, we now seem to have enough knowledge to make it worth looking again for a primary cause.

ACKNOWLEDGMENTS

Thanks are due to the Academic Press Incorporated, Blackwell Scientific Publications Limited, the Cana-dian Medical Association Journal, the Journal of Endocrinology and Springer-Verlag for permission to reproduce Fig. 12, Fig. 8, Figs. 2 and 11, Fig. 9 and Fig. 10 respectively.

References

ARMSTRONG, M. D., MCMILLAN, A. & SHAW, K. N. F. (1957). *Biochim. biophys. Acta.*, **25**, 442.

AXELROD, J., WHITBY, L. G., HERTTING, G. & KOPING, I. L. (1960). *Hypertension*, **9**. "Proceedings of the Council for High Blood Pressure Research", p. 715. American Heart Association, November 1960.

BARAJAS, L. & LATTA, H. (1963). *Lab. Invest.*, **12**, 1046.

BARRACLOUGH, M. A., BACCHUS, B., BROWN, J. J., DAVIES, D. L., LEVER, A. F. & ROBERTSON, J. I. S. (1965). *Lancet*, **2**, 1310.

BEER, E., KING, F. H. & PRINZMETAL, M. (1937). *Ann. Surg.*, **106**, 85.

BERGSTRÖM, S., DUNER, H., EULER, U. S. VON, PERNOW, B. & SJÖVALL, J. (1959). *Acta physiol. scand.*, **45**, 145.

BIGLIERI, E. G. (1965). *J. clin. Endocrin.*, **25**, 884.

BIGLIERI, E. G. & McILROY, M. B. (1966). *Circulation*, **33**, 78.

BLAIR-WEST, J. R., COGHLAN, J. P., DENTON, D. A., GODING, J. R., MUNRO, J. A., PETERSON, R. E. & WINTOUR, M. (1962). *J. clin. Invest.*, **41**, 1606.

BLASCHKO, H. (1942). *J. Physiol.*, Lond., **101**, 337.

BOCK, K. D. & KRECKE, H.-J. (1958). *Klin. Wschr.*, **36**, 69.

BORST, J. G. G. & BORST-DE GEUS, A. (1963). *Lancet*, **1**, 677.

BOUCHER, R., VEYRAT, R., DE CHAMPLAIN, J. & GENEST, J. (1964). *Canad. med. Ass. J.*, **90**, 194.

BOYD, G. W., ADAMSON, A. R., FITZ, A. E. & PEART, W. S. (1969). *Lancet*, **1**, 213.

BOYD, G. W., FITZ, A., ADAMSON, A. R. & PEART, W. S. Protein and Polypeptide Hormones, Part 3, Proceedings of the International Symposium held in Liege, Belgium, 19–25 May 1968, Ed. M. Margoulies. Excerpta Medica Foundation.

BOYD, G. W., LANDON, J. & PEART, W. S. (1967). *Lancet*, **2**, 1002.

BOYD, G. W., LANDON, J. & PEART, W. S. (1968). Protein and Polypeptide Hormones, Part 2, Proc. Internat. Symp., Liege, Belgium, 19–25 May 1968, Ed. M. Margoulies, Excerpta Medica Foundation.

BOYD, G. W. & PEART, W. S. In preparation.

BRODSKY, W. A. & GRAUBARTH, H. N. (1953). *J. lab. clin. Med.*, **41**, 43.

BROWN, J. J., DAVIES, D. L., DOAK, P. B., LEVER, A. F. & ROBERTSON, J. I. S. (1963). *Lancet*, **2**, 900.

BROWN, J. J., DAVIES, D. L., DOAK, P. B., LEVER, A. F., ROBERTSON, J. I. S. & TREE, M. (1964). *Lancet*, **2**, 64.

BROWN, J. J., DAVIES, D. L., LEVER, A. F., McPHERSON, D. & ROBERTSON, J. I. S. (1966). *Clin. Sci.*, **30**, 279.

BROWN, J. J., DAVIES, D. L., LEVER, A. F., PEART, W. S. & ROBERTSON, J. I. S. (1964). *Brit. med. J.*, **2**, 1636.

BROWN, J. J., DAVIES, D. L., LEVER, A. F., PEART, W. S. & ROBERTSON, J. I. S. (1965). *J. Endocrin.*, **33**, 279.

BROWN, J. J., DAVIES, D. L., LEVER, A. F. & ROBERTSON, J. I. S. (1964*a*). *Canad. med. Ass. J.*, **90**, 201.

BROWN, J. J., DAVIES, D. L., LEVER, A. F. & ROBERTSON, J. I. S. (1964*b*). *Brit. med. J.*, **2**, 1114.

BROWN, J. J., DAVIES, D. L., LEVER, A. F. & ROBERTSON, J. I. S. (1965*a*). *Proc. Soc. Endocrin.*, **32**, v.

BROWN, J. J., DAVIES, D. L., LEVER, A. F. & ROBERTSON, J. I. S. (1965*b*). *Brit. med. J.*, **2**, 1215.

BROWN, J. J., DAVIES, D. L., LEVER, A. F. & ROBERTSON, J. I. S. (1965*c*). *Brit. med. J.*, **2**, 144.

BROWN, J. J., DAVIES, D. L., LEVER, A. F. & ROBERTSON, J. I. S. (1966*a*). *J. Endocrin.*, **34**, 129.

BROWN, J. J., DAVIES, D. L., LEVER, A. F. & ROBERTSON, J. I. S. (1966*b*). *Postgrad. med. J.*, **42**, 153.

BROWN, J. J., DAVIES, D. L., LEVER, A. F., ROBERTSON, J. I. S. & PEART, W. S. (1964). "Aldosterone". A Symposium organized by the Council for International Organizations of Medical Sciences established under the joint auspices of UNESCO and WHO. Ed. Baulieu, E. E. & Robel, P. p. 417. Oxford, Blackwell.

BROWN, J. J., DAVIES, D. L., LEVER, A. F., ROBERTSON, J. I. S. & TREE, M. (1964). *Biochem. J.*, **93**, 594.

BROWN, J. J. & PEART, W. S. (1962). *Clin. Sci.*, **22**, 1.

BRUNJES, S., JOHNS, V. J. & CRANE, M. G. (1960). *New Engl. J. Med.*, **262**, 393.

BURN, G. P. (1953). *Brit. med. J.*, **1**, 697.

CATT, K. J., CAIN, M. C. & COGHLAN, J. P. (1967). *Lancet*, **2**, 1005.

COHEN, E. L., ROVNER, D. R., CONN, J. W. & BLOUGH, W. M. (1964). *Clin. Res.*, **12**, 362.

CONN, J. W. (1955). *J. lab. clin. Med.*, **45**, 661.

CONN, J. W. (1964). *J. Amer. med. Ass.*, **190**, 222.

CONN, J. W. (1965). *New Engl. J. Med.*, **273**, 1135.

CONN, J. W., COHEN, E. L. & ROVNER, D. R. (1964). *J. Amer. med. Ass.*, **190**, 213.

CONN, J. W., COHEN, E. L., ROVNER, D. R. & NESBIT, R. M. (1965). *J. Amer. med. Ass.*, **193**, 200.

CORCORAN, A. C. & PAGE, I. H. (1942). *Amer. J. Physiol.*, **135**, 361.

COTTIER, P. T., WELLER, J. M. & HOOBLER, S. W. (1958). *Circulation*, **17**, 750.

CROUT, J. R., PISANO, J. J. & SJOERDSMA, A. (1961). *Amer. Heart J.*, **61**, 375.

DAHL, L. K. (1960). "Essential Hypertension". An International Symposium. Ed. Bock, K. D. & Cottier, P. p. 61. Berlin, Göttingen, Heidelberg, Springer-Verlag.

DAVIS, J. O. (1963). "Hormones and the Kidney", Mem. Soc. Endocrin., No. 13. Ed. Williams, P. C. p. 325. London, Academic Press.

DE BONO, E., LEE, G. DE J., MOTTRAM, F. R., PICKERING, G. W., BROWN, J. J., KEEN, H., PEART, W. S. & SANDERSON, P. H. (1963). *Clin. Sci.*, **25**, 123.

DE CAMP, P. T. & BIRCHALL, R. (1958). *Surgery*, **43**, 134.

DEMING, Q. B. (1954). *Arch. intern. Med.*, **93**, 197.

DOLLERY, C. T., SHACKMAN, R. & SHILLINGFORD, J. (1959). *Brit. med. J.*, **2**, 1367.

EBERLEIN, W. R. & BONGIOVANNI, A. M. (1956). *J. biol. Chem.*, **223**, 85.

ELLIOTT, D. F. & PEART, W. S. (1956). *Nature*, Lond., **177**, 527.

ELLIOTT, D. F. & PEART, W. S. (1957). *Biochem. J.*, **65**, 246.

ENGEL, A. & EULER, U. S. VON (1950). *Lancet*, **2**, 387.

EULER, U. S. VON (1951). *Ann. Surg.*, **134**, 929.

EULER, U. S. VON (1956). "Noradrenaline". Springfield, Ill., Charles C. Thomas.

EULER, U. S. VON & FLODING, I. (1955). *Acta physiol. scand.*, **33**, Suppl. 118, 57.

EULER, U. S. VON, FRANKSSON, C. & HELLSTRÖM, J. (1954). *Acta physiol. scand.*, **31**, 6.

EULER, U. S. VON & LUFT, R. (1951). *Brit. J. Pharmacol.*, **6**, 286.

FARNSWORTH, E. B. & BARKER, M. H. (1943). *Proc. Soc. exp. Biol.*, N.Y., **52**, 74.

FELDBERG, W. & LEWIS, G. P. (1964). *J. Physiol.*, Lond., **171**, 98.

FITZ, A., BOYD, G. W. & PEART, W. S. In preparation.

FITZGEARLD, M. G., FOURMAN, P., JAMES, A. H. & SCARBOROUGH, H. (1957). *Scot. med. J.*, **2**, 473.

FOLKOW, B., JOHANSSON, B. & MELLANDER, S. (1961). *Acta physiol. scand.*, **53**, 99.

FRASER, R., JAMES, V. H. T., BROWN, J. J., ISAAC, P., LEVER, A. F. & ROBERTSON, J. I. S. (1965). *Lancet*, **2**, 989.

GENEST, J., BOUCHER, R., NOWACZYNSKI, W., KOIW, E., DE CHAMPLAIN, J., BIRON, P., CHRÉTIEN, M. & MARC-AURÈLE, J. (1964). "Aldosterone". A Symposium organized by the Council for International Organizations of Medical Sciences established under the joint auspices of UNESCO and WHO. Ed. Baulieu, E. E. & Robel, P. p. 393. Oxford, Blackwell.

GENEST, J., NOWACZYNSKI, W., KOIW, E., SANDOR, T. & BIRON, P. (1960). "Essential Hypertension". An International Symposium. Ed. Bock, K. D. & Cottier, P. p. 126. Berlin, Göttingen, Heidelberg, Springer-Verlag.

GITLOW, S. E., MENDLOWITZ, M., KRUK, E. & KHASSIS, S. (1960). "Hypertension", **9**. Proceedings of the Council for High Blood Pressure Research, p. 746. American Heart Association, November 1960.

GOLDBLATT, H. (1937). *Ann. intern. Med.*, **11**, 69.

GOLDENBERG, M. (1951). *Amer. J. Med.*, **10**, 627.

GOLDENBERG, M. & ARANOW, H., Jr. (1950). *J. Amer. med. Ass.*, **143**, 1139.

GOLDENBERG, M., ARANOW, H., Jr., SMITH, A. A. & FABER, M. (1950). *Arch. intern. Med.*, **86**, 823.

GOLDENBERG, M. & RAPPORT, M. M. (1951). *J. clin. Invest.*, **30**, 641.

GOLDENBERG, M., SERLIN, I., EDWARDS, T. & RAPPORT, M. M. (1954). *Amer. J. Med.*, **16**, 103.

GORDON, R. D., WOLFE, L. K., ISLAND, D. P. & LIDDLE, G. W. (1966). *J. clin. Invest.*, **45**, 1587.

GOWENLOCK, A. H. & WRONG, O. (1962). *Quart. J. Med.*, **31**, 323.

GROLLMAN, A., WILLIAMS, J. R., Jr. & HARRISON, T. R. (1940). *J. biol. Chem.*, **134**, 115.

GROSS, F. (1960). "Essential Hypertension". An International Symposium. Ed. Bock, K. D. & Cottier, P. p. 92. Berlin, Göttingen, Heidelberg, Springer-Verlag.

GROSS, F., LOUSTALOT, P. & SULSER, F. (1956). *Arch. exp. Path. Pharmak.*, **229**, 381.

GROSS, F., REGOLI, D. & SCHAECHTELIN, G. (1963). "Hormones and the Kidney". Mem. Soc. Endocrin., No. 13. Ed. Williams, P. C. p. 293. London, Academic Press.

HAMILTON, J. G. & GROLLMAN, A. (1958). *J. biol. Chem.*, **233**, 528.

HAMILTON, M., LITCHFIELD, J. W., PEART, W. S. & SOWRY, G. S. C. (1953). *Brit. Heart J.*, **15**, 241.

HICKLER, R. B., SAROVIS, C. A., MOWBRAY, J. F., LAULER, D. P., VAGNUCCI, A. I. & THORN, G. W. (1963). *J. clin. Invest.*, **42**, 942.

HILDEN, T. & KROGSGAARD, A. R. (1958). *Amer. J. med. Sci.*, **236**, 487.

HODGE, R. L., LOWE, R. D. & VANE, J. R. (1966). *J. Physiol.*, Lond., **185**, 613.

HOLLANDER, W., CHOBANIAN, A. V. & BURROWS, B. A. (1956–57). *Proc. New Engl. Cardiovasc Soc.*, **15**, 19.

HOLTON, P. (1949). *J. Physiol.*, Lond., **108**, 525.

HOOD, B., FALKHEDEN, T., AURELL, M., OLANDERS, S. & BJÖRK, S. (1967). "Stroke", Proceedings of the Thule International Symposium held in Stockholm, 19–21 April 1966. Ed. Engel, A. & Larsson, T. p. 253. Stockholm, Nordiska Bokhandelns Förlag.

JEFFERS, W. A., ZINTEL, H. A., HAFKENSCHIEL, J. H., HILLS, A. G., SELLERS, A. M. & WOLFERTH, C. C. (1953). *Ann. intern. Med.*, **39**, 254.

KAPLAN, N. M. & SILAH, J. G. (1964). *J. clin. Invest.*, **43**, 659.

KLIMAN, B. & PETERSON, R. E. (1960). *J. biol. Chem.*, **235**, 1639.

LABBÉ, M., AZÉRAD & VIOLLE (1929). *Bull. Soc. méd. Hôp.*, Paris, **53**, 952.

LARAGH, J. H. (1961). "Hypertension, Recent Advances", Second Hahnemann Symposium on Hypertensive Disease. Ed. Brest, A. N. & Moyer, J. H. p. 95. Philadelphia, Lea & Febiger.

LARAGH, J. H., ANGERS, M., KELLY, W. G. & LIEBERMAN, S. (1960). *J. Amer. med. Ass.*, **174**, 234.

LARAGH, J. H., ULICK, S., JANUSZEWICZ, V., DEMING, Q. B., KELLY, W. G. & LIEBERMAN, S. (1960). *J. clin. Invest.*, **39**, 1091.

LEATHER, H. M., SHAW, D. B., CATES, J. E. & MILNES WALKER, R. (1962). *Brit. med. J.*, **1**, 1373.

LEE, J. B., COVINO, B. G., TAKMAN, B. H. & SMITH, E. R. (1965). *Circulat. Res.*, **17**, 57.

LEVER, A. F., MOWBRAY, J. F. & PEART, W. S. (1961). *Clin. Sci.*, **21**, 69.

LEVER, A. F. & PEART, W. S. (1962). *J. Physiol.*, Lond., **160**, 548.

LEVER, A. F. & ROBERTSON, J. I. S. (1964). *J. Physiol.*, Lond., **170**, 212.

LEWIS, T. & PICKERING, G. W. (1931). *Heart*, **16**, 33.

LITCHFIELD, J. W. & PEART, W. S. (1956). *Lancet*, **2**, 1283.

LOEB, R. F., ATCHLEY, D. W., FERREBEE, J. W. & RAGAN, C. (1939). *Trans. Ass. Amer. Physicians*, **54**, 285.

LUFT, R. & EULER, U. S. VON (1953). *J. clin. Invest*, **32**, 1065.

McCUBBIN, J. W. & PAGE, I. H. (1963*a*). *Circulat. Res.*, **12** (Part 2), 553.

McCUBBIN, J. W. & PAGE, I. H. (1963*b*). *Science*, **139**, 210.

McCULLAGH, E. P. & RYAN, E. J. (1940). *J. Amer. med. Ass.*, **114**, 2530.

MACKEITH, R. (1944). *Brit. Heart J.*, **6**, 1.

MARGOLIN, E. G., MERRILL, J. P. & HARRISON, J. H. (1957). *New Engl. J. Med.*, **256**, 581.

MASSANI, Z. M., FINKIELMAN, S., WORCEL, M., AGREST, A. & PALADINI, A. C. (1966). *Clin. Sci.*, **30**, 473.

MILES, B. E. & DE WARDENER, H. E. (1953). *Lancet*, **2**, 539.

MILLIEZ, P., LAGRUE, G. & MEYER, P. (1963). *Gaz. méd. France*, **70**, 3663.

MOORE, F. D., EDELMAN, I. S., OLNEY, J. M., JAMES, A. H., BROOKS, L. & WILSON, G. M. (1954). *Metabolism*, **3**, 334.

MOWBRAY, J. F. & PEART, W. S. (1960). *J. Physiol., Lond.*, **151**, 261.

MUIRHEAD, E. E., BROOKS, B., KOSINSKI, M., DANIELS, E. G. & HINMAN, J. W. (1966). *J. lab. clin. Med.*, **67**, 778.

MUIRHEAD, E. E., DANIELS, E. G., PIKE, J. E. & HINMAN, J. W. (1967). "The Prostaglandins", Ed. Bergstrom, S. & Samuelson, B. Uppsala, Almqvist & Wicksells.

MUNRO, A. F. & ROBINSON, R. (1958). *J. Physiol., Lond.*, **141**, 4P.

NG, K. K. F. & VANE, J. R. (1967). *Nature, Lond.*, **216**, 762.

ØSTER, J. (1947). *Acta med. scand.*, **128**, 42.

PEART, W. S. (1954). CIBA Foundation Symposium on Hypertension, Humoral and Neurogenic Factors. Ed. Wolstenholme, G. E. W. & Cameron, M. P. p. 104. London, Churchill.

PEART, W. S. (1955). *Biochem. J.*, **60**, vi

PEART, W. S. (1956). *Biochem. J.*, **62**, 520.

PEART, W. S. (1959a). *Brit. med. J.*, **2**, 1353 & 1421.

PEART, W. S. (1959b). Lectures on the Scientific Basis of Medicine, VII, 1957–58. p. 182. London, Athlone Press, University of London.

PEART, W. S. (1960). "Essential Hypertension". An International Symposium. Ed. Bock, K. D. & Cottier, P. p. 112. Berlin, Göttingen, Heidelberg, Springer-Verlag.

PEART, W. S. (1965a). *Rec. Progr. Hormone Res.*, **21**, 73.

PEART, W. S. (1965b). *Pharmacol. Rev.*, **17**, 143.

PEART, W. S. (1966). "Antihypertensive Therapy". Proceedings of Symposium held in Siena, Italy, 28 June–3 July 1965, sponsored by CIBA. Ed. Gross, F. p. 468. Berlin, Heidelberg, Springer-Verlag.

PEART, W. S., LLOYD, A. M., THATCHER, G. N., LEVER, A. F., PAYNE, N. & STONE, N. (1966). *Biochem. J.*, **99**, 708.

PICKERING, G. W. (1936). *Clin. Sci.*, **2**, 209.

PICKERING, G. W. & HESS, W. (1933). *Clin. Sci.*, **1**, 213.

Proceedings of Second Catecholamine Symposium held in Milan, July 1965. Pharmacol. Rev., **18**, No. 1, 1966.

PRUNTY, F. T. G. & SWAN, H. J. C. (1950). *Lancet*, **1**, 759.

RABIN, C. B. (1929). *Arch. Path.*, **7**, 228.

RAPPELLI, A. & PEART, W. S. (1968). *Circulat. Res.*, **23**, 531.

"Renal Hypertension" (1968). Ed. I. H. Page & J. W. McCubbin. Chicago, Year Book Medical Publishers, Inc.

ROBINSON, R., SMITH, P. & WHITTAKER, S. R. (1964). *Brit. med. J.*, **1**, 1422.

ROSS, E. J. (1956). *Clin. Sci.*, **15**, 81.

SCORNIK, O. A. & PALADINI, A. C. (1961). *Amer. J. Physiol.*, **201**, 526.

SCRIBNER, B. H., FERGUS, E. B. & BOEN, S. T. (1965). *Ann. Rev. Medicine*, **16**, 285.

SCROOP, G. C. & WHELAN, R. F. (1966). *Clin. Sci.*, **30**, 79.

SEN, S., SMEBY, R. R. & BUMPUS, F. M. (1967). *Biochemistry*, **6**, 1572.

SHALDON, S. (1966). "Scientific Basis Med. Ann. Rev.", p. 201. London, Athlone Press, University of London.

SIMS, E. A. H., MEEKER, C. I., GRAY, M. J., WATANABE, M. & SOLOMON, S. (1964). "Aldosterone". A Symposium organized by the Council for International Organizations of Medical Sciences established under the joint auspices of UNESCO and WHO. Ed. Baulieu, E. E. & Robel, P. p. 499. Oxford, Blackwell.

SKEGGS, L. T., KAHN, J. R., LENTZ, K. E. & SHUMWAY, N. P. (1957). *J. exp. Med.*, **106**, 439.

SKEGGS, L. T., KAHN, J. R. & SHUMWAY, N. P. (1956). *J. exp. Med.*, **103**, 295.

SKEGGS, L. T., LENTZ, K. E., HOCHSTRASSER, H. & KAHN, J. R. (1963). *J. exp. Med.*, **118**, 73.

SKEGGS, L. T., LENTZ, K. E., KAHN, J. R. & SHUMWAY, N. P. (1958). *J. exp. Med.*, **108**, 283.

SKEGGS, L. T., LENTZ, K. E., KAHN, J. R., SHUMWAY, N. P. & WOODS, K. R. (1956). *J. exp. Med.*, **104**, 193.

SKEGGS, L. T., MARSH, W. H., KAHN, J. R. & SHUMWAY, N. P. (1955). *J. exp. Med.*, **102**, 435.

SKINNER, S. L., MCCUBBIN, J. W. & PAGE, I. H. (1963). *Circulat. Res.*, **13**, 336.

THOMPSON, J. E., SILVA, T. F., KINSEY, D. & SMITHWICK, R. H. (1954). *Circulation*, **10**, 912.

THORN, G. W. & FIROR, W. M. (1940). *J. Amer. med. Ass.*, **114**, 2517.

THORN, G. W., HARRISON, J. H., MERRILL, J. P., CRISCITIELLO, M. G., FRAWLEY, T. F. & FINKENSTAEDT, J. T. (1952). *Ann. intern. Med.*, **37**, 972.

THURAU, K. (1964). *Amer. J. Med.*, **36**, 698.

TIGERSTEDT, R. & BERGMAN, P. G. (1898). *Skand. Arch. Physiol.*, **8**, 223.

TOBIAN, L. (1960). *Physiol. Rev.*, **40**, 280.

VALLOTTON, M. B., PAGE, L. B. & HABER, E. (1967). *Nature, Lond.*, **215**, 714.

VANDER, A. J. & MILLER, R. (1964). *Amer. J. Physiol.*, **207**, 537.

WEST, G. B., SHEPHERD, D. M., HUNTER, R. B. & MACGREGOR, A. R. (1953). *Clin. Sci.*, **12**, 317.

WILKINS, L., CRIGLER, J. F., Jr., SILVERMAN, S. H., GARDNER, L. I. & MIGEON, C. J. (1952). *J. clin. Endocrin.*, **12**, 1015.

WILSON, C. & BYROM, F. B. (1941). *Quart. J. Med.*, **10**, 65.

Chapter 10

DISEASES OF THE KIDNEY AND GENITO-URINARY TRACT

by

M. D. MILNE

Westminster Medical School, London

A RATIONAL approach to the study of the chemical pathology of the kidney necessitates a preliminary account of modern concepts of renal physiology. Cushny (1926), in his classical monograph "The Secretion of the Urine", described his filtration-reabsorption theory of kidney function. He considered that the first step in the formation of urine was a process of plasma ultrafiltration through the glomerular membrane with the production of an almost protein-free filtrate, energy being derived from the hydrostatic pressure of the blood within the glomerular capillaries. The solutes contained in this ultrafiltrate were classified as "threshold substances", e.g. glucose, amino acids, and electrolytes, and "non-threshold substances", e.g. urea, creatinine and uric acid. The former were considered to be completely reabsorbed by the tubular cells provided that their plasma concentration was below a fixed "threshold" level, whilst the latter were excreted without tubular reabsorption at all plasma levels. Cushny considered that this process of reabsorption of "threshold" substances and the concentration of "non-threshold" substances was effected by the reabsorption of an "ideal fluid" of constant composition. He denied the existence of any mechanism of active tubular secretion of solutes. This theory has since been considerably modified in that tubular secretion has been proved to occur, and the concept of reabsorption of a fluid of constant composition has been shown to be quantitatively inadmissible.

The brilliant researches of Richards & Walker (1937) and of Walker, Bott, Oliver & MacDowell (1941) furnished a direct proof of the filtration–reabsorption mechanism. By micro-puncture of the renal tubules of the frog and various mammalian species, it was shown that the glomerular filtrate contained less than 30 mg. protein/100 ml. Glucose and phosphate were shown to be reabsorbed in the proximal tubule, whilst acidification of the urine and ammonia formation took place in the distal tubule. The osmotic pressure of the tubular fluid remained equal to that of plasma throughout the proximal tubule, water and solute being reabsorbed proportionately.

Renal clearances. The introduction of the conception of renal clearance by van Slyke, and its development by Homer Smith and his co-workers, has been of fundamental importance in modern renal physiology. As the methods are readily applicable to human subjects, they have proved of equal value in the elucidation of disordered renal function in disease. Standard abbreviations will be used throughout this chapter in description of renal clearance, and all numerical values are corrected to refer to adult subjects of average surface area of 1·73 sq. m. The renal clearance of any substance X is referred to as C_x, and is defined by the simple formula $\dfrac{U_x \cdot V}{P_x}$, where V is the rate of urine flow expressed as ml./min., and U_x and P_x are the concentrations of the substance X in urine and plasma respectively. These concentrations must be in the same units, and are usually expressed as mg./ml. in the case of non-electrolytes, and as μ-equiv./ml. in the case of electro-

lytes. Since $U_x \cdot V$ measures the actual mass of the substance X excreted each minute, the factor $\dfrac{U_x \cdot V}{P_x} = C_x$ gives the volume of plasma in ml. which could be theoretically "cleared" of substance X in 1 min.

The glomerular filtration rate. Determination of the clearance of a substance which is neither reabsorbed nor secreted by the tubule cells gives a measure of the volume of glomerular filtrate produced each minute (glomerular filtration rate or GFR). This value is as fundamental in renal physiology as is determination of the cardiac output in the physiology of the heart. Creatinine is the substance usually used in the experimental animal, and the polysaccharide inulin in the human subject. The latter must be given either as a subcutaneous depot injection, or better by steady intravenous infusion. Details of the techniques of clearance methods are well described by Goldring & Chasis (1944). The reasons for the assumption that inulin is neither secreted nor reabsorbed by the tubule cells will be given later. The amount of inulin excreted each minute ($U_{in} \cdot V$) is equal to the amount filtered at the glomeruli. Since the concentration of inulin in the glomerular filtrate is equal to that in the plasma (P_{in}), the factor $\dfrac{U_{in} \cdot V}{P_{in}} = C_{in}$ gives the volume of filtrate per minute (GFR). The mean value of this and other

TABLE 10.1

Value and significance of renal clearance tests. Most values are quoted from H. W. Smith:
"The Kidney. Structure and Function in Health and Disease", and are corrected to standard surface area of 1·73 sq. m.

Clearance or other test	Average value	Renal function measured
Inulin Clearance. C_{in} (GFR)	125 ml./min.	Glomerular filtration rate
PAH Clearance. C_{PAH} (ERPF)	633 ml./min.	Effective renal plasma flow
Extraction Ratio PAH (E_{PAH})	0·92	Fraction of RPF perfusing functional nephrons
Filtration Fraction. C_{in}/C_{PAH}	19·8%	Fraction of plasma filtered at glomeruli
Renal Plasma Flow. C_{PAH}/E_{PAH} (RPF)	690 ml./min.	Renal circulation (plasma)
Renal Blood Flow	1280 ml./min.	Renal circulation (blood)
Cardiac Output (C.O.)	5300 ml./min.	Total cardiac output
Renal Circulatory Fraction RBF/C.O.	24%	Fraction of cardiac output supplying the kidneys
Tubular Maximal Reabsorptive Capacity for Glucose. Tm_G	305 mg./min.	Proximal tubular reabsorptive function
Tubular Maximal Secretory Capacity for PAH. Tm_{PAH}	79 mg./min.	Proximal tubular secretory function
Ratio C_{in}/Tm_{PAH}	1·58 ml./mg.	Ratio of glomerular to proximal tubular function
Ratio C_{PAH}/Tm_{PAH}	8·0 ml./mg.	Relative blood supply of functioning renal tissue

clearance values in the normal adult are given in Table 10.1.

The technical difficulties in the analysis of inulin make the use of inulin clearances unacceptable for routine clinical work. There has, therefore, been considerable recent interest in alternative methods for accurate estimation of the glomerular filtration rate. Nelp, Wagner & Reba (1964) found that [57]Co-cyanocobalamin clearance correlated well with inulin clearances in man, but later workers (Foley, Jones & Clapham, 1966) have found inaccuracies due to the protein-binding of vitamin B_{12}. Breckenridge & Metcalfe-Gibson (1965) reduced but did not completely eliminate this source of error by giving a large dose of unlabelled vitamin to saturate the binding sites on plasma albumin. The method obviously relies on a low rate of exchange between bound unlabelled B_{12} and labelled B_{12} which is free in plasma. Most workers have, in fact, found it necessary to estimate the degree of B_{12} binding at the mid-point of a clearance period (Ekins, Nashat, Portal & Sgherzi, 1966).

Obviously, a substance which is not protein-bound is both theoretically and practically preferable. Garnett, Parsons & Veall (1967) showed that ^{51}Cr-EDTA is not significantly bound to plasma proteins and does not enter the red cell. Stacey & Thorburn (1966) found that the clearance of ^{51}Cr-EDTA agreed well with the inulin clearance in sheep, and Garnett et al. (1967) obtained similar close correspondence of the two clearances in man. An alternative substance is ^{125}I-sodium iothalamate (Elwood, Sigman & Tregar, 1967) which also has a clearance agreeing well with that of inulin. If simultaneous renal plasma flows are desired using an isotope technique, ^{131}I-iodopyracet can be given (Elwood et al., 1967). Probably, however, ^{51}Cr-EDTA is the most satisfactory substance used to date as it is easy to prepare and the total dosage is extremely small and far below any possible toxic level, both from the pharmacological and radiation points of view.

CLEARANCES OF SUBSTANCES REABSORBED OR SECRETED BY THE RENAL TUBULES

No substance which occurs naturally in human plasma has a clearance value exactly equal to that of the glomerular filtration rate. Most substances are reabsorbed by the tubule cells and the clearance is lower than that of inulin; a few are secreted and the clearance is higher. Glucose is the classical example of the former group. Creatinine, urobilin, and N-methyl-nicotinamide (a metabolic product

of nicotinic acid) are naturally occurring substances with clearance values in man somewhat higher than that of inulin. The clearances of certain foreign substances, e.g. diodrast and p-aminohippuric acid (PAH) are still higher. These are the best examples of compounds actively secreted by tubule cells. The latter compound is more often used in assessing renal function owing to the ease of its chemical estimation.

No compound with a higher clearance than that of diodrast or PAH is known. The clearance of these substances, when present at low plasma concentration, is limited only by the rate of renal plasma flow. Many investigators have combined the determination of C_{PAH} in normal human subjects with the analysis of blood obtained from the right renal vein by means of a cardiac catheter. The PAH concentration of plasma from the renal vein averages only 8% of that of plasma obtained simultaneously from a peripheral vein. It is usually assumed that blood having circulated through normal functioning renal tissue has been completely cleared of PAH, and that the 8% found on analysis represents that portion of blood which has supplied peri-renal fat and inert fibrous tissue within the kidney. The factor $\frac{(P_x - R_x)}{P_x}$ where P_x and R_x are the concentrations of X in peripheral and renal venous plasma respectively, is known as the extraction ratio of the substance X (E_x), and for PAH (E_{PAH}) is equal to 0·92 in the normal subject.

The renal blood flow. The renal plasma flow (RPF), and from this the renal blood flow (RBF), may be directly determined from renal clearances by application of the Fick principle. Let P_x represent the concentration of substance X in renal arterial plasma in mg./ml., and R_x the concentration in renal venous plasma. The amount of substance X entering the kidneys by the renal arteries is $P_x . RPF$; the amount leaving in the urine is $U_x . V$, and the amount leaving in the renal veins is $R_x . (RPF - V)$, since the volume of plasma leaving the kidneys must be less than the amount entering by a volume V equal to that of the urine formed.

$$P_x . RPF = U_x . V + R_x . (RPF - V)$$

Solving for RPF:

$$RPF = \frac{(U_x - R_x) . V}{(P_x - R_x)} \text{ (Wolf, 1941).}$$

In practice PAH is used as the substance X. The clearance of this compound is so high that R_{PAH} is negligible as compared to U_{PAH} and the equation becomes:

$$RPF = \frac{U_{PAH} . V}{P_{PAH} - R_{PAH}}$$

The PAH clearance (C_{PAH}) measures the plasma flow which has perfused functioning renal tissue, and is known as the effective renal plasma flow (ERPF). Total renal plasma flow is given by the fraction $\dfrac{C_{PAH}}{E_{PAH}}$, and total renal blood flow by $\dfrac{C_{PAH}}{E_{PAH}.\,(1-\text{haematocrit})}$. Average normal values are given in Table 10.1. It will be seen that the renal blood flow is normally between 20 and 25% of the resting cardiac output. Since the measurement of E_{PAH} by renal vein catheterization considerably complicates the procedure, the assumption is usually made that E_{PAH} is 92%. This leads to no significant error provided that C_{in} and C_{PAH} are above 50% of the expected normal figure. If renal function is depressed further, E_{PAH} steadily falls and must be determined if an accurate estimate of renal plasma flow is desired (Cargill, 1949).

The PAH method for determination of renal blood flow becomes inaccurate when extraction ratios are low. The method depends on the difference of concentration of PAH in arterial and renal venous blood, and errors obviously increase as the two values tend to approximate as renal function and blood flow is progessively reduced. By contrast, a method based on the diffusibility of inert gases becomes of greater accuracy with reduced renal blood flows. Brun, Crone, Davidson, Fabricius, Hansen, Lassen & Munck (1955) used radioactive krypton (^{85}Kr) to give the first accurate measurement of renal blood flow in acute tubular necrosis. Similar results have been obtained more recently by use of a dye (Shaldon, Higgs, Chiandussi, Walker, Garsenstein & Ryder, 1962) indocyanin green, which is neither excreted nor metabolized by the kidney. If the dye is infused at constant rate into a renal artery until the concentration in the corresponding renal vein becomes constant, the blood flow through the kidney can be calculated if the renal vein concentration and rate of infusion are known. As

$$RPF = \frac{\text{amt. infused/min.}}{\text{Conc. in renal vein plasma}}$$

it is clear that accuracy increases with fall of RPF. The disadvantage of the method is that it necessitates renal arterial as well as venous catheterization, and gives the blood flow in one kidney rather than the sum of both. However, if renal function is grossly different in the two kidneys, intubation of one renal vein to measure extraction ratio for PAH will give a further source of inaccuracy as E_{PAH} will not be equal in the two kidneys.

Tubular maximal reabsorptive and secretory capacity. Whilst determination of the glomerular filtration rate gives the best assessment of glomerular function, and renal blood flow of the circulation in the kidneys, proximal tubular function is best measured by the tubular maximal reabsorptive capacity for glucose (Tm_G), and the maximal secretory capacity for PAH (Tm_{PAH}). These values expressed in mg./min. give the maximum amount of each compound that can be transferred each minute between plasma and tubular fluid.

Although glucose has been studied in most detail, many other compounds that are reabsorbed by the proximal tubules have Tm values, e.g. other carbohydrates, some amino acids, ascorbic and lactic acids, and phosphate. The following general mathematical relationships are applicable: the amount of a substance excreted is equal to the amount filtered at the glomeruli less the amount reabsorbed,

$$U_x . V = P_x . C_{in} - Tm_x \qquad . \qquad . \quad (1)$$

Since C_{in} and Tm_x are almost of constant value, the graph of the equation relating the amount of a substance excreted to the plasma level is a straight line of gradient equal to C_{in}, and is illustrated for glucose by line AB (Fig. 10.1). When $U_x . V = 0$, $P_x = \dfrac{Tm_x}{C_{in}}$. This is the true mathematical expression of the "threshold" level of a substance X. Any factor which separately alters either the glomerular filtration rate or the tubular reabsorptive capacity will change the so-called "threshold" level of plasma concentration at which the substance first appears in the urine. If equation (1) is divided throughout by P_x, the following relationships are obtained:

$$\frac{U_x . V}{P_x} = C_{in} - \frac{Tm_x}{P_x} \qquad . \qquad . \quad (2)$$

The expression on the left is the clearance of substance X, and therefore the graph of the equation relating clearance to plasma level is a portion of a rectangular hyperbola with the line $y = C_{in}$ as one asymptote. The graph for glucose is shown by curve AB (Fig. 10.2).

Similar considerations apply to a substance secreted by the proximal tubule cells. e.g. PAH. The equations in this case are:

$$U_x . V = P_x . C_{in} + Tm_x \qquad . \qquad . \quad (3)$$

$$\frac{U_x . V}{P_x} = C_{in} + \frac{Tm_x}{P_x} \qquad . \qquad . \quad (4)$$

The line CD, relating excretion to plasma level, is given for PAH in Fig. 10.1, and the portion of the rectangular hyperbola CD relating clearance to plasma level in Fig. 10.2. There is no

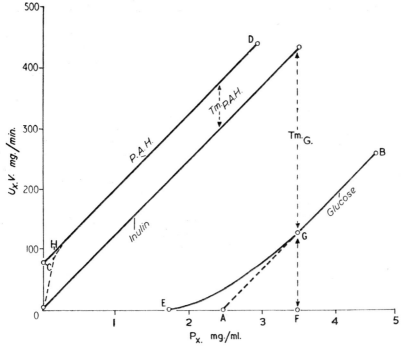

FIG. 10.1. Graphs of equations $U_x . V = P_x . C_{in}$ (Inulin).

$U_x . V = P_x . C_{in} - Tm_G$ (Glucose).

$U_x . V = P_x . C_{in} + Tm_{PAH}$ (PAH).

Assumed constants are $C_{in} = 125$ ml./min., $Tm_G = 305$ mg./min., and $Tm_{PAH} = 79$ mg./min. Point A is "Mean Threshold", point E is "Appearance Threshold", and point F is "Maximal Threshold" for glucose. Below plasma levels of PAH of about 0·16 mg./ml., the excretion of PAH is limited by the renal plasma flow. Actual excretion is indicated by the broken line OH.

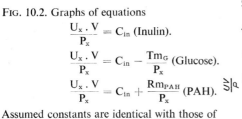

FIG. 10.2. Graphs of equations

$$\frac{U_x . V}{P_x} = C_{in} \text{ (Inulin).}$$

$$\frac{U_x . V}{P_x} = C_{in} - \frac{Tm_G}{P_x} \text{ (Glucose).}$$

$$\frac{U_x . V}{P_x} = C_{in} + \frac{Rm_{PAH}}{P_x} \text{ (PAH).}$$

Assumed constants are identical with those of Fig. 10.1.

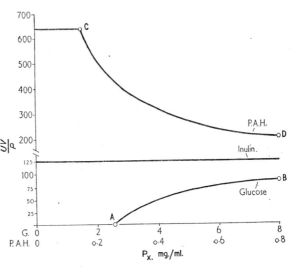

"threshold" plasma level for a substance secreted by tubule cells, considerable amounts being excreted at all plasma concentrations. The maximal clearance value is, however, limited by the effective renal plasma flow. From equation (4), when C_{PAH} equals ERPF, the following relationship applies:

$$ERPF = C_{in} + \frac{Tm_{PAH}}{P_{PAH}}$$

whence $P_{PAH} = \frac{T_{PAH}}{REPF - C_{in}}$

This value of plasma level of PAH defines the point C (Fig. 10.2). It is a plasma level which should be avoided in determination of ERPF or Tm_{PAH}. Plasma levels of PAH well below this should be used for the determination of the ERPF, and values considerably above for determination of Tm_{PAH}.

Fig. 10.2 shows that the clearance of a substance reabsorbed by the tubule cells increases with rising plasma levels, and that of a substance secreted decreases. Both clearances approach that of inulin at very high plasma concentrations. The clearance of a substance such as inulin, which is neither secreted nor reabsorbed, remains constant at widely differing plasma concentrations. The validity of the use of inulin clearance as an index of the glomerular filtration rate in man has been reinvestigated by Kennedy & Kleh (1953). They found that the inulin clearance was constant at plasma levels ranging from 3 to 175 mg./100 ml.

Variation between individual nephrons. The equations above relating renal clearances to tubular maximal reabsorptive or secretory capacity are considerably more ideal than are found in actual fact. They assume that the kidneys are made up of many identical nephrons, amounting to almost two million in man (Moore, 1931). Nephrons are in fact far from identical, and vary widely in details of size, structure and functional capacity. This is especially well seen in relation to glucose excretion (Govaerts, 1952). Calculation from the fraction $\frac{Tm_G}{C_{in}}$ gives the mean "threshold" plasma level of glucose of 245 mg./100 ml. (point A in Fig. 10.1). Some nephrons have a lower $\frac{Tm_G}{C_{in}}$ ratio than the average, and most individuals will show a significant glycosuria at plasma levels of glucose of 170 mg./100 ml. (the minimal or "appearance" threshold, point E in Fig. 10.1). Conversely, many nephrons have a higher ratio, and all the tubules will not be reabsorbing glucose to a maximum degree until plasma concentrations

of 350 mg. glucose/100 ml. are reached (maximal threshold, point F in Fig. 10.1). This plasma level must be exceeded in determination of Tm_G. The correct relationship between glucose excreted and plasma glucose concentration is not, therefore, the theoretical straight line AB, but the curvilinear relation EG at plasma concentrations below the "maximal" threshold, and the straight line GB at higher plasma levels.

Renal glycosuria. This may be defined as a condition in which there is significant glycosuria at plasma concentrations of glucose below the normal "appearance" threshold of 170 mg./100 ml. It is usually a completely harmless anomaly, of importance only in that it may lead to a false diagnosis of diabetes mellitus. Two separate types are known to occur. In the more severe variety there is an abnormally low Tm_G, but the "splay" of tubular variation between minimal and maximal threshold levels is not increased. Glucose excretion is therefore excessive both at high and low plasma concentrations. This type of proximal tubular abnormality is the cause of the glycosuria seen in the Fanconi syndrome (Lambert & de Heinzelin, 1951; Robertson & Gray, 1953), and after the injection of phlorrhizin.

The other variety is due to an increased "splay" of nephrons with regard to glucose reabsorption. The "appearance" threshold of glucose is reduced, but the mean threshold and the Tm_G value are perfectly normal. Excessive urinary loss of glucose is therefore only present at low plasma concentrations of glucose, the excretion at plasma levels above the "maximal threshold" being normal.

The amount of "splay" in the glucose titration curve has been found to correlate well with heterogeneity of the structural dimensions of nephrons by micro-dissection technique (Oliver & MacDowell, 1961). In the normal kidney "splay" is minimized by a close relationship between the surface area of the glomerular tuft and the mass of the corresponding proximal tubule cells (Bradley, Laragh, Wheeler, MacDowell & Oliver, 1961). The former is claimed to determine the glomerular filtration rate of the nephron, and the latter to parallel the tubular Tm_G.

EXCRETION OF END-PRODUCTS OF PROTEIN METABOLISM

One of the main homeostatic functions of the kidney is the elimination of nitrogenous end-products of protein metabolism. Protein intake is very variable in different individuals and races. It is usually recommended that the adult diet should contain at least 1 g. of protein/kg. body weight each day. This corresponds to a daily intake of about 11 g. of protein nitrogen. Some of this nitrogen, averaging 1·3 g./day, is lost in the faeces, and about 0·3 g. in the sweat. The remainder is excreted in the urine, chiefly as urea, ammonia, creatinine and uric acid, together with small quantities of amino acids and other nitrogenous compounds.

Urea is the only constituent which varies considerably with the protein intake. On high-protein diets, urea nitrogen may account for 90% of the total urinary nitrogen, but may fall to 20% of the total on a diet composed almost entirely of carbohydrates and fats. Ammonia excretion is primarily influenced by changes in acid-base balance, uric acid by the intake of purines and nucleoproteins, while creatinine excretion remains constant despite gross variation in diet. The urinary amino-nitrogen is slightly influenced by the protein intake but is relatively far more constant than urea.

Urea excretion. In normal adults the blood urea varies according to the protein intake from 12 to 47 mg./100 ml. (Wootton, King & Smith, 1951). The actual value is approximately equal to twice the nitrogen intake in g./day, e.g. if the nitrogen intake is 11 g./day, the blood urea averages 22 mg./100 ml. Urea is freely diffusible throughout the body water. Owing to the high concentration of haemoglobin in the erythrocytes, the plasma urea concentration is slightly higher than the blood urea, and it is preferable to use the former value in determinations of urea clearance. The urea clearance ranges from 30 to 60% of the simultaneous inulin clearance, depending on the rate of urine flow. Its value is uninfluenced by the level of plasma urea, except in so far as this affects the urine flow due to osmotic diuresis. This type of clearance, where the value is less than the glomerular filtration rate but is independent of plasma concentration, is typical of a substance which is not actively reabsorbed by the tubules, but which diffuses across the cellular membrane. Other substances resembling urea in this respect are lithium (Foulks, Mudge & Gilman, 1952) and iodide (Childs, Keating, Rall, Williams & Power, 1950). The ratio, urea clearance/inulin clearance, falls with diminishing rates of urine flow, since there is then more time available for back-diffuson to take place.

Austin, Stillman & van Slyke (1921) claimed that urea clearance remained constant at rates of urine flow above 2 ml./min., whilst at lower rates the clearance diminished proportionately to the square root of the flow. Expressed mathematically, at flows more than 2 ml./min.,

$$C_{urea} = \frac{U_{urea} \cdot V}{P_{urea}} = constant = 0.60 \times C_{in}$$
$$= 75 \; ml./min.$$

At flows less than 2 ml./min.,

$$\frac{U_{urea} \cdot V}{P_{urea}} \times \frac{I}{\sqrt{V}} = \frac{U_{urea} \cdot \sqrt{V}}{P_{urea}} = constant$$
$$= 0.43 \times C_{in} = 54 \; ml./min.$$

The rate of urine flow of 2 ml./min. at which urea clearance was assumed to become constant was termed the "augmentation limit". Later work by Shannon (1936) in the dog, and by Chasis & Smith (1938) in man, has failed to show any evidence of an "augmentation limit", the urea clearance increasing linearly with urine flow at all values from extreme oliguria to maximal water diuresis. In man it was found that urea clearance averaged 60% of the inulin clearance at flows of 10 ml./min., and 40% at flows of 0·5 ml./min. The original formula introduced by Van Slyke (1943) and his colleagues of $\frac{U_{urea} \cdot \sqrt{V}}{P_{urea}}$ for rates of urine flow below 2 ml./min. cannot strictly be defined as a clearance value, and it is not consistent with modern views of renal physiology. It remains, however, of much more than mere historical interest, since it is still used in routine chemical clinical pathology for the calculation of urea clearance.

Urea excretion is of great importance in relation to mechanisms of urinary concentration. The kidney is capable of excreting a urine of higher osmolality if large amounts of urea are being excreted (Levinsky & Berliner, 1959). Urea is present in high concentration in the fluids of the papillary tip and together with sodium chloride accounts for the hyperosmolality of the tissues of this specialized portion of the kidney substance.

Estimation of the blood urea or plasma non-protein nitrogen may be grossly misleading as an index of renal function if uraemic patients are being treated on low-protein diets. Treatment with the Giovannetti-Giordano regime (Giordano, 1963; Giovannetti & Maggiure, 1964; Berlyne & Shaw, 1965; Shaw, Bazzard, Booth, Nilwarangkur & Berlyne, 1965) involves a dietary intake of only 10 g. high class protein daily. On such regimes the blood urea may fall to about 20% of its value on a normal protein diet, and the plasma creatinine becomes a more reliable index of renal functional impairment.

The excretion of creatinine. In many experimental animals, including the dog, the clearance of exogenous creatinine gives a measure of the glomerular filtration rate. This has been confirmed by Selkurt (1952), who found that the discrepancy between simultaneous creatinine and inulin clearances in the dog was always less than 10%.

Unfortunately, creatinine is secreted by the tubules in the higher apes and in man, and therefore the exogenous creatinine clearance is invariably higher than that of inulin. Ratios of creatinine to inulin clearance (C_{cr}/C_{in}) varying from 1·25 to 1·40 have been reported by many workers. The endogenous creatinine clearance much more nearly approximates to the inulin clearance in man (Brod & Sirota, 1948), but there is evidence that this identity is fortuitous. Plasma creatinine, as estimated by the Jaffé colorimetric method, ranges from 0·9 to 1·7 mg./100 ml. in the normal subject. Miller & Dubos (1937), using a specific enzymic method for creatinine, found that between 0 and 20% of the chromogenic material in plasma was not creatinine. The endogenous creatinine clearance is therefore under-estimated if the plasma chromogen is considered to be entirely creatinine. At normal plasma levels this error tends to compensate for the fact that the true creatinine clearance is higher than that of inulin. In uraemia the plasma chromogen increases and a higher proportion of it is creatinine. The endogenous creatinine clearance is then substantially higher than that of inulin (Mattar, Barnett, McNamara & Lauson, 1952). Apparently then, this clearance cannot be regarded as a convenient means of giving a true estimate of the glomerular filtration rate, but it has proved of great value in indicating a change of filtration over periods which are too prolonged for the continuous infusion of inulin solutions.

The excretion of uric acid. The concentration of uric acid in normal human plasma varies from 2·0 to 6·0 mg./100 ml. and averages 4·0 mg./100 ml. (Bulger & Johns, 1941).

Uric acid is excreted by a triple process of glomerular filtration, and both tubular secretion and reabsorption. Normally, there is considerable net tubular reabsorption of uric acid, the clearance being much lower than that of inulin, the ratio C_u/C_{in} averaging 0·08. There is a maximal tubular reabsorptive capacity of about 15 mg./min. (Berliner, Hilton, Yü & Kennedy, 1950) which is not saturated at ordinary plasma levels either in the normal subject or in the gouty individual. Gutman, Yü & Berger (1959), by a combination of urate infusion and mannitol diuresis in human subjects, have proved that the urate clearance may exceed that of inulin, indicating net tubular secretion. Nugent & Tyler (1959) have shown that the high plasma urate in gout is at least partially due to diminished urate excretion and excessive tubular urate reabsorption in gouty subjects. When plasma urate is raised in normal subjects by urate infusion to values typical of clinical gout, urinary output of uric acid is considerably higher than in cases of gout.

Reabsorption of uric acid may be reduced in certain disorders of the proximal renal tubules associated with amino-aciduria. Thus Sirota, Yü & Gutman (1952) found a C_u/C_{in} ratio of 0·98, which was unaffected by probenecid, in a case of the Fanconi syndrome, and Bishop, Zimdahl & Talbott (1954) found a similar value in a case of hepatolenticular degeneration. In such cases, the plasma uric acid is abnormally low owing to excessive urinary loss.

Yü, Berger & Gutman (1962) present evidence that tubular reabsorption of urate is virtually complete, and that almost all excreted urate is derived from tubular secretion at a more distal site in the nephron. This gives a unified view of the action of many acidic drugs on urate excretion. Both secretion and reabsorption of urate are competitively reduced by many organic acids, but inhibition of secretion is the more sensitive and therefore is the sole effect at low dosage. Drugs which increase serum urate, e.g. thiazide diuretics and pyrazinamide, inhibit urate secretion at therapeutic doses and the clearance may fall to very low values. By contrast, uricosuric drugs, e.g. salicylates, probenecid, phenylbutazone and sulphinpyrazone, at small dosage inhibit urate secretion and thus increase serum urate, but at larger therapeutic doses prevent the quantitatively more important urate absorption and therefore lower serum urate.

Urate excretion is competitively reduced by lactate and β-hydroxybutyric acid. Hyperlactic-acidaemia occurs in ethanol intoxication (Lieber, Jones, Losowsky & Davidson, 1962), toxaemia of pregnancy (Handler, 1960) and after severe muscular exercise (Nichols, Miller & Hiatt, 1951) and in surgical shock with reduced oxygenation of venous blood. Increased blood lactate and associated raised plasma urate is invariable in glycogenosis Type I due to glucose-6-phosphatase deficiency (Howell, Ashton & Wyngaardens, 1962). Increase of plasma β-hydroxybutyrate accounts for the hyperuricaemia found in starvation (Murphy & Shipman, 1963) and in diabetic ketosis (Padova & Bendersky, 1962). All of these conditions may be associated with attacks of clinical gout.

WATER AND SALT EXCRETION

Variation in rate of urine flow. The normal kidney can alter the rate of urine flow through wide limits and maintain homeostasis despite variation of fluid intake and of extrarenal fluid loss in the sweat, expired air and faeces. The proportion of water in the glomerular filtrate which is not reabsorbed by the tubules and therefore lost in the urine can best be measured by determination of the plasma/urine concentration ratio of a substance such as inulin, which is neither reabsorbed nor secreted. The average rate of urine flow in the normal adult is about 1 ml./min., and thus over 99% of the water in the glomerular filtrate is usually reabsorbed by the tubules. In maximum water diuresis, or in the most severe grades of clinical diabetes insipidus, the rate of urine flow rarely exceeds 16 ml./min., with an inulin U/P ratio of 8 (Chasis & Smith, 1938; Winer, 1942). This indicates that seven-eighths of the water in the glomerular filtrate have been reabsorbed, and one-eighth excreted.

In the opposite condition of hydropenia, the minimum rate of urine flow is limited only by the capacity of the tubules to maintain an osmotic gradient between urine and plasma, and by the total amount of solute requiring excretion. The maximal total solute concentration in human urine averages 1·4 osmol./l. (Gamble & Butler, 1944). Since the plasma solute concentration is about 0·33 osmol./l., the average maximum osmotic urine/plasma ratio $\left(\dfrac{U_{osm}}{P_{osm}}\right)$ is 4·2. This factor varies considerably in different mammalian species; e.g. it is 6·0 in the dog and as high as 17·0 in the desert rat (Schmidt-Nielsen, Schmidt-Nielsen & Brokaw, 1948), a species which has become adapted to chronic water deprivation. Maximum urinary concentration is not obtained by relatively short periods of hydropenia, such as a mere 16 hr. of fluid deprivation, as used in the usual clinical maximum urinary specific gravity test. Gamble (1951a) found that a maximum urinary concentration of 1·4 osmol./l. was not attained until the second or even third day of complete water deprivation. The actual minimal rate of urine flow is therefore proportional to the amount of solute to be excreted. On an average diet, an adult excretes about 1200 m-osmol. of solute daily. This is almost entirely composed of urea, which amounts to about 500 m-osmol., and the three univalent cations Na, K, and NH₄, with their associated anions. A minimal solute excretion is obtained after a few days on an electrolyte-free and protein-free diet, e.g. a diet consisting entirely of glucose. Under these circumstances the daily solute excretion may fall to 200 m-osmol. each day. In Fig. 10.3, the relationship between urinary volume and urinary concentration is

shown for this artificial diet, and for low, average and high protein diets with solute excretion of 500 1200 and 1700 m-osmol./day. It is seen that the lowest possible urine volume compatible with renal sufficiency is about 150 ml./day, equivalent to 0·1 ml. each minute, with a theoretical inulin U/P ratio of over 1000.

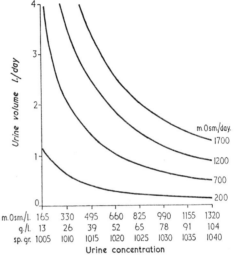

Fig. 10.3. Relationship between the daily urine volume and the average urinary concentration at varying levels of solute output.

The classical experiments of Verney (1947) have shown that this wide variation in permissible rates of urine flow is controlled by the secretion of the antidiuretic hormone (ADH) by the posterior pituitary gland. Hypertonicity of the plasma stimulates intra-cranial osmo-receptors which cause a maximal secretion of antidiuretic hormone, and the reverse occurs in states of hypotonicity. In addition, hypertonicity stimulates the thirst mechanism, with correction of the abnormality provided that fluid is freely available (Wolf, 1950). This homeostatic mechanism is both sensitive and rapid in taking effect. The osmo-receptors respond to a change of about 1% in the tonicity of the blood (Verney, 1947), and the equilibrium level is usually restored within an hour or two.

Osmotic diuresis. Increasing the urinary solute excretion above the normal level of approximately 1 m-osmol./min. greatly increases the rate of urine flow, the excretion of NaCl, and to a lesser extent of K. Osmotic diuresis may be produced experimentally by intravenous infusion of various solutes including urea, hypertonic NaCl, Na salts of non-reabsorbable anions such as thiosulphate and *p*-aminohippurate, and carbohydrates such as glucose, sucrose and mannitol. Rapoport, Brodsky, West & Mackler (1949) have shown that the effect is independent of the actual substance used, being influenced only by the osmotic effect of excreted solute. Mannitol is the most popular substance for producing experimental osmotic diuresis, since it is non-toxic and does not affect the acid-base balance of the urine. Examples of osmotic diuresis occurring in human pathology are those produced by glucose in severe diabetes mellitus, and by NaCl after mercurial injections, and the polyuria of chronic renal failure where urea is the main loading solute.

The maximal rate of urine flow may be much higher in osmotic diuresis than is possible in maximum water diuresis. Inulin U/P ratios as low as 3·5, with urine flows of 41 ml./min., have been obtained in man during glucose osmotic diuresis (Smith, Goldring, Chasis, Ranges & Bradley, 1943). In the dog, still lower ratios of 2·0 have been recorded, indicating that only half of the water of the glomerular filtrate was reabsorbed (Mudge, Foulks & Gilman, 1949). Osmotic diuresis has been most studied in the hydropenic state since variation from a simultaneous water diuresis is thereby avoided. Although osmotic diuresis is associated with an increased urinary volume and total solute excretion, the power of the tubules to maintain an osmotic gradient between urine and plasma is progressively diminished, and the osmolarity of the urine asymptotically approaches that of the plasma (Fig. 10.4).

Mechanism of water and salt reabsorption. Previously the most widely accepted theory of water reabsorption by the renal tubules was that advanced by Homer Smith and his colleagues (Wesson, Anslow & Smith, 1948). Walker *et al.* (1941) showed that the fluid in the proximal tubules remained isotonic with plasma, and, as stated above, under normal conditions at least seven-eighths of filtered water is reabsorbed. It was postulated that this was effected by a process of passive reabsorption of water in the proximal tubule consequent to active tubular reabsorption of Na with its main associated anions, Cl and bicarbonate. This passive reabsorption of water is necessarily impeded if there is excess of unreabsorbed solute as in osmotic diuresis, and therefore a greater than normal volume of isotonic fluid passes into the distal tubules.

Views on the mechanisms of water and Na reabsorption by the renal tubules have been considerably modified in the last decade by the description and subsequent elaboration of the counter-current theory of urinary concentration and dilution (Wirz, Hargitay & Kuhn, 1951). This theory has provided alternative explanations for previous views which were difficult to reconcile with basic thermodynamic principles, i.e. active transport of water in a predominantly aqueous medium, and the production and maintenance of considerable osmotic gradients over very short lengths of renal tissue. Water transport is now considered to be a completely passive physico-chemical process due to the osmotic effects from movement of solute. Renal tubule cells are freely permeable to water with the exception of the cells of the collecting ducts which are impermeable in the absence of circulating anti-diuretic hormone, but freely permeable in its presence. Osmotic gradients are thought to be developed gradually over the whole thickness of the renal medulla and not abruptly across a single renal tubular cell.

The loop of Henle acts as a counter-current multiplier system, osmotic work being performed by the extrusion of Na from the tubular lumen to the interstitial fluid of the medulla. By contrast the *vasa recta* act as a passive counter-current exchanger, no work being performed by the system. The principles of counter-current exchange are more easily understood in relation to alterations of temperature than to changes in osmolality as in the renal medulla. Fig. 10.4 shows a simple type of counter-current exchanger relating to temperature. Cold water flowing through the simple U-tube on the left rapidly removes heat from the hot water in the container, and therefore the hot water is rapidly cooled. The counter-current exchanger on the right only slowly removes heat from the hot water in the container. Cold water in the descending limb of the loop is warmed by the fluid in the outgoing limb, and conversely the warm water in the ascending limb is cooled by contact with the descending limb. Obviously the larger the loop and the slower the flow in the system, the greater will be the efficiency in maintaining the heat in the water within the vessel.

Similarly, in the renal medulla, the counter-current exchange system of the *vasa recta* maintains the hyperosmolality of the papillary tip and prevents dissipation of the unusually high concentration of NaCl and urea within the tissue. Species with unusually long loops of Henle, e.g. the desert rat, are most efficient in building up high levels of osmolality within the renal medulla, and thus in producing highly concentrated urine. The counter-current exchange effect of the *vasa recta* would, however, be ineffective if the blood supply of the medulla of the kidney were as high as that of the renal cortex. In fact, the outer medulla probably only receives about 10% of blood per equal mass of tissue as the cortex, and the papillary tip only 2%.

The development of hyperosmolality of the tissues and fluids within the medulla depends on extrusion of Na from the tubular lumen to the interstitial fluid by the cells of the ascending limb of Henle's loop. This generates an electro-chemical gradient and causes chloride ion to accompany the transported sodium. The counter-current system of the *vasa recta* is most efficient in maintaining the high concentration of NaCl at the papillary tip and least efficient in the outer zone of the medulla. In this way layers of renal tissue of

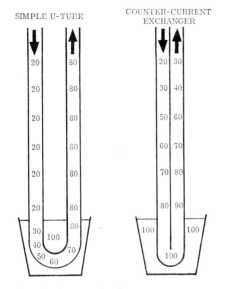

FIG. 10.4. Simple example of counter-current exchange applied to heat. In the U-tube on the left, water in the descending limb remains cool until it enters the vessel of hot water. The water in the ascending limb remains hot and therefore heat is rapidly removed from the contents of the vessel. In the counter-current tube on the right, water in the descending limb is heated by the outgoing stream and is already hot before it enters the vessel. The hot water in the ascending limb is cooled by the ingoing stream. Little heat is therefore removed from the contents of the vessel.

gradually increasing osmolality are built up from the portions of medulla immediately adjacent to the cortex to the papillary tip, where the osmolality in man may be four times that of plasma and other body fluids and tissues.

Details of water and salt reabsorption have recently been clarified by many investigators using micro-puncture techniques, usually in the

rat and the dog. The results in most respects agree well between these two species, suggesting that the results are probably applicable to man. It has been confirmed that proximal tubular Na and water reabsorption is strictly iso-osmolar, the tubular epithelium being freely permeable to water. (Clapp, Watson & Berliner, 1963). The fact that Na reabsorption is against a constant electro-chemical gradient of about 20 m.v. (Watson, Clapp & Berliner, 1964) indicates that the process involves active transport presumably mediated by a cellular "sodium pump" involving ATP and ATP-ase. During osmotic diuresis from substances poorly absorbed from the tubular lumen, e.g. mannitol, a considerable fraction of the osmolality of the tubular fluid is due to the diuretic, and the sodium concentration may be reduced to a minimum of 30% below that of plasma (Ullrich, Schmidt-Nielsen, O'Dell, Pehling, Gottschalk, Lassiter & Mylle, 1963). Diffusion of sodium from plasma to lumen prevents reduction below this minimum value.

The proximal tubular electro-chemical gradient is enough to account for all chloride reabsorption at this site. Bicarbonate is transported chiefly by ionic exchange of H^+ for Na^+ and thus is partially dependent on carbonic anhydrase activity. Fall of pH in the proximal tubule is considerable in the rat (Gottschalk, Lassiter & Mylle, 1960) but much less in the dog (Clapp *et al.*, 1963). Secondary accumulation of ammonia by non-ionic diffusion is, therefore, considerable in the rat, but quantitatively unimportant in the dog. Bicarbonate is removed somewhat more rapidly than chloride, and luminal chloride concentration often considerably exceeds that of plasma.

In the descending limb of Henle's loop, water is continuously reabsorbed by the hyperosmolality of the medulla. The free permeability to water of this segment allows almost complete equilibration of osmolality and at the tip of the loop the tubular contents reach the same high osmotic pressure as that of the environment. By contrast, the wall of the ascending limb is impermeable to water and continuous extrusion of Na continually reduces the osmolality of the contents to values considerably below that of plasma.

In the distal convoluted tubules, the tubular fluid is invariably hypotonic as compared to plasma (Gottschalk & Mylle, 1959), the Na and Cl concentrations being below that of blood. Permeability of the distal convoluted tubule to water is, however, influenced by vasopressin. In the presence of ADH, the hypo-osmolality lessens along the length of the tubule and becomes isotonic with plasma at the upper part of the collecting ducts. By contrast, in the absence of the hormone the hypotonicity persists unchanged.

The electro-chemical gradient in the distal tubules is usually two to three times that of the proximal tubule, and may occasionally be as much as six times as great (Solomon, 1957). The sodium concentration gradient between plasma and luminal fluid is also higher, indicating that the membrane is less permeable than that of the proximal tubule for back-diffusion of Na. Chloride is chiefly reabsorbed by the high electro-chemical gradient in this part of the nephron, but there may be active transport in addition (Rector & Clapp, 1962).

trast, the collecting ducts of *all* nephrons pass through the medullary tissue, and therefore the mechanisms of urinary concentration apply equally to tubular fluid derived from the glomeruli of the outer cortex and the juxta-medullary nephrons provided with a long Henle's loop (Figs. 10.5 and 10.6).

The hyperosmolality of the papillary tip is produced by high concentrations of urea as well as of NaCl. Urea concentrations are more affected by rate of urinary flow than are concentrations of NaCl. Free availability of urea increases the maximal osmolality of urine whether produced by water deprivation or injection of exogenous

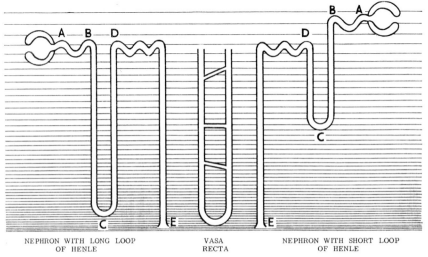

NEPHRON WITH LONG LOOP OF HENLE   VASA RECTA   NEPHRON WITH SHORT LOOP OF HENLE

FIG. 10.5. Diagram of a nephron from a juxta-medullary glomerulus—left; nephron from a glomerulus in the outer cortex—right; and of a *vasa recta*—centre. In the nephron on the left the long loop of Henle BCD dips into an area of high osmolality represented by the density of the shading, whilst the short loop of Henle only dips for a short distance into the medulla and is not exposed to an area of high osmolality. The collecting tubules of both nephrons DE pass through the whole thickness of the medulla. The high osmolality of the medulla is maintained by the counter-current exchange system of the *vasa recta*.

The above simplified account of water reabsorption by the tubules does not fully explain the large variation in urine volume from 0·3 to 15 ml./min. The maximum volume possible by the system described would be only 5% of the glomerular filtration rate, i.e. about 6 ml./min. This discrepancy is explained by the fact that all nephrons do not have a long loop of Henle extending deep into the inner layers of the renal medulla (Figs. 10.5 & 10.6). About 75% of nephrons are derived from glomeruli within the outer cortex and have a short loop of Henle. These nephrons are therefore not concerned with the development of medullary hyperosmolality, and there is no loss of water within the descending limb of the loop. By con-

ADH. Thus urinary concentrating power is decreased on a low-protein diet or after prolonged water diuresis which increases urea excretion, and is increased on a high-protein diet or after ingestion of large doses of pre-formed urea. The high concentration of urea within the renal medulla explains some curious features of urea excretion (Schmidt-Nielsen, 1958). If fluid intake is suddenly increased, urea excretion temporarily rises to very high values, and then falls. Conversely, on stopping a maintained diuresis, urea output becomes temporarily very low as the concentration within the renal papilla rises.

Disorders which affect the efficiency of the medullary counter-current system reduce the

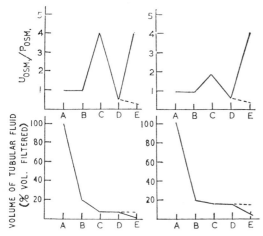

FIG. 10.6. Diagram of the ratio of the osmolality of the tubular fluid to that of plasma—top, and of the ratio of the volume of tubular fluid to the volume filtered—bottom, in the proximal tubule—AB; descending limb of Henle's loop—BC; ascending limb—CD; and collecting tubule—DE. The graphs on the left represent the situation in a nephron from a juxtamedullary glomerulus with a long loop of Henle, and those on the right that in a nephron from a glomerulus of the outer cortex with a short loop of Henle. In the collecting tubule the continuous line represents the situation with maximal action of ADH, whilst the broken line represents the situation in maximal water diuresis with no secretion of ADH.

power of the kidney to produce a highly concentrated urine, e.g. pyelonephritis which particularly involves the medulla, K deficiency which reduces the power of the ascending limb of Henle's loop to extrude Na, hypercalcaemia and hypercalcuria where the medullary tissue is damaged by calcific deposits, and sickle-cell anaemia in which thromboses occur in the *vasa recta*. The countercurrent exchange system of the *vasa recta* also affects gas tensions within the medulla. The tissue of the papillary tip has an unusually high pCO_2 and a very low pO_2, features which are also typical of excreted urine. The low partial pressure of oxygen combined with the relatively low blood supply of the papillary tip explains the peculiar liability of this tissue to ischaemic papillary necrosis.

Excreted water can be divided into three moieties:

(a) that which is equal to the volume of water required to contain the urinary solutes in a solution iso-osmotic with the concomitant plasma (C_{osm}),

(b) that which accounts for the excess water in a hypotonic urine (C_{H_2O}) and

(c) the deficit in a hypertonic urine ($T^c_{H_2O}$).

The following mathematical relations hold:

$$C_{osm} = \frac{U_{osm}}{P_{osm}} . \, V,$$ where U_{osm} and P_{osm} are the osmotic concentrations of urine and plasma, and V is the urinary volume in ml./min.

The urine flow $V = C_{osm} + C_{H_2O}$ if the urine is hypotonic and $V = C_{osm} - T^c_{H_2O}$ if the urine is hypertonic.

Therefore $C_{H_2O} = V \left(I - \dfrac{U_{osm}}{P_{osm}} \right)$ in a hypotonic urine

and $T^c_{H_2O} = V \left(\dfrac{U_{osm}}{P_{osm}} - I \right)$ in a hypertonic urine.

Wesson & Anslow (1948) showed that in maximum water diuresis C_{H_2O} is approximately constant in any individual whatever the osmotic solute load. Zak, Brun & Smith (1954) have similarly shown that $T^c_{H_2O}$ is almost constant in osmotic diuresis in the hydropenic state, provided the urinary volume is more than 4–5 ml./min.

Fig. 10.4 gives the relationship between $\dfrac{U_{osm}}{P_{osm}}$ (urinary concentration factor) and the urinary volume during osmotic diuresis in the hydropenic state (upper curve), and after a large water load (lower curve), assuming that $T^c_{H_2O} = 5$ ml./min. and $C_{H_2O} = 12$ ml./min. It is seen that the range of urinary concentration is wide at low rates of flow, but becomes progressively reduced in osmotic diuresis with high rates of urine flow, and that the osmolarity of the urine becomes almost fixed at a level equal to that of the plasma.

Excretion of salt. The intake of NaCl varies considerably in different individuals and in different races, usually ranging from 60 to 350 m-equiv./day. Ashe & Mosenthal (1937) found that there was a corresponding variation in daily urinary excretion. The normal kidney is very efficient in the conservation of Na, and after a month on a very low Na diet, e.g. the Kempner (1948) rice and fruit diet containing only 7 m-equiv. Na/day, less than 0·5 m-equiv./day of Na is lost in the urine, the balance appearing in the sweat and faeces.

Since the plasma Na averages 140 m-equiv./l., approximately 17 m-equiv. of Na are filtered through the glomeruli each minute. The mean rate of Na excretion is about 0·1 m-equiv./min., and therefore only 0·6% of the filtered Na is excreted, the remainder being reabsorbed by the tubules as described in the section on water excretion. The control of Na excretion is of especial importance in clinical medicine since it is the means by which the extracellular fluid volume is maintained within normal limits. The familiar pathological conditions of dehydration and oedema are examples of failure of homeostatic control. Although Cl excretion usually parallels that of Na, it is the excretion of the latter ion which is primarily important. Administration of $NaHCO_3$ in cases of congestive heart failure increases the oedema, whilst NH_4Cl does not.

Even in health, the control of the extracellular fluid volume is neither so rapid nor so sensitive as control of its osmolality by the antidiuretic hormone. Ingestion of a litre of water leads to a brisk

for the total change in Na excretion. This small variation is well within the limits of experimental error of the methods available, and thus it is impossible to be certain whether any given change in Na excretion is secondary to change in glomerular or tubular function or both. The glomerular filtration rate is more labile in the dog than in man, which probably accounts for the greater ability of the dog to excrete excess Na loads. Variation of tubular function is almost certainly of greater importance in man.

The following are factors known to influence Na excretion in man:

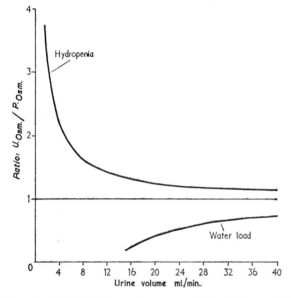

FIG. 10.7. Graphs of equations

$$C_{H_2O} = V \left(I - \frac{U_{osm}}{P_{osm}} \right) \text{ water load.}$$

$$T^c_{H_2O} = V \left(\frac{U_{osm}}{P_{osm}} - I \right) \text{ hydropenia.}$$

$T^c_{H_2O}$ is assumed to be 5 ml./min. and C_{H_2O} 12 ml./min.

diuresis which eliminates the excess fluid within 4 hr., whilst a litre of normal saline results in a slow and incomplete diuresis. The ADH homeostatic mechanism is sensitive to a change of 1% in body fluid tonicity, whilst an alteration of as much as 6% in the volume of extracellular fluid invokes no immediate regularizing response (Black, 1953).

The controlling mechanisms of Na excretion are complex and ill-understood. Variation can occur from changes in glomerular or tubular function, or both.

Na excretion = $U_{Na} . V = P_{Na} . C_{in} - T_{Na}$ where T_{Na} is the amount of Na reabsorbed by the tubules. The normal range of variation of $U_{Na} . V$ is from almost zero to 400 μ-equiv./min. Since the amount of Na filtered at the glomeruli ($P_{Na} . C_{in}$) is normally about 17 m-equiv./min., it follows that if T_{Na} remains constant, variations of as little as 2·5% in the amount of Na filtered can account

(a) *Variation in Na load* (*i.e. change in* $C_{in} . P_{Na}$). Change of excretion in relation to dietary intake has already been discussed. Infusion of hypertonic NaCl causes a brisk Na diuresis by increase of P_{Na}. Infusion of isotonic saline results in a much slower response since there is no change in P_{Na} and increased Na excretion then depends on a gradual slight increase of glomerular filtration rate, and possibly on alterations in tubular function.

(b) *Influence of the associated anion.* Various anions differ considerably in their diffusibility across cells including those of the renal tubules. Chloride is freely diffusible, whereas bicarbonate, sulphate, phosphate, and some foreign anions, e.g. *p*-aminohippurate and ferrocyanide, diffuse either very slowly or not at all. In the proximal tubule sodium is reabsorbed by two mechanisms: direct Na transport which generates an electrochemical gradient of up to 35 m-volts causing secondary passive chloride reabsorption, and ion-exchange of H+ for the Na+ which is present as NaHCO₃.

The presence of non-diffusible anions has the most effect on distal tubular Na+ reabsorption which occurs by three methods:

   (a) Direct Na+ transport generating an electro-chemical gradient of up to 70 m-volts causing secondary passive Cl⁻ reabsorption.

   (b) Exchange of H+ for Na+.

   (c) Exchange of K+ for Na+.

All three of these mechanisms are potentiated by aldosterone, whereas only the last is potentiated by cortisol (Mills, Thomas & Williamson, 1961). The first mechanism can only occur if Na+ within the tubular lumen is accompanied by Cl⁻. If Na+ is chiefly combined with a non-diffusible anion, Na+ reabsorption results in a highly acid urine containing large amounts of K+, and a maximal electro-chemical gradient is generated from the tubular lumen to the interstitial fluid.

(c) *Influence of an osmotic diuresis.* Na excretion is not significantly influenced by water diuresis, but is increased by osmotic diuresis whatever the loading solute. The actual increase is always proportionally less than the rise in water excretion; e.g. Wesson & Anslow (1948) found that, in mannitol diuresis in dogs, whilst 63% of the water of the glomerular filtrate was excreted, there was still only 26% excretion of the filtered Na. Proximal tubular reabsorption of Na is therefore an active process which is independent of water reabsorption. Na salts may themselves be the loading osmotic solute, e.g. Brodsky & Graubarth (1953) have shown that the diuresis produced by mercurials is an example of an osmotic diuresis with NaCl as the excess solute. A particularly striking example is that obtained by inhibition of renal carbonic anhydrase, when NaHCO₃ is the loading osmotic agent. Schwartz & Relman (1954) have given acetazolamide, a potent inhibitor of carbonic anhydrase, to normal dogs at a dosage of 500 mg./kg. body weight, which is about 50 times the usual therapeutic dose in man. An extreme diuresis resulted, with 50 to 60% of the filtered water, 80 to 90% of the filtered bicarbonate, 50 to 67% of the filtered Na and 20 to 40% of the filtered Cl being excreted.

(d) *Adrenal cortical hormones.* Tubular reabsorption of Na is profoundly modified by the action of adrenal cortical hormones. Previously deoxycortone was considered to be the steroid causing maximal increase of Na reabsorption. Aldosterone, which is the active mineralocorticoid actually secreted by the adrenal cortex

(Simpson, Tait & Bush, 1952), has been shown to have a Na-retaining potency of over 30 times that of deoxycortone (Desaulles, Tripod & Schuler, 1953). There is evidence that increased secretion of aldosterone may explain the excess tubular reabsorption of Na in clinical conditions associated with generalized oedema.

Secondary hyperaldosteronism, with increased aldosterone production and urinary excretion, is more important in causing salt retention and clinical oedema in cases of the nephrotic syndrome and in cirrhosis of the liver than in congestive heart failure. Spironolactones, which inhibit the action of aldosterone on the distal tubule cells, are therefore less effective as diuretics in cardiac than in nephrotic oedema or that associated with hepatic cirrhosis.

The effect of cortisone and corticotropin on Na excretion is less dramatic and more variable. These hormones have a comparatively weak effect on the tubules causing increased Na reabsorption. In some cases, however, they increase the glomerular filtration rate and thus raise the tubular load of Na with a tendency to increased Na excretion. This may occur in Addison's disease where the filtration rate is almost always reduced, but is specifically increased by cortisone (Burston & Garrod, 1952). The Na diuresis seen in cases of the nephrotic syndrome successfully treated by ACTH or cortisone is associated with a rise of glomerular filtration rate (Eder, Lauson, Chinard, Greif, Cotzias & Van Slyke, 1954).

Aldosterone secretion rates are chiefly influenced by angiotensin produced by the action of renin, an enzyme formed in the juxta-glomerular apparatus (Tobian, 1960; Cook & Pickering, 1959). Probably the macula densa, a specialized part of the distal convoluting tubule, and adjacent to the juxtaglomerular apparatus, monitors renin production by a "feed-back" mechanism triggered by the degree of hypo-osmolality of the fluid in the distal tubular lumen. It has been suggested that angiotensin produced locally may alter the glomerular filtration rate of the same nephron by action on glomerular arterioles (Guyton, 1963). Such an action would ensure rapid auto-regulation, in addition to the slower effects produced by aldosterone release.

In addition to the renin—angiotensin—aldosterone mechanism which reduces sodium output, there is considerable experimental evidence for a mechanism which increases urinary sodium output if there is an abnormally high body sodium content, and which can counteract the sodium-retaining effects of both reduction of glomerular filtration rate and of increased adrenal steroid production (de Wardener, Mills, Clapham & Hayter, 1961; Levinsky & Lalone, 1963).

POTASSIUM EXCRETION

The relationship of potassium to intracellular fluid is somewhat similar to that of Na to extracellular fluid. Loss of K leads to reduction of intracellular fluid volume, and to a decreased concentration of K therein, with progressive replacement by extracellular Na. Plasma K ranges from 3·5 to 5·5 m-equiv./l., and the daily urinary excretion is approximately 60 m-equiv. The K clearance is therefore about 9 ml./min., and 92% of the filtered load is apparently reabsorbed.

Potassium clearance is normally considerably below that of inulin, indicating net tubular reabsorption, but in certain circumstances the clearance can exceed that of inulin, indicating net tubular secretion.

Potassium excretion in excess of that filtered at the glomeruli, with a C_K/C_{in} ratio greater than unity, has been observed in the normal kidney after infusion of K salts (Berliner, Kennedy & Hilton, 1950), after large doses of a carbonic anhydrase inhibitor in dogs (Schwartz & Relman, 1954) and after hyperventilation combined with the ingestion of K salts in man (Franglen, McGarry & Spencer, 1953). In the diseased human kidney, clearance ratios C_K/C_{in} above unity are frequently observed when the glomerular filtration rate is grossly reduced as in chronic uraemia (Leaf & Camara, 1949; Platt, 1950; Nickel, Lowrance, Leifer & Bradley, 1953), or in the early diuretic phase of acute tubular necrosis (Sirota & Kroop, 1951).

In primary aldosteronism and K-losing tubular syndromes, e.g. Fanconi syndrome and renal tubular acidosis, the K clearance is abnormally high. There is a normal or high urinary K loss despite abnormally low plasma K concentration and gross total body K depletion. A K-losing renal state may be defined as a condition in which the urinary K loss in an adult patient is above 25 m-equiv. K/day despite a plasma K of less than 3·0 m-equiv./l.

Berliner, Kennedy & Orloff (1951) have shown that tubular secretion of K is more strictly a process of cation-exchange for Na in the distal tubular lumen. In this exchange process there is an inverse relationship between the rate of excretion of K and that of hydrogen ion. Thus, when K excretion is increased after ingestion of K salts, the urine becomes temporarily more alkaline. When excretion of hydrogen ion is diminished by hyperventilation, ingestion of $NaHCO_3$, or administration of an inhibitor of carbonic anhydrase, e.g.

acetazolamide, K excretion is increased. Berliner et al. (1951) consider that these facts are best explained by a hypothesis that K and hydrogen ion share a single transport mechanism in cation-exchange for Na, and that there is a competition between the two ions in the exchange process. Rate of K excretion is in fact much more dependent on the total quantity of body K rather than on the plasma concentration.

Micro-puncture evidence has now proven that all filtered K is reabsorbed in the proximal tubules of both the rat and the dog (Bloomer, Rector & Selding, 1963; Malnic & Giebisch, 1963; Watson et al., 1964). This complete reabsorption persists despite K loading with considerable hyperkalaemia. Control of K output is, therefore, entirely due to variation in K secretion in the distal tubules. This is mediated by K and Na exchange in which transfer of K is chiefly due to the distal tubular electro-chemical gradient. It cannot, however, be a purely passive process as K secretion is not directly proportional to the distal tubular K gradient, and is specifically inhibited by mercurial diuretics (Berliner, 1961).

It has been shown that the kidney is extremely efficient in the conservation of Na and Cl in states of salt depletion. By contrast, K is only conserved moderately well in states of K deficiency. Thus, in a study of an individual on a diet containing only 14 m-equiv./day (Blahd & Bassett, 1953), there was still a urinary loss of K in excess of that ingested after two months. After a similar period on an extremely low-salt diet, e.g. the Kempner rice-fruit diet (1948), Na and Cl excretion in the urine is negligible.

Potassium excretion is increased by the action of adreno-cortical steroids. With corticotropin, cortisone and hydrocortisone, loss of K is considerable, and it is wise to administer oral potassium supplements during prolonged treatment with these hormones (Liddle, Bennett & Forsham 1953). The mineralo-corticoids have a much greater sodium-retaining effect (Fourman, Reifenstein, Kepler, Dempsey, Bartter & Albright, 1952). The natural hormone, aldosterone, is more active in this respect than is deoxycortone. Desaulles et al. (1953) claim that aldosterone is 30 times as active as deoxycortone in promoting Na retention, but only five times as active in increasing K excretion.

ACID-BASE BALANCE AND EXCRETION OF HYDROGEN ION

The hydrogen ion concentration of plasma and extracellular fluid is kept almost constant at about pH 7·4 by the buffering action of salts of weak acids, and by the homeostatic action of the lungs and kidneys. The principal extracellular buffers are bicarbonate and plasma proteins. In addition, hydrogen ion readily diffuses into the cells, and therefore the intracellular buffers, including protein and phosphate esters, are of equal or even greater importance in maintaining a fixed pH (Schwartz, Jenson & Relman, 1954). The actual hydrogen ion concentration of plasma is defined by the Henderson-Hasselbalch equation:

$$pH = 6\cdot1 + \log \left[\frac{BHCO_3}{H_2CO_3} \right]$$

The concentration of carbonic acid is kept constant by adjustment of the depth and rate of pulmonary ventilation, which maintains the partial pressure of CO_2 in the alveoli, and therefore in the arterial blood, at a value of about 40 mm. Hg. The kidney maintains the plasma bicarbonate at 25 to 28 m-equiv./l. by appropriate alteration of hydrogen ion or bicarbonate excretion.

Constant adjustment of acid-base balance has to be maintained both by the lungs and the kidneys. In the general processes of metabolism about 20 mol. of volatile acid in the form of CO_2 are formed daily by oxidation of carbohydrate, fat and protein. In addition, from 50 to 100 m-equiv. of H^+ are produced by the metabolism of phospholipids and sulphur-containing amino-acids. The CO_2 is eliminated by the lungs and the H^+ by the kidney. In starvation, and to a much greater extent in diabetic ketosis, additional acid in the form of oxo-acids has to be excreted. In severe diabetic ketosis, despite a 5–10 fold increase of acid excretion, the capacity of the kidney to maintain homeostasis becomes overwhelmed and a fatal acidosis may result.

Excretion of hydrogen ion. In the healthy subject, the pH of urine may vary between the limits of 4·6 and 8·0, but on an average diet is usually about 6·0. This means that the urine/plasma concentration ratio of hydrogen ion may vary from 800 to 0·33. To maintain homeostasis, the kidney has to excrete from 50 to 100 m-equiv. hydrogen ion daily, this being the usual amount produced in normal metabolism. This excretion is represented partly by titratable acid and partly by ammonia. The former averages 10–40 m-equiv./day and the latter 30–60 m-equiv./day. Ammonia excretion is almost always greater than that of titratable acid, the ratio varying from 1·0 to 2·5. Titratable acid within the permissible pH range of urine can only be formed of weak acids. Normally, phosphate accounts for almost the whole of the titratable acidity of the urine, the remainder being accounted for by creatinine and organic acids, especially citric acid. In diabetic ketosis,

increase of titratable acidity far above normal levels results from excretion of excess organic acid, especially β-hydroxybutyric acid. In urine of maximum acidity phosphate occurs entirely as the monobasic salt, which reduces excretion of metallic cations by 0·8 m-equiv. for every m-mol. of phosphate excreted. Similarly, in ketosis, the excretion of β-hydroxybutyric acid, partly as the free acid, results in retention of 0·45 m-equiv. of metallic cations for every m-mol. of organic acid excreted.

The classical experiments of Pitts and his colleagues (Pitts & Alexander, 1945; Pitts, Lotspeich. Schiess & Ayer, 1948) have shown that the mechanism of excretion of hydrogen ion is almost certainly a process of cation exchange, hydrogen ion being exchanged for Na in the tubular lumen. Both in man and in the dog, large quantities of phosphate were infused after an acidosis had been induced by NH_4Cl. The phosphate was excreted entirely as the acid salt with a consequent large increase of the titratable acidity. In one human subject, the rate of excretion of titratable acid was 330 μ-equiv./min., which is three or four times the highest rate recorded in diabetic ketosis. This extremely rapid rate of excretion of hydrogen ion could only be satisfactorily explained by secretion of hydrogen ion with exchange for Na.

The only available source of the hydrogen ion is carbonic acid which is produced by the hydration of CO_2 in the tubular cells:

$$CO_2 + H_2O \rightleftharpoons H_2CO_3 \rightleftharpoons H^+ + HCO_3^-.$$

The actual hydration of CO_2 is slow in reaching equilibrium, but the reaction rate is greatly increased by the action of the enzyme carbonic anhydrase.

Excretion of bicarbonate. Experiments involving the production of a metabolic acidosis or alkalosis in dogs and in human subjects (Pitts & Lotspeich, 1946; Pitts, Ayer & Schiess, 1949) have shown that there is a threshold plasma level for bicarbonate of from 25 to 27 m-equiv./l. At lower levels during metabolic acidosis, all the bicarbonate in the glomerular filtrate is reabsorbed with excretion of an acid urine. At higher levels during metabolic alkalosis, large quantities of bicarbonate are excreted in an alkaline urine. Further observations have, however, shown that the plasma level of bicarbonate is by no means the sole determinant of bicarbonate excretion. During hyperventilation (Stanbury & Thomson, 1952), and following the ingestion of potassium salts (Roberts, Magida & Pitts, 1953) or carbonic anhydrase inhibitors (Berliner et al., 1951), the urine is alkaline despite a reduction of plasma bicarbonate in each instance. Conversely, in respiratory acidosis (Longson & Mills, 1953), and in K depletion (Black & Milne, 1952), the urine is acid with little bicarbonate excretion, despite a raised plasma bicarbonate.

Pitts & Lotspeich (1946) originally considered that there were two distinct processes in bicarbonate reabsorption. They postulated that 80% of the filtered bicarbonate was reabsorbed isohydrically with Na in the proximal tubule, whilst 20% was reabsorbed in the distal tubule by a process of ion-exchange:

$$Na^+ + HCO_3^- + H^+ = Na^+ + H_2CO_3$$
$$H_2CO_3 = CO_2 + H_2O$$

By use of large doses of a potent inhibitor of carbonic anhydrase, acetazolamide, Schwartz & Relman (1954) have shown that all the filtered bicarbonate is reabsorbed by this ion-exchange process both in the proximal and distal tubules. At doses of acetazolamide used therapeutically in man, i.e. 3–12 mg./kg. body weight, less than 20% of the filtered bicarbonate is excreted (Counihan, Evans & Milne, 1954), but with higher doses in the experimental animal up to 50% of filtered bicarbonate may appear in the urine. This suggests that the tubular carbonic anhydrase is only partially inhibited at the lower dosage, and that the whole of bicarbonate reabsorption is dependent on the exchange of hydrogen ion for Na in the tubular lumen.

As previously described, exchange of H^+ for Na in the proximal tubule causes a considerable fall in the pH of the tubular fluid in the rat, but a much smaller reduction in the dog.

It seems, therefore, that bicarbonate excretion is determined by the balance between the amount of bicarbonate filtered at the glomeruli and the hydrogen ion exchanged in the tubules. The bicarbonate filtered is equal to the product of plasma concentration and glomerular filtration rate. The availability of hydrogen ion for exchange is dependent upon the intracellular hydrogen ion concentration and on the rate of production of hydrogen ion from carbonic acid. In hyperventilation and in respiratory acidosis, bicarbonate reabsorption has been shown to be proportional to the partial pressure of CO_2 in plasma and extracellular fluid (Brazeau & Gilman, 1953; Relman, Etsten & Schwartz, 1953; Dorman, Sullivan & Pitts, 1954). The higher the partial pressure of CO_2, the greater is the concentration of substrate for hydration of CO_2 under the influence of renal carbonic anhydrase, and therefore the greater the amount of available hydrogen ion. Potassium depletion causes an intracellular acidosis (Gardner, MacLachlan & Berman, 1952; Cooke, Seger, Cheek, Coville &

Darrow, 1952) with increased intracellular hydrogen ion, and the reverse occurs after ingestion of K salts. Iacobellis, Muntwyler & Griffen (1954) have shown that the amount of carbonic anhydrase in the renal tubular cells is increased in K-depleted rats. More hydrogen ion is therefore available for exchange in depleted states and less after K ingestion.

Ammonia excretion. Urinary ammonia usually accounts for about 2 to 5% of the total urinary nitrogen. Ammonia is similar to hydrogen ion in that the amount excreted is far in excess of the amount filtered. It is doubtful whether arterial blood contains any free ammonium ion (Conway, 1950). Pitts (1936) showed that the urea + ammonia nitrogen excreted in states of metabolic acidosis in dogs gave a clearance which was greater than that of creatinine, whilst the urea clearance maintained its normal relation to the glomerular filtration rate. It was inferred, therefore, that urinary ammonia was derived from some other nitrogenous precursor than urea. Van Slyke, Phillips, Hamilton, Archibald, Futcher & Hiller (1943) found that in dogs glutamine N was removed from the blood by the kidney in amounts far greater than that appearing as glutamine in the urine. They considered that about 60% of urinary ammonia was derived from the amide N of glutamine, and the remainder from the amino N of various amino acids. Lotspeich & Pitts (1947) found that infusion of glycine, alanine, leucine and aspartic acid increased urinary ammonia, but arginine, lysine and glutamic acid did not. There was shown to be a correlation between the ability of the tubular cells to produce ammonia from amino acids and to reabsorb them from the tubular lumen. The ammonia is formed in the tubular cells by means of the enzymes glutaminase and amino-acid oxidase:

$$COOH.CH(NH_2).CH_2.CH_2.CO.NH_2 + H_2O$$
$$\rightleftharpoons COOH.CH(NH_2).CH_2.CH_2.COOH + NH_3$$
$$2R.CH(NH_2).COOH + O_2 \rightleftharpoons 2R.CO.COOH + 2NH_3.$$

Some of the ammonia thus produced is excreted in the urine as ammonium ion, the necessary H^+ being derived from carbonic acid. The remainder passes into the renal vein blood, which always contains an appreciable quantity of ammonia (Nash & Benedict, 1921). This is due to purely physico-chemical factors (Orloff & Berliner, 1955; Milne, Scribner & Crawford, 1958), the NH_3 fraction being freely diffusible and ionized NH_4^+ almost completely undiffusible across the renal tubular cells.

More recent investigations (Pitts, Pilkington &

De Hanz, 1965) by use of ^{15}N-labelled amino-acids in the acidotic dog have shown that a mean of 43 % of urinary ammonia is derived from the amide nitrogen of glutamine and 18 % from the amino-nitrogen. Alanine, glycine and glutamic acid account for a much smaller fraction, about 73 % of urinary ammonia being derived from these four amino acids. Of the remainder, a considerable amount is probably due to plasma ammonia in arterial blood, and is therefore derived from a true form of excretion rather than from a process of intrarenal synthesis.

The amount of ammonia produced by the kidney is clearly limited by the quantity of N available for its synthesis. The average concentration of plasma glutamine is 8·3 mg./100 ml. (Waelsch, 1951) and the average renal plasma flow in the adult is 690 ml./min. Only 5·4 mg. of amide N are therefore available to the kidney each minute. If it can be assumed that 60 % of urinary ammonia is derived from glutamine in man, as has been proved to occur in the dog, it can be calculated that the theoretical maximal ammonia production is 650 μ-equiv./min. Even in severe prolonged diabetic acidosis, ammonia excretion is in fact rarely greater than 250 μ-equiv./min. Titratable acidity is limited by the amount of urinary buffer excreted, which in the case of diabetic acidosis is chiefly β-hydroxybutyric acid, and is almost always less in amount than the ammonia excretion. Excretion of hydrogen ion has therefore a limiting value which is often exceeded in diabetic ketosis, leading to a progressive and eventually fatal metabolic acidosis unless appropriate treatment is given.

The actual amount of ammonia excreted is dependent on at least three separate factors:

(a) *The reaction of the urine.* More ammonia is excreted in an acid than in an alkaline urine. Ammonia diffuses from the tubule cells into the tubular lumen as undissociated and freely diffusible NH_3. It then combines with H^+ to form ionized $NH_4{}^+$, which is either indiffusible or only diffuses across the tubular cells extremely slowly. More $NH_4{}^+$ is therefore "trapped" in highly acid urine where there is free availability of H^+. The logarithm of the rate of ammonia excretion is inversely proportional to the urinary pH (Stanbury & Thomson, 1952). When plasma and urinary pH are dissociated, as after the administration of carbonic anhydrase inhibitors, it is the urinary and not the plasma reaction which determines ammonia excretion (Ferguson, 1951).

(b) *The rate of ammonia formation.* This is dependent on the concentration of the enzymes glutaminase and amino-acid oxidase and of their substrates. Increase of plasma amino acids, as in acute hepatic necrosis or after infusions of casein hydrolysates, will increase the substrate for ammonia production. Increase of renal glutaminase and amino-acid oxidase is, however, of greater practical importance, as their concentration rises during chronic metabolic acidosis when a high ammonia production is essential to maintain homeostasis (Davies & Yudkin, 1952). Sartorius, Calhoon & Pitts (1952) found that the ability to excrete ammonia was greatly reduced in the adrenalectomized animal, and it seems likely that the ability to increase enzyme content in conditions of acidotic stress is dependent on cortical hormones, thus accounting for the poor tolerance of the patient with Addison's disease to metabolic acidosis. Increase of enzyme concentration is a relatively slow process and takes several days to reach a maximum. This explains the continued rise of ammonia excretion during the first few days of an acidosis. The high ammonia excretion persists for some time after restoration of normal acid-base balance, because the enzyme only slowly falls to its original concentration.

(c) *The simultaneous excretion of Na and K.* Increased excretion of ammonia not explained by the previous factors has been observed in both K and Na depletion (Schwartz & Relman, 1953; Schwartz et al., 1954). The increase during K depletion may possibly be explained by the intracellular acidosis which accompanies hypokalaemia. The intracellular rather than the extracellular reaction is more likely to be the main determinant of increased production of cellular enzymes. Seldin, Rector, Carter & Copenhaver (1954) report that hypokalaemic alkalosis produced in rats by injections of adrenal steroids is associated with a three-fold increase of renal glutaminase. Increase of ammonia excretion in acidosis superimposed on states of Na depletion (Schwartz et al., 1954) is a much more doubtful entity. There is an unequivocal relative increase of ammonia excretion as compared to Na and Cl. The absolute amount of ammonia excreted, however, appears to be normal, and therefore the difference in renal response appears to be a retention of Na and Cl rather than increase of ammonia output.

CLINICAL TESTS OF RENAL FUNCTION

Clearance methods involving infusions of inulin and p-aminohippurate are easy to interpret, but too laborious and time-consuming to be used in the routine investigation of cases of renal disease. They are therefore reserved for research and for cases of especial interest when the more precise information provided is of importance in diagnosis or management. Clinical tests of renal function are more difficult to interpret exactly, but are much easier to apply in ordinary routine hospital practice.

The *urea clearance test* is the most popular method of assessment of glomerular function. It is theoretically incorrect to give urea by mouth prior to the test, as is recommended by some authorities, since the clearance is then performed during varying plasma levels, which is always an undesirable feature. Plasma urea should if possible be determined in preference to blood urea, since the latter is influenced by the haematocrit and by haemoglobin concentration. The clearance value obtained is always less than the glomerular filtration rate, and is usually expressed as a percentage of an assumed normal value. As previously described, the formula $\dfrac{U_{urea} \cdot \sqrt{V}}{P_{urea}}$ introduced by Van Slyke and his colleagues (Austin *et al.*, 1921) is used for rates of urine flow below 2 ml./min. with an assumed normal value of 54 ml./min., whilst the usual clearance formula is used for higher flows, with a normal value of 75 ml./min. The former cannot be described as a true clearance and is based on the misconception of an "augmentation limit". It is therefore better to avoid the use of this formula altogether, and endeavour to obtain rates of urine flow of above 2 ml./min. by giving excess fluid before the test. This has the further practical advantage of reducing collection errors, which are the main source of inaccuracy in clearances performed without bladder wash-outs, as used in determination of inulin or PAH clearances. Results should preferably be reduced to standard surface area of 1·73 sq. m., and this is obviously essential in children. McCance & Widdowson (1952) have advanced arguments that in clearance values in infancy a standard based on total body water is preferable to the use of surface area.

The *endogenous creatinine clearance* has been used in many centres as a means of giving a closer estimate of the glomerular filtration rate. This clearance has the advantage that, provided collection errors are avoided, the result is not appreciably affected by the rate of urine flow. The main disadvantage of the method arises from inaccuracies in determination of plasma creatinine. A variable proportion of plasma chromogen is not true creatinine, and since the plasma concentration in the normal is only about 1·3 mg./100 ml. there is considerable experimental error. As previously stated the clearance gives a fortuitous approximation of the glomerular filtration rate if renal function is normal or only slightly depressed. In uraemia the clearance is higher than the simultaneous inulin clearance (Mattar *et al.*, 1952). This clearance has been of value in renal research as it is a useful indication of long-term change in glomerular filtration rate. There is a common tendency to express the results of special clearances, e.g. phosphate, as a ratio of the simultaneous endogenous creatinine clearance. This has the advantage that collection errors are eliminated, but chemical errors are considerable, since the value depends on four separate chemical estimations. The plasma level of the substance being considered should always be given, since the clearance will vary automatically with plasma concentration, as previously described.

In general, in the clinical assessment of cases of renal disease, the urea clearance is more often used than the endogenous creatinine clearance. A very good approximation to the urea clearance can usually be obtained from a simple determination of the plasma urea (Fig. 10.8). On a fixed

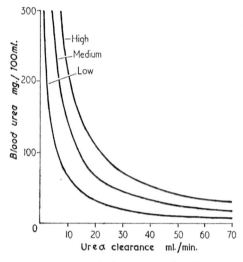

FIG. 10.8. Relationship between the blood urea concentration and the urea clearance during states of high, medium and low protein intake.

protein intake, the product of plasma urea and the urea clearance is a constant. Determination of the clearance is, however, a more sensitive indication in the early stages of renal failure. The blood urea may remain within the accepted normal limits, although the glomerular filtration rate has fallen to 50% of normal value. Roscoe (1952) has shown that in cases in which anaemia is due to renal failure, the level of haemoglobin is inversely proportional to the blood urea. An estimation of the degree of anaemia is probably the most useful single observation in purely clinical assessment of uraemia in renal disease.

The *phenolsulphonphthalein (phenol red) excretion test* gives a value which is dependent on the renal plasma flow. The clearance of phenol red is intermediate between that of inulin and *p*-aminohippurate, being about 394 ml./min. (Smith, Goldring & Chasis, 1938). A considerable quantity is therefore secreted by the tubule cells, and usually as much as 94% of injected dye is eliminated by tubular secretion (Goldring, Clarke & Smith, 1936). In the usual phenol red test, a solution containing 6 mg. of the dye is injected either intravenously or intramuscularly, and samples of urine are obtained 1 and 2 hr. after the injection. Normally, 40 to 60% of the dye is excreted in the first hour and 20 to 25% in the second hour. The test is made more sensitive if more frequent catheter specimens are obtained in the first hour, e.g. three specimens at 20-min. intervals. Goldring & Chasis (1944) give the following values in normal subjects: 1st 20 min., $30.0 \pm 6.1\%$ excretion; 2nd 20 min., $16.9 \pm 5.8\%$ excretion; 3rd 20 min., $9.2 \pm 4.2\%$ excretion; 1st hour, $55.4 \pm 9.2\%$ excretion. The phenol red excretion is early reduced in varieties of renal disease with a high filtration fraction where renal plasma flow is impaired more than glomerular filtration rate, e.g. the heart failure kidney, severe hypertension, and pyelonephritis. In extreme uraemia the concentration of plasma phenol red may be above the critical value at which clearance becomes reduced with rising plasma concentration. In such cases the phenol red test is more closely related to tubular maximal secretory capacity than to renal plasma flow.

The *urinary specific gravity test* (Addis & Shevky, 1922) is the most useful clinical test of distal tubular function. The maximum specific gravity of the urine is measured after at least 16 hr. fluid deprivation, and the minimum specific gravity after the rapid ingestion of 1 l. of fluid. This test is an attempt to measure the power of the tubules to maintain a concentration gradient of solute between urine and plasma. It has been shown that the limiting factor in the concentration test is the maximum osmotic urine/plasma ratio, which is 4·2 in man, and in the dilution test the maximum rate of urine flow during water diuresis of about 16 ml./min. The test would be easier to interpret if depression of freezing point, which gives a measure of the osmolality of plasma and urine, were available in assessing the concentration gradient. This method is unfortunately too difficult for routine practice, and other methods

of estimating total solute concentration have therefore to be used, including determination of urinary specific gravity, refractive index, and surface tension. The last property is unsatisfactory since, whilst some solutes increase surface tension, others, such as proteins and bile salts, reduce it. Specific gravity and refractive index are of equal value, but the former is universally used since simple apparatus is sufficient for its determination, whilst expensive refractometers are essential for the latter. Price, Miller & Hayman (1940) have shown that urinary specific gravity is an additive function of that of the separate solutes. Unfortunately, iso-osmotic solutions of the various solutes are not of equal specific gravity. In general, solutions of smaller molecules including urea and chlorides are of less than average specific gravity, whilst solutions of larger molecules including phosphates and sulphates are of greater than average. The abnormal constituents glucose, protein and diodone are of especial interest. These are all of comparatively large molecular weight, and therefore have a large effect on specific gravity but little effect on osmotic pressure. It is usual to correct the specific gravity if glucose or protein are present. A subtraction of 0·001 should be applied to the observed figure for a glucose concentration of 2·7 g./l. and for a protein concentration of 3·9 g./l. A proportionate correction should be made for other concentrations of these two abnormal constituents. Readings of specific gravity are completely meaningless after intravenous pyelography when the urine may contain large amounts of excreted diodone; a specific gravity as high as 1065 has been recorded under such circumstances (Baumrucker, 1943). The total solute of urine may be roughly determined by multiplying the last two figures of the specific gravity by 2·6 (Long's coefficient, 1903), e.g. if the specific gravity is 1010, the concentration of total solute is approximately 26 g./l.

Addis & Shevky (1922), in their first description of the clinical concentration test, obtained a maximum specific gravity of between 1029 and 1035 in healthy medical students after 24 hr. fluid deprivation. As previously stated maximum concentration is not obtained until the second or third day of complete hydropenia, and many young individuals can attain a specific gravity of slightly over 1040. The usual convention is that the concentrating power is considered to be normal if a value of over 1026 is reached. The concentration power steadily declines over the age of 40. There is an average decrease of 0·0015 for every decade of increasing age (Lewis & Alving, 1938).

In renal failure, urinary concentrating power is usually lost before diluting power. In some cases, the maximum urinary specific gravity is 1010, whilst water excretion is perfectly normal with a minimum specific gravity of 1001. This agrees with the data in Fig. 10.3 showing the relationship between urinary concentrating power and urine flow in osmotic diuresis, and supports Platt's opinion (1952) that the isosthenuria of renal failure is usually due to a relative osmotic diuresis, a normal osmotic load being excreted by a grossly diminished number of nephrons. This cannot be the explanation in cases where there is failure of urinary concentrating power, although the GFR is normal or only slightly depressed, e.g. some cases of pyelonephritis, K deficiency, hypercalcaemic states, and the heterozygous case of sickle cell anaemia. In such cases the disease specifically damages the counter-current multiplier system of the renal medulla, which is responsible for the production of concentrated urine. In adrenal failure, concentrating power is normal or only slightly reduced, whilst the capacity to excrete an excess water load and attain a normal minimum specific gravity is greatly diminished (Slessor, 1951; Garrod & Burston, 1952). The defect is specifically corrected by cortisone.

The renal function tests described measure the composite function of the two kidneys. Measurement of separate renal function is usually of greater importance to the urological surgeon than the physician, since an assessment of separate function is essential before any operation which may possibly involve nephrectomy. *Intravenous pyelography* is the simplest differential functional test. A rough idea of the function of each kidney can be obtained by comparing the density of the radiological pelvic shadows at various times after the injection of diodone. A satisfactory pyelogram is unlikely to be obtained if the blood urea is more than twice the upper limit of normal, with the one exception of the condition of uretero-sigmoidostomy, where satisfactory pyelograms may often be obtained despite gross elevation of the urea level. Cystoscopy with observation of the time and amount of excretion of injected phenol red from each separate ureteric orifice is another useful but relatively insensitive differential functional test. More precise methods necessitate bilateral ureteric catheterization and obtaining separate specimens of urine from each kidney. Injection of phenol red helps in the recognition of leakage of urine around the catheters, since appearance of the dye in the bladder cavity can be observed through the cystoscope. Chasis & Redish (1942) have found that there may be considerable variation in reab-

sorption of water by the tubules on the two sides, causing unequal specific gravity of the two specimens. This may explain the discrepancy of radiological density of the renal pelves seen in many pyelograms of apparently healthy subjects. Divided renal function tests, including separate determination of inulin, urea, creatinine and PAH clearances, and comparison of urinary concentrations of Na^+, Cl^-, and K^+ have proved useful in assessment of unilateral ischaemia in the investigation of severe hypertension (Graber & Shackman, 1956; Connor, Thomas, Haddock & Howard, 1960). Modification of the usual renal function tests for use in patients with ureterosigmoidostomy, in whom timed urine specimens cannot be obtained, are described later.

Measurement of external radioactivity after intravenous injection of ^{131}I-labelled hippuran has now become well established as a divided renal function test. Direct measurement has the advantage of plotting external radioactivity against time. It thus gives a measure of peak activity which is roughly proportional to glomerular filtration rate and renal blood flow, and of the rate of fall-off of activity which may be impaired in surgical renal disease, e.g. hydronephrosis or ureteric obstruction. Organ accumulation of the isotope is not entirely specific for the kidney, and higher values on the right side may be influenced by counts from the liver. The alternative procedure of external scanning gives better information of local abnormalities of the kidney, and of the shape and size of the organ, but has the disadvantage that no data are obtained of the rate of decay of radioactivity with time.

PROTEINURIA

Urine normally contains a small quantity of protein, but not sufficient to give a positive reaction to routine clinical tests. Rigas & Heller (1951) have shown by concentration of urine using an ultrafiltration method that the normal adult excretes 30–50 mg. protein daily, about one-third being albumin and two-thirds globulin. Electrophoretic separation showed an excess of α_1- and α_2-globulin fractions.

There has been considerable controversy with regard to the mechanism of production of pathological proteinuria. One view is that normally the glomerular filtrate is protein-free, and that proteinuria is entirely due to an increase of glomerular permeability. The alternative view is that normally the glomerular filtrate contains small amounts of protein, and that this is almost entirely reabsorbed by the tubule cells. It seems unlikely that the normal glomerulus should be completely impermeable to protein. The micro-puncture experiments of Walker *et al.* (1941) showed that some samples of filtrate contained less than 30 mg. protein/100 ml., but it could not be guaranteed that any specimen was absolutely protein-free.

The protein content of proximal tubular fluid in the dog has been re-assessed by Dirks, Clapp & Berliner (1964), using a more refined immuno-chemical method. In 90% of samples the albumin concentration was less than 3 mg./100 ml., a value considerably less than that of human cerebro-spinal fluid. The volume of glomerular filtrate per day in the normal adult is, however, about 170 l. so that even these extremely small concentrations of protein are more than sufficient to account for the normal daily urinary protein loss.

Proteinuria is readily produced by infusion of concentrated homologous plasma protein both in the dog (Terry, Hawkins, Church & Whipple, 1948) and in man (Waterhouse & Holler, 1948). The rate of protein excretion is directly propor-tional to the plasma level, which suggests a com-bination of glomerular filtration and tubular reabsorption. Similar results have been obtained in the case of haemoglobin. Both in the dog (Lichty, Havill & Whipple, 1932) and in man (Gilligan, Altschule & Katersky, 1941), haemo-globin is not excreted until its plasma concentra-tion exceeds a "threshold" level of about 135 mg./100 ml. Once haemoglobinuria has been induced, it may persist until the plasma concentration has fallen to 30–50 mg./100 ml. The demonstration that certain plasma proteins with the electro-phoretic mobility of α_2-globulins have the pro-perty of binding extra-corpuscular haemoglobin (Polonovski & Jayle, 1938; Jayle, Boussier & Bodin, 1952), has led to a re-examination of the mechanisms involved in haemoglobinuria (Van-derveiker, Gueritte, de Myttenaere & Lambert, 1958; Latham, 1959; Lowenstein, Faulstick, Yiengst & Shock, 1961). No unbound haemo-globin can occur in plasma unless the plasma haptoglobins are fully saturated, and haemoglobin is not excreted in the urine in the absence of free plasma haemoglobin. Myohaemoglobin is of much lower molecular weight, this being only one-quarter that of haemoglobin. Yuile & Clark (1941) found that the greatest myohaemoglobin/creatinine clearance ratio was 0·58 as compared to 0·023 in the case of haemoglobin. Myohaemoglobinuria is not usually associated with any increase in colour of the concomitant plasma, whilst in the case of haemoglobinuria there is obviously a considerable quantity of free plasma haemoglobin present. This distinction is useful in their clinical recog-nition, since otherwise spectrographic or electro-phoretic methods are necessary in the differential diagnosis. In general, glomerular permeability to proteins is roughly inversely proportional to their molecular weight. Further examples will be de-scribed later in relation to protein excretion in the nephrotic syndrome.

Proteinuria has been classified into the three classes of transitory, orthostatic, and continuous (King & Gronbeck, 1952). Transitory proteinuria never indicates permanent renal disease. It may occur in fever, after intense physical exertion, and in some individuals after relatively minor emo-tional stimuli. Continuous proteinuria is always pathological and is usually indicative of glomerulo- or pyelonephritis. In other cases, intravenous pyelography may reveal congenital or acquired renal defects.

Orthostatic proteinuria is caused by the two factors of the erect posture and lumbar lordosis, and is much commoner in adolescence than in any other age group. It can hardly be termed patho-logical, as Bull (1948) was able to induce it in 77% of normal adolescents between the ages of 14 and 16. It is often accompanied by the presence of considerable numbers of hyaline and granular casts. The assumption of the erect lordotic posture is associated with a fall of glomerular filtration rate, renal plasma flow, salt and water excretion and a rise of pressure in the inferior vena cava and the renal veins, King & Baldwin (1954), however, consider that the fall in inulin and PAH clearances is no greater in cases of orthostatic proteinuria than in non-proteinuric controls. Bull considered that the usual cause of the proteinuria was a constriction of the inferior vena cava between the vertebrae and the liver in the erect lordotic posture. The protein usually originates from both kidneys, but occasionally is only found in urine obtained from the left ureter (Sonne, 1921; Beer, 1937). In such cases it has been suggested that the left renal vein is constricted in erect lordosis as it lies anterior to the abdominal aorta.

Wolman (1944) has recorded a maximum urinary protein concentration of 3 g./100 ml. in this condition, but usually the protein loss is much less than in glomerulonephritis. About one-third of cases of continuous proteinuria show an orthostatic element, the rate of protein excretion being greater whilst ambulant than whilst recum-bent (King, 1954). Orthostatic proteinuria is almost invariably a benign anomaly, and disap-pears spontaneously after adolescence. This type of proteinuria may occur in the convalescent stage after an attack of acute glomerulonephritis, when it usually clears after 3–4 months (Derow, 1942). Very occasionally, however, it persists (King, 1954), and in such cases a guarded prognosis should be given, especially if function tests suggest renal damage.

Although Rigas & Heller (1951) claimed the protein in urine in orthostatic proteinuria to be almost entirely albumin, more recent investigators (Rowe & Soothill, 1961) found rather poor selectivity of the glomerulus with excretion of a considerable fraction of higher-molecular-weight globulins. By contrast, the increased protein output produced by violent exercise was more selective, the urinary protein being chiefly albumin.

NEPHRITIS

Primary nephritis can be classified into the two main types of glomerulo- and pyelonephritis. The former as its name suggests, primarily affects the glomeruli, and at the onset is diffuse and fairly uniform throughout both kidneys. At some stage of the disease proteinuria is usually of severe degree, the urine contains large numbers of casts, and in most cases there is an oedematous phase. Some cases of glomerulonephritis show the clini-

scanty, and oedema never occurs unless it is secondary to hypertensive cardiac failure. Pyuria and bacteriuria are present in the acute stage and during exacerbations, but may be completely absent for long periods during the chronic stage.

All varieties of chronic bilateral renal disease may finally pass into a stage of terminal renal failure with uraemia. The biochemical and clinical features may then be very similar, whatever the cause, and an accurate diagnosis is dependent on the patient's history. A summary of the biochemical abnormalities found in these various types of renal disease is given in Table 10.2.

Acute Glomerulonephritis

This condition has been termed "Type I nephritis" by Ellis (1942). It usually occurs from one to three weeks after streptoccocal tonsillitis, and is characterized by the cardinal symptoms and signs of haematuria, oedema, hypertension and oliguria. It is considered to be due to an abnormal immune response, as the serum antistreptolysin titre is generally high (Lyttle, Seegal, Loeb & Jost, 1938), and the serum complement is low (Lange, Graig, Oberman, Slobody, Ogur &

TABLE 10.2

Typical biochemical findings in acute glomerulonephritis, the nephrotic syndrome, chronic pyelonephritis and chronic uraemia

	Acute glomerulo-nephritis	Nephrotic syndrome	Chronic pyelo-nephritis	Chronic uraemia
Blood urea	N or +	N or +	N or +	+ + +
Plasma albumin	N or −	− − −	N or −	N or +
Plasma cholesterol	N or +	+ + +	N	N
Proteinuria	+ +	+ + +	+	+
Casts	+ +	+ + +	+	+
Inulin clearance C_{PAH}	− early	N or −	− late	− − −
PAH clearance C_{In}	N or −	N or −	−	− − −
Filtration fraction	− −	N or −	N or +	Variable
C_{In}/Tm_{PAH}	−	−	+	Variable

(N = normal, + = increased, − = decreased.)

cal features of the nephrotic syndrome with gross oedema and severe proteinuria, but, as will be described later, this syndrome can be produced by many other diseases.

Pyelonephritis primarily affects the pelvis, and the collecting and distal tubules, although the glomeruli may be involved later. It is patchy in distribution, and in some cases may be unilateral. Proteinuria is mild, almost always amounting to less than 2 g. daily, and it may be completely absent in some cases (Raaschou, 1945). Casts are

LoCasto, 1951; Kellett, 1952). Most cases make a complete recovery, but some die in the acute stage, whereas others pass into either a slowly or rapidly progressive chronic stage of the disease. In the latter type, the oedema steadily increases and the patient passes into a nephrotic phase before dying of uraemia, usually within a year of the onset. In the more chronic type, all symptoms and signs except the proteinuria and the presence of casts gradually disappear, but there is a slowly progressive renal failure which finally causes death from hypertension and uraemia, often many years after the onset of the nephritis.

The most characteristic functional abnormality in the acute stage is a reduction of the glomerular filtration rate (Earle, Taggart & Shannon, 1944; Black, Platt, Rowlands & Varley, 1948) which results in a corresponding fall in urea clearance, and an increase of the blood urea. The clearance ratios C_{in}/C_{PAH} and C_{in}/Tm_{PAH} are both reduced, indicating that the glomerular filtration rate is lowered out of proportion to reduction of renal blood flow or failure of tubular function. The ratio C_{PAH}/Tm_{PAH} tends to be increased, suggesting hyperaemia of functioning renal tissue. The extraction ratio of PAH is often reduced (Bradley, 1949), and therefore estimation of renal blood flow from C_{PAH} is unreliable without renal vein catheterization. There is no correlation between the clearance ratios C_{in}/Tm_{PAH} and C_{PAH}/Tm_{PAH} and the increase of blood pressure, which shows that the hypertension is not a compensatory circulatory adjustment to attempt to correct a lowered glomerular filtration rate or renal blood flow.

The reduced glomerular filtration rate leads to a decreased filtration of NaCl and water. Since tubular function is less affected, an abnormally high proportion of water and salt is reabsorbed causing the characteristic oliguria and oedema of the disease. The oliguria tends to increase the passive reabsorption of urea with decrease of the ratio C_{urea}/C_{in}, and further rise of the blood urea. Resolution of the glomerular lesion is associated with increase of filtration rate and a critical diuresis with rise of salt output, and disappearance of the hypertension and oedema. The condition cannot be considered to be cured until the urine is protein-free. A period of orthostatic proteinuria is often seen during convalescence (Derow, 1942).

The Nephrotic Syndrome

The nephrotic syndrome is characterized by massive proteinuria, gross oedema usually associated with serous effusions, hypoalbuminaemia and hypercholesterolaemia. It may be caused by any renal disease which results in severe urinary protein loss, and almost always occurs if there is a long continued proteinuria of more than 10 g./day. The various causes of the syndrome may be classified as follows:

(a) General disease which secondarily affects the kidneys, e.g. diabetes mellitus, amyloidosis, disseminated lupus erythematosus and secondary syphilis.

(b) The toxic action of certain drugs, e.g. troxidone (Barnett, Simons & Wells, 1948),

and inorganic mercurials, e.g. calomel (Wilson, Thomson & Holzel, 1952).

(c) Obstruction of renal veins usually from inferior vena caval thrombosis (Derow, Schlesinger & Savitz, 1939).

(d) The rapidly progressive type of nephritis following acute glomerulonephritis.

(e) The nephrotic syndrome of unknown causation termed "pure lipoid nephrosis" or "Type II nephritis" (Ellis, 1942).

Classification of cases of the nephrotic syndrome has been made more logical and exact by the wide use of percutaneous renal needle biopsy (Iverson & Brun, 1951; Kark & Muehrcke, 1954). Cases of glomerulonephritis causing a nephrotic syndrome may be divided into:

(a) Those showing no glomerular abnormality on light microscopy, but showing abnormalities and obliteration of the podocytes of glomerular epithelial cells on electron microscopy.

(b) Those showing thickening of the glomerular basement membrane (membranous glomerulonephritis).

(c) Those showing proliferative changes in the glomerular tuft or in Bowman's capsule (proliferative glomerulonephritis).

Types (a) and (b) roughly correspond to "Type II nephritis" and type (c) to "Type I nephritis". Cases of the nephrotic syndrome in childhood almost invariably show no glomerular change on light microscopy, whilst adult cases may show changes typical of any of the three histological types. The prognosis both regarding the chances of final cure and satisfactory response to steroid therapy is much better in patients with no glomerular abnormality on light microscopy.

Some authorities exclude cases which are complicated by haematuria, hypertension or retention of non-protein nitrogen. This is an artificial distinction, since cases which originally show none of these complications may develop them as the disease progresses, and it is difficult to draw a rigid boundary between complicated and uncomplicated cases. Although the prognosis is grave in the majority of cases of the nephrotic syndrome, it is much worse in patients showing unequivocal haematuria, hypertension or urea retention. Cases secondary to known toxic agents usually recover when administration of the drug is stopped, and the cases secondary to amyloidosis often resolve if the primary disease responsible for the amyloid deposition can be adequately treated. The nephrotic syndrome in secondary syphilis is now extremely rare, but it is reported that the prognosis was good when effective anti-syphilitic therapy was given (Munk, 1913). A certain percentage of cases of "Type II nephritis" recover completely. The condition is most common in the age group 2–5 years, and at this age the prognosis is better than in older patients, as many as 25% of cases recovering with complete disappearance of the oedema and proteinuria (Barnett, Forman & Lauson, 1952). In all other types of the nephrotic syndrome the prognosis is uniformly poor.

Proteinuria and protein metabolism. The single most important biochemical abnormality in the nephrotic syndrome is the proteinuria. Although the correlation is by no means absolute, the proteinuria, hypoalbuminaemia and severity of the oedema tend to vary in parallel (Squire, 1953). Oedema often occurs at a daily protein excretion of between 5 and 10 g., and is usually present if there is a prolonged protein loss of more than 10 g./day. There has previously been considerable controversy with regard to the causation of the proteinuria. There is no evidence that the excreted protein in the nephrotic syndrome is chemically abnormal. Gitlin & Janeway (1952) have shown that albumin obtained from plasma, urine and serous effusions is immunologically identical. There is now clear proof that increased glomerular permeability is the main cause of the proteinuria, but diminished tubular reabsorption of filtered protein cannot be excluded as a possible additional factor. Chinard, Lauson, Eder, Grief & Hiller (1954), using immunological methods for determination of albumin, have measured the minimal possible concentration of albumin in the glomerular filtrate (min. G_{alb}) in cases of the nephrotic syndrome.

The amount of albumin filtered/min. $= G_{alb} \times$ GFR $= G_{alb} \times C_{In}$, where G_{alb} is the concentration of albumin in the glomerular filtrate. The amount of albumin excreted/min. $= U_{alb} \times V = G_{alb} \times C_{In} -$ albumin reabsorbed by the tubules. The minimal possible value of G_{alb} (min. G_{alb}) is obtained if it is assumed that no albumin is reabsorbed.

Therefore   min. $G_{alb} = \dfrac{U_{alb} \times V}{C_{In}}$

It was found that during the infusion of concentrated serum albumin, the excretion of albumin ($U_{alb} . V$), the albumin clearance $\left(\dfrac{U_{alb} . V}{P_{alb}}\right)$, and the minimum G_{alb} all increased proportionately to the plasma albumin concentration. This relationship is typical of a substance actively reabsorbed by the tubules. The actual value of minimum G_{alb}, obtained when the plasma concentration of albumin was within normal limits, was considerably higher than the maximum

normal level of protein in the glomerular filtrate, i.e. greater than 30 mg./100 ml. This proves that, in the nephrotic syndrome, the albumin of the glomerular filtrate is abnormally high, and therefore the glomeruli must be excessively permeable to macro-molecules of the size of plasma albumin.

Further evidence of the importance of glomerular permeability in the production of the proteinuria is furnished by electrophoretic separation of plasma and urinary proteins (Slater & Kunkel, 1953; Lagrue, Mozziconacci & Vialatte, 1954). Approximate values of the molecular weights of plasma protein fractions are as follows:

Albumin—65,000 (Charlwood, 1952);
α_1-globulin—200,000 (Gutman, 1948), α_2-globulin —300,000 (Squire, 1953);
β-globulin—two main fractions: the metal-carrying globulin, transferrin—90,000 (Surgenor, Koechlin & Strong, 1949), and β-lipoprotein—1,300,000 (Oncley, Gurd & Melin, 1950);
γ-globulin—156,000 (Oncley, Scatchard & Brown, 1947);
fibrinogen—400,000 (Oncley et al., 1947).

The glomerular membrane appears to be permeable to proteins roughly in inverse proportion to the size of their molecules. Most of the protein found in the urine in cases of the nephrotic syndrome is of molecular weight less than 200,000, and includes albumin, α_1-globulin, transferrin and γ-globulin. These results obtained from electrophoretic data have been confirmed by use of the ultracentrifuge. Jahnke & Scholtan (1953) found that fractions above molecular weight 1,000,000 never occurred in urine, the fraction of M.W. 300,000—1,000,000 was found in very small amounts in 50% of cases of proteinuria, and by far the greatest amount was made up of the fraction of M.W. below 70,000. Differential permeability of the glomerular basement membrane to proteins of increasing molecular weight has been found to correlate well with the structural abnormalities of the glomerulus found at percutaneous renal biopsy (Blainey, Brewer, Hardwicke & Soothill, 1960). The urine of cases showing no glomerular abnormalities on light microscopy contains albumin and the smaller molecular weight globulins, especially transferrin, γ-globulin, and complement. Larger molecular weight globulins, e.g. α_2-glycoproteins and some β-lipoprotein, are present in the urine of cases of proliferative or of membranous glomerulonephritis, indicating more severe glomerular leak. Usually the membranous types show more severe glomerular functional abnormality than the cases of proliferative glomerulonephritis. Patients with diabetic glomerulosclerosis, lupus nephritis, and renal amyloidosis often excrete considerable quantities of the larger molecular weight proteins, correlating with the relatively poor prognosis of these types of renal disease. The plasma concentration of all of the smaller M.W. fractions is reduced, but there is some increase of the larger fractions. Albumin and α_1-globulin are greatly decreased, whilst α_2-globulin, β-lipoprotein and fibrinogen are all increased. The plasma γ-globulin concentration may be either increased or decreased according to the aetiology of the condition. It is usually very low in "Type II nephritis" owing to chronic urinary loss, but it is raised in cases secondary to lupus erythematosus or amyloidosis where there is a primary increase of plasma γ-globulin. Urinary γ-globulin is high in such cases, since the amount filtered at the glomeruli is increased.

In "non-selective" proteinuria, the γ-globulin clearance/albumin clearance ratio can be up to 50%, but is below 10% in the "selective" type. "Non-selective" proteinuria occurs in acute glomerulo-nephritis, nephrotic syndrome with a proliferative or membranous type of glomerular damage, renal involvement in collagen diseases, amyloid disease and diabetic glomerulo-sclerosis, whilst the less common "selective" type is found in the nephrotic syndrome with minimal glomerular lesions, i.e. no change on light microscopy and obliteration of the podocytes of epithelial cells on electron microscopy.

Proteins can be separated in relation to molecular size by column chromatography using Sephadex gel G 200. Simultaneous determinations on plasma and urine allow a calculation of U/P concentration ratios over a wide range (Hardwicke, 1965). When the logarithms of the ratios are plotted against the logarithms of the estimated radii of the molecules, an approximately linear relationship is obtained. The slope gives an estimate of the glomerular permeability to macromolecules. Comparable determinations can be made after infusions of polyvinylpyrrolidone (PVP) of graded polymer size. Similar results are obtained, but the glomerulus is somewhat more permeable to the foreign colloid than to protein of apparently similar molecular diameter (Hulme & Hardwick, 1966).

The reduction of plasma albumin greatly decreases the plasma colloid osmotic pressure with a consequent shift of water and smaller diffusible solutes from plasma to the interstitial spaces. Although oedema formation in the nephrotic syndrome is roughly proportional to the hypoalbuminaemia, the final deciding factor is the rate of water and salt excretion by the kidney. Diuresis with relief of oedema can occur without any change in the plasma protein concentration. The increase of large molecular weight globulins is not sufficient to have any appreciable effect on plasma osmotic pressure. Solutions of these proteins are very viscous, and therefore plasma viscosity in the nephrotic syndrome is usually increased despite a reduction of the total concentration of plasma proteins.

Most cases reach a condition of equilibrium, the plasma protein concentration and the daily urinary protein loss often remaining constant over long periods. The utilization of plasma albumin in the normal subject is about 0.25 g./kg. body weight/day (Sterling, 1951), whilst urinary wastage of albumin in severe cases of the syndrome may actually exceed this amount. It follows therefore that the rate of protein synthesis is likely to be increased. It has been shown that the rate of incorporation into plasma albumin of methionine labelled with ^{35}S (Kelley, Ziegler, Doeden & McQuarrie, 1950), and of ^{15}N-labelled glycine (Spector, 1954) is much higher than in normal subjects. An increase of protein intake usually raises the urinary protein loss to some extent. Some protein may be retained and a positive N balance may be achieved with high-protein diets (Squire, 1953).

The notorious susceptibility to infection shown by the nephrotic patient may in part be due to loss of immune proteins in the γ-globulin fraction. Rytand, Rantz & Randall (1950) found that the serum anti-streptolysin titre was low in nephrotics due to loss of this fraction of γ-globulin in the urine. Nephrotic subjects require larger doses of γ-globulin in measles prophylaxis owing to urinary loss of immune body.

Many previously unexplained features regarding thyroid function in the nephrotic syndrome have now been clarified. It has long been known that nephrotic patients are unusually tolerant to oral thyroid extract (Epstein, 1926). The plasma protein-bound iodine is as low in many cases of the nephrotic syndrome as in severe myxoedema (Peters & Man, 1948). Circulating thyroxine is chiefly bound to α_1-globulin (Gordon, Gross, O'Connor & Pitt-Rivers, 1952), and thus there is considerable urinary loss of organic iodine in nephrotic patients. Recant & Riggs (1952), however, have found this to be less than 40 μg. iodine in 24 hr. and considered that the low protein-bound iodine was principally due to a reduction in binding capacity of the plasma proteins for organic iodine. Other tests of thyroid function are consistently normal. The BMR appears low if calculated on an actual body-weight basis, but is normal if allowance is made for excess extracellular fluid (Farr, 1938). It has been shown that the uptake of radioactive iodine by the thyroid glands of nephrotic children is normal or even somewhat increased (Farr, Gamble, Foster & Robertson, 1951). The low protein-bound iodine often returns to normal concentration when clinical improvement occurs after ACTH therapy (Emerson, Roche, Kahn, Moser & Jenkins, 1951).

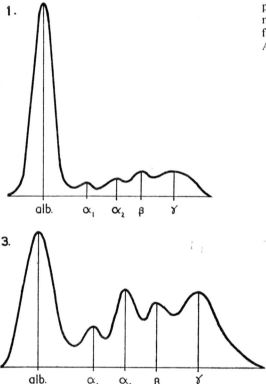

amount which is roughly proportional to the degree of the proteinuria. Hypoferraemia is a relatively common biochemical abnormality, but hypocupraemia is uncommon, being found only in the nephrotic syndrome, in hepatolenticular degeneration, and in the new-born infant (Cartwright et al., 1954). There is no proof to date that the abnormalities of Fe and Cu metabolism are of clinical importance in the nephrotic syndrome. An iron-deficiency type of anaemia is not a clinical feature of the nephrotic syndrome.

Hyperlipaemia in the nephrotic syndrome. The plasma lipids are increased in most cases of the nephrotic syndrome to such an extent that the fasting plasma has an opaque, milky appearance. All the lipid fractions are involved (Page, Kirk &

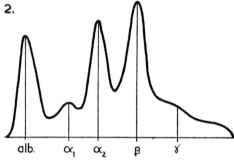

FIG. 10.9. Paper electrophoresis data of serum proteins in (1) a normal subject, (2) a case of "Type II" nephritis, and (3) a case of secondary amyloidosis with the nephrotic syndrome.

The metal-binding proteins of plasma, transferrin and caeruloplasmin, are also excreted in the nephrotic syndrome (Cartwright, Gubler & Wintrobe, 1954). Transferrin is contained in the low molecular-weight fraction of β-globulin (M.W.90,000), and carries the whole of plasma Fe. Caeruloplasmin, although an α_2-globulin, is of comparatively low molecular weight (M.W. 151,000), and accounts for almost all the plasma Cu (Holmberg & Laurell, 1948). The plasma Fe, the plasma Fe-binding capacity and the plasma Cu are all abnormally low in the nephrotic syndrome owing to urinary wastage of these proteins. Urinary Fe and Cu are greatly increased in an

Van Slyke, 1936), but neutral fat is increased most, and cholesterol more than the phospholipid fraction. There is a rough correlation between the degree of hypoalbuminaemia and the hyperlipaemia (Thomas, Rosenblum, Lander & Fisher, 1951). Total lipids may rise as high as 5000 mg./ 100 ml. (average normal 620 mg./100 ml.), and plasma cholesterol to higher than 1000 mg./100 ml., but more often to about two to three times the normal value, ranging from 450 to 600 mg./ 100 ml. The ratio of free to esterified cholesterol is normal, but the cholesterol/phospholipid ratio is raised, averaging 1·28 (mean normal value is 0·95).

These changes in plasma lipids are associated with primary changes in plasma lipoprotein fractions. Using the Cohn fractionation technique (Oncley et al., 1947), the plasma lipoproteins may be separated into α- and β-fractions, α-lipoprotein contains only 35% lipid with a cholesterol/phospholipid ratio of 0·52, whilst β-lipoprotein has both a higher proportion of lipid (75%), and a higher cholesterol/phospholipid ratio (1·28). Gofman, Glazier, Tamplin, Strisower & de Lalla (1954), using the ultracentrifuge, have shown that these fractions are far from uniform, and contain a spectrum of lipoproteins of varying flotation rates. All fractions separated by the ultracentrifuge were found to be increased in amount in nephrotic sera, whilst the increase in many other conditions associated with hyperlipaemia was more selective, some fractions remaining perfectly normal (Gofman et al., 1954).

A fractionation of lipoproteins may be obtained more simply by paper electrophoresis (Fasoli, 1953). α-lipoprotein has the mobility characteristic of α_1-globulin, whilst β-lipoprotein separates in association with the α_2- and β-globulin fractions, the maximum concentration being near the β-globulin peak. Kunkel & Slater (1952), using a zone electrophoresis technique, have shown that the lipoproteins in the nephrotic syndrome are often abnormal, and migrate in a single irregular peak between the α and β peaks of normal serum. Spontaneous diuresis was associated with a return of the pattern to normal. Barr, Russ & Elder (1951) found that, in the nephrotic syndrome, α-lipoprotein is decreased both relatively and absolutely, whilst β-lipoprotein is enormously increased. The changes are qualitatively similar to those seen in atherosclerosis and in diabetes mellitus, but are of much greater degree. Atherosclerosis of great vessels is a common complication of long-standing cases of the nephrotic syudrome.

Intravenous heparin reduces the turbidity of lipaemic serum by increasing the concentration of high-density α-lipoproteins with decrease of the low-density β-lipoproteins, and by causing disappearance of chylomicrons. Nikkila & Grasbeck (1954) found that only a slight reduction of the turbidity of fasting nephrotic serum was produced by this means. Electrophoretic mobility of the lipoproteins was, however, increased to a position between the α_1- and α_2-globulin peaks. Although there was a slight reduction of total lipid, cholesterol and phospholipid after each injection, no permanent biochemical or clinical improvement was produced by prolonged heparin therapy. Gordon, Boyle, Brown, Cherkes & Anfinsen

(1953) have shown that plasma albumin potentiates the action of heparin in reducing the turbidity of lipaemic sera, and therefore the comparatively small effect in nephrotic sera may be due to the hypoalbuminaemia.

The mechanism of production of the hyperlipaemia is still not fully elucidated. Observations in patients usually have to be carried out during a steady state of hyperlipaemia. The actual development of the hyperlipaemia has been studied in experimental nephrosis in rats. This condition produced by the injection of anti-rat-kidney serum closely resembles the nephrotic syndrome in man (Heymann & Lund, 1951). Plasma lipids are increased within 2–4 hr, and cholesterol within 6–8 hr. after the injection (Heymann & Hackel, 1952). These changes slightly precede the development of hypoproteinaemia. Friedman, Roseman & Byers (1954) found that the hypercholesterolaemia develops despite the animals being on a completely lipid-free diet. It was concluded that the increase is due to a diminished rate of removal of endogenous lipid by the liver. In patients with the nephrotic syndrome, Stanley & Thannhauser (1949) found that fat labelled with ^{131}I was utilized more slowly than in normal controls. London, Sabella & Yamasaki (1951), using cholesterol labelled with deuterium, found that the half-life and turn-over time of cholesterol was prolonged proportionately to the plasma cholesterol concentration, indicating that the absolute rates of addition and removal of the lipid were normal. The rate of removal would, however, normally be raised at increased plasma concentration. More recent investigations however (Baxter, Goodman & Allen, 1961) suggest that the hyperlipaemia is secondary to fall of plasma albumin. These investigators showed that repeated infusions of plasma albumin, in cases of the nephrotic syndrome, cause an increase of plasma and urinary albumin with loss of oedema and a fall of plasma cholesterol, phospholipids and of the cholesterol/phospholipid ratio. In addition, there was a simultaneous fall of plasma triglyceride and of lipoproteins, together with diminution of plasma lactescence. The authors point out that hyperlipaemia is not a feature of other varieties of hypo-albuminaemia, e.g. cirrhosis of the liver, malnutrition and kwashiorkor or protein-losing enteropathy. In these conditions, however, there are secondary nutritional abnormalities which are not present in uncomplicated cases of the nephrotic syndrome.

Oedema formation in the nephrotic syndrome. Oedema formation is roughly correlated with the reduction of the colloid osmotic pressure of the plasma, but it can only be produced and maintained by the failure of the kidney to excrete an appropriate amount of water and salt to conserve a normal extracellular volume. In some cases of the nephrotic syndrome, especially if secondary to acute glomerulonephritis, the glomerular filtration rate is decreased. In many cases of "Type II nephritis" it is normal or even above normal. In all cases, however, there is evidence of "glomerular tubular imbalance", with a reduction of the clearance ratio, C_{in}/Tm_{PAH} (Bruck, Rapoport & Rubin, 1954). This is shown clinically by excess reabsorption of Na and Cl with the excretion of an almost salt-free urine. The abnormality of Na reabsorption is especially well-demonstrated by the infusion of a Na salt of a non-reabsorbable anion such as p-aminohippurate or thiosulphate (Metcoff, Nakasone & Rance, 1954). In a normal subject this is quantitatively excreted in the urine. In a nephrotic patient, a considerable proportion of the infused Na is retained, the anion being excreted partly as the Na and partly as the K salt. During stages of spontaneous or induced remission, the proportion of Na excreted increases to normal levels.

The excess Na reabsorption is usually due to an increased secretion of mineralo-corticoid by the adrenal cortex. Luetscher & Johnson (1954) have demonstrated the presence of excess Na-retaining steroid in the urine of cases of the nephrotic syndrome. More recently Luetscher, Neher & Wettstein (1954) have isolated pure crystalline aldosterone from nephrotic urine. Increased secretion of aldosterone is more important in the genesis of nephrotic oedema than in the oedema of congestive heart failure. One of the most potent stimuli to increased secretion of aldosterone is diminution in the circulating blood volume. This is often reduced in the nephrotic syndrome secondary to reduction of plasma colloid osmotic pressure.

Treatment of the nephrotic syndrome. Treatment consists chiefly in the adoption of symptomatic measures to reduce oedema and avoid infection. In patients in whom the glomerular filtration rate is normal or only moderately depressed, a low-salt and high-protein diet remains the essential basis of therapy. There is still controversy with regard to the use of mercurial diuretics. The efficacy of these drugs in the nephrotic syndrome is far below that in congestive heart failure, and in general it would seem desirable to avoid the use of a nephrotoxic drug in a primary renal disease. There is no doubt that *intravenous* mercurials are strongly contra-indicated in the nephrotic syndrome. The toxicity of intravenous mer-

curials is inversely proportional to the plasma albumin concentration, and the incidence of sudden death after this method of administration is much higher in the nephrotic syndrome than in congestive heart failure (Vogl, 1953). Salt restriction can be reinforced by the use of cation-exchange resins by mouth (Spencer & Lloyd-Thomas, 1954). These should be given charged with 75% NH_4 ion and 25% K ion, and should be used only if the glomerular filtration rate is not greatly reduced. In severe renal failure the kidney is incapable of forming ammonia or of secreting an acid urine and a severe acidosis may be produced by use of ammonium-charged cation-exchange resins.

The use of "plasma-expanders", and in particular salt-free concentrated plasma albumin or dextran, has usually proved disappointing. These agents increase the plasma volume and secondarily raise the glomerular filtration rate (Eder *et al.*, 1954; James, Gordillo & Metcoff, 1954). This is almost invariably associated with a diuresis and increased salt excretion, but unfortunately the beneficial effect is usually short-lived. Concentrated plasma albumin causes an increase of proteinuria due to a rise both of the plasma albumin concentration and of the glomerular filtration rate.

Artificial infection with malaria or measles has proved to be of benefit in many cases, but the rationale is not fully understood. The influence of the fever on renal haemodynamics may be of importance in the production of a diuresis and consequent clinical improvement. Bradley, Chasis Goldring & Smith (1945) have shown that an uncomplicated pyrexia causes an increase of renal blood flow with a reduced filtration fraction, but little change in the glomerular filtration rate. This was considered to indicate reduction of vasomotor tone in both the afferent and efferent glomerular arterioles. In general, the use of corticotropin or cortisone is a more reliable and less troublesome method of treatment than induced infections.

A single course of corticotropin results in diuresis in about 80% of nephrotic children (Rapoport, McCrory, Barbero, Barnett, Forman & McNamara, 1951). The diuresis may occur during administration of the hormone, but more commonly begins immediately the course of treatment is stopped. The improvement sometimes proves to be temporary and the oedema rapidly re-accumulates, although in other more favourable cases a sustained remission occurs. This may lead to complete recovery with disappearance of the proteinuria, but some patients show a late exacerbation with recurrence of the oedema. Diuresis due to corticotropin or cortisone is invariably associated with increase of the glomerular filtration rate (Lauson, Forman, McNamara, Mattar & Barnett, 1954). A sustained improvement is accompanied by reduction of glomerular permeability and proteinuria, and of T-1824 (Evans blue) clearance (Lauson et al., 1954). This blue dye when injected intravenously becomes attached to plasma albumin, and Chinard, Lauson & Eder (1952) have shown that C_{T-1824} is almost identical with the true albumin clearance. The latter can be accurately determined only by difficult immunological procedures. The ratio C_{T-1824}/C_{in} decreased more than 10-fold in 8 out of 10 nephrotic children after treatment with corticotropin. There was a relatively much greater change in C_{T-1824} than in C_{in}. Other biochemical evidence of improvement is furnished by a fall of plasma lipids (Barnett, McNamara, McCrory, Forman, Rapoport, Michie & Barbero, 1950), and a return to normal of the electrolyte excretory pattern after infusion of sodium p-aminohippurate (Metcoff et al., 1954). With greater experience of the use of steroids in the nephrotic syndrome longer courses of therapy are now recommended. Steroid therapy in favourable cases reduces the daily protein loss by diminishing glomerular permeability to plasma proteins. This allows albumin synthesis to exceed the loss of albumin in the urine, with steady improvement in the plasma protein electrophoretic pattern. Steroids should at least be continued until the electrophoretic pattern is virtually normal, and preferably until there is no proteinuria. Cases with no glomerular abnormalities on light microscopy respond more satisfactorily to steroids than those with more severe glomerular pathology. This explains the better response in nephrotic children in whom the disease is almost invariably of the milder type.

A recent large controlled trial has proved that steroids are the treatment of choice for the nephrotic syndrome with minimal glomerular lesions. In other types, complications and mortality due to the secondary effects of steroid therapy were at least as important as the rather dubious effects of the medication on the glomerular lesion.

Complications may arise during corticotropin or cortisone therapy (Metcoff, Rance, Kelsey, Nakasone & Janeway, 1952). The nephrotic subject is extremely liable to infection, pneumococcal peritonitis being an especially frequent complication. This tendency is increased by corticotropin or cortisone, and evidence of infection may be masked. Treatment should always be combined with the use of prophylactic courses of antibiotics, especially penicillin. Potassium depletion may be produced by corticotropin or cortisone therapy in any condition, but is more liable to develop in the treatment of the nephrotic syndrome, where there is an abnormal tendency to retain Na and excrete K in its place. Potassium supplements should always be given as a routine and should be controlled by frequent determinations of the serum K level. Cardiac failure and the production or exacerbation of hypertension are not infrequent complications, and are indications that the treatment should be immediately discontinued.

There is no doubt that hormonal treatment and the efficient control of intercurrent infections by antibiotics has greatly improved the prognosis of the nephrotic syndrome. Luetscher, Deming, Johnson & Piel (1953) report complete recovery in 43% of a series of 30 patients. Of the remainder, 10% were symptomless and oedema-free, 30% were still oedematous after one year, and 17% had died.

Pyelonephritis

Acute pyelonephritis is characterized by lumbar pain, frequency of micturition, dysuria, pyrexia, pyuria and bacteriuria. Chronic pyelonephritis may follow an incompletely treated acute attack, but in some cases no history of an acute stage is obtainable. Bacteriuria and pyuria are present during acute exacerbations, but the urine may be almost normal in the remissions of the disease. The urine may be completely protein-free in some cases (Raaschou, 1945). Many different varieties of renal disease predispose to the development of pyelonephritis. Obstructive lesions of the ureters and renal pelvis, e.g. renal calculi, stricture and the ureteric dilatation and stasis of late pregnancy, have long been recognized as increasing the incidence of haematogenous urinary infection. Ascending infection may occur from abnormalities at the uretero-vesical junction causing urinary reflux during micturition (Edwards, 1960). In addition, distal tubular abnormalities causing lesions of the renal medulla and collecting tubules greatly increase the incidence of haematogenous infection, e.g. the lesions of chronic potassium depletion (Muehrcke, 1960), nephrocalcinosis, the nephropathy of gout, and the nephropathy due to prolonged ingestion of phenacetin (Zollinger, 1955).

There is clear pathological evidence that tubular damage precedes involvement of the glomeruli (Staemmler & Dopheide, 1930). It is to be expected, therefore, that failure of tubular function should precede any fall in inulin clearance and increase of the blood urea. Urinary concentrating power may be lost in the early stages, producing complete isosthenuria at a time when the blood urea is within normal limits (Raaschou, 1943). The ratio of inulin clearance to maximal tubular secretory capacity (C_{in}/Tm_{PAH}) is always increased (Raaschou, 1945). The functional derangement is the reverse of that of the nephrotic syndrome, the predominant tubular failure tending to cause a salt-losing state. Oedema is never seen unless hypertensive cardiac failure complicates the clinical picture.

No satisfactory explanation has been given to account for the variable functional and clinical effects of chronic pyelonephritis. In some cases recurrent relapsing urinary infection is the main disability, whilst others develop severe hypertension before there is any obvious renal functional impairment. This is of great practical importance if the disease is unilateral, since nephrectomy may reduce the blood pressure to normal levels (Pickering & Heptinstall, 1953). In other cases the disease is not recognized until the patient is already uraemic, either with or without a complicating hypertension. Some cases develop striking electrolyte abnormalities which will be discussed in a later section.

URAEMIA

The pathological state of uraemia includes any condition in which the blood urea is raised above the upper limit of normal. Levels of blood urea between 40 and 50 mg./100 ml. sometimes occur in healthy subjects on a high-protein diet, but values above 50 mg./100 ml. are always pathological. Acute uraemia is associated with anuria or severe oliguria, whilst chronic uraemia is more commonly accompanied by polyuria, although there may be a terminal oliguric phase.

Chronic Uraemia

Chronic uraemia can be caused by almost any chronic bilateral renal disease. The terminal clinical state may be very similar in cases of widely different primary cause, and accurate diagnosis is then entirely dependent on a good history of the symptoms during the earlier stages of the disease. Cases differ clinically especially with regard to associated oedema or hypertension. Some cases of the nephrotic syndrome die of uraemia without ever losing their oedema, whilst others develop a salt-losing state with complete loss of oedema before death occurs. Chronic uraemia without hypertension is often an insidious and prolonged syndrome, the condition persisting for many years. The main clinical evidence of the disease is a chronic normochromic and refractory anaemia, and polyuria with isosthenuria. Pericarditis and uraemic convulsions may occur in the later terminal stages. Uraemia associated with hypertension is a much more acute and rapidly progressive condition. The clinical picture is often dominated by symptoms and signs primarily due to the increased blood pressure, such as failure of vision from hypertensive retinopathy, left ventricular failure, or evidence of cerebro-vascular disease.

Platt (1952) has described how efficiently the kidney maintains a biochemical state compatible with continued existence despite extreme damage from chronic renal disease. All renal clearances are grossly lowered, and the urinary concentrating power and ability to secrete an acid urine are reduced or lost. In order to preserve homeostasis, the kidneys in uraemia have to maintain a solute excretion equal to that in health despite the disadvantage of a greatly reduced glomerular filtration rate.

The amount of a substance x excreted $= U_x . V = P_x . C_{in} - T_x$, where T_x is the amount reabsorbed by the tubules. If the glomerular filtration rate (C_{in}) is reduced, the amount excreted ($U_x . V$) can be maintained either by increase of the plasma concentration of x (P_x) or by reduction of the amount reabsorbed (T_x). Increase of P_x alters the chemical composition of plasma and extracellular fluid, and is therefore only compatible with life if the substance x is relatively innocuous. The amount of solute reabsorbed by the tubules (T_x) is automatically reduced in chronic uraemia owing to destruction of nephrons, but it is decreased proportionately more than the glomerular filtration rate, resulting in a greater fraction of the filtered load of solute being excreted. This reduction of reabsorption of the filtered solute load is typical of osmotic diuresis, since isosmotic proximal tubular solute reabsorption is impeded by the effect of excess solute. Platt (1952) considers that in uraemia there is a constant state of osmotic diuresis, urea and NaCl being the main loading solutes. The total osmotic load is normal, but, owing to the gross reduction in functioning nephrons, the amount of solute handled by each single nephron is much greater in the uraemic than in the normal kidney.

In Table 10.3 the excretion of various solutes and of water is compared in a normal subject with glomerular filtration rate of 120 ml./min. and in a uraemic patient in whom filtration rate has been reduced by bilateral renal disease to the very low figure of 6 ml./min. The assumption is made that both subjects are taking a similar diet and that

TABLE 10.3

Comparison of the excretion of water and various solutes in the normal individual and in a patient in whom bilateral renal disease has reduced the glomerular filtration rate to 6 ml./min.

Substance x	P_x	C_x ml./min.	Amount filtered/24 hr.	Amount excreted/24 hr.	% reabsorbed or secreted
Urea					
(normal)	24 mg./100 ml.	72·0	41·5 g.	25 g.	40% reab.
(uraemia)	360 mg./100 ml.	4·8	31·0 g.	25 g.	20% reab.
Creatinine					
(normal)	1·0 mg./100 ml.	144·0	1·72 g.	2·06 g.	20% secr.
(uraemia)	20·0 mg./100 ml.	7·2	1·72 g.	2·06 g.	20% secr.
Sulphate					
(normal)	0·5 m-mol./l.	30·0	86 m-mol.	21·5 m-mol.	75% reab.
(uraemia)	3·3 m-mol./l.	4·5	28·6 m-mol.	21·5 m-mol.	25% reab.
Phosphate					
(normal)	1·0 m-mol./l.	18·0	172 m-mol.	30 m-mol.	85% reab.
(uraemia)	4·6 m-mol./l.	4·5	40 m-mol.	30 m-mol.	25% reab.
Potassium					
(normal)	4·5 m-equiv./l.	9·2	780 m-equiv.	60 m-equiv.	92% reab.
(uraemia)	4·5 m-equiv./l.	9·2	39 m-equiv.	60 m-equiv.	54% secr.
Sodium					
(normal)	140 m-equiv./l.	0·75	24,000 m-equiv.	150 m-equiv.	99·4% reab.
(uraemia)	140 m-equiv./l.	0·75	1200 m-equiv.	150 m-equiv.	87·5% reab.
Chloride					
(normal)	100 m-equiv./l.	1·04	17,300 m-equiv.	150 m-equiv.	99·1% reab.
(uraemia)	100 m-equiv./l.	1·04	865 m-equiv.	150 m-equiv.	82·7% reab.
Water					
(normal)	—	—	172,000 ml.	1500 ml.	99·1% reab.
(uraemia)	—	—	8600 ml.	2500 ml.	71% reab.

both are in chemical equilibrium, and therefore each kidney is excreting the same amount of solute. The details of the physiological adaptation vary according to the substance concerned, and it is convenient to classify these into four separate groups:

(a) *Creatinine and urea.* The tubular secretion of creatinine persists in uraemia, and its clearance therefore remains higher than that of inulin (Mattar *et al.*, 1952). The passive tubular reabsorption of urea is slightly diminished in uraemia owing to the increased average rate of urine flow, and the clearance value approximates more closely to the glomerular filtration rate (Chasis & Smith, 1938). Since the variation in the amount secreted or reabsorbed cannot be greatly varied in the case of either substance, the amount excreted can be maintained only by a great increase of the plasma level (P_x). Fortunately this is compatible with continued existence since both substances are non-toxic. Values of blood urea much higher than the one given in Table 10.3 are, however, usually obtained only in the last few days of chronic uraemia, and are therefore of extremely grave prognostic import. The cause of death is not directly related to the height of the blood urea, but

this serves as an indication that renal function has fallen to levels where electrolyte homeostasis can no longer be maintained.

The increase of plasma non-protein N in uraemia is almost entirely due to rise of urea. In the normal subject urea N accounts for only about 55% of the total plasma non-protein N, but this rises to over 80% in renal failure. Peters & Van Slyke (1946) have shown that the relationship between plasma non-protein N and urea N in uraemia agrees closely with the regression line of the formula: plasma N.P.N. = 10 + 1·07 × plasma urea N, where both values are expressed in mg./100 ml.

(b) *Sulphate and phosphate.* Excess retention of the two fixed anions sulphate and phosphate is one of the most important biochemical abnormalities of uraemia. Diminution of tubular reabsorption (T_x) is insufficient to maintain adequate excretion, and the plasma levels inevitably rise. The sum of the increased concentration of the two anions expressed in m-equiv./l. is almost exactly equal to the fall in plasma bicarbonate in the same units (Briggs, 1947). In the case shown in Table 10.3, plasma concentration has increased to about five times the normal value. The increase of sulphate is 2·8 m-mol./l. (equal to 5·6 m-equiv./l.), and increase of phosphate is 3·6 m-mol./l. (equal to 6·5 m-equiv./l.). The increase of fixed anion would therefore be expected to be associated with a fall of plasma bicarbonate of approximately 12 m-equiv./l., a reduction to almost half the normal value. Severe symptoms of acidosis are not usually seen until the plasma bicarbonate is less than half the normal level, but as the acidosis becomes more severe, obvious hyperpnoea develops and the patient passes into uraemic coma. Death can only be delayed by a reduction of the dietary intake of phosphate and sulphate. This is equivalent to a low-protein diet. Such diets have been shown to prolong life in experimental uraemic states (Addis, 1948).

Administration of sulphate or phosphate should clearly be avoided in uraemia. The use of intra-venous Na_2SO_4 as a diuretic agent is anathema to most nephrologists, but is still unfortunately used in some centres. Saline aperients containing these anions are undesirable, as considerable absorption from the gut occurs. Magnesium sulphate is particularly contra-indicated, since both the anion and cation are toxic and are eliminated with great difficulty in renal failure. Hirschfelder (1934) found very high plasma levels of Mg after purgative doses of Epsom salts in uraemic subjects.

(c) *Potassium*. Increase of the K concentration of plasma and extracellular fluid above 10 m-equiv./l. usually results in death from cardiac arrest in diastole. Fortunately, plasma K is not usually increased in chronic uraemia provided the urine volume is well maintained. Excretion suffi-cient to maintain a normal plasma level is possible only by means of the ion-exchange process already described. The amount of K excreted is consistently above the quantity in the glomerular filtrate in all cases of severe uraemia (Leaf & Camara, 1949; Platt, 1952; Nickel *et al.*, 1953). Homeostasis is preserved provided the urine flow is adequate, but if oliguria supervenes the plasma K rises and the patient may die of cardiac arrest. Potassium salts should be administered with great caution in chronic uraemia, and only if there is unequivocal evidence of K depletion.

(d) *Sodium chloride and water*. In the normal subject, over 99% of the amount of Na, Cl, and water is reabsorbed by the tubules. Excretion in uraemia can therefore be maintained without rise in plasma levels and consequent change of osmo-tic equilibrium, simply by reduction of the pro-portion reabsorbed. This may be reduced to 80% or even less (Platt, 1952; Nickel *et al.*, 1953). Since concentrating power is lost, a greater urinary

volume than in health is required to excrete the same quantity of solute. The average daily volume in uraemic adults varies from 2 to 3 l. This polyuria causes increased thirst and a correspond-ing increase of fluid intake. Uraemic patients can-not tolerate fluid deprivation except for very limited periods, and easily develop water intoxi-cation if given excess fluid. Vomiting usually prevents dangerous excess fluid absorption after ingestion of large quantities of water by mouth, but death can easily be produced by injudicious parenteral infusions or retention enemata. Salt depletion rather than excess retention is a common and dangerous complication of uraemia. The normal kidney is extremely efficient in conserva-tion of salt in states of Na depletion. In contrast, urinary excretion of NaCl persists during uraemia despite salt depletion from inadequate dietary intake or excess loss in gastro-intestinal secretions or in the sweat. This is of especial importance, since a state of acute renal circulatory failure due to salt depletion is added to the existing chronic uraemia, with further reduction of the inadequate glomerular filtration rate (Nickel *et al.*, 1953). The final fatal termination in uraemic patients is often due to acute salt deficiency from an attack of vomiting or diarrhoea. The dietary salt intake should be liberal unless severe oedema complicates the clinical picture.

(e) *Other substances less easily classified.* Striking temporary clinical improvement in chronic uraemia occurs after haemodialysis by the artificial kidney, in many cases without any signi-ficant change in electrolyte balance. This suggests that a diffusible or dialysable toxic substance (or substances) has been removed from the body. Although Grollman & Grollman (1959) have suggested that this may be urea itself, it is prob-able that other toxic substances are also of importance in the causation of clinical uraemia. Substances removed by dialysis include phenols and their sulphate conjugates, phenolic acids and their conjugates, indican, indolic acids and conjugates, amines, and guanido-derivatives. There is considerable current research on the more detailed biochemical changes in uraemia and the effect of haemodialysis, but it is too early to be certain of the importance of these metabolites in the clinical syndrome of uraemia.

Biochemical aspects of renal transplantation. Uraemia considerably reduces the immunological response against foreign tissue, and thus prolongs homograft survival even without use of immuno-suppressive drugs and steroids (Hume, Merrill, Miller & Thom, 1955). This is shown by the slowness of rejection of skin homografts in the uraemic patient (Dammin, Couch & Murray, 1957), by the decreased incidence of delayed cutaneous hypersensitivity (Kirkpatrick, Wilson & Talmage, 1964) and a reduced capacity to synthesize immune γ-globulins (Wilson, Kirkpatrick & Talmage, 1964).

Diagnosis of rejection of a homografted kidney is best made by a combination of clinical and biochemical evidence. There is usually pyrexia, although this may not be present in patients receiving large doses of prednisone. The transplanted organ becomes tender, and there may be hypertension or increase of an already high blood pressure. Oliguria or even anuria, proteinuria, the presence of lymphocytes and casts in the urinary deposit, a rising blood urea and creatinine with a corresponding fall in their clearances are later and ominous signs of overt rejection. Urinary sodium often falls causing sodium retention, oedema formation and gain in weight. Serum and urinary lactic dehydrogenase may rise (Prout, Macalalag & Hume, 1964) and there is often a fall in serum complement. There is also an early fall in p-aminohippurate or ^{131}I-hippuran clearances indicating a corresponding reduction of renal blood flow, a sign which correlates well with the histological abnormalities of the rejected transplant (Kountz, Lauf & Cohn, 1965).

The present status of transplantation results (Hume, Lee, Williams, White, Ferre, Wolf, Prout, Slapak, O'Brien, Kilpatrick, Kauffman & Cleveland, 1966) is that about 40% of cadaver transplants and 65% of those from a living donor should be functioning three years after the operation. Renal function in successful cases is good, the inulin clearance sometimes being higher than the remaining kidney of the donor indicating good functional hypertrophy in the recipient. Slight proteinuria is usual, but heavy protein loss usually indicates either a rejection episode or the development of membranous glomerulonephritis in the transplanted kidney.

Autonomous hyperparathyroidism requiring parathyroidectomy has been reported after renal transplantation (McPhaul, McIntosh, Hammond & Park, 1964), presumably due to continuation of the secondary hyperparathyroidism from the original uraemia. Diabetes mellitus due to the large doses of prednisone required for immunological suppression is not uncommon. Most clinicians with experience both of continued intermittent dialysis and renal transplantation consider that the latter method, if successful, results in a patient in better health and with much less inconvenience in relation to treatment of the problems. Unfortunately, the current rate of success in cadaver transplantation is not equivalent to the survival of cases treated by dialysis. The two methods, however, are not mutually incompatible, and the modern clinic should be fully equipped for both methods with facilities for transfer of patients from one method to the other.

Acute Renal Failure

Acute renal failure is a term applied to any condition in which uraemia is directly due to a grossly reduced rate of delivery of urine from the ureters to the bladder. This definition includes cases caused by renal disease and bilateral ureteral obstruction, but excludes cases in which oliguria and renal failure are secondary to urethral obstruction, e.g. prostatic hypertrophy or urethral stricture. This distinction is clinically convenient, since the latter type of case is associated with distension of the bladder and difficulty of micturition. Some patients with acute renal failure have complete anuria, but more commonly there is severe oliguria, small quantities of urine being secreted each day.

Acute renal failure due to bilateral ureteric obstruction is usually termed surgical anuria, a name which emphasizes the fact that the treatment is essentially surgical with a view to relief of the obstruction. In this type of case there is more commonly an absolute anuria, no urine whatsoever entering the bladder. The commonest cause is calculous anuria due to simultaneous blockage of both ureters, or of one ureter when the contralateral kidney is either functionless or absent. Anuria following the administration of sulphonamides may occasionally be due to ureteral blockage from crystalluria, but more commonly arises from direct renal damage. Carcinoma sometimes involves both ureters, the most common primary site being the uterine cervix. Cystoscopy and ureteric catheterization should be performed if there is any possibility of surgical anuria, since delay in relieving the ureteric obstruction may gravely prejudice recovery.

The cases not due to surgical anuria but secondary to renal damage may be classified as follows:

(1) *Cases due to renal ischaemia of varying degrees of severity.*

(*a*) *Acute renal circulatory failure.* This term is applied to cases without any structural parenchymatous renal damage. The group may be distinguished clinically by the fact that adequate renal function is immediately restored when the cause of the renal ischaemia is removed. The less satisfactory term "pre-renal azotaemia" has been used in the past to describe this type of case.

(*b*) *Acute tubular necrosis.* There is definite

structural renal damage, the lesion consisting of a patchy necrosis of short segments of both proximal and distal tubules. The necrosis involves the whole thickness of the tubule including the basement membrane (Oliver, MacDowell & Tracy, 1951). Renal failure persists for a considerable period after the cause of the ischaemia has been removed, but, if death from uraemia is averted, recovery is eventually complete.

(c) *Renal cortical necrosis.* This is an ischaemic necrosis which may involve the whole or scattered portions of the renal cortex (Sheehan & Moore, 1952). The distinguishing feature of this severe type of ischaemic renal necrosis is destruction of glomeruli, and therefore the affected nephrons are permanently and irretrievably damaged. Lesions typical of acute tubular necrosis are found in the less severely affected areas where a more adequate blood supply has been preserved. Death is inevitable if a major portion of the renal cortex is involved, but recovery may occur if the necrosis of glomeruli is limited to scattered portions of cortex.

(2) *Toxic necrosis of tubules. Proximal tubular necrosis.* This is due to a specialized type of renal damage from nephrotoxic drugs or poisons. The necrosis affects relatively long segments of *all* proximal tubules, but affects only the tubular cells with sparing of the basement membrane (Oliver *et al.*, 1951). By contrast, the lesions of acute tubular necrosis are distributed at random among separate nephrons and in any portion of a single nephron, and the basement membrane is damaged and ruptured. The segment of tubule affected in proximal tubular necrosis is determined by the point of maximal concentration of the necrotizing agent. With higher dosage the segment of tubule involved becomes more extensive, and ischaemic lesions causing acute tubular necrosis are seen in addition to the characteristic proximal tubular damage. Different toxic agents are maximally concentrated in varying portions of the proximal tubule, and therefore produce characteristic areas of cellular necrosis. Typical areas involved are: proximal third—bichromate; middle third—uranium salts; distal third—mercury, carbon tetrachloride, mushroom (*Amanita phalloides*) poisoning, serine; middle and distal thirds—tartrates, chlorates, diethylene glycol; all segments of the proximal tubule—sulphonamides (Oliver *et al.*, 1951). It should be noted that these selective lesions are best seen in experimental cases in animals where the dosage can be accurately adjusted. In cases seen in man, a higher dose has usually been taken with greater lengths of proximal tubule involved and with the ischaemic

lesions of acute tubular necrosis in the distal tubules.

(3) *Acute glomerulonephritis.* Acute glomerulonephritis (Type I, Ellis) is usually associated with moderate oliguria, but occasionally there is either complete anuria or very severe oliguria. The incidence of complete anuria is higher than in cases due to renal ischaemia.

(4) *Acute deterioration of renal function in cases of chronic uraemia.* In some cases of chronic uraemia the characteristic polyuria is replaced by severe oliguria, with consequent rapid deterioration of the clinical state and further rise of the blood urea. In many cases this is due to acute renal circulatory insufficiency from NaCl depletion, but it may indicate an acute exacerbation of the disease responsible for the glomerular damage with almost complete cessation of glomerular filtration.

(5) *Lesions involving both renal arteries*, e.g. bilateral embolism or a dissecting aortic aneurysm involving the main renal arterial trunks.

Causes of renal ischaemic lesions. The commonest type of acute renal failure is that due to renal ischaemia. It is possible that the three classes of acute renal circulatory failure, acute tubular necrosis, and renal cortical necrosis represent grades of severity of the ischaemic process, and many cases show pathological features of more than a single class. The differential diagnosis in the early stages of the oliguria may be impossible without biopsy evidence. The clinical differentiation is that whilst acute renal circulatory failure causes only temporary oliguria, acute tubular necrosis results in an oliguria which recovers from one to three weeks after the onset, and renal cortical necrosis is irrecoverable unless only small areas of cortex are involved.

The possible causes of renal ischaemia are legion and include:

(a) *Lesions causing haemorrhage and surgical shock*, e.g. severe traumatic injuries, especially those involving severe injury or crushing of muscle, severe burns or scalds, complications of pregnancy including septic abortion, concealed accidental haemorrhage and post-partum haemorrhage, and haematemesis or melaena.

(b) *Disorders involving electrolyte imbalance or dehydration*, e.g. severe vomiting from pyloric stenosis or intestinal obstruction, severe diarrhoea as in cholera or acute bacillary dysentery, Addison's disease, and diabetic ketosis.

(c) *Renal vaso-constriction due to extra-corpuscular haemoglobin, or to sensitivity reactions*, e.g. incompatible blood transfusion, blackwater fever, intravascular haemolysis from hypotonic infusions, sulphonamide sensitivity and overwhelming bacterial infections.

Functional abnormalities in renal ischaemia. Lauson, Bradley & Cournand (1944) investigated renal haemodynamics in states of severe surgical shock. They found a depression of glomerular filtration rate and renal blood flow greater than could be accounted for by the fall of arterial blood pressure, suggesting an active renal vaso-constriction. The renal blood flow was reduced proportionately more than the fall in cardiac output, and the calculated renal arteriolar resistance was consistently increased. The renal circulation often failed to improve during the period of emergency treatment at times when cardiac output and arterial blood pressure had been restored to normal. Phillips, Dole, Hamilton, Emerson, Archibald & Van Slyke (1946), investigating massive acute haemorrhage in dogs, found that for a time the kidneys were favoured at the expense of the rest of the circulation, but if the haemorrhage was both too severe and too prolonged renal vaso-constriction developed. The renal blood flow was then reduced more than the flow to more vital organs, e.g. the heart and the brain, and ischaemic damage could be produced. Dole, Emerson, Phillips, Hamilton & Van Slyke (1946), found that the normally small arterio-venous O_2 difference of the kidney persists after haemorrhage, unlike most organs where the oxygen consumption is maintained by an increased abstraction of oxygen from the circulating haemoglobin. De Wardener, Miles, Lee, Churchill-Davidson, Wylie & Sharpey-Schafer (1952) found that after a rapid venesection of 1400 ml. of blood in adult patients, there was usually no change in glomerular filtration rate and renal plasma flow for periods of 80 min. or less. This confirmed the impression from the animal experiments that the haemorrhagic shock had to be prolonged for several hours before renal vaso-constriction occurred. Determinations of renal blood flow by the radio-krypton or dye dilution methods (Brun *et al.*, 1955; Shaldon *et al.*, 1962), indicate that this is reduced to about one-third the normal value in the oliguric stage, and to approximately two-thirds during the early diuretic stage.

The oliguria associated with incompatible blood transfusions or severe haemoglobinuria has recently been found to be associated with similar renal ischaemia. The formation of intratubular pigment casts had for long been considered to be the most important factor in the production of oliguria. Maegraith (1944) showed that in black-water fever there was little correlation between the degree of tubular blockage found at necropsy and the severity of the oliguria, and often the obstruction observed was quite insufficient to account for fatal renal failure. Many conflicting opinions on the effect of extracorpuscular haemoglobin on renal function have resulted from a failure to realize that stimuli causing renal vaso-constriction are additive. Thus severe renal damage may be produced in states of shock by a quantity of free haemoglobin which would be innocuous in the normal subject. Miller & McDonald (1951) found that doses of up to 15 g. of free haemoglobin injected intravenously into normal adults definitely reduced the inulin and *p*-aminohippurate clearances and the rate of urine flow, but no permanent renal damage occurred. Blackburn, Hensley, Grant & Wright (1954) injected distilled water intravenously at a rate of 4 ml./min. for periods of several hours. The haemolysis caused a severe oliguria which was closely correlated with the fall in renal blood flow and less closely correlated with a similar fall of glomerular filtration rate. Renal function was rapidly restored after cessation of the infusion. In clinical cases, haemoglobinuric renal failure is usually associated with other conditions which predispose to renal ischaemia, e.g. surgical shock or anaemia, and in these circumstances less severe degrees of haemolysis might well result in acute tubular necrosis. One familiar example is the oliguria which may be produced during transurethral prostatectomy by irrigation of the operative field with sterile tap-water.

Bull, Joekes & Lowe (1950) have reported on a study of renal function in acute tubular necrosis, based on experience of over 100 cases. They divide the illness into the four stages of onset, anuric or oliguric, early diuretic, and late diuretic phases. The onset phase is the stage of shock associated with renal vaso-constriction, and a rapidly falling rate of urine flow. In the anuric or oliguric phase, there is a rapidly increasing uraemia. Definition of the end of this phase is arbitrary, but is usually taken as the day when the urine volume becomes greater than 400 ml. in the 24 hr. During the diuretic phases there is a period of recovery of renal function which is rapid at first, but becomes more gradual later. Follow-up studies (Lowe, 1952; Finkenstaedt, O'Meara, Weller & Merrill, 1953) have shown that no further recovery occurs after three to six months from the onset. Thereafter, there is apparent full clinical recovery, but inulin, PAH, and urea clearances remain slightly below normal limits. It seems certain, therefore, that some nephrons are destroyed by the ischaemic process, and that the renal reserve remains somewhat reduced. Theoretically, a greater degree of permanent functional impairment is to be expected in cases where there has been some element of renal cortical necrosis with ischaemic destruction of glomeruli.

A subdivision of the recovery period into early and late diuretic phases is not justified on purely theoretical grounds, but is of great clinical convenience. During the early diuretic phase, the life of the patient remains at considerable risk, at least 25% of deaths occurring during this stage, and meticulous biochemical control of treatment is as essential as in the oliguric phase. In the late diuretic phase convalescence is well established, the patient can take a reasonably normal diet, and biochemical control becomes only of prognostic

centres is very much higher (Bluemle, Webster & Elkington, 1959), averaging 40% in the surgical group and less than 10% in the medical and obstetrical cases. The rate of rise of blood urea is much more rapid in the surgical cases due to a hypercatabolic response due to tissue injury (Milne, Loughridge, Shackman & Struthers, 1960), and secondary infection is more serious and more common.

During the oliguric and early diuretic stages, inulin and PAH clearances, Tm_{PAH} and Tm_G, and extraction ratio of PAH are all grossly reduced. The renal arterio-venous O_2 difference tends to be increased, arguing against the participation of any intrarenal vascular shunt as a cause of the oliguria. As in chronic uraemia, there is a raised blood urea, plasma creatinine and uric acid, and increase

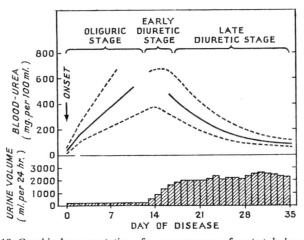

FIG. 10.10. Graphical representation of an average case of acute tubular necrosis.

The regression lines of blood urea and the upper limit at twice the standard deviation for the oliguric and late diuretic stages are not continuous in this series of cases, because many of the patients were treated by haemodialysis in the last few days of the oliguric stage. Reproduced by permission of the Editor of the *Lancet*.

or research interest. Loughridge, Milne, Shackman & Wootton (1960) have reinvestigated the course of uncomplicated acute tubular necrosis. They define the early diuretic phase as the period of increasing urinary output, without any fall of the blood urea. The late diuretic stage is associated with a maintained and almost constant diuresis and a progressive fall of blood urea. The average durations of the various stages of the disease (Fig. 10.10) were found to be as follows:

(a) Oliguric stage—12 days;
(b) Early diuretic stage—15 days;
(c) Late diuretic stage—18 days.

Acute tubular necrosis due to surgical trauma is more serious than cases due to medical or obstetric causes, and the mortality rate in most

of plasma sulphate and phosphate with consequent fall of plasma bicarbonate and production of a metabolic acidosis. Because of the oliguria, the ionic exchange mechanism of K excretion is ineffective, and the plasma K increases. Hyperkalaemia of a severity sufficient to endanger life occurs in at least one-quarter of the cases (Swan & Merrill, 1953). Serum Na and Cl are almost invariably reduced and there is increase of the total body water, both intra- and extracellular compartments being involved (Swan & Merrill, 1953; Hamburger & Mathé, 1954). This increase of body water occurs despite meticulous care in fluid balance and is derived from excessive catabolism of body fat. Moore, Edelman, Olney, James, Brooks & Wilson (1954) have shown that there is invariably a rise of total exchangeable Na and a fall of total exchangeable K, even in cases with severe hyponatraemia and hyperkalaemia.

In the early diuretic phase, the urinary daily volume rapidly increases until several litres of dilute urine are being formed each 24 hr. The osmolarity of the urine is similar to that of plasma and the specific gravity is 1010. Urine/plasma ratios of urea, creatinine, and uric acid are abnormally low at first, but steadily increase to near normal values throughout the whole of the diuretic stage. Salt and water previously retained are now excreted, and there is progressive weight loss with restoration to normal of the increased body water (Swan & Merrill, 1953). This loss may be excessive and a generous intake of water and salt should be allowed at this stage, but no attempt should be made to maintain exact salt and water balance, since this only serves to perpetuate the diuresis. The ionic exchange process of K excretion is now highly effective and the K clearance becomes considerably higher than that of inulin (Sirota & Kroop, 1951). This results in K depletion and hypokalaemia, and K supplements are necessary until the late diuretic phase is reached. The urinary abnormalities of the early diuretic phase are typical of a state of osmotic diuresis, urea being the chief loading solute.

Functional abnormalities in other types of acute renal failure. Minor variations are seen in cases of acute renal failure not due to renal ischaemia. In some cases of proximal tubular necrosis there may be more evidence of specific proximal tubular damage, as is to be expected in view of the distribution of the lesion. Thus, renal glycosuria and amino-aciduria are especially prominent in cases of kidney damage from uranium poisoning (Rothstein & Berke, 1949), and have also been described in oliguria from lysol poisoning (Spencer & Franglen, 1952). Lowe, Moodie & Thomson (1954) have described an excess excretion of glucose and amino acids during the oliguric phase of acute tubular necrosis, but the abnormality is minute and can be detected only by somewhat refined chromatographic methods. Anuria from acute glomerulonephritis is more liable to be absolute and tends to persist longer than in cases of acute tubular necrosis, there often being an oliguric phase of three to four weeks or even longer. In many of these cases there is total glomerular destruction and fibrosis, and diuresis never occurs. The mortality of cases of oliguric glomerulonephritis is therefore much higher than that of acute tubular necrosis. There are usually other signs of nephritis, especially oedema and hypertension. The urinary specific gravity remains high for several days, whilst in acute tubular necrosis it rapidly falls to 1010. The urine remains acid in reaction, whereas in the ischaemic lesions it becomes neutral or only slightly acid. The Cl concentration is of especial diagnostic importance. In glomerulonephritis there is excess salt reabsorption and the urinary concentration is below 30 m-equiv./l., whilst in tubular necrosis there is an approximation to the plasma concentration, and urinary levels are above 30 m-equiv./l. (Swan & Merrill, 1953).

Treatment. The therapeutic objective in acute renal failure is to prolong life until adequate renal function is spontaneously restored. Renal ischaemic lesions can often be prevented by rapid correction of general states of circulatory failure by blood transfusion, restoration of electrolyte balance and the maintenance of an adequate systolic arterial blood pressure. After ingestion of a nephrotoxic drug or poison, renal damage may be minimized by water diuresis produced either by drinking 1 l. of fluid by mouth, or by infusion of a similar volume of 5% glucose intravenously, as the diuresis reduces the concentration of the toxic agent in the tubular lumen. This excess fluid should not be given if the oliguria is already established, since by then the damage has been done, and excess fluid will not be excreted.

In the anuric or oliguric phase, elimination of excess electrolyte becomes impossible, and water is only lost in the expired air and sweat. In temperate conditions extrarenal water loss is about 600–800 ml./day, and as water is produced from metabolism of ingested carbohydrate and from body fat, only 400–500 ml. of fluid should be given to the patient in addition to an amount equal to the previous 24 hr. urinary volume. No electrolyte should be administered unless the patient is vomiting or has diarrhoea, or is in a Na-depleted state, when the loss should be made good. It is not considered that the hyponatraemia of the oliguric phase is an indication for giving NaCl, because it is due to dilution of body fluids in association with an increased extracellular fluid volume. There is no doubt that death from pulmonary oedema, secondary to excess retention of both salt and water, is a much greater risk than is dehydration.

Provided Na and water balance is maintained, the other important causes of death are cardiac arrest from hyperkalaemia, and metabolic acidosis from retention of excess phosphate and sulphate. In rare cases, hyperkalaemic paralysis of voluntary muscle may precede cardiac arrest (Bull, Carter & Lowe, 1953), and in such cases artificial respiration may be necessary. The steady increase of blood non-protein N, which is principally urea N, and of plasma K, phosphate and sulphate, is secondary to protein catabolism. This arises chiefly from breakdown of endogenous protein, with transfer of N and of intracellular electrolytes to the extracellular phase. Gamble (1951b) has shown that the average endogenous consumption of protein by the starving adult is 70 g. each day. If 100 g. of glucose are taken, this is reduced to 40 g./day, but no further decrease occurs with greater carbohydrate intake. It can be assumed, therefore, that in the anuric patient there is a theoretical minimum catabolism of protein of 40 g. each day, equivalent to 6·4 g. nitrogen. Unfortunately, owing to breakdown of damaged tissue, fever, or infection, the actual protein catabolism is usually higher than the theoretical minimum. This variation accounts for the extremely different rates of clinical deterioration in patients with acute renal failure.

One gram of protein N is associated in muscle tissue with 2·7 m-equiv. K, 4·25 m-equiv. sulphate, 3·9 m-equiv. phosphate and 0·6 m-equiv. Mg (Reifenstein, Albright & Wells, 1945). Assuming that 40 g. of protein are broken down daily and that the extracellular fluid volume is 20% of the body weight, it is to be expected that there would be the following daily changes in the composition of extracellular fluid; urea, 28 mg./100 ml. increase; K, 1·25 m-equiv./l. increase; sulphate, 1·95 m-equiv./l. increase; phosphate, 1·8 m-equiv./l. increase; Mg, 0·3 m-equiv./l. increase; bicarbonate, 3·75 m-equiv./l. decrease. The actual increase in urea is usually higher, and the change in electrolyte concentration less. The electrolytes may be transferred back to the cells as a result of the considerable glycogen synthesis which occurs with the use of high glucose diets in the treatment of anuria. The figures, although theoretical, serve to illustrate how rapid may be the deterioration in some cases, and emphasize the liability to fatal hyperkalaemia or metabolic acidosis.

Diet in anuria should therefore consist of an electrolyte-free and low protein régime, should contain large amounts of carbohydrate, and fluid should be restricted to about 400–500 ml./day. The fluid is best given by mouth either as 20% lactose or fructose, as these sugars are less nauseating and better tolerated than glucose. Administration of sterile 40% glucose by a drip cannula inserted via the median basilic and subclavian veins into the superior vena cava is now a less popular method than it was some years ago, as secondary infection with septicaemia often occurs. If vomiting is severe enough to prevent administration of the fluid by mouth, either 5%

glucose or, preferably, 10% fructose should be given by infusion into a peripheral vein. More concentrated solutions of these sugars are liable to cause local venous thrombosis.

The incidence of severe hyperkalaemia has been greatly reduced by administration of cation-exchange resins in the Na phase (Evans et al., 1954). Berlyne (1965) considers that resin charged with calcium is preferable. This type of resin exchanges rather less completely than a sodium type as the affinity of calcium for resin is higher than that of sodium. It is, however, certainly indicated in cases where there is already evidence of excess sodium retention. Resin therapy both by mouth and by retention enemata should be instituted as soon as the plasma K rises above 6 m-equiv./l. and continued until the level has fallen below 5 m-equiv./l. The resin by mouth takes up approximately 0·5 m-equiv. K/g. of resin administered, and therefore, since 60 g. of resin can be given daily, approximately 30 m-equiv. K may be removed every 24 hr. The method fails in cases where there is severe vomiting and where there is uraemic ileus with retention of the resin in the stomach. Resin given by enemata is not so efficacious as when given by mouth. Meroney & Herndon (1954), from extensive experience in Korea, have found that resin treatment is inadequate when there is considerable damage to muscle. They found that intravenous infusions of calcium gluconate and hypertonic $NaHCO_3$ were of great value in reducing intoxication as shown by improvement in the electrocardiogram.

Treatment by dialysis is indicated if conservative methods are insufficient to prevent rapid clinical deterioration, or in cases with a prolonged oliguric stage. Either haemodialysis with an artificial kidney or peritoneal dialysis may be used, but the former method is preferable. An efficient artificial kidney will produce the same degree of clinical and biochemical improvement within six hr. as peritoneal dialysis lasting two or three days. The indications for dialysis in medical or obstetrical cases are as follows:

(a) Clinical signs and symptoms of uraemic toxaemia, e.g. fits, jactitations, hiccough, vomiting, and stupor or coma.

(b) A blood urea above 300 mg./100 ml.

(c) Uraemic acidosis with a plasma bicarbonate less than 12 m-equiv./l.

(d) Hyperkalaemia with a plasma K above 7·0 m-equiv./l. despite therapy with ion-exchange resins.

A blood urea above 300 mg./100 ml. is the commonest indication for dialysis in clinical practice (Milne, Loughridge, Shackman &

Struthers, 1960). Hyperkalaemia is more important in patients who have been badly controlled during the early oliguric stage of the disease, or in cases with extensive damage or injury to voluntary muscle. Cases of acute tubular necrosis of surgical cause should be dialysed more frequently, and the blood urea should not be allowed to rise above 250 mg./100 ml. (Scribner, Magid & Burnell, 1960). The average rise of blood urea in the surgical cases is 60 mg./100 ml./day, as compared to a figure of 34 mg./100 ml./day in the medical or obstetrical cases (Milne *et al.*, 1960). Haemodialysis, therefore, is often necessary every two or three days, and is made technically easier by use of the extracorporeal arterio-venous fistula introduced by Scribner, Buri, Caner, Hegstrom & Burnell (1960). With more modern methods, including timely and frequent haemodialysis, the recovery rate should be over 90% in cases of acute tubular necrosis due to medical and obstetrical conditions, and over 60% in the surgical cases.

Prognosis. The recovery rate of cases of acute renal failure varies according to the aetiology and to the efficiency of the treatment. One of the largest series has been reported by Dérot & Legrain (1954) with a recovery rate of 62% of 226 cases. In this series, the prognosis was better than the average in cases due to abortion, or to ingestion of nephrotoxic drugs, but was more serious in cases due to incompatible blood transfusion, post-operative cases and in association with serious liver disease and jaundice (the so-called hepato-renal syndrome). A grave view should be taken of cases following concealed accidental haemorrhage of pregnancy, since this is the usual cause of severe renal cortical necrosis with massive glomerular damage (Sheehan & Moore, 1952).

Biochemical   problems   during   dialysis. Haemodialysis using the twin coil dialyser (Kolff & Watschinger, 1956) or the parallel plate dialyser (Kiil, 1960), or peritoneal dialysis are now widely used in the management of acute and chronic renal failure and in removal of dialysable poisons or toxins from the body. Dialysis primarily results in equilibration of the composition of diffusible substances in the plasma and extracellular fluid, and the fluid used in the method adopted. Equilibration between the intracellular and extracellular compartments may be delayed for considerable periods, and during this time complications can arise owing to differences in rate of diffusion of various substances across the cell membranes. Water is more rapidly diffusible than urea and therefore if plasma urea is reduced

rapidly by dialysis there may be a high concentration gradient of urea between the intra- and extracellular compartments. This is well shown by delay in equilibration of cerebrospinal fluid and muscle urea with the level in plasma (Kennedy, Linton & Eaton, 1962). Water will move into the cells to preserve equality of osmotic pressure across the cell membrane causing temporary cellular over-hydration. In the central nervous system this will cause headache, twitching of muscle, or even major fits. In the heart, dangerous arrhythmias may result. The effects of this dysequilibration syndrome can be reduced by less vigorous dialysis for the first two hr. when removal of urea is most rapid, and in more frequent dialysis choosing a time when the plasma urea is not above 200 mg./100 ml. Obviously, this complication will be more frequent using the artificial kidney than in peritoneal dialysis where removal of urea is slower and more gradual.

Considerable quantities of protein and amino-acid nitrogen are removed during dialysis. Both peritoneal and haemodialysis cause an undesirable outflow of amino acids from the blood resulting in body protein breakdown. In addition, during peritoneal dialysis large amounts of plasma protein leak into the dialysis fluid. There is frequently an accumulation of protein-rich ascitic fluid between successive dialyses as a result of peritoneal irritation. This is of little significance in the treatment of acute oliguric renal failure, but becomes very important in the repeated dialyses involved in the therapy of chronic uraemia. If an adequate diet, sufficient to maintain good nutrition, is allowed, frequent dialyses, three or four times weekly are necessary. This is usually only practical in a home dialysis scheme. Most patients treated by bi-weekly hospital dialysis are in a less satisfactory clinical state than those who have been fortunate enough to receive a well-functioning homotransplanted kidney.

BIOCHEMICAL CHANGES
FOLLOWING
URETERO-SIGMOIDOSTOMY

This operation is now commonly performed in cases of ectopia vesicae, in cystectomy for carcinoma of the bladder, and for intractable vesico-vaginal fistulae. There has therefore been considerable interest in the metabolic abnormalities which frequently follow this procedure. They may occur at any time after the operation, but become more common the longer the patient survives, and are especially liable to develop if renal function becomes impaired. Ferris & Odel (1950) found that there was a reduced plasma bicarbonate and a raised plasma Cl in about 80% of cases one year after the operation. Jacobs & Stirling (1952) found that a raised blood urea was equally common, and recorded a significant reduction in plasma K in 30% of cases. These biochemical changes do not invariably cause untoward symptoms, but a proportion of cases complain of tiredness, weakness, anorexia, nausea and vomiting, a salty taste in the mouth, and thirst with consequent polydipsia.

The usual tests of renal function are inapplicable after uretero-sigmoidostomy since it is impossible to obtain a timed specimen of urine, and in most cases to obtain any specimen which is not contaminated with faeces. Some studies have, however, been made after modified operations in which the ureters are implanted into an artificial bladder formed from rectum and lower sigmoid, the faeces escaping by means of a terminal colostomy (Parsons et al., 1952). Even that useful and simple procedure, the determination of the blood urea, is less informative than in other renal diseases. A raised blood urea after uretero-sigmoidostomy does not necessarily indicate reduction of the glomerular filtration rate. Urea is reabsorbed from the urine within the bowel lumen and thus a high blood urea may occur without any renal dysfunction. The most useful simple functional test is intravenous pyelography. Usually this method is inapplicable in the presence of a significant raised blood urea, but satisfactory delineation of the renal pelves may be obtained in cases of uretero-sigmoidostomy despite apparent uraemia, since this does not necessarily indicate impairment of renal function. Renal clearances may be calculated despite the impossibility of obtaining timed urinary specimens. Inulin and p-aminohippurate are infused intravenously at steady rates until a stable plasma concentration is obtained. It can then be assumed that the rate of excretion by the kidneys is equal to the known speed of infusion. This method is more time-consuming and less accurate than the classical methods, but is the only one applicable in this type of case as urinary analyses are not involved.

There has been considerable controversy with regard to the relative importance of renal and colonic factors in the causation of the biochemical disorders. There is now little doubt that both are of importance in most cases, but some may show no evidence of renal impairment, the changes being entirely due to differential reabsorption of solutes from the urine by the colonic mucosa.

Evidence in favour of disordered colonic function.

(*a*) The biochemical changes and the symptoms are relieved, either partially or completely, by colonic drainage by means of an in-dwelling rectal tube, or by frequent voluntary evacuations which reduce the time of contact of the urine with the colonic mucosa.

(*b*) Improvement occurs on a low-salt diet which reduces the excretion of salt, and therefore diminishes differential colonic reabsorption of Na and Cl ions.

(*c*) Transplantation of the ureters into the caecum of dogs often proves fatal (Boyce, 1951), but the mortality rate is progressively reduced if the anastomosis is performed at lower levels of the colon. Reabsorption of Cl and urea was shown to be greater in the caecum than the rectum. Kekwick et al. (1951) found that the mortality rate was high after operations in man in which the right ureter was anastomosed to the caecum and the left to the sigmoid colon.

(*d*) Parsons et al. (1952) studied the effect of transplantation of the ureters into an isolated artificial bladder. They found that as much as 30% of urea, 70% of Cl, 50% of Na, and 20% of water could be reabsorbed from the urine by the colonic mucosa. There was simultaneously a 15% increase of K content. Conclusive proof of a more rapid reabsorption of Cl than of Na was obtained by use of salt solutions containing ^{24}Na and ^{38}Cl. The plasma concentration of the former ion rose more slowly than the latter.

(*e*) Mitchell & Valk (1953) found that the biochemical changes with hyperchloraemic acidosis could still occur in cases whose renal function measured by C_{in}, C_{PAH}, and Tm_{PAH} was within normal limits.

Evidence in favour of disordered renal tubular function. (*a*) Pathological evidence of infection can be found in many kidneys shortly after ureteric transplantation, and after some years there is almost invariably histological evidence of chronic pyelonephritis often associated with hydronephrosis (Pool & Cook, 1950; Graves & Buddington, 1950).

(*b*) Creevy & Reiser (1952) found that hyperchloraemic acidosis was two and a half times as common if there was pyelographic evidence of gross bilateral renal disease, and that symptoms in such patients occurred ten times as frequently as in cases where one or both kidneys showed a normal pyelogram.

(*c*) The tendency to develop K deficiency sometimes severe enough to cause a flaccid quadriplegia (Diefenbach et al., 1951) and the development in some patients of renal osteodystrophy with osteomalacia (Pines & Mudge, 1951), are identical with changes seen in some cases of pyelonephritis.

The evidence therefore suggests that the increase of blood urea may be due to colonic reabsorption, and that the hyperchloraemic acidosis is due to preferential reabsorption of Cl to Na with replacement by bicarbonate ion to neutralize the unabsorbed Na. The K deficiency appears to be chiefly due to renal tubular dysfunction, but there is also evidence of passage of K into the colonic contents. In view of the efficiency of the normal kidney in preserving biochemical homeostasis, it is not surprising that the changes should be more frequent and more severe when there is an associated pyelonephritic renal failure.

The treatment of this condition should include advice with regard to frequent evacuations of the colonic bladder, salt restriction combined with unrestricted fluid intake, and the use of potassium citrate supplements if there is evidence of K depletion. One difficulty in the biochemical control of treatment is that, whilst the anastomosis primarily causes an acidosis with fall of plasma bicarbonate, an associated K depletion may result in a hypokalaemic alkalosis with opposite biochemical changes. This may obviously result in confusion if one aspect of the disordered biochemistry is corrected before the other.

RENAL TUBULAR SYNDROMES

These are metabolic disorders, either hereditary or acquired, in which there is an anomaly of one or several specialized tubular functions. They may be classified as follows:

(1) *Disorders of proximal tubular function.*
(a) Renal glycosuria due to reduced glucose reabsorption.
(b) Vitamin D resistant rickets or osteomalacia due to decreased phosphate reabsorption.
(c) Fanconi syndrome in which there is a mixed reabsorption defect involving many amino acids, glucose, phosphate and uric acid, with renal osteodystrophy and in some cases hypokalaemia and disturbance of acid-base balance.
(d) Cystinuria with reduced reabsorption of cystine, lysine, arginine and ornithine, and associated in some cases with renal calculi.
(e) Hartnup disease, where there is reduced reabsorption of many of the amino acids derived from protein with the exception of the dibasic amino acids involved in cystinuria, and also of glycine and proline.
(f) The amino-aciduria of hepatolenticular degeneration and infantile galactosaemia possibly due to the toxic influence of excess Cu and galactose-1-phosphate respectively on proximal tubular function.

(2) *Disorders of distal tubular function.* (a) Renal tubular acidosis of infants—Lightwood type (1935).
(b) Renal tubular acidosis—Albright, Consolazio, Coombs, Sulkowitch & Talbott type (1940) —with or without an associated nephrocalcinosis.
(c) Salt-losing nephritis (Thorn, Koepf & Clinton, 1944).
(d) Potassium-losing nephritis (Earle et al., 1951; Evans & Milne, 1954).
(e) Water-losing nephritis or nephrogenic diabetes insipidus.

Abnormalities associated with renal osteodystrophy and with amino-aciduria are described in other chapters, and therefore only the disorders of distal tubular function will be considered. Infantile renal acidosis was first described by Lightwood (1935) and shortly afterwards by Butler, Wilson & Farber (1936). It occurs most commonly in the first 18 months of life, and is characterized by a metabolic acidosis with lowering of the plasma bicarbonate and increase of plasma Cl. The urine is alkaline, neutral, or only faintly acid, the fundamental tubular disorder being a failure to produce a normal concentration gradient of hydrogen ion between urine and plasma. In some late cases there is radiological evidence of nephrocalcinosis, the Ca being deposited in the renal medulla. Symptoms usually start between the fourth and seventh month of life, and consist of anorexia, vomiting, and constipation with wasting and failure to thrive. The chronic acidosis leads to salt depletion with clinical evidence of dehydration, and to K depletion with hypotonia of muscle. Improvement takes place on an alkalinizing régime of sodium bicarbonate or citrate, and complete clinical recovery usually occurs after several months of therapy. Potassium salts may be added if there is clear evidence of K depletion.

The aetiology of the condition is unknown, although pyelonephritis has been considered as a possible cause. In many cases the urine is sterile on culture, but this does not exclude damage from previous infection. Latner & Burnard (1950) found that infusion of sodium phosphate resulted in a temporary amelioration of the inability of the tubules to produce an acid urine and form ammonia. In addition it was found that the partial pressure of CO_2 in the urine was higher than that of plasma. Basing their arguments on the original theories of Pitts & Alexander (1945) with regard to the mechanism of acidification of the urine, they considered that the defect lay in the proximal tubular reabsorption of bicarbonate, the distal ion-exchange mechanism being intact. More recent advances in renal physiology have proved these arguments to be completely invalid. The high urinary P_{CO_2} is now fully explained by the counter-current circulation of the *vasa recta* of the renal medulla, and is unrelated to proximal tubular function. In addition, the observations of Schwartz & Relman (1954), which have been previously described, have shown that both proximal and distal bicarbonate reabsorption is due to the hydrogen ion exchange mechanism. Pathological evidence from the distribution of the tubular damage and nephrocalcinosis indicates a predominantly distal tubular disturbance. The severe Na depletion present in this condition may possibly explain the temporary urinary acidification produced by sodium phosphate infusions. Schwartz, Jenson & Relman (1955) have shown that infusions of sodium phosphate and sulphate, whilst not causing any marked change in urinary pH in normal subjects, produced a strongly acid urine in salt depletion because of enhanced exchange of hydrogen ion for Na.

The renal tubular acidosis described by Albright *et al.* (1940) appears to be a different condition to the infantile type. The disorder usually starts in adolescence and may present either with bone pain or deformity from renal osteodystrophy, or with attacks of hypokalaemic paralysis from excess urinary K loss. The severe dehydration and wasting of the infantile condition are never seen. Although the effects of the tubular disease can be kept in abeyance by treatment with alkaline Na and K salts, the underlying disease is not cured and treatment must be continued indefinitely. Milne, Stanbury & Thomson (1952) applied the same arguments as Latner & Burnard (1950) with regard to the high P_{CO_2} found in the alkaline or neutral urines of this condition. The arguments with regard to localization of the defect in the nephron are equally invalid, and again pathological and radiological evidence favours a predominantly distal tubular abnormality. The aetiology is unknown, but chronic pyelonephritis has been suspected in some cases. Schreiner, Smith & Kyle (1953) have reported three cases in which the condition seemed to be due to a dominant hereditary factor.

"Salt-losing nephritis" was first described by Thorn *et al.* (1944) and several other cases have been reported since. There appears to be a specific tubular defect of reabsorption of Na and Cl. The urine contains large quantities of salt despite considerable body depletion as shown by dehydration, hypotension, hyponatraemia and hypochloraemia. The Na loss results in a secondary reduction of glomerular filtration rate with increase of the blood urea. There is often a brownish pigmentation of the skin which is frequently seen in chronic renal disease. The condition therefore closely simulates Addison's disease, and the true diagnosis is usually only made when the abnormal salt loss is found to be resistant to treatment with adrenal cortical steroids. The only effective therapy is direct replacement of NaCl by saline infusions followed by a high-salt diet. Enticknap (1952) has presented evidence that the condition is almost always secondary to chronic pyelonephritis.

Although most cases of renal failure show a tendency to urinary loss of salt, and an inability to reduce Na and Cl excretion during conditions of salt depletion, the defect is not so severe as in true cases of "salt-losing nephritis". Most cases of chronic uraemia will maintain Na and Cl balance provided there is adequate salt intake, and there is no undue gastro-intestinal Na and Cl loss from uraemia. By contrast, true cases of "salt-losing nephritis" are in negative balance for Na and Cl on an average daily salt intake, and can only remain in reasonable health if excess salt is given in the diet. The tendency to salt depletion in the disease causes a reduction of the circulating blood volume leading to secondary hyperaldosteronism and abnormally high levels of urinary aldosterone. The adrenal cortical hypertrophy may persist even if the disease has been adequately treated with excess NaCl (Stanbury & Mahler, 1959).

Abnormal loss of K in the urine sufficient to cause hypokalaemic paralysis can occur in renal tubular acidosis (Brown, Currens & Marchand, 1944) and in both the adult and juvenile types of the Fanconi syndrome (Milne *et al.*, 1952; Bickel, Smallwood, Smellie & Hickmans, 1952). Primary or secondary aldosteronism causes more severe degrees of K deficiency. Unlike the cases due to primary renal tubule disorders, there is usually a severe alkalosis with rise of plasma bicarbonate and arterial blood pH. This is partly due to the K depletion and partly to the fact that aldosterone enhances tubular exchange of H^+ for Na^+, and thus increases loss of H^+ from the body. Loss of K alone can cause complete isosthenuria, and reduction of the glomerular filtration rate, renal plasma flow, and Tm_{PAH} (Schwartz & Relman, 1953). In addition, there is impaired ability to secrete a maximally acid urine (Clarke *et al.*, 1955). These functional defects are associated with vacuolization of the cytoplasm and pyknosis of nuclei of tubular cells (Spargo, 1954). The abnormalities, which may progress to patchy cellular necrosis, are more prominent in the proximal tubule.

"Water-losing nephritis" or "nephrogenic diabetes insipidus" may closely simulate true diabetes insipidus due to lack of antidiuretic hormone. The distinguishing feature is that the diuresis is unaffected by injections of pitressin, and antidiuretic hormone can be demonstrated by bioassay in the urine. The condition may be congenital or acquired. The congenital form appears to be due to a sex-linked recessive hereditary factor, and therefore the disease only affects males and is transmitted by apparently normal females (Forssman, 1945; Williams & Henry, 1947). The female heterozygotes, however, invariably show some reduction of urinary concentration below the normal maximum. Forssman has directly compared three families with sex-linked diabetes insipidus, in two of which the condition was pitressin-sensitive and, in one, pitressin-resistant. The condition was more severe in the renal type, all the adult cases having urine volumes of over 7 l./day. The adults learn to maintain homeostasis by adequate fluid intake, but in infants severe haemoconcentration with hypernatraemia and hyperchloraemia may occur unless the condition is recognized and sufficient fluid given. The acquired disease has been reviewed by Roussak & Oleesky (1954). The condition seems to occur particularly in association with nephrocalcinosis and hypercalcaemia. It has been described in hyperparathyroidism (Albright & Reifenstein, 1948; Snapper, 1952) and in multiple myelomatosis (Roussak & Oleesky, 1954). Diagnosis of this condition depends on the demonstration that there is an obligatory hyposthenuria considerably below the level seen in the isosthenuria of renal failure. Determination of the maximal urinary osmolality is obviously a much more satisfactory method than use of urinary specific gravity, since the latter is influenced by variation in the proportion of excreted solutes. If the condition causing the hypercalcaemia can be cured, e.g. hyperparathyroidism, the abnormality may completely resolve and the tubules regain their ability to reabsorb water and form a hypertonic urine.

URINARY LITHIASIS

Urinary lithiasis is a recurrent condition. From the figures given by Pyrah (1954), it can be calculated that the mean ipsilateral recurrence rate is 23 % after pyelolithotomy, 29 % after ureterolithotomy and 38 % after nephrolithotomy. The contralateral recurrent rate is 14 % both after nephrectomy and after more conservative operations. About one-third of patients with renal stone eventually lose the function of the affected kidney either from pyelonephritis or from unavoidable nephrectomy. Modern post-operative treatment

can probably improve these rather pessimistic figures.

Urinary stones may be classified into four main groups according to their chemical composition:

(a) Stones composed of *calcium phosphate*, *magnesium ammonium phosphate, calcium carbonate*, or varying mixtures of these three insoluble salts. These stones usually, but not invariably, are formed in an alkaline and infected urine and account for about one-third of all urinary calculi.

(b) *Calcium oxalate calculi*. These stones are much smaller in diameter and account for about one-quarter of urinary calculi. They usually, but not invariably, occur in an acid and uninfected urine.

(c) *The mixed stone*, which is equally common, is chemically a mixture of calcium oxalate and one or several of the insoluble salts listed as forming stones of the first group.

(d) Stones composed of *insoluble organic compounds* of which the most important is *uric acid*. *Cystine* stones are much less common and account for less than 1 % of calculi, whilst *xanthine* stones are extremely rare, only about 25 authenticated examples having been described. Uric acid and xanthine stones are radio-translucent, but cystine stones are radio-opaque even if they contain no calcium. Their radiological density is approximately equivalent to stones formed of magnesium ammonium phosphate, and is considerably less than that of stones formed predominantly of calcium salts.

The most important aetiological factor in the formation of calculi of the first group is urinary infection with "urea-splitting" organisms which actively form ammonia with increased alkalinity of the urine. This type of calculus is especially common in certain Asiatic countries where the combination of a tropical climate resulting in a concentrated and scanty urine, and a vitamin A-deficient diet, is especially conducive to stone formation. Any disease resulting in a high excretion of Ca and phosphate may be complicated by stones of this type. These conditions include hyperparathyroidism, carcinomatosis of bone, multiple myelomatosis, vitamin D intoxication, some cases of sarcoidosis with hypercalcaemia, excessive milk and alkali intake in the treatment of duodenal ulcer, immobilization osteoporosis and idiopathic hypercalciuria. Many of these conditions are associated with hypercalcaemia, and determinations of serum and urinary Ca should always be made in cases of urinary lithiasis. In immobilization osteoporosis two separate factors are conducive to formation of calculi. Lack of movement and change of position results in stasis of urine within the renal pelves, with greater tendency to crystallization of insoluble salts and consequent stone formation. The osteoporosis produced by the immobilization leads to about 50% increase of Ca excretion (Cordonnier & Talbot, 1948). Idiopathic hypercalciuria (Flocks, 1940) is a condition in which there is increased Ca excretion despite a normal serum Ca, and in which all other causes have been excluded. It is naturally rarely diagnosed except in cases of renal stones.

Calcium oxalate stones tend to occur in individuals excreting increased quantities of oxalate. The metabolism of oxalic acid has been reviewed in detail by Jeghers & Murphy (1945). Urinary oxalate is both exogenous and endogenous in origin. The normal blood oxalate ranges from 0·25 to 0·75 mg./100 ml. (Barrett, 1943), and the average urinary excretion is 33 mg. each day. The amount excreted increases after ingestion of vegetables of high oxalate content, e.g. spinach and rhubarb, and is reduced by a high-Ca diet which tends to precipitate insoluble calcium oxalate in the gut. Oxalate calculi are therefore especially common with vegetarian diets deficient in high-Ca dairy foods. These calculi were frequent in central European countries soon after World War I, when they accounted for as many as 65 to 90% of all urinary stones (Grossmann, 1938).

Uric acid calculi are common in gout which is associated with an increased excretion of uric acid. About 10% of cases have urinary complications from uric acid stones or from renal failure secondary to deposition of urates in the region of the distal tubules. A high fluid intake is especially desirable in cases of gout at the commencement of therapy with uricosuric drugs. The use of probenecid (Benemid) is particularly liable to be associated with a high urinary uric acid content at the start of treatment. Diseases of the haemopoietic system associated with increased cellular turnover, e.g. leukaemia and polycythaemia vera, are also occasionally liable to be complicated by uric acid calculi. The related radio-translucent xanthine stones are extremely rare, and the metabolic anomaly which causes a high excretion of this very insoluble purine is not fully understood. Dent & Philpot (1954) have reported a case in which the blood uric acid was found to be very low and almost all the urinary purine was xanthine, only traces of uric acid being found. It was concluded that the disorder could be explained either by a renal abnormality of diminished tubular reabsorption of xanthine or by a general metabolic anomaly with deficiency of the enzyme, xanthine oxidase. The recent studies of Dickinson &

Smellie (1959) suggest that there is a combination of absence of xanthine oxidase, and absence of the renal tubular reabsorptive mechanism for xanthine. Xanthine oxidase is present in high concentration in human milk, but there has been no opportunity to date for examination of a lactating female with this anomaly. If the condition is hereditary, it must be due to a recessive factor, since the parents of cases are normal. Cystine stones occur in most examples of homozygous cystinuria. They are never found in other conditions associated with increase of urine cystine, e.g. Fanconi syndrome and Wilson's disease, since the amount of cystine excreted is much less than in cystinuria. In particular, the condition of cystinosis in which cystine crystals occur in various organs, e.g. liver, lymph glands and bone marrow, is never complicated by cystine lithiasis.

Cystine calculi are liable to occur if the urine contains more than 250 mg. cystine/g. creatinine, corresponding to a daily output in adults of more than 400 mg. cystine (Harris & Warren, 1953). This high level of excretion only occurs in homozygous individuals, heterozygotes excreting either lower or normal amounts of cystine. The solubility of cystine is less in acid solutions, and therefore precipitation occurs particularly at night when the urine is both highly acid and more concentrated than in the day. The maintenance of a high urinary output at night is therefore of especial importance in therapy (Dent & Senior, 1955).

Medical measures are usually of little value in the treatment of calculi that have already formed, but are of great importance in preventing recurrence after surgery. The single most important item is a constant large fluid intake producing a dilute urine which should preferably be kept below a specific gravity of 1010. Urinary infection should always be adequately treated, and any anatomical abnormality interfering with free urinary drainage should be corrected. Patients kept in bed for long periods, and especially patients immobilized in plaster casts, etc., should be treated by physiotherapy and their position should be frequently changed to prevent stasis. All urinary calculi should be analysed, since recurrent stones are usually of similar composition. Calculi of the first group are best prevented by keeping the urine acid in reaction. Treatment with NaH_2PO_4 at a dosage of 1 g. four times daily is preferable to the use of NH_4Cl. The former tends to diminish Ca absorption by precipitation of calcium phosphate in the gut, whilst NH_4Cl always increases urinary Ca output. Any condition tending to produce hypercalciuria should be treated, and the intake of high calcium foods should be avoided. Shorr

(1945) has recommended the use of aluminium hydroxide gels which diminish phosphate absorption by precipitation of aluminium phosphate in the gut. This cannot be used in conjunction with NaH_2PO_4, and adequate doses are extremely constipating. In the prevention of recurrence of oxalate calculi, vegetables of high oxalate content should be avoided, but control of the urinary reaction is unimportant. Uric acid and cystine are both more soluble in alkaline urines, and therefore the urine should be kept alkaline by prescription of sodium citrate. Dietary measures are of no importance in the case of cystine lithiasis, but a high-purine diet should be avoided in uric acid and xanthine lithiasis.

Scott, Huggins & Selman (1943) considered that a reduction in the excretion of citrate was of importance in production of Ca stones, since citrate forms a soluble chelation compound with Ca. Conway, Maitland & Rennie (1949) confirmed that urinary lithiasis was often associated with reduction of urinary citrate, but showed that this occurred only in infected urines. Urinary citrate was found to be rapidly destroyed by many organisms, and it appears therefore that citrate is of no importance in the causation or prevention of calculi. Butt, Hauser & Seifter (1952) considered that urinary colloids were of especial importance in prevention of stone formation, and that they could be increased by injections of hyaluronidase with consequent alteration of urinary surface tension. This work has not been confirmed, and one case has been reported in which use of hyaluronidase appeared to encourage recurrence (Prien, 1954). Smiddy (1954) has shown that urinary surface tension is very variable, being inversely proportional to the specific gravity, and that it is not influenced by hyaluronidase. The development of experimental urinary stones in rats was not significantly affected by hyaluronidase.

PRIMARY HYPEROXALURIA

Primary hyperoxaluria is a rare metabolic abnormality probably due to recessive heredity, and is characterized clinically by bilateral calcium oxalate nephrocalcinosis and urolithiasis. Death invariably occurs from renal failure in childhood or early adult life. There is an increased urinary output of oxalate, usually from 100 to 400 mg. daily, as compared to the normal maximum of 40 mg./day. At necropsy there is destruction of renal tubular cells with secondary renal fibrosis, and deposits of calcium oxalate are present both in the renal cortex and medulla. Bilateral calcium oxalate calculi with secondary hydronephrosis and pyelonephritis are frequently present. Calcium

oxalate crystals are usually also found in extrarenal sites, especially in cartilage, myocardium, bone marrow, lymph nodes, spleen, and in the walls of blood vessels.

The urinary oxalate is endogenous and not exogenous in origin. Normally glycine is the precursor of at least 40% of urinary oxalate (Elder & Wyngaarden, 1959; Crawhall, de Mowbray, Scowen & Watts, 1959), and the conversion is approximately the same in hyperoxaluria. The clearance of oxalate is higher than the glomerular filtration rate, there being proximal tubular secretion of the acid (Spencer, 1962). The plasma level of oxalate in normal subjects has been estimated as less than 0·8 mg./100 ml. (Crawhall & Watts, 1961). The defect is presumably related to glyoxylate metabolism, this being derived from glycine by transamination. Glyoxylate is normally metabolized in four separate ways:

(a) transamination to glycine,
(b) reduction to glycollic acid,
(c) oxidative degradation to formate and CO_2,
(d) oxidation to oxalic acid.

Presumably in hyperoxaluria there is depression of one or more of the first three pathways with corresponding excess conversion of glycine to oxalate. High concentrations of oxalate in body fluids lead to deposition of crystals of calcium oxalate, and tissue damage, especially to the renal tubular cells.

There is no effective therapy known, the disease being uniformly fatal. In the terminal uraemic stage of the disease urinary oxalate falls to normal levels or less, and the diagnosis may therefore be difficult or impossible if patients are first investigated in the later stages of the condition.

The metabolic defect in primary hyperoxaluria has recently been clarified, but no advances in treatment have been made. It now seems probable that there are two distinct varieties of the condition, which are indistinguishable on clinical grounds alone (Williams & Smith, 1968). The type I variety is due to absence of the enzyme 2-oxoglutarate:glyoxylate carboligase in liver, kidney and spleen (Koch, Stokstad, Williams & Smith, 1967). In this disease the urinary oxalate averages 250 mg./24 hr./1·73 sq. m. surface area, and the urinary glycollic acid 250 in the same units (normal figures are below 50 and 60 mg./24 hr./ 1·73 sq. m. surface area). The type II disease is due to absence of D-glyceric dehydrogenase. In this disorder urinary oxalate averages 150 and urinary L-glyceric acid 400 mg./24 hr./1·73 sq. m. surface area. Only small amounts of L-glyceric acid occur in normal urine. In type II oxaluria glycollate output is below normal values, indicating a reduced conversion of glyoxylate to glycollate. The reason for the increased urinary output of oxalate in the Type II disease is not certain, but probably D-glyceric dehydrogenase and the enzyme involved in the reduction of glyoxylate to glycollic acid are identical. Thus more glyoxylate is available for conversion to oxalate. As would be expected in a generalized metabolic disorder, transplanted kidneys in patients with terminal renal failure from hyperoxaluria become involved in the disease process, and deposition of calcium oxalate rapidly occurs.

CARCINOMA OF THE PROSTATE

Kutscher & Wolbergs (1935) showed that prostatic tissue is rich in acid phosphatase. Gutman & Gutman (1938) found that this enzyme was present in increased amounts in the serum of 11 out of 15 cases of prostatic carcinoma with metastases. They noted that the serum alkaline phosphatase was also raised in most cases with skeletal metastases. Huggins & Hodges (1941) found that castration or the administration of oestrogens to such patients resulted in a prompt fall in the serum acid phosphatase with clinical improvement. The administration of androgens was shown to have the opposite effect. The serum alkaline phosphatase often temporarily increased during phases of remission, owing to increased osteoblastic activity with new bone formation. These classical observations have stimulated a vast amount of work on the therapy of prostatic carcinoma, and endocrine control remains the best example of effective chemotherapy for malignant disease.

The most satisfactory method for determination of serum acid phosphatase is the modification by Gutman & Gutman (1938) of the King & Armstrong (1934) phenyl phosphate method. Normal serum contains 1–5 King-Armstrong units/100 ml. Since similar figures are found in serum from females, it is obvious that a proportion of the phosphatase is not of prostatic origin. There are at least two acid phosphatases in normal serum of non-prostatic origin, one of which is derived from erythrocytes. Methods which differentiate prostatic phosphatase by specific inactivation techniques have therefore proved of great value in diagnosis. Herbert (1946) found that incubation with 40% alcohol for 30 min. inactivated prostatic phosphatase, whilst Abul-Fadl & King (1948) showed that 0·5% formaldehyde completely inactivates erythrocyte phosphatase, but has no effect on the prostatic enzyme. The latter workers give the following figures for values of formaldehyde-stable serum acid phosphatase: Normal—0–3 units/100 ml.; "suspicious"—3–5 units/100 ml.; diagnostic of prostatic carcinoma—above 5 units/100 ml.

Woodard & Dean (1947) found that determination of the serum acid phosphatase was of no value in the early diagnosis of prostatic carcinoma before metastasis had occurred. Although no false positive diagnoses were observed, false negative results were recorded in 60% of cases clinically free from metastasis. Even in cases with obvious skeletal metastases, as many as 28% false negative results were recorded. It was thought that only fairly well-differentiated prostatic carcinomata were capable of production of the enzyme, the highly anaplastic forms accounting for the false negative figures. Nesbit & Baum (1950) have reported on an extensive statistical survey of the results of endocrine therapy. They found that general well-being, and both 3- and 5-year survival rates were improved by therapy. In cases with metastasis, castration alone and use of oestrogens alone were of about equal value, but combined therapy gave more favourable survival rates. In the cases with metastasis, oestrogen therapy was less effective than castration, and in fact did not significantly improve the 5-year survival figures despite symptomatic relief. About 30% of cases with metastasis showed no response to endocrine therapy, the tumour being completely androgen-independent.

After a period of satisfactory control by castration and oestrogens, most cases eventually relapse with increase of symptoms and a rising serum acid phosphatase. Huggins & Scott (1945) considered that the tumour was then being stimulated by androgens produced by the adrenal cortex, and attempted to prolong the remission by bilateral adrenalectomy. The results were unsatisfactory owing to the inadequate steroid maintenance therapy available at that time. More success was obtained seven years later when cortisone was available for post-operative maintenance. Six cases were treated (Huggins & Bergenstal, 1952), and four improved with relief of intractable bone pain, gain of weight and decrease of the raised serum acid phosphatase.

Some cases of prostatic carcinoma with skeletal metastases are complicated by a haemorrhagic tendency which may be secondary to thrombocytopenia associated with leuco-erythroblastic anaemia from bone marrow involvement. In other cases the platelet count is normal and the presence of an abnormal fibrinolysin with fibrinogenopenia has been demonstrated in the blood (Tagnon, Schulman, Whitmore & Leone, 1953).

The fibrinolysin is produced by the prostatic tissue in the same manner as is the acid phosphatase, and is similarly reduced by oestrogens and in-creased by androgens. Operative procedures should preferably be postponed if a circulating fibrinolysin is demonstrated.

References

ABUL-FADL, M. A. M. & KING, E. J. (1948). *J. clin. Path.*, **1**, 80.

ADDIS, T. (1948). "Glomerulo-nephritis". New York, Macmillan.

ADDIS, T. & SHEVKY, M. C. (1922). *Arch. intern. Med.*, **30**, 559.

ALBRIGHT, F., CONSOLAZIO, W. V., COOMBS, F. S., SULKOWITCH, H. W. & TALBOTT, J. H. (1940). *Bull. Johns Hopk. Hosp.*, **66**, 7.

ALBRIGHT, F. & REIFENSTEIN, E. C. (1948). "The Parathyroid Glands and Metabolic Bone Disease". London, Bailliere, Tindall & Cox.

ALWALL, N. (1947). *Acta med. scand.*, **128**, 317.

ASHE, B. I. & MOSENTHAL, H. O. (1937). *J. Amer. med. Ass.*, **109**, 1160.

AUSTIN, J. H., STILLMAN, E. & VAN SLYKE, D. D. (1921). *J. biol. Chem.*, **46**, 91.

BARNETT, H. L., FORMAN, C. & LAUSON, H. D. (1952). *Advanc. Pediat.*, **5**, 53.

BARNETT, H. L., MCNAMARA, H., MCCRORY, W., FORMAN, C., RAPAPORT, M., MICHIE, A. & BARBERO, G. (1950). *Amer. J. Dis. Child.*, **80**, 519.

BARNETT, H. L., SIMONS, D. J. & WELLS, R. E. (1948). *Amer. J. Med.*, **4**, 760.

BARR, D. P., RUSS, E. M. & EDER, H. A. (1951). *Amer. J. Med.*, **11**, 480.

BARRETT, J. F. B. (1943). *Biochem. J.*, **37**, 254.

BAUMRUCKER, G. O. (1943). *J. Urol.*, **50**, 290.

BAXTER, J. H., GOODMAN, H. C. & ALLEN, J. C. (1961). *J. clin. Invest.*, **40**, 490.

BEER, E. (1937). *J. Mt. Sinai Hosp.*, **3**, 193.

BERLINER, R. W. (1961). *Harvey Lect.*, **55**, 141.

BERLINER, R. W., HILTON, J. G., YU, T. F. & KENNEDY, T. J. (1950). *J. clin. Invest.*, **29**, 396.

BERLINER, R. W., KENNEDY, T. J. & HILTON, J. G. (1950). *Amer. J. Physiol.*, **162**, 348.

BERLINER, R. W., KENNEDY, T. J. & ORLOFF, J. (1951). *Amer. J. Med.*, **11**, 274.

BERLYNE, G. M. (1965). *Amer. Heart J.*, **70**, 143.

BERLYNE, G. M., JANABI, K., SHAW, A. B. & HOCKEN, A. G. (1966). *Lancet*, **1**, 169.

BERLYNE, G. M. & SHAW, A. B. (1965). *Lancet*, **2**, 7.

BICKEL, H., SMALLWOOD, W. C., SMELLIE, J. M. & HICKMANS, E. M. (1952). *Acta paediatr.* (Stockh.), Suppl. 90, 27.

BISHOP, C., ZIMDAHL, W. T. & TALBOTT, J. H. (1954). *Proc. Soc. exp. Biol.* (N.Y.), **86**, 440.

BLACK, D. A. K. (1953). *Lancet*, **1**, 305.

BLACK, D. A. K. & MILNE, M. D. (1952). *Clin. Sci.*, **11**, 397.

BLACK, D. A. K., PLATT, R., ROWLANDS, E. N. & VARLEY, H. (1948). *Clin. Sci.*, **6**, 295.

BLACKBURN, C. R. B., HENSLEY, W. J., GRANT, D. K. & WRIGHT, F. B. (1954). *J. clin. Invest.*, **33**, 825.

BLAHD, W. H. & BASSETT, S. H. (1953). *Metabolism*, **2**, 218.

BLAINEY, J. D., BREWER, D. B., HARDWICKE, J. & SOOTHILL, J. F. (1960). *Quart. J. Med.*, n.s., **29**, 235.

BLOOMER, H. A., RECTOR, F. C., Jr. & SELDIN, D. W. (1963). *J. clin. Invest.*, **42**, 277.

BLUEMLE, L. W., Jr., WEBSTER, G. D., Jr., ELKINTON, J. R. (1959). *Arch. intern. Med.*, **104**, 180.

BOTT, P. A. (1953). Transactions of the Fifth Conference on Renal Function. New York. Josiah Macy Jr. Foundation.

BOYCE, W. H. (1951). *J. Urol.*, **65**, 241.

BRADLEY, S. E. (1949). *Amer. J. Med.*, **7**, 382.

BRADLEY, S. E., CHASIS, H., GOLDRING, W. & SMITH, H. W. (1945). *J. clin. Invest.*, **24**, 749.

BRADLEY, S. E., LARAGH, J. H., WHEELER, H. O., MACDOWELL, M. & OLIVER, J. (1961). *J. clin. Invest.*, **40**, 1113.

BRAZEAU, P. & GILMAN, A. (1953). *Amer. J. Physiol.*, **175**, 33.

BRECKENRIDGE, A. & METCALFE-GIBSON, A. (1965). *Lancet*, **2**, 265.

BRIGGS, A. P. (1947). *Exp. Med. Surg.*, **5**, 128.

BROD, J. & SIROTA, J. H. (1948). *J. clin. Invest.*, **27**, 645.

BRODSKY, W. A. & GRAUBARTH, H. N. (1953). *Amer. J. Physiol.*, **172**, 67.

BROWN, M. R., CURRENS, J. H. & MARCHAND, J. F. (1944). *J. Amer. med. Ass.*, **125**, 545.

BRUCK, E., RAPOPORT, M. & RUBIN, M. I. (1954). *J. clin. Invest.*, **33**, 699.

BRUN, C., CRONE, C., DAVIDSEN, H. G., FABRICIUS, J., HANSEN, A. T., LASSEN, N. A. & MUNCK, O. (1955). *Proc. Soc. Exper. Biol. & Med.*, **89**, 687.

BULGER, H. A. & JOHNS, H. E. (1941). *J. biol. Chem.*, **140**, 427.

BULL, G. M. (1948). *Clin. Sci.*, **7**, 77.

BULL, G. M., CARTER, A. B. & LOWE, K. G. (1953). *Lancet*, **2**, 60.

BULL, G. M., JOEKES, A. M. & LOWE, K. G. (1950). *Clin. Sci.*, **9**, 379.

BURSTON, R. A. & GARROD, O. (1952). *Clin. Sci.*, **11**, 129.

BUTLER, A. M., WILSON, J. L. & FARBER, S. (1936). *J. Pediat.*, **8**, 489.

BUTT, A. J., HAUSER, E. A. & SEIFTER, J. (1952). *J. Amer. med. Ass.*, **150**, 1096.

CARGILL, W. H. (1949). *J. clin. Invest.*, **28**, 533.

CARTWRIGHT, G. E., GUBLER, C. J. & WINTROBE, M. M. (1954). *J. clin. Invest.*, **33**, 685.

CHARLWOOD, P. A. (1952). *Biochem. J.*, **51**, 113.

CHASIS, H. & REDISH, J. (1942). *Arch. intern. Med.*, **70**, 738.

CHASIS, H. & SMITH, H. W. (1938). *J. clin. Invest.*, **17**, 347.

CHILDS, D. S., Jr., KEATING, F. R., RALL, J. E., WILLIAMS, M. M. D. & POWER, M. H. (1950). *J. clin. Invest.*, **29**, 726.

CHINARD, F. P., LAUSON, H. D. & EDER, H. A. (1952). *J. clin. Invest.*, **31**, 895.

CHINARD, F. P., LAUSON, H. D., EDER, H. A., GREIF, R. L. & HILLER, A. (1954). *J. clin. Invest.*, **33**, 621.

CLAPP, J. R., WATSON, J. F. & BERLINER, R. W. (1963). *Amer. J. Physiol.*, **205**, 273.

CLARKE, E., EVANS, B. M., MACINTYRE, I. & MILNE, M. D. (1955). *Clin. Sci.*, **14**, 421.

CONN, J. W. (1955). *J. Lab. clin. Med.*, **45**, 3 & 661.

CONNOR, T. B., THOMAS, W. C., HADDOCK, L. & HOWARD, J. E. (1960). *Ann. intern. Med.*, **52**, 544.

CONWAY, E. I. (1950). "Microdiffusion Analysis and Volumetric Error". 3rd Ed. London, Lockwood.

CONWAY, N. S., MAITLAND, A. I. L. & RENNIE, J. B. (1949). *Brit. J. Urol.*, **21**, 30.

COOK, W. F. & PICKERING, G. W. (1959). *J. Physiol.*, **149**, 526.

COOKE, R. E., SEGAR, W. E., CHEEK, D. B., COVILLE, F. E. & DARROW, D. C. (1952). *J. clin. Invest.*, **31**, 798.

CORDONNIER, J. J. & TALBOT, B. S. (1948). *J. Urol.*, **60**, 316.

COUNIHAN, T. B., EVANS, B. M. & MILNE, M. D (1954). *Clin. Sci.*, **13**, 583.

CRAWHALL, J. C., DE MOWBRAY, R. R., SCOWEN, E. F. & WATTS, R. W. E. (1959). *Lancet*, **2**, 810.

CRAWHALL, J. C. & WATTS, R. W. E. (1961). *Clin. Sci.*, **20**, 357.

CREEVY, C. D. & REISER, M. P. (1952). *Surg. Gynec. Obstet.*, **95**, 589.

CUSHNY, A. R. (1926). "The Secretion of the Urine". 2nd Ed. London, Longmans Green.

DAMMIN, G., COUCH, N. P. & MURRAY, J. E. (1957). *Ann. N.Y. Acad. Sci.*, **64**, 967.

DAVIES, B. M. A. & YUDKIN, J. (1952). *Biochem. J.*, **52**, 407.

DENT, C. E. & PHILPOT, G. R. (1954). *Lancet*, **1**, 182.

DENT, C. E. & SENIOR, B. (1955). *Brit. J. Urol.*, **27**, 317.

DÉROT, M. & LEGRAIN, M. (1954). *Bull. Acad. nat. Méd.*, (Paris), **138**, 37.

DEROW, H. A. (1942). *New Engl. J. Med.*, **227**, 827.

DEROW, H. A., SCHLESINGER, M. J. & SAVITZ, H. A. (1939). *Arch. intern. Med.*, **63**, 626.

DESAULLES, P., TRIPOD, J. & SCHULER, W. (1953). *Schweiz. med. Wschr.*, **83**, 1088.

DICKINSON, C. J. & SMELLIE, J. M. (1959). *Brit. med. J.*, **2**, 1217.

DIEFENBACH, W. C. L., FISK, S. C. & GILSON, S. B. (1951). *New Engl. J. Med.*, **244**, 326.

DIRKS, J. H., CLAPP, J. R. & BERLINER, R. W. (1964). *J. clin. Invest.*, **43**, 916.

DOLE, V. P., EMERSON, K., Jr., PHILLIPS, R. A., HAMILTON, P. & VAN SLYKE, D. D. (1946). *Amer. J. Physiol.*, **145**, 337.

DORMAN, P. J., SULLIVAN, W. J. & PITTS, R. F. (1954). *J. clin. Invest.*, **33**, 82.

EARLE, D. P., Jr., TAGGART, J. V. & SHANNON, J. A. (1944). *J. clin. Invest.*, **23**, 119.

EDER, H. A., LAUSON, H. D., CHINARD, F. P., GREIF, R. L., COTZIAS, G. C. & VAN SLYKE, D. D. (1954). *J. clin. Invest.*, **33**, 636.

EDWARDS, D. (1960). In "Recent Advances in Renal Disease". Ed. Milne, M. D. p. 145. Pitman Medical Publishing Co.

EKINS, R. P., NASHAT, F. S., PORTAL, R. W. & SGHERZI, A. M. (1966). *J. Physiol.*, **186**, 347.

ELDER, T. D. & WYNGAARDEN, J. B. (1959). *J. clin. Invest.*, **38**, 1001.

ELLIS, A. (1942). *Lancet*, **1**, 1.

ELWOOD, C. M., SIGMAN, E. M. & TREGER, C. (1967). *Brit. J. Radiol.*, **40**, 581.

EMERSON, K., ROCHE, M., KAHN, S. S., MOSER, H. W. & JENKINS, D. (1951). *J. clin. Invest.*, **30**, 637.

ENTICKNAP, J. B. (1952). *Lancet*, **2**, 458.

EPSTEIN, A. A. (1926). *J. Amer. med. Ass.*, **87**, 913.

EVANS, B. M., HUGHES JONES, N. C., MILNE, M. D. & STEINER, S. (1954). *Clin. Sci.*, **13**, 305.

EVANS, B. M. & MILNE, M. D. (1954). *Brit. med. J.*, **2**, 1067.

FARR, L. E. (1938). *Amer. J. Dis. Child.*, **56**, 309.

FARR, L. E., GAMBLE, J. L., FOSTER, C. G. & ROBERTSON, J. S. (1951). *Amer. J. Dis. Child.*, **82**, 247.

FASOLI, A. (1953). *Acta med. scand.*, **145**, 233.

FERGUSON, E. B. (1951). *J. Physiol.*, **112**, 420.

FERRIS, D. O. & ODEL, H. M. (1950). *J. Amer. med. Ass.*, **142**, 634.

FINKENSTAEDT, J. T., O'MEARA, M. P., WELLER, J. M. & MERRILL, J. P. (1953). *J. clin. Invest.*, **32**, 567.

FLOCKS, R. H. (1940). *J. Urol.*, **44**, 183.

FOLEY, T. H., JONES, N. F. & CLAPHAM, W. F. (1966). *Lancet*, **2**, 86.

FORSSMAN, H. (1945). *Acta med. scand.*, Suppl. 159.

FOULKS, J., MUDGE, G. H. & GILMAN, A. (1952). *Amer. J. Physiol.*, **168**, 642.

FOURMAN, P., REIFENSTEIN, E. C., KEPLER, E. J., DEMPSEY, E., BARTTER, F. & ALBRIGHT, F. (1952). *Metabolism*, **1**, 242.

FRANGLEN, G. T., McGARRY, E. & SPENCER, A. G. (1953). *J. Physiol.*, **121**, 35.

FREIDMAN, M., ROSEMAN, R. H. & BYERS, S. O. (1954). *J. clin. Invest.*, **33**, 1103.

GAMBLE, J. L. (1951a). "Chemical Anatomy, Physiology, and Pathology of Extracellular Fluid". 5th Ed. Cambridge, Mass., Harvard University Press.

GAMBLE, J. L. (1951b). *Lane Medical Lectures*, **5**, 9.

GAMBLE, J. L. & BUTLER, A. M. (1944). *Trans. Ass. Amer. Physns.*, **58**, 157.

GARDNER, L. I., MACLACHLAN, E. A. & BERMAN, H. (1952). *J. gen. Physiol.*, **36**, 153.

GARNETT, E. S., PARSONS, V. & VEALL, N. (1967). *Lancet*, **1**, 818.

GARROD, O. & BURSTON, R. A. (1952). *Clin. Sci.*, **11**, 113.

GILLIGAN, D. R., ALTSCHULE, M. D. & KATERSKY, E. M. (1941). *J. clin. Invest.*, **20**, 177.

GIORDANO, C. (1963). *J. Lab. clin. Med.*, **62**, 231.

GIOVANNETTI, S. & MAGGIORE, Q. (1964). *Lancet*, **1**, 1000.

GITLIN, D. & JANEWAY, C. A. (1952). *J. clin. Invest.*, **31**, 223.

GOFMAN, J. W., GLAZIER, F., TAMPLIN, A., STRISOWER, B. & DE LALLA, O. (1954). *Physiol. Rev.*, **34**, 589.

GOFMAN, J. W., RUBIN, L., MCGINLEY, J. P. & JONES, H. B. (1954). *Amer. J. Med.*, **17**, 514.

GOLDRING, W. & CHASIS, H. (1944). "Hypertension and Hypertensive Disease". N.Y. Commonwealth Fund.

GOLDRING, W., CLARKE, R. W. & SMITH, H. W. (1936). *J. clin. Invest.*, **15**, 221.

GORDON, A. H., GROSS, J., O'CONNOR, D. & PITT-RIVERS, R. (1952). *Nature*, **169**, 19.

GORDON, R. S., BOYLE, E., BROWN, R. K., CHERKES, A. & ANFINSEN, C. B. (1953). *Proc. Soc. exp. Biol. (N.Y.)*, **84**, 168.

GOTTSCHALK, C. W., LASSITER, W. E. & MYLLE, M. (1960). *Amer. J. Physiol.*, **198**, 581.

GOTTSCHALK, C. W. & MYLLE, M. (1959). *Amer. J. Physiol.*, **196**, 927.

GOVAERTS, P. (1952). *Brit. med. J.*, **2**, 175.

GRABER, I. G. & SHACKMAN, R. (1956). *Brit. med. J.*, **1**, 1321.

GRAVES, R. C. & BUDDINGTON, W. T. (1950). *J. Urol.*, **63**, 261.

GROLLMAN, E. F. & GROLLMAN, A. (1959). *J. clin. Invest.*, **38**, 749.

GROSSMAN, W. (1938). *Brit. J. Urol.*, **10**, 46.

GUTMAN, A. B. (1948). *Advanc. Protein Chem.*, **4**, 155.

GUTMAN, A. B. & GUTMAN, E. B. (1938). *J. clin. Invest.*, **17**, 473.

GUTMAN, A. B., YÜ, T. F. & BERGER, L. (1959). *J. clin Invest.*, **38**, 1778.

GUYTON, A. C. (1963). *Physiologist*, **6**, 194.

HAMBURGER, J. & MATHÉ, G. (1964). In Ciba Foundation Symposium on The Kidney. London, Churchill.

HANDLER, J. S. (1960). *J. clin. Invest.*, **39**, 1526.

HARDWICKE, J. (1965). *Clin. Chim. Acta*, **12**, 89.

HARRIS, H. & WARREN, F. L. (1953). *Ann. Eugen.*, **18**, 125.

HERBERT, F. K. (1946). *Quart. J. Med.*, **15**, n.s., 221.

HEYMANN, W. & HACKEL, D. B. (1952). *J. Lab. clin. Med.*, **39**, 429.

HEYMANN, W. & LUND, H. Z. (1951). *Pediatrics*, **7**, 691.

HIRSCHFELDER, A. D. (1934). *J. Amer. med. Ass.*, **102**, 1138.

HOLMBERG, C. G. & LAURELL, C. B. (1948). *Acta chem. scand.*, **2**, 550.

HOWELL, R. R., ASHTON, D. M. & WYNGAARDEN, J. B. (1962). *Pediatrics*, **29**, 553.

HUGGINS, C. & BERGENSTAL, D. M. (1952). *Cancer Res.*, **12**, 134.

HUGGINS, C. & HODGES, C. V. (1941). *Cancer Res.*, **1**, 293.

HUGGINS, C. & SCOTT, W. W. (1945). *Ann. Surg.*, **122**, 1031.

HULME, B. & HARDWICKE, J. (1966). *Proc. Roy. Soc. Med.*, **59**, 509.

HUME, D. M., LEE, H. M., WILLIAMS, G. M., WHITE, H. J. O., FERRE, J., WOLF, J. S., PROUT, G. R., Jr., SLAPAK, M., O'BRIEN, J., KILPATRICK, S. J., KAUFFMAN, H. M., Jr. & CLEVELAND, R. J. (1966). *Ann. Surg.*, **164**, 352.

HUME, D. M., MERRILL, J. P., MILLER, B. F. & THORN, G. W. (1955). *J. clin. Invest.*, **34**, 327.

IACOBELLIS, M., MUNTWYLER, E. & GRIFFEN, G. E. (1954). *Amer. J. Physiol.*, **178**, 477.

IVERSEN, P. & BRUN, C. (1951). *Amer. J. Med.*, **11**, 324.

JACOBS, A. & STIRLING, W. B. (1952). *Brit. J. Urol.*, **24**, 259.

JAHNKE, K. & SCHOLTAN, W. (1953). *Dtsch. Arch. klin. Med.*, **200**, 821.

JAMES, J., GORDILLO, G. & METCOFF, J. (1954). *J. clin. Invest.*, **33**, 1346.

JAYLE, M. F., BOUSSIER, G. & BADIN, J. (1952). *Bull. Soc. Chim. Biol.* (Paris), **34**, 1063.

JEGHERS, H. & MURPHY, R. (1945). *New Engl. J. Med.*, **233**, 208 & 238.

KARK, R. M. & MUEHRCKE, R. C. (1954). *Lancet*, **1**, 1047.

KEKWICK, A., PAULLEY, J. W., RICHES, E. W. & SEMPLE, R. (1951). *Brit. J. Urol.*, **23**, 112.

KELLETT, C. E. (1952). *Lancet*, **2**, 911.

KELLEY, V. C., ZIEGLER, M. R., DOEDEN, D. & MCQUARRIE, I. (1950). *Proc. Soc. exp. Biol. (N.Y.)*, **75**, 153.

KEMPNER, W. (1948). *Amer. J. Med.*, **4**, 545.

KENNEDY, T. J. & KLEH, J. (1953). *J. clin. Invest.*, **32**, 90.

KENNEDY, A. C., LINTON, A. L. & EATON, J. C. (1962). *Lancet*, **1**, 410.

KIIL, F. (1960). *Acta chir. scand. supp.*, **253**, 142.

KING, E. J. & ARMSTRONG, A. R. (1934). *Canad. med. Ass. J.*, **31**, 376.

KING, S. E. (1954). *J. Amer. med. Ass.*, **155**, 1023.

KING, S. E. & BALDWIN, D. S. (1954). *Proc. Soc. exp. Biol. (N.Y.)*, **86**, 634.

KING, S. E. & GRONBECK, C. (1952). *Ann. intern. Med.*, **36**, 765.

KIRKPATRICK, C. H., WILSON, W. E., TALMAGE, D. W. (1964). *J. Exp. Med.*, **119**, 727.

KOCH, J., STOKSTAD, E. L. R., WILLIAMS, H. E. & SMITH, L. H. (1967). *Proc. Nat. Acad.*, **57**, 1123.

KOLFF, W. J. & WATSCHINGER, B. (1956). *J. Lab. clin. Med.*, **47**, 969.

KOUNTZ, S. L., LAUB, D. R. & COHN, R. (1965). *J. Amer. Med. Assoc.*, **191**, 997.

KUNKEL, H. G. & SLATER, R. J. (1952). *J. clin. Invest.*, **31**, 677.

KUTSCHER, W. & WOLBERGS, H. (1935). *Hoppe-Seyl. Z.*, **236**, 237.

LAGRUE, G., MOZZICONACCI, P. & VIALATTE, J. (1954). *Ann. Méd.*, **55**, 196.

LAMBERT, P. P. & DE HEINZELIN DE BRAUCOURT, C. (1951). *Acta clin. belg.*, **6**, 13.

LANGE, K., GRAIG, F., OBERMAN, J., SLOBODY, L., OGUR, G. & LOCASTO, F. (1951). *Arch. intern. Med.*, **88**, 433.

LATHEM, W. (1959). *J. clin. Invest.*, **38**, 652.

LATNER, A. L. & BURNARD, E. D. (1950). *Quart. J. Med.*, **19**, 285.

LAUSON, H. D., BRADLEY, S. E. & COURNAND, A. (1944). *J. clin. Invest.*, **23**, 381.

LAUSON, H. D., FORMAN, C. W., MCNAMARA, H., MATTAR, G. & BARNETT, H. L. (1954), *J. clin. Invest.*, **33**, 657.

LEAF, A. & CAMARA, A. A. (1949). *J. clin. Invest.*, **28**, 1526.

LEVINSKY, N. G. & BERLINER, R. W. (1959). *J. clin. Invest.*, **38**, 741.

LEVINSKY, N. G. & LALONE, R. C. (1963). *J. clin. Invest.*, **42**, 1261.

LEWIS, W. H., Jr. & ALVING, A. S. (1938). *Amer. J. Physiol.*, **123**, 500.

LICHTY, J. A., Jr., HAVILL, W. H. & WHIPPLE, G. H. (1932). *J. exp. Med.*, **55**, 603.

LIDDLE, G. W., BENNETT, L. L. & FORSHAM, P. H. (1953). *J. clin. Invest.*, **32**, 1197.

LIEBER, C. S., JONES, D. P., LOSOWSKY, M. S. & DAVIDSON, C S. (1962). *J. clin. Invest.*, **41**, 1863.

LIGHTWOOD, R. (1935). *Arch. Dis. Childh.*, **10**, 205.

LONDON, I. M., SABELLA, G. F. & YAMASAKI, M. M. (1951). *J. clin. Invest.*, **30**, 657.

LONG, J. H. (1903). *J. Amer. chem. Soc.*, **25**, 257.

LONGSON, D. & MILLS, J. N. (1953). *J. Physiol.*, **122**, 81.

LOWE, K. G. (1952). *Lancet*, **1**, 1086.

LOWE, K. G., MOODIE, G. & THOMSON, M. B. (1954). *Clin. Sci.*, **13**, 187.

LOTSPEICH, W. D. & PITTS, R. F. (1947). *J. biol. Chem.*, **168**, 611.

LOUGHRIDGE, L. W., MILNE, M. D., SHACKMAN, R. & WOOTTON, I. D. P. (1960). *Lancet*, **1**, 351.

LOWENSTEIN, J., FAULSTICK, D. A., YIENGST, M. J. & SHOCK, N. W. (1961). *J. clin. Invest.*, **40**, 1172.

LUETSCHER, J. A., Jr., DEMING, Q. B., JOHNSON, B. B. & PIEL, C. F. (1953). *J. Amer. med. Ass.*, **153**, 1236.

LUETSCHER, J. A., Jr., HALL, A. D. & KREMER, V. L. (1950). *J. clin. Invest.*, **29**, 896.

LUETSCHER, J. A., Jr. & JOHNSON, B. B. (1954). *J. clin. Invest.*, **33**, 1441.

LUETSCHER, J. A., Jr., NEHER, R. & WETTSTEIN, A. (1954). *Experientia*, **10**, 456.

LYTTLE, J. D., SEEGAL, D., LOEB, E. N. & JOST, E. L. (1938). *J. clin. Invest.*, **17**, 631.

MCCANCE, R. A. & WIDDOWSON, E. M. (1952). *Lancet*, **2**, 860.

MCPHAUL, J. J., MCINTOSH, D. A., HAMMOND, W. S. & PARK, O. K. (1964). *New England J. Med.*, **271**, 1342.

MAEGRAITH, B. G. (1944). *Trans. R. Soc. trop. Med. Hyg.*, **38**, 1.

MALNIC, G. & GIEBISCH, G. (1963). *Federation Proc.*, **22**, 631.

MATTAR, G., BARNETT, H. L., MCNAMARA, H. & LAUSON, H. D. (1952). *J. clin. Invest.*, **31**, 938.

MERONEY, W. H. & HERNDON, R. F. (1954). *J. Amer. med. Ass.*, **155**, 877.

METCOFF, J., NAKASONE, N. & RANCE, C. P. (1954). *J. clin. Invest.*, **33**, 665.

METCOFF, J., RANCE, C. P., KELSEY, W. M., NAKASONE, N. & JANEWAY, C. A. (1952). *Pediatrics*, **9**, 543.

MILLER, B. F. & DUBOS, R. (1937). *J. biol. Chem.*, **121**, 457.

MILLER, J. H. & MCDONALD, R. K. (1951). *J. clin. Invest.*, **30**, 1033.

MILLS, J. N., THOMAS, S. & WILLIAMSON, K. S. (1961). *J. Physiol.*, **156**, 415.

MILNE, M. D., SCRIBNER, B. H. & CRAWFORD, M. A. (1958). *Amer. J. Med.*, **24**, 709.

MILNE, M. D., LOUGHRIDGE, L., SHACKMAN, R. & STRUTHERS, N. J. (1960). In "Recent Advances in Renal Disease". Ed. Milne, M.D. Pitman Medical Publishing Co. Ltd.

MILNE, M. D., STANBURY, S. W. & THOMSON, A. E. (1952). *Quart. J. Med.*, **21**, 61.

MITCHELL, A. D. & VALK, W. L. (1953). *J. Urol.*, **69**, 82.

MOORE, F. D., EDELMAN, I. S., OLNEY, J. M., JAMES, A. H., BROOKS, L. & WILSON, G. M. (1954). *Metabolism*, **3**, 334.

MOORE, R. A. (1931). *Anat. Rec.*, **48**, 153.

MUDGE, G. H., FOULKS, J. & GILMAN, A. (1949). *Amer. J. Physiol.*, **158**, 218.

MUEHRCKE, R. C. (1960). In "Biology of Pyelonephritis". p. 581. Eds. Quinn, E. L. & Kass, E. H. London, J. & A. Churchill, Ltd.

MUNK, F. (1913). *Z. klin. Med.*, **78**, 1.

MURPHY, R. & SHIPMAN, K. H. (1963). *Arch. int. Med.*, **112**, 954.

NASH, T. P. & BENEDICT, S. R. (1921). *J. biol. Chem.*, **48**, 463.

NELP, W. B., WAGNER, H. N. & REBA, R. C. (1964). *J. Lab. clin. Med.*, **63**, 480.

NESBIT, R. M. & BAUM, W. C. (1950). *J. Amer. med. Ass.*, **143**, 1317.

NICHOLS, J., MILLER, A. T., Jr. & HIATT, E. P. (1951). *J. appl. Physiol.*, **3**, 501.

NICKEL, J. F., LOWRANCE, P. B., LEIFER, E. & BRADLEY, S. E. (1953). *J. clin. Invest.*, **32**, 68.

NIKKILA, E. & GRASBECK, R. (1954). *Acta med. scand.*, **150**, 39.

NUGENT, C. A. & TYLER, F. H. (1959). *J. clin. Invest.*, **38**, 1890.

OLIVER, J. & MACDOWELL, M. (1961). *J. clin. Invest.*, **40**, 1093.

OLIVER, J., MACDOWELL, M. & TRACY, A. (1951). *J. clin. Invest.*, **30**, 1307.

ONCLEY, J. L., GURD, F. R. N. & MELIN, M. (1950). *J. Amer. chem. Soc.*, **72**, 458.

ONCLEY J. L., SCATCHARD, G. & BROWN, A. (1947). *J. phys. Chem.*, **51**, 184.

ORLOFF, J. & BERLINER, R. W. (1955). *J. clin. Invest.*, **35**, 223.

PADOVA, J. & BENDERSKY, G. (1962). *New Engl. J. Med.*, **267**, 530.

PAGE, I. H., KIRK, E. & VAN SLYKE, D. D. (1936). *J. clin. Invest.*, **15**, 101.

PARSONS, F. M., PYRAH, L. N., POWELL, F. J. N., REED, G. W. & SPIERS, F. W. (1952). *Brit. J. Urol.*, **24**, 317.

PETERS, J. P. & MAN, E. B. (1948). *J. clin. Invest.*, **27**, 397.

PETERS, J. P. & VAN SLYKE, D. D. (1946). "Quantitative Clinical Chemistry". Vol. I: Interpretations, 2nd Ed. London, Bailliere, Tindall & Cox.

PHILLIPS, R. A., DOLE, V. P., HAMILTON, P. B., EMERSON, K., ARCHIBALD, R. M. & VAN SLYKE, D. D. (1946). *Amer. J. Physiol.*, **145**, 314.

PICKERING, G, W. & HEPTINSTALL, R. H. (1953). *Quart. J. Med.*, n.s., **22**, 1.

PINES, K. L. & MUDGE, G. H. (1951). *Amer. J. Med.*, **11**, 302.

PITTS, R. F. (1936). *J. clin. Invest.*, **15**, 571.

PITTS, R. F. (1948). *Fed. Proc.*, **7**, 418.

PITTS, R. F. & ALEXANDER, R. S. (1945). *Amer. J. Physiol.*, **144**, 239.

PITTS, R. F., AYER, J. L. & SCHIESS, W. A. (1949). *J. clin. Invest.*, **28**, 35.

PITTS, R. F. & LOTSPEICH, W. D. (1946). *Amer. J. Physiol.*, **147**, 138.

PITTS, R. F., LOTSPEICH, W. D., SCHIESS, W. A., & AYER, J. L. (1948). *J. clin. Invest.*, **27**, 48.

PITTS, R. F., PILKINGTON, L. A. & DE HANS, J. C. M. (1965). *J. clin. Invest.*, **44**, 731.

PLATT, R. (1950). *Clin. Sci.*, **9**, 367.

PLATT, R. (1952). *Brit. med. J.*, **1**, 1313 & 1372.

POLONOWSKI, M. & JAYLE, M. (1938). *C.R. Soc. Biol. Paris*, **129**, 457.

POOL, T. L. & COOK, E. N. (1950). *J. Urol.*, **63**, 228.

PRICE, J. W., MILLER, M. & HAYMAN, J. M. (1940). *J. clin. Invest.*, **19**, 537.

PRIEN, E. L. (1954). *J. Amer. med. Ass.*, **154**, 744.

PROUT, G. R., Jr., MACALALAG, E. V., Jr. & HUME, D. M. (1964). *Surgery*, **56**, 283.

PYRAH, L. N. (1954). *Brit. med. J.*, **2**, 963.

RAASCHOU, F. (1943). *Acta med. scand.*, **114**, 414.

RAASCHOU, F. (1945). *Nord. Med.*, **25**, 457.

RAASCHOU, F. (1948). *Acta med. scand.*, (Suppl. 206), **130**, 217.

RAPOPORT, M., MCCRORY, W. W., BARBERO, G., BARNETT, H. L., FORMAN, C. W. & MCNAMARA, H. (1951). *J. Amer. med. Ass.*, **147**, 1101.

RAPOPORT, S., BRODSKY, W. A., WEST, C. D. & MACKLER, B. (1949). *Amer. J. Physiol.*, **156**, 433.

RECANT, L. & RIGGS, D. S. (1952). *J. clin. Invest.*, **31**, 789.

RECTOR, F. C., Jr. & CLAPP, J. R. (1962). *J. clin. Invest.*, **41**, 101.

REIFENSTEIN, E. C., ALBRIGHT, F. & WELLS, S. L. (1945). *J. clin. Endocrin.*, **5**, 367.

RELMAN, A. S., ETSTEN, B. & SCHWARTZ, W. B. (1953). *J. clin. Invest.*, **32**, 972.

RICHARDS, A. N. & WALKER, A. (1937). *Amer. J. Physiol.*, **118**, 111.

RIGAS, D. A. & HELLER, C. G. (1951). *J. clin. Invest.*, **30**, 853.

ROBERTS, K. E., MAGIDA, M. G. & PITTS, R. F. (1953). *Amer. J. Physiol.*, **172**, 47.

ROBERTSON, J. A. & GRAY, C. H. (1953). *Lancet*, **2**, 15.

ROSCOE, M. H. (1952). *Lancet*, **1**, 444.

ROTHSTEIN, A. & BERKE, H. (1949). *J. Pharmacol.*, **96**, 179.

ROUSSAK, N. J. & OLEESKY, S. (1954). *Quart. J. Med.*, **23**, 147.

ROWE, D. S. & SOOTHILL, J. F. (1961). *Clin. Sci.*, **21**, 87.

RYTAND, D. A., RANTZ, L. A. & RANDALL, E. (1950). *J. clin. Invest.*, **29**, 843.

SARTORIUS, O. W., CALHOON, D. & PITTS, R. F. (1952). *Endocrinology*, **51**, 444.

SCHMIDT-NIELSON, B. (1958). *Physiol. Rev.*, **38**, 139.

SCHMIDT-NIELSON, K., SCHMIDT-NIELSON, B. & BROKAW, A. (1948). *J. cell. comp. Physiol.*, **32**, 361.

SCHREINER, G. E., SMITH, L. H. & KYLE, L. H. (1953). *Amer. J. Med.*, **15**, 122.

SCHWARTZ, W. B. & RELMAN, A. S. (1953). *J. clin. Invest.*, **32**, 258.

SCHWARTZ, W. B. & RELMAN, A. S. (1954). *J. clin. Invest.*, **33**, 965.

SCHWARTZ, W. B., JENSON, R. L. & RELMAN, A. S. (1954). *J. clin. Invest.*, **33**, 587.

SCHWARTZ, W. B., JENSON, R. L. & RELMAN, A. S. (1955). *J. clin. Invest.*, **34**, 673.

SCOTT, W. W., HUGGINS, C. & SELMAN, B. C. (1943). *J. Urol.*, **50**, 202.

SCRIBNER, B. H., BURI, R., CANER, J. E. Z., HERGSTOM, R. & BURNELL, J. M. (1960). *Trans. Amer. Soc. artif. intern. Org.*, **6**, 114.

SCRIBNER, B. H., MAGID, G. J. & BURNELL, J. M. (1960). *Clin. Res.*, **8**, 136.

SELDIN, D. W., RECTOR, F., CARTER, N. & COPENHAVER, J. (1954). *Amer. J. Med.*, **16**, 608.

SELKURT, E. E. (1952). *Proc. Soc. exp. Biol. (N.Y.)*, **81**, 374.

SHALDON, S., HIGGS, B., CHIANDUSSI, L., WALKER, G., GARSENSTEIN, M. & RYDER, J. (1962). *J. Lab. clin. Med.*, **60**, 954.

SHANNON, J. A. (1936). *Amer. J. Physiol.*, **117**, 206.

SHAW, A. B., BAZZARD, F. G., BOOTH, E. M., NILWARANGKUR, S. & BERLYNE, G. M. (1965). *Quart. J. Med.*, **34**, 237.

SHEEHAN, H. L. & MOORE, H. C. (1952). "Renal Cortical Necrosis and the Kidney of Concealed Accidental Haemorrhage". Oxford University Press.

SHORR, E. (1945). *J. Urol.*, **53**, 507.

SIMPSON, S. A., TAIT, J. F. & BUSH, I. E. (1952). *Lancet*, **2**, 226.

SIROTA, J. H. & KROOP, I. G. (1951). *J. clin. Invest.*, **30**, 1082.

SIROTA, J. H., YÜ, T. F. & GUTMAN, A. B. (1952). *J. clin. Invest.*, **31**, 692.

SLATER, R. J. & KUNKEL, H. G. (1953). *J. Lab. clin. Med.*, **41**, 619.

SLESSOR, A. (1951). *J. clin. Endocrinol.*, **11**, 700.

SMIDDY, F. G. (1954). *Proc. R. Soc. Med.*, **47**, 807.

SMITH, H. W. (1951). "The Kidney: Structure and Function in Health and Disease". New York, Oxford University Press.

SMITH, H. W., GOLDRING, W. & CHASIS, H. (1938). *J. clin. Invest.*, **17**, 263.

SMITH, H. W., GOLDRING, W., CHASIS, H., RANGES, H. A. & BRADLEY, S. E. (1943). *J. Mt. Sinai Hosp.*, **10**, 59.

SNAPPER, I. (1952). "Rare Manifestations of Metabolic Bone Disease". Springfield, Ill., Charles C. Thomas.

SOLOMON, S. (1957). *J. Cell. Comp. Physiol.*, **49**, 351.

SONNE, C. (1921). *Z. klin. Med.*, **90**, 1.

SPARGO, B. J. (1954). *J. Lab. clin. Med.*, **43**, 802.

SPECTOR, W. G. (1954). *Clin. Sci.*, **13**, 1.

SPENCER, A. G. (1962). *Clin. Sci.*, **22**, 43.

SPENCER, A. G. & FRANGLEN, G. T. (1952). *Lancet*, **1**, 190.

SPENCER, A. G. & LLOYD-THOMAS, H. G. L. (1954). *Brit. med. J.*, **1**, 597.

STACEY, B. D. & THORBURN, G. D. (1966). *Science*, **152**, 1076.

SQUIRE, J. R. (1953). *Brit. med. J.*, **2**, 1389.

STAEMMLER, M. & DOPHEIDE, W. (1930). *Virchow's Arch.*, **277**, 713.

STANBURY, S. W. & MAHLER, R. F. (1959). *Quart. J. Med.*, n.s., **28**, 425.

STANBURY, S. W. & THOMSON, A. E. (1952). *Clin. Sci.*, **11**, 357.

STANLEY, M. M. & THANNHAUSER, S. J. (1949). *J. Lab. clin. Med.*, **34**, 1634.

STERLING, K. (1951). *J. clin. Invest.*, **30**, 1228.

SURGENOR, D. M., KOECHLIN, B. A. & STRONG, L. E. (1949). *J. clin. Invest.*, **28**, 73.

SWAN, R. C. & MERRILL, J. P. (1953). *Medicine*, **32**, 215.

TAGNON, H. J., SCHULMAN, P., WHITMORE, W. F. & LEONE, L. A. (1953). *Amer. J. Med.*, **16**, 875.

TERRY, R., HAWKINS, D. R., CHURCH, E. H. & WHIPPLE, G. H. (1948). *J. exp. Med.*, **87**, 561.

THOMAS, E. M., ROSENBLUM, A. H., LANDER, H. B. & FISHER, R. (1951). *Amer. J. Dis. Child.*, **81**, 207.

TOBIAN, L. (1960). *Ann. intern. Med.*, **52**, 395.

THORN, G. W., KOEPF, G. F. & CLINTON, M. (1944). *New Engl. J. Med.*, **231**, 76.

ULLRICH, K. J., SCHMIDT-NIELSEN, B., O'DELL, R., PEHLING, G., GOTTSCHALK, C. W., LASSITER, W. E. & MYLLE, M. (1963). *Amer. J. Physiol.*, **204**, 527.

VANDERVEIKEN, F., GUERITTE, F., DE MYTTENAERE, M. & LAMBERT, P. P. (1958). *J. Urol. Med. Chir.*, **64**, 136.

VAN SLYKE, D. D., PHILLIPS, R. A., HAMILTON, P. B., ARCHIBALD, R. M., FUTCHER, P. H. & HILLER, A. (1943). *J. biol. Chem.*, **150**, 481.

VERNEY, E. B. (1947). *Proc. roy. Soc. London, B.*, **135**, 25.

VOGL, A. (1953). "Diuretic Therapy". Baltimore, Williams & Wilkins.

WAELSCH, H. (1951). *Advanc. Protein Chem.*, **6**, 299.

WALKER, A. M., BOTT, P. A., OLIVER, J. & MAC-DOWELL, M. C. (1941). *Amer. J. Physiol.*, **134**, 580.

DE WARDENER, H. E., MILES, B. E., LEE, G. DE J., CHURCHILL-DAVIDSON, H., WYLIE, D. & SHARPEY-SCHAFER, E. P. (1952). *Clin. Sci.*, **12**, 175.

DE WARDENER, H. E., MILLS, I. H., CLAPHAM, W. F. & HAYTER, C. J. (1961). *Clin. Sci.*, **21**, 249.

WATSON, J. F., CLAPP, J. R. & BERLINER, R. W. (1964). *J. clin. Invest.*, **43**, 595.

WATERHOUSE, C. & HOLLER, J. (1948). *J. clin. Invest.*, **27**, 560.

WESSON, L. G. & ANSLOW, W. P. (1948). *Amer. J. Physiol.*, **153**, 465.

WESSON, L. G., ANSLOW, W. P. & SMITH, H. W. (1948). *Bull. N.Y. Acad. Med.*, **24**, 586.

WILLIAMS, R. H. & HENRY, C. (1947). *Ann. intern. Med.*, **27**, 84.

WILLIAMS, H. F. & SMITH, L. H. (1968). *New Engl. J. Med.*, **278**, 233.

WILSON, W. E., KIRKPATRICK, C. H. & TALMAGE, D. W. (1964). *J. clin. Invest.*, **43**, 1881.

WILSON, V. K., THOMSON, M. L. & HOLZEL, A. (1952). *Brit. med. J.*, **1**, 358.

WINER, N. J. (1942). *Arch. intern. Med.*, **70**, 61.

WIRZ, H., HARGITAY, B. & KUHN, W. (1951). *Helv. physiol. Acta*, **9**, 196.

WOLF, A. V. (1941). *Amer. J. Physiol.*, **133**, 496.

WOLF, A. V. (1950). *Amer. J. Physiol.*, **161**, 75.

WOLF, A. V., REMP, D. G., KILEY, J. E. & CURRIE, G. D. (1951). *J. clin. Invest.*, **30**, 1062.

WOLMAN, I. J. (1944). *Amer. J. med. Sci.*, **208**, 767.

WOODARD, H. Q. & DEAN, A. L. (1947). *J. Urol.*, **57**, 158.

WOOTTON, I. D. P., KING, E. J. & SMITH, J. M. (1951). *Brit. med. Bull.*, **7**, 307.

YÜ, T. F., BERGER, L. & GUTMAN, A. B. (1962). *Amer. J. Med.*, **33**, 829.

YUILE, C. L. & CLARK, W. F. (1941). *J. exp. Med.*, **74**, 187.

ZAK, G. A., BRUN, C. & SMITH, H. W. (1954). *J. clin. Invest.*, **33**, 1064.

ZOLLINGER, H. U. (1955). *Schweiz. med. Wsch.*, **85**, 746.

Chapter 11

DISEASES OF THE ADRENAL GLANDS

by

A. H. Gowenlock and Donald Longson
University of Manchester and Manchester Royal Infirmary

THE secretions of the adrenal cortex and medulla clearly demonstrate the inextricable involvement of chemical structure and physiological function. The adrenal cortex, essential for the maintenance of life, is now recognized as an important mediator between the environment and the organism, as a regulator of homeostasis under resting and emergency conditions, as a provider of one of many mechanisms designed to conserve sodium and water, and as a participant in the supply of certain androgenic hormones. For all these physiological actions the adrenal cortex supplies specific categories of steroid substances. Minute differences in the structure of these steroid hormones often confer major differences in type or degree of physiological action. The various sympathomimetic amines secreted by the adrenal medulla are similarly specific in their effects upon the cardio-vascular system and upon metabolism, specificities again dependent upon small alterations of chemical structure. In human disease of the adrenal cortex and medulla, one sees clearly the effects of lack (Addison's disease) or excess (Cushing's syndrome, phaeochromocytoma) of these chemical substances, and in disorders such as congenital adrenal virilism, one observes the effects upon the organism of abnormal biosynthesis or catabolism of glandular products. Studies of these pathological conditions have contributed much to knowledge of normal as well as abnormal processes involved in the synthesis and degradation of steroids and amines, and have emphasized the impossibility of understanding these disorders without detailed information concerning their chemical basis.

THE ADRENAL CORTEX

The Biosynthesis of Steroid Hormones

The adrenal cortex exerts its regulatory effects upon carbohydrate, protein and mineral metabolism by a sustained release of steroid hormones into the circulation under resting conditions; certain of these substances are secreted in increasing quantities as a result of such noxious stimuli as surgical intervention, fever, haemorrhage, exposure to cold, heat, and the administration of various toxic substances (Sayers & Sayers, 1949). This hypersecretion is mediated via an increased secretion or release of adrenocorticotropin from the adenohypophysis. In man, the adrenal vein has been shown to contain principally cortisol and corticosterone (Romanoff, Hudson & Pincus, 1953; Bush & Sandberg, 1953) with smaller amounts of dehydroepiandrosterone (and its sulphate), androstenedione, 11β-hydroxyandrostenedione, 11-deoxycortisol, pregnenolone, 17-hydroxypregnenolone and aldosterone. Cortisol, corticosterone and dehydroepiandrosterone are secreted by the gland in increased amounts in response to a noxious stimulus or to the administration of ACTH. In this response, steroid hormones assume a regulatory rather than an initiating role in the biochemical responses to stress, although the precise homeostatic role of each of the steroid hormones thus hypersecreted is unknown.

The adrenal cortex was shown to be essential for the maintenance of life (Rogoff & Stewart, 1927; Swingle et al., 1930, 1934) as indicated by prolongation of survival in bilaterally adrenalectomized dogs and cats treated with crude adrenal cortical extracts. It soon became apparent that such extracts contained several steroid substances, the isolation and chemical structures of which were the subject of intensive investigation. By 1943, 28 steroids had been isolated and characterized (Reichstein & Shoppee, 1943). The present number exceeds 40 and includes both biologically active and inactive substances. They may be classified by the number of C atoms present. The C_{18} steroids include the oestrogens, oestrone and oestradiol-17β. The C_{19} steroids include the androgens, androst-4-ene-3:17-dione and 3β-hydroxy-androst-5-ene-17-one (dehydroepiandrosterone). The C_{21} steroids (Fig. 11.1) include the corticoids: 11β:17α:21-trihydroxypregn-4-ene-3:20-dione (hydrocortisone, cortisol, Kendall's compound F), 17α:21-dihydroxypregn-4-ene-3:11:20-trione (cortisone, Kendall's compound E), 11β:21-dihydroxy-18-oxopregn-4-ene-3:20-dione (aldosterone), 17α:21-dihydroxypregn-4-ene-3:20-dione (cortexolone, 11-deoxycortisol, Reichstein's compound S), 11β:21-dihydroxypregn-4-ene-3:20-dione (corticosterone, Kendall's compound B), 21-hydroxypregn-4-ene-3:11:20-trione (dehydrocorticosterone, Kendall's compound A) and pregn-4-ene-3:20-dione (progesterone). All these steroids have a methyl group at position C-18 except for aldosterone in which it is replaced by an aldehyde group. The C_{18} steroids lack the angular methyl group at position C-19 present in all the other steroids. In addition to the biologically active steroids in Fig. 11.1, there are closely related C_{21} corticoids with reduced A rings or with hydroxy groups at positions 3α, 3β, 6β, 16α, 19, 20α and 20β. Some of these more polar compounds have weak biological activity. Some have been

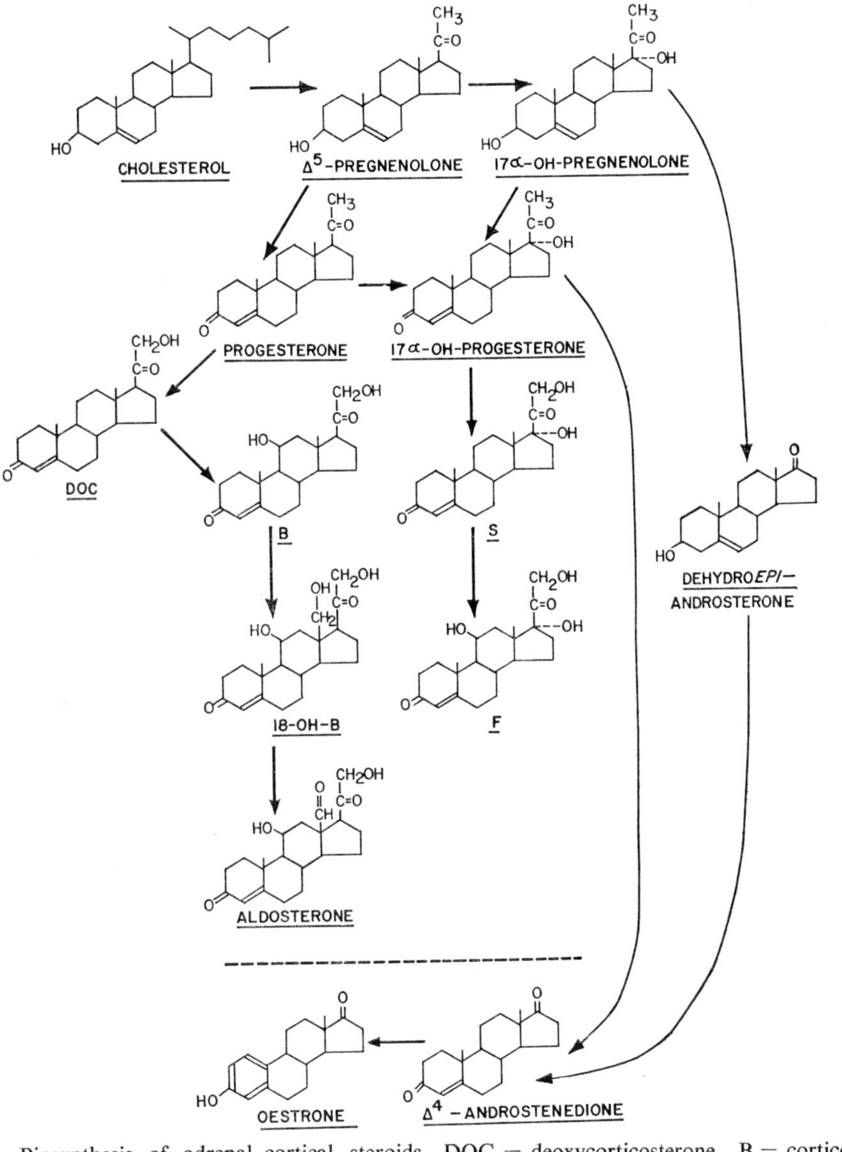

FIG. 11.1. Biosynthesis of adrenal cortical steroids. DOC = deoxycorticosterone, B = corticosterone, S = 11-deoxycortisol, F = cortisol.

isolated from adrenal cortical tissue, others are formed during metabolism in extra-adrenal sites.

The biosynthesis of adrenal steroids involves a number of enzymes which have been identified in adrenal corticoid tissue. The starting substance may be acetate, a cholesterol precursor, or cholesterol itself which is present in high concentration in the cortex. The beef adrenal converts ^{14}C-cholesterol into labelled cortisol and corticos-

terone (Hechter *et al.*, 1951, 1953; Hayand *et al.*, 1956). Administration of ^{14}C-cholesterol in man is followed by the excretion of labelled tetra-hydrometabolites of cortisol in urine (Werbin & Le Roy, 1954). A similar pattern of labelled products is found when ^{14}C-acetate is used as the starting material (Hechter *et al.*, 1953; Caspi *et al.*, 1956, 1957) and conversion of acetate to cholesterol is well established. The specific activity of the final products may be higher than that of the cholesterol isolated from the gland (Hechter et al., 1953). This difference disappears once all the adrenal cholesterol has reached a constant specific activity and is considered to be due to a slow exchange rate of part of the adrenal cholesterol. Cholesterol is believed to be an intermediate in the synthetic pathway and the distribution of labelled C atoms in the steroid nucleus is the same for cholesterol, cortisol and corticosterone when ^{14}C-acetate is used as precursor (Caspi et al., 1962).

The biosynthesis of cholesterol from acetate involves many intermediates several of which have been identified. The partial sequence at present is considered to be: acetate → acetyl CoA and acetoacetyl CoA → mevalonic acid → isopentenyl pyrophosphate → farnesyl pyrophosphate → squalene → lanosterol → 14-desmethyllanosterol → zymosterol → desmosterol → cholesterol. The further breakdown of cholesterol has been shown to proceed through 20α-hydroxycholesterol (Solomon et al., 1956) and 20α, 22-dihydroxycholesterol (Shimizu et al., 1961). Scission of the side chain between the hydroxy groups yields 3β-hydroxypregn-5-ene-20-one (pregnenolone) and isocaproic aldehyde. An alternative pathway has been demonstrated through 20α-hydroxycholesterol to 17α, 20α-dihydroxycholesterol (Shimizu et al., 1965). Scission in this case leads to 17-hydroxypregnenolone and isocaproic aldehyde. These two C_{21} steroids, pregnenolone and 17-hydroxypregnenolone, are the intermediates in the biosynthesis of other C_{21} steroids and of the C_{19} and C_{18} steroids.

Pregnenolone, which has been isolated from adrenal tissue, can be converted to progesterone by the microsomal enzyme β-hydroxysteroid dehydrogenase and the cytoplasmic enzyme Δ^5-3-keto-isomerase. In the zona fasciculata the microsomal enzyme steroid 17α-hydroxylase catalyses the incorporation of molecular oxygen into either progesterone or pregnenolone with the formation of 17α-hydroxyprogesterone and 17α-hydroxypregnenolone respectively (Fig. 11.1). The human adrenal can convert the latter compound into 17α-hydroxyprogesterone (Lipsett & Hökfelt, 1961). The introduction of hydroxy groups at positions 11β and 21 is brought about by the two enzymes steroid 11β (and 21) hydroxylase and oxygen. The precise order of addition of these hydroxy groups is not certain but the route indicated for cortisol is probably the major one, with other minor pathways representing the various alternative orders. Aberrations of these pathways are discussed in

relation to congenital adrenal virilism. The major route for aldosterone synthesis, which occurs in the zona glomerulosa, is through cortexone, corticosterone and 18-hydroxycorticosterone (Fig. 11.1). The androgen, androst-4-ene-3,17-dione, is produced by the action of a desmolase on 17α-hydroxyprogesterone, an identical pathway to that occurring in testis. In the adrenal, however, further conversion to testosterone is relatively slight and 11β-hydroxylation leads to 11β-hydroxyandrostenedione, a steroid also produced during the metabolism of cortisol. The important androgen, dehydroepiandrosterone, is not derived from progesterone but from 17α-hydroxypregnenolone (Kahnt et al., 1961) and undergoes further conversion to androstenedione. Also, dehydroepiandrosterone may be reduced to give androst-5-ene-3β,17β-diol which is converted to testosterone (Baulieu et al., 1963; Colla et al., 1964). These conversions are indicated in Figs. 11.1 and 11.4. Most of the dehydroepiandrosterone is converted to the 3-sulphate, which may also be produced from sulphated precursors. The production of oestrogens by the adrenal is discussed later. The conversion of androstenedione to 19-hydroxyandrostenedione (Meyer, 1955a) and thence to oestrone (Meyer, 1955b) is indicated in Fig. 11.4.

The adrenal cortex of the human foetus shows a well defined foetal zone which disappears within a few days of birth. Although the foetal cortex can synthesize the usual steroids, it has a relatively low β-hydroxysteroid dehydrogenase activity and produces a preponderance of 3β-hydroxy-Δ^5-steroids (Bloch & Benirschke, 1962), at least 11 of which have been identified in umbilical cord blood (Eberlein, 1964). Some of these are hydroxylated in the 16α-position, probably in the foetal liver, and appear to be important precursors for the formation of oestriol in the placenta. Such Δ^5-16α-hydroxylated steroids are excreted in neonatal urine for a few days but disappear with involution of the foetal cortex. The importance of the foetal adrenal steroids as oestriol precursors is indicated by the low oestriol excretion by women bearing an anencephalic foetus, without pituitary tissue (Frandsen & Stakemann, 1964). In such a foetus, the adrenals are atrophic and the circulating Δ^5-C_{19}-steroids are reduced in amount (Colás & Heinrichs, 1965).

Categories of Adrenal Cortical Secretion: Action of Adrenocortical Steroids

The active secretory products of the human adrenal cortex may be functionally divided into four groups: (1) C_{21}-steroids chiefly influencing carbohydrate and protein metabolism, and essential for the maintenance of life (cortisol); (2) C_{21}-steroids chiefly influencing renal conservation of Na and also essential for maintenance of life (aldosterone); (3) C_{19}-17-oxosteroids with androgenic properties (dehydroepiandrosterone, androstenedione); and (4) C_{18}-oestrogens (oestrone).

Cortisol. This is quantitatively the chief circulating C_{21} adrenocortical steroid of man (Romanoff et al., 1953; Bush & Sandberg, 1953). The biological function in man of corticosterone, the next most abundant steroid of this class, is unknown. Cortisol secretion increases in response to many environmental stimuli and its blood concentration is a principal regulator of the rate of adenohypophyseal release of ACTH (Ingle, 1938). Cortisol and other oxygenated corticosteroids maintain the glycogen stores of the liver (Britton & Silvette, 1934), principally by increasing gluconeogenesis. This accounts for the low urinary N output of adrenalectomized animals and patients with Addison's disease. When animals are given phlorrhizin followed by cortisol-like steroids, increasing glycosuria is parallelled by an elevation of urinary N (Wells & Kendall, 1940; Segaloff & Many, 1951), indicating the formation of glucose from protein as an important action of cortisol. Cortisol has profound effects upon the metabolism of proteins and amino acids. Long-term administration of cortisol results in major loss of body protein. Experiments with ^{14}C-labelled amino acids show an inhibitory effect of cortisol upon protein anabolism and an acceleration of catabolic processes (Hoberman, 1950). Similar conclusions may be derived from studies of the inhibitory effect of cortisol upon tissue response to injury (Ragan et al., 1950) and upon antibody formation (Bjorneboe et al., 1951; Fischel, 1961). The hepatic uptake of amino acids released by such protein catabolism is increased by cortisol (Riggs, 1964) and is apparent within 2 hr. of administration. Metabolic breakdown of these amino acids can contribute to increased formation of urea and glucose. Unlike most other tissues, there is an increase in the synthesis of RNA and, later, of protein in the liver following cortisol administration (Feigelson & Feigelson, 1964). Protein synthesis is blocked by puromycin and actinomycin suggesting that the effect is mediated by nucleic acid synthesis. The earliest change seems to be an increase in the activity of liver RNA nucleotidyltransferase (Lang & Sekeris, 1964), followed by an increase in the synthesis of messenger RNA and then by increased protein synthesis by ribosomes. The activities of a number of hepatic enzymes are increased at varying times

after glucocorticoid administration and early increased synthesis of enzyme protein has been demonstrated in some cases (Kenny, 1962). These effects are antagonized by insulin. In some cases the enzyme increase is delayed until after marked changes in glucose metabolism have occurred. The general pattern of enzymic change observed is such as to facilitate the conversion of amino acids to glucose and urea.

In carbohydrate metabolism the effects of cortisol are opposed to those of insulin. The improvement of glycosuria in the diabetic animal after adrenalectomy and the production of diabetes by steroid therapy or in Cushing's syndrome are well known. One of the earliest changes produced by cortisol in fasting adrenalectomized animals is a rise in blood glucose (Long et al., 1960). At least part of this rise is attributable to increased hepatic production of glucose. This may be demonstrated in the whole animal (Welt et al., 1952) and also in liver slices removed 2–4 hr. after glucocorticoid administration (Koepf et al., 1941). Although the effect cannot be observed by addition of cortisol to tissue slices direct, this is probably due to catabolism of the steroid by hepatic enzymes. Using triamcinolone, a potent synthetic glucocorticoid less readily inactivated in the liver, it is possible to observe the direct conversion by liver slices of a number of substances, including pyruvate and alanine, into glucose (Haynes, 1962; Eisenstein et al., 1964). In the whole animal, the increased hepatic output of glucose is followed by a rise in the liver glycogen content at the time the output of non-protein nitrogen is increasing (Long et al., 1960). This effect is inhibited by actinomycin D and may therefore depend on preliminary nucleic acid synthesis. The peripheral utilization of glucose is increased by insulin and inhibited by glucocorticoids, but the effect is not always easy to observe. Long et al. (1960) reported little effect in the intact rat but a reduction has been found in studies using skin (Overell et al., 1960), lymphoid tissues (Jedeikin & White, 1958), heart muscle (Morgan et al., 1959) and adipose tissue (Munck, 1962). The reduction in peripheral utilization in man by glucocorticoids is made use of in the cortisone tolerance test for the detection of prediabetes.

In addition to these important effects on carbohydrate and protein metabolism, cortisol has a number of other actions which are of importance in human disease. These have been reviewed by Grant (1967). Cortisol is essential for the mobilization of free fatty acids from adipose tissue by catecholamines (see later). Suppression of inflammatory responses is an important therapeutic effect. It has been claimed (Cline & Melmon, 1966) that cortisol interferes with the release of plasma kinins by leucocytes or kallikrein. Part of this effect may be attributable to stabilization of leucocyte lysosomes. Such an effect on lysosomal membranes (Weissman & Thomas, 1964) has been invoked to explain other anti-inflammatory effects. Cortisol reduces granulocyte "stickiness", diapedesis and phagocytosis. The inhibition by glucocorticoids in connective tissue of fibroblast growth and acid mucopolysaccharide formation are important in tissue repair. Gastric ulceration is a recognized complication of steroid therapy. The relative importance of increased gastric secretion, reduced mucosal protection by alteration of mucus and delayed healing of damaged mucosa is still uncertain. Cortisol inhibits vitamin D-induced calcium absorption from the intestine, an effect made use of clinically in the treatment of the hypercalcaemia of sarcoidosis or hypervitaminosis D. Its effect on the hypercalcaemia of multiple myelomatosis has been attributed to a reduction in bone resorption. Cortisol causes involution of lymphoid tissue, destroying small lymphocytes and producting lymphopenia. Eosinopenia, long used as an index of glucocorticoid activity, is probably due to destruction of eosinophils.

Cortisol has important effects upon Na and water metabolism. It is synergistic to the Na-retaining effect of aldosterone exerting a "permissive" effect (Nelson & August, 1958). Continued administration of glucocorticoids in high dosage is well known to cause oedema. Cortisol produces a K diuresis (Sprague et al., 1950) by a variety of effects (Bartter & Fourman, 1957). The failure of water diuresis in adrenal cortical insufficiency is restored by cortisol but not by cortexone (Oleesky & Stanbury, 1951; Wynn & Garrod, 1955). The mechanism is complex. The defect does not appear to be due to alterations in ADH activity (Kleeman et al., 1965) or to reduction in glomerular filtration rate. Kleeman et al., (1965) have speculated that cortisol decreases the permeability of the distal tubular epithelium to water. Glucocorticoids appear to be necessary to maintain the hyperosmolarity of the renal papilla. This is reduced in adrenal insufficiency and is not restored by aldosterone alone (Crabbé & Nichols, 1959). Studies on the effect of glucocorticoids on the internal distribution of water between different fluid compartments have given contradictory results, and it is not certain that an abnormal distribution is a significant factor.

Aldosterone. Aldosterone is the principal "mineralocorticoid" of the adrenal cortex and accounts for the Na-retaining activity of the so-called "amorphous fraction" of adrenal extracts. It is present in adrenal venous blood (Grundy et al., 1952; Simpson et al., 1952) and has been isolated from adrenal extracts (Simpson et al., 1953) and from the urine of patients with the nephrotic syndrome (Luetscher et al., 1955). The Na-retaining activity of aldosterone is some 10-30 times that of deoxycorticosterone (Gross & Gysel, 1954), and both steroids restore to normal the defective tubular Na re-absorption of adrenal insufficiency (Pitts, 1951; Mach & Fabre, 1954). Aldosterone shows weak glucocorticoid activity but is greatly overshadowed by cortisol in normal physiological situations (Gaunt et al., 1955). It plays an important role in the regulation of Na and K excretion and may be involved in the formation of oedema.

The chief effect is on the renal tubule, commencing about an hour after administration and lasting up to 8 hr. (Barger et al., 1958; Ganong & Mulrow, 1958). Aldosterone promotes reabsorption of sodium chloride in the distal convoluted tubule and also facilitates the ionic exchange of Na^+ for K^+, H^+ and, possibly Mg^{++} at this site. (Vander et al., 1960; Bartter & Fourman, 1962; Horton & Biglieri, 1962; Yunis et al., 1964). The stimulation of K excretion depends on an adequate supply of Na being delivered to the distal tubular site and disappears on low Na intakes. After several days of aldosterone administration with Na retention and expansion of the ECF volume, the kidney 'escapes' from the Na-retaining action by a mechanism which remains obscure, but the K diuresis persists and leads to K deficiency (August et al., 1958). Some oedematous patients secrete increased amounts of aldosterone (secondary hyperaldosteronism) but do not lose K. It is presumed that proximal tubular reabsorption of Na is enhanced and less is available for the exchange process. Substances such as the spironolactones and 17-hydroxyprogesterone can block the renal tubular actions of aldosterone. The K-excreting action is enhanced by cortisol. Aldosterone also affects the transport of Na and K at other sites. It retards the entry of Na into erythrocytes (Spach & Streeten, 1964) and stimulates Na reabsorption and K excretion by intestinal mucosa (Davis et al., 1959; Levitan & Ingelfinger, 1965; Wrong et al., 1961). In saliva it causes a fall in Na and some increase in K secretion (August et al., 1958) and the effect is used in bioassay procedures in the sheep. In sweat, a similar effect occurs (Collins, 1966) and is probably of importance in restricting Na loss during heat acclimatization. In the case of saliva and sweat the effect is delayed for about 24 hr., slowly reaches a maximum and is not subject to the 'escape' mechanism noted in the renal tubule. Aldosterone has a hypertensive effect once Na retention has occurred but the mechanism is obscure.

The details of the mechanism of aldosterone action have been the subject of several recent investigations in which the aldosterone-stimulated transport of Na by the toad bladder *in vitro* has been used as the experimental model (Porter & Edelman, 1964; Edelman *et al.*, 1964; Sharp & Leaf, 1964). The concept which emerges is that aldosterone and other steroids with mineralo-corticoid activity stimulate the synthesis of messenger RNA which directs the synthesis of an enzyme active in Na transport. The transport depends on the availability of pyruvate whose reaction with the enzyme provides the energy required. Such a requirement for protein synthesis would explain the delay in onset of aldosterone action.

Androgens. Analysis of adrenal venous blood gives evidence of the secretion of several weak androgens in the normal, and in cases of adrenal tumour and congenital adrenal hyperplasia. These substances are: dehydroepiandrosterone (Bush *et al.*, 1956) and its sulphate (Baulieu, 1963), androstenedione (Pincus & Romanoff, 1955) and 11β-hydroxyandrostenedione (Romanoff *et al.*, 1953). The secretion rate of dehydroepiandro-sterone (10–30 mg./day) is comparable with that of cortisol (Van de Wiele & Lieberman, 1960) but this substance has only weak androgenic activity, about 5 % that of testosterone. The corresponding figures for androstenedione and 11-hydroxy-androstenedione are 20 % and 1 %. The importance of their androgenic effect in the normal human is uncertain. In the castrate rat, prolonged stimu-lation of adrenal androgen production by ACTH fails to maintain normal structure and function of the seminal vesicles and prostate. The relative anabolic effects of adrenal androgens is not cer-tain, but such effects are observed as growth stimulation, positive N balance and counteraction of the catabolic effect on protein of cortisol. Reduction of muscle mass in Addison's disease and increased muscular development and skeletal growth in the adrenogenital syndrome are discussed later. Normal human peripheral plasma has been shown to contain the androgens appa-rently secreted by the adrenal, and their metabo-lites, androsterone and aetiocholanolone. The steroids found in highest concentration and present as their sulphates are dehydroepiandro-sterone (12–131 μg./100 ml.) and androsterone

(0–52 μg./100 ml.). Lower concentrations are found for glucuronides (2·6 μg./100 ml.) and especially for the unconjugated steroids (0–0·4 μg./100 ml.) (Migeon, 1960). Such figures are similar in males and females and fall with age. Since the active androgens are the unconjugated forms, the biological effect on target tissues is difficult to assess.

Oestrogens. Oestrone and oestradiol-17β have been isolated from beef adrenals and the adrenal has been shown to possess the biochemical path-ways for the formation of these substances from androstenedione, 19-hydroxyandrostenedione and testosterone (Engel, 1957; Ryan, 1958; Vinson & Jones, 1964). Hardy & Ward (1958) reported higher levels of oestrogens in adrenal venous blood than in peripheral blood, and West *et al.* (1958) found increased oestrogen excretion after ACTH administration to a patient with a func-tioning adrenal carcinoma. Adrenal oestrogens have practical importance in the rare cases of feminizing adrenal tumours in animals (Christy *et al.*, 1951) and man, and in the uncommon instances of detectable oestrogenic activity, pre-sumably adrenal cortical in origin, occurring in post-menopausal or ovariectomized women with metastatic carcinoma of the breast.

Control of Adrenal Cortical Function

Although ACTH usually augments adrenal androgen secretion, the control of androgens and oestrogens is not understood and its physiological importance is uncertain. This section is thus con-fined to a consideration of factors influencing the secretory rates of cortisol and aldosterone.

Cortisol. At least four mechanisms are known to influence cortisol secretion. These are (1) the condition of the anterior pituitary as this affects the secretion of ACTH; (2) the influence of the hypothalamus upon the release of ACTH; (3) the circulating level of cortisol itself; and (4) a direct stimulation of the adrenal cortex by vasopressin.

Hypopituitarism or hypophysectomy results in atrophy of the adrenal cortex, thyroid and gonads. In animals and man, hypophysectomy is followed within hours by a sharp fall in adrenal cortical secretion of cortisol. In hypopituitarism a reduced concentration in urine and plasma of cortisol and its metabolites is well established (Perkoff *et al.*, 1954; Wallace, Christy & Jailer, 1955). These deficiencies, due to deficiency or total absence of ACTH secretion, can be corrected by administra-tion of anterior pituitary extracts or of purified ACTH. ACTH administration to normal human subjects, in doses as small as 0·1 I.U. (Eik-Nes *et al.*, 1954), rapidly increases the urinary excretion and plasma concentration of corticosteroids. This increase is subnormal in patients with hypopituitarism, and is the basis for a diagnostic test of adrenal function in pituitary disease. Prolonged administration of ACTH results in sustained hypersecretion of cortisol, and in hyperplasia, hyperaemia, and increased water content of the adrenal cortex. In animals, prolonged administration of ACTH also alters the ratio of corticosterone to cortisol; and in man an increased production of compound S results. These data suggest that ACTH may alter the concentration, stability or activity of the enzymes, steroid 11β-hydroxylase and steroid 17α-hydroxylase.

In man, it is not clear which part of the cortex is chiefly under ACTH influence or responsible for cortisol secretion. In animals (rat, dog) hypophysectomy is followed by atrophy of the fascicular and reticular zones of the cortex, with little anatomical change in the zona glomerulosa (Greep & Deane, 1949). Early data indicated that pituitary ACTH does not influence aldosterone secretion in man (Luetscher & Johnson, 1954) as it does cortisol secretion; and patients with hypopituitarism have some preservation of aldosterone secretory function (Muller et al., 1958). Since ACTH administration caused widening of the fascicular zone without much change in the glomerulosa or in the excretion of aldosterone, it was assumed that the glomerulosa was the site of aldosterone production (Giroud et al., 1956) and was largely independent of ACTH control, while the fasciculata was the zone chiefly influenced by ACTH and the site of production of cortisol and corticosterone. This is an over-simplified view for man, as Sheehan & Summers (1949) showed that patients with prolonged, severe hypopituitarism have nearly complete fibrous replacement of the zona glomerulosa with at least partial preservation of the fasciculata. ACTH has in fact been shown to cause at least transient increases in aldosterone excretion, and patients with hypopituitarism have some difficulty in conserving Na (Wynn & Garrod, 1955; Muller et al. 1958). In one patient, hyperaldosteronism with a unilateral adrenal tumour was associated with narrowing of the fascicular, not the glomerular, zone of the contralateral gland (Conn, 1955). In short, functional localization of steroid secretion in specific zones of the human adrenal cortex is not so clearly demarcated as in certain animal species.

ACTH stimulation of the secretion of adrenal cortical steroids is the result of increased synthesis, not increased release from the gland, and occurs independently of such vegetative or nutritive functions of the gland as incorporation of amino acids into its substance. Haynes et al. (1960) have pointed out the possible importance of ACTH in increasing energy metabolism of the gland by specifically activating an adrenal phosphorylase through stimulation of synthesis of cyclic 3′, 5′ adenosine monophosphate, and by making available increased amounts of NADPH, essential for steroid biosynthesis.

Recent advances in techniques of biological assay for ACTH (reviewed by Munson, 1960) permit its detection in the peripheral blood of man under certain circumstances. In the normal subject, the concentrations are probably lower than 0·2 milliunits/100 ml. (Munson, 1960), and are consistently increased only in Addison's disease (mean concentration 8 mU./100 ml.) and in congenital adrenal virilism with adrenal insufficiency. Although Bornstein & Trewhella (1950) and others reported high blood ACTH levels in various kinds of "stress", their values are so high and so inconsistent with more recent determinations that the results must be viewed with some scepticism.

The second major control of adrenal cortical secretion of cortisol is exerted by the central nervous system (reviewed by Jailer & Christy, 1957). Many noxious stimuli activate the adrenal cortex, stimulating ACTH release by neural or humoral mechanisms. The central nervous system structures that are concerned are incompletely understood: they include the cerebrum (hippocampus, amygdala, anterior thalamic nucleus, anterior cingulate gyrus, limbic system), the brain stem ("reticular activating system"), the hypothalamus (posterior tuber cinereum, mammillary bodies, eminentia mediana) and the pituitary stalk. The work of Harris (1955) and others shows that electrical stimulation of hypothalamic nuclei results in ACTH release from the pituitary, and that localized injury to these nuclei or section of the pituitary stalk blocks the expected release of ACTH in response to numerous stimuli. Although neural connections exist between the hypothalamus and the pars distalis, it is unlikely that the functional connection is neural, as nerve fibres are few and electrical stimulation of the stalk itself fails to elicit ACTH. This "corticotropin-releasing factor" (CRF) is not adrenaline, vasopressin, serotonin or histamine, but a chemically distinct peptide, isolated from hypothalamic extracts (Guillemin, 1964). Clinical evidence on CNS control of ACTH release arises from the presence of pituitary-adrenal functional abnormalities in extrahypophyseal disease of the brain (Kahana et al., 1962). Further, various external stimuli activate the pituitary-adrenal system in man, presumably via the CNS, increasing the plasma corticosteroid concentration in such situations as major surgery, tissue trauma, burns, etc.

The circulating cortisol concentration controls the rate of release, or synthesis, of ACTH, thereby affecting the rate of cortisol release from the adrenal. Ingle (1938) and others later showed that administration of adrenal cortical extract, cortisone or cortisol resulted in adrenal atrophy which could be prevented by exogenous ACTH administration. The inference that high circulating concentrations of corticosteroid suppress pituitary ACTH release is borne out by animal studies showing reduced pituitary ACTH content after cortisol administration (Kitay et al., 1959), and by clinical data indicating anatomical and functional hypoadrenalism after prolonged administration of cortisol (Sprague et al., 1950; Salassa et al., 1953; Christy et al., 1956). The converse is seen in Addison's disease in which high ACTH figures are rapidly suppressed to normal by administration of cortisol (Bethune et al., 1957).

The fourth mechanism controlling, at least potentially, the secretory rate of cortisol is the direct stimulatory effect of vasopressin upon adrenal production of cortisol in the absence of the pituitary (Anderson & Egdahl, 1964). Vasoconstriction does not appear to be an important factor, since noradrenaline has no such stimulatory effect. The physiological significance of this direct stimulating action is obscure.

Another factor, the importance of which is becoming apparent, is that the plasma cortisol is not constant throughout the 24 hr. and the simple notion of a feed-back mechanism sensitive to fluctuations in cortisol levels inadequately defines the pituitary-adrenal relationship. A diurnal rhythm occurs with peak values between 05.00 and 08.00 hr. Thereafter, values fall, rapidly at first and reach their lowest levels around midnight in individuals following a normal sleep-wake schedule. The range of these variations is quite large, from 15–25 μg./100 ml. in the morning to 2–8 μg./100 ml. by late evening. These fluctuations are the consequence of changes in the rate of secretion of cortisol, not of altered cortisol catabolism and are reflected by similar but delayed fluctuations in the urinary excretion of metabolites. This time lag, approximately 2 hr., represents the rate of inactivation of the hormone in peripheral tissues (Migeon et al., 1956). Variations in posture, muscular activity and the visual effects of daylight are not immediate causal factors; a relationship to sleep-wake schedules is established but is not a direct influence of sleep on adrenal function. Reversed day/night schedules, or those based on an experimental "day" differing from 24 hr., result after several "days" in the establishment of an appropriate cortisol rhythm with peak values occurring on awakening and the lowest values shortly after the onset of sleep (Orth et al., 1967). Observations on the behaviour of plasma cortisol levels during sleep are not numerous but generally suggest a fairly rapid and regular rise from the moment of mid-sleep. However, Weitzman, Schaumburg & Fishbein (1966) reported a succession of peaks in relation to periods of irregular respirations, rapid eye movements and low voltage high frequency E.E.G. changes. These events are normal phenomena, recurring with a periodicity of 1–2 hr. in the second half of normal sleep and their association with short bursts of adrenal secretion suggests a neural basis for the morning tide of pituitary-adrenal activity.

An ACTH secretory rhythm is apparent in Addisonian patients maintained on sub-optimal doses of cortisol (less than 10 mg. per day). Their high plasma ACTH levels show a clear diurnal change with peak values at 06·00 hr. Similarly, patients recovering from prolonged pituitary-adrenal suppression after glucocorticoid therapy, but who still have subnormal plasma cortisol levels, show a clear diurnal ACTH rhythm (Graber et al., 1965). Slight variations in adrenal sensitivity to ACTH occur, but are probably of little importance and may be a direct result of the preceding intensity of ACTH stimulation; infusion of ACTH increases the sensitivity of the gland to further stimulation. The point of reference of the hypothalamo-pituitary feed-back mechanism appears to be a variable one which adjusts itself to the low levels of plasma cortisol in the later part of the day. The feed-back mechanism apparently never escapes from the influence of the plasma cortisol level and if this is varied experimentally at any time of day, an appropriate ACTH response is elicited. However, a decrease in plasma cortisol in the evening, produced by metyrapone, produces a much smaller rise in ACTH secretion than when the same experiment is conducted in the morning, thus providing further evidence that the ACTH secretory rhythm is a basic characteristic of hypothalamo-pituitary function (Martin & Hellman, 1964).

The cortisol rhythm may disappear in the presence of gross abnormalities of the sleep rhythm, in prolonged coma, heart failure, and possibly in renovascular hypertension (Cade et al., 1967). Leaving aside the importance of carefully relating plasma cortisol levels to a precise time of day, certain other practical clinical consequences emerge from the fact that ACTH secretion is mainly confined to the forenoon.

The inhibition of the morning increase in adrenal secretory activity arises only if suppressive levels of administered glucocorticoids are active during those nocturnal and early morning hours when the rise occurs. Similar doses administered after 08.00 hr. and during the middle of the day cause some decrease in endogenous cortisol levels, but do not prevent the secretion of ACTH the following morning. It is therefore possible that *small* doses of glucocorticoids administered in the early part of the day may not lead to cortical atrophy. Conversely, when adrenal inhibition is specifically desired, the therapeutic objective may be attained with smaller doses if they are taken in the late evening (Nichols *et al.*, 1965).

Aldosterone. Since the discovery of aldosterone, many investigators have explored the physiological control of its secretion. A number of factors have emerged but they have gradually been placed in perspective. The current view is that the renin-angiotensin system is the major one, that ACTH may have an important supplementary action and that changes in the plasma concentrations of Na and K are of secondary importance.

The renin-angiotensin system may be viewed as a self-regulating mechanism for the maintenance of a normal blood volume. A fall in the mean renal arterial pressure stimulates the juxta-glomerular (JG) apparatus to release renin, an enzyme which acts on a plasma globulin, angiotensinogen, forming angiotensin I which is then converted to angiotensin II. This substance stimulates the adrenal production of aldosterone which causes renal conservation of Na and consequent increase in ECF volume and hence in blood volume, provided the exchange of fluid between the plasma and interstitial fluid is normal. There is a considerable body of evidence to support this scheme and only an outline can be given here. The JG cells are granular, myo-epithelioid cells occurring in the walls of the afferent arterioles of the glomeruli. They are in very close anatomical relationship to the epithelial cells of the macula densa, the first part of the proximal convoluted tubule. That the granules in the JG cells are renin is indicated by the correspondence between granularity and kidney content of renin (reviewed by Tobian, 1960), the localization of renin to the vascular pole of isolated glomeruli (Cook, 1960) and to the JG cells themselves by a fluorescent antibody technique (Edelman & Hartroft, 1961). Hypergranularity of JG cells has been noted in human

kidneys in various hypertensive states, reviewed later. The release of renin by the JG cells is not mediated through a nervous mechanism (Davis, 1964) but is a direct consequence of a fall in mean perfusing arterial pressure; changes in pulse pressure and renal blood flow seem to be less important (Tobian, 1960; Skinner *et al.*, 1964). The concept is thus that of a baroreceptor mechanism. The close relationship of the JG cells and the macula densa suggests the possibility that the chemical composition of the glomerular filtrate or of the fluid reabsorbed in the proximal tubule may control renin release. The evidence for such a mechanism is less satisfactory (Thurau, 1964). The existence of an aldosterone-stimulating humoral factor was suggested by the cross perfusion experiments of Yankopoulos *et al.* (1959). Such a factor is present in kidney extracts and behaves like renin (Davis, 1963). The stimulation of aldosterone secretion by purified renin has been shown in animals and in man (Bryan *et al.*, 1964). Renin is present in the blood and lymph leaving the kidney, and angiotensin I, a decapeptide, is formed in both fluids (Lever & Peart, 1962). The conversion to angiotensin II, an octapeptide, is brought about by a "converting enzyme" present in plasma (Skeggs *et al.*, 1956) and lymph (Higgins *et al.*, 1964). Angiotensin II is effective in man in increasing aldosterone secretion; the secretion is sustained for many days with continuous infusion of angiotensin II (Laragh *et al.*, 1960, 1964). Similar activity is shown in animals and in the isolated dog adrenal. Very small doses produce an increase in aldosterone and corticosterone output within 5 min. suggesting that release as well as synthesis may be affected (Ganong *et al.*, 1962). Angiotensin II increases aldosterone and corticosterone synthesis in beef adrenal slices, but no rise in circulating glucocorticoid is apparent during angiotensin infusions in the intact organism. It is possible that inhibition of ACTH production occurs and limits the overall production of glucocorticoids. Abnormalities in the concentrations of renin and angiotensin in human pathological states are considered later. The release of aldosterone brings about conservation of Na, provided the renal tubule is capable of responding, and the extracellular fluid volume increases. If capillary fluid exchange is normal, the blood volume increases and the JG cells are no longer stimulated to produce renin. There does not appear to be any evidence for the direct suppression of aldosterone secretion by a rise in circulating aldosterone concentration (Blair-West *et al.*, 1962). Complicating factors in secondary hyperaldosteronism arise from abnormalities of capillary fluid balance or delayed catabolism of the hormone. These are discussed later.

The place of the renin-angiotensin system is now accepted in pathological states. It does, however, seem to be an important regulating mechanism under physiological conditions. Variations in the daily intake of Na are accompanied by the expected changes in aldosterone secretion and in plasma renin. The acute alterations in aldosterone and Na excretion following a change from recumbency to the upright posture are compatible with such a controlling system (Gowenlock *et al.*, 1959), and plasma renin increases under such circumstances (Conn, 1964). Renin is necessary for the maintenance of aldosterone production in normal adrenals in an analogous fashion to the action of ACTH in maintaining cortisol production. In cases of primary hyperaldosteronism, the circulating renin content is very low. Following removal of the adenoma, the remaining adrenal tissue has a subnormal capacity to secrete aldosterone which persists for several weeks and may be associated with the usual symptoms of such deficiency (Brown *et al.*, 1964; Conn, 1964). Furthermore, pregnancy is associated with a rise in plasma renin (Brown *et al.*, 1964) and increased aldosterone production (Sims *et al.*, 1964).

It is now clear that ACTH produces some stimulation of aldosterone secretion. Interpretation of some animal experiments on the effect of acute hypophysectomy has been confused by the fact that operative stress stimulates ACTH production in non-hypophysectomized animals and that undue blood loss during collection of adrenal venous samples stimulates aldosterone secretion by the renin mechanism even after hypophysectomy (Mulrow & Ganong, 1961). In chronic experiments in dogs, where such effects are inoperative, hypophysectomy reduces aldosterone secretion (Davis *et al.*, 1960). Hypophysectomy reduces aldosterone excretion rate in man also (Dingman *et al.*, 1960). In a number of experimental circumstances in which hyperaldosteronism occurs, the response is reduced in the absence of the adenohypophysis, or by the administration of cortisone in its presence. The only pituitary hormone which is active in stimulating aldosterone secretion by injection is ACTH although it is less effective, on a dose for dose basis, for aldosterone than for cortisol (Mulrow & Ganong, 1961). This stimulant effect on steroidogenesis is considered to assist angiotensin in maintaining a high aldosterone output. In some circumstances, ACTH may be the major factor involved. This appears to be the case for the stress of laparotomy (Holzbauer, 1964), or acute carotid

artery occlusion (Biglieri & Ganong, 1961).

The reciprocal relationship between Na intake and aldosterone secretion is well known and appears to result from activation of the renin-angiotensin system. Na restriction increases plasma renin and angiotensin levels and the reverse is demonstrable on a high Na intake. A low concentration of Na in the blood perfusing the isolated adrenal has, however, been shown to have an independent direct action in stimulating aldosterone secretion (Davis *et al.*, 1963). It is unlikely that such a change of Na concentration would occur in human pathology without associated changes in ECF volume and the importance of such stimulation is thus not clear. The effects of K on aldosterone secretion have also been studied extensively. Increased aldosterone excretion in man was observed in man following K loading by Laragh & Stoerk (1957) and has been confirmed by others. Reduction of aldosterone output was noted in K depletion (Johnson *et al.*, 1957). A direct stimulant action on the isolated adrenal of a high plasma K concentration occurs (Davis *et al.*, 1963). It is possible that this direct action of K plays a role in man in regulating K excretion in accordance with K intake. In man, however, there is often a complicating factor in that a K load often induces a Na diuresis (von Bunge, 1873) and thus activates the renin-angiotensin system.

Metabolism of Adrenocortical Steroids

Metabolism of the steroid hormones brings about their biological inactivation, changing them to forms more readily excreted in the urine, During this process, the steroid nucleus remains intact and the chemical modifications to its substituent groups, or those of the side chain, are few and common to many steroids. A common occurrence is the reduction of ketone groups and double bonds, and the introduction of additional hydroxyl groups. This produces a more water-soluble steroid and this property is further accentuated by the formation of glucuronides (or sulphates less commonly). These materials are not bound to plasma proteins, are readily excreted by the kidney, and appear in the urine as major products. Unconjugated steroids are excreted in small quantities only.

Most of the reductive and conjugative processes occur in the liver. The reductive steps are NADPH dependent. The importance of an intact hepatic parenchyma for steroid metabolism is apparent in liver disease, in which their catabolism is considerably slowed. The activity of the thyroid is also of importance; hyperactivity increases the activity of some enzymes, and their activity is

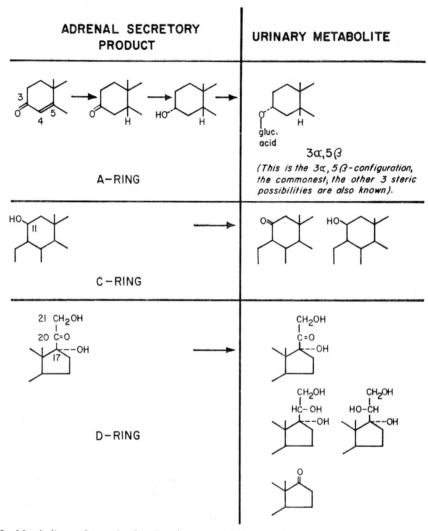

FIG. 11.2. Metabolism of certain functional groups of the steroid nucleus (gluc. acid = β-glucuronic acid residue).

reduced in myxoedema. Steroid metabolism has been extensively studied following improvements in analytical techniques and methods for the hydrolysis and extraction of steroid conjugates and by the use of isotopically labelled steroids.

Cortisol metabolism has been widely studied; the reactions involved are indicated in Fig. 11.2. Tracer studies with ^{14}C-cortisol show that its biological life is short. In the normal subject over 90% of the dose is excreted within 24 hr. (Hellman *et al.*, 1954), and the plasma "half-life" is 80-120 min. The normal secretory rate of cortisol, derived from isotopic dilution studies, is of the

order 10–25 mg./day, with a miscible body pool of about 1·8 mg. (Peterson & Wyngaarden, 1956; Cope & Pearson, 1965). The secretory rate agrees well with the best estimates of total adrenocortical steroid metabolite excretion (approx. 20 mg./24 hr.).

The concentration of cortisol in peripheral plasma is lower than that in adrenal venous plasma owing to hepatic removal. The physicochemical state of cortisol in blood has aroused interest. A small portion (10–30%) is associated with erythrocytes and the remainder is largely bound to plasma proteins. There are two separate binding systems in plasma; one with high affinity for a few steroids but of low binding capacity, and one of lower affinity but with a higher total binding capacity for a wider range of steroids (Daughaday, 1958; Slaunwhite & Sandberg, 1959). The first is represented by the α-globulin, transcortin, isolated by Seal & Doe (1962) and shown to be an acid glycoprotein with a single binding site per molecule with highest affinity for cortisol and corticosterone. The second protein system is albumin which is the more important binding agent for oestrogens and androgens. Even for cortisol it probably accounts for about 30% of bound hormone under basal conditions. In normal plasma, the average transcortin-binding capacity is 20–25 μg. cortisol/100 ml. (Daughaday et al., 1962; Doe et al., 1964). The concentration of transcortin increases in pregnancy and after oestrogen administration. Such increased binding power would explain the absence of hyperadrenal effects in association with the high plasma cortisol concentration found in these states, if the assumption is made that only the non-protein-bound form is biologically active. The renal excretion of cortisol is compatible with the glomerular filtration of the unbound moiety and the passive tubular reabsorption of about two-thirds of that filtered (Beisel et al., 1964). Table 11.1 gives typical concentrations of plasma cortisol in different conditions. A rise in total cortisol concentration can exceed the transcortin-binding capacity resulting in a marked increase in the unbound fraction. This is associated with increased physiological effects and a rise in the urinary excretion of cortisol which is thus a sensitive indicator of biologically active cortisol concentration (Cope & Black, 1959).

In its passage through the liver, cortisol undergoes reduction and conjugation to produce a group of metabolites which are excreted in the urine (see Fig. 11.2) and are determined as a group in some laboratory measurements of 17-hydroxy-corticoid excretion. Reduction of the double bond in the A ring is important and virtually irreversible. Two separate NADPH-dependent enzymes are concerned in the reduction of the double bond, and determine the configuration of the 5-hydrogen atom. The enzyme producing the 5β form is predominant and the 5α form (allo derivatives) is only found in a small fraction of cortisol metabolites. This reduction is probably the rate-limiting one and the high biological activity of some synthetic glucocorticoids is attributable to impaired reduction of this double bond (Bush, 1962). The dihydrocortisol derivatives are probably physiologically inactive but are rapidly further reduced at the 3-ketone group to form the tetrahydro derivatives, which are then conjugated with glucuronic acid. In man the configuration of the 3-hydroxy group is largely 3α. Major metabolites in urine are thus tetrahydrocortisone and tetrahydrocortisol (Fig. 11.3) with allotetrahydrocortisol in smaller quantities (Bush & Willoughby, 1957). The 5β-steroids also readily undergo reduc-

TABLE 11.1

Plasma "cortisol" concentrations in normal and pathological states

	Plasma "cortisol" (μg./100 ml.)		
	Range	Mean	Method
New-born infants	0–4	2	PS
Normal adults	5–20	13	PS
Normal adults	6–26	14	F
Adults, after prednisolone	1–22	10	PS
Adults, after prednisolone	0–8	3	F
Adults, after oestrogen	31–72	56	PS
Pregnancy, third trimester	27–44	33	PS
Addison's disease	0–8	3	PS
Hypophysectomy	0–4	2·5	F
Cushing's syndrome	16–68	28(H), 43(T)	PS
Cushing's syndrome	22–120	42	F
Adults, after ACTH	63–86	70	F
Congenital adrenal hyperplasia	0–20	9	PS
Terminal illness	22–80	30	PS

PS = Porter-Silber chromogens, Christy et al. (1956)
F = Fluorimetric method of Mattingly (1962)
H = hyperplasia;　T = tumour.

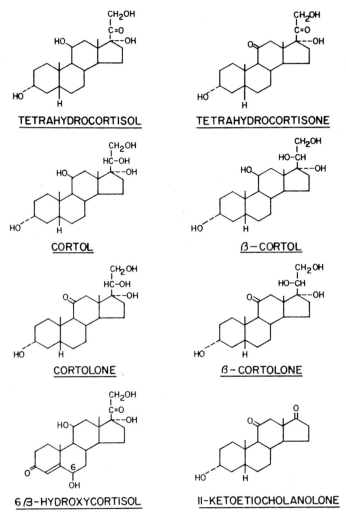

FIG. 11.3. Some urinary metabolites of cortisol. Tetrahydrocortisol, tetrahydrocortisone and allotetrahydro-cortisol make up 25 to 30% of the excretory product of administered cortisol; the cortols and cortolones comprise a further 30 to 40%.

tion of the keto group at C-20 producing 20α and 20β hydroxy groups giving rise to α and β cortols and cortolones (Fig. 11.3) whereas the 5α-steroids are only slightly reduced further to allocortols and allocortolones (Fukushima *et al.*, 1960). Reduction at C-20 also occurs with cortisone and cortisol themselves. The products are minor metabolites in urine and undergo further reduction in ring A to the cortols and cortolones (Bradlow *et al.*, 1962). Whereas all these reductions are virtually irreversible, there is easy exchange between ketone and 11β-hydroxy groups at C-11 (Fig. 11.2) in parent steroids and in their metabolites. This system is responsible for conversion of the bio-logically inactive cortisone given therapeutically into cortisol. Under normal conditions the equilibrium cortisol ⇌ cortisone is slightly in favour of cortisone (Bush & Willoughby, 1957) and this preponderance is increased in hyperthyroidism and reduced in hypothyroidism (Hellman *et al.*, 1961). The enzyme system is easily overloaded and increased endogenous or exogenous release of cortisol results in increased output of 11β-hydroxy derivatives (Baulieu & Jayle, 1957). It is of interest that, whereas allotetrahydrocortisone is almost fully converted to allotetrahydrocortisol, there is little interconversion between tetrahydrocortisone and tetrahydrocortisol (Bush & Mahesh, 1959*a*).

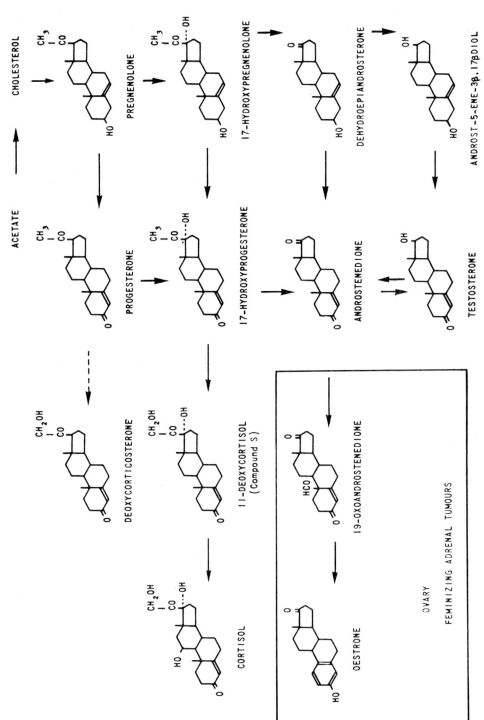

Fig. 11.4. Pathways of synthesis of androgens and oestrogens.

The cleavage of the side chain (Fig. 11.2) is a feature of 17α-hydroxycorticosteroids and is used as such in their laboratory determination. The reaction as it occurs *in vivo* involves the reduced 5β-steroids, tetrahydrocortisone and -cortisol, cortols and cortolones to produce 11β-hydroxy- and 11-oxo-aetiocholanolone (Fig. 11.3). The 17-oxosteroids derived from cortisone and cortisol themselves, namely, adrenosterone and 11β-hydroxyandrostenedione are mainly metabolized to the 5α or androstane series. Although most of the cortisol metabolites are excreted as the 3-glucuronides, small amounts are excreted as the 21-sulphates (Pasqualini & Jayle, 1961; Tamm *et al.*, 1964) and this is especially so in neonatal urines (Drayer & Giroud, 1965). The substance 6β-hydroxycortisol (Fig. 11.3) is sufficiently polar to be excreted unconjugated. Although normally a minor metabolite, its excretion is increased in infancy, pregnancy, toxaemia, cirrhosis, and in terminal illnesses, conditions in which the biological half-life of cortisol is increased (Frantz *et al.*, 1961).

Prolongation of this half-life has a variety of causes. In cirrhosis, the major defect is in reduction of ring A and, to a lesser extent, in conjugation. In hypothyroidism, both steps are slowed. In pregnancy, the increase in transcortin binds cortisol more avidly. These factors impose restrictions on the clinical interpretation of values of plasma cortisol. Thus, in pregnancy, or after administration of oestrogens or of oral contraceptive agents, high values do not signify hyperadrenocorticism but increased cortisol-binding. High values in the terminal state do not necessarily imply over-production of cortisol; its disposal from plasma is exceedingly slow. In hypothyroidism and hepatic disease, the generally normal plasma cortisol figures probably do not mean a normal cortisol secretion rate; this is often reduced and the urinary excretion of metabolites is similarly subnormal. In thyrotoxicosis, a normal plasma cortisol level may be associated with increased secretion and excretion rates. Correct assessment of plasma cortisol figures depends, therefore, upon detailed knowledge of the clinical state. For practical purposes it is usually advisable to obtain figures for both urinary and plasma corticosteroids, and, where necessary, to study the secretion rate of cortisol. Glucuronide metabolites of cortisol appear to be excreted at least partly by tubular secretion and in renal failure the plasma concentration of steroid glucuronides is greatly increased.

Corticosterone metabolism has been less well studied but follows similar lines. The peripheral plasma level is of the order of 1–2 μg./100 ml., the secretion rate is about 2–4 mg./day, both figures appreciably less than those for cortisol; the half life is, however, only slightly lower at 60–100 min. (Peterson, 1959). The equilibrium of 11-oxo ⇌ 11β-hydroxy groups is predominantly in favour of the alcohol. Reduction of ring A and at C-20 occurs in a similar fashion to cortisol but, unlike cortisol, the greater proportion of the tetrahydrometabolites are of the allo (5α) form; the major product is allotetrahydrocorticosterone, with smaller quantities of tetrahydrocorticosterone and its 11-oxo derivative (Peterson & Pierce, 1960). In the hexahydro derivatives, analogous to cortol, an even greater proportion is in the allo form and the 11β-hydroxy-5α-isomer predominates (Exley, 1965). Side chain cleavage and other hydroxylations have not been reported. Although most of the conjugated metabolites are glucuronides, small quantities of sulphates occur. In the neonate, the formation of corticosterone sulphate may occur in the adrenal and some is probably secreted as such and then reduced (Drayer & Giroud, 1965). It is also claimed that this may occur in the adult and that the amount so secreted is about 5 mg./day (Lebeau & Baulieu, 1964). The biological significance of these findings remains to be seen.

11-Deoxycortisol (substance S) is produced in states where 11-hydroxylation is inhibited. Its principal metabolites in urine are its tetrahydro and α- and β-hexahydro derivatives, corresponding to tetrahydrocortisol and α- and β-cortols, and the allotetrahydro compound corresponding to allotetrahydrocortisol.

C-21 Deoxysteroids are important in various enzyme defects in that their metabolites appear in the urine and may be identified (Figs. 11.5 & 11.6). 17-Hydroxyprogesterone undergoes reduction to tetrahydro and hexahydro derivatives of the 5β series, the main products being 3α, 17α-dihydroxy-5β-pregnane-20-one and 5β-pregnane-3α,17α,20α-triol (pregnanetriol). 17-Hydroxypregnenolone also produces pregnanetriol but in addition the product, pregn-5-ene-3β,17α,20α-triol, occurs, in which the rings A and B are unchanged from those of the parent steroid. Likewise, 21-deoxycortisol is converted to 3α,17α-dihydroxypregnane-11,20-dione; 3α, 17α, 20α-trihydroxypregnane-11-one (11-oxopregnanetriol) and pregnane-3α,11β,17α,20α-tetrol (11β-hydroxypregnanetriol). In this case, the 11-oxo compounds predominate and there seems to be very little conversion to 17-oxosteroids by loss of the side chain.

Aldosterone has also been shown to be metabolized along the usual lines but there are modifications in that the molecule exists with the 11β-

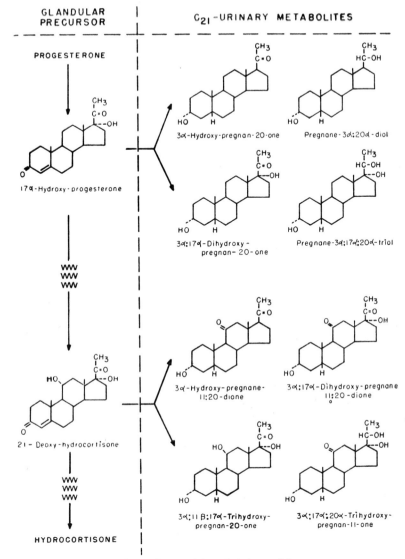

GLANDULAR PRECURSOR

C_{21}-URINARY METABOLITES

PROGESTERONE

17α-Hydroxy-progesterone

3α-Hydroxy-pregnan-20-one

Pregnane-3α:20α-diol

3α:17α-Dihydroxy-pregnan-20-one

Pregnane-3α:17α:20α-triol

21-Deoxy-hydrocortisone

3α-Hydroxy-pregnane-11:20-dione

3α:17α-Dihydroxy-pregnane-11:20-dione

3α:11β:17α-Trihydroxy-pregnan-20-one

3α:17α:20α-Trihydroxy-pregnan-11-one

HYDROCORTISONE

FIG. 11.5. Urinary C_{21} steroids and their possible precursors.

hydroxy and 18-aldehyde groups linked together to form a stable cyclic hemiacetal. The usual transformations of the 11β-hydroxy group are not seen and the 18-aldehyde does not undergo oxidation. The normal plasma level is very low at 0·04–0·08 μg./l. and the normal secretory rate is about 100–150 μg./day, only 1 % of that of cortisol (Tait *et al.*, 1961; Cope *et al.*, 1961; Siegenthaler *et al.*, 1962). Aldosterone is less bound to protein than is cortisol, and transcortin-binding is probably not an important factor as there is no increase in pregnancy; the binding is probably to albumin

and plasma fraction IV-4 (Meyer *et al.*, 1961). Aldosterone is excreted as a unique acid-labile conjugate of the hormone itself as well as undergoing reduction before conjugation. The acid-labile conjugate is probably a glucuronide involving the hemiacetal hydroxy group at C-18 (Underwood & Tait, 1964). The 4,5β-dihydrometabolite has been isolated as have three tetrahydro compounds. Of these the 3α-hydroxy-5β derivative, analogous to tetrahydrocortisol is present in the largest amount. The minor products are the 3α-hydroxy-5α derivative, analogous to

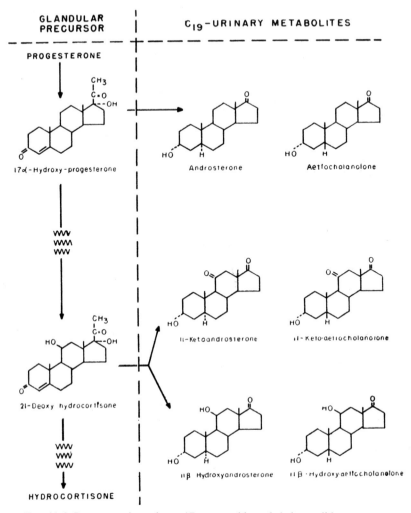

FIG. 11.6. Representative urinary 17-oxosteroids and their possible precursors.

allotetrahydrocortisol, and the 3β-hydroxy-5β derivative. Further reduction at C-20 can occur with the 3α-hydroxy-5β steroid to form the 20β-hydroxy derivative, analogous to β-cortol. Loss of the 21-hydroxy group from the commonest tetrahydro compound and from the hexahydro compound has also been demonstrated, but loss of the side chain at C-17 does not occur. The reduced products are mainly excreted as the glucuronides conjugated at C-3 (Kelly *et al.*, 1962*a*, *b*, 1963; Pasqualini *et al.*, 1963; Ulick *et al.*, 1962).

Androgen metabolism is still being clarified. Dehydroepiandrosterone is secreted as such and as its 3-sulphate. Further conversion to the sulphate occurs in peripheral tissues, but normally the amount of this substance in the urine is only a small fraction of that secreted as the free and conjugated steroid. The major part undergoes oxidation by β-hydroxysteroid dehydrogenase (Bradlow *et al.*, 1964) to the corresponding Δ^5-3-oxosteroid which is converted by an isomerase to androstenedione (Talalay & Wang, 1955), a substance also secreted by the adrenal and produced by oxidation of the 17β-hydroxy group of testosterone. Androstenedione undergoes reduction in ring A similar to that seen in other steroids to produce 3α-hydroxy-5α-androstane-17-one (androsterone), 3α-hydroxy-5β-androstane-17-one (aetiocholanolone) and small amounts of the corresponding 3β-hydroxy compounds. The adrenal also secretes 11βhydroxyandrostenedione which can undergo the usual oxidation at C-11 to produce adrenosterone (11-oxoandrostenedione). Both steroids then undergo reduction of ring A with an emphasis on the production of tetrahydro compounds with the 3α-hydroxy-5α configuration. The major product is 11β-hydroxyandrosterone with lesser amounts of 11-oxoandrosterone, 11β-hydroxy- and 11-oxo-aetiocholanolone (Savard et al., 1953; Bradlow & Gallagher, 1957). 11β-Hydroxyandrostenedione is also converted to the rather unusual metabolite 3α-hydroxyandrost-4-ene-3:17-dione, in which the double bond of ring A is preserved. Excretion of this metabolite is increased in myxoedema.

These metabolites are excreted as the glucuronides and, in lesser amounts, as the sulphates and contribute to the 17-oxosteroid fraction of urine. Aetiocholanolone can undergo further reactions. Reduction of the ketone group to the 17β-hydroxy group yields aetiocholane-3α-17β-diol, a metabolite also produced by ring A reduction of testosterone. Testosterone glucuronide is converted virtually exclusively to aetiocholane-3α,17β-diol (Robel et al., 1966). Further hydroxylation of aetiocholanolone can also occur yielding the 7β-hydroxy and 18-hydroxy derivatives. Androsterone can likewise produce androstane-3α,17β-diol, a minor reduction product of testosterone, and 18-hydroxyandrosterone.

Further hydroxylation of dehydroepiandrosterone and its sulphate has also been described, leading to such products as 7α-hydroxydehydroepiandrosterone (Sulcova & Starka, 1963), 7-oxo-dehydroepiandrosterone (Baulieu et al., 1961), 16α-hydroxydehydroepiandrosterone and 7α,16α-dihydroxyepiandrosterone (Okada et al., 1959). The conversion of the 16α-hydroxy compound to oestriol has been mentioned earlier. The conversion of dehydroepiandrosterone, its sulphate and androstenedione to testosterone is of importance in virilizing conditions (see later). This conversion can occur in the liver where the testosterone can be further converted to the biologically inactive products: testosterone glucuronide, androsterone and aetiocholanolone. About 5% of the testosterone is converted to the glucuronide and about 15% of this appears in the urine as such, the rest being further reduced (Robel et al., 1966).

Laboratory Investigation of Adrenal Cortical Disease

The details of laboratory techniques will not be considered here, but certain general principles are worthy of mention. A large number of adrenal cortical steroids, including metabolites, are now recognized, and it will be apparent that there are only a limited number of different substituents in the steroid nucleus. Their chemical properties are thus not very different so that specific chemical methods for their determination are not easy to devise. Furthermore, a single hormone is usually represented by a number of different metabolites in urine, all having slightly different chemical and physical properties. In general, methods for the determination of a hormone and its metabolites involve either the application of a relatively specific chemical method to detect a whole group of metabolites with a common feature, or the application of a relatively non-specific method to a carefully isolated single hormone or metabolite. Methods of the second type are usually laborious and for rapid routine determinations, those of the first type are preferred.

Another consideration is the nature of the specimens to be analysed. In practice the choice is between plasma and urine; this is also true when secretion rate studies are being considered. In the case of plasma, the only steroid commonly determined is cortisol. The determination of cortisol metabolites and corticosterone, aldosterone, adrenal androgens or their metabolites is more difficult and, although such investigations have been performed, they are not available in most centres; the same is true for determinations on adrenal venous plasma. Determinations on plasma only give information about the circulating hormone concentration at the time of sampling and the importance of this in the case of substances showing a diurnal rhythm has been discussed earlier. Determinations of urinary steroids are usually performed on a 24 hr. sample and give an average picture of steroid excretion over this period. Such a specimen contains a much larger quantity of steroid than any plasma sample, but the number of different steroids is much greater and most of them are excreted in conjugated form. The conjugates have to be hydrolysed at some stage before final assessment.

Plasma cortisol methods fall into two main groups; colorimetric and fluorimetric. Unconjugated steroids in plasma are extracted into an organic solvent such as methylene dichloride. This extract may be washed before the final stage. In the colorimetric procedure, the extract is mixed with sulphuric acid—phenylhydrazine mixture and the intensity of the yellow colour in the acid layer is measured. Substances giving this reaction (Porter-Silber chromogens) include steroids bearing an α-ketol side chain and a hydroxy group at position C-17. The major steroid in the extract possessing this feature is cortisol. Corticosterone does not react, but Compound S and any un-conjugated reduction products of this substance or of cortisol will interfere as they possess the required features. Interference can also occur with such non-steroidal substances as aldehydes, ketones and various pharmaceutical preparations if they are extracted. The method, despite its limitations, is suitable for routine use provided the possible errors are remembered. It has been particularly used in the United States and a number of variants of the basic procedure are available. An alternative approach involves mixing the plasma extract with sulphuric acid—alcohol mixture, and measuring the intensity of fluorescence in the acid layer, a reaction given by 11-hydroxysteroids. Corticosterone gives a fluorescence 2·5 times as intense as that from cortisol and is the main interfering substance. Reduction products of cortisol, compound S itself and various synthetic steroids give much less interference than with the Porter-Silber technique. Although modifications may be introduced to reduce corticosterone interference, the method as usually used determines cortisol plus cortico-sterone, i.e. 11-hydroxycorticosteroids. Under normal circumstances the mean plasma corticosterone level is 1·3 μg./100 ml., so the interference is not great. Figures comparing the two methods have been given in Table 11.1. Other factors affecting the interpretation of plasma "cortisol" figures are discussed earlier.

The determination of 17-oxosteroids (17-OS) in urine has been carried out for over 30 years. Androgens derived from the adrenal and the testis are, in large measure, excreted as reduction products bearing a 17-oxo group. Determination of 17-OS is therefore an indication of the production of total androgen from two glands. As a large part of the 17-OS is derived from substances of relatively low androgenic potency, the 17-OS excretion is a poor indicator of biological androgenic activity. The 17-OS in urine comprise a group of steroids present as glucuronides and sulphates. The principle of the method is to hydrolyse the conjugates, to extract the steroids and to determine them as a group by taking advantage of the purple colour given by the 17-oxo group with m-dinitrobenzene (Zimmermann reaction). Ketones substituted at other positions can occur and these and certain non-steroidal substances interfere in the reaction. The conjugates of 17-OS are relatively stable, but the traditional hydrolysis procedure with hot hydrochloric acid produces some artefacts. Enzymic hydrolysis is milder but more time-consuming. The method has been extended to the examination of the individual 17-oxo-steroids by

combining further fractionation of the crude steroid extract with the Zimmermann reaction.

The other major group of steroids in urine are the metabolites of cortisol. These are excreted mainly as conjugated reduction products, mostly as glucuronides. These conjugates are much more susceptible to damage by drastic hydrolytic procedures than are those of 17-OS. A type of method in common use in the United States involves preliminary hydrolysis of the conjugates with β-glucuronidase, extraction of the free steroids into an organic solvent and application of the colour reaction for Porter-Silber chromogens, (see above). The major reactants are tetrahydro-cortisol, tetrahydrocortisone and allotetrahydro-cortisol; cortols and cortolones, although important metabolites, do not react. The metabolites of corticosterone and 21-deoxycortisol also do not react but those of 11-deoxycortisol (Compound S) do. Difficulties may thus arise in cases of enzyme defect discussed later. In Europe one of the methods measuring 17-oxogenic steroids (17-OGS) is more commonly employed. These make use of the fact that steroids bearing at C-17 a hydroxy group and one of the side chains: —CO . CH$_2$OH, —CH(OH) . CH$_2$OH, —CH-(OH).CH$_3$, are oxidized by sodium bismuthate or metaperiodate to produce a ketone group at C-17, hence the name 17-OGS. The increment in 17-OS as determined by the Zimmermann reaction is measured. The method avoids enzymic hydrolysis of the rather delicate C$_{21}$ steroid conjugates by converting them to the more stable 17-OS conjugates and hydrolysing these with hot acid. Even this step can be avoided if the oxidizing agent is metaperiodate; it oxidizes the glucuronide residue also. The reaction is given by all the usual cortisol metabolites including the cortols and cortolones. Metabolites of 11-deoxycortisol also react as do some of those from 21-deoxycortisol (those with a —CO . CH$_3$ side chain do not react) but corticosterone metabolites do not. These additional substances from 21-deoxycortisol may be determined by a modification in which all ketone groups in the urinary steroids are firstly reduced to the corresponding alcohol with sodium borohydride. This step thus removes the original 17-OS and produces side chains of the form: —CH(OH) . CH$_2$OH and —CH(OH).CH$_3$. These are oxidized to the corresponding 17-oxosteroids with metaperiodate and determined in the usual way. This gives a measure of "total 17-hydroxy-corticosteroids".

The metabolites of corticosterone and especially those of aldosterone are present in smaller amounts than the 17-OS and 17-OGS. Their measurement involves hydrolysis of conjugates, extraction and somewhat laborious chromatographic separation of the individual steroids before application of a relatively non-specific method for the final determination. Details of these procedures will be found in specialized works. Such methods are much more time-consuming and are less frequently employed.

The common techniques for the determination of plasma "cortisol", and urinary cortisol metabolites, are frequently combined with some method of stimulating or suppressing adrenal cortical function. Such tests as the ACTH-stimulation test and dexamethasone suppression test are discussed later. Similarly an assessment of the ability of the pituitary to produce ACTH is possible by using metyrapone (Metopirone), an 11β-hydroxylase inhibitor to suppress circulating cortisol concentration and thus to stimulate the hypothalamic-adenohypophyseal mechanism.

Mention should finally be made of the use of secretion rate studies to supplement the information on the circulating plasma concentration and excretion rate of metabolites. This involves the administration of a known amount of the required hormone labelled with ^{14}C or ^{3}H. The rate of disappearance of the labelled hormone from plasma is determined by repeated sampling over the next hour or so and can be used to derive the secretion rate over the period of the test. Alternatively, urine may be collected for 24 hr. following the introduction of the labelled hormone into the body's metabolic pathways. The isolation of a particular metabolite, e.g. tetrahydrocortisone, aldosterone, and determination of the specific activity of that metabolite permits the calculation of the 24 hr. secretion rate. Such studies are more complex than the usual routine steroid determinations, but have yielded valuable additional information in interpreting abnormalities of steroid metabolism in difficult cases.

HYPOADRENOCORTICISM (ADDISON'S DISEASE)

Aetiology

Adrenal insufficiency, or Addison's disease, is an uncommon condition. Destruction of both glands by tuberculosis is still encountered in Great Britain, though its importance in the aetiology of the disease will naturally vary according to the prevalence of tuberculosis in the community. Non-tuberculous cases are associated with an atrophy of the cortices, hitherto described as "idiopathic" but which may be the result of auto-immune processes. In about half these cases,

antibodies directed against the adrenal cortex may be demonstrated in the blood (Anderson et al., 1966). Occasionally, these patients can also be shown to produce antibodies directed against the thyroid gland, thus providing a possible explanation for the known association between idiopathic Addison's disease and hypothyroidism. A similar pathological mechanism may explain the association between Addison's disease and hypoparathyroidism (Blizzard et al., 1963; Blizzard & Kyle, 1963). Although neoplasms frequently spread to the adrenals, and are found at autopsy, they rarely produce Addison's disease; a few well-documented instances of adrenal cortical insufficiency have been reported in association with metastatic lung carcinoma and widespread lymphoma (Hagtvet, 1963). Most cases of pigmentation, asthenia and hyponatraemia observed in the presence of neoplastic disease are associated with normal adrenal cortical function; when vomiting is not the cause, the production of anti-diuretic hormone by the neoplasm should be suspected. It must be emphasized that adrenal insufficiency occurs only after the removal of at least 90% of the total cortical tissue and that, in many cases, death from malignant disease probably occurs before adrenal disease becomes clinically evident.

Other causes of adrenal destruction are of great rarity but include amyloidosis, histoplasmosis and blastomycosis. There is no evidence that exposure to a violent "stress" causes adrenal atrophy, and there is no recorded instance of a case of the Waterhouse-Friderichsen syndrome that went on to chronic adrenal insufficiency.

The diagnosis of Addison's disease is a matter of the utmost gravity. It implies lifelong replacement therapy and a constant threat to life from infections, surgical operations and severe trauma. Although the classical clinical syndrome is widely known, great difficulty may be experienced in establishing the diagnosis in certain patients. The potential hazards to life in these cases are no less serious than in the classical type, and no effort should be spared in reaching a firm conclusion concerning the state of the adrenal function. None of the individual signs or symptoms of Addison's disease may be considered as pathognomonic of adrenal insufficiency. For example, pigmentation, asthenia, hyponatraemia and hyperkalaemia are all found in a wide variety of conditions unassociated with adrenal disease. An understanding of the basic disturbances in adrenal physiology is essential for a full appreciation of the clinical and biochemical features, and for a rational therapeutic approach.

Renal and electrolyte disturbances. Loss of body Na is the cardinal feature of the adrenal-deficient state. It occurs after adrenalectomy in laboratory animals (Marine & Baumann, 1927) and in naturally occurring Addison's disease (Loeb *et al.*, 1933). Although the major route of Na loss is through the urine, the defect in electrolyte metabolism is widespread, since increased amounts of Na are found in the sweat and the gastro-intestinal secretions. Vomiting and diarrhoea, which occur at times of crisis, aggravate the dehydration and electrolyte depletion. Renal blood flow and glomerular filtration rate decrease as a result of the contraction of the extracellular space and lead to azotaemia.

The failure of the kidney to conserve Na is only one of several renal defects found in Addison's disease; others lead to hyperkalaemia and acidosis. The intimate mechanisms of these abnormalities are not known, but there is a large body of evidence which points to major renal tubular defects. The effects of adrenal cortical steroids upon the renal handling of Na has been mentioned. The ion-exchange mechanisms seem to be implicated in further abnormalities in Addison's disease, since both H^+ and NH_4^+ secretion by the tubules is also impaired after adrenalectomy in laboratory animals (Sartorius *et al.*, 1952, 1953); under conditions of acid loading, there is an inadequate renal response, the urinary acidification being suboptimal. Herein lies a plausible explanation for the metabolic acidosis seen in Addisonian crises. Deoxycorticosterone corrects this abnormality, but adrenalectomized animals maintained in good condition with salt alone may exhibit some degree of acidosis. It is of interest, but probably of no direct relevance to the electrolyte abnormalities, that T_m (*p*-aminohippuric acid) has been found reduced in some female Addisonian patients. A similar change in T_m (glucose) has been observed. Apparently, multiple facets of tubular function are affected.

The problem of plasma electrolyte, acid-base and water changes in Addison's disease is more complicated, however, than a simple study of renal function would indicate. Certain extra-renal effects of steroids influence the distribution of electrolytes between the various body fluid compartments. The administration of deoxycorticosterone to nephrectomized dogs leads to an increase in the distribution space of ^{24}Na. Following adrenalectomy, there is a greater loss of Na from the extracellular space than can be explained on the basis of the negative external balance of this ion. Conversely, during recovery from Addisonian crises, more Na is added to this space

than is present in the food. Since the intracellular content of Na is decreased in Addison's disease, another source of this ion must be postulated. Bone has been suggested as a large reservoir in which Na might be sequestered in larger than normal amounts under these conditions, but proof of this phenomenon is still awaited. Similar extra-renal effects are observed in relation to K (Pitts, 1951). It may be observed that the acid-base disturbances of Addison's disease may also be partly due to an extra-renal effect. The infusion of KCl into normal dogs leads to a shift of bicarbonate into the cells and hence to acidosis. The exchange of K^+ for H^+ across the cell membrane works in the reverse direction in K depletion and in overdosage with steroids. Acidosis may therefore have a dual origin: renal and extra-renal. Although these extra-renal effects are of great physiological interest, the magnitude of their contribution to the clinical abnormalities in Addison's disease is not known. Knowledge of their existence should not be allowed to overshadow the major role of the renal defects, nor should it in any way minimize the imperative need for massive saline therapy in the dehydrated patient.

A gross deficiency in circulating cortisol is also characterized by abnormalities in the renal handling of water. The free water clearance falls but the defect is abolished following the administration of glucocorticoids (Oleesky & Stanbury, 1951). Conversely, glucosteroids increase the clearance of free water in normal individuals and thereby increase the maximal water diuresis (Kleeman *et al.*, 1960). Despite evidence implicating a direct effect of steroids on the tubular epithelium and conflicting information concerning the role of the anti-diuretic hormone, the evidence now favours a direct effect of glucocorticoids on the secretion of vasopressin by the neurohypophysis. Ahmed *et al.* (1967) have shown that the plasma arginine vasopressin is increased to unusual values during dehydration and remains elevated despite haemodilution in patients with untreated adrenocortical insufficiency, demonstrating a delayed water diuresis. Glucocorticoid therapy lowered the vasopressin values to normal on dehydration; zero values were recorded during diuresis tests on treated patients.

Disturbances of carbohydrate and protein metabolism. The most important evidence of organic metabolic derangement in Addison's disease is the occurrence of hypoglycaemia. In the presence of an adequate food intake, or during replacement therapy with cortisone, marked hypoglycaemia is rarely seen; however, during fasting or under stress, hypoglycaemia may supervene. A diet deficient in carbohydrate is also capable of unmasking the hypoglycaemic tendency; the dietary treatment of obesity in the Addisonian patient may be very difficult. Insulin sensitivity is exaggerated, though not to the same degree as is observed after hypophysectomy or with hypopituitarism. Adrenaline fails to induce the customary hyperglycaemic response in the adrenal-deficient state. A defect of glucose absorption from the intestine in Addison's disease is also readily recognizable on comparison between the oral and intravenous glucose tolerance curves, but this defect cannot adequately account for the observed abnormalities which arise chiefly from deficient gluconeogenesis. The overall effect of adrenal insufficiency is to deprive the metabolic pool of those intermediary products from protein which serve as substrates for glycogen synthesis. Although adrenal steroids can be demonstrated to accelerate gluconeogenesis from fat, this has only been achieved under carefully selected experimental conditions, and there is no evidence at present to indicate the quantitative importance of this process in relation to the hypoglycaemia of Addison's disease.

The reciprocal relationship between the circulating level of cortisol upon the release of MSH (melanocyte-stimulating hormone) from the anterior pituitary is analogous to that between cortisol and ACTH. The high circulating levels of MSH in Addison's disease appear to account satisfactorily for the increased dermal pigmentation. As is the case with ACTH, the elevated titre of MSH in plasma is restored to normal by the pituitary-inhibiting effect of administered cortisol.

The Diagnosis of Addison's Disease

It cannot be over-emphasized that the diagnosis of Addison's disease must rest upon impeccable evidence, which includes the laboratory confirmation of the clinical impression. There is no *single* diagnostic test for adrenal failure; as in other clinical states, a battery of tests must be performed and evaluated before a conclusion can be reached.

(1) *Electrolyte studies.* Adrenal insufficiency is accompanied by hyponatraemia, hyperkalaemia and an increase in the urea and haematocrit of the blood. However, these findings are non-specific. Many patients with chronic diseases, e.g. cancer, tuberculosis, salt-losing nephritis, may show decreased concentrations of Na in the blood, whilst there are patients with Addison's disease whose serum Na or K may be normal. Normal serum electrolyte concentrations may be found in Addisonian crisis, especially if this has occurred rapidly in a patient who is maintained on steroid hormone therapy. A low serum Na concentration is in itself not diagnostic of Addison's disease.

(2) *Salt deprivation or salt withdrawal test.* This is perhaps the most rigorous test of adrenal function. On a low-salt diet the patient with adrenal insufficiency fares poorly. He loses weight, develops anorexia, nausea and later vomits, and easily slips into adrenal crisis. The serum Na falls, the serum K and haematocrit rise. Obviously, this is a dangerous diagnostic test and must be done under close medical supervision *in the hospital.* The test need not be carried out to the point of overt adrenal crisis. Once the patient complains of weakness, anorexia and possibly nausea, blood should be drawn for Na, K, urea and haematocrit determinations. The diagnostic findings are: a fall in serum Na concentration of 4 or 5 meq./l., a rise in serum K of 0·5–1·0 meq./l. and a rise in blood urea of 5–15 mg./100 ml. This test should not be carried out to the point of severe hypotension, since an adrenal crisis may supervene quite suddenly; definite evidence is usually elicited within 72 hr. and the procedure should be terminated by the administration of 100 mg. cortisone acetate orally or 100 mg. cortisol intravenously, and liberal amounts of salt.

(3) *Water-loading test.* The patient with adrenal insufficiency cannot excrete a water load as readily as a normal individual because of the inappropriate secretion of vasopressin. Several tests of water-loading have been described. In brief, they test the percentage of a given water-load excreted over a specific time (normal excretion in one such test, over 50% of 1000 ml. water within 4 hr.) The adrenalectomized or adrenal-deficient patient will retain the water for an abnormally long period of time (Kepler *et al.*, 1948).

The water-loading test may be hazardous and, together with the salt-depletion test, should be avoided in those cases in which other evidence of Addison's disease is already conclusive. Acute water intoxication is a real danger. Both these tests are, of course, non-specific, and in the case of a faulty water diuresis, similar results may be obtained in hypothyroidism, hypopituitarism, advanced renal and hepatic disease and in oedematous conditions generally. The value of an abnormal result is greatly enhanced if the test is repeated, at the same time of day, following the oral administration of 100 mg. cortisone acetate. Correction of a faulty water diuresis in this way is very strong evidence of hypocortisolaemia.

The tests of adrenal steroid production, especially in response to ACTH, are far more specific and generally safe; they should be used as the principal diagnostic procedures, the provocative tests being reserved for doubtful cases, or when other tests are not available. The results in these latter circumstances should be interpreted with great caution in the light of the total clinical picture.

(4) *Steroid studies.* In adrenal insufficiency, the 24 hr. urinary 17-oxosteroid excretion is low, i.e. less than 5 mg./24 hr. However, the procedure lacks chemical specificity at low values and further difficulties arise because of the diverse origins of these steroids from adrenal and gonadal sources and in the peripheral metabolism (e.g. liver) of C_{21} steroids, a process which may be altered in liver disease, hypothyroidism, malnutrition and in many chronic non-endocrine illnesses. The methods which measure urinary cortisol metabolites are rather more specific (e.g. 17-oxogenic steroids, 17-hydroxycorticoids), but even they may occasionally give low values for non-specific reasons. Anti-convulsant therapy with phenobarbitone and diphenylhydantoin must be cited in addition to the previously mentioned factors since it appears to cause a deviation in cortisol metabolism to 2α- and 6β-hydroxycortisol metabolites which may not be estimated by the analytical method in current use (Burstein *et al.*, 1967).

17-Oxogenic steroids below 7 mg./day are compatible with Addison's disease but certainly not diagnostic; values of 1 mg. or under are highly suggestive. In cases of low 17-OGS without endocrine disease, plasma cortisol will be found to be within the normal range, allowing for the usual diurnal variations.

The measurement of plasma corticosteroid provides a much more direct estimate of adrenal secretory function, and values are usually low in primary adrenal insufficiency. Values lying between 0–5 μg./100 ml. at 09.00 hr. are highly suggestive—for reasons connected with the circadian rhythm such values later in the day would be of no value. However, patients with Addison's disease are encountered with plasma corticosteroid figures overlapping the normal range (6–24 μg./100 ml.).

(5) *ACTH tests.* Whilst abnormal values in the above-mentioned tests play an important part in the diagnosis of Addison's disease, the chemical hallmark of the disease is the failure of the adrenals to respond to ACTH.

(1) The intramuscular administration of ACTH gel, 40 units b.d. for 3 days is satisfactory but time-consuming and inconvenient. The response is judged from the 24 hr. urinary 17-OGS or 17-OHCS output which, in normal patients, should rise to values above the normal range. In Addisonian individuals there is no significant change in the urinary value.

(2) An infusion of 25 units ACTH over a fixed period, usually 4 hr., causes a significant rise in plasma corticosteroids in normal individuals; in patients with adrenal insufficiency, no such rise occurs. In very rare instances, the intravenous administration of ACTH has appeared to cause an adrenal crisis (chills, fever, hypotension and hyponatraemia) in patients with adrenal insufficiency, even with the relatively pure preparations which are available commercially; some protection may be obtained by dissolving the ACTH in isotonic saline instead of 5% dextrose. Alternatively, the prior oral administration of 0·2 mg. fludrocortisone has been suggested.

The critical feature of this test is the duration of the infusion rather than the precise quantity of ACTH administered to the patient since the dose is designed to provide a supra-maximal stimulus to the adrenal cortices. The procedures may be standardized at will, on the basis of a 4, 6 or 8 hr. infusion, provided the response of normal individuals is ascertained in the same manner. The infusions should always be commenced at the same time of day, preferably around 09.00 hr. when the adrenal sensitivity is at its highest. The response is measured as the change in plasma corticosteroids before and immediately after the infusion.

(3) Synthetic β^{1-24} corticotropin (Synacthen) may be used intramuscularly or intravenously. Freedom from impurities and allergic reactions is a considerable advantage. An intravenous infusion rate of 3 μg./hr. provides a maximal stimulus, but amounts of up to 100 μg./hr. may be employed with safety, in tests of 4–6 hr. An intramuscular test (Wood *et al.*, 1965) is convenient and rapid. β^{1-24} Corticotropin (250 μg.) is injected intramuscularly at 09.00 hr.; blood is withdrawn before the injection and 30 min. afterwards. In normal individuals, a doubling of the basal plasma corticosteroid level is observed. Using the Mattingly method, the figures are: mean resting level 14·7 μg. $\pm$ 3·95; at 30 min. 31·4 μg. $\pm$ 5·17. In view of the urgency in establishing or refuting the diagnosis of Addison's disease, the rapidity of this method is a considerable advantage, results being obtained the same day.

Careful assessment of the clinical situation usually permits a clear distinction to be made between cases of primary adrenal and pituitary disease. Rarely, some doubt may exist and it may be advisable to confirm negative results in the rapid intravenous tests by more prolonged stimulation of the adrenals using ACTH gel over several days.

Treatment of Addison's Disease

The treatment of Addison's disease resolves itself into the management of the patient from day to day and the treatment of the acute episode of adrenal insufficiency ("adrenal crisis").

Day-to-day management. Steroid therapy. Cortisone or cortisol are the drugs of choice in the treatment of Addison's disease. Prednisone and other synthetic glucocorticoid analogues lack the salt-retaining effects which are physiological and desirable in substitution therapy. Cortisone, 25 to 50 mg./day, by mouth, provides adequate treatment in the majority of cases. Hyperthyroidism leads to an increased rate of metabolic destruction of steroids and the dose may have to be increased. Conversely, untreated hypothyroidism would decrease the requirement. The most gratifying aspect of cortisone treatment in patients with adrenal insufficiency is its extraordinary and consistent effect upon the feeling of well-being and the appetite of the patients. Patients experience an increase in weight, but this rarely becomes excessive. The 11-oxygenated steroids are effective in protecting against hypoglycaemia and stress of all sorts. Nevertheless, intercurrent infections and trauma require a temporary increase in dosage to twice the usual amount and parenteral therapy is occasionally necessary in these circumstances. However, the effect of cortisone or cortisol on electrolyte metabolism varies from patient to patient; some may be maintained on cortisone alone; others, even on large doses of cortisone, continue to show loss of urinary Na together with a fall in the serum Na, and may even experience mild adrenal crises. Many patients with Addison's disease thus require a mineralocorticoid in addition to cortisone.

The cortisol analogue, fludrocortisone, has replaced deoxycorticosterone in the treatment of this aspect of Addison's disease. This steroid is 10–13 times more potent as a glucocorticoid than cortisone, but is more than 50 times as potent in its Na-retaining action. (Table 11.2.) Very small doses, 0·1 to 0·2 mg. of fludrocortisone, may be given by mouth daily in addition to cortisone and as a substitute for injection of deoxycorticosterone acetate. Great care must be exercised to avoid overdosage indicated by hypertension and hypokalaemia. Still greater caution is obviously necessary in older patients with existing or potential cardiac disease.

The deleterious effects of large doses of cortisone in patients with tuberculosis have been noted. Cortisone must be used with great caution and in minimal doses in patients whose Addison's disease is due to tuberculosis, but is certainly not contra-indicated. The beneficial effects of cortisone on the appetite and the weight gain noted in these patients may actually help the patient to deal more effectively with the tuberculous infection.

Sodium chloride. Whether the patient be maintained on cortisone alone, or on cortisone plus a mineralocorticoid, exogenous NaCl must sometimes be added to the regimen. The dosage of NaCl can be varied more readily than that of fludrocortisone, and with quicker response;

TABLE 11.2

Relative biological activities of certain natural and synthetic corticosteroids

(Cortisol = 1·0)

Steroid	Liver glycogen deposition	Granuloma pouch	Anti-inflammatory	Na retention
Cortisol	1	1	1	1
Cortisone	0·5–1	0·5–1	0·5	—
Prednisolone	4–5	3–4	4–5	1
6α-Methylprednisolone	10	6	3–4	none
Fludrocortisone	11	13	10	50
16α-Methyl-9α-fluoro-prednisolone	17	170	28	none
Aldosterone	0·3	—	0·25	50
Corticosterone	0·5	—	0·3	2

Modified from Fried, J. & Borman, A. (1958). Vitamins and Hormones, **16**, 303.

when the patient shows signs of excess salt-retention, the amount can be decreased; if hyponatraemia is observed, the amount of salt can easily be increased.

Treatment of adrenal crisis. The clinical symptoms of adrenal crisis may vary widely from patient to patient. One may see shock or coma, or the patient's mental status may be normal and fever the only symptom. The crisis may have a gradual onset or, when vomiting and diarrhoea have been prominent, dehydration (as evidenced by an increase in the haematocrit and the blood urea) may come on precipitously. Often the serum Na is depressed and the K elevated, but the electrolyte concentrations may be normal.

The treatment of adrenal crisis requires rapid emergency measures. After blood is drawn for Na, K, haematocrit, glucose and urea determinations, an infusion of glucose and saline should be given in large quantities. Soluble cortisol preparations are available which can be given intravenously for a more rapid response (the 21-phosphate or hemisuccinate). A good practice is to administer 100 mg. of such a preparation over a 2 min. period via the infusion tubing, then to add another 100 mg. to the infusion bottle. Although treatment must be indivualized, too much cortisol is better than too little. In the authors' experience, most Addisonian crises can be successfully managed with 200–300 mg. of cortisol within the first 24 hr. Occasionally, one needs doses as large as 600 mg. to reverse shock, often with the addition of a sympathomimetic amine (noradrenaline, neosynephrine). Rarely, unpleasant emotional reactions are encountered, but, generally speaking, side effects are not serious in the *short-term* administration of large doses of cortisol. In the presence of shock, intramuscular cortisone is almost useless; if the shock is severe, supplementary blood or plasma expander infusions may be required. Intravenous steroids should be continued until the patient can take drugs by mouth, together with treatment of infection or other underlying cause of the crisis; thereafter, treatment gradually goes over into the day-to-day management. Then, the doses should be kept minimal, because patients with Addison's disease seem to be more susceptible than normal subjects to such effects of overdose as facial rounding, hirsutism and emotional instability.

HYPERADRENOCORTICISM (CUSHING'S SYNDROME)

Hyperfunction of the adrenal cortex occurs in three forms: glucocorticoid, mineralocorticoid and androgenic. Excessive secretion of cortisol, aldosterone and androgen is responsible for these three types of adrenal cortical over-function; in some instances, mixed types of hypersecretion are encountered.

Aetiology

The symptoms and signs of Cushing's syndrome are generally agreed to be the result of hypersecretion of cortisol. Cushing himself believed that the disorder was a form of hyperpituitarism associated with basophilic adenoma of the anterior pituitary (1932). It later became apparent that classic forms of the disease occurred without primary neoplasms of the pituitary or the adrenal cortex, and that the syndrome was usually accompanied by the laboratory finding of a high concentration of adrenal cortical steroids in the urine. With the advent of cortisone and cortisol in 1948, it became clear that typical Cushing's syndrome could be produced by an overdose of these steroids. Attention was thus drawn away from pituitary hyperfunction as an important aetiological basis for Cushing's syndrome. There appears to be no doubt that adrenal cortical adenoma and carcinoma are autonomous disorders like other neoplastic diseases; there is a large body of evidence that such tumours generally behave independently of anterior pituitary control. The aetiology of adrenocortical hyperplasia is controversial. Despite data to the contrary, the weight of present evidence appears to favour the anterior pituitary; it seems unlikely that adrenal hyperplasia can be satisfactorily explained on the basis of a primary adrenocortical dysfunction (Jailer *et al.*, 1956).

Following the discovery that the clinical manifestations of Cushing's syndrome are due to hypercortisolaemia, and bearing in mind the relative rarity of the basophilic adenomata described by Cushing (1932), many arguments were adduced suggesting that the adrenal hyperplasia is a primary adrenal disorder (Horwith & Stokes, 1960). Whereas Cushing believed that pituitary tumours occurred in all cases, the incidence is, in fact, much lower. In the series published by Plotz, Knowlton & Ragan (1952), the incidence was 30%. Sharpening of diagnostic tools in recent years has resulted in the detection of milder cases and the present incidence of such tumours is in the region of 10–15%; this figure includes a number of cases in which the tumour was observed after adrenalectomy. Other evidence included the facts that basophilic adenomata are occasionally found in conditions other than Cushing's syndrome, and the failure to detect abnormal plasma ACTH concentrations. These latter observations probably resulted from poor sensitivity of assay methods which only detected the grossly increased values found in untreated Addison's disease and following adrenalectomy. With improvement in techniques and the study of more cases, there are now sufficient data to suggest the existence of an abnormal ACTH secretion in adrenal hyperplasia.

(1) ACTH assays now show elevated values in a small number of cases at the time of the diagnosis. Subsequent follow-up studies of patients whose condition has relapsed following partial adrenalectomy demonstrate in each case an abnormally high value, i.e. 1–90 mu./100 ml. The level in normal individuals is < 1 mu./100 ml. Patients in remission following total adrenalectomy, but maintained on the usual substitution dosage, yet showing some increase in pigmentation, have consistently elevated values (range 1–400 mu./100 ml.). Although it is possible that adrenalectomy in these cases may have stimulated ACTH secretion, the general picture presented by these figures suggests that there is a progressive increase in ACTH levels, at least in some cases, and that this may be a function of the duration of the illness. The lowest levels would, in general, be found at the time of the original diagnosis when the duration of the illness is relatively short (Nelson et al. 1966).

(2) Slight increases in plasma ACTH levels, insufficient to be detected by present methods, but maintained by infusion throughout the 24 hr., produce a state of hyperadrenocorticism (Nugent et al., 1960), so failure to detect elevated levels by present methods in the early stage of the disease does not exclude an ACTH mechanism.

(3) Loss of the diurnal rhythm of cortisol secretion appears to be the earliest manifestation of this type of adrenal hyperplasia. In normal individuals, a large part of the daily cortisol secretion occurs during a limited period of time during the morning. Maintenance of cortisol secretion at morning rates throughout the 24 hr. by a level of ACTH which is "normal" but inappropriate to the time of day would account for a marked hypercortisolaemia in the early stages of the disease.

(4) Improvement in, or cure of, the disease, by procedures directed at the anterior pituitary, (radiation, electrocoagulation, implantation of radioactive material or hypophysectomy) is compatible with the idea of the pituitary playing a sustaining or supporting role, but many studies testify to the pituitary dependence of the adrenal in this disease. Administration of ACTH causes

adrenal hyper-response in adrenal hyperplasia, not in adrenal tumour (Christy et al., 1957); and administration of cortisone, cortisol or more potent analogues generally results in a fall in urinary corticosteroid excretion, presumably mediated via suppression of endogenous ACTH in hyperplasia but not in tumours (Jailer et al., 1954; Liddle, 1960). An abnormal adrenocorticotropin has been detected in the blood of patients with hyperplasia but not with a tumour (Jailer et al., 1957), which disappears after successful pituitary radiation (Christy & Drucker, 1961). ACTH is more difficult to suppress with exogenous cortisol in patients bilaterally adrenalectomized for this form of Cushing's syndrome than in patients with Addison's disease (Williams et al., 1961).

The cause of the loss of diurnal rhythm and absolute increase in ACTH secretion is not known. Degranulation of the pituitary basophil cells with some increase in their number is often found in adrenocortical hyperplasia (Crooke, 1935). At first glance, this finding appears to favour a pituitary aetiology; however, such changes in the basophils occur after administration to animals and man of cortisol or ACTH. The Crooke changes found in spontaneously occurring adrenal hyperplasia may thus be only secondary to hypersecretion of cortisol, and if this be the case, are compatible with a primary adrenal cortical disorder. If, however, Crooke's changes are to be interpreted as primary hyperpituitarism, this would imply hypersecretion by the pituitary of ACTH.

Heinbecker (1944) claimed that it was possible to produce hyperpituitarism by creating lesions in the hypothalamus. This is unconfirmed, and Maren (1953) was unable to find histological evidence of hypothalamic disease in autopsied patients with Cushing's syndrome and adrenal hyperplasia.

The role of the pituitary tumours, present at onset, or developing later, is not understood. Presumably, they secrete ACTH, but it is not possible to state if there are other differences between cases with and without such pituitary lesions. It is suspected that when a tumour becomes clinically obvious years after the adrenalectomy, one is witnessing the progression of a lesion which was already present but undetectable at the time of the original diagnosis. Alternatively, steroid deprivation resulting from adrenalectomy may accelerate the growth of the tumour. The matter is complicated by a lack of uniformity in the histological picture shown by such lesions. For instance, Montgomery (1963) reviewed 43 cases from the literature and found 34 tumours occurring before or at the time of the endocrine disorder and 9 following adrenalectomy. Histologically, 28 were chromophobe tumours, 9 basophil, 1 eosinophil and 5 mixed chromophobe-basophil.

If these pituitary tumours secrete ACTH, they would seem to lack the autonomy usually associated with adenomata. The administration of dexamethasone or other potent glucocorticoid may suppress ACTH secretion as judged by urinary steroid analyses, and a response to metyrapone has also been observed. The resistance to suppression is, of course, abnormally great and large doses of dexamethasone may be required to achieve it in some instances. Nevertheless, the occurrence of adenomata susceptible to the mechanisms for the control of secretion in normal glands is a matter of some interest. A practical consequence of these observations is that there is no biochemical method of differentiating cases with a pituitary tumour and those without (Nelson & Sprunt, 1964).

Ectopic secretion of "ACTH". The occurrence of non-endocrine neoplasms in patients with Cushing's syndrome is not a fortuitous association. Bilateral adrenal hyperplasia and the clinical and biochemical manifestations of hypercortisolaemia have been observed particularly with the oat-cell carcinoma of the lung. Other reported cases include non-functioning islet-cell carcinoma of the pancreas, carcinoma of the ovary, prostate, thyroid and breast, phaeochromocytoma, thymoma, malignant and benign carcinoid tumours and neuroblastoma. Removal of these tumours, when possible, has led to a remission of the endocrine syndrome suggesting an aetiological relationship; the presence of increased plasma ACTH, unresponsive to suppression with dexamethasone, and a subnormal content of ACTH in the pituitary, have focused attention on the possibility that these tumours may secrete ACTH rather than a corticotropin-releasing factor. Liddle *et al.* (1963, 1964) examined 30 such tumours of diverse non-endocrine origins, without histological similarities and in no way resembling pituitary tissue. In all instances, ACTH activity was found in extracts of these neoplasms, whereas non-malignant tissues from the same patients showed no activity. Full chemical identification of this material as ACTH has not yet been achieved. Immunological studies, however, provide abundant evidence of a close similarity of the tumour "ACTH" and the pituitary hormone. Antibodies raised in rabbits against human and porcine ACTH react with tumour "ACTH" and pituitary

ACTH in precisely the same way. Using antiserum specific to porcine ACTH and a fluorescent antibody technique, it has also been possible to demonstrate specific staining in an islet-cell carcinoma, a carcinoid, and a parotid gland tumour. When the same technique was applied to the pituitary gland from these patients, less than normal activity was found (Jarett *et al.*, 1964). The antigenic properties common to both imply chemical similarity in the C-terminal portion of the molecule, i.e. amino acids 24 to 39. The steroidogenic properties of ACTH observed in assay procedures appear to reside in the N-terminal sequence (amino acids 1–20) (Imura *et al.*, 1965). The similarities between the two molecules thus appear to apply to the whole 39 amino acid sequence of the pituitary hormone and the recently discovered material is unlikely to be a short polypeptide chain. It is of considerable interest that "ACTH"-producing neoplasms are also found to contain a fraction with strong resemblance to pituitary melanocyte stimulating hormone (MSH). In some cases, the secretion of "ACTH" and "MSH" has been associated with the vicarious secretion of substances with the properties of gastrin, vasopressin, parathyroid hormone, thyrotropin, insulin, erythropoietin, gonadotropin (for references: see editorial, *Lancet*, 1967, **1**, 86, which also includes discussion of possible genetic mechanisms).

The clinical manifestations of Cushing's syndrome due to adrenal hyperplasia are the result of hypercortisolaemia and the cortisol secretion rate is necessarily raised above the normal. Many of the features are predictable from an understanding of the pharmacological effects of glucocorticoids, though it should be noted that polycythaemia, diabetic glucose tolerance curves and definite plasma electrolyte changes are perhaps not so common as is frequently stated. A fine growth of downy facial hair is frequently seen, but more severe androgenic manifestations are rather unusual. Occasionally, a mixed syndrome occurs in which the adrenal androgens are also increased with correspondingly severe hirsutism. Hyperaldosteronism is not a feature of the condition and when a hypokalaemic alkalosis supervenes, a severe hypersecretion of cortisol is usually held responsible. Nevertheless, the secretion of deoxycorticosterone may be elevated in this condition and this could contribute to the development of hypokalaemia (Crane & Harris, 1966). This is particularly noticeable when the source of the "ACTH" is a non-endocrine neoplasm. The highest cortisol secretion rates have been observed in this syndrome, a figure of

550 mg./24 hr. having been recorded in one instance (O'Riordan *et al.*, 1966).

Diagnosis

There are three principal diagnostic problems in spontaneous Cushing's syndrome: establishing the existence of the disease in mild or atypical form; distinguishing adrenal tumour from hyperplasia; and excluding hyperplasia due to a non-endocrine neoplasm. There is now a great variety of diagnostic procedures aimed at detection of hypercortisolism, but it must be emphasized that no one of these manoeuvres provides absolute grounds upon which to base the diagnosis or the aetiology. Several tests must be done and interpreted in the light of the clinical circumstances. Occasionally, surgical exploration is the only diagnostic recourse, even after full biochemical and radiological investigation.

(1) *Plasma cortisol.* Consistently elevated plasma cortisol values are strong evidence in favour of the diagnosis. Much valuable information is to be gained from relating plasma levels to the time of day, since abolition of the diurnal rhythm of cortisol secretion is a characteristic feature of the condition (Ekman *et al.*, 1961). Values in the upper normal morning range, maintained throughout the 24 hr., imply a considerably increased secretion and are suggestive of the diagnosis. As a screening procedure, blood should be drawn at 24.00 hr. and 09.00 hr., at which times a normal rhythm should be immediately apparent. Care should be taken to exclude patients with severe head injuries, a profoundly disturbed sleep rhythm or congestive heart failure, since the diurnal variations may be abolished in these circumstances.

(2) *Urinary free cortisol.* Only a minute proportion of the total daily cortisol secretion reaches the urine in unchanged form. Using methods based upon double isotope dilution derivative assay (Peterson, 1960), the normal urinary output is less than 100 μg./day. This fraction is derived from the non-protein-bound plasma cortisol which is filtered at the glomerulus and 80 to 90% reabsorbed in the renal tubules (Daughaday, 1956; Schedl *et al.*, 1959). Since the α-globulin transcortin, which plays a major role in binding cortisol in the plasma, reaches saturation at plasma cortisol levels of about 20 μg./100 ml., amounts of cortisol greater than this spill over on to albumin-binding sites. These display a much lower affinity for cortisol, a greater proportion of which now remains unbound and available for filtration in the kidney. The urinary free cortisol therefore rises disproportionately as the total plasma cortisol reaches the upper limits of normal and moves

into the pathological range. Accordingly, the determination of this fraction in urine has proved particularly valuable in detecting hypercortisolism though the method is too involved for routine use. Using glass fibre chromatography for the determination, the mean free cortisol excretion was 71 μg./24 hr. (range 0–181 μg.) whereas in nine patients with Cushing's syndrome, the values ranged from 297 to 3605 μg./24 hr. (Rosner *et al.*, 1963). In thyrotoxic and obese patients with high 17-hydroxysteroids, the free cortisol excretion was normal. A screening test based on the Mattingly method as applied to urine, may be found convenient (Mattingly & Tyler, 1967).

(3) *Estimation of cortisol metabolites in urine.* A substantial fraction of the available cortisol undergoes metabolism to the tetrahydro-derivatives; a further fraction is also reduced at the 20-keto grouping forming the 20-hydroxy compounds cortol and cortolone. In their water soluble glucuronide form, these are the main excretory products found in urine and may be measured by a variety of methods. The 17-OGS procedure and that measuring total 17-OHCS are widely available in the United Kingdom. Variations of the Porter-Silber reaction are commonly used in the U.S.A. A significant limitation of these methods is the poor correlation between the results obtained and the cortisol secretion rates derived from isotope studies, especially in mild cases of hypersecretion. Although the urinary metabolites determined by the previously mentioned methods usually account for 40 to 50% of the total adrenal secretion, wide variations do occur quite frequently. It is claimed, however, that for any one subject, the relationship between secretion rate and 17-OGS is constant, thus allowing the secretion rate to be inferred from subsequent urinary assays. Malnutrition, liver disease and other factors might interfere with this relationship over long periods of time (Brooks *et al.*, 1963). In a series of 33 cases of Cushing's syndrome with secretion rates of over 35 mg. daily, 17-OGS secretion in seven was below 15 mg./24 hr., the usually accepted upper limit of the normal range; in borderline cases with secretion rates lying between 25 and 35 mg./day, the urinary values ranged from 4–17 mg./day. The problem is fully discussed by Cope (1964). When the possibility of Cushing's syndrome is a serious consideration, the patient should be hospitalized for the collection of several 24 hr. specimens of urine; this tends, not only to eliminate errors in timing of specimens, but also the effect of accidental stress on adrenocortical function. Despite these precautions, however, considerable

TABLE 11.3

The figures show the results of urinary steroid analyses on the first 24 hr. specimen of urine collected in hospital, when the diagnosis of Cushing's syndrome was suspected.

Patient	Diagnosis	mg./24 hr. Oxosteroid	Oxogenic steroid
Bs	Hyperplasia	6·0	33·0
Jn	,,	16·0	36·0
Bh	,,	10·0	12·0
Bl	,,	5·0	24·0
Fr	,,	10·0	20·0
Hs	,,	20·0	30·0
Ay	,,	60·0	30·5
Cs	,,	10·0	30·0
Tn	,,	11·0	12·0
Sk	,,	7·0	18·0
By	,,	14·0	52·0
Hl	,,	22·0	31·0
Bw	,,	13·0	21·0
Wy	,,	25·0	27·5
Py	,,	9·0	14·5
Dh	Adenoma	6·0	25·0
Hys	,,	18·0	27·5
Mh	,,	3·5	14·5
Hay	,,	6·0	21·0
Pd	Carcinoma	9·0	21·0
Fil	,,	40·0	68·0
Rs	,,	50·0	74·0

variation in output may occur on a day-to-day basis and this can cause difficulties in interpretation of results. Simple obesity may cause a consistent and moderate increase in 17-OHCS and 17-OGS excretion, and in these patients cortisol secretion rates may be elevated (Migeon *et al.*, 1963). Since the diagnostic exercise frequently entails the differentiation of obesity from Cushing's syndrome, recourse will have to be made to other techniques for conclusive evidence, i.e., the presence or absence of a diurnal rhythm and the results of the suppression tests.

(4) *Cortisol secretion rates.* The determination of the cortisol secretion rate necessitates the administration of ^{14}C- or ^{3}H-labelled cortisol to the patient and the determination of the specific activity of a unique urinary metabolite (tetrahydrocortisone or tetrahydrocortisol). The normal range is $16·2 \pm 5·7$ mg./day and values are elevated, by definition, in Cushing's syndrome (Cope & Black, 1958). In adrenal hyperplasia due to pituitary ACTH, values of 36–138 mg./day have been reported by Cope & Pearson (1965). The effect of severe obesity on the cortisol secretion rate has already been noted.

(5) *Dexamethasone suppression test.* The pre-sence of an increased blood level of ACTH in adrenal hyperplasia implies insensitivity of the hypothalamo-pituitary apparatus to the usual inhibitory effects of normal levels of plasma cortisol. This insensitivity is relative, and in each case there is a supranormal level of cortisol which will inhibit the secretion of ACTH. Attempts to demonstrate a marked fall in plasma ACTH by the administration of cortisone or cortisol are frustrated, as the administered steroid meets the same metabolic fate as endogenous hormones and its metabolites in the urine will be qualitatively and quantitatively similar. The advent of potent analogues, i.e. dexamethasone or fludrocortisone removed this obstacle since, in the doses used, the metabolites are present in minute quantities or are not estimated by the relevant analytic methods.

When dexamethasone is administered in suit-able amounts to a normal individual over a period of several days, the plasma cortisol falls to zero and the urinary 17-OGS and 17-OHCS excretion to levels of 0–2 mg./day. The fall in plasma cortisol level is very rapid, but the urinary values may not fall to their nadir until the second or third day because of the time taken to clear the body of accumulated metabolites. In adrenal hyperplasia, all grades of resistance to the sup-pressive effects of dexamethasone are encountered; however, complete resistance is unusual and difficult to establish; the administration of very large doses of dexamethasone to severe cases of Cushing's syndrome is dangerous. The usual clinical procedure follows the recommendations of Liddle (1960). Dexamethasone administered orally (0·5 mg. 6-hourly for 72 hr.) leads to a profound depression of urinary 17-OGS to values of 2 mg./day or less; in Cushing's syndrome, little or no fall in output is observed. It must be empha-sized that since the abnormality of ACTH secre-tion appears to be a graded one, no single dose of glucosteroid can be credited with the power to discriminate with absolute certainty between physiological and pathological states. Neverthe-less, the method is of considerable value.

(6) *Miscellaneous tests.* Stimulation of the adrenal cortices by ACTH contributes nothing to the diagnosis of hypercortisolism. The measure-ment of the urinary 6β-hydroxycortisol may provide useful information, but demands special facilities. Normally, the urinary output of this steroid is inferior to 500 μg./day, but in hyper-cortisolism, much higher values are achieved. 6β-Hydroxylation also plays an increased role in the disposal of cortisol when alternative pathways are inadequate (in infancy and in pregnancy) and

during the administration of oestrogens and barbiturates.

Despite the use of these procedures, it is often impossible to be certain that a given patient with borderline symptoms and signs has Cushing's syndrome, and, in such instances, a prolonged period of observation is required, the diagnostic tests being repeated at intervals. When the diagnosis is established, attention must be turned to the problem of aetiology. Studies of the diurnal rhythm and plasma and urinary steroid estimations are not helpful in this respect. The major differences in behaviour between adrenal hyperplasia and tumour are related to the independence of the latter from ACTH control. The sensitivity of ACTH assays does not permit the ascertainment of zero levels which must exist in the presence of an autonomous tumour and of which contralateral adrenal atrophy is clear evidence. Failure of suppression of cortisol secretion during high dexamethasone dosage is an inevitable consequence of autonomy, but could equally be the result of extreme refractoriness to suppression in ACTH-dependent adrenal hyperplasia. Diagnostic conclusions from such an observation should be drawn with great care. A practical method is to administer dexamethasone 8 mg./day for 3 days (2 mg. 6-hourly). It is generally agreed that a definite fall in urinary steroid excretion is a very strong indication of ACTH dependence, i.e. adrenal hyperplasia. Failure of suppression or an ambiguous result strengthens the suspicion that a tumour is present, but the conclusion is only tentative and recourse must be made to radiographic technique (pre-sacral aerography, aortography, venography). Great care must be taken in the interpretation of apparently positive suppression tests in patients whose base line urinary steroids fluctuate widely and spontaneously. An alternative procedure is to use the plasma corticosteroid level at 09.00 hr. as an index of adrenal suppression. The inability of these tests to suggest the presence of a pituitary tumour has already been mentioned.

The sensitivity of the adrenal cortex to exogenous ACTH is a useful test. In most cases of adrenal tumour, the plasma corticosteroid does not increase, or increases minimally after ACTH administration. Patients with adrenal hyperplasia demonstrate an exaggerated response (Christy *et al.*, 1957), but this is not specific since the same phenomenon may be observed in obesity and when the adrenal cortex is under chronic stimulation as a part of the response to stress. An abnormal rise in urinary pregnanetriol and pregnanediol following ACTH is said to be characteristic of hyperplasia; in neoplasms, the slightly raised base line values remain constant (Martin & Hamman, 1966).

Metyrapone, (2-methyl-1,2-bis(3'-pyridyl)-1-propanone), a compound which causes a reversible block in cortisol synthesis (Liddle *et al.*, 1958) and the effects of which are only detectable in the presence of a normal ACTH secreting mechanism, is employed primarily in the study of pituitary and hypothalamic conditions. However, when applied to cases of Cushing's syndrome, a negative response, or even a fall in adrenal activity (Daniels *et al.*, 1964) is obtained in the presence of an adrenal tumour, whereas hyperplasia leads to an exaggerated response. It is doubtful if this approach adds significantly to the information elicited in direct suppression and inhibition tests. The presence of unusually high concentrations of dehydroepiandrosterone in the urine is not, as was formerly believed, a reliable indication of adrenal tumour.

Treatment

Since the natural history of Cushing's syndrome is short, half the patients being dead within five years (Plotz *et al.*, 1952), definitive cure is mandatory. Adrenal tumours must be removed surgically; since the contralateral adrenal is atrophied, it is a good plan to administer intramuscular ACTH 40–80 I.U./day in the gelatin or zinc form for several days pre-operatively. During the surgical procedure, 100–200 mg. of cortisol are given intravenously; intravenous steroid therapy is continued as needed until the patient can take cortisone or cortisol by mouth; the steroid dosage is tapered slowly over a period of days to weeks. Despite ACTH stimulation, the remaining adrenal may not return to a normal functional state for periods as long as one year after operation (Kyle *et al.*, 1957). Intermittent stimulation with ACTH during this period results in an adequate adrenal response, but basal secretion falls to low levels when treatment is stopped, indicating inadequate pituitary function. The surgical results in adrenal adenoma are good; in adrenal carcinoma, the likelihood that the patient will survive operation is reasonably good, but the rate of cure is negligible, almost all patients dying of recurrence and metastatic disease within 12–18 months. Temporary anatomical and chemical remissions have been brought about by administration of a chemical related to the insecticides, *o,p'*-DDD (Bergenstal *et al.*, 1960), but the results of this treatment are disappointing (Hutter & Kayhoe, 1966).

The ideal treatment for adrenal hyperplasia is

not yet at hand. Complete adrenalectomy cures the majority of cases, but partial adrenalectomy, whilst usually inducing an immediate remission, is contra-indicated because of the frequency of regrowth of the remnant and relapse of the disease. The very rare failure of total adrenalectomy is due to incomplete operation or to the growth of accessory adrenal tissue (Kozak *et al.*, 1966). The operation may be carried out in one (transabdominal) or two stages (flank approach); the former method permits inspection of the abdominal cavity for an ectopic and neoplastic source of ACTH, and allows a satisfactory examination of both adrenals in cases resistant to dexamethasone suppression. No special preparation is necessary for the removal of the first adrenal in a two-stage operation, but careful medication and supervision is essential in all other circumstances. Prior administration of cortisone acetate intramuscularly is not of proved value. Prior to induction of anaesthesia, cortisol (100 mg.) is administered by rapid intravenous injection followed by constant intravenous infusion of saline or dextrose solutions containing 200 to 400 mg. cortisol/24 hr. The exact amount is determined by the clinical condition of the patient; in favourable circumstances, cortisol (100 mg.) may be injected intramuscularly or intravenously twice or thrice on the second day. Oral therapy with cortisone acetate is commenced as soon as possible and the dose gradually reduced, the rate of reduction being guided by blood pressure and electrolyte levels. A maintenance dose of 25–50 mg. may not be reached for several weeks in contrast to requirements of patients adrenalectomized for other reasons.

The realization that the cause of the disease usually resides in the pituitary gland and that tumours develop in a significant number of cases (10%) has shifted the emphasis of therapy to this gland. Surgical hypophysectomy is mandatory when evidence of a pituitary tumour is obtained at the time of the initial diagnosis, and careful exclusion of such a lesion is of great importance. However, despite careful assessment by clinical and radiological methods, small tumours may be missed or may develop months or years later. Surgical hypophysectomy involves intrinsic hazards and may fail because very small remnants of pituitary tissue may sustain abnormal ACTH secretion when revascularization from the hypophyseal portal circulation has taken place. External radiation to the pituitary (3000–4000 rads) may induce remission in up to 40% of cases, but many "remissions" are partial or transient. [198]Au and radon seeds have been abandoned because of

damage to the optic nerves by gamma radiation. Cryogenic pituitary ablation has not been widely used, but [90]yttrium implanted transnasally into the gland offers some advantages (Forrest, Blair & Valentine, 1958). The method can be used in patients too ill to withstand major surgery; by suitable choice of dosage, it is claimed that growth and gonadotropic function can be preserved, an important consideration in young patients.

Cushing's Syndrome induced by Exogenous Steroids

The physiological and structural changes of Cushing's syndrome are reproduced by prolonged administration of large doses of cortisone, cortisol or synthetic analogues. Table 11.2 lists some of the synthetic compounds and compares their potency to that of cortisol and cortisone. The structural basis for their greater anti-inflammatory effect (per weight unit) is not known. Most of the analogues are metabolized more slowly (i.e. plasma half-time is longer) than cortisol; this difference may account for their augmented effect. The argument could equally well be advanced that their slower metabolic rate impedes access to sites of cellular action. Preliminary studies of the binding of cortisol analogues to plasma protein suggest that certain of them are bound only weakly to transcortin, thus allowing readier egress from plasma into cells. Most of the metabolic reactions of the analogues, so far as they have been studied, are essentially the same as those cortisol undergoes. An interesting difference from the cortisol pattern has been found in the cases of 9α-fluorocortisol and 9α-fluorocortisone, almost all of the metabolites of which have the 11β-hydroxyl group (Bush, 1956). This apparent favouring of the 11β-ol grouping (more potent biologically than the 11-ketone) by the 9α-fluoro substituent may perhaps explain the increased "glucocorticoid" activity of 9α-fluoroderivatives of cortisol; it does not explain the vastly greater augmentation of mineralocorticoid than of glucocorticoid potency.

No matter which anti-inflammatory steroid has been administered, the influence on the pituitary-adrenal system is the same and is due to the inhibiting effect on ACTH synthesis and release. There is no good evidence of a dissociation of therapeutic and ACTH-inhibiting properties in any of the potent cortisol analogues. The administration of such a preparation leads to a very rapid fall in plasma cortisol level; even quite small doses will achieve this, but their effect will vary according to the time of administration. Nichols *et al.* (1965), have shown that dexamethasone 0·5 mg.

ingested at 0.900 hr. when the matutinal tide of adrenal activity is nearing its zenith, will have little effect; the same dose given at midnight will almost completely abolish the rise of plasma cortisol the following day and profoundly affect the amount of circulating cortisol for 24 hr. More prolonged therapy leads to adrenal atrophy, the degree of which depends mainly on its duration. Salassa et al. (1953) found a mean total adrenal weight of 7·9 g. in patients who died following long-term therapy, compared with 12·6 g. in untreated patients. Functionally, the effect is detectable as a diminished response to exogenous ACTH. Prednisone, 25 mg./day for one week interferes markedly with adrenal responsiveness (Christy et al., 1956) and smaller doses of 5–10 mg./day exert similar effects over longer periods of time.

The problems which face the steroid patient are of two kinds: the dangers of a therapeutically-induced Cushing's syndrome and those following the cessation of treatment. From the chemical standpoint, the iatrogenic "Cushingoid" state is easy to distinguish from the spontaneous conditions, since the plasma cortisol is low on withdrawal of therapy and the adrenals respond poorly to exogenous ACTH. Sudden, and even sometimes gradual, withdrawal of therapy may lead to a recrudescence of previously suppressed non-endocrine disease. Other events are more specifically related to endocrine phenomena. A "deprivation syndrome" consisting of malaise, myalgia, stiffness, nausea and mild circulatory collapse occurs after prolonged therapy without a concomitant depression of plasma cortisol; its mechanism is obscure but, since the symptoms are relieved by resuming treatment, habituation of the tissues to abnormal steroid levels may be a factor. True adrenal insufficiency, however, may result from abnormally low plasma cortisol levels, but differs from the true Addisonian crisis in that aldosterone secretion is not impaired. Although the cardiovascular collapse may be accompanied by a low serum Na, raised serum K values are not observed. Finally, patients who have been given prolonged therapy are exposed to the risk of cardiovascular collapse during surgery or intercurrent illness; the period of risk is ill-defined but may be as long as one to two years. It is customary to regard such occurrences as a consequence of hypocortisolaemia in the face of stress, but evidence on the subject is not complete; nevertheless, the intravenous administration of cortisol is usually helpful.

Despite the undoubted occurrence in some cases of profound adrenal atrophy, the plasma cortisol

level and the secretion rate return to normal with remarkable speed in a substantial proportion of patients (Robinson et al., 1962). The recovery of adrenal function does not necessarily give complete protection against sudden collapse during stress, since this involves hypothalamic centres and pathways not involved in the maintenance of base-line function. There is evidence that even when adrenal responsiveness is not yet impaired by steroid therapy, defects in the hypothalamo-pituitary mechanisms may be revealed by appropriate tests such as insulin-induced hypoglycaemia and metyrapone administration (Jasani et al., 1967). The importance of pituitary factors is clearly seen in observations of patients with unilateral adrenal atrophy following removal of the other adrenal which contained a functioning adenoma. Despite successful stimulation of the gland by exogenous ACTH on several occasions base-line function returned to a low and symptomatic level, indicating the lack of endogenous stimulation. The eventual recovery of ACTH secretion was indicated by rising urinary oxogenic steroids and an increasing response to metyrapone.

Little is known concerning the changes in the pituitary resulting from steroid therapy. It is known that cortisone or cortisol administration to animals is associated with depletion of pituitary ACTH (Lacqueur, 1950), but it cannot yet be stated with certainty whether this depletion is a function of altered synthesis, storage or release of ACTH. In experimental situations, ACTH administration increases the pituitary content of ACTH, but does not appear to accelerate, and in fact, may partially prevent pituitary ACTH depletion in response to an acute stimulus (Kitay et al., 1959). However, as Armatruda and associates (1960) have shown, the administration of ACTH concomitantly with cortisol or prednisone results in the retention of adrenal responsiveness to ACTH and of responsiveness of the pituitary and adrenal to the stress of hypoglycaemia. One study in human subjects has purported to show that the ability of the pituitary to release ACTH returns to normal more quickly after long-term steroid administration than does adrenal responsiveness to ACTH, but the data are inconclusive.

These controversial findings bear on the management of patients treated for long periods with steroids and steroid analogues, and on the question of whether or not ACTH prevents functional hypoadrenalism (or hypopituitarism). There is no good clinical evidence that ACTH administration after a course of steroid accelerates the return to normal of pituitary-adrenal responsiveness (Christy *et al.*, 1956, Fleisher *et al.*, 1967). There is some evidence that ACTH administration *during* the course of steroid therapy may aid in the prevention of hyporesponsiveness of the pituitary-adrenal system, but this procedure does not necessarily preclude unpleasant "withdrawal symptoms" (Armatruda *et al.*, 1960).

In this clinic, a patient who has been treated with large doses of steroid and whose treatment is to be stopped, is usually reduced abruptly to a "physiological" dose, that is, a steroid dose equivalent to 20–30 mg. of cortisol/day. The steroid is then gradually reduced over a period of one to two weeks *without* ACTH, as the underlying disease permits. This regimen is rarely associated with evidence of serious adrenal insufficiency such as electrolyte disturbances, hypoglycaemia and the like. For the patient whose course of steroid therapy is interrupted by an acute intercurrent illness, or a surgical emergency, *whether or not supplementary ACTH has been given*, the treatment of the acute situation should be replacement of steroids at high dose levels, as in Addisonian crisis (q.v.). The use of ACTH alone is inadequate and possibly therefore dangerous, since the responsiveness of the adrenal in the steroid-treated individual is extremely variable, and cannot be counted upon to provide adequate endogenous steroid replacement for an acute clinical emergency (Christy *et al.*, 1956).

VIRILISM

Hypersecretion by the adrenal cortex may give rise to the syndrome of pure virilism which is usually not attended by disturbances of carbohydrate and electrolyte metabolism. Masculinization of the female and precocious puberty in the male are considered to be virilizing phenomena. Although such changes may occur in gonadal and hypothalamic disease, the commonest underlying abnormality is altered adrenal function. The clinical manifestations of the syndrome depend on the severity of the adrenal abnormality, the age of onset and the sex of the patient.

Adrenal Neoplasms

Virilizing adrenal carcinoma and adenoma. High urinary oxosteroid values are characteristic in functional adrenal tumours. Values frequently range from 30–200 mg./24 hr. and occasionally reach levels of several hundred milligrams. Chromatography may reveal certain important qualitative abnormalities which are not observed in adrenal hyperplasia. There is commonly, but

not always, an excessive secretion of dehydroepiandrosterone and other C_{19} steroids with the Δ^5-3-β-hydroxy configuration. This abnormality is due to a relative deficiency in tumour tissue of the enzyme 3β-ol dehydrogenase which converts the Δ^5-3-β-hydroxy precursors to the usual Δ^4-3-ketone compounds. Other enzyme deficiencies may occur; a deficiency in the 11-β-hydroxylase results in the secretion of 11-deoxycortisol (compound S) (see Fig. 11.4). In such cases, the urinary assays for cortisol metabolites which depend on the dihydroxyacetone side chain (17-OGS and 17-OHCS) will yield high values. The features of Cushing's syndrome will be absent, nevertheless, since the 11-deoxycortisol measured by these procedures has virtually no biological activity. Many carcinomas are diagnosed at a fairly late stage, probably because of inefficient steroid production by malignant tissue which has lost some of its more specialized synthetic functions. Lipsett *et al.* (1963) studied such a tumour which synthesized 0·1–0·2 mg. of steroids/g. of tissue compared with 1 mg./g. from normal adrenals under similar conditions. Although non-functioning tumours probably occur, the lack of clinically observable endocrine effects may be due to the lack of biological activity of the steroids released from the tumour. In one case, Δ^5-pregnene-3β,20α-diol and pregnane-3α,20α-diol were produced in large quantities suggesting that the tumour was only capable of the first step in the synthesis of pregnenolone from cholesterol (Fukushima & Gallagher, 1963).

Feminizing carcinoma. The occurrence of feminization is a rare but well-recorded event in adrenal cortical carcinoma. In a careful study of such a case (West *et al.*, 1964), it was demonstrated that oestrogen excretion may be increased at a time when oxosteroid and oxogenic steroid output is still normal, the increment including the three usual oestrogens: oestrone, 17β-oestradiol and oestriol. The results of *in vivo* studies and incubation of the tumour tissue with various substrates suggested that the usual defect in 11β-hydroxylation was present; additionally, there was an abnormally active aromatizing enzyme system. The formation of oestrogens is currently thought to proceed from androstenedione via the 19-oxo derivative and this substrate is present in excessive amounts in the presence of an 11-hydroxylation block (West *et al.*, 1964). (See Fig. 11.4.)

Diagnosis. The differentiation between hyperplasia and neoplasia is clearly of the utmost importance. A marked elevation of the oxosteroid values will arouse suspicion of a neoplasm, but considerable overlap occurs and further techniques are indicated.

(*a*) The predominance of dehydroepiandrosterone is strong evidence in favour of a tumour. Several tests exist for the detection of this compound, avoiding the need for chromatography. Such a method as that proposed by Allen *et al.* (1950) may be employed, though the specificity of the method is not great.

(*b*) *Adrenal suppression tests.* The administration of a potent cortisol analogue should have no effect on the steroid production by these tumours. Dexamethasone (8 mg./day) should be used (see under "Cushing's syndrome") and the response evaluated from urinary steroid assays. The plasma corticosteroid level, estimated by the Mattingly method, is not a suitable guide to suppression, since the plasma cortisol may originate in remaining non-malignant cortical tissue.

(*c*) *X-ray evidence.* In many cases adrenal tumours may be located by tomography of the adrenal areas, following insufflation of O_2 by the presacral route. In difficult cases, aortography may reveal small tumours not otherwise detectable.

Simple Virilism

Leaving aside racial considerations, there is little doubt that frequently, the immediate cause of hirsutism is an increased plasma testosterone concentration (Finkelstein *et al.*, 1961; Hudson *et al.*, 1963) and that the excess steroid arises from ACTH-responsive tissue. Estimation of urinary testosterone glucuronide excretion leads to the same conclusion, not only in idiopathic hirsutism, but also in arrhenoblastoma, lipoid ovarian tumours and carcinoma of the adrenal cortex. Testosterone secretion rate studies, however, have not confirmed an increase over normal (Korenman *et al.*, 1965); these studies, based on the isotope dilution method, may not be valid, since urinary testosterone glucuronide is not a unique metabolite of testosterone. Androstenedione and dehydroepiandrosterone are converted peripherally to testosterone glucuronide (Mahesh & Greenblatt, 1962; Horton & Tait, 1966), thus contributing to the excretion of this substance in the urine without necessarily providing the biological action of free testosterone in the tissues. Nevertheless, conversion of androstenedione to free testosterone also occurs, and in normal females, approximately 60% of circulating testosterone may arise from this source; the remainder arises directly from the adrenals and possibly from the ovaries (Burger *et al.*, 1964). Thus, there are two pathways from the adrenals

to circulating free testosterone and there is evidence that both may be involved in producing the high blood testosterone levels in hirsutism. The problem is complicated by the overlap between simple hirsutism and the polycystic ovary syndrome (Stein-Leventhal syndrome). The polycystic ovary has been shown to be the site of a partial block in the formation of oestrogens from androstenedione; the androgen/oestrogen ratio is increased in ovarian venous blood because of the accumulation of androgenic precursors (Mahesh, 1964). The defect is presumably not a genetic one, since it may be abolished by the induction of ovulation (Crooke *et al.*, 1963). In these cases, the increase of ovarian androstenedione may provide a further source of substrate for the peripheral formation of testosterone. Increased pilosity, whilst frequently an adrenal disorder, may also have an ovarian origin and, in certain cases, both causes may co-exist.

Simple virilism usually affects females in early reproductive life. Whilst the aetiology remains doubtful, there is much evidence to incriminate an adrenal abnormality in many instances. The constitutional aspect of the problem has been emphasized by several workers. Ferriman *et al.* (1957) demonstrated the increased incidence of hirsuties in both mothers and sisters of patients complaining of the same condition. Although many of these women excrete amounts of 17-oxosteroids within the normal range, these authors showed that, taken as a group, these patients have a higher output than non-hirsute controls. Moreover, the frequency distribution curve of 17-oxosteroid excretion rates is skew, with the hirsute members of the community occupying the upper end of the curve. Fractionation of the oxosteroids by chromatography lends further weight to the possibility of an adrenal abnormality. In a series of 13 consecutive patients referred to the Sloan-Kettering Institute, chromatography revealed a consistent increase in the excretion of androsterone and aetiocholanolone with mean values three times greater than in non-hirsute controls. The output of 11-oxygenated C_{19} steroids was also increased, but to a much lesser degree (Gallagher *et al.*, 1958). Since androsterone and aetiocholanolone are metabolites of precursors which are more markedly androgenic than the precursors of the 11-hydroxy C_{19} steroids, it is obvious that normal figures for total "crude" oxosteroid output may conceal qualitative differences of considerable importance.

Bush & Mahesh (1959*b*) showed the similarity of the oxosteroid pattern in monozygotic twins, suggesting that the androgen/cortisol ratio may be genetically determined, and that hirsutism occurs when the ratio is high. This theory could explain the sudden development of hirsuties following severe emotional stress or shock. Individuals with a high androgen/cortisol ratio would show no evidence of virilism at moderate secretion rates; however, as a result of severe stress, the androgen secretion would rise to high levels and produce hirsutism, acne and possibly menstrual abnormalities.

In many cases, treatment with small suppressive doses of prednisone (7·5 mg./day) may restore a regular ovulatory menstrual cycle and fertility, when hirsutism is accompanied by ovarian disturbances. The effect of treatment on hirsutism is disappointing. Biochemically, it has been shown that this treatment depresses the excretion of 11-deoxy C_{19} steroids and restores to normal the elevated urinary testosterone excretion (Nichols et al., 1966).

Congenital Adrenal Hyperplasia

This condition makes itself manifest at birth in most cases. Occasionally, the clinical onset does not occur until shortly before puberty. In the female, varying degrees of pseudo-hermaphroditism are seen, ranging from simple enlargement of the clitoris to an associated fusion of the labial folds; in these more severe cases, the external appearance may resemble that of the hypospadiac male and occasionally, a true "penile" urethra is seen. In males, no abnormality may be seen for several months, or years, after birth, when precocious isosexual development occurs, but without accompanying testicular enlargement. The clinical features are well described elsewhere (Prader, 1954; Forsham, 1962; Wilkins, 1957). The disease is a genetically determined inborn error of metabolism probably associated with an autosomal recessive gene (Childs et al., 1956).

It has been demonstrated that the adrenals of patients with congenital adrenal hyperplasia respond differently from normal individuals when stimulated with exogenous ACTH; for example, it has been shown that ACTH administration does not lead to a normal increase in urinary or plasma corticoids, or to renal salt retention. On the other hand, a definite rise occurs in the already elevated values of the urinary pregnanediol, pregnanetriol and 17-oxosteroids. The data were interpreted as meaning that such adrenals are having difficulty in increasing the secretion of cortisol, but can secrete very readily a steroid or steroids which are precursors of the urinary 17-oxosteroids (Jailer et al., 1955). Subsequent work, which has confirmed and elaborated this view,

may be summarized as follows: the synthesis of cortisol by the adrenal is dependent on the hydroxylation of progesterone at the 17α, 11β and 21-positions (see Fig. 11.4). In the normal gland, the intermediate compounds presumably have a short existence before passing on to the next step in the synthetic pathway, since they only reach the systemic circulation in very small quantities. The majority of C_{21} compounds isolated from normal blood and urine are metabolites of cortisol, corticosterone and 11-deoxycortisol, and hence possess an O function at C-21. On the other hand, in congenital adrenal hyperplasia, the C_{21} steroids isolated from the urine consist almost entirely of 21-deoxy compounds, of which pregnanetriol and its 11-oxo derivative, pregnanetriolone (3α, 17α, 20α-trihydroxypregnane-11-one in Fig. 11.5) are the most characteristic. It will be observed that these compounds are metabolites of the two major cortisol precursors, and their presence in large quantities suggests the possibility of a lack, relative or absolute, of the enzyme 21-hydroxylase. A block at this site would lead to a low cortisol secretion rate; Jailer et al. (1959a) estimated the secretion rates in two patients, and obtained the low values 5·5 and 7·7 mg./day. As a result of the impairment of cortisol synthesis at the stage of 21-hydroxylation, the immediate and penultimate precursors, 21-deoxycortisol and 17-hydroxyprogesterone respectively, would be expected to accumulate in the adrenal cells and eventually be excreted into the circulation to yield the final metabolites depicted in Figs. 11.5 and 11.6. The experimental administration of large quantities of these precursors to patients with Addison's disease, in fact, leads to a urinary C_{21} steroid pattern which resembles closely that found in congenital adrenal hyperplasia thus providing further evidence of the correctness of the hypothesis. Similarly, the anticipated rise in plasma ACTH has been confirmed by Sydnor et al. (1953). There is no doubt that the degree of impairment of 21-hydroxylation varies from case to case. This classical explanation of the usual form of congenital adrenal hyperplasia must now be modified to the extent that the enzyme deficiency may be more complex than was previously postulated. The fact that 17-hydroxyprogesterone is the major steroid in the adrenals in these cases suggests a deficiency of 11-hydroxylase in addition to 21-hydroxylase deficiency, though this may be a functional defect due to a high circulating androgen level (Sharma & Dorfman, 1963). Birke et al. (1958) also produced evidence of multiple enzyme deficiencies. The claim that the virilizing agent is 17-hydroxyprogesterone itself cannot be upheld since there is clear evidence that the plasma testosterone level is elevated. In infants and children with the simple virilizing and salt-losing forms of the disorders, plasma testosterone levels varied between 110 and 600 μg./100 ml. plasma (normal adult males 374–917 μg./100 ml.; normal adult females 25–68 μg./100 ml.). Whilst the secretion rate of testosterone was clearly elevated, a considerable part of the circulating material arose from peripheral conversion of androstenedione; the plasma levels of the latter were particularly high (Rivarola et al., 1967).

The rare occurrence of periodic fever in this condition has been thought to be the result of high plasma oxosteroids (Cara & Gardner, 1960), producing one form of aetiocholanolone fever. The view held by earlier workers that the 17-oxosteroids arise solely from the peripheral metabolism of the C_{21} steroids is also not in concordance with recent data. Detailed studies of the chromatographic pattern of 17-oxosteroids, following the administration of 17-hydroxy-progesterone, reveal patterns which differ in a significant way from those found in patients suffering from the disease (Fukushima et al., 1957; Axelrod & Goldzieher, 1960; Brooks, 1960). It seems likely that adrenal androgen secretion is increased per se and that the major steroids in this group are dehydroepiandrosterone, Δ^4-androstene-3,17-dione, and 11β-hydroxy-Δ^4-androstene-3,17-dione.

Variants of congenital adrenal hyperplasia. (*a*) *Hypertensive form.* This is the rarest presentation of the condition. Eberlein & Bongiovanni (1955) have studied in detail the urinary steroid pattern and failed to find any 11-oxygenated steroids of either C_{21} or C_{19} steroids, and, therefore, postulated a single enzymic defect at the stage of 11β-hydroxylation. The consequences of such a block in the synthetic pathway are the formation of abnormal amounts of 11-deoxy-corticosterone (DOC, cortexone) and 11-deoxy-cortisol (compound S). The former compound is presumed to cause the hypertension.

(*b*) *Salt-losing form.* Patients belonging to this group present the usual clinical and biochemical evidence of abnormal adrenal activity as previously described. In addition, they manifest abnormalities of electrolyte metabolism which are typical of the Addisonian state, i.e., Na loss and K retention. There is a positive correlation between salt loss and adrenal activity; increased adrenal activity, whether induced by exogenous ACTH or stress, leads to an increase in salt loss, leading to dehydration and collapse. The mechanism leading to this abnormality is not well

understood. Eberlein & Bongiovanni (1958), on the basis of comparative studies of the excretion of cortisol metabolites in urine (i.e., tetrahydro-cortisol and tetrahydrocortisone) in the uncomplicated disease and the salt-losing form, attributed the electrolyte defect in the latter to a more complete block (i.e., enzyme deficiency). Other investigators considered the possibility of a "salt-losing steroid", antagonistic to aldosterone, the secretion of which would depend on the general level of adrenal activity and thus *v* plain the paradoxical effect of ACTH on the external salt balance of these patients. The matter was partially resolved by the discovery that 17-hydroxyproges-terone itself caused sodium loss (Jacobs et al., 1961); since the excretion of this precursor depends on the severity of the enzymic defect, the findings of Eberlein & Bongiovanni, and the "salt-losing steroid" theory can be reconciled. However, the net effect of a sodium-losing steroid on the external balance must depend on the response of the aldosterone-secreting mechanism, and the pertinent observations are of considerable interest. Prader (1954) and Jailer et al. (1959a) found high aldosterone secretion rates in the pure form of congenital adrenal hyperplasia and normal values in the salt-losing form. More recent work generally confirms these findings. The aldosterone secretion rates are normal in "non-salt losers" and rise satisfactorily during salt deprivation in contrast to the findings in "salt-losers" whose secretion rates are extremely low and do not increase during salt deprivation. Furthermore, during ACTH stimulation, cortisol secretion rates rise appreciably in "non-salt losers" but remain constant in "salt-losers" emphasizing once more the difference in the degree of enzymic block between the two groups (Cost & Visser, 1964). It is to be noted, however, that these cases of congenital adrenal hyperplasia segregate clearly into one or other of these categories clinically and genetically; also, in biochemical studies, there is no clear evidence of the existence of intermediate grades of the defect. It is possible to envisage the existence of two separate genetic defects of 21-hydroxylation, the synthesis of aldosterone being impaired only in the more severe form. The low aldosterone secretion rates in this variant of the disease probably occur in spite of an adequate physiological stimulus, since there is evidence of hypertrophy of the juxtaglomerular cells in the kidney and of the zona glomerulosa (Cara & Gardner, 1963).

(*c*) *Hypoaldosteronism: C-18 dehydrogenase block.* This condition has been recognized in infants suffering from salt wastage which is corrected by the administration of DOCA. Dehydration accompanied by hyponatraemia and hyperkalaemia are characteristic features. In the original case (Visser & Cost, 1964), aldosterone was not detected in the urine, but corticosterone, a precursor of aldosterone was present in increased amounts. A genetic basis for the condition was revealed by the occurrence of three affected patients in the same family. Subsequent studies on a similar case have helped to define the condition in more detail. In this infant, the secretion rate of aldosterone was 40 μg./day/m^2 (normal adult 40–130 μg./day/m^2), a figure which was obtained during gross Na depletion when a much higher value would have been expected. However, the more striking abnormality was the excretion of 2420 μg./day of 18-hydroxycorticosterone and 6800 μg. of corticosterone. The biosynthetic pathway to aldosterone which involves the preliminary hydroxylation of corticosterone at C-18 is followed by dehydrogenation at the same site. In normals, the secretion of 18-hydroxycorticosterone has been shown to vary in response to the same factors which influence aldosterone secretion; the 18-hydroxycorticosterone/aldosterone ratio averages 2·26. In the above-mentioned case, the ratio was 300. The high cost of inadequate aldosterone secretion, in terms of precursor release, seems to justify the presumption of a partial defect of 18-dehydrogenation. It is to be noted that no defect in cortisol synthesis occurs in this disease and that pituitary-adrenal mechanisms are not disturbed; there are, therefore, no abnormalities in the excretion of oxosteroids and cortisol metabolites. Likewise, pregnanetriol excretion is not increased. The estimation of urinary 18-hydroxytetrahydrocorticosterone may prove to be a sensitive diagnostic procedure (Ulick *et al.*, 1964; Ulick & Vetter, 1965).

(*d*) *3β-Hydroxysteroid dehydrogenase deficiency.* This variant of congenital adrenal hyperplasia, described by Bongiovanni (1962) appears to lead to less intense virilization of the female and, in males, surprisingly, hypospadias has been observed. The urinary steroids retain the Δ^5-3β-ol configuration of cholesterol and the early intermediates of the adrenal synthetic pathway, indicating a deficiency of the enzyme 3β-hydroxysteroid dehydrogenase which converts the Δ^5-3β-ol to the Δ^4-3-ketone grouping. The oxosteroids are raised owing to the excretion of the 3β steroid dehydroepiandrosterone and the pregnenetriol and 11-oxopregnenetriol are also of the Δ^5 configuration. Cortisol synthesis is impaired and, since salt loss is an integral part of the syndrome, aldosterone secretion is presumably abnormally low. The milder virilization is probably related to the lowered androgenicity of Δ^5 C$_{19}$ compounds and the inability to convert Δ^5-androstenediol to testosterone.

(*e*) *Congenital lipoid hyperplasia.* An even rarer variant of the disease, in which a defect occurs before the formation of any biologically active hormone, has been described by Prader & Grutner (1955). The absence of hormonal activity in the foetal testes ensures the development of the Müllerian system even in males whose phenotype develops along female lines. The adrenals are enlarged and filled with lipid and the reported cases have all died.

(*f*) *17-Hydroxylase deficiency.* Hypertension, hypokalaemic alkalosis and low plasma renin activity due to hyperaldosteronism and reversible by glucosteroid therapy have been described in a case report by New & Peterson (1967), who have suggested the possibility of a 17-hydroxylase deficiency. Such a defect would lead to a relative cortisol deficiency and increased ACTH secretion; the authors tentatively suggest that, in the circumstances, the known marginal effects of ACTH on aldosterone secretion might over-ride the normal renin-angiotensin mechanism and lead to abnormal secretion rates. Such an explanation must remain conjectural until further cases of the syndrome are studied. An increased secretion of corticosterone should be sought in this syndrome.

Diagnosis and treatment. In the new-born female child, the condition must be differentiated from other forms of pseudo-hermaphroditism. Sex chromatin determination is obviously a useful preliminary investigation, since the diagnosis implies the presence of an ambiguous gonadal sex and a female chromatin pattern. For further discussion of this problem, see Chapter 23. The diagnosis is ultimately based on the finding of urinary steroid abnormalities. The results of oxosteroid determinations must be compared with normal values for infants of the same age. Amounts of 17-OS exceeding 2 mg./day in infants aged 3–4 weeks are highly suggestive. In older children and in young adults, high oxosteroid values do not differentiate between congenital adrenal hyperplasia and neoplasms of the adrenal. Whilst suppression tests are clearly valuable as an aid to diagnosis, the determination of pregnanetriol in urine is of the greatest assistance (Bongiovanni, 1954, Martin *et al.*, 1961). Normal adults may excrete up to 2 mg./24 hr. Untreated patients with congenital adrenal hyperplasia in the same age group usually excrete more than 10 mg./24 hr., and frequently values may range between 20 and 50 mg./24 hr. In infants, values of over 0·2 mg./day are significant. Confirmation of the diagnosis is particularly urgent in infants suffering from the salt-losing variant. Bell & Varley (1960) have published a method, suitable for routine laboratories, which is applicable to small volumes of urine. Concentrations of pregnanetriol exceeding 10 μg./10 ml. are significant. It must be emphasized that slight elevation of the pregnanetriol output above normal values has been observed in cases of adrenal carcinoma and in hirsutism. Finkelstein & Shoenberger (1959) claim that the excretion of pregnanetriolone (pregnane-3,17,20-triol-11-one) is specific for congenital adrenal hyperplasia, and therefore differentiates this condition from adrenal carcinoma. Values for urinary pregnanetriol may be misleading in the diagnosis of the hypertensive adrenogenital syndrome, for these may be within normal limits even though virilization and hypertension are progressing. The pre-natal diagnosis of congenital adrenal hyperplasia has been achieved through the estimation of pregnanetriol in amniotic fluid (Jeffcoate *et al.*, 1965).

The treatment of congenital adrenal hyperplasia is by the administration of cortisone or cortisone-like steroids. It should be emphasized that the aim of therapy is to replace a missing adrenal secretion and not to produce a state of hypercortisolism as is done in the treatment of certain non-endocrine diseases. If our understanding of the pathogenesis of the condition were entirely correct, it might be expected that the dosage of cortisone or other steroid would never exceed the equivalent normal range of secretion rate for cortisol. However, in practice, the dose is frequently higher than this, particularly in the salt-losing variant; in infants, the equivalent of 25–37·5 mg. cortisone is often found to be necessary, whereas the normal cortisol secretion rate is of the order of 3 or 4 mg. The best guide to dosage is the maintenance of the urinary 17-OS at a level which is close to what would be considered normal for the age and sex of the patient. Alternatively, virtual elimination of pregnanetriol from the urine may be the logical goal of therapy. The steroids may be administered orally or intramuscularly (Wilkins, 1957). Dosage varies with age; prednisone, 1–2 mg. daily, may suffice in the new-born, whilst older children or adolescents may require 10–12·5 mg. In infants, injections of a depot preparation of prednisone, at intervals of three weeks, may afford adequate control (Komrower & Longson, 1961). The use of intramuscular preparations in older children is advocated by some workers on the grounds that it ensures regular supervision by the physician.

Dexamethasone and fludrocortisone have been used successfully, though the latter compound, unfortunately, may cause excessive salt retention and hypertension. Patients with the salt-losing syndrome require, in addition to the foregoing therapy, regular administration of a mineralocorticoid. Implants of DOCA have been widely employed, but the injection of deoxycorticosterone trimethylacetate at intervals of approximately one month is particularly convenient. Parenteral therapy with mineralocorticoids is desirable in infants since oral administration of drugs may be erratic. When oral treatment is desired, adequate control of renal salt loss may be achieved by fludrocortisone in a dose of 0·1 mg./day or thereabouts, but close supervision is necessary to avoid an undesirable increase in blood pressure.

The restraining influence of treatment on ACTH release and on adrenocortical hyperactivity leads to the disappearance of abnormal androgen production. Virilization is arrested, acceleration of skeletal maturation no longer occurs, and previously inhibited gonadal development is allowed to proceed to a stage which corresponds to the skeletal age rather than to the true age of the patient. Glucocorticoid therapy also diminishes renal salt wastage in salt-losers, and reduces the blood pressure in the hypertensive kind of disease. In older patients, ovulatory menses may occur and successful pregnancy is reported; in such cases, the infants have been normal. In the 18-dehydrogenase block, there is no requirement for glucosteroid therapy; DOCA would seem to be the agent of choice.

PRIMARY HYPERALDOSTERONISM

This condition, first described by Conn (1955), is the result of the excessive secretion of aldosterone by an autonomous adrenal tumour. In the vast majority of cases, a single cortical adenoma is present, but multiple adenomata have been observed; a similar syndrome has been observed in an adrenal carcinoma (Santander *et al.*, 1965) but may have been due to the excessive secretion of deoxycorticosterone. Case reports attributing the primary role to adrenal hyperplasia are open to doubt in view of more recently acquired information. Adrenal hyperplasia and hyperaldosteronism occur in malignant hypertension and renovascular disease, secondarily to activation of the renin-angiotensin mechanism. Furthermore, Bartter and his colleagues have described a syndrome of hyperaldosteronism with hyperplasia of the juxtaglomerular apparatus and macula densa which also suggests a primary renal cause (Bartter *et al.*, 1962). There is widespread agreement that the normal physiological control of aldosterone secretion operates through the renin-angiotensin mechanism, and that renin is produced by the juxtaglomerular apparatus or the macula densa in response to hypovolaemia and other less defined physiological needs. An increase in this trophic influence leads to hyperplasia of the zona glomerulosa in a variety of renal disorders and can be detected by plasma renin assays. Conversely, a primary adrenal hyperplasia of this type cannot be accepted as an entity unless the plasma renin level has been shown to be consistently and severely depressed. In primary hyperaldosteronism, plasma renin activity is not detectable even during salt deprivation; in normal individuals, salt depletion, presumably operating through hypovolaemia, is a potent stimulus to renin secretion and plasma levels rise sharply (Conn, 1965). The upright position, which is also a strong stimulus to renin secretion in normal individuals, is ineffective in this disorder. The suppression of renin in these various circumstances, together with the hypervolaemia which is a usual finding (Biglieri & Forsham, 1961) suggests that adrenal adenomata function independently of trophic control.

The increase in extracellular and plasma volumes due to sodium retention does not lead to oedema unless other factors are present (i.e. heart failure); following the retention of 2–3 kg. of fluid, an "escape" mechanism ensures the rapid elimination of additional electrolytes and the phenomenon is similar to that observed during mineralocorticoid administration to normal individuals (August *et al.*, 1958) in essential hypertension and in Cushing's syndrome. Aldosterone appears to play no role in this rapid disposal of electrolytes, but a local humoral mechanism ensuring decreased proximal tubular reabsorption of sodium has been suggested (de Wardener *et al.*, 1961; Rovner *et al.*, 1965).

The clinical features of primary hyperaldosteronism are, broadly speaking, those which one would have predicted from a knowledge of the effects of overdosage with deoxycorticosterone.

(*a*) *Hypertension.* This may vary in severity but the malignant phase is very strong evidence against the diagnosis and in favour of secondary hyperaldosteronism. The mechanism of its production is not understood, but probably involves the interaction of Na and K with aldosterone at the level of the arterial wall.

(*b*) *Sodium retention.* Renal Na reabsorption is excessive and the resultant expansion of the extracellular space has already been mentioned (*v. supra*).

(*c*) *Potassium metabolism.* K depletion is an essential feature of the disorder. It arises from excessive secretion of K in the distal tubule, in exchange for Na. The deficiency may be of the order of 100 m-eq. and serum K levels below 2 m-eq./l. are common. The level of K in the serum is sensitive to the Na intake, since Na/K exchange in the distal tubule is dependent upon the amount of Na delivered to the site of the ion-exchange mechanism, i.e. an increase in Na intake will augment renal K loss. Alkalosis is usually present.

The renal consequences of K deficiency may play an important role in the clinical picture. Anatomically the lesions consist of hydropic and vacuolar changes, particularly in the proximal tubules (Relman & Schwartz, 1956; Milne *et al.*, 1957). The functional consequences of renal K depletion consist of a defect in urinary concentrating ability manifested clinically by polyuria and polydipsia. Nocturia is a common symptom; the specific gravity of the urine cannot be raised above 1·010, or its osmolarity above that of plasma. Other changes in renal function consist of inversion of the diurnal excretory rhythm and the excretion of an alkaline urine. In hypokalaemia, the extracellular alkalosis is accompanied by an intracellular acidosis and K deficiency. When the condition is due to extra-renal losses of K (i.e. gastro-intestinal loss), the distal tubular cells secrete hydrion in preference to K, with the result that the urine is paradoxically acid. In hyperaldosteronism however, the secretion of K by the tubular cells is specifically stimulated at the expense of urinary acidification, with the consequence that the urine is alkaline. The subject has been reviewed by Stanbury *et al.* (1958). Mg deficiency may occur as described by Mader & Iseri (1955) and may be a factor in the production of tetany.

Muscular weakness may mimic that seen in familial periodic paralysis. Its onset may be sudden and unpredictable.

Diagnosis. The possibility of primary hyperaldosteronism should be considered in the presence of a combination of the following: (1) hypertension with hypokalaemic alkalosis, (2) polyuria and polydipsia when accompanied by pitressin-resistant hyposthenuria, (3) hypernatraemia, (4) neutral or alkaline urine resistant to acidification with NH_4Cl, (5) reduced urinary Na/K ratio.

Measurement of the urinary aldosterone excretion rate has been reported as normal in several authentic cases, and it is generally agreed to be an unsatisfactory way of confirming the diagnosis,

On the other hand, secretion rate studies are much more dependable though unavailable to many physicians. The published figures of Laragh *et al.* (1960) may be taken as representative; in five cases of Conn's syndrome values ranged from 520 to 1690 μg./day (controls 180–330 μg./day). The secretion rates in primary aldosteronism may be lower than those observed in secondary disorder. A survey of published values for secretion rates in primary hyperaldosteronism reveals that minimal increases are not uncommonly found and that normal values (i.e. 100–200 μg./day) may be compatible with the diagnosis, particularly when the serum potassium level is very low. Hypokalaemia is known to depress aldosterone secretion (Cannon *et al.*, 1966) from normal glands; in primary aldosteronism, the lower secretion may be adequate to maintain potassium depletion and absolute values should probably be interpreted in the light of the prevailing potassium concentration. (Biglieri *et al.*, 1967). The measurement of 18-hydroxycorticosterone in urine (Ulick & Vetter, 1965) and aldosterone in blood (Brodie *et al.*, 1967) may provide useful indices of mineralocorticoid activity but results using these methods have not been reported in aldosterone-producing tumours.

The differentiation of this syndrome from other forms of renal K-wasting disease does not present great difficulties since these disorders usually present a metabolic acidosis apart from other substantial differences. However, the greatest difficulty may be experienced in separating primary hyperaldosteronism from cases of hypertension with hypokalaemic alkalosis, although the finding of the gross retinal changes of the malignant phase is itself a strong argument against the diagnosis. Hypokalaemia in essential hypertension occurs with sufficient frequency to create a diagnostic problem. Wrong (1961), in a study of 64 patients with severe hypertension, found 13 patients with a low serum potassium (plasma K 2·7–3·4 m.eq./l.) often accompanied by alkalosis. In patients with papilloedema, the incidence was 43% and a similar finding is to be made in some cases of renal artery obstruction. Aldosterone secretion rates have been measured in hypertensive patients (Laragh *et al.*, 1960). In eight patients with benign essential hypertension, the secretion rate was found to be normal (180–330 μg./day) and was also normal in two patients with unilateral renal disease. In three of eight patients with severe hypertension, and in 14 out of 15 patients with malignant hypertension, the secretion rate was significantly raised (520–2730 μg./day) and high values were usually associated with low serum K levels and alkalosis. Later work has generally confirmed these findings; hyperaldosteronism is not present in the majority of hypertensives but occurs with increasing frequency as cases with higher pressures are considered. Conn (1964) has suggested an aetiological role for aldosterone in the genesis of essential hypertension and drawn attention to the frequent discovery of small adrenal adenomata in this condition; the view generally held now is that the hyperaldosteronism is secondary to the renal consequences of a raised blood pressure. Furthermore, *in vitro* studies of these adenomata have shown a lower rate of aldosterone secretion than the normal surrounding adrenal tissue (Kaplan, 1967). Similarly, although there seems little doubt that the renin-angiotensin mechanism is responsible for the stimulation of aldosterone secretion in some cases of hypertension, its role in the production of the hypertension itself is not certain. This latter subject has been reviewed by Peart (1965*a,b*).

In order to differentiate between primary aldosteronism and those cases in which the condition arises secondarily from hyperactivity of the juxtaglomerular cells, certain other procedures may be helpful.

(*a*) Failure to detect renin activity in plasma, especially during salt deprivation and the upright posture (Conn, 1965) is most helpful, especially if associated with increased sensitivity to angiotensin II (Kaplan & Silah, 1964; Biglieri *et al.*, 1966).

(*b*) The persistence of abnormal aldosterone secretion rates during salt-loading procedures can be employed as a diagnostic method. However, effective expansion of the extracellular volume may be difficult because of the rapid elimination of electrolytes by the kidney ("escape mechanism"). When secretion rate methods are not available, the same conclusion may be reached indirectly from an observation of urinary potassium behaviour. The intravenous infusion of 2 litres of isotonic saline in 4 hr. on 2 successive days to normal individuals and patients with secondary aldosteronism on a low salt diet (Na 10 m.eq., K 60 m.eq./day) leads to a fall in aldosterone secretion, a slow rise in urinary Na output and a moderate increase in potassium excretion; the plasma potassium does not change. In primary aldosteronism, the aldosterone secretion is unchanged, the sodium output rises rapidly and because of the high rate of aldosterone induced Na/K change in the distal tubule, the potassium excretion rises rapidly, producing a drop in serum K level. The procedure should be avoided when cardiac failure is present and in patients whose control plasma potassium is already markedly depressed and electrocardiographic control is desirable (Espiner *et al.*, 1967).

(*c*) Acute volume expansion may be achieved by the use of DOCA (10 mg. intramuscularly for 3 days); the suppression of aldosterone secretion is not observed in the adenomatous condition. The use of spironolactone in large amounts will correct the electrolyte abnormalities and control the hypertension; the peripheral antagonism between this compound and aldosterone results in the reappearance of plasma renin (Brown *et al.*, 1967). The value of spironolactone in the differentiation between primary and secondary aldosteronism is limited (Ross, 1965).

The usual X-ray techniques applicable to the adrenal areas may help in localizing these tumours but, owing to their small size, many escape detection pre-operatively.

Following the removal of an aldosterone-producing tumour, hyperkalaemia and hyponatraemia are frequently observed and are the consequences of an abnormally low rate of secretion of aldosterone. The suppression of secretion from the remaining zona glomerulosa is due to inactivation during the active phase of the disease through chronic expansion of the extracellular space. The mechanism appears to be different from the direct feed-back inhibition of ACTH secretion which leads to cortical atrophy in the cortisol-secreting tumours of the adrenal; in this instance, a third factor, hypervolaemia, intervenes between the adrenal secretion and the inhibition of the trophic factors. The postoperative hypoaldosteronism may last 4–8 weeks (Biglieri *et al.* 1966) and appears to be due to a true atrophy of the zona glomerulosa since the administration of large doses of ACTH fails to cause a temporary increase in secretion of aldosterone as it does in normal individuals; hypovolaemia is also present. The plasma renin activity rises to supranormal values during a period of 1–2 weeks and during this period the very low aldosterone secretion rates suggest a lack of adrenal responsiveness to stimulation (Conn, 1965). Temporary mineralocorticoid therapy is rarely necessary at this stage, but salt restriction in the treatment of hypertension or heart failure may be hazardous. The change in plasma renin activity from undetectable to supranormal levels permits observations on angiotensin II pressor sensitivity to be made in the same patient under different conditions and confirms the current views on the interpretation of this investigation. In the pre-operative low-renin phase pressor sensitivity is enhanced, whereas when high levels prevail post-operatively, a more

normal or low sensitivity is observed (Kaplan & Silah, 1964; Biglieri *et al.*, 1966).

Exceptionally, a syndrome is encountered similar to primary aldosteronism with respect to electrolyte abnormalities, but without hypertension (Bartter *et al.*, 1962) and in which juxtaglomerular hyperplasia is found. The associated aldosteronism may have been a consequence of an unexplained and persistent hypovolaemia. A juvenile and possibly congenital form of aldosteronism associated with malignant hypertension has been described (Van Buchem *et al.*, 1956). However, this may be a variant of the syndrome described by New & Peterson (1967) in which hypertension, hypokalaemic alkalosis, low plasma renin and hypervolaemia were rectified by glucosteroid therapy. (See congenital adrenal hyperplasia: 17-hydroxylase deficiency).

SECONDARY HYPERALDOSTERONISM

An increase in aldosterone production may occur during the oedematous phase of cardiac, renal and hepatic disease, or following surgical operations and trauma. The abnormality in hormone production is a consequence of the disease and not its cause; on the other hand, the effects of hyperaldosteronism may play an important role in the clinical picture. There can be no serious doubt concerning the influence of aldosterone on the formation of oedema in the nephrotic syndrome and cirrhosis of the liver with ascites even though other factors play a primary role; Ulick *et al.* (1958) determined the secretion rates in both these conditions, and obtained values of 1570–6600 μg./day (normal 300 μg./day); similarly, Petersen (1959) found a secretion rate of 3000 μg./day in a patient with decompensated hepatic cirrhosis. Subsequent work has confirmed these observations. It seems certain that the excessive sodium retention is partly attributable to aldosterone since it is diminished by spironolactone (Kerr *et al.*, 1958); the incompleteness of the block is strong evidence that other factors also operate to produce abnormal sodium reabsorption. The discovery of high plasma renin values (Brown *et al.*, 1964) suggests that when ascites occurs as a result of portal hypertension and hypoproteinaemia, the following sequence of events is initiated: ascites → diminished plasma volume → renin → angiotensin → aldosterone secretion → sodium retention → ascites. In cardiac failure, the events are much more obscure and it is certain that oedema may occur without increase in aldosterone secretion; however, later in the evolution of the disease, and especially following the use of diuretics, high values may be found. Clearly, these have arisen in the face of hypervolaemia rather than hypovolaemia, and if the renin-angiotensin mechanism operates, a serious derangement of trophic control must be postulated. It is interesting to note that the administration of salt to an oedematous cardiac patient inhibits aldosterone secretion, suggesting that the juxtaglomerular system is active in this condition, despite the expanded plasma volume (Cope, 1964). The matter is complicated by the abnormalities in the hepatic extraction and inactivation of aldosterone in heart failure (Tait *et al.*, 1965). A secondary role must be attributed to aldosterone in all these conditions, since there is clear evidence of the influence of other sodium-retaining mechanisms, probably acting on the proximal renal tubule (Nelson & August, 1959).

Post-operative hyperaldosteronism. Retention of Na and increased excretion of K are familiar features of the metabolic response to surgery. The excretion of aldosterone also rises in the same circumstances (Llaurado *et al.*, 1956). There is strong evidence, however, that the two phenomena are not related, since Addisonian patients receiving constant substitution therapy exhibit the same changes during and following surgery as normal individuals. Furthermore, there is a discordance between the timing and duration of the salt retention and the increase in aldosterone. For the same reasons, it is not possible to incriminate the glucocorticoid secretion of the adrenal cortex for the electrolyte changes or the negative N balance which accompanies it (Dudley *et al.*, 1957).

Pregnancy. There is a considerable body of evidence which suggests that the sex hormones influence the secretion of aldosterone, though the clinical importance of the phenomenon is not clear. Landau & Lugibihl (1961) have described the catabolic and natriuretic effect of physiological doses of progesterone. The electrolyte effect was more marked in Addisonian patients on constant therapy with cortisone and deoxycorticosterone than in normal individuals. No effect was observed when progesterone was administered to Addisonian patients prior to therapy, but, following treatment in normal individuals, there occurred a period of salt-retention suggestive of enhanced secretion of salt-retaining hormone. It was suggested, therefore, that progesterone induced salt loss by virtue of a peripheral (renal tubular) competitive inhibition of the adrenal mineralocorticoid. Gornall (1961), using progesterone, observed increased aldosterone secretion rates in subjects

receiving a constant salt intake, whilst similar results have been observed using the synthetic progestational compound norethynodrel (Layne *et al.*, 1962). The observation that plasma renin is elevated from an early stage of pregnancy (Brown *et al.*, 1963) is compatible with these views; in later trimesters, when a hypervolaemic state exists, other mechanisms must be involved. There is some doubt concerning the origin of plasma renin in pregnancy, since a high level of activity is to be found in amniotic fluid; recent evidence, however, favours involvement of the maternal kidneys. These findings are of considerable interest in relation to the aetiology of the salt-losing phenomenon in congenital adrenal hyperplasia (see p. 345). Oestrogens usually do not increase aldosterone secretion but simultaneously cause a positive Na balance, thus suggesting a completely different mechanism. Similar processes may operate in pregnancy, since some women at least show an increase in aldosterone secretion which is not associated with electrolyte abnormalities. There is little correlation between the plasma and urinary electrolytes or the amount of oedema and the urinary aldosterone in pregnant subjects. There is, however, a good correlation between aldosterone secretion rate and pregnanediol output, and, by inference, with progesterone production; nevertheless, the aldosterone secretion rate responds to variations in dietary sodium intake. These observations could be explained by competitive inhibition between progesterone and aldosterone (Jones *et al.*, 1959). In mild pre-eclampsia, the aldosterone values remain within the normal pregnancy range, or fall slightly. With the onset of severe pre-eclampsia, or following intra-uterine foetal death, the values are depressed to non-pregnant levels (Watanabe *et al.*, 1965). These authors also showed that the administration of 200 mg. of progesterone/day during normal or abnormal pregnancy leads to an increase in aldosterone secretion, thus confirming previous work.

Idiopathic oedema. Chronic oedema, in the absence of cardiac, renal, hepatic or local causes, occurs almost always in females. Although the primary disorder is presumably a capillary leak, posture plays an important part in determining the clinical picture. The blood pressure and electrolyte concentrations are normal. Secondary hyperaldosteronism occurs, presumably in response to the loss of fluid from the vascular compartment. Salt restriction and synthetic aldosterone antagonists (e.g. spironolactone) may be of benefit to these patients, but, in many cases, oedema persists despite therapy (Streeten *et al.*, 1960; Mach, 1958).

HYPOALDOSTERONISM

Whilst hypoaldosteronism occurs together with other steroid deficiencies in Addison's disease, and, to a less severe degree, in prolonged and severe hypopituitarism, its existence as a sole defect is a very rare occurrence. By contrast, cortisol deficiency occurs as a solitary major deficiency in hypopituitarism and in congenital adrenal hyperplasia. Selective failures of secretion are not described as a result of recognized primary acquired disease of the adrenal glands. However, selective aldosterone deficiency of unknown aetiology has been described, the important clinical manifestation being the result of the cardiac effects of hyperkalaemia (Hudson et al., 1957; Lambrew et al., 1961). Autopsy information is scarce, but in one case at least, the zona glomerulosa was found to be abnormally thin (Wilson & Goetz, 1964). There was no evidence of an association with tuberculosis or other inflammatory process, but the atrophic state of the zona glomerulosa suggests a failure of the trophic mechanism controlling aldosterone secretion. One possible but unusual cause for such a failure may have been the use of heparin. Heparin is known to inhibit aldosterone secretion (Veyrat et al., 1962; Schlatmann et al., 1964) and induce sodium diuresis in oedematous states. There is now further evidence, derived from in vitro studies, that heparin inhibits the production of angiotensin by renin (Sealey et al., 1967).

A solitary defect in aldosterone secretion has already been described in the C-18 dehydrogenase deficiency syndrome (see congenital adrenal hyperplasia). An inadequate secretion of aldosterone occurs in the syndrome of autonomic insufficiency. The important features of this condition are: hypotension, anhidrosis and impotence, but renal conservation of sodium is also impaired. During salt deprivation and angiotensin infusions, the rise in aldosterone secretion is subnormal (Slaton & Biglieri, 1967) though prolonged stimulation by either of these methods is more effective, suggesting an atrophy of the zona glomerulosa rather than a biosynthetic defect. The above-mentioned authors have suggested a suppression of juxtaglomerular release of renin mediated by defective autonomic control of tone in the afferent glomerular arterioles. This view is supported by the low catecholamine excretion found in these patients (Luft & von Euler, 1953), the increased pressor response to infusions of noradrenaline (Barnett & Wagner, 1958) and the increased plasma renin and aldosterone secretion which follows noradrenaline

infusion (Gordon et al., 1966). Aldosterone deficiency has also been described in relation to the regrowth of the adrenal remnant following partial adrenalectomy for Cushing's syndrome in a patient whose glucosteroid syndrome recurred (Hartog et al., 1967).

PERIODIC (AETIOCHOLANOLONE) FEVER

The thermogenic influence of progesterone and its role in the temperature changes during the menstrual cycle are well known. A different and more dramatic phenomenon has been described following the intramuscular or intravenous injection of aetiocholanolone and some related compounds (Kappas et al., 1960a, 1960b), both of the C_{19} and C_{21} series, especially in men (Kimball et al., 1966). These compounds belong to the 5β series and arise from the normal metabolism of adrenocortical and gonadal hormones; they are found, in conjugated form, in the oxosteroid fraction of normal urine. Following their injection, there occurs a marked pyrogenic reaction after a latent period which varies from 4–8 hr. Symptoms consist of severe rigors, local heat and swelling at the site of the injection, muscular aches, headaches, anorexia and fever of up to 103° F. These symptoms usually disappear within 18 hr. of onset. The prior administration of cortisone mitigates these effects, but this benefit may be simply a manifestation of the usual antipyretic effect of glucocorticoids. Attempts to ward off attacks by adrenal suppression with exogenous steroid have met with some success and, in certain individuals, administration of ACTH may bring on a febrile episode. It seems unlikely that the pyrexia is caused directly by the steroid, since the half-life is of the order of 1 hr.; the latent period before pyrexia develops suggests an intermediate mechanism. An "endogenous pyrogen", comparable to the leucocytic pyrogen induced by bacterial endotoxin, has been sought, but not found (Kappas et al., 1960a). These experiments appear to have a bearing on the cause of the pyrexia in two cases described by Bondy et al. (1958). Both these patients experienced periodic attacks of fever and malaise, in association with a marked change in oxosteroid pattern in both blood and urine. Whereas, during afebrile periods, plasma contained dehydroepiandrosterone and androsterone in conjugated form, these compounds disappeared during the febrile phase and were replaced by non-conjugated (i.e. free) aetiocholanolone. The mechanism which produces this steroid abnormality is not understood. One of the cases reported by these authors, and a further case reported by Gonzales & Gardner (1956) also had congenital adrenal hyperplasia, but the syndrome has been described in the absence of this abnormality. A plausible, but unproved theory suggests that there may not be simple hypersecretion of aetiocholanolone, but rather that a hepatic disorder leads to the over-production of aetiocholanolone in the course of the abnormal degradation of adrenal hormones, and that a further failure of conjugation allows the free compound to escape into the general circulation. It is not known whether or not the precursor of aetiocholanolone is secreted in excess during episodes of fever. It should be pointed out that raised levels of aetiocholanolone have been found in the blood of some patients with cirrhosis of the liver who were apyrexial (Tisdale & Klatz-kin, 1960); nevertheless, aetiocholanolone may conceivably play a role in some diseases (Bondy et al., 1965).

References

AHMED, A. B. J., GEORGE, B. C., GONZALEZ-AUVERT, C. & DINGMAN, E. F. (1967). *J. clin. Invest.*, **46**, 111.

ALLEN, W. M., HAYWARD, S. J. & PINTO, A. (1950). *J. clin. Endocr. Metab.*, **10**, 54.

ANDERSON, R. N. & EGDAHL, R. H. (1964). *Endocrinology*, **74**, 538.

ANDERSON, J. R., GOUDIE, R. B., GRAY, K. & WHITE, W. G. (1966). *Lancet*, **1**, 1173.

ARMATRUDA, T. T., JNR., HOLLINGSWORTH, D. R., D'ESOPO, N. D., UPTON, G. V. & BONDY, P. K. (1960). *J. clin. Endocr. Metab.*, **20**, 339.

AUGUST, J. T., NELSON, D. H. & THORN, G. W. (1958). *J. clin. Invest.*, **37**, 1549.

AXELROD, B. J. & GOLDZIEHER, J. (1960). *J. clin. Endocr. Metab.*, **20**, 238.

BARGER, A. C., BERLIN, R. D. & TULENKO, J. F. (1958). *Endocrinology*, **62**, 804.

BARNETT, A. J. & WAGNER, G. R. (1958). *Am. Heart J.*, **56**, 412.

BARTTER, F. C. & FOURMAN, P. (1957). *J. clin. Invest.*, **36**, 872.

BARTTER, F. C. & FOURMAN, P. (1962). *Metabolism*, **11**, 6.

BARTTER, F. C., PRONOVE, P., GILL, J. R. & MacCARDLE, R. C. (1962). *Am. J. Med.*, **33**, 811.

BAULIEU, E. E. (1963). *Rec. Progr. Horm. Res.*, **19**, 306.

BAULIEU, E. E., EMILIOZZI, R. & CORPECHOT, C. (1961). *Experientia*, **17**, 110.

BAULIEU, E. E. & JAYLE, M. F. (1957). *Bull. Soc. Chim. Biol.*, **39**, 37.

BAULIEU, E. E., WALLACE, E. & LIEBERMAN, S. (1963). *J. biol. Chem.*, **238**, 1316.

BEISEL, W. R., DI RAIMONDO, V. C. & FORSHAM, P. H. (1964). *Ann intern. Med.*, **60**, 641.

BELL, M. & VARLEY, H. (1960). *Clin. Chim. Acta*, **5**, 396.

BERGENSTAL, D. M., LIPSETT, M. B., MOY, R. H. & HERTZ, R. (1960). In "Biological Activities of Steroids in Relation to Cancer." Eds. Pincus & Vollmer. p. 463. New York, Academic Press.

BETHUNE, J. E., NELSON, D. H. & THOM, G. W. (1957). *J. clin. Invest.*, **36**, 1701.

BIGLIERI, E. G. (1965). *J. clin. Endocr. Metab.*, **25**, 884.

BIGLIERI, E. G. & FORSHAM, P. H. (1961). *Am. J. Med.*, **30**, 564.

BIGLIERI, E. G. & GANONG, W. F. (1961). *Proc. Soc. exp. Biol. Med.*, **106**, 806.

BIGLIERI, E. G., SLATON, P. E., KRONFIELD, S. J. & DECK, J. B. (1967). *J. clin. Endocr. Metab.*, **27**, 715.

BIGLIERI, E. G., SLATON, P. E., Jnr., SILEN, W. S., GALANTE, M. & FORSHAM, P. H. (1966). *J. clin. Endocr. Metab.*, **26**, 554.

BIRKE, G., DICZFALUSY, E., PLANTIN, L.-O., ROBBE, H. & WESTMAN, A. (1958). *Acta Endocr.*, *Kbh.*, **29**, 55.

BJORNEBOE, M., FISCHEL, E. E. & STOERCH, H. C. (1951). *J. exp. Med.*, **93**, 39.

BLAIR-WEST, J., COGHLAN, J. P. & DENTON, D. A. (1962). *Acta Endocr.*, *Kbh.*, **41**, 61.

BLIZZARD, R. M. & KYLE, M. (1963). *J. clin. Invest.*, **42**, 1653.

BLIZZARD, R. M., TOMASI, T. B. & CHRISTY, N. P. (1963). *J. clin. Endocr. Metab.*, **23**, 1179.

BLOCH, K. & BENIRSCHKE, K. (1962). In "The Human Adrenal Cortex". p. 589. Eds. Currie, A. R., Symington, T. & Grant, J. K. Baltimore, Wilkins & Wilkins.

BONDY, P. K., COHN, G. L. & GREGORY, P. B. (1965). *Medicine* (Baltimore), **44**, 249.

BONDY, P. K., COHN, G. L., HERRMAN, W. & CHRISPELL, K. R. (1958). *Yale J. Biol. Med.*, **30**, 395.

BONGIOVANNI, A. M. (1954). *J. clin. Endocr. Metab.*, **14**, 341.

BONGIOVANNI, A. M. (1962). *J. clin. Invest.*, **41**, 2086.

BORNSTEIN, J. & TREWHELLA, P. (1950). *Lancet*, **2**, 678.

BRADLOW, H. L., FUKUSHIMA, D. K., ZUMOFF, B., HELLMAN, L. & GALLAGHER, T. F. (1962). *J. clin. Endocr. Metab.*, **22**, 748.

BRADLOW, H. L., FUKUSHIMA, D. K., ZUMOFF, B., HELLMAN, L. & GALLAGHER, T. F. (1964). *Acta Endocr. Kbh.*, **45**, 26.

BRADLOW, H. L., & GALLAGHER, T. F. (1957). *J. biol. Chem.*, **229**, 505.

BRITTON, S. W. & SILVETTE, H. (1934). *Am. J. Physiol.*, **107**, 190.

BRODIE, A. H., SHIMIZU, N., TAIT, S. A. S. & TAIT, J. F. (1967). *J. clin. Endocr. Metab.*, **27**, 997.

BROOKS, R. V. (1960). *J. Endocr.*, **21**, 277.

BROOKS, R. V., DUPRÉ, J., GOGATE, A. N., MILLS, I. H. & PRUNTY, F. T. G. (1963). *J. clin. Endocr. Metab.*, **23**, 725.

BROWN, J. J., DAVIES, D. L., DOAK, P. B., LEVER, A. F. & ROBERTSON, J. I. S. (1963). *Lancet*, **2**, 900.

BROWN, J. J., DAVIES, D. L., LEVER, A. F., PEART, W. S. & ROBERTSON, J. I. S. (1964). *Br. med. J.*, **2**, 1636.

BROWN, J. J., DAVIES, D. L., LEVER, A. F. & ROBERTSON, J. I. S. (1967). *Canad. med. Ass. J.*, **90**, 201.

BRYAN, G. T., KLIMAN, B., GILL, J. R., Jnr. & BARTTER, F. C. (1964). *J. clin. Endocr. Metab.*, **24**, 729.

BURGER, H. G., KENT, J. R. & KELLIE, A. E. (1964). *J. clin. Endocr. Metab.*, **24**, 432.

BURSTEIN, S., KIMBALL, H. L., KLAIBER, E. L. & GUT, M. (1967). *J. clin. Endocr. Metab.*, **27**, 491.

BUSH, I. E. (1962). *Pharmac. Rev.*, **14**, 317.

BUSH, I. E. (1956). *Experientia*, **12**, 325.

BUSH, I. E. & MAHESH, V. B. (1959a). *Biochem. J.*, **71**, 705.

BUSH, I. E. & MAHESH, V. B. (1959b). *J. Endocr.*, **18**, 1.

BUSH, I. E. & SANDBERG, A. A. (1953). *J. biol. Chem.*, **205**, 783.

BUSH, I. E., SWALE, J. & PATTERSON, J. (1956). *Biochem. J.*, **62**, 16P.

BUSH, I. E. & WILLOUGHBY, M. (1957). *Biochem. J.*, **67**, 689.

BUNGE, G. VON (1873). *Ztschr. f. Biol.*, **9**, 104.

CADE, R., SHIRES, D. L., BARROW, M. V. & THOMAS, W. C., Jnr. (1967). *J. clin. Endocr. Metab.*, **27**, 800.

CANNON, P. J., AMES, R. P. & LARAGH, J. H. (1966). *J. clin. Invest.*, **45**, 865.

CARA, J. & GARDNER, L. I. (1960). *J. Pediat.*, **57**, 461.

CARA, J. & GARDNER, L. I. (1963). *Pediatrics*, **32**, 825.

CASPI, E., DORFMAN, R. I., KHAN, B. T., ROSENFELD, G. & SCHMID, W. (1962). *J. biol. Chem.*, **237**, 2085.

CASPI, E., ROSENFELD, G. & DORFMAN, R. I. (1956). *J. org. Chem.*, **21**, 814.

CASPI, E., UNGAR, F. & DORFMAN, R. I. (1957). *J. org. Chem.*, **22**, 326.

CHILDS, B., GRUMBACH, M. M. & WYCK, J. J. VAN (1956). *J. clin. Invest.*, **35**, 213.

CHRISTY, N. P., DICKIE, M. M., ATKINSON, W. B. & WOOLLEY, G. W. (1951). *Cancer Res.*, **11**, 413.

CHRISTY, N. P. & DRUCKER, W. D. (1961). *J. clin. Invest.*, **40**, 1029.

CHRISTY, N. P., LONGSON, D. & JAILER, J. W. (1957). *Am. J. Med.*, **23**, 910.

CHRISTY, N. P., WALLACE, E. Z. & JAILER, J. W. (1956). *J. clin. Endocr. Metab.*, **16**, 1059.

CLINE, M. J. & MELMON, K. L. (1966). *Science*, **153**, 1135.

COLÀS, A. & HEINRICHS, W. L. (1965). *Steroids*, **5**, 753.

COLLA, J. C., COHN, M. L. & UNGAR, F. (1964). *Proc. Soc. exp Biol. Med.*, **117**, 717.

COLLINS, K. J. (1966). *Clin. Sci.*, **30**, 207.

CONN, J. W. (1955). *J. lab. clin. Med.*, **45**, 3.

CONN, J. W. (1964). *J. Am. med. Ass.*, **190**, 222.

CONN, J. W. (1965). *Rec. Prog. Horm. Res.*, **21**, 101.

COOK, W. F. (1960). *J. Physiol. (Lond.)*, **152**, 27P.

COPE, C. L. (1964). In "Adrenal Steroids and Disease", pp. 134, 493. Pitman. London.

COPE, C. L. & BLACK, E. G. (1958). *Br. med. J.*, **1**, 1020.

COPE, C. L. & BLACK, E. G. (1959). *Br. med. J.*, **2**, 5160.

COPE, C. L., NICOLIS, G. & FRASER, B. (1961). *Clin. Sci.*, **21**, 367.

COPE, C. L. & PEARSON, J. (1965). *J. clin. Path.*, **18**, 82.

COST, W. S. & VISSER, H. K. A. (1964). "Proceedings 2nd International Congress of Endocrinology, 1964." p. 870.

CRABBÉ, J. & NICHOLS, G., Jnr. (1950). *Proc. Soc. exp. Biol. Med.*, **101**, 168.

CRANE, M. G. & HARRIS, J. J. (1966). *J. clin. Endocr. Metab.*, **26**, 1135.

CROOKE, A. C. (1935). *J. Path. & Bact.*, **41**, 339.

CROOKE, A. C., BUTT, W. R., PALMER, R., MORRIS, R., EDWARDS, R. L., TAYLOR, C. W. & SHORT, R. V. (1963). *Br. med. J.*, **1**, 1119.

CUSHING, H. (1932). *Bull. Johns Hopk. Hosp.*, **50**, 137.

DANIELS, H., VAN AMSTEL, W. J., SCHOPMAN, W. & VAN DOMMELEN (1964). *Acta Endocr. Kbh.*, **44**, 346.

DAUGHADAY, W. H. (1956). *J. clin. Invest.*, **35**, 1428.

DAUGHADAY, W. H. (1958). *J. clin. Invest.*, **37**, 519.

DAUGHADAY, W. H., ADLER, R. F., MARIZ, I. K. & RASINSKI, D. C. (1962). *J. clin. Endocr. Metab.*, **22**, 704.

DAVIS, J. O. (1963). *Yale J. Biol. Med.*, **35**, 402.

DAVIS, J. O. (1964). *Circulation*, **30**, 1.

DAVIS, J. O., BALL, W. C., Jnr., BAHN, R. C. & GOODKIND, M. J. (1959). *Am. J. Physiol.*, **196**, 149.

DAVIS, J. O., CARPENTER, C. C. J., AYERS, C. R. & BAHN, R. C. (1960). *Am. J. Physiol.*, **199**, 212.

DAVIS, J. O., URQUHART, J. & HIGGINS, J. T., Jnr. (1963). *J. clin. Invest.*, **42**, 597.

DE WARDENER, H. E., MILLS, I. H., CLAPHAM, W. F. & HAYTER, C. J. (1961). *Clin. Sci.*, **21**, 249.

DINGMAN, J. F., GAITAN, E., STAUB, M. C., ARIMURA, A. & PETERSON, R. E. (1960). *J. clin. Invest.*, **39**, 981.

DOE, R. P., FERNANDEZ, R. & SEAL, H. S. (1964). *J. clin. Endocr. Metab.*, **24**, 1029.

DRAYER, N. M. & GIROUD, C. J. P. (1965). *Steroids*, **5**, 289.

DUDLEY, H. A., ROBSON, J. S., SMITH, M. & STEWART, C. P. (1957). *Clin. Chim. Acta*, **2**, 461.

EBERLEIN, W. R. (1964). *J. clin. Invest.*, **43**, 1255.

EBERLEIN, W. & BONGIOVANNI, A. M. (1955). *J. clin. Endocr. Metab.*, **15**, 1531.

EBERLEIN, W. & BONGIOVANNI, A. M. (1958). *Pediatrics*, **21**, 667.

EDELMAN, I. S., BOGOROCH, R. & PORTER, G. A. (1964). *Trans. Ass. Am. Phycns.*, **77**, 307.

EDELMAN, R. & HARTROFT, P. M. (1961). *Circulation Res.*, **9**, 1069.

EIK-NES, K., SANDBERG, A. A., NELSON, D. H., TYLER, F. H. & SAMUELS, L. T. (1954). *J. clin. Invest.*, **33**, 1502.

EISENSTEIN, A. B., BERG, E., GOLDENBERG, D. & JENSEN, B. (1964). *Endocrinology*, **74**, 123.

EKMAN, H., HÅKANSSON, B., McCARTHY, J. D., LEHMANN, J. & SJÖGREN, B. (1961). *J. clin. Endocr. Metab.*, **21**, 684.

ENGEL, I. L. (1957). *Cancer*, **10**, 711.

ESPINER, E. A., TUCCI, J. R., JAGGER, P. I. & LAULER, D. P. (1967). *New Engl. J. Med.*, **277**, 1.

EXLEY, D. (1965). *Biochem. J.*, **94**, 271.

FEIGELSON, P. & FEIGELSON, M. (1964). In "Action of Hormones on Molecular Processes". Eds. Litwack, G. & Kritchevsky, D. p. 218. New York, Wiley.

FERRIMAN, D., THOMAS, P. K. & PURDIE, A. M. (1957). *Br. med. J.*, **2**, 1410.

FINKELSTEIN, M., FORCHIELLI, E. & DORFMAN, R. I. (1961). *J. clin. Endocr. Metab.*, **21**, 98.

FINKELSTEIN, M. & SHOENBERGER, J. (1959). *J. clin. Endocr. Metab.*, **19**, 608.

FISCHEL, E. E. (1961). In "Inflammation and Diseases of Connective Tissue". Eds. Mills, L. C. & Moyer, J. H. p. 472. Philadelphia, Saunders.

FLEISHER, N., ABE, K., LIDDLE, G. W., ORTH, D. N. & NICHOLSON, W. F. (1967). *J. clin. Invest.*, **46**, 196.

FORREST, A. P., BLAIR, D. W. & VALENTINE, J. M. (1958). *Lancet*, **2**, 192.

FORSHAM, P. H. (1962). Chapter 5 in "Textbook of Endocrinology". Ed. Williams, R. H. Philadelphia, Saunders.

FRANDSEN, V. A. & STAKEMANN, G. (1964). *Acta Endocr. Kbh.*, **47**, 265.

FRANTZ, A. G., KATZ, F. H. & JAILER, J. W. (1961). *J. clin. Endocr. Metab.*, **21**, 1290.

FUKUSHIMA, D. K., BRADLOW, H. L., HELLMAN, L., ZUMOFF, B. & GALLAGHER, T. F. (1960). *J. biol. Chem.*, **235**, 2246.

FUKUSHIMA, D. K. & GALLAGHER, T. F. (1957). *J. biol. Chem.*, **229**, 85.

FUKUSHIMA, D. K. & GALLAGHER, T. F. (1963). *J. clin. Endocr. Metab.*, **23**, 923.

GALLAGHER, T. F., KAPPAS, A., HELLMAN, L., LIPSETT, M. B., PEARSON, O. H. & WEST, C. D. (1958). *J. clin. Invest.*, **37**, 794.

GANONG, W. F. & MULROW, P. J. (1958). *Am. J. Physiol.*, **195**, 337.

GANONG, W. F., MULROW, P. J., BORYCZKA, A. & CERA, A. (1962). *Proc. Soc. exp. biol. Med.*, **109**, 381.

GAUNT, R., RENZI, A. A. & CHART, J. J. (1955). *J. clin. Endocr. Metab.*, **15**, 621.

GIROUD, C. J. P., STACHENKO, J. & VENNING, E. N. (1956). *Proc. Soc. Exp. Biol.* (N.Y.), **92**, 154.

GONZALES, R. F. & GARDNER, L. I. (1956). *Pediatrics*, **17**, 524.

GORDON, R. D., KUCHEL, O., ISLAND, D. P. & LIDDLE, G. W. (1966). 58th Annual Meeting of the American Society for Clinical Investigation, May, 1966.

GORNALL, A. G. (1961). *Rec. Progr. Horm. Res.*, **17**, 282.

GOWENLOCK, A. H., MILLS, J. N. & THOMAS, S. (1959). *J. Physiol.* (Lond.), **146**, 133.

GRABER, A. L., GIVENS, J. R., NICHOLSON, W. E., ISLAND, D. P. & LIDDLE, G. W. (1965). *J. clin. Endocr. Metab.*, **25**, 804.

GRANT, N. (1967). In "The Adrenal Cortex". Ed. Eisenstein, A. B., p. 269. London, Churchill.

GREEP, R. O. & DEANE, H. W. (1949). *Ann. N. Y. Acad. Sci.*, **50**, 596.

GROSS, F. & GYSEL, H. (1954). *Acta endocr. Kbh.*, **15**, 199.

GRUNDY, H. M., SIMPSON, S. A., TAIT, J. F. & WOODFORD, M. (1952). *Acta endocr. Kbh.*, **11**, 199.

GUILLEMIN, R. (1964). *Rec. Prog. Horm. Res.*, **20**, 89.

HAGTVET, J. (1963). *Acta Med. Scand.*, **174**, 1.

HARDY, J. D. & WARD, V. B. (1958). *Am. J. Med.*, **25**, 122.

HARRIS, G. W. (1955). "Neural Control of the Pituitary Gland". London, E. Arnold Ltd.

HARTOG, M., HARRISON, R. J., JOPLIN, G. F. & SLATER, J. D. H. (1967). *J. clin. Endocr. Metab.*, **27**, 843.

HAYAND, M., SABA, N., DORFMAN, R. I. & HECHTER, O. (1956). *Rec. Progr. Horm. Res.*, **12**, 79.

HAYNES, R. C., Jnr., SUTHERLAND, E. W. & RALL, T. W. (1960). *Rec. Progr. Horm. Res.*, **16**, 121.

HAYNES, R. C., Jnr. (1962). *Endocrinology*, **71**, 399.

HECHTER, O., SOLOMON, M M., ZAFFARONI, A. & PINCUS, G. (1953). *Archs. Biochem. Biophys.*, **46**, 201.

HECHTER, O., ZAFFARONI, A., JACOBSEN, R. P., LEVY, H., JEANLOZ, R. W., SCHENKER, V. & PINCUS, G. (1951). *Rec. Progr. Horm. Res.*, **6**, 215.

HEINBECKER, P. (1944). *Medicine*, **23**, 225.

HELLMAN, L., BRADLOW, H. L., ADESMAN, J., FUKUSHIMA, D. K., KULP, L. & GALLAGHER, T. F. (1954). *J. clin. Invest.*, **33**, 1106.

HELLMAN, L., BRADLOW, H. L., ZUMOFF, B. & GALLAGHER, T. F. (1961). *J. clin. Endocr. Metab.*, **21**, 1231.

HIGGINS, J. T., Jnr., DAVIS, J. O. & URQUHART, J. (1964). *Am. J. Physiol.*, **207**, 814.

HOBERMAN, H. D. (1950). *Yale, J. Biol. Med.*, **22**, 341.

HOLZBAUER, M. (1964). *J. Physiol.* (Lond.), **172**, 138.

HORTON, R. & BIGLIERI, E. G. (1962). *J. clin. Endocr. Metab.*, **22**, 1187.

HORTON, R. & TAIT, J. F. (1966). *J. clin. Invest.*, **45**, 301.

HORWITH, M. & STOKES, P. E. (1960). *Adv. intern. Med.*, **10**, 259.

HUDSON, J. B., CHOBANIAN, A. V. & RELMAN, A. S. (1957). *New Engl. J. Med.*, **257**, 529.

HUDSON, B., COGHLAN, J., DULMANIS, A., WINTOUR, M. & EKKEL, I. (1963). *Aust. J. exp. Biol. Med. Sci.*, **41**, 235.

HUTTER, A. M., Jnr., & KAYHOE, D. E. (1966). *Am. J. Med.*, **41**, 581.

IMURA, H., SPARKS, L. L., GRODSKY, G. M. & FORSHAM, P. H. (1965). *J. clin. Endocr. Metab.*, **25**, 1361.

INGLE, D. J. (1938). *Am. J. Physiol.*, **124**, 369.

JACOBS, D. R., VAN DER POLL, J., GABRILOVE, J. L. & SOFFER, L. J. (1961). *J. clin. Endocr. Metab.*, **21**, 909.

JAILER, J. W. & CHRISTY, N. P. (1957). *Ann. Rev. Med.*, **8**, 193.

JAILER, J. W., GOLD, J. J. & WALLACE, E. Z. (1954). *Am. J. Med.*, **16**, 340.

JAILER, J. W., GOLD, J. J., VAN DE WIELE, R. & LIEBERMAN, S. (1955). *J. clin. Invest.*, **34**, 1639.

JAILER, J. W., LONGSON, D. & CHRISTY, N. P. (1956). *J. clin. Endocr. Metab.*, **16**, 1276.

JAILER, J. W., LONGSON, D. & CHRISTY, N. P. (1957). *J. clin. Invest.*, **36**, 1608.

JAILER, J. W., ULICK, S. & LIEBERMAN, S. (1959a). *Trans. Ass. Am. Phycns.*, **72**, 149.

JAILER, J. W., VAN DE WIELE, R. L., CHRISTY, N. P. & LIEBERMAN, S. (1959b). *J. clin. Invest.*, **38**, 357.

JARRETT, L., LACY, P. E. & KIPNIS, D. M. (1964). *J. clin. Endocr. Metab.*, **24**, 543.

JASANI, M. J., BOYLE, J. A., GREIG, W. R., DALAKOS, T. G., BROWNING, M. C. K., THOMPSON, A. & BUCHANAN, W. W. (1967). *Quart. J. Med.*, **36**, 261.

JEDEIKIN, L. A. & WHITE, A. (1958). *Endocrinology*, **63**, 226.

JEFFCOATE, T. N. A., FLIEGNER, J. R. H., RUSSELL, S. H., DAVIS, J. C. & WADE, A. P. (1965). *Lancet*, **2**, 553.

JOHNSON, B. B., LIEBERMAN, A. H. & MULROW, P. J. (1957). *J. clin. Invest.*, **36**, 757.

JONES, K. M., LLOYD-JONES, R., RIONDEL, A., TAIT, J. F., TAIT, S. A. S., BULBROOK, R. D. & GREENWOOD, F. C. (1959). *Acta Endocr. Kbh.*, **30**, 321.

KAHANA, L., LEBORITZ, H., LUSK, W., MCPHERSON, H. T., DAVIDSON, E. T., OPPENHEIMER, J. H., ENGEL, F. L., WOODHALL, B. & ODOM, G. (1962). *J. clin. Endocr.*, **22**, 304.

KAHNT, F. W., NEHER, R., SCHMID, K. & WETTSTEIN, A. (1961). *Experientia*, **17**, 19.

KAPLAN, N. M. (1967). *J. clin. Invest.*, **46**, 728.

KAPLAN, N. & SILAH, J. G. (1964). *J. clin. Invest.*, **43**, 659.

KAPPAS, A., GLICKMAN, P. B. & PALMER, R. H. (1960a). *Trans. Ass. Am. Phycns.*, **73**, 176.

KAPPAS, A., SOYBEL, W., GLICKMAN, P. & FUKUSHIMA, D. K. (1960b). *Arch. intern. Med.*, **105**, 701.

KELLY, W. G., BANDI, L., SHOOLERY, J. N. & LIEBERMAN, S. (1962a). *Biochemistry* (Wash.), **1**, 172.

KELLY, W. G., BANDI, L. & LIEBERMAN, S. (1962b & 1963). *Biochemistry* (Wash.), **1**, 792; **2**, 1243, 1249.

KENNY, F. T. (1962). *J. biol. Chem.*, **237**, 3495.

KEPLER, E. J., SPRAGUE, R. G., MASON, H. L. & POWER, M. H. (1948). *Rec. Progr. Horm. Res.*, **2**, 345.

KERR, D. N. S., READ, A. E., HASLAM, R. M. & SHERLOCK, S. (1958). *Lancet*, **2**, 1084.

KIMBALL, H. R., WOLFF, S. M., VOGEL, J. M. & PERRY, S. (1966). *J. clin. Endocr. Metab.*, **26**, 222.

KITAY, J. I., HOLUB, D. A. & JAILER, J. W. (1959). *Endocrinology*, **64**, 475.

KLEEMAN, C. R., CZACKZES, J. W. & CUTLER, R. (1965). *J. clin. Invest.*, **44**, 1641.

KLEEMAN, C. R., KOPLOWITZ, J., MAXWELL, M. H., CUTLER, R. & DOWLING, J. T. (1960). *J. clin. Invest.*, **39**, 1472.

KOEPF, G. F., HORN, H. W., GEMMILL, C. L. & THORN, G. W. (1941). *Am. J. Physiol.*, **135**, 175.

KOMROWER, G. M. & LONGSON, D. (1961). *Acta endocr. Kbh.*, **36**, 157.

KORENMAN, S. G., KIRSCHNER, M. A. & LIPSETT, M. B. (1965). *J. clin. Endocr. Metab.*, **25**, 798.

KOZAK, G. P., PAUK, G. L., VAGNUCCI, A. I., LAULER, D. P. & THORN, G. W. (1966). *Ann. intern. Med.*, **64**, 778.

KYLE, L. H., MEYER, R. J. & CANARY, J. J. (1957). *New Engl. J. Med.*, **257**, 57.

LACQUEUR, G. L. (1950). *Science*, **112**, 429.

LAMBREW, C. T., CARVER, S. T., PETERSON, R. E. & HORWITH, M. (1961). *Am. J. Med.*, **31**, 81.

LANDAU, R. L. & LUGIBIHL, K. (1961). *Rec. Progr. Horm. Res.*, **17**, 249.

LANG, N. & SEKERIS, C. E. (1964). *Z. physiol. Chem.*, **339**, 238.

LARAGH, J. H., ANGERS, M., KELLY, W. G. & LIEBERMAN, S. (1960). *J. Am. med. Ass.*, **174**, 234.

LARAGH, J. H., CANNON, P. J. & AMES, R. P. (1964). *Canad. med. Ass. J.*, **90**, 248.

LARAGH, J. H. & STOERK, H. C. (1957). *J. clin. Invest.*, **36**, 383.

LAYNE, D. S., MEYER, C. J., VAISHWANER, P. S. & PINCUS, G. (1962). *J. clin. Endocrin.*, **22**, 107.

LEBEAU, M. C. & BAULIEU, E. E. (1964). *Compt. rend. Acad. Sci.*, **258**, 6265.

LEVER, A. F. & PEART, W. S. (1962). *J. Physiol.* (Lond.), **160**, 548.

LEVITAN, R. & INGELFINGER, F. J. (1965). *J. clin. Invest.*, **44**, 801.

LIDDLE, G. W. (1960). *J. clin. Endocr. Metab.*, **20**, 1539.

LIDDLE, G. W., GIVENS, J. R., NICHOLSON, W. E. & ISLAND, D. P. (1964). "Proceedings 2nd Int. Congr. Endocrinology". p. 1063.

LIDDLE, G. W., ISLAND, D., LANCE, E. M. & HARRIS, A. P. (1958). *J. clin. Endocr. Metab.*, **18**, 906.

LIDDLE, G. W., ISLAND, D. P., NEY, R. L., NICHOLSON, W. E. & SHIMIZU, N. (1963). *Arch. intern. Med.*, **111**, 471.

LIPSETT, M. B., HERTZ, R. & ROSS, G. T. (1963). *Am. J. Med.*, **35**, 374.

LIPSETT, M. B. & HÖKFELT, B. (1961). *Experientia*, **17**, 449.

LLAURADO, J. G., NEHER, R. & WETTSTEIN, A. (1956). *Clin. Chim. Acta*, **1**, 236.

LOEB, R. F., ATCHLEY, D. W., BENEDICT, E. M. & LELAND, J. (1933). *J. exp. Med.*, **57**, 775.

LONG, C. N. H., SMITH, O. K. & FRY, E. G. (1960). In "Metabolic Effects of Adrenal Hormones" (CIBA Foundation Study Group, 6.), p. 4. Boston, Little, Brown.

LUETSCHER, J. A., DOWDY, A., HARVEY, J., NEHER, R. & WETTSTEIN, A. (1955). *J. biol. Chem.*, **217**, 505.

LUETSCHER, J. A. & JOHNSON, B. B. (1954). *J. clin. Invest.*, **33**, 276.

LUFT, R. & EULER, U. S. VON (1953). *J. clin. Invest.*, **32**, 1065.

MACH, R. S. (1958). In "Internat. Symp. on Aldosterone". Eds. Muller, A. F. & O'Connor, C., pp. 186ff. London, J. & A. Churchill.

MACH, R. S. & FABRE, J. (1954). *Bull. Soc. Méd. Hôp. Paris*, **70**, 353.

MADER, I. J. & ISERI, L. T. (1955). *Am. J. Med.*, **19**, 976.

MAHESH, V. B. (1964). "Proceedings 2nd Int. Congress of Endocrinology". p. 944.

MAHESH, V. B. & GREENBLATT, R. B. (1962). *Acta Endocr. Kbh.*, **41**, 400.

MAREN, T. (1953). *J. clin. Endocr. Metab.*, **13**, 884.

MARINE, D. & BAUMANN, E. J. (1927). *Am. J. Physiol.*, **81**, 86.

MARTIN, M. M. & HAMMAN, B. L. (1966). *J. clin. Endocr. Metab.*, **26**, 257.

MARTIN, M. M. & HELLMAN, D. E. (1964). *J. clin. Endocr. Metab.*, **24**, 253.

MARTIN, M. M., REDDY, W. J. & THORN, G. W. (1961). *J. clin. Endocr. Metab.*, **21**, 923.

MATTINGLY, D. (1962). *J. clin. Path.*, **15**, 374.

MATTINGLY, D. & TYLER, C. (1967). *Br. med. J.*, **2**, 394.

MEYER, A. S. (1955a). *Experientia*, **11**, 99.

MEYER, A. S. (1955b). *Biochem. biophys. Acta*, **17**, 441.

MEYER, C. J., LAYNE, D. S., TAIT, J. F. & PINCUS, G. (1961). *J. clin. Invest.*, **40**, 1663.

MIGEON, C. J. (1960). In "Hormones in Human Plasma". (Ed. Antoniades, H.), p. 297. Boston, Little, Brown & Co.

MIGEON, C. J., GREEN, O. C. & ECKERT, J. P. (1963). *Metabolism*, **12**, 718.

MIGEON, C. J., TYLER, F. H., MAHONEY, J. P., FLORENTIN, A. A., CASTLE, H., BLISS, E. L. & SAMUELS, L. T. (1956). *J. clin. Endocr. Metab.*, **16**, 622.

MILNE, M. D., MUEHRCKE, R. C. & HEARD, B. E. (1957). *Brit. Med. Bull.*, **13**, 15.

MONTGOMERY, D. A. D. (1963). *Q. Jl. Med.*, **32**, 365.

MORGAN, H. E., HENDERSON, M. J., REGEN, D. M. & PARK, C. R. (1959). *Ann. N.Y. Acad. Sci.*, **82**, 387.

MULLER, A. F., MANNING, E. L. & RIONDEL, A. M. (1958). In "Internat. Symp. on Aldosterone". Eds. Muller, A. F. & O'Connor, C., pp. 111ff. London, J. & A. Churchill.

MULROW, P. J. & GANONG, W. F. (1961). *J. clin. Invest.*, **40**, 579.

MUNCK, A. (1962). *Biochim. biophys. Acta*, **57**, 318.

MUNSON, P. L. (1960). In "Hormones in Human Plasma". Ed. Antoniades, H., pp. 149ff. Boston, Little, Brown & Co.

NELSON, D. H. & AUGUST, J. T. (1958). *J. clin. Invest.*, **37**, 919.

NELSON, D. H. & AUGUST, J. T. (1959). *Lancet*, **2**, 883.

NELSON, D. H. & SPRUNT, J. G. (1964). "Proceedings 2nd Int. Congress of Endocrinology". p. 1053.

NELSON, D. H., SPRUNT, J. G. & MIMS, R. B. (1966). *J. clin. Endocr. Metab.*, **26**, 722.

NEW, M. I. & PETERSON, R. E. (1967). *J. clin. Endocr. Metab.*, **27**, 301.

NICHOLS, T., NUGENT, C. A. & TYLER, F. H. (1965). *J. clin. Endocr. Metab.*, **25**, 343.

NICHOLS, T., NUGENT, C. A. & TYLER, F. H. (1966). *J. clin. Endocr. Metab.*, **26**, 79.

NUGENT, C. A., EIK-NES, K., KENT, H. S., SAMUELS, L. T. & TYLER, F. H. (1960). *J. clin. Endocr. Metab.*, **20**, 1259.

OKADA, M., FUKUSHIMA, D. K. & GALLAGHER, T. F. (1959). *J. biol. Chem.*, **234**, 1688.

OLEESKY, S. & STANBURY, S. W. (1951). *Lancet*, **2**, 664.

O'RIORDAN, J. L. H., BLANSHARD, G. P., MOXHAM, A. & NABARRO, J. D. N. (1966). *Q. Jl. Med.*, **35**, 137.

ORTH, D. N., ISLAND, D. P. & LIDDLE, G. W. (1967). *J. clin. Endocr. Metab.*, **27**, 549.

OVERELL, B. G., CONDEN, S. E. & PETROW, V. (1960). *J. Pharm. Pharmac.*, **12**, 150.

PASQUALINI, J. R. & JAYLE, M. F. (1961). *Biochem. J.*, **81**, 147.

PASQUALINI, J. R., LEGRAND, J. C. & JAYLE, M. F. (1963), *Acta Endocr. Kbh*, **43**, 67.

PEART, W. S. (1965a). *Pharmac. Rev.*, **17**, 143.

PEART, W. S. (1965b). *Rec. Progr. Horm. Res.*, **21**, 73.

PERKOFF, G. T., SANDBERG, A. A., NELSON, D. H. & TYLER, F. H. (1954). *Arch. intern. Med.*, **93**, 1.

PETERSON, R. E. (1960). In "Lipids and the Steroid Hormones in Clinical Medicine". Eds. Sunderman, F. W. & Sunderman, F. W., Jr., p. 141. Lippincott, Philadelphia.

PETERSON, R. E. (1959). *Ann. N.Y. Acad. Sci.*, **82**, 846.

PETERSON, R. E. & PIERCE, C. E. (1960). *J. clin. Invest.*, **39**, 741.

PETERSON, R. E. & WYNGAARDEN, J. B. (1956). *J. clin. Invest.*, **35**, 552.

PINCUS, G. & ROMANOFF, E. B. (1955). *Ciba Foundation Colloq. Endocr.*, **8**, 97.

PITTS, R. F. (1951). Trans. 3rd Conf. Josiah Macy, Jr. Foundation. p. 204.

PLOTZ, C. M., KNOWLTON, A. I. & RAGAN, C. (1952). *Am. J. Med.*, **13**, 597.

PORTER, G. A. & EDELMAN, I. S. (1964). *J. clin. Invest.*, **43**, 611.

PRADER, A. (1954). *Helv. Acta paed.*, **9**, 231.

PRADER, A. & GRUTNER, H. P. (1955). *Helv. Acta paed.*, **10**, 397.

RAGAN, C., HOWES, E. L., PLOTZ, C. M., MEYER, K. K., BLUNT, J. W. & LATTES, R. (1950). *Bull. N.Y. Acad. Med.*, **26**, 254.

REICHSTEIN, T. & SHOPPEE, C. W. (1943). *Vitamins & Hormones*, **1**, 345.

RELMAN, A. S. & SCHWARTZ, W. R. (1956). *New Engl. J. Med.*, **255**, 195.

RIGGS, T. R. (1964). In "Actions of Hormones on Molecular Processes". Eds. Litwack, G. & Kritchevsky, D., p. 1. New York, Wiley.

RIVAROLA, M. A., JAEZ, J. M. & MIGEON, C. J. (1967). *J. clin. Endocr. Metab.*, **27**, 624.

ROBEL, P., EMILIOZZI, R. & BAULIEU, E. E. (1966). *J. biol. Chem.*, **241**, 20.

ROBINSON, B. H. B., MATTINGLY, D. & COPE, C. L. (1962). *Br. med. J.*, **1**, 1579.

ROGOFF, J. M. & STEWART, G. N. (1927). *Science*, **66**, 327.

ROMANOFF, E. B., HUDSON, P. B. & PINCUS, G. (1953). *J. clin. Endocr. Metab.*, **13**, 1546.

ROSNER, J. M., COS, J. J., BIGLIERI, E. G., HANE, S. & FORSHAM, P. H. (1963). *J. clin. Endocr. Metab.*, **23**, 820.

ROSS, E. J. (1965). *Clin. Pharmac. Ther.*, **6**, 65.

ROVNER, D. R., CONN, J. W., KNOPF, R. F., COHEN, E. L. & HSUEH, M. T.-Y. (1965). *J. clin. Endocr. Metab.*, **25**, 53.

RYAN, K. J. (1958). *Biochim. biophys. Acta.*, **27**, 658.

SALASSA, R. M., BENNETT, W. A., KEATING, F. R., Jr. & SPRAGUE, R. G. (1953). *J. Am. med. Ass.*, **152**, 1509.

SANTANDER, R. S., GONZALEZ, A. & SUAREZ, J. A. (1965). *J. clin. Endocr. Metab.*, **25**, 1429.

SARTORIUS, O. W., CALHOON, D. & PITTS, R. F. (1952). *Endocrinology*, **51**, 444.

SARTORIUS, O. W., CALHOON, D. & PITTS, R. F. (1953). *Endocrinology*, **52**, 256.

SAVARD, K., BURSTEIN, S., ROSENKRANTZ, H. & DORFMAN, R. I. (1953). *J. biol. Chem.*, **202**, 717.

SAYERS, G. & SAYERS, M. A. (1949). *Ann. N.Y. Acad. Sci.*, **50**, 522.

SCHEDL, H. P., CHEN, P. S., GREENE, G. & REDD, D. (1959). *J. clin. Endocr. Metab.*, **19**, 1223.

SCHLATMANN, R. J. A. F., JANSEN, A. P., PRENEN, H., VAN DER KORST, J. K. & MAJOOR, C. L. H. (1964). *J. clin. Endocr. Metab.*, **24**, 35.

SEAL, U. S. & DOE, R. P. (1962). *J. biol. Chem.*, **237**, 3136.

SEALEY, J. E., GERTEN, J. N., LEDINGHAM, J. G. G. & LARAGH, J. H. (1967). *J. clin Endocr. Metab.*, **27**, 699.

SEGALOFF, A. & MANY, A. S. (1951). *Endocrinology*, **49**, 390.

SHARMA, D. C. & DORFMAN, R. I. (1963). *Fed. Proc.*, **22**, 530.

SHARP, G. W. G. & LEAF, A. (1964). *Nature* (Lond.), **202**, 1185.

SHEEHAN, H. L. & SUMMERS, V. K. (1949). *Q. Jl. Med.*, **18**, 319.

SHIMIZU, K., GUT, M. & DORFMAN, R. I. (1961). *J. biol. Chem.*, **237**, 699.

SHIMIZU, K., SHIMAO, A. S. & TANAKA, M. (1965). *Steroids*, **1** (Suppl.), 85.

SIEGENTHALER, W. E., DOWDY, A. J. & LUETSCHER, J. A. (1962). *J. clin. Endocr. Metab.*, **22**, 172.

SIMPSON, S. A., TAIT, J. F. & BUSH, I. E. (1952). *Lancet*, **2**, 226.

SIMPSON, S. A., TAIT, J. F., WETTSTEIN, A., NEHER, R. VON EUW, J., SCHINDLER, O. & REICHSTEIN, T., (1953). *Experientia*, **9**, 333.

SIMS, E. A. H., MEEKER, C. I., GRAY, M. J., WATANABE, M. & SOLOMON, S. (1964). In "Aldosterone". p. 499. Oxford, Blackwell.

SKEGGS, L. T., KAHN, J. R. & SHUMWAY, N. P. (1956). *J. exp. Med.*, **103**, 295.

SKINNER, S. L., McCUBBIN, J. W. & PAGE, I. H. (1964). *Circulation Res.*, **15**, 64.

SLATON, P. E. & BIGLIERI, E. G. (1967). *J. clin. Endocr. Metab.*, **27**, 37.

SLAUNWHITE, W. R., Jr. & SANDBERG, A. A. (1959). *J. clin. Invest.*, **38**, 384.

SOLOMON, S., LEVITAN, P. & LIEBERMAN, S. (1956). *Rev. Canad. Biol.*, **15**, 282.

SPACH, C. & STREETEN, D. H. P. (1964). *J. clin. Invest.*, **43**, 217.

SPRAGUE, R. G., POWER, M. H., MASON, H. L., ALBERT, A., MATHIESON, D. R., HENCH, P. S., KENDALL, E. C., SLOCUM, C. H. & POLLEY, H. F. (1950). *Arch. intern. Med.*, **85**, 199.

STANBURY, S. W., GOWENLOCK, A. H. & MAHLER, R. F. (1958). In "International Symposium on Aldosterone". Eds. Muller, A. F. & O'Connor, C. Boston, Little, Brown & Co.

STREETEN, D. H. P., LAWRENCE, H. L. & CONN, J. W. (1960). *Trans. Ass. Amer. Phycns.*, **78**, 227.

SULCOVA, J. & STARKA, L. (1963). *Experientia*, **19**, 632.

SWINGLE, W. W. & PFIFFNER, J. J. (1930). *Science*, **71**, 321.

SWINGLE, W. W., PFIFFNER, J. J., VARS, H. M. & PARKINS, W. M. (1934). *Am. J. Physiol.*, **108**, 144.

SYDNOR, K. L., KELLEY, V. C., RAILE, R. B., ELY, R. S. & SAYERS, G. (1953). *Proc. Soc. exp. Biol. N.Y.*, **82**, 605.

TAIT, J. F., BOUGAS, J., LITTLE, B., TAIT, S. A. S. & FLOOD, C. (1965). *J. clin. Endocr. Metab.*, **25**, 219.

TAIT, J. F., TAIT, S. A. S., LITTLE, B. & LAUMAS, K. R. (1961). *J. clin. Invest.*, **40**, 72.

TALALAY, P. & WANG, V. S. (1955). *Biochim. biophys. Acta*, **18**, 300.

TAMM, J., VOLKWEIN, D. & VOIGT, K. D. (1964). *Experientia*, **20**, 601.

THURAU, K. (1964). *Am. J. Med.*, **36**, 698.

TISDALE, W. A. & KLATSKIN, G. (1960). *Yale J. Biol. Med.*, **33**, 94.

TOBIAN, L. (1960). *Physiol. Rev.*, **40**, 280.

ULICK, S., GAUTIER, E., VETTER, K. K., MARKELLO, J. R., YAFFE, S. & LOWE, C. U. (1964). *J. clin. Endocr. Metab.*, **24**, 669.

ULICK, S., LARAGH, J. H. & LIEBERMAN, S. (1958). *Trans. Ass. Am. Phycns.*, **71**, 225.

ULICK, S. & VETTER, K. K. (1965). *J. clin. Endocr. Metab.*, **25**, 1015.

ULICK, S., VETTER, K. K. & AUGUST, J. T. (1962). *J. biol. Chem.*, **237**, 3364.

UNDERWOOD, R. H. & TAIT, J. F. (1964). *J. clin. Endocr. Metab.*, **24**, 1110.

VAN BUCHEM, F. S. P., DOORENBOS, H. & ELINGS, H. S. (1956). *Lancet*, **2**, 335.

VANDER, A. J., WILDE, W. S. & MALVIN, R. L. (1960). *Proc. Soc. exp. Biol. Med.*, **103**, 235.

VAN DE WIELE, R. L. & LIEBERMAN, S. (1960). In "Biological Activities of Steroids in Relation to Cancer". Eds. Pincus, G. & Vollmer, E. P., p. 93. New York, Academic Press.

VEYRAT, P. R., FABRE, J. & MULLER, A. F. (1962). *Helv. Med. Acta.*, **29**, 543.

VINSON, G. P. & JONES, I. C. (1964). *J. Endocr.*, **29**, 185.

VISSER, H. K. A. & COST, W. E. (1964). *Acta endocr. Kbh.*, **45**/Suppl. 89, 31.

WALLACE, E. Z., CHRISTY, N. P. & JAILER, J. W. (1955). *J. clin. Endocrin.*, **15**, 1073.

WATANABE, M., MEEKER, C. I., GRAY, M. J., SIMS, E. A. H. & SOLOMON, S. (1965). *J. clin. Endocr. Metab.*, **25**, 1665.

WEISSMAN, G. & THOMAS, L. (1964). *Rec. Progr. Horm. Res.*, **20**, 215.

WEITZMAN, E. D., SCHAUMBURG, H. & FISHBEIN, W. (1966). *J. clin. Endocr. Metab.*, **26**, 12.

WELLS, B. B. & KENDALL, E. C. (1940). *Proc. Staff Meet. Mayo Clin.*, **15**, 565.

WELT, I. D., STETTEN, D., Jr., INGLE, D. J. & MOR-
LEY, E. H. (1952). *J. biol. Chem.*, **197**, 57.

WERBIN, H. & LE ROY, G. V. (1954). *J. Am. chem.
Soc.*, **76**, 5260.

WEST, C. D., DAMAST, B. S. & PEARSON, O. H. (1958).
J. clin. Endocr, Metab., **18**, 15.

WEST, C. D., KUMAGAI, L. F., SIMONS, E. L., DOMIN-
GUEZ, O. V. & BERLINER, D. L. (1964). *J. clin.
Endocr. Metab.*, **24**, 567.

WILKINS, L. (1957). "The Diagnosis and Treatment of
Endocrine Disorders in Childhood and Adolescence". Springfield, Ill. C. C. Thomas.

WILLIAMS, W. C., Jr., ISLAND, D., OLDFIELD, R. A. A.,
Jr. & LIDDLE, G. W. (1961). *J. clin. Endocr.
Metab.*, **21**, 426.

WILSON, I. D. & GOETZ, F. C. (1964). *Am. J. Med.*, **36**,
635.

WOOD, J. B., FRANKLAND, S. W., JAMES, V. H. T. &
LANDON, J. (1965). *Lancet*, **1**, 243.

WRONG, O. (1961). *Br. med. J.*, **2**, 419.

WRONG, O., MORRISON, R. B. I. & HURST, P. E. (1961).
Lancet, **1**, 1208.

WYNN, V. & GARROD, O. (1955). *Br. med. J.*, **1**, 505.

YANKOPOULOS, N. A., DAVIS, J. O., KLIMAN, B. &
PETERSON, R. E. (1959). *J. clin. Invest.*, **38**, 1278.

YUNIS, S. L., BERCOVITCH, D. D., STEIN, R. M.,
LEVITT, M. F. & GOLDSTEIN, M. H. (1964). *J. clin.
Invest.*, **43**, 1668.

THE ADRENAL MEDULLA

Nature of the Secretion

The adrenal medulla secretes catecholamines,
a generic term applied to *o*-dihydric phenols with
a side chain carrying an amino group. Catecholamines occur also in sympathetic nerves and in the
brain, and consideration of such extra-adrenal
sources is necessarily involved in any discussion of
the chemical pathology of catecholamines. The
recognition of adrenaline (epinephrine) as an
active catecholamine secreted by the adrenal
medulla dates back to the end of the nineteenth
century. From work on the frog heart it was later
regarded as the transmitter substance at sympathetic nerve endings (Loewi, 1921), but this
position was challenged with the recognition that
noradrenaline (norepinephrine) was an important
physiological catecholamine. More recently it has
been realized that dopamine (3-hydroxytyramine)
is concerned in physiological and pathological
conditions as an active catecholamine rather than
solely as the precursor of noradrenaline. Increasing fundamental knowledge of the physiology and
chemistry of the catecholamines has led to a greater
understanding of their role in disease.

Noradrenaline has been detected in mammalian nerves and tissues and is currently regarded
as the sole peripheral sympathetic neurotrans-
mitter in mammals. Practically all peripheral
tissue noradrenaline is located at the ends of
sympathetic nerves (Falck & Torp, 1962).
Adrenaline may be the sympathetic neurotrans-
mitter in non-mammalian species, and has been
identified histochemically in sympathetic nerve
endings in the frog heart (Falck *et al.*, 1963), an
interesting confirmation of Loewi's (1921) findings. Noradrenaline occurs in normal bovine
adrenal glands (Goldenberg *et al.*, 1949; Tullar,
1949; Bergström *et al.*, 1949), constituting 12 to 18%
of the total pressor activity of the gland. Similar

results have been reported for surgically removed
human adrenal glands (von Euler *et al.*, 1954).
The adrenaline-noradrenaline ratio in the adrenal
medulla varies between mammalian species (von
Euler, 1965) but in the human gland is approximately 4:1. Foetal medullary tissue secretes
almost exclusively noradrenaline (Shepherd &
West, 1951). Small amounts of adrenaline appear
in late foetal life, but the adult adrenaline/
noradrenaline ratio is not attained until the end
of the first year of post-natal life (West, 1955).
The small amount of adrenaline found in the
urine of new-born infants may be produced in
extra-adrenal chromaffin tissue (organ of Zucker-
kandl), which differentiates, structurally and functionally, earlier than the adrenal medulla.

The dopamine and noradrenaline contents of
brain are similar but the localization differs,
dopamine being present in the caudate and lenti-
form nuclei and in the striatum in concentrations
20–100 times that of noradrenaline, whose highest
concentration is in the hypothalamus. The localization in nerve terminals in such areas suggests
that both noradrenaline and dopamine function
as neurotransmitters (Carlsson *et al.*, 1962a;
Hornykiewicz, 1966). Dopamine has been found
in relatively large amounts in tissue extracts
especially in liver, lung and intestine, where it can
account for over 90% of the total catecholamine
content. Most peripheral tissue dopamine is now
believed to be located in a special type of mast cell
(Bertler *et al.*, 1959; Falck *et al.*, 1964) whose
function is obscure. Dopamine accounts for
about 2% of the catecholamine content of adrenal
medulla (Dengler, 1957; Shepherd & West, 1953).
Its association with neural crest tumours and its
occurrence in normal urine suggest that it may
have some peripheral role also. Small amounts
of 3,4-dihydroxyphenylalanine (dopa) have been

detected in sheep adrenals (Goodall, 1951) and the phenylethylamine derivatives, octopamine, *o*-, *m*- and *p*-tyramine and synephrine have been recorded in some tissues and occur in human urine.

Biosynthesis of Catecholamines

Following the identification of the enzyme L-dopa decarboxylase (Holtz *et al.*, 1938), a bio-

adrenal glands after administration of radioactive phenylalanine to the intact animal. Later workers fully established the validity of adrenal conversion of tyrosine or dopa into dopamine, noradrenaline and adrenaline (Demis *et al.*, 1955; Hagen, 1956; Masuoka *et al.*, 1956; Udenfriend & Wyngaarden, 1956; Goodall & Kirshner, 1957; Pellerin & D'Iorio, 1957). A similar synthetic pathway from tyrosine to noradrenaline was later demonstrated

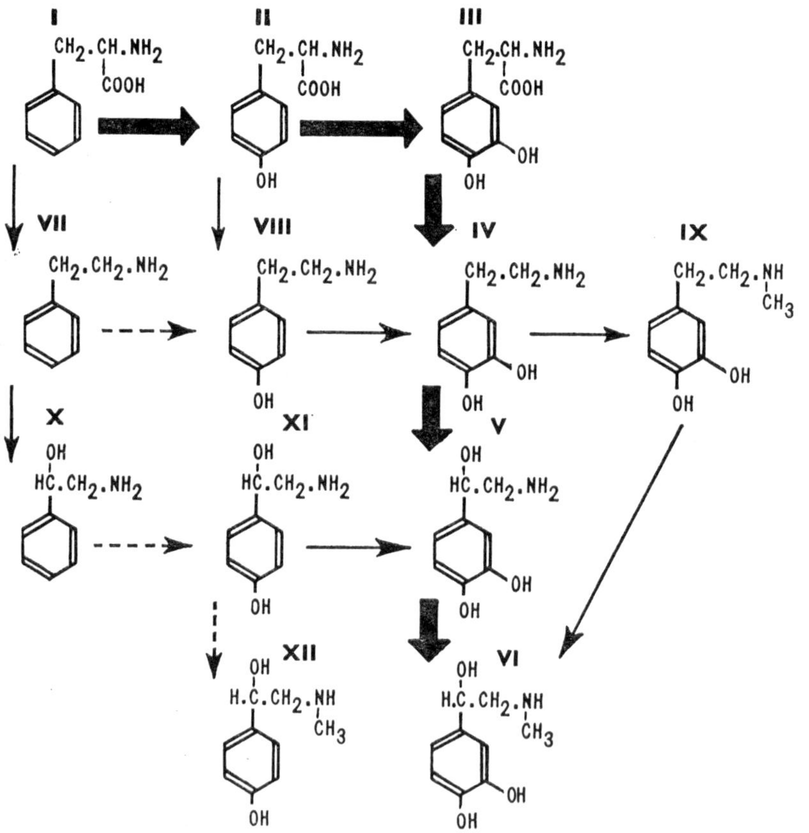

FIG. 11.7. Biosynthesis of catecholamines. Major pathways are indicated by heavy arrows, minor pathways demonstrated *in vivo* by continuous arrows, and pathways only demonstrated *in vitro* by broken arrows. The substances are: phenylalanine (I), tyrosine (II), dopa (III), dopamine (IV), noradrenaline (V), adrenaline (VI), β-phenylethylamine (VII), *p*-tyramine (VIII), epinine (IX), β-phenylethanolamine (X), octopamine (XI), synephrine (XII). The same numerals are used, where appropriate in Figs. 11.8 and 11.9.

synthetic pathway for the conversion of tyrosine to noradrenaline and adrenaline was proposed by Blaschko (1939) which is still accepted as the major route (Fig. 11.7). Pathways have been studied by *in vivo* or *in vitro* techniques frequently using radioisotopic methods. Gurin & Delluva (1947) were able to isolate labelled adrenaline from rat

in sympathetic nerves and ganglia (Goodall & Kirshner, 1958), brain (Masuoka *et al.*, 1961, 1963) and in the heart (Goldstein *et al.*, 1962; Chidsey *et al.*, 1963; Musacchio & Goldstein, 1963; Spector *et al.*, 1963). In such tissues adrenaline is not formed but appreciable quantities of dopamine may be found.

The enzymes concerned in these conversions have been investigated and many found to act on substrates other than those in the main metabolic pathway. The enzyme system hydroxylating phenylalanine occurs in the cell cytoplasm, requires reduced NADP and pteridine co-factors and also converts tryptophan into 5-hydroxytryptophan (Mitoma, 1956; Kaufman, 1957; Renson et al., 1961). Tyrosine hydroxylase which converts L-tyrosine to L-dopa has been identified in the adrenal medulla (in the cell cytoplasm) and in sympathetic nervous tissue and brain (particulate). It requires tetrahydropteridine co-factors with Fe^{2+} and appears specific for L-tyrosine (see Udenfriend, 1966). L-Dopa is converted into dopamine by dopa decarboxylase (Holtz et al., 1938) which also decarboxylates a number of aromatic amino acids including 5-hydroxytryptophan and is better described as "aromatic L-amino acid decarboxylase". Like other decarboxylases it requires pyridoxal phosphate as a co-factor. It is widely distributed and occurs in the adrenal medulla, sympathetic nerves and brain, in which it occurs in the soluble fraction of the cell, although Stjärne (1966) has reported its presence in noradrenaline storage particles in splenic nerve tissue. The properties of this enzyme are reviewed by Sourkes (1966). Conversion of dopamine to noradrenaline is catalysed by dopamine-β-hydroxylase (see Kaufman & Friedman, 1965). This copper-containing enzyme has been found in the adrenal medulla, brain, and heart in association with catecholamine storage particles and requires ascorbic acid and oxygen for activity. It is capable of β-hydroxylating other phenylethylamine derivatives including tyramine, β-phenylethylamine and N-methyldopamine (epinine). The final step involves the N-methylation of noradrenaline to form adrenaline, the methyl donor being S-adenosylmethionine. The enzyme, phenylethanolamine N-methyl transferase (see Axelrod, 1966), is virtually confined to the supernatant fraction of the adrenal medulla, but very low levels are demonstrable in the rat heart and rabbit mid-brain. It catalyses the N-methylation of a number of β-phenylethanolamine compounds and can also add a second N-methyl group to form e.g. N-methyladrenaline. Most of the biosynthetic steps take place in the cell cytoplasm, the exception being the conversion of dopamine to noradrenaline which occurs in the chromaffin granules which are also the site of storage of the catecholamines. The rate-limiting step in the reaction sequence appears to be the conversion of tyrosine to dopa by tyrosine hydroxylase (Kaufman & Friedman, 1965; Levitt et al., 1965) and

there is the possibility of a negative feedback control in that this enzyme is inhibited by noradrenaline (Udenfriend, 1966).

The relatively wide specificity of several of the enzymes (but not tyrosine hydroxylase) in the major pathway provides a number of possible alternative routes (Fig. 11.7). Some reactions have been demonstrated in vivo and others have occurred under in vitro conditions. The conversion of monophenols other than tyrosine to the corresponding catechols is achieved by an enzyme detected in rabbit liver (Axelrod, 1963), but it is not certain what role this plays in man. Tyramine, octopamine, synephrine and epinine have been found to occur normally. Although such pathways are of biochemical interest they are quantitatively unimportant in normal metabolism. Their existence is of importance when considering the mode of action of drugs of the phenylethylamine group.

Inhibitors of the enzymes involved in the main pathway have been studied in the hope of developing drugs of therapeutic value. Inhibitors of dopa decarboxylase such as α-methyl-dopa reduce tissue noradrenaline content. More potent inhibitors of this widespread enzyme have no such effect and the mechanism of action may be indirect. Although in vitro inhibitors of dopamine-β-hydroxylase have been described (Van der Schoot & Creveling, 1965), the only one used in man is disulphiram. Recent recognition of α-methyltyrosine and iodotyrosine derivatives as in vivo inhibitors of the rate-limiting step due to tyrosine hydroxylase (Spector et al., 1965) offers the possibility of effective blocking of catecholamine synthesis (Sjoerdsma et al., 1965). It is of interest that the natural thyroxine precursors, 3-iodo-L-tyrosine and 3,5-diiodo-L-tyrosine act as inhibitors as does phenylalanine. The latter may account for the reduced brain catecholamine content seen in phenylketonuria.

Physiological Actions

The physiological actions of adrenaline and noradrenaline have been studied in great detail. They are most active in the laevo form, exerting their peripheral and cardiac actions after combination with a receptor mechanism in the end-organ. These "adrenotropic receptors" have been divided into two broad groups: α and β, identified by the selective inhibition of sympathomimetic amine activity by specific blocking agents for the two types (see later). Cells of sympathetically innervated tissues usually have a preponderance of one type of receptor. The α-receptors are mainly associated with excitatory mechanisms, i.e. vasoconstrictor, stimulation of the uterus, nictitating membrane and the pupillary dilator muscle, although α-receptors causing inhibition in intestinal muscle have been identified (Ahlquist & Levy, 1959). On the other hand, the β-receptors are concerned primarily, but not exclusively, with inhibitory functions (vasodilation, inhibition of the uterus in certain species and bronchodilation). Differences between amines in their ability to stimulate α-receptors are not accompanied by parallel variations in their influence on β-receptors (Ahlquist, 1948). Indeed, synthetic sympathomimetic amines show a spectrum of activity ranging from pure α to pure β activity. The mechanism of the direct action in smooth or cardiac muscle has not been elucidated but several theories have been put forward (Innes & Nickerson, 1965). The catecholamines have marked actions on the cardiovascular system, but the details of action differ significantly. Adrenaline produces tachycardia, increased cardiac output and stroke volume and increased coronary blood flow. Blood flow in skeletal muscle and the splanchnic area is increased following vasodilation (β-receptors) but the skin vessels are constricted. The overall effect on peripheral resistance is a reduction unless the dose is high. The net result is an increase in the systolic and mean blood pressures with little effect on the diastolic pressure. If α-receptor blocking agents are given, the vasodilation is sufficient to produce a fall in blood pressure despite the increased cardiac output. Noradrenaline acts mainly on α-receptors and on cardiac β-receptors. The coronary arteries are dilated but direct stimulatory effects are not seen; indeed reflex bradycardia may occur. Cardiac output is usually unchanged but may be reduced if hypertension is marked. Widespread peripheral vasoconstriction greatly increases peripheral resistance with resultant increase in systolic, diastolic and mean blood pressures. The opposing effects of the hypertension and vasoconstriction usually result in little change in tissue blood flow. The use of α-receptor blocking agents indicates that vasodilatory effects are weak (Nickerson & Nomaguchi, 1953). Noradrenaline is more effective than adrenaline in producing sweating, piloerection and mydriasis. Noradrenaline also has the effect when given repeatedly of reducing blood volume by loss of fluid from the plasma into the interstitial fluid probably effected by postcapillary vasoconstriction.

Dopamine also shows activity in the cardiovascular system (Hornykiewicz, 1966). It increases splanchnic and renal blood flow with a fall in blood pressure in experimental animals, but also shows α-receptor activity. However, the effects of dopamine are not blocked by the usual α or β-receptor blockers, suggesting that separate peripheral dopamine receptors may exist.

The metabolic effects of adrenaline are much more marked than with noradrenaline and are concerned with providing sufficient metabolic fuel to meet fluctuating energy requirements, by very rapid activation of enzymes concerned in carbohydrate and fat metabolism. They are concerned in the responses to cold or muscular exercise. The catecholamines produce glycogenolysis in liver and muscle with a rise in circulating glucose and lactate. This is brought about by increased activity of phosphorylase resulting in formation of glucose-1-phosphate. This is further converted into glucose-6-phosphate which is hydrolysed by glucose-6-phosphatase in the liver with release of glucose. In muscle this enzyme is lacking, and further metabolism occurs to form lactate. Breakdown of glycogen is associated with release of intracellular K^+ and a rise in plasma K^+ concentration. Adrenaline stimulates the formation of cyclic 3′,5′-adenosine monophosphate (cyclic 3′,5′-AMP) which increases the activity of phosphorylase b kinase. This enzyme converts phosphorylase b into phosphorylase a, the active but rate-limiting enzyme in the conversion of glycogen to glucose (review by Sutherland & Robison, 1966). The effect of adrenaline on the formation of cyclic 3′,5′-AMP has also been invoked to explain this catecholamine's action on myocardial contraction (Sutherland & Robison, 1966) and on glyconeogenesis from lactate (Exton & Park, 1966). The effect on fat metabolism was demonstrated much later than that on carbohydrate metabolism. Adrenaline stimulates the release of non-esterified fatty acids (NEFA) from adipose tissue (Gordon & Cherkes, 1958; White & Engel, 1958). The metabolic consequence (Steinberg, 1966) of NEFA liberation is the increased turnover of a fatty acid transport cycle, as indicated by increased uptake and utilization of NEFA in the tissues with increase of fatty deposits in the liver, increased plasma lipoprotein concentration with increase in cholesterol, phospholipid and triglyceride components and increased uptake of triglycerides in adipose tissue. The increase in NEFA may also account for the rise in basal metabolic rate which is a well recognized effect of adrenaline. The liberation of NEFA is attributed to activation of a specific lipase in adipose tissue and it is currently believed that this activation is mediated through cyclic 3′,5′-AMP (Butcher, 1966). β-Adrenergic blocking agents inhibit the lipolytic and glycogenolytic actions of adrenaline, and are believed to act by competitively blocking the action of adrenaline on adenyl cyclase, the enzyme occurring in all tissues and responsible for cyclic 3′,5′-AMP formation (Brodie *et al.*, 1966).

Metabolic Breakdown of Catecholamines

Two enzymes play a major role in the catabolism of catecholamines namely, monoamine oxidase (MAO) and catechol-O-methyl transferase (COMT).

The widely distributed mitochondrial enzyme, MAO, is a flavoprotein converting a wide variety of monoamines to the corresponding aldehydes. The aldehyde is usually converted to the corresponding carboxylic acid by a dehydrogenase but may also undergo reduction to the alcohol. COMT, discovered by Axelrod (1957), occurs in

the cell sap of most tissues, especially liver and kidney (Axelrod & Tomchick, 1958), and catalyses methyl group transfer from S-adenosylmethionine to the *m*-phenolic group of a number of substituted catechols.

Oral or intravenous administration of radioactive adrenaline or noradrenaline and subsequent examination of urinary metabolites has shown that O-methylation in the liver is a major pathway in the inactivation of these amines. Available evidence suggests that O-methylation is also a major pathway in the metabolism of noradrenaline released in peripheral tissues from sympathetic nerve endings or injected into the brain. Adrenaline and noradrenaline are converted into metadrenaline (metanephrine) and normetadrenaline (normetanephrine) respectively. These products, which have little pressor activity, occur

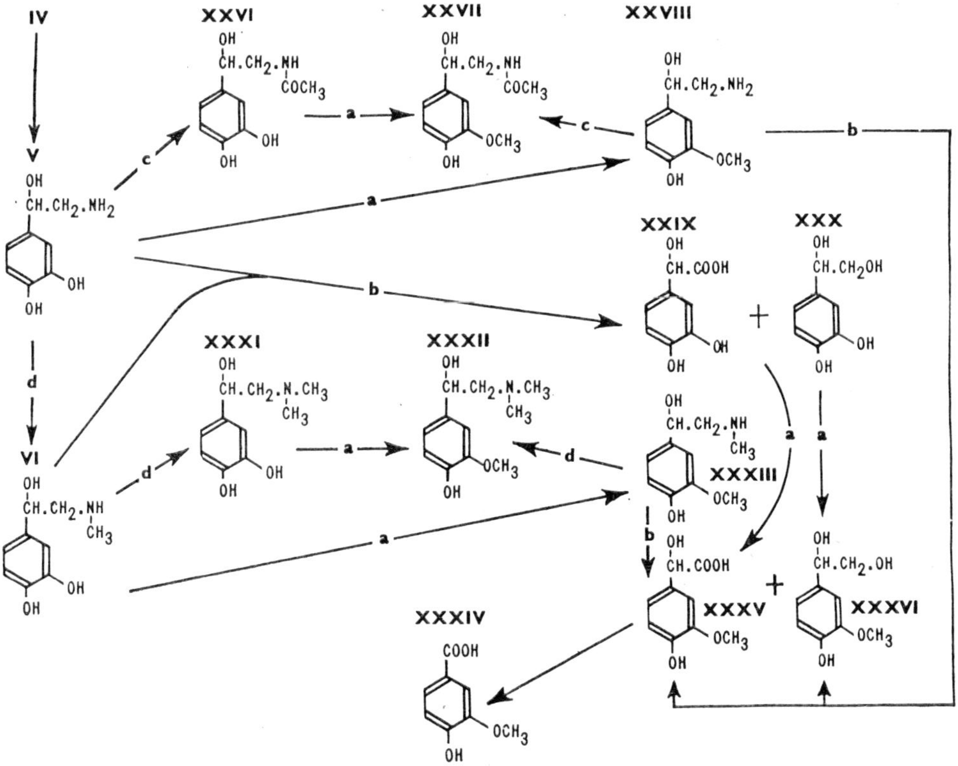

FIG. 11.8. Metabolites of noradrenaline and adrenaline in normal and pathological urines. The main processes are: O-methylation (a); deamination with further oxidation or reduction (b); acetylation (c); N-methylation (d).

The substances, many of which are excreted partly as conjugates are: dopamine (IV), noradrenaline (V), adrenaline (VI), N-acetylnoradrenaline (XXVI), N-acetylnormetadrenaline (XXVII), normetadrenaline (normetanephrine, XXVIII), 3,4-dihydroxymandelic acid (XXIX), 3,4-dihydroxyphenyl glycol (XXX), N-methyladrenaline (XXXI), N-methylmetadrenaline (XXXII), metadrenaline (metanephrine, XXXIII), vanillic acid (XXXIV), 4-hydroxy-3-methoxymandelic acid (HMMA, VMA, XXXV) and 4-hydroxy-3-methoxyphenyl glycol (HMPG, XXXVI).

in normal urine both free and as the sulphate or glucuronide. Deamination of the O-methylated amines by MAO and further oxidation or reduction of the aldehyde product yields as a major product, 4-hydroxy-3-methoxymandelic acid (HMMA) also known, erroneously, as vanillyl-mandelic acid (VMA); 4-hydroxy-3-methoxy-phenyl glycol (HMPG) is a minor product. Adrenaline and noradrenaline can also be converted by MAO to 3,4-dihydroxymandelic acid and 3,4-dihydroxyphenyl glycol which occur in small amounts in urine partly in conjugated form, and which are capable of O-methylation in tissues to form HMMA and HMPG. In addition, adrenaline and noradrenaline occur in urine either unchanged or in conjugated form. Other minor metabolites identified are N-methyladrenaline, N-methylmetadrenaline, N-acetylnormetadrenaline and 4-hydroxy-3-methoxy-benzoic acid (vanillic acid) (Fig. 11.8).

In the brain and in certain tumours, dopamine undergoes metabolic transformations other than the usual conversion to noradrenaline or epinine outlined earlier. The two enzymes mainly concerned are again MAO and COMT. Methylation produces 3-methoxytyramine and deamination forms 3,4-dihydroxyphenyl-acetic acid and, to a lesser extent, 3,4-dihydroxyphenyl glycol. These metabolites have been detected in urine but mostly they undergo further reactions forming homo-vanillic acid (HVA, 4-hydroxy-3-methoxyphenyl-acetic acid) the overall process being entirely analogous to the formation of HMMA from adrenaline and noradrenaline. In some pathological states dopa metabolites appear in the urine. As indicated in Fig. 11.9, these involve either "O-methylation" or amine group oxidation or both.

The relative amounts of the different noradrenaline and adrenaline metabolites in urine varies

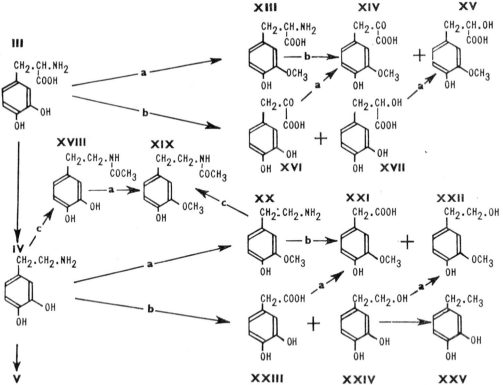

Fig. 11.9. Metabolites of dopa and dopamine in normal and pathological urines. The main processes are: O-methylation (a); deamination with further oxidation or reduction (b); acetylation (c). The substances, many of which are excreted partly as conjugates are: dopa (III), dopamine (IV), noradrenaline (V), 4-hydroxy-3-methoxyphenylalanine (XIII), 4-hydroxy-3-methoxyphenyl pyruvic (XIV) and lactic (XV) acids, 3,4-dihydroxyphenyl pyruvic (XVI) and lactic (XVII) acids, N-acetyldopamine (XVIII), N-acetyl-3-methoxytyramine (XIX), 3-methoxytyramine (XX), homovanillic acid (HVA, XXI), 4-hydroxy-3-methoxyphenyl ethanol (XXII), 3,4-dihydroxyphenylacetic acid (XXIII), 3,4-dihydroxyphenyl ethanol (XXIV) and 3,4-dihydroxyphenylethane (XXV).

with the physiological circumstances (Crout, 1966). With normal endogenous secretion the percentage excretions of adrenaline + noradrenaline, metadrenaline + normetadrenaline and HMMA are 1·1, 7·6 and 91 respectively. Intravenous infusion of radioactive catecholamines has been useful in delineating pathways of metabolism, but has distorted the proportions above. This is especially obvious when dl-catecholamines are used. Even with l-adrenaline, however, this route gives the following results: catecholamines (4%), metadrenalines (34%), HMMA (55%), other metabolites (7%). Tumours which release catecholamines into the circulation in spurts usually show an intermediate pattern.

Circulation and Storage of Catecholamines

Significant but variable concentrations of adrenaline and noradrenaline are present in arterial blood and rise markedly in response to appropriate physiological stimuli. Circulating catecholamines may originate from the adrenal medulla or sympathetic nerve endings in peripheral tissues, but not from brain (Glowinski et al., 1965). Release of noradrenaline in peripheral tissues is quantitatively the more important. Bilateral adrenalectomy in man causes rapid reduction of adrenaline excretion in the urine to very low levels, but urinary noradrenaline values are virtually unchanged. Adrenaline excretion after adrenalectomy may return slowly suggesting that extra-adrenal tissue can develop the capacity to convert noradrenaline into adrenaline (Henkin & Bartter, 1965). The adrenal medulla releases catecholamines in response either to stimulation of its preganglionic cholinergic fibres, as in emotional stress or in response to circulating substances such as insulin and histamine. Nervous stimulation releases both adrenaline and noradrenaline (Lund, 1951), and involves the entry of calcium ions through the cell membrane (Douglas, 1966). Insulin may selectively release adrenaline implying the existence of two types of medullary cell (Eranko, 1960). The venous blood level of noradrenaline exceeds that of arterial blood indicating its continuous release from tissues. This is considerably increased in an organ following stimulation of its sympathetic nerve supply and is well demonstrated in the heart. Increased noradrenaline secretion occurs in trauma, physical stress and emotional situations with a strong active, aggressive component.

Adrenaline and noradrenaline are released into the circulation from intracellular storage granules together with ATP (Douglas, 1966). The granules occur in the chromaffin cells of the medulla in which both amines are stored in high concentration (600 mM) giving rise to the characteristic histochemical staining reactions. Noradrenaline storage granules are found in the varicosities occurring on terminal sympathetic nerve fibres in peripheral tissues and in nerve endings in the brain. Such storage granules have been studied by density gradient centrifugation and by electron microscopy. They possess an outer limiting membrane, contain the enzyme dopamine-β-hydroxylase and have a central core of catecholamine combined with ATP in a molecular ratio of approximately 4:1 (Potter & Axelrod, 1963; von Euler et al., 1963). They vary in diameter, medullary chromaffin granules (500-4000 Å) being the largest and sympathetic nerve granules (400–500 Å) the smallest, with hypothalamic granules (1300 Å) occupying an intermediate position. Their density and sedimentation velocities also differ similarly. Whereas the catecholamines in medullary particles are virtually all bound, some of the noradrenaline in sympathetic nerves and in the uterus is apparently unattached to particles and greater quantities of non-particulate noradrenaline and dopamine are present in brain tissue. These differences have been reviewed by Wurtman (1965) and Stjarne (1966).

Although the intact granules show only weak pressor activity, a variety of physico-chemical agents can disrupt the limiting membrane and release the catecholamines in active form. The main functions of the storage granules are to take up dopamine from the cytoplasm, convert it to noradrenaline and store this amine or its further conversion product, adrenaline. Storage in this way protects the catecholamines from destruction by other cell enzymes and also permits release of the active substances by various stimuli. They are also capable of removing catecholamines from their surroundings by re-storing. The details of these processes and the effect of various drugs on them have been the subject of numerous publications in the last few years, and present concepts are still in danger of undergoing marked modification in the future. The account which follows is a resumé of present thinking but the reader should consult recent reviews for details (Wurtman, 1965; Acheson, 1966; Iversen, 1967).

Studies using isotopically labelled adrenaline and noradrenaline show that when these amines are infused intravenously they are rapidly removed from the circulation, the initial half-life being of the order of 10–30 seconds. Tissue extraction ratios are usually 75% or more, and the uptake of various organs is mainly determined by the proportion of the cardiac output which perfuses them.

Any circumstance, physiological or pharmacological, which alters relative perfusion rates therefore influences the fate of circulating catecholamines. The fate of the material taken up depends on the organ. The kidney excretes some catecholamines unchanged. The liver and also the kidney convert them mainly to their O-methylated derivatives, normetadrenaline and metadrenaline and thence to HMMA as these organs are rich in the enzymes MAO and COMT. Sympathetic nerve endings and the adrenal medulla take up the catecholamines into their storage granules chemically unchanged. This process involves both diffusion and an active transport mechanism and accounts for almost all of the catecholamine uptake by most organs, parenchymal uptake being small. The physiological effects of infused catecholamines are only seen when circulating concentrations are increased and tissue receptors are stimulated. Re-binding by storage particles removes the amines from the receptor sites and thus limits the effects even though no chemical change has occurred. Thus drugs which interfere with the uptake process potentiate the action of adrenaline and noradrenaline. Inhibition of COMT can also lead to prolongation of action but less markedly. It is possible that the level of sensitivity of receptor sites may vary but such changes are difficult to measure.

The tissue catecholamine content usually remains constant but there is a continuing turnover. Release of catecholamines from stores is balanced by re-accumulation. Catecholamines in tissues may be synthesized locally or taken up from the circulation. Adrenaline is mainly synthesized in the adrenal medulla but can enter tissue storage sites. Brain takes up little circulating catecholamine and synthesis is thus important. The heart has been found to derive up to 20% of its catecholamine content from circulating material. The available evidence suggests that the catecholamine of storage granules exists in two physiological "pools". One has a rapid turnover rate (half life about 2 hr.), the catecholamine is released by tyramine and other sympathomimetic amines and by nerve stimulation, emerges from the nerve ending and acts on receptors. Angiotensin is particularly potent in releasing *adrenal* catecholamines. Only a minor part of the noradrenaline released acts on receptors. Most of it re-enters the sympathetic nerve endings and is converted to bound form in the same pool from which it was liberated. A lesser proportion is inactivated by COMT in surrounding parenchymal cells (the enzyme is absent from nerve endings themselves). Depending on the amount of nor-

adrenaline released and on the local blood flow, a varying proportion leaves the organ in the blood unchanged. The enzyme MAO appears to have no role in the physiological inactivation of adrenaline or noradrenaline and inhibition of this enzyme does not alter the physiological response to endogenous or exogenous catecholamine.

The other pool has a slower turnover rate (half-life about 1 day) and is relatively refractory to stimulation. Catecholamines released are mainly metabolized by MAO in mitochondria within the nerve cell and effects on receptors are small. The deaminated products, dihydroxymandelic acid and dihydroxyphenylglycol emerge from the nerve and are either excreted unchanged or undergo further methylation to HMMA and HMPG respectively before excretion. The major part of the daily turnover of stored catecholamine is through the second pool. There is some blurring of definition of "pools" depending on the stimulating agent and no anatomical difference has been defined although it is postulated that the more labile pool is in the particles closest to the nerve ending.

The action of a wide range of drugs can be considered under various headings although some drugs have more than one action.

(*a*) *Agents interfering with the synthesis of catecholamines.* These have been discussed in the section on biosynthesis.

(*b*) *Agents causing release of catecholamine from storage sites.* Tyramine and other indirect-acting sympathomimetic amines exert their effects indirectly by releasing noradrenaline from the "labile" pool and become less effective as this pool is depleted. Reserpine appears to have a destructive effect on the storage vesicles releasing catecholamines from both pools. The released material is mainly deaminated within the nerve before entering the circulation. Reserpine thus greatly reduces tissue catecholamine concentrations and the response to indirect-acting sympathomimetic agents or nerve stimulation.

(*c*) *Agents blocking the release of catecholamines from storage sites.* Bretylium and guanethidine probably block conduction in preterminal sympathetic fibres, and block the release of catecholamines either by nerve stimulation or by reserpine. Ganglion-blocking drugs interfere with transmission of impulses from preganglionic sympathetic fibres through sympathetic ganglia and thus block the release normally achieved by nervous stimulation.

(*d*) *Agents blocking the action of released catecholamines on tissue receptors.* Tissue receptors are classified as α and β and are associated with the two types of action of catecholamines mentioned earlier. Some drugs (dibenzyline, phentolamine) block the action on α-receptors and others (pronethalol, propranalol) block β-receptors. The physiological consequences are those of unbalanced action of the unblocked type of response.

(*e*) *Agents interfering with uptake and binding of catecholamines in storage particles.* Some drugs interfere with the re-entry of catecholamine into nerve endings either by altering diffusion or blocking active transport mechanisms. Cocaine, imipramine and some MAO inhibitors have this effect. Others (e.g. reserpine) block the accumulation of catecholamine within the storage granule by interfering with the binding mechanism rather than with entry into the cell. A group of substances act as "false transmitters" and compete with noradrenaline for binding sites in the storage granules. They are released by the usual mechanisms but are less physiologically active and thus reduce the usual effects of stimulation. Some false transmitter amines (metaraminol) are administered as such. In other cases precursors are given and release the desired amine intracellularly. Thus α-methyl dopa produces α-methyl noradrenaline and α-methyl-*m*-tyrosine produces metaraminol. Tyramine is similarly converted to octopamine if its normal metabolism is inhibited.

(*f*) *Agents interfering with MAO and COMT.* Inhibition of these enzymes interferes with metabolism of native catecholamines and of other amines either of dietary origin or administered therapeutically. MAO is mainly concerned with the intraneuronal disposal of catecholamine released from the less labile store. Adrenaline and noradrenaline are poorer substrates than tyramine or dopamine. A number of MAO inhibitors have been used therapeutically including the long acting hydrazine drugs such as iproniazid and the shorter acting harmala alkaloids (Pletscher, 1963). Inhibition is associated with increased noradrenaline content of the brain and peripheral tissues; the dopamine content of brain is also increased. MAO inhibitors have little effect on physiological actions of adrenaline and noradrenaline, but potentiate the action of such substances as tyramine which are normally rapidly deaminated. Thus serious hypertensive episodes may occur in patients taking MAO inhibitors subjected to increased dietary intake of tyramine in cheese and wine. Inhibition of tyramine deamination may also lead to its conversion to octopamine, a false transmitter. MAO inhibitors also depress the release of noradrenaline from stores by various agents, possibly because MAO is required for

rupture of the storage particles of the less labile pool.

A number of inhibitors of COMT belonging to the tropolone, dopacetamide and papaverine series have been investigated (Belleau & Burba, 1961; Carlsson et al., 1962b; Ross & Haljasmaa, 1961; Burba & Murnaghan, 1965). COMT has a greater affinity for adrenaline and other N-alkylnoradrenalines. Crout (1961) reported no great prolongation of noradrenaline activity in the presence of inhibitors of MAO and COMT. The effect of COMT inhibitors alone has little effect in increasing the action of noradrenaline, but prolongs or potentiates the effect of adrenaline and other N-alkyl noradrenalines (Bacq et al., 1959; Wylie et al., 1960; Murnaghan & Mazurkiewicz, 1963; Izquiredo & Kaumann, 1963; Ross, 1963). However, disposal of released catecholamines by COMT action is not the major route and any effects are usually only slight.

Routine Laboratory Methods for the Investigation of Disorders of Catecholamine Metabolism

Only the principles involved are discussed here. More detailed accounts appear elsewhere (Varley & Gowenlock, 1963; Whitby, 1965). Most investigations are performed on urine which is best collected with added mineral acid and which can be preserved frozen for many weeks unchanged. Plasma is sometimes used for catecholamine determinations.

Catecholamines. Most methods measure unconjugated catecholamines which are mainly noradrenaline, adrenaline and dopamine. Hydrolysis increases the figures up to threefold. One or more of these amines may occur in increased concentration in pathological urines. Methods are mainly fluorimetric and differ in that some do not measure dopamine. These may either record total adrenaline plus noradrenaline excretion or each separately. Methods are available for "total catecholamines" which include all three catecholamines.

The "trihydroxyindole" methods involve oxidation of the catecholamines and subsequent conversion by alkali into fluorescent trihydroxyindoles. Dopamine usually gives only traces of fluorescent product but adrenaline and noradrenaline form adrenolutine and noradrenolutine. These may either be determined together or separately. In the latter case differential oxidation or differential fluorimetry is employed. All three catecholamines after oxidation form intensely fluorescent derivatives with ethylenediamine, as do a number of interfering substances. Preliminary purification of extracts and, if necessary, separation of catecholamines is usually needed.

Normal ranges vary somewhat with methods but in general terms the noradrenaline + adrenaline output is less than 100 μg./24 hr. or 25–50 μg./g. creatinine with a noradrenaline/adrenaline ratio of about 3 to 1. Dopamine excretion is 100–200 μg./24 hr. or 130–260 μg./g. creatinine and "total catecholamines" may be taken as up to 200 μg./24 hr. It is important to remember that certain fruits and vegetables, especially bananas, are rich sources of catecholamines. They should be excluded from the diet before collecting urine. Catecholamine excretion is sometimes used as a "screening" test (Hingerty, 1957). False positive tests may occur from dietary factors.

Plasma catecholamine concentrations are much lower, 2.4 ± 1.1 μg./l. Noradrenaline accounts for about 85% of the total, but dopamine has not been detected.

Metadrenaline and normetadrenaline. The urine is first hydrolysed with acid to break down sulphate conjugates and frequently metadrenaline and normetadrenaline are determined together. The commonest method involves oxidation with periodate to convert both substances into vanillin which is determined spectrophotometrically. Modifications in which the two methylated metabolites are determined individually are less often used but yield estimates of the separate secretion of adrenaline and noradrenaline.

Normal figures are 0.6 ± 0.3 mg./24 hr. with an upper limit of normal at 1.3 mg./24 hr. In children the range is 0.5–1.0 mg./g. creatinine. About one quarter of the total is metadrenaline. The figures are increased in patients receiving MAO inhibitors or α-methyldopa and such drugs should be withdrawn before carrying out the test.

HMMA (VMA). This major metabolite of both adrenaline and noradrenaline is excreted in free form and hydrolysis of urine is therefore not necessary. A colorimetric method was used as a screening test by Gitlow *et al.* (1960). The result was expressed as the ratio of the colorimeter reading at 450 mμ to that at 530 mμ. The figure is normally greater than 1.30. The test is subject to false positive results from dietary causes, notably vanilla products. More refined methods are usually employed, the most popular involving periodate oxidation of the separated HMMA to form vanillin which is determined spectrophotometrically. Such methods are not affected by diet. Patients receiving MAO inhibitors have reduced HMMA output, but this is not seen with α-methyldopa.

Normal ranges vary somewhat with the method used but 1.5 to 6.5 mg./24 hr. is representative. In children the upper limit is 5–10 mg./g. creatinine, the upper figure being for children under 3 years old.

Other substances. The above three groups of tests are currently the basis of most routine diagnostic work. Many other substances have been identified and quantified, but these are mainly for research purposes. The only exception is homovanillic acid (HVA) which has been used fairly often in investigating dopamine-secreting tumours. A variety of methods have been employed but the average upper limit of normal is 8 mg./24 hr.

CATECHOLAMINE PRODUCTION BY NEURAL CREST TUMOURS

During embryonic development sympathogonia migrate from the neural crest to form the adrenal medulla and sympathetic ganglia. In the medulla they develop into phaeochromoblasts and then into phaeochromocytes, the mature medullary cells. In the ganglia they become sympathoblasts and then mature into sympathetic ganglion cells. Tumours derived from the mature cell types or from their precursors are known and might be expected to be active endocrinologically. The next sections review the important clinicobiochemical correlations which have been established.

Phaeochromocytoma

A phaeochromocytoma is a tumour, usually benign, of chromaffin tissue (phaeochromocytes). Most tumours are unilateral and originate in the adrenal medulla, but about 15% derive from extra-adrenal sources of chromaffin tissue usually in the para-aortic region but intrathoracic and intravesical forms are well documented. A multicentric origin is sometimes seen (6.5%) and bilateral adrenal tumours or simultaneous adrenal and extra-adrenal tumours are well recognized and may cause confusion with the metastasing malignant variant (6.5%) derived from phaeochromoblasts. The tumour occurs mainly in adults without sexual discrimination, but when it develops in children, multiple and extra-adrenal tumours are commoner than in adults and there is a male preponderance (Evans, 1963; Hermann & Mornex, 1964). A familial form of the disease often with bilateral tumours has been described on a number of occasions (Evans, 1963; Hermann & Mornex, 1964; Crout, 1966). The familial form has been found to be significantly associated with neuroectodermal dyplastic conditions such as neurofibromatosis and von Hippel-Landau's disease, with thyroid carcinoma and with para-thyroid adenoma (Crout, 1966). The form of inheritance is usually that of an autosomal Mendelian dominant. Such associations should be borne in mind whenever the diagnosis of phaeochromoctyoma is made.

The name, phaeochromocytoma, is derived from the darkening in colour of tumour cells occurring in the presence of dichromate. This formation of a brown pigment and other histo-chemical reactions result from the oxidation of adrenaline or noradrenaline which occur in abnormal amounts in such tumours. These reactions are non-specific and the chromaffin reaction is given by 5-hydroxytryptamine in carcinoid tumours (Evans, 1963).

Although first recorded as an autopsy finding, phaeochromocytoma was later found to be associated with the clinical syndrome of paroxysmal hypertension. Analysis of tumour tissue has established beyond doubt that phaeochromocytomas synthesize catecholamines often in considerable quantities. The normal human medulla contains less than 1 mg. of catecholamine/g. of tissue (von Euler et al., 1954), predominantly as adrenaline. Phaeochromocytomas may contain up to 73 mg./g. of catecholamine, but usually the figure is less than 10 mg./g. The relative amounts of adrenaline to noradrenaline vary widely but, in general, noradrenaline predominates and may account for virtually all the catecholamine, whereas tumours containing only adrenaline are much rarer (Robinson, 1963; Evans, 1963; Hermann & Mornex, 1964; Käser, 1966; Bell, 1968). Extramedullary tumours usually, but not invariably, contain a very high proportion of noradrenaline.

The tumours contain storage particles but catecholamine storage is abnormal in that the ratio of catecholamine to ATP is often as high as 30 and in some cases the percentage of particle-bound catecholamine is low. These variations from normal may account for the varying pattern of urinary metabolites seen in phaeochromocytoma, and suggest that metabolites are produced within some tumours and enter the circulation as such (Crout, 1966). The enzymology of phaeochromoctyoma tissue appears to have attracted little attention but the conversion of dopa or dopamine to noradrenaline by tumour tissue has been demonstrated, as has the presence of COMT and MAO (Sjoerdsma et al., 1959).

Dopamine has not often been detected in phaeochromocytomas, and the belief that the malignant variant produces dopamine is not substantiated from the few tumour analyses recorded and the difficulty of establishing adequate criteria

for malignancy (Evans, 1963). The highest dopamine figure, 1970 μg./g., was recorded for a locally invasive tumour (McMillan, 1956), but dopamine was absent in other malignant tumours (Manger et al., 1954; Kennedy et al., 1961) or present in lower concentration than in non-malignant tumours (Donath et al., 1965; Käser, 1966). In other tumours in which dopamine was detected (Weil-Malherbe, 1956; Manger et al., 1954) the status of the tumour was unknown. Dopa has also been reported in one dopamine-containing tumour (Weil-Malherbe, 1956).

As might be expected from tumours secreting noradrenaline and adrenaline, the clinical findings involve cardiovascular and metabolic disturbances. Among the former, paroxysmal hypertension was first associated with phaeochromocytoma. During the hypertensive episodes, which can be initiated by a wide variety of physical and mental stimuli and which may last from a few minutes to several days, there may occur headache, palpitations, sensations of terror, marked sweating, pallor and other vasomotor phenomena. Following the episode the blood pressure returns to normal. Later investigations have shown that paroxysmal hypertension is present only in about one quarter of the cases. Most of the remainder have a more sustained hypertension, about half of them with episodes of more severe hypertension (Hermann & Mornex, 1964). In some cases the picture closely resembles essential hypertension, sometimes of the malignant type especially if the tumour occurs in childhood.

It has been suggested that the sustained release of even small amounts of noradrenaline from the tumour may eventually produce sustained hypertension (Dickinson & De Swiet, 1967). There is no difference in the mean size of tumours occurring in patients with sustained hypertension compared with those with the paroxysmal type (Gifford et al., 1964). As a cause of hypertension, phaeochromocytoma is uncommon, the incidence is estimated as about 0·5 %. There is, however, little evidence to implicate increased circulating catecholamines in the usual types of hypertension. Still more recently, cases have been described in which marked hypotensive episodes occurred, either in isolation or after hypertensive attacks, (Richmond et al., 1961; Leather et al., 1962; Ramsey et al., 1962; Hamrin, 1962; Mackenzie & Pearson, 1967). It has been suggested that in such cases excessive secretion of adrenaline produces vasodilatation (β-receptors), but β-adrenergic blockers do not improve the hypotension and the syndrome has been reported in tumours which appear to be noradrenaline secretors. It is possible that dopamine may be exerting a peripheral effect in such cases and the reduction of plasma volume known to occur during continued noradrenaline infusions has been considered as an important factor. About 9% of phaeochromocytoma patients are normotensive and about 5% are symptomless, the finding of the tumours often being by chance (Hermann & Mornex, 1964).

The metabolic effects are best seen in tumours secreting adrenaline or large quantities of noradrenaline. Increase in the basal metabolic rate is common and its association with thyroid swelling and the vasomotor phenomena mentioned above may cause diagnostic confusion with thyrotoxicosis. Protein-bound iodine concentration is, however, normal. Disturbances of glucose metabolism occur and plasma glucose and, sometimes, potassium concentrations may be increased. Glucose tolerance is disturbed, leading to curves of the diabetic type in about 10% of cases. Usually this state disappears after removal of the tumour, but in some cases it persists probably due to associated true diabetes mellitus, the incidence of which may be increased in phaeochromocytoma (Evans, 1963). Disturbances of lipid metabolism have been studied less, but patients with phaeochromocytoma are often thin (Kvale et al., 1957) and there is an increase in plasma NEFA concentration (Engleman et al., 1964).

Diagnosis of phaeochromocytoma. The increased knowledge of the metabolism of adrenaline and noradrenaline, and the development of methods for determination of various metabolites in urine to supplement the older methods of catecholamine determination in plasma or urine has altered the emphasis in diagnostic procedures. Biochemical investigations are now the mainstay and pharmacological tests are less frequently employed than formerly. In general, the presence of a phaeochromocytoma is suspected on the basis of unusual features such as sweating, glycosuria or hypermetabolism in a hypertensive patient whose blood pressure may be paroxysmal. The routine screening of all hypertensive patients is laborious and only rarely rewarding. When the diagnosis is confirmed, radiological investigation (pyelography, air insufflation and tomography) of the adrenal areas reveals the tumour in about half the cases. For extra-adrenal tumours, determination of the catecholamine content of blood obtained from different sites by venous catheterization has been helpful (Crout & Sjoerdsma, 1960).

Urinary determinations are most frequently used in the biochemical investigation of patients with suspected phaeochromocytoma. The parameters most often measured have been: unconju-
gated catecholamines, either *in toto* or with separate assessment of adrenaline, noradrenaline and, sometimes, dopamine; conjugated metadrenaline and normetadrenaline, either separately or together; HMMA (VMA). A diagnostic index more useful than absolute excretion of any metabolite is the percentage increase in excretion above the upper limit of the normal range. In the majority of cases of phaeochromocytoma there is a significant increase in total catecholamines, total metadrenalines and HMMA. The relative increases have varied (Crout et al., 1961), but in 15 out of 23 cases this rise was most marked for total catecholamines, less so for total metadrenalines and least for HMMA. Indeed, in three cases the catecholamine excretion alone was abnormal. In the remaining eight cases the relative increase was greatest for total metadrenalines. Although the two other parameters were increased in all cases there was no consistent preference. Bell (1968) investigated 11 cases similarly and found two of the first type and seven of the second type, of which three had normal catecholamine excretion. In another case the order was catecholamines, HMMA, metadrenalines, but all were abnormal, and in the remaining case all were within normal limits. Bell found that either metadrenalines or HMMA were increased in 15 out of 16 cases, in 12 of which the preference was for metadrenalines. In general there is no single test which is invariably positive in cases of phaeochromocytoma. Although increased HMMA excretion has been the basis of the most commonly used screening test (Gitlow et al., 1960), this procedure is prone to dietary interference and one of the more specific methods is desirable. The results are then not affected by vanillin or by drugs such as α-methyl dopa, and the excretion is normal in essential hypertension. MAO inhibitors should be withdrawn before the test is performed. Figures recorded in phaeochromocytoma vary from normal up to 528 mg./day, but most patients are below 50 mg./day. The measurement of total metadrenalines is no more technically demanding than the better methods for HMMA, and some workers prefer to use this as a first test (Crout et al., 1961). However the excretion of metadrenalines is increased in patients taking α-methyl dopa and drugs of this type should be withdrawn before a hypertensive patient is assessed. Figures of over 100 mg./day are recorded, but mostly they are under 20 mg./day. The assessment of catecholamine excretion by the Hingerty (1957) test has been found troublesome owing to a number of false positive and negative tests. Other methods are technically more demanding but catechola-

mine excretion is often the most sensitive indicator of abnormality. Figures of 2000 μg./day are not uncommon. It has a place specially in the patient with paroxysmal attacks of hypertension. Infusion of catecholamines increases their urinary excretion for a few hours only and a sharp rise in excretion often follows a paroxysmal attack in patients even when the excretion of metabolites is only equivocally abnormal.

Pharmacological tests. The use of pharmacological tests in diagnosing phaeochromocytoma still has a place. They fall into two main groups; in the provocative tests the aim is to initiate a burst of catecholamine secretion by the tumour, whereas the use of adrenergic blocking agents is designed to counteract the effect of an increased concentration of catecholamines in the circulation.

Provocative tests. Mecholyl and tetraethylammonium chloride have been abandoned in favour of histamine, an agent known to cause the release of adrenaline from the adrenal medulla. An extensive review of the use of this test (Gifford *et al.*, 1964) indicates that it is most suitable for patients whose blood pressure is not too high or sustained. The test should be preceded by a cold pressor test and is carried out by injecting 0·025–0·05 mg. of histamine base intravenously and recording the blood pressure at 30 sec. intervals. The blood pressure falls during the first minute, with accompanying facial flush and throbbing headache. In a positive test the blood pressure then rises sharply and a positive test is indicated by a rise of systolic pressure greater than 20 mm Hg. and of diastolic pressure greater than 10 mm. Hg. over the maximum figures obtained during the cold pressor test. This rise of pressure is usually maximal about 2 min. after injection, and should then be counteracted by the intravenous injection of 5 mg. of phentolamine. The test is not without the hazard of initiating a violent hypertensive attack and has the additional disadvantage that it may be falsely negative in 20% of cases (Hermann & Mornex, 1964). Some of the false negative reactions have been associated with hypertensive therapeutic agents. The test is probably most useful in those patients with paroxysmal hypertension who show normal urine chemistry between attacks. In these cases the urinary catecholamine excretion increases during the period after a positive test.

More recently tyramine has been advocated as a safer and more reliable provocative agent (Engelman & Sjoerdsma, 1964; Sheps & Maher, 1966).

The use of adrenergic blocking agents. A number of substances have been investigated for this purpose. Dibenamine and benzodioxane are now mainly of historical interest, whereas phentolamine is still in use. According to Gifford *et al.* (1964), the test is most suitable for patients whose blood pressure is at least 170/110 mm. Hg. at the time of testing and is not satisfactory in the paroxysmal type of hypertension. The test is carried out by rapidly injecting 5 mg. of phentolamine intravenously after making base-line readings of blood pressure. Readings are continued at $\frac{1}{2}$ min. intervals for 10 min. Normal subjects frequently respond with a fall in systolic blood pressure of 10–15 mm. Hg during the first 1–2 min. For a positive result the blood pressure should fall by at least 35/25 mm. Hg. This usually occurs 2–3 min. after injection and lasts for 10 min. False negative tests are not common but have been related to antihypertensive therapy and this should be discontinued 8–10 days before the test. A number of tests give doubtful or variable results. False positive tests have occurred with the use of sedatives; barbiturates, tranquillisers and especially Rauwolfia derivatives are well recognized and such therapy should be discontinued for several days previously. Opinion as to the value of this test in modern practice varies. Gifford *et al.* (1964) feel that it still has a useful place whereas others consider it to be only occasionally useful (Delarue & O'Brien, 1963; Crout, 1966).

Malignant phaeochromocytomas and dopamine. The suggestion that malignant phaeochromocytomas are secretors of dopamine has aroused interest in the biochemistry of this variant. In six malignant phaeochromocytomas there has been evidence of increased urinary excretion of dopamine or one or more of its metabolites, as follows: dopamine, homovanillic acid (HVA) and 3,4-dihydroxyphenylacetic acid (Sankoff & Sourkes, 1963), N-acetyldopamine and 3,4-dihydroxyphenylethane (Karlson *et al.*, 1963), dopamine, 3-methoxytyramine and HVA (Robinson *et al.*, 1964; Donath *et al.*, 1965), dopamine and HVA (Ruthven & Sandler, 1964; von Studnitz, 1966). Although HVA excretion has usually been found to be normal in cases of benign phaeochromocytoma, increased excretion of dopamine and HVA were noted in two cases (Ruthven & Sandler, 1964; Page & Jacoby, 1964) as was increased dopamine excretion in an apparently benign case (Weil-Malherbe, 1956) and in a tumour only locally invasive (McMillan, 1956). Furthermore Sato & Sjoerdsma (1965) were able to find increased HVA excretion in only one of five patients with proven malignant phaeochromocytoma. It appears that further experience is necessary before the precise inter-relationship in phaeochromocytoma of dopamine secretion and metastasizing ability is clarified.

Management of phaeochromocytoma. Although surgical removal of the tumour is the only satisfactory long-term procedure, there are patients unsuitable for surgery, either because of their general condition or because of the existence of active metastases. Such patients have been successfully managed by using α-adrenergic blocking agents such as phenoxybenzamine (Engelman & Sjoerdsma, 1964). Attempts to use inhibitors of enzymes in the biosynthetic pathway have generally been disappointing (Crout, 1966) but the use of α-methyl tyrosine, an inhibitor of the rate-limiting enzyme tyrosine hydroxylase appears more effective in reducing catecholamine synthesis and alleviating the hypertension, even in patients with malignant phaeochromocytoma (Sjoerdsma *et al.*, 1965).

Surgical removal of the tumour is not without hazard to the patient, and a surgical mortality rate of 13% for published cases has been recorded (Crout, 1966). The major hazards during removal are the development of severe hypertension or serious sinus tachycardia and arrhythmias attributable to marked catecholamine release from the tumour. The post-operative period has been complicated by the development of hypotensive shock. Control of hypertensive attacks is possible by using α-adrenergic blocking agents such as phenoxybenzamine or phentolamine either by oral administration during the pre-operative period or by using the latter drug intravenously during operation when an attack occurs. The control of tachycardia and arrhythmias has been more recently achieved using the β-adrenergic blocking agents pronethalol or propranolol in addition to α-blockers. Pre-operative oral treatment with additional intravenous doses during the operation is recommended (Dornhorst & Laurence, 1963; Ross *et al.*, 1967). The choice of anaesthetic merits attention. Cyclopropane is best avoided as it sensitizes the myocardium to β-adrenergic stimulation. Halothane has less action of this type and is claimed to antagonize peripheral vasoconstriction. It has been widely used and is the subject of conflicting reports as to its suitability (Annotation, 1967; Mann, 1967).

The hypotension occurring after removal of the tumour, especially in patients with the sustained form of hypertension, suggests that endogenous production of noradrenaline is temporarily inadequate and noradrenaline infusions have been used with some success in controlling this undesirable development following successful excision of the tumour. It is known that continuous noradrenaline infusion reduces the blood volume in animals and the recognition that hypovolaemia occurs in the patient with phaeochromocytoma (Brunjes *et al.*, 1960) led to the recognition of the importance of this factor in the pathogenesis of the post-removal shock. Blood transfusion either pre-operatively (De Blasi, 1966) or at the onset of hypotension (Mackenzie & Pearson, 1967) reduces the incidence of post-operative circulatory collapse as does the use of α-adrenergic blocking agents (Johns & Brunjes, 1962; Ross *et al.*, 1967), or α-methyl tyrosine (Mann, 1967) pre-operatively to reduce the effect of noradrenaline on blood volume. With such procedures the need for noradrenaline infusions has been reduced which is desirable as they may maintain the hypovolaemic state.

It is probable that the greater understanding of the problems involved in the management of patients with phaeochromocytoma subjected to operation will reduce the surgical mortality rate considerably.

Neuroblastoma

This is another important neural crest neoplasm. The recognition that such tumours are associated with catecholamine production came much later than for phaeochromocytoma, but the biochemical abnormalities are now recognized to be of assistance in diagnosis, prognosis and assessing the response to therapy.

The tumour is one of the more frequent solid tumours of childhood occurring especially during the first five years of life, although cases in adults are known (Marsden, 1963). It is a malignant tumour with a tendency to form secondary deposits in bone, liver and lymph nodes, and originates either from sympathogonia or sympathoblasts. Neuroblastoma may arise along the lines of migration of sympathogonia and a number originate in the adrenal medulla whereas others are found in abdominal, thoracic and pelvic sites often in a paravertebral position.

Clinical features associated with neuroblastomas are often attributable to widespread metastases. Abdominal pain, pain in the limbs and general malaise are common. Hypertension occurs in about half the cases and chronic diarrhoea is sometimes present and may be severe (Marsden, 1963; von Studnitz, 1966; Käser, 1966). The hypertension and diarrhoea regress after removal of the tumour, and the realization that neuroblastomas secrete catecholamines has led to the suggestion that these two symptoms arise from the biological activity of the secretions. There is, however, no clear relation between catecholamine excretion and the incidence of hypertension, nor is diarrhoea a feature of phaeochromocytoma. Neuroblastomas are known to produce dopamine and, in some cases, dopa, and the biological activity of these substances and their metabolites is less clearly defined than for adrenaline and noradrenaline. The pathogenesis of the hypertension and diarrhoea thus remains obscure.

The realization that neuroblastomas secrete catecholamines originates from the observation of Mason *et al.* (1957) of pressor activity in the urine of an infant with an intrathoracic neuroblastoma. Later work has established the presence of noradrenaline precursors such as dopa and dopamine and of metabolites of dopa, dopamine and noradrenaline in the urine of such cases. Dopa metabolites detected include 4-hydroxy-3-methoxyphenylalanine, 3,4-dihydroxyphenyl pyruvic and lactic acids and 4-hydroxy-3-methoxyphenyl pyruvic and lactic acids (Fig. 11.9). The major dopamine metabolite is 4-hydroxy-3-methoxyphenylacetic acid (homovanillic acid, HVA), but in addition 3-methoxytyramine and its N-acetyl derivative, 3,4-dihydroxyphenylacetic acid and 4-hydroxy-3-methoxyphenylethanol have been identified (Fig. 11.9). The major noradrenaline metabolite present is HMMA but 4-hydroxy-3-methoxyphenylglycol and 3,4-dihydroxymandelic acid and N-acetyl noradrenaline occur in small amounts (Gjessing, 1964; von Studnitz, 1966). Adrenaline excretion does not appear to be increased. There is therefore good evidence to indicate a disturbance of catecholamine metabolism at a stage of biosynthesis earlier than noradrenaline. However the whole spectrum of metabolites has only been investigated in a few cases (Gjessing, 1964). The number of patients showing increased excretion of dopa or its metabolites is uncertain as this has not been investigated in most cases. von Studnitz *et al.* (1963) reported increased dopa excretion in 17 of 20 cases, whereas Gjessing (1964) found increased dopa metabolites in all of 10 cases examined. In a group of 51 cases, increased excretion of HVA was observed in 41 (von Studnitz, 1966; Käser, 1966). Increased dopamine excretion was reported in 32 out of 34 cases (Käser, 1966) and increased total catecholamines, mainly dopamine in 26 out of 32 cases (Bell, 1968). For the noradrenaline metabolites increased excretion of HMMA has been recorded in 119 out of 130 cases (von Studnitz, 1966; Käser, 1966; Bell, 1968), and increased normetadrenaline and metadrenaline excretion in 45 out of 48 cases (von Studnitz *et al.*, 1963; Bell, 1968). The presence of a neuroblastoma, especially if of adrenal origin, is associated

with the excretion of cystathionine and β-amino-*iso*-butyric acid (Gjessing, 1964). Cystathionine is sometimes replaced by homoserine (von Studnitz, 1965). A minority of neuroblastoma cases excrete increased amounts of tyramine (von Studnitz *et al.*, 1963). The significance of these unusual findings has yet to be established. Some neuroblastomas are difficult to differentiate histologically from Ewing's tumour, which is not a catecholamine-producing tumour. The occasional report of biochemically inactive neuroblastomas may really be examples of Ewing's tumour.

For routine diagnosis it is probably most satisfactory to use screening tests for increased HMMA and increased total catecholamine excretion (Bell, 1968). The catecholamine method should be of the type which includes dopamine amongst the amines measured. Suspicious results should be followed up by quantitative determination of metadrenalines and HMMA. Although the common pattern is an increase in total catecholamines, HMMA and metadrenalines the relative increases in the three measurements vary. There is a smaller group of cases in which the relative excretion of dopamine is greatly increased, but increases in metadrenalines and HMMA are much less or absent. Such cases show increased output of HVA and dopa metabolites and may represent dopa secretors (Bell, 1968; Käser, 1966). There is a suggestion that the prognosis in such cases is poor. In a further subgroup, catecholamine excretion is not increased, HVA excretion is relatively little increased but the excretion of metadrenalines and HMMA is definitely increased. Such tumours may be secreting mainly noradrenaline and there is some evidence that such cases have a better prognosis (Bell, 1968). Biochemical investigations of urinary catecholamines and metabolites thus play a role in diagnosis and assessing prognosis in neuroblastoma. The same parameters are helpful in assessing the response of the patient to surgery, radiotherapy or chemotherapy. Reduction in tumour mass is associated with a fall in output of catecholamine products eventually to normal amounts in cases who survive. Recurrence of tumour deposits is associated with a rise in metabolite excretion.

Investigation of neuroblastoma tissue by histochemical techniques reveals only weak colour reactions for reducing substances of the catecholamine type (Marsden, 1963). This is probably due to lack of any storage mechanism (Page & Jacoby, 1964), and from the relatively few determinations available it appears that total catecholamine content is usually less than 100 μg./g., a figure much below that found for phaeochromocytomas, In some tumours dopamine has predominated but this is not invariable; dopa has been detected. It is possible that there is a constant release of catecholamine, especially dopamine, from the tumour cell and that this is metabolized peripherally sufficiently rapidly to make hypertension a not inevitable consequence of catecholamine release. The tumour has been shown to contain enzymes: tyrosine hydroxylase, COMT, MAO, aldehyde reductase and a sulphate conjugase have been identified. Thus it is possible that in some tumours a considerable part of the catecholamines are metabolized within the tumour protecting the peripheral tissues from the pressor effects of the native catecholamines. Metabolism within tumours has also been invoked in some cases of phaeochromocytoma.

Ganglioneuroma

The term ganglioneuroma is best reserved for a benign tumour of the mature sympathetic ganglion cell. Such tumours are related to neuroblastoma, the malignant tumour of the ganglion cell precursor. Some authors also recognize an intermediate form, the ganglioneuroblastoma.

There is evidence that this neural crest tumour is also associated with catecholamine production. Hypertension and chronic diarrhoea may be related clinical symptoms which occur more frequently than in neuroblastoma and which regress after removal of the tumour (Rosenstein & Engelman, 1963; Käser, 1966).

The excretion pattern is qualitatively and quantitatively similar to that seen in neuroblastoma and unlike that of phaeochromocytoma, the other benign neural crest tumour. Increased excretion of HMMA and normetadrenaline has been recorded in most cases reported. Where dopamine or its metabolites have been investigated, they have been found to be excreted in increased amounts. Increased excretion of dopa was recorded in two cases investigated (von Studnitz et al., 1963; Smellie & Sandler, 1961), but dopa metabolites were not increased in two other cases (Gjessing, 1964). The excretion of adrenaline or metadrenaline is not increased. Tumour tissue has only occasionally been analysed. Noradrenaline and dopamine have been detected qualitatively (Smellie & Sandler, 1961; Greenberg & Gardner, 1960), found in low concentration (Rosenstein & Engelman, 1963) or not detected (Gjessing, 1964). Smellie and Sandler also found evidence of dopa. The enzymology of these tumours does not appear to have been investigated.

There is a tendency to report unexpected biochemical findings in relation to this tumour and

the incidence in unselected cases of ganglioneuroma of increased production of catecholamines is uncertain. Käser (1966) reported that two out of eight cases had increased HMMA excretion and one out of six cases had increased dopamine and HVA excretion, while Young et al. (1963) found increased HMMA output in three out of six cases. It is certain that some ganglioneuromas show increased output of catecholamines (particularly dopamine) or their metabolites. In such cases the excretion of these substances post-operatively should permit assessment of the adequacy of the surgical procedure.

CATECHOLAMINE METABOLISM IN NON-NEOPLASTIC CONDITIONS

Increased production of noradrenaline and adrenaline has been recorded in circumstances where a physiological increase would be expected. Plasma and urinary noradrenaline concentrations increase on tilting from the recumbent to the vertical position and after exercise and physical and mental stress. Adrenaline in plasma and urine increases in hypoglycaemia and following muscular exertion and severe mental or physical stress. Urinary catecholamine excretion may increase 10-fold in some cases. A 10 to 20 fold increase in urinary excretion of noradrenaline and adrenaline has been reported in severe thermal burns. In fatal cases adrenaline excretion fell in the terminal stages without change in noradrenaline excretion suggesting that adrenal medullary failure is a factor (Goodall & Haynes, 1960). Reduction in noradrenaline excretion and to a lesser extent in adrenaline excretion has been recorded in some cases of postural hypotension (Luft & von Euler, 1953).

Disorders of dopamine metabolism have been postulated to occur in Parkinsonism. The dopamine content of the striatum, substantia nigra and pallidum is reduced (Hornykiewicz, 1966), as is the excretion of dopamine in the urine of such patients (Barbeau et al., 1961; Bischoff & Torres, 1962), although the excretion of HVA is normal (Greer & Williams, 1963). The di-O-methylated derivative of dopamine; 3,4-dimethoxyphenyl ethylamine produces a hypokinetic rigid syndrome in many animals (but not in man) and has been detected in human Parkinsonism (Barbeau et al., 1963), suggesting a disturbance of dopamine metabolism. This work needs extension and confirmation. The same dimethoxy compound was claimed to occur in the urine of schizophrenic patients (Friedhoff & van Winkle, 1962) but not of normal subjects. Conversion of dopamine to 3,4-dimethoxyphenylacetic acid was claimed in schizophrenia (Friedhoff & van Winkle, 1963). Confirmatory reports of the existence of dimethoxyphenylethylamine in schizophrenic urine appeared, but more recently it has been realized that it occurs in the urine of normal and schizophrenic subjects and is of dietary origin. Further attempts to demonstrate conversion of dopamine to dimethoxyphenylethylamine have been unsuccessful. The topic has been reviewed recently by Howorth (1966).

INTERRELATIONSHIPS BETWEEN THE ADRENAL CORTEX AND MEDULLA

The close anatomical relationship between cortex and medulla has a physiological counterpart. The enzyme, phenylethanolamine N-methyl transferase which converts noradrenaline to adrenaline in the medulla is activated by glucocorticoids (Wurtman & Axelrod, 1966). Hypophysectomy reduces adrenaline production in the rat medulla, and adrenaline is only produced in the chromaffin tissue of those species in which it is anatomically surrounded by cortical tissue. The production of adrenaline in response to insulin hypoglycaemia is dependent on a hypothalamic mechanism (Duner, 1953), is reduced in hypophysectomized humans (Luft & von Euler, 1956) and is restored by the administration of ACTH (Green & Ingbar, 1961).

Mobilization of glucose and NEFA by catecholamines is dependent on corticosteroids. The mode of action seems to involve maintenance of a proper electrolyte balance between intracellular and extracellular fluids which determines the formation of the activator substance, cyclic-3′,5′-AMP by catecholamines (Brodie et al., 1966). Noradrenaline has reduced pressor activity in corticosteroid insufficiency and this has been claimed to be due to reduction of the Na content of the arteriolar wall (Ross, 1961).

Some neural crest tumours contain adrenocortical cells throughout their substance (Marsden, 1963), and cortisol has been detected in some of them (Mulrow et al., 1959; Ramsey & Langlands, 1962). In some cases suppression of the cortex has occurred.

References

ACHESON, G. H. (1966). *Pharmac. Rev.*, **18**, 1.

AHLQUIST, R. P. (1948). *Am. J. Physiol.*, **153**, 586.

AHLQUIST, R. P. & LEVY, B. (1959). *J. pharmac. tox.*, **127**, 146.

ANNOTATION, (1967). *Lancet*, **1**, 717.

AXELROD, J. (1957). *Science*, **126**, 400.

AXELROD, J. (1963). *Science*, **140**, 499.

AXELROD, J. (1966). *Pharmac. Rev.*, **18**, 95.

AXELROD, J. & TOMCHICK, R. (1958). *J. biol. Chem.*, **233**, 702.

BACQ, Z. M., GOSSELIN, L., DRESSE, A. & RENSON, J. (1959). *Science*, **130**, 453.

BARBEAU, A., GROOT, J.-A., JOLY, J.-G., RAYMOND-TREMBLAY, D. & DONALDSON, J. (1963). *Revue can. Biol.*, **22**, 469.

BARBEAU, A., MURPHY, C. F. & SOURKES, T. L. (1961). *Science*, **133**, 1706.

BELL, M. (1968). In "Tumours in Children". Eds. Marsden, H. B. & Steward, J. K. Ch. 6. Heidelberg, Springer-Verlag.

BELLEAU, B. & BURBA, J. (1961). *Biochim. biophys. Acta*, **54**, 195.

BERGSTRÖM, S., EULER, U. S. VON & HAMBERG, V. (1949). *Acta chem. scand.*, **3**, 305.

BERTLER, A. FALCK, B., HILLARP, N. Å., ROSENGREN, E. & TORP, A. (1959). *Acta physiol. scand.*, **47**, 251.

BISCHOFF, F. & TORRES, A. (1962). *Clin. Chem.*, **8**, 370.

BLASCHKO, H. (1939). *J. Physiol.* (Lond.), **96**, 50P.

BRODIE, B. B., DAVIES, J. I., HYNIE, S., KRISHNA, G. & WEISS, B. (1966). *Pharmac. Rev.*, **18**, 273.

BRUNJES, S., JOHNS, V. J. & CRANE, M. G. (1960). *New Engl. J. Med.*, **262**, 393.

BURBA, J. & MURNAGHAN, M. F. (1965). *Biochem. Pharmac.*, **14**, 823.

BUTCHER, R. W. (1966). *Pharmac. Rev.*, **18**, 237.

CARLSSON, A., FALCK, B. & HILLARP, N. Å. (1962a). *Acta physiol. scand.*, **56**, Suppl. 196.

CARLSSON, A., LINQVIST, M., FILA-HROMADKO, S. & CORRODI, H. (1962b). *Helv. chim. Acta*, **45**, 270.

CHIDSEY, C. A., KAISER, G. A. & BRAUNWALD, E. (1963). *Science*, **139**, 828.

CROUT, J. R. (1961). *Proc. Soc. exp. Biol. Med.*, **108**, 482.

CROUT, J. R. (1966). *Pharmac. Rev.*, **18**, 651.

CROUT, J. R., PISANO, J. J. & SJOERDSMA, A. (1961). *Am. Heart J.*, **61**, 375.

CROUT, J. R. & SJOERDSMA, A. (1960). *Circulation*, **22**, 516.

DE BLASI, S. (1966). *Br. J. Anaesth.*, **38**, 740.

DELARUE, N. C. & O'BRIEN, D. (1963). *Can. J. Surg.*, **6**, 259.

DEMIS, D. J., BLASCHKO, H. & WELCH, A. D. (1955). *J. Pharmac. exp. Ther.*, **113**, 14.

DENGLER, H. (1957). *Arch. exp. Path. Pharmak.*, **231**, 373.

DICKINSON, C. J. & DE SWIET, M. (1967). *Lancet*, **1**, 986.

DONATH, A., KÄSER, H., ROOS, B., ZIEGLER, W., OETLIKER, O., COLOMBO, J. P. & BETTEX, M. (1965). *Helv. paediat. Acta*, **20**, 1.

DORNHORST, A. C. & LAURENCE, D. R. (1963). *Br. med. J.*, **2**, 1250.

DOUGLAS, W. W. (1966). *Pharmac. Rev.*, **18**, 471.

DUNER, H. (1953). *Acta physiol. scand.*, **28**, Suppl. 102.

ENGELMAN, K., MÜLLER, P. S. & SJOERDSMA, A. (1964). *New Engl. J. Med.*, **270**, 865.

ENGELMAN, K. & SJOERDSMA, A. (1964). *J. Am. med. Ass.*, **189**, 81.

ERANKO, O. (1960). "Symposium on Adrenergic Mechanisms". p. 103. London, Ciba Foundation.

EULER, U. S. VON (1965). "Noradrenaline". Springfield, Illinois. Chas. C. Thomas.

EULER, U. S. VON, FRANKSSON, C. & HELLSTRÖM, J. (1954). *Acta physiol. scand.*, **31**, 6.

EULER, U. S. VON, LISHAJKO, F. & STJARNE, L. (1963). *Acta physiol. scand.*, **59**, 495.

EVANS, R. W. (1963). In "The Clinical Chemistry of Monamines". Eds. Varley H. & Gowenlock, A. H., p. 48. Amsterdam, Elsevier.

EXTON, J. H. & PARK, C. R. (1966). *Pharmac. Rev.*, **18**, 181.

FALCK, B., HAGGENDAL, J. & OWMAN, C. (1963). *Q. Jl. exp. Physiol.*, **48**, 253.

FALCK, B., NYSTEDT, T., ROSENGREN, E. & STENFLO, J. (1964). *Acta pharmac. tox.*, **21**, 51.

FALCK, B. & TORP, A. (1962). *Medna exp.*, **6**, 169.

FRIEDHOFF, A. J. & WINKLE, E. VAN (1962). *J. nerv. ment. Dis.*, **135**, 550.

FRIEDHOFF, A. J. & WINKLE, E. VAN (1963). *Nature*, (Lond.), **199**, 1271.

GIFFORD, R. W., KVALE, W. F., MAHER, F. T., ROTH, G. M. & PRIESTLEY, J. T. (1964). *Proc. Staff Meet. Mayo Clin.*, **39**, 281.

GITLOW, S. E., ORNSTEIN, L., MENDLOWITZ, M., KHASSIS, S. & KRUK, E. (1960). *Am. J. Med.*, **28**, 921.

GJESSING, L. R. (1964). *Scand. J. clin. Lab. Invest.*, **16**, 661.

GLOWINSKI, J., KOPIN, I. J. & AXELROD, J. (1965). *J. Neurochem.*, **12**, 25.

GOLDENBERG, M., FABER, M., ALSTON, E. S. & CHARCOFF, E. C. (1949). *Science*, **109**, 534.

GOLDSTEIN, M., MUSACCHIO, J. M. & CONTRERA, J. F. (1962). *Biochem. Pharmac.*, **11**, 809.

GOODALL, McC. (1951). *Acta physiol. scand.*, **24**, Suppl. 85.

GOODALL, McC. & HAYNES, B. W. (1960). *J. clin. Invest.*, **39**, 1927.

GOODALL, McC. & KIRSHNER, N. (1957). *J. biol. Chem.*, **226**, 213.

GOODALL, McC. & KIRSHNER, N. (1958). *Circulation*, **17**, 366.

GORDON, R. S. & CHERKES, A. (1958). *Proc. Soc. exp. Biol. Med.*, **97**, 150.

GREEN, W. L. & INGBAR, S. H. (1961). *Arch intern. Med.*, **108**, 945.

GREENBERG, R. E. & GARDNER, L. I. (1960). *J. clin. Invest.*, **39**, 1729.

GREER, M. & WILLIAMS, C. M. (1963). *Neurology*, (Minneap.), **13**, 73.

GURIN, S. & DELLUVA, A. M. (1947). *J. biol. Chem.*, **170**, 545.

HAGEN, P. (1956). *J. Pharmac. exp. Ther.*, **116**, 26.

HAMRIN, B. (1962). *Lancet*, **2**, 123.

HENKIN, R. I. & BARTTER, F. C. (1965). *Fedn. Proc. Fedn. Am. Socs. exp. Biol.*, **24**, 133.

HERMANN, H. & MORNEX, R. (1964). "Human Tumours Secreting Catecholamines". London, Pergamon Press.

HINGERTY, D. (1957). *Lancet*, **1**, 766.

HOLTZ, P., HEISE, R. & LUDTKE, K. (1938). *Arch. exp. Path. Pharmak.*, **191**, 87.

HORNYKIEWICZ, O. (1966). *Pharmac. Rev.*, **18**, 925.

HOWORTH, P. J. N. (1966). *Hospital Med.*, **1**, 115.

INNES, I. R. & NICKERSON, M. (1965). In "The Pharmacological Basis of Therapeutics". Ed. Goodman, L. S. & Gilman, A. Ch. 24. New York, Macmillan.

IVERSEN, L. L. (1967). "The Uptake and Storage of Noradrenaline in Sympathetic Nerves". Cambridge, University Press.

IZQUERIDO, J. A. & KAUMANN, A. J. (1963). *Arch int. Pharmacodyn. Thér.*, **144**, 437.

JOHNS, V. J. & BRUNJES, S. (1962). *Am. J. Cardiol.*, **9**, 120.

KARLSON, P., SEKERIS, C. E. & HERRLICH, P. (1963). *Dt. med. Wschr.*, **88**, 1873.

KÄSER, H. (1966). *Pharmac. Rev.*, **18**, 659.

KAUFMAN, S. (1957). *J. biol. Chem.*, **226**, 511.

KAUFMAN, S. & FRIEDMAN, S. (1965). *Pharmac. Rev.*, **17**, 71.

KENNEDY, J. S., SYMINGTON, T. & WOODGER, B. (1961). *J. Path. Bact.*, **81**, 409.

KVALE, W. F., ROTH, G. M., MANGER, W. M. & PRIESTLEY, J. T. (1957). *J. Am. med. Ass.*, **164**, 854.

LEATHER, H. M., SHAW, D. B., CATES, J. E. & MILNES WALKER, R. (1962). *Br. med. J.*, **1**, 1373.

LEVITT, M., SPECTOR, S., SJOERDSMA, A. UDENFRIEND, S. (1965). *J. Pharmac. exp. Ther.*, **148**, 1.

LOEWI, O. (1921). *Pflügers Arch. ges. Physiol.*, **189**, 239.

LUFT, R. & EULER, U. S. VON (1953). *J. clin. Invest.*, **32**, 1065.

LUFT, R. & EULER, U. S. VON (1956). *J. clin. Endocr. Metab.*, **16**, 1017.

LUND, A. (1951). *Acta pharmac. tox.*, **7**, 309.

MACKENZIE, A. & PEARSON, D. T. (1967). *Br. J. Anaesth.*, **39**, 592.

MANGER, W. M., FLACK, E. V., BERKSON, J., BOLLMANN, J. L., ROTH, G. M., BALDES, E. J. & JACOBS, A. (1954). *Circulation*, **10**, 641.

MANN, P. E. G. (1967). *Lancet*, **1**, 1004.

MARSDEN, H. B. (1963). In "The Clinical Chemistry of Monamines". Eds. Varley, H. & Gowenlock, A. H., p. 71. Amsterdam, Elsevier.

MASON, G. A., HART-MERCER, J., STRANG, L. B. & WYNNE, N. A. (1957). *Lancet*, **2**, 322.

MASUOKA, D. T., CLARK, W. G. & SCHOTT, H. F. (1961). *Revue can. Biol.*, **20**, 1.

MASUOKA, D. T., SCHOTT, H. F., AKANIE, R. I. & CLARK, W. G. (1956). *Proc. Soc. exp. Biol. Med.*, **93**, 5.

MASUOKA, D. T., SCHOTT, H. F. & PETRIELLO, L. (1963). *J. Pharmac. exp. Ther.*, **139**, 73.

MCMILLAN, M. (1956). *Lancet*, **2**, 284.

MITOMA, C. (1956). *Archs Biochem. Biophys.*, **60**, 476.
MULROW, P. J., COHN, G. L. & YESNER, R. (1959). *Yale J. Biol. Med.*, **31**, 363.
MURNAGHAN, M. F. & MAZURKIEWICZ, I. M. (1963). *Revue can. Biol.*, **22**, 99.
MUSACCHIO, J. M. & GOLDSTEIN, M. (1963). *Biochem. Pharmac.*, **12**, 1061.
NICKERSON, M. & NOMAGUCHI, G. N. (1953). *J. Pharmac. exp. Ther.*, **107**, 284.
PAGE, L. B. & JACOBY, G. A. (1964). *Medicine* (Baltimore), **43**, 379.
PELLERIN, J. & D'IORIO, A. (1957). *Can. J. Biochem. Physiol.*, **35**, 151.
PLETSCHER, A. (1963). In "The Clinical Chemistry of Monamines". Eds. Varley, H. & Gowenlock, A. H., p. 191. Amsterdam, Elsevier.
POTTER, L. T. & AXELROD, J. (1963). *J. Pharmac. exp. Ther.*, **142**, 299.
RAMSAY, I. D. & LANGLANDS, J. H. M. (1962). *Lancet*, **2**, 126.
RENSON, J., GOODWIN, F., WEISSBACH, H. & UDENFRIEND, S. (1961). *Biochem. biophys. Res. Commun.*, **6**, 20.
RICHMOND, J., FRAZER, S. C. & MILLAR, D. R. (1961). *Lancet*, **2**, 904.
ROBINSON, R. (1963). In "The Clinical Chemistry of Monoamines". Eds. Varley, H. & Gowenlock, A. H., p. 63. Amsterdam, Elsevier.
ROBINSON, R., SMITH, P. & WHITTAKER, S. R. F. (1964). *Br. med. J.*, **1**, 1422.
ROSENSTEIN, B. R. & ENGELMAN, K. (1963). *J. Pediat.*, **63**, 217.
ROSS, E. J. (1961). *Q. Jl. Med.*, **30**, 285.
ROSS, S. B. (1963). *Acta pharmac. tox.*, **20**, 267.
ROSS, E. J., PRICHARD, B. N. C., KAUFMAN, L., ROBERTSON, A. I. G. & HARRIES, B. J. (1967). *Br. med. J.*, **1**, 191.
ROSS, S. B. & HALJASMAA, Ö. (1964). *Acta pharmac. tox.*, **21**, 205, 215.
RUTHVEN, C. R. J. & SANDLER, M. (1964). *Analyt. Biochem.*, **8**, 282.
SANKOFF, I. & SOURKES, T. L. (1963). *Can. J. Biochem. Physiol.*, **41**, 1381.
SATO, T. L. & SJOERDSMA, A. (1965). *Br. med. J.*, **2**, 1472.
SHEPHERD, D. M. & WEST, G. B. (1951). *Br. J. Pharmac. Chemother*, **6**, 665.
SHEPHERD, D. M. & WEST, G. B. (1953). *J. Physiol.*, (Lond.), **120**, 15.
SHEPS, S. G. & MAHER, F. T. (1966). *J. Am. med. Ass.*, **195**, 265.
SJOERDSMA, A., ENGELMAN, K., SPECTOR, S. & UDENFRIEND, S. (1965). *Lancet*, **2**, 1092.
SJOERDSMA, A., LEEPER, L. C., TERRY, L. L. & UDENFRIEND, S. (1959). *J. clin. Invest.*, **38**, 31.
SMELLIE, J. M. & SANDLER, M. (1961). *Proc. R. Soc. Med.*, **54**, 327.
SOURKES, T. L. (1966). *Pharmac. Rev.*, **18**, 53.
SPECTOR, S., MATER, R. O., SJOERDSMA, A. & UDENFRIEND, S. (1965). *Life Sciences*, **4**, 1307.
SPECTOR, S., SJOERDSMA, A. & UDENFRIEND, S. (1965). *J. pharmac. exp. Ther.*, **147**, 86.
SPECTOR, S., SJOERDSMA, A., ZALTMAN-NIRENBERG, P., LEVITT, M. & UDENFRIEND, S. (1963). *Science*, **139**, 1299.
STEINBERG, D. (1966). *Pharmac. Rev.*, **18**, 217.
STJARNE, L. (1966). *Pharmac. Rev.*, **18**, 425.
STUDNITZ, W. VON (1965). *Scand. J. clin. Lab. Invest.*, **17**, 558.
STUDNITZ, W. VON (1966). *Pharmac. Rev.*, **18**, 645.
STUDNITZ, W. VON, KÄSER, H. & SJOERDSMA, A. (1963). *New Engl. J. Med.*, **269**, 232.
SUTHERLAND, E. W. & ROBISON, G. A. (1966). *Pharmac. Rev.*, **18**, 145.
TULLAR, B. F. (1949). *Science*, **109**, 586.
UDENFRIEND, S. (1966). *Pharmac. Rev.*, **18**, 43.
UDENFRIEND, S. & WYNGAARDEN, J. B. (1956). *Biochim. biophys. Acta.* **20**, 48.
VAN DER SCHOOT, J. B. & CREVELING, C. R. (1965). *Adv. Drug Res.*, **2**, 47.
VARLEY, H. & GOWENLOCK, A. H. (1963). "The Clinical Chemistry of Monoamines". Amsterdam, Elsevier.
WEIL-MALHERBE, H. (1956). *Lancet*, **2**, 282.
WEST, G. B. (1955). *Q. Rev. Biol.*, **30**, 116.
WHITBY, L. G. (1965). *Scot. med. J.*, **10**, 269.
WHITE, J. E. & ENGEL, F. L. (1958). *Proc. Soc. exp. Biol. Med.*, **99**, 375.
WURTMAN, R. J. (1965). "Catecholamines". London, J. & A. Churchill.
WURTMAN, R. J. & AXELROD, J. (1966). *J. Biol. Chem.*, **241**, 2301.
WYLIE, D. W., ARCHER, S. & ARNOLD, A. (1960). *J. Pharmac. exp. Ther.*, **130**, 239.
YOUNG, R. B., STECKER, D. D., BONGIOVANNI, A. M. KOOP, C. E. & EBERLEIN, W. R. (1963). *J. Pediat.*, **62**, 844.

Chapter 12

DISORDERS OF IODINE METABOLISM

by

J. WOLFF

National Institute of Arthritis and Metabolic Diseases, Bethesda

IODIDE ABSORPTION AND DISTRIBUTION

THE thyroid gland is a structure peculiar to vertebrates. It accumulates iodine, synthesizes, stores and secretes its hormones by processes which are extraordinarily efficient considering the scarcity of iodine on the earth's land surface. So avid is the thyroid gland for iodine that measurement of the radioactivity of commercial beef thyroid serves as a very sensitive test for fall-out from nuclear and atomic weapons tests (Van Middlesworth, 1963). [131]I is a relatively abundant fission product and its short half-life permits the study of the dates of, and dissemination from, such tests.

Ingested iodine is reduced to iodide in the gastro-intestinal tract, perhaps as a pre-requisite for absorption (Small, Bezman, Longarini, Fennell & Zamcheck, 1961). Thereafter it is rapidly absorbed, largely from the intestine. The stomach may also play a role since iodine deficiency has been reported after total gastrectomy

(Harden & Adams, 1964). Despite the fact that secretion toward the mucosal side occurs (Pastan, 1957), the absorption appears to be nearly complete as judged by the essentially quantitative appearance of ingested ^{131}I in the urine of athyroid subjects (Riggs, 1952).

Radioiodide rapidly attains distribution volumes of 27 to 28% of the body weight excluding thyroid, urine and gastro-intestinal contents (Hays & Solomon, 1965). This volume then expands more slowly until, at equilibrium, the extrathyroidal diffusion space amounts to about 35 to 39% of the body weight (Myant, Corbett, Honour & Pochin, 1950; Riggs, 1952).

Cellular I^- distribution can be divided into three classes. Red cells equilibrate rapidly to about 0·56 of the plasma concentration (the value varying with the degree of chloride shift) (Owen & Power, 1953), whereas most other cells equilibrate more slowly and to values less than 0·5 (Hamilton *et al.*, 1953). It has been suggested that these low values result from mediated efflux of iodide

(Salvatore, Salvatore & Wolff, 1966). A third group consists of iodide-concentrating tissues to be discussed below.

Renal Excretion

The two main organs competing for the circulating iodide are the thyroid and the kidney. The renal clearance of iodide amounts to 20 to 50 ml. (mean 35 ml.) of plasma per minute at normal glomerular filtration rates. Occasional values outside this range have been reported for normal individuals, and the values are depressed in renal disease. Changes produced by variations in thyroid status appear to parallel changes in the glomerular filtration rate, i.e. the $^{131}I^-$ clearance varies as a linear function of the inulin clearance (Bricker & Hlad, 1955). Except for a small amount that may be lost in sweat and faeces, most of the iodine that leaves the body as iodide does so via the kidney.

The mechanism of renal I^- excretion has been the subject of controversy. In the dog I^- reabsorption is mainly passive and occurs in the same portion of the tubule where Cl^- is absorbed. The discrimination factor between these two anions is constant over a wide range of anion concentrations. However, at very low excretion fractions ("clearances") of Cl^-, I^- reabsorption becomes more efficient. This suggests a separate mechanism, possibly "active" transport, which is readily saturated by a halide load (Walser & Rahill, 1965). In man the ratio of iodide to chloride clearances is greater. Increasing urine flow decreases discrimination slightly (Walser & Rahill, 1965) but this ratio is not changed by mercurial diuretics. There is a circadian pattern to renal iodide excretion with a nocturnal decrease which may, in part, be due to changes in glomerular filtration induced by changes in corticosteroid secretion (Fisher, Oddie & Epperson, 1965).

A probable example of the role of competition between kidney and thyroid is that described by Cassano, Baschieri & Andreani (1959) who studied cases of simple goitre that were apparently caused by increased renal clearance of $^{131}I^-$ (> 41 ml./min.). It is important that this be further studied. It is also possible to increase renal clearance of $^{131}I^-$ in rats by imposing a Cl^- load. This eventually leads to goitre formation (Isler, Leblond & Axelrod, 1958; Isler, 1959).

Nonthyroidal Concentrating Mechanism

Iodide may be temporarily accumulated in other iodide concentrating tissues or their secretions (Brown-Grant, 1961). These include:

(1) Salivary glands and saliva.
(2) Gastric mucosa or juice.
(3) Mammary gland and milk.
(4) Placenta (not certain in man). Possibly the ovary.
(5) Tracheal endothelium (unconfirmed).
(6) Skin (young rat).
(7) Uterus of rat (induced by progesterone and inhibited by oestrogens (Brown-Grant, 1966).
(8) The choroid plexus actively pumps I^- out of the cerebrospinal fluid.
(9) Ciliary body.

Except for lactating mammary tissue and the placenta, this iodide ultimately returns to the circulation and thus becomes available for the biosynthesis of the thyroid hormones. These tissues do contribute significantly to the iodide pool. At early times 23% of the injected dose of $^{131}I^-$ may be cleared by the gastrointestinal tract. The combined salivary-gastric clearance is 40 ml./min. (Hays & Solomon, 1965). In contrast to earlier opinions, the salivary iodide concentrating mechanism is relatively independent of thyroid function (Harden, Mason & Buchanan, 1965).

THE IODIDE CONCENTRATING MECHANISM

Accumulation of $^{131}I^-$ by the thyroid follows a regular curvilinear, although not simple, pattern for some hours thus permitting easy measurement of an effective thyroid clearance. This is about half the renal iodide clearance, with a mean of ~ 18 ml./min. Little I^- accumulates in the gland at the usual iodide loads, and the effective clearance represents largely organic iodine formation. To what extent trapped iodide will leak out in the same chemical form is not precisely known. This relative lack of reversibility accounts for the fact that thyroid iodine represents about 80% of the total body iodine, whereas thyroid mass amounts to only 1/2500 to 1/10,000 of the body weight. The iodine concentrations in the thyroids of various species range from 30 to 250 mg. of total iodine/100 g. of tissue, depending on the iodine supply (Wolff & Chaikoff, 1947). When organic iodine formation does not occur, accumulation would not be expected to follow the same regular curve for very long. Except to the extent that such glands may be goitrous, the maximum amount of I^- so trapped will be less than can be accumulated as organic iodine (Fig. 12.1).

Although organic iodine formation does not require functioning iodide transport in man, enough thyroid hormones cannot be formed at prevailing blood iodide levels from iodide entering the thyroid by diffusion alone. Evidence for this stems from mouse thyroid tumours (Wollman, Scow, Wagner & Morris, 1953), and from several cases of congenital goitres that have lost the ability to concentrate iodide but have an otherwise intact biosynthetic apparatus (Stanbury & Chapman, 1960; Wolff, Thompson, & Robbins, 1964). These patients were hypothyroid but could be treated with large doses of iodide alone, allowing adequate iodide to "diffuse" into the gland. A concentrating mechanism for I^- thus seems to be necessary under conditions of normal I^- supply.

The thyroidal iodide-concentrating mechanism has been extensively reviewed (Halmi, 1961; Wolff, 1964) and only an outline of this subject will be given here. Although iodide accumulation occurs in the binding thyroid (Wollman & Reed, 1962), high I^- concentrations are not attained and artefacts from de-iodination are difficult to rule out since recently made organic iodine is also the most rapid fraction to be excreted and de-iodinated. That is, the gland operates on a "last come-first served" basis (Schneider, 1964), because of marked heterogeneity in the organic iodine pool (Pitt-Rivers, 1963).

The study of iodide accumulation *per se* is easier if the synthesis of organic iodine is blocked. It was first shown in "blocked" thyroid slices (Franklin, Chaikoff & Lerner, 1944) that iodide accumulated in considerable amounts. This suggested that the concentrating mechanism was not dependent upon the further fate of iodide in the gland. Thyroid glands of various species including man accumulate iodide to as much as several hundred times the plasma I^- concentration. The process is not instantaneous and equilibration with plasma or medium requires 30 to 90 min. Thereafter the concentration gradient is maintained quite constant as the plasma $^{131}I^-$ level falls following injection of a single dose indicating that these two compartments are in rapid equilibrium with each other. Thus, as iodide is cleared by the kidney, the plasma level of iodide drops and thyroid iodide follows, while their ratio, (T/S[I]), remains constant.

The Mechanism

The mechanism of iodide concentration may be conveniently divided into those properties relating to the energetics of the system and those supplying specificity for iodide and related anions. A list of the most important properties is presented here (for details see Wolff, 1964):

(1) The concentrated $^{131}I^-$ behaves like iodide by all presently available criteria although activity coefficients are not known.

(2) Although the follicular architecture is not necessary since isolated thyroid cells prepared by trypsinization (Tong, Kerkhof, & Chaikoff, 1962) or with collagenase (Wolff & Alexander, unpublished observations) concentrate iodide, the cell membrane must be intact. Homegenates do not concentrate iodide, so a simple adsorption process is not likely, although binding or adsorption to "catalytic" amounts of a carrier may well contribute to the overall process. Agents known to alter various properties of the membranes interfere with iodide accumulation by thyroid slices (Larsen & Wolff, 1967).

(3) Energy production must be intact: Iodide "pumping" is abolished at low temperatures, in the absence of O_2, or by agents that uncouple oxidative phosphorylation, etc.

(4) External Na^+ and K^+ are required and the Na^+ pump must be functioning. Ouabain and other cardiac glycosides inhibit iodide concentration apparently via the Na^+ and K^+-requiring ATPase. This effect can be reversed by excess K^+ (Wolff, 1960; Wolff & Halmi, 1963; Iff & Wilbrandt, 1963; Alexander & Wolff, 1964). The nature of this coupling to the Na^+ pump is entirely unknown and a choice between dependence on cation concentrations and fluxes is not yet possible.

(5) The trap is saturated at external iodide concentrations of 1–5×10^{-3}M. Fifty per cent. saturation occurs at about 3×10^{-5}M I^- in thyroids of various species as well as in the non-thyroidal iodide concentrating tissues such as salivary glands, mammary gland and choroid plexus (Wolff & Maurey, 1962). At very high iodide concentrations the thyroidal iodide space approaches 0·4 of the thyroid weight, i.e. like non-pumping cells.

(6) Transport against an electrical gradient has only recently been demonstrated (Woodbury & Woodbury, 1963). The cell is negative by about 50 mV with respect to both the outside and the lumen. This suggests that the active step of inward transport occurs at the basal membrane. This conclusion is supported by radio-autographs made by Andros and Wollman (1967) in which *cellular* $^{125}I^-$ accumulation could be shown to precede I^- accumulation in the *lumen*. Thereafter lumen I^- exceeds cell I^- concentration several fold. The apical membrane must also be a diffusion barrier since free diffusion of I^- is too fast ($\sim$65 μ/sec.) to permit demonstration of *cellular* $^{125}I^-$ concentration. The concentration difference is less than would be expected from the 50 mV potential difference in the direction of luminal movement (downhill), hence this process is not likely to be "active".

(7) Selectivity for iodide resembles an ion-exchange process. Although the thyroid displays very high preference for I^- as compared to other halides, certain other monovalent anions are concentrated and/or inhibit I^- transport. These are, in decreasing order of potency or avidity (the range here is $>10^4$): $ClO_4^- \simeq TcO_4^- > ReO_4^- > BF_4^- > SeCN^- > SO_3F^- > SCN^- > I^- > NO_3^- > NO_2^-$ $OCN^- > Br^-$. Thiocyanate is the only anion tested so far that is not significantly concentrated; this may be due to the rapid metabolism of this substance. Certain anions are probably too unstable in biological systems to be fitted easily into the above scheme ($ClO_3^-, IO_3^-, NO_2^-, OCN^-, PO_2F_2^-$). The anions of the above series are mutually competitive for accumulation; thus I^- inhibits ReO_4^- accumu-

lation and ReO_4^- inhibits I^- accumulation, etc. They appear thus to use the same or similar "carriers". These anions can be related to each other as a function of their size in solution (partial molal ionic volumes). The above *order* of anions also expresses their relative affinity for the quarternary ammonium class of anion-exchange resins (Wolff, 1964). This suggests that ion pair formation may be important in I^- transport.

(8) Present evidence, though very incomplete, suggests that the quarternary N of choline in lecithin or a closely related substance may play an anion-exchanger role in the thyroid gland (Vilkki, 1962; Schneider & Wolff, 1965). The whole phospholipid molecule must be intact since activity is abolished by treatment with phospholipases (Schneider & Wolff, 1965). Recently Vilkki and Jaakonmäki (1966) have presented evidence that the β-fatty acid may be nervonic acid.

effectiveness is very sensitive to dietary iodine intake. Despite an essentially total block of hormone synthesis the goitres so obtained are smaller than obtained with thiocarbamide antithyroid compounds (see below). The origin of this difference is not clear (Alexander & Wolff, 1966).

Control of Iodide Concentration

A number of factors are known to influence the iodide-concentrating capacity of the thyroid. Foremost among these is the state of activity of the gland, which is largely a reflection of the level of thyrotropic (TSH) stimulation. Thyroids made hyperplastic by the chronic administration of a goitrogen exhibit very high iodide levels. This is largely the result of increased endogenous TSH

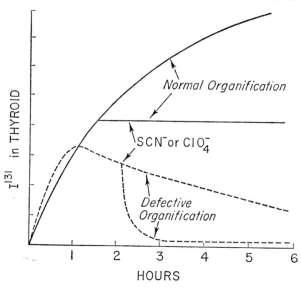

FIG. 12.1. Hypothetical kinetics of radioiodine accumulation in the thyroid gland when organification is permitted (—) and when it is blocked (- -). Absolute uptake values are not listed. Both the maximum uptakes and the rates of attaining them will vary with the activity of the gland. The effect of perchlorate or SCN^- would be mimicked by ReO_4^-, large doses of I^-, etc.

(9) The monovalent anions have certain useful properties. Iodide accumulated in the gland can be rapidly discharged by the administration of large doses of SCN^- or ClO_4^-. In the normal thyroid there is little iodide and the anions merely stop further ^{131}I accumulation. However, when much of the thyroidal ^{131}I is iodide the anions compete effectively and $^{131}I^-$ is discharged from the gland (Fig. 12.1). This phenomenon is of considerable diagnostic value for certain congenital defects in organic iodine formation or as a measure of the efficiency of treatment with antithyroid drugs (see below). If these drugs are acting maximally to block hormone synthesis, all of the injected dose of ^{131}I accumulated by the thyroid gland should remain in the inorganic form and should thus be dischargeable; if not, part of it must have been converted to organic forms (Stanley & Astwood, 1948).

In addition, the anions are goitrogenic. Because they are competitive inhibitors of iodide transport their

production. After a single dose of TSH (injected into the rat), the T/S ratio first drops, presumably because de-iodination is stimulated, then reaches a peak in 24 to 48 hr. and the effect has subsided by 72 hr. (Halmi, Spirtos, Bogdanove & Lipner, 1953). Hypophysectomy reduces the T/S $[I^-]$ and exogenous TSH returns the ratio to normal or higher levels before histological changes can be demonstrated (Vanderlaan & Greer, 1950). Although hypophysectomy in man lowers most of the parameters of thyroid function, changes in the T/S $[I^-]$ ratio have not been measured. Whatever the mechanism, TSH effects on I^- transport are late responses to the hormone.

The iodine content of the diet has a regulatory effect on the T/S $[I^-]$. Even in the absence of histological evidence for thyrotropic stimulation, thyroids of iodine-deficient rats show increased ratios. High-iodine diets give the reverse picture (Halmi, 1954). Factors which have in common the tendency to lower the total thyroidal iodine increase the T/S [I⁻] and vice versa (Vanderlaan & Caplan, 1954). The potentiating effect of anti-thyroid drugs on the TSH response in hypophy-sectomized rats (Halmi *et al*. 1953) may occur because the drug tends to empty the gland of iodine. Species, sex, age and especially thyroid blood flow may influence iodide concentrating ability of thyroid tissue. These are, however, not well understood as yet (for details see Wolff, 1964).

A second iodide pool, not in rapid equilibrium with circulating iodide has been proposed (Halmi & Pitt-Rivers, 1962; Nagataki & Ingbar, 1963). This iodide appears to derive from labile organic iodine (Rosenberg, Athans & Behar, 1960; Pitt-Rivers, 1963) but to what extent this "pool" is an artefact or may represent a single pool with two fluxes (Simon, 1963) has been very difficult to determine.

FORMATION OF ORGANIC IODINE COMPOUNDS

When a tracer dose of ¹³¹I is administered, the maximum uptake by the normal human thyroid varies from ∼ 15 to ∼ 40% of the dose, depend-ing on the amounts of iodine (¹²⁷I) available, the presence of drugs, etc. When only iodide is per-mitted to accumulate (in glands treated with anti-thyroid drugs) the peak thyroidal ¹³¹I content is attained in several hours and falls off rapidly. Under otherwise identical conditions the total amount is less than that in a gland not blocked by

antithyroid agents. Thyroidal accumulation rates in the normal unblocked gland are greatest during the first 4 to 8 hr.; the uptakes slowly reach a peak at 24 to 48 hr. Continued large uptakes of iodide are possible only because iodide taken up by the thyroid is converted to forms no longer in equilibrium with plasma iodide. This is the orga-nic iodine of the thyroid which is found largely in the protein thyroglobulin and which amounts to ∼ 99% of the total thyroid iodine. The amount of hormone (in terms of daily hormone require-ments) stored in the gland shows tremendous species variations. It is small in the rat but large in man. Thus, accumulated ¹³¹I leaves the thyroid slowly in man and rapidly in the rat. Because of heterogeneity of the organic iodine pool the rate of loss of ¹³¹I cannot serve directly as a measure of the stores.

The iodine concentration of thyroids of various species shows wide variations (Wolff & Chaikoff, 1947), and in thyroglobulin a similar spread has been found (0·05 to ∼ 1·0% I) (Rall, Robbins & Lewallen, 1964). Approximately equal numbers of MIT and DIT residues are found. Thus there is twice as much iodine present as DIT than MIT (Table 12.1). Together the iodinated tyrosines con-stitute 2/3 to 3/4 of the thyroid iodine. The thyro-nines make up nearly all of the remaining iodine. Recent evidence suggests that (contrary to earlier opinions) T_3 is an important fraction of the iodothyronines and T_4:T_3 ratios vary from 7–8:1 in the rat to 2:1 in porcine desiccated thyroid (Wiberg, Devlin, Stephenson, Carter & Bayne, 1962; Simon & Lissitzky, 1964; Pileggi, Golub &

TABLE 12.1

Approximate distribution of thyroidal iodine
(Average for various species*)

Compound	Relative abundance	
	(% of total thyroid iodine)	Moles/mole thyroglobulin
3-Monoiodotyrosine	15–30	6–12
3:5-Di-iodotyrosine	35–42	6–10
Thyroxine (3:5:3′:5′-Tetra-iodothyronine)	15–30	2–5
3:5:3′-Tri-iodothyronine	3–17	<1–2
3:3′:5′-Tri-iodothyronine	trace	
3:3′-Di-iodothyronine	trace	
4-Mono-iodohistidine	< 0·3	
Iodide	≤ 1**	
(Thyronine)	(not found to date)	

(The exact percentages vary with the iodine supply and the state of thyrotropic stimulation.)
* Taken from data of Edelhoch, 1962; Rall *et al.*, 1964; Simon & Lissitzky, 1964; Wolff, unpublished.
** Larger values probably result from methodological artefacts.

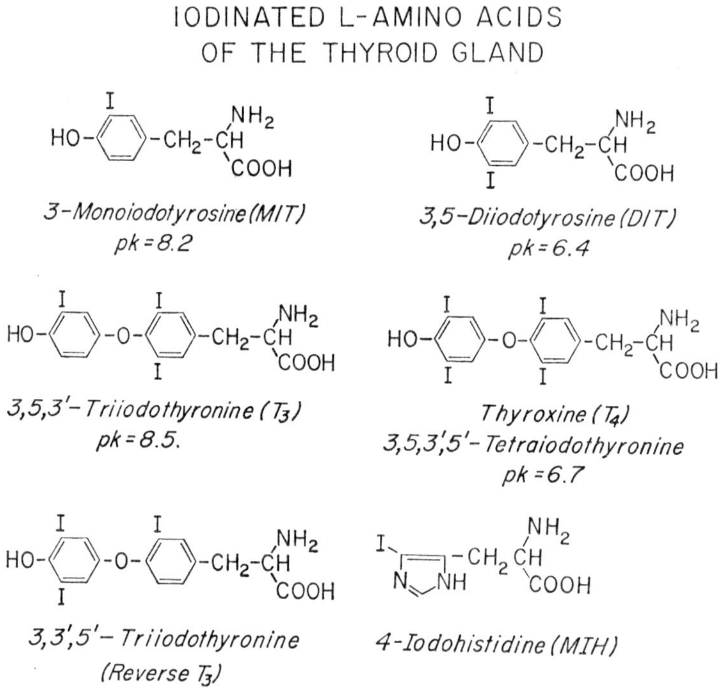

IODINATED L-AMINO ACIDS
OF THE THYROID GLAND

HO-⟨⟩-CH₂-CH(NH₂)(COOH), I

3-Monoiodotyrosine (MIT)
pk = 8.2

HO-⟨⟩-CH₂-CH(NH₂)(COOH), I (two I)

3,5-Diiodotyrosine (DIT)
pk = 6.4

HO-⟨⟩-O-⟨⟩-CH₂-CH(NH₂)(COOH)

3,5,3'-Triiodothyronine (T₃)
pk = 8.5.

HO-⟨⟩-O-⟨⟩-CH₂-CH(NH₂)(COOH)

Thyroxine (T₄)
3,5,3',5'-Tetraiodothyronine
pk = 6.7

HO-⟨⟩-O-⟨⟩-CH₂-CH(NH₂)(COOH)

3,3',5'-Triiodothyronine
(Reverse T₃)

I-⟨N⟩-CH₂-CH(NH₂)(COOH)

4-Iodohistidine (MIH)

FIG. 12.2. The common iodinated amino acids. Abbreviations are listed in parentheses. pK values obtained by spectrophotometric titration.

Lee, 1965; Devlin & Watanabe, 1966). No data exist for the normal human thyroid. Iodide constitutes less than 1.0% of thyroid iodine, and mono-iodohistidine less than 0.3%. Di-iodohistidine and the other iodothyronines exist only as traces. The structural formulae for some of the iodoamino acids are given in Fig. 12.2.

The Oxidizing System

Perhaps nothing in the thyroid field is more controversial than the problem of I^- oxidation and the site of the iodination reaction. It is agreed that iodide must be oxidized to permit substitution reactions in positions *ortho* to the phenol, and it is agreed that the bulk of the iodinated protein resides in the follicular lumen.

Present evidence suggests that, in model systems, the iodinating species is probably I_2 but chemical forms in equilibrium with this form of iodine, such as I^+ or H_2OI^+ or enzyme-bound iodine, cannot be ruled out *in vivo*.

The rather high redox potential for the couple $2I^- \rightarrow I_2 + 2e^- = +0.535V$ limits the number of available oxidizing agents in biological systems. In *in vitro* systems the following have stimulated iodination reactions (see Pitt-Rivers & Cavalieri, 1964; and Rall *et al.* 1964 for details):

Cu^{++} hematin
Mn^{++} quinones
flavins   peroxide

Peroxide is a product common to most of the above and the most widely held view is that a peroxidative reaction, either of the type $H_2O_2 + 2I^- + 2H^+ \rightleftharpoons I_2 + 2H_2O$ or $2H_2O_2 + 2I^- \rightleftharpoons I_2 + O_2 + 2H_2O$ (Alexander, 1959) is probably involved. The most nearly physiological system is probably that of Kondo (1961), in which thyroglobulin is iodinated at reasonable iodide concentrations.

The peroxide-producing reaction *in vivo* has not been identified. Provided metals do not play a major role, the most likely agent would be a flavin-linked oxidation, and pyridine nucleotides and amines may be so oxidized by thyroid tissue. With the former substrates an iodide dependence has been demonstrated (De Groot & Davis, 1961). Xanthine oxidase and polyphenol oxidase have also been suggested.

Because various peroxidases ($+ H_2O_2$) can iodinate various proteins (Nunez, Pommier, El Hilali & Roche, 1965; Taurog & Howells, 1966) and because the rate of oxidation of low concentrations of I^- by H_2O_2 is slow, it appears probable that a peroxidase is involved in I_2 formation. A number of groups have described peroxidases in the thyroid and most, but not all, believe these contain haem, probably ferriprotoporphyrin IX (e.g. Alexander, 1959; Klebanoff, Yip & Kessler, 1962; Alexander & Corcoran, 1962; Maloof & Soodak, 1964; Hosoya & Morrison, 1967). It is found in small particles of the cell, perhaps the peroxisomes (De-Duve & Baudhuin, 1966). It is likely that there are several different peroxidases in the thyroid, and since a variety of peroxidases can oxidize I^- it may prove difficult to identify a specific iodide peroxidase. Furthermore, for a human gland oxidizing about $2\ \mu$moles of I^-/day or approximately 1 to 2 nanomoles/ g./hr. and, given the usual high turnover numbers of peroxidases and 10% saturation, the amount of enzyme that need be present is indeed very small (of the order of $0 \cdot 1$ nanogram/g.). It is of interest that pathological thyroid tissue has been described that was unable to form organic iodine even after H_2O_2 supplementation (Haddad & Sidbury, 1959).

Since I_2 will, by itself, iodinate any number of proteins, usually to the detriment of biological activity, a distinct enzyme, called "tyrosine iodinase", has been proposed to direct iodination toward the thyroglobulin molecule (Fawcett & Kirkwood, 1954). No firm evidence for its existence has been produced. Since peroxidase catalyzes transiodinations (Saunders & Stark, 1958) it is not unreasonable to suppose that peroxidase may fulfill an iodinase role, and some evidence for this has been presented by Klebanoff, Yip & Kessler (1962). Random iodination may be restricted also by the particulate nature of thyroid peroxidases and their location. As an alternative, indirect evidence has been presented that iodination may proceed via an active carrier in the sulphenyl iodide form (Cunningham, 1964):

$$RSH + I_2 \rightleftharpoons RSI + I^- + H^+$$
$$RSI + Protein \rightarrow I\text{-}Protein + RSH$$

The Iodination Mechanism

The mechanism of tyrosine iodination has recently been reinvestigated by Mayberry et al. (1964). The important points for this discussion are:

(1) There is a marked pH dependence determined (a) by the dissociation to the phenolate and (b) because the removal of the proton is rate-limiting (thus leading to base catalysis).

(2) Iodide inhibits iodination in a second order concentration dependence. One term represents the equilibrium $I_2 + I^- \rightleftharpoons I_3^-$, while the other represents the substitution step. Thus:

In model compounds the ratio of the corrected rate constants for tyrosyl and mono-iodotyrosyl iodination in water is 30:1. This accounts for the high yield of MIT at relatively low degrees of iodination. In less aqueous (polar) environments this ratio of rates is smaller and Van Zyl and Edelhoch (1967) suggest that the hydrophobic environment of the tyrosyl residues may account for the relatively small proportion of MIT normally found in thyroglobulin, in contrast to the more nearly normal behaviour of the tyrosyl residues of some other proteins (Covelli & Wolff, 1966, 1967). It must be pointed out that iodination with peroxidases shows differences in reaction kinetics and the behaviour of MIT residues that throw some doubt on the validity of the chemical models (Hosoya, unpublished; Taurog, unpublished).

The Site of Iodination

While there is little doubt that thyroglobulin is synthesized in the thyroid cell a great deal of difficulty has been encountered in localizing the site of iodination of this protein. Radio-autographic evidence (see review by Wollman 1965) shows organic iodine in the follicular lumen near the apical cell border within seconds after injection of labelled I^-. While iodide can diffuse rapidly into a follicle (65 μ/sec.) (Andros & Wollman, 1967), there is no evidence for oxidizing systems in the luminal contents (De Robertis & Grasso, 1946). The assumption most often made is that iodination occurs at the apical cell border; apical fragments can iodinate although not better than mitochondrial or microsomal fractions (Benabdeljlil, Michel-Bechet & Lissitzky, 1967). Objections to this concept are: (1) the facts that peroxidases are particulate and are not especially concentrated near the apex of the cell (Dempsey, 1944), and no granule accumulation is found at the apical microvilli. Vesicles surrounded by small particles are however found near the cell apex (Wissig, 1964); (2) that in some laboratories but not others, particulate iodine is thought to be a precursor for thyroglobulin (Nunez, Jacquemin, Brun & Roche, 1965; Sellin & Goldberg, 1965). The question of the site of iodination had thus best be left open for the moment.

Iodination is one of several examples of changes that can be produced in the native protein *after* the primary structure has been completed. Protein synthesis can be completely blocked in the thyroid without affecting iodination (Seed & Goldberg, 1965; Nunez, Mauchamp, Macchia & Roche 1965).

IODOPROTEINS

The main substrate iodinated in the thyroid is the protein thyroglobulin. It constitutes about

70 to 80% of the soluble protein and nearly all of the organic iodine in normal thyroids. It is defined as: (1) possessing a sedimentation coefficient of ~ 19S, (2) having an electrophoretic mobility of $- 5 \times 10^{-5}$ cm.²/v/sec. in veronal buffer at pH 8·6, and (3) salting out sharply at 38% $(NH_4)_2SO_4$ (for details see review by Edelhoch, 1965). Thyroglobulin has a molecular weight of *ca.* 670,000. Small differences in density, electrophoretic and chromatographic behaviour can be demonstrated within the 19S fraction. This appears to be due to differences in iodine content which in turn will influence phenolic ionization (Robbins, Salvatore, Vecchio & Ui, 1966). The protein has an iso-electric point of 4·6 and a high content of arginine (~ 8%) and of the dicarboxylic acids (~ 21%). The tyrosine content amounts to about 3·1%, which is equivalent to ~ 125 tyrosyl residues per molecule (see Robbins & Rall, 1960; Rolland, Bismuth, Fondarai & Lissitzky, 1966). A portion of these tyrosyl residues is "buried" and cannot be iodinated in native thyroglobulin but becomes available in 8M urea (Edelhoch, 1965). Thyroglobulin is a glycoprotein containing about 8 to 10% carbohydrate probably joined to the protein by the β-carboxyl group of aspartic acid in two types of carbohydrate chains (Spiro & Spiro, 1965). The hexose components in human thyroglobulin are chiefly mannose (3·1%) and *N*-acetyl glucosamine (3.9%). Other constituents are galactose, fucose and sialic acids.

Thyroglobulin may be considered a mixture of two types of tetramers made up of monomers of 160,000 (8S) which are rather large for protein subunits. In one class all four monomers appear to be joined by disulphide bridges. In the other two monomers are joined by disulphide bridges into dimers (12S) which in turn are joined by noncovalent interactions to yield the tetramer. Studies using amino-acid pulse labelling, although incomplete, suggest that these subunits, especially the 12S dimer, are precursors in the biosynthesis of the 19S protein. Iodination occurs probably in the 12S and certainly in the 19S moieties. Iodinated amino acids are not incorporated into protein as such (Seed & Goldberg, 1965). Furthermore, iodination is not dependent on concomitant protein synthesis and, conversely, amino-acid incorporation proceeds when iodinations are blocked. The carbohydrate portion is attached after synthesis of the peptide chain (Spiro & Spiro, 1966).

Several thyroglobulin-like proteins are minor constituents of thyroid tissue. They are larger and have sedimentation coefficients of 27S and 33S.

The former may be a dimer of the 19S thyroglobulin although it has also been claimed to have a higher I/N ratio (Salvatore, Vecchio, Salvatore, Cahnmann & Robbins, 1965; Vecchio, Edelhoch, Robbins & Weathers, 1966). In this case a simple reversible dimerization seems unlikely. Abnormal thyroglobulins will, no doubt, be found in pathological human thyroids, but so far this has been described only in congenital goitre of cattle (Robbins, Van Zyl & Van der Walt, 1966), and in transplantable rat thyroid tumours (DeNayer, Weathers & Robbins, 1967). The amino-acid composition of thyroglobulin from various pathological human thyroids is normal (Bismuth, Rolland & Lissitzky, 1966).

Other soluble iodinated proteins may occasionally be identified in thyroid tissue (see review by Rall *et al.*, 1964). The most important of these is an albumin-like protein found in various states of thyroid dysfunction. It will be discussed below.

In addition small amounts of particulate iodine occur in thyroid tissue (see Rall *et al.*, 1964). This fraction may constitute 50% of the iodine of some tumours. Evidence regarding the precursor nature of these particle-bound iodoproteins is conflicting (Nunez, Jacquemin, Brun & Roche, 1965; Sellin & Goldberg, 1965).

The Coupling of Iodinated Tyrosyl Residues

Harington (1926) first suggested that thyroxine was formed by the coupling of two di-iodotyrosine molecules with elimination of one alanine side chain. This coupling was shown by von Mutzenbecher (1939) and by Harington & Pitt-Rivers (1945). In thyroid tissue the early studies of Chaikoff's laboratory and subsequently of many other groups have led to a similar picture:

mono-iodotyrosine → di-iodotyrosine →
thyroxine

and other iodinated thyronines. This has been shown both by the progressive appearance of label (^{131}I) in the amino acids and by specific activity-time relationships. Recent data show these to be more complicated (Rosenberg, Goldman, LaRoche & Dimick, 1964), and the problem of heterogeneity causes difficulties here. Nevertheless, monoiodotyrosine is the probable precursor of di-iodotyrosine and the iodinated tyrosines are the likely precursors of the iodinated thyronines (Taurog, Tong & Chaikoff, 1950; Roche, Lissitzky, Michel & Michel, 1951; Roche, Lissitzky & Michel, 1952b). These events occur *in vivo* and, less efficiently, in tissue slices or isolated thyroid cells (Tong, 1964). In homogenates of the thyroid gland (and in salivary and mammary homogenates) mono-iodotyrosine is readily formed whereas di-iodotyrosine is formed in poor yield and thyroxine not at all. This suggests that cellular organization is required for hormone synthesis in systems other than the purely chemical (Taurog, Potter & Chaikoff, 1955; Potter, Tong & Chaikoff, 1959). The reaction requires oxygen or an oxidizing system or agent, and it has been suggested that the oxidized form of iodine may be instrumental in *this* reaction as well as the iodination. A peroxidase-linked reaction could be involved since this enzyme can catalyse the formation of the diphenyl ether linkage (Westerfeld & Lowe, 1942). However, practically nothing is known of actual events in the thyroid.

In model systems it was found that coupling occurred in much better yield when both the —COOH and the —NH$_2$ groups were bound in peptide linkage (Pitt-Rivers, 1948; Pitt-Rivers & James, 1958), and it is generally assumed that *in vivo* coupling of iodotyrosyl residues occurs in the intact, preformed thyroglobulin molecule. The evidence for this stems from the failure to find thyronine in this protein, from the increased efficiency of the coupling reaction when the di-iodotyrosine is in peptide linkage, and from the finding that di-iodotyrosine and thyroxine have higher specific activities in the protein than in the free form at very high tyrosine content (10 to 11 %). This may be because the di-iodotyrosyl residues are sterically hindered from coupling (Michel & Pitt-Rivers, 1948). However, thyroxine *is* formed during the chemical iodination of poly-L-tyrosine (Sela & Sarid, 1956).

Although thyroxine formation in pure thyroglobulin and other proteins suggests intramolecular coupling of two iodotyrosyl residues, the possibility that the phenolic ring derives from free di-iodotyrosine or a derivative thereof has been extensively investigated. It has been shown that 4-hydroxy-3,5-di-iodophenylpyruvic acid couples rapidly and efficiently (20% + yield) with DIT to form thyroxine (Hillmann, 1956; Meltzer & Stanaback, 1961; Shiba & Cahnmann, 1962). With thyroglobulin *in vitro* the yield of T$_4$ is low (Toi, Salvatore & Cahnmann, 1965). The reaction may proceed by an intermediate peroxide which is converted to a free radical that can couple with DIT in the absence of oxygen (Nishinaga *et al.*, 1968). Compounds such as 2,6-di-iodobenzo-quinone or reduced congeners thereof, although formed as a bi-product of this reaction and also during the breakage of the diphenyl ether bond (Wynn & Gibbs, 1964), appear not to be involved. Traces of the ketoacid can probably be formed in thyroid tissue (Covelli & Wolff, unpublished). Furthermore, at intervals of one hour or more after ^{131}I injection the labelling is said to be uniformly distributed between both benzene rings (Plaskett, 1961).

early intervals after I^{131} injection. Furthermore, thyroxine in peptide linkage can be formed by chemical iodination of thyroglobulin and other proteins.

The native structure of thyroglobulin seems to confer considerable efficiency on the coupling process since thyroxine is not formed upon iodination of fragments of thyroglobulin (Edelhoch, 1962), and the efficiency of thyroxine synthesis is reduced when the molecule is unfolded with guanidine (Van Zyl & Edelhoch, 1967). It is of interest that thyroxine formation does not occur during the iodination of silk fibroin, despite the

Thyroxine and Tri-iodothyronine (T$_4$ & T$_3$)

No unanimity exists regarding the metabolic inter-relationships of T$_3$ and T$_4$ in the thyroid. The most widely held concept is that both thyronines are formed by the coupling reaction, T$_3$ from one MIT + one DIT, etc. and T$_4$ from two DIT residues. This is supported by the findings that the ratio of labelled T$_3$/T$_4$ varies in proportion to changes in the MIT/DIT ratio (Leloup & Lachiver 1955; Pitt-Rivers, 1962). Furthermore, labelled T$_3$ and T$_4$ either appear simultaneously after ^{131}I injection (Roche, Michel & Tata, 1953), or T$_3$

may precede T$_4$ (Feuer, 1959). The opposite suggestions that T$_3$ derives from de-iodination of T$_4$ (Plaskett, 1961) would not be consistent with the above, nor with the difficulty in de-iodinating iodothyronines and protein-bound iodine (Yagi, Michel & Roche, 1953; Pitt-Rivers, 1966). Thus the coupling concept appears to be the best substantiated at present. Although the evidence is indirect TSH seems to exert an effect on the coupling reaction (Rosenberg et al., 1964).

The contribution of T$_3$ to the total metabolic response of the animal is greater than initially thought. For the rat it has been calculated that endogenously produced tri-iodothyronine contributes about 40% of the total thyroid hormone-maintained oxygen consumption (Pitt-Rivers & Rall, 1961). The fraction may be higher in other species in whom the T$_3$/T$_4$ ratio in thyroid tissue is higher (up to 1/2 as opposed to 1/7 or so in the rat (Wiberg et al., 1962; Pileggi et al., 1965; Devlin & Watanabe, 1966)). The fraction of T$_3$ in the plasma is lower than these ratios ($\sim$ 3%, see below) whereas that of the peripheral tissues may be higher (Albright et al., 1965). Since most investigators have looked in plasma, evidence for conversion of T$_3$ to T$_4$, e.g. in the athyreotic subject, is quantitatively inconclusive. Such conversion can occur and has been demonstrated by biliary excretion of T$_3$ and T$_3$ conjugates after T$_4$ administration (Flock, Bollman, Grindlay & Stobie, 1961). It is clear in any event that T$_3$ contributes more to the hormone effect than heretofore suspected; its role has been calculated (from pool size and fractional turnover) to be equal to that of T$_4$ in man (Nauman, Nauman & Werner, 1967).

It might reasonably be supposed that combinations of any des-, mono, or di-iodotyrosine should lead to the formation of thyronine derivatives with all degrees of iodination. All the iodinated combinations have been synthesized (Roche, Michel & Wolf, 1954), yielding 3- or 3'-mono-iodothyronine, 3:5- or 3':5'- or 3:3'-di-iodothyronine and 3:3':5'-tri-iodothyronine. Neither of the mono-iodo derivatives has been isolated from thyroid tissue. The labelled 3:3' congener and traces of 3:3':5'-tri-iodothyronine have been found in thyroid tissue after ^{131}I (iodide) administration and in bile (Flock et al., 1961). The former compound can also be demonstrated in the circulation (Roche, Michel, Wolf & Nunez, 1956).

HORMONE RELEASE

Hydrolysis

Contrary to earlier opinion it now seems fairly certain that small amounts of thyroglobulin are normally present in the circulation. In peripheral blood of experimental animals this protein contributes only a few per cent. to the total iodine but in thyroid lymph more than half of the iodine may be present as thyroglobulin (Daniel, Pratt, Roitt & Torrigiani, 1967). More may appear after trauma such as surgery, irradiation or in subacute thyroiditis (see review by Robbins & Rall, 1967). Nevertheless, considerable evidence supports the conclusion that the bulk of the thyroxine and tri-iodothyronine present in the periphery derives from thyroglobulin hydrolysed within the thyroid gland.

The older literature has been reviewed (Rall et al., 1964; Lundblad, Bernbäck & Widemann, 1965), but recent findings have helped to clarify this confusing picture (Wetzel, Spicer & Wollman, 1965; Wollman, 1965). Histological evidence now suggests that colloid is taken up by apical pseudopods projecting into the lumen. The pinocytotic droplets so formed move toward the interior of the cell and are now called the intracellular colloid droplets. They can be shown to contain protein-bound ^{125}I presumably still as thyroglobulin (Stein & Gross, 1964). Subsequently they fuse with dense, acid phosphatase-rich granules and progress toward the basal cytoplasm, becoming smaller. These granules are likely to be the lysosomes which contain, among many other acid hydrolases, cathepsins with a pH optimum of 3·5 to 4·0. The isolated enzymes hydrolyse thyroglobulin slowly and appear to proceed via high molecular weight intermediates before iodoamino acids are released (Alpers, Robbins & Rall, 1955; Balasubramaniam & Deiss, 1965; Herveg, Beckers & De Visscher, 1966). It seems likely that the whole thyroglobulin molecule must be broken down to liberate the iodinated amino acids. However, release of free iodoamino acids is more efficient with intact particles and proteolysis is much faster when these are derived from TSH-stimulated thyroid glands (Deiss, Balasubramaniam, Peake, Starrett & Powell, 1966).

The enzyme has been purified and the substrate specificity has been partially determined (Haddad & Rall, 1960; Kress, Peanasky & Klitgaard, 1966), but so far no specificity toward iodoamino acids has been established. A similar enzyme has been demonstrated in human thyroid tissue (Shapland, 1964; Lundblad et al., 1965).

Because of the very acidic pH optimum of the cathepsins, attempts have been made to find proteases and peptidases with more alkaline pH optimum. Although not invariably found, two additional activities, less potent than the cathepsins, have been repeatedly reported with optima near pH 5·5 and pH 8·5

(Haddad & Rall, 1960; Lundblad *et al.*, 1965). Furthermore, various peptidases have been described (Loughlin, McQuillan & Trikojus, 1960) but the role of these is not yet clear.

Free Iodothyronines

Probably as a result of hydrolysis small quantities of the free iodinated amino acids are found in the gland. Free iodothyronines account for about 0·5 to 1·0% and free iodotyrosines for another 0·5 to 1·0% of the total thyroid iodine (Tong, Taurog & Chaikoff, 1951; Gross & Leblond, 1951). At early intervals after the administration of ^{131}I the specific activity of thyroglobulin-thyroxine is greater than that of free thyroxine, suggesting that iodination probably occurred in the protein molecule. Free thyroxine, and presumably tri-iodothyronine, are not dehalogenated significantly, and can build up a concentration gradient over plasma of about 100-fold. This facilitates delivery of the hormone to the circulation (Leblond & Gross, 1949; Tong *et al.*, 1951). Free thyroxine is increased by TSH treatment. Part of this gradient appears to be due to binding of T_4 (and perhaps T_3) to thyroglobulin and probably other tissue proteins of the thyroid gland (Ingbar & Freinkel, 1957). To what extent this binding controls release of the hormones into the blood is not known. Binding of the iodothyronines to plasma proteins (see below) may facilitate the release of these substances from the gland by mass action; this may also increase specificity of removal since di-iodotyrosine is less firmly bound (Tong *et al.*, 1954). A significant fraction of the iodine leaving the thyroid does so via the lymphatics and the concentration in lymph may be higher than in venous plasma (Daniel *et al.*, 1967).

Intrathyroidal De-iodination

Normally little MIT or DIT appear in the peripheral blood whereas the iodothyronines are readily secreted into the circulation. The problem of the selectivity of the release mechanism has been clarified by Roche, Michel, Michel & Lissitzky (1952a). Mono- and di-iodotyrosines are de-iodinated when incubated with thyroid tissue; thyroxine and tri-iodothyronine are dehalogenated at very much smaller rates. However, de-iodination can occur only when the iodotyrosines exist as free amino acids (Tong, Taurog & Chaikoff, 1954; Roche & Michel, 1954). Peptides of di-iodotyrosine are not de-iodinated unless they are first hydrolysed to free di-iodotyrosine (Wolff & Pitt-Rivers, 1959, unpublished). The enzyme responsible for de-iodination of mono- and di-iodotyrosine is found in the microsomal fraction

and has a TPNH requirement (Stanbury & Morriss 1958). Although TPNH consumption has not been directly shown, TPNH concentration is rate-limiting for de-iodination in the gland (Maayan & Rosenberg, 1963). The I$^-$ thus liberated can re-enter the cycle of thyroxine synthesis in the gland and some will leak to the circulation. The process is accelerated within a half-hour after TSH injection (Bastomsky, Rosenfeld & Rosenberg, 1966). Thus in addition to acting as hormone precursors, the iodotyrosines store iodine in the gland. Since iodotyrosine cannot be incorporated into protein as such, failure to de-iodinate then would entail a sizeable loss of iodine. This appears to occur in a certain type of congenital goitre (see below).

The fraction of ^{131}I normally released from the thyroid as iodide is difficult to quantitate but may be considerable. While some may be I$^-$ from the trap, the larger portion appears to be derived from organic ^{131}I. The amount appearing in the venous thyroid blood thus depends on the ratio of the de-iodination and iodination capacities of the tissue. If internal recycling is prevented by the use of an antithyroid agent it can be shown that a substantial portion of the ^{131}I released is iodide. The many attempts to measure the amount (µg.) of thyroxine released from the thyroid gland by means of radioactive isotopes come to grief because of this problem, and Lewallen (Rall *et al.*, 1964) has estimated that thyroxine secretion rates so derived over-estimate true rates by a factor of 2–3. Furthermore, Triantaphyllidis (1958) was able to show that in the first few days after ^{131}I administration the specific activity of the secreted iodine was three to four times greater than that of the thyroidal iodine. More recent evidence on the extensive heterogeneity of the thyroid iodine (Pitt-Rivers, 1963; Schneider, 1964; Wollman, 1965) precludes all simple quantitative interpretations from short term labelling experiments.

THYROTROPIN (TSH)

The importance of TSH in the release of iodine from the thyroid gland has already been alluded to. Blood flow to the gland increases one minute after intravenous TSH injection (Söderberg, 1958). Within 10 minutes apical pseudopods and colloid droplets may be seen (Nadler, Sarkar & Leblond, 1962; Wetzel *et al.*, 1965)). Release of organic and inorganic ^{131}I into the circulation is accelerated by TSH after a similarly short latent period (Nagataki, Shizume & Okinaka, 1961; Rosenberg, Athans & Isaacs, 1965). There is also an increase of the free thyroxine of the gland (Tong *et al.*, 1951). It is of some interest that the morphological effects occur at least as fast as the biochemical consequences of TSH action.

When TSH is given either to the normal or hypophysectomized animal, release of organic iodine may occur to such an extent that synthesis of new organic iodine cannot keep up with release, and the gland becomes depleted of iodine and especially thyroxine (Wolff & Chaikoff, 1947). The rate of release of T_4 and probably tri-iodothyronine is, to a certain extent, independent of the rate of synthesis. A similar independence is also shown by preparations blocked with antithyroid agents, where rates of release can be varied by TSH, etc. (Wolff, 1951). Manipulation of the TSH level such as chronic administration of antithyroid agent, hypophysectomy or thyroxine injection influence ^{131}I release from the thyroid in the expected manner. Iodine depletion is thus a useful index of thyrotropic stimulation and has been extensively used as an assay (Bates & Condliffe, 1966).

The release of iodine from the *human* thyroid has also been shown to be under TSH control. Although the normal thyroid iodine has an inconveniently long biological half-life (~ 60 to 100 days), this can be markedly shortened by TSH (Goldsmith et al., 1951). The effect can be seen also as an increase in the $PB^{131}I$ or the $PB^{127}I$ of serum and is highly significant in less than 90 min. (Einhorn & Larsson, 1959; Becker, Rall, Peacock & Rawson, 1953). Kinetic evidence suggests that a sizeable fraction of ^{131}I leaving the gland is iodide, which is in excess of any iodide that can be accounted for by the trap. Thus the uptake greatly exceeds the release of calculated "hormone" iodine (Riggs, 1952; Ermans, Dumont & Bastenie, 1963; Berman et al., 1968), and the specific activity of urine iodide exceeds that of the PBI. This is difficult to explain otherwise (Ermans et al., 1963). In some cases, an acute *rise* in serum iodide can be imposed on an otherwise rapidly falling curve by TSH injection (Deiss, O'Shaughnessy & Wynn, 1959).

The mechanism of action of TSH is unknown but extensive work on various metabolic effects has been carried out in recent years and has been abundantly reviewed (Freinkel, 1964; Dumont, 1965; Pastan, 1966; Bates & Condliffe, 1966). The highlights of these studies are summarized below.

(1) TSH leads to a cation-dependent stimulation of glucose oxidation, primarily of the hexose monophosphate pathway and to a lesser extent via glycolysis. Although originally thought to be due to an increase in TPN levels, the relation between these two changes is not obligatory and the mechanism remains obscure. Glycogenolysis may also be stimulated.

(2) Thyroidal phospholipid synthesis, primarily of phosphatidyl inositides, is increased by TSH.

(3) TSH leads to an early increase in $^{24}Na^+$ and water uptake and a later stimulation of the Na^+ pump.

(4) RNA synthesis is stimulated by TSH treatment. This may be secondary to an increase in ribose.

(5) Protein synthesis is stimulated later according to some reports. These data are complicated by the extensive early proteolysis caused by TSH.

The current view is that many of these changes result from increases in the production of cyclic $3',5'$-AMP which is then supposed to lead to the numerous metabolic and anatomical changes characteristic of TSH stimulation. Preliminary evidence suggests that the increase in nucleotide level results from a rapid stimulation of adenyl cyclase by TSH (Pastan & Katzen, 1967). The precise interplay with iodine metabolism, except for a TPNH requirement in de-iodination, is rather vague at present.

Thyroid Pituitary Relations

The control of TSH secretion is, among other things, under thyroid hormone control. It has been shown that the thyroid hormone, thyroidectomy or antithyroid drugs lead to changes in anterior-pituitary cytology (Griesbach & Purves, 1945; Goldberg & Chaikoff, 1951), and thyroid administration decreases pituitary thyrotropin (TSH) content. On the basis of an abundance of such indirect evidence it has been assumed that there is an inverse relationship (of the feed-back variety) between the level of circulating thyroid hormone and thyrotropin output by the anterior pituitary. Tri-iodothyronine is concentrated in the posterior, and to a lesser extent in the anterior, pituitary gland of rabbits, rats and guinea pigs in amounts well above the plasma level. There is also a slight preferential concentration in the diencephalon when compared with the rest of the brain. Labelled thyroxine is less well concentrated, mostly in the posterior pituitary gland (Courrier, Horeau, Marois & Morel, 1951; Jensen & Clark, 1951; Ford & Gross, 1958) and a fair portion of this may actually be present as T_3 (Reichlin, Volpert & Werner, 1966). Whether or not this results from local de-iodination or concentration of T_3 made elsewhere is uncertain but current evidence favours mono-deiodination of T_4—an unusual reaction in the body. The significance of such data is strictly inferential, since concentration of these hormones may not be necessary. Nevertheless, indirect evidence suggests that it may play a role in TSH release. Propylthiouracil, which can inhibit peripheral de-iodination of T_4, enhances the latter's suppressive effect on "TSH output" (Mouriz, Morreale de Escobar & Escobar del Rey, 1966). TSH output suppression by T_3 is not so influenced by the antithyroid drug. Evidence that similar reactions control the *peripheral* effects of T_4 is lacking.

There are two types of control of TSH secretion—that occurring at the level of the pituitary (true feed-back control), and neural influences from the hypothalamus. The former can be demonstrated by direct injection or in pituitary transplants (see Reichlin, 1963). It appears to be produced by changes in serum *free* T_4 (or T_3). The rapid response of TBPA (see below) may be of importance. Agents which raise the free-T_4 by displacement (Wolff, Rubin & Chaikoff, 1950; Austen, Meroney, Rubin & Wolff, 1958; Wolff & Austen, 1958; Wolff, Standaert & Rall, 1961) may inhibit thyroid function transiently at this locus. However, nothing is known of hormone displacement from cellular binding proteins by these agents. Whatever the site of action, it has been shown that salicylate and several congeners probably depress circulating TSH in the rat, apparently by raising the level of free T_4 (Good, Hetzel & Hogg, 1965).

Although considerable controversy existed in the past regarding the need for an intact connection to the median eminence, hypothalamus, etc. via the pituitary stalk, reasonable evidence exists today that the hypothalamus produces a thyrotropin-released factor (TRF) which reaches the pituitary via the portal circulation (Guillemin, Yamazaki, Gard, Jutisz & Sakiz, 1963; Schally, Bowers & Redding, 1966). Various neural stimuli are transmitted by this route. These are electric stimulation of certain hypothalamic areas, and local cooling of the pre-optic areas. The high temperature co-efficient of hormone binding to proteins may prove to be of interest in this respect. However, evidence as to whether there is a feed-back at the hypothalamic level as well is controversial (Reichlin, 1963). In general, TRF stimulates and T_4 and T_3 inhibit pituitary thyrotropin.

It must be remembered that despite the dominant role of thyrotropin in thyroid activation, the metabolic rate and protein-bound iodine of hypophysectomized rats are not generally as low as after thyroidectomy. This difference is encountered when comparing primary with pituitary myxoedema. Furthermore, mild responses to typical stimuli (e.g. cold, iodine-deficient diet) can be evoked in the thyroid glands of hypophysectomized animals (Wolf & Greep, 1937; Goldberg, Nay & Greep, 1953). That is, the thyroid functions at a low level in the absence of the pituitary, and can make minor adaptive responses.

In addition to the above, cold increases the release of thyroidal ^{131}I, and heat tends to slow it down (Brown-Grant, von Euler, Harris & Reichlin, 1954; Goldberg, Wolff & Greep, 1957). The decrease in hormone "requirements" produced by heat are such that goitre formation with antithyroid drugs can be hindered at elevated environmental temperatures (Dempsey & Astwood, 1943).

ACTH or cortisone decreases, or may temporarily abolish, ^{131}I release in the rabbit (Brown-Grant et al., 1954). This may be due to a change in the peripheral metabolism of TSH, but the responses of the thyroid to adrenal steroids may be far more complicated (Ackerman, Smith & Miller, 1961; Ingbar & Freinkel, 1955).

Physical and emotional stresses decrease the release of thyroidal ^{131}I even in the absence of the adrenals. Rabbits "escape" from the emotional stresses and tend to resume normal release rates (Brown-Grant et al., 1954). In other hands opposite results have been obtained. Nervous stimuli, acetylcholine, serotonin, adrenaline and noradrenaline all can alter ^{131}I secretion. These effects appear to be independent of blood flow but are dependent on the level of TSH stimulation and dosage. Large doses of adrenaline or noradrenaline suppress ^{131}I release from the thyroid (Söderberg, 1958).

Many drugs may, when given acutely, inhibit release of iodine from the gland. Among these are:

2,4-Dinitrophenol (Goldberg, Wolff & Greep, 1957).

Salicylate (Wolff & Austen, 1958).

Lysine vasopressin, γ and β MSH (see Schally et al., 1966).

Morphine and chlorpromazine (Samel, 1958).

BLOOD IODINE

Nature of Compounds

Most of the iodine of normal plasma or serum can be precipitated with the usual protein-precipitating agents, even though it is not present in peptide linkage, and has therefore been called the protein-bound iodine or PBI.

A small but significant fraction of the total blood iodine is present as iodide. The exact level is a function of several variables, notably the dietary iodine intake. Average values for different localities have been summarized by Rosen, Ezrin & Volpe (1967) and range from 0·19 to 0·63 μg./100 ml. of serum or plasma. The level is of little diagnostic importance *per se*, but in conjunction with the thyroid iodide clearance determines the absolute iodine uptake as discussed below.

The extensive recent literature on the circulating organic iodine has been reviewed (Robbins & Rall, 1967) and only a summary of these findings is suitable here. Thyroxine constitutes the major portion of the organic iodine of the blood. Tri-iodothyronine constitutes about 3 to 4% of the serum iodine in rats and man (Pitt-Rivers & Rall, 1961; Nauman et al., 1967). There may be up to 15% iodoprotein iodine (Rall & Conard, 1966), and part of this can be thyroglobulin (Daniel et al., 1967). Thyroxine metabolites (see below) are seen only in biliary obstruction. Traces of the iodo-tyrosines are agreed to be present but the larger amounts claimed by some cannot usually be demonstrated and seem kinetically unlikely because of their rapid disposal (Block, Werner, Mandl, Low & Radichevich, 1960; Whitehead & Beale, 1959, 1960; Wynn, 1960). Labelled di-iodotyrosine has been reported in some hyperthyroid patients (Farran, Lea, Goolden & Abbatt, 1959). The latter findings do not necessarily imply any measurable amounts of stable di-iodotyrosine. Traces of other labelled iodinated thyronines have been demonstrated in the blood of experimental animals (Roche et al., 1956).

The "normal" levels of organic iodine, measured as PBI, show considerable species variation and also a rather wide spread in the range of concentrations. In man the normal PBI is considered to be 3·5 to 8·0 μg./100 ml. which is approximately 1×10^{-7}M expressed as thyroxine. Thyroxine iodine amounts to 2·9 to 6·4 μg./100 ml. and on the average makes up 82% of the PBI (Robbins & Rall, 1967). Preliminary results for tri-iodothyronine iodine are 0·14 to 0·19 μg./100 ml. (Nauman et al., 1967). The small fraction present as tri-iodothyronine does not reflect its true importance since in the tissues the T_3/T_4 ratio may vary from 0·03 to as much as 0·5 or more (Albright, Heninger & Larson, 1965). This is seen also in the larger T_3 than T_4 spaces. Furthermore, the faster disappearance of T_3 indicates that relative secretion rates are not the same as relative blood levels.

Transport of Blood Iodine

Although thyroxine (and probably tri-iodothyronine) is precipitated with the plasma protein, it is not bound in peptide linkage but in a specific, but poorly understood, attachment to the transport protein which involves the phenolate form of the hormones. Affinity constants are high so that at physiological hormone levels essentially all of the iodothyronine is associated. Nevertheless, the best current evidence suggests that these bound forms of T_4 and T_3 act primarily as reservoirs and that the tiny fraction of free T_4 and T_3 in equilibrium with them determines the action and the disposal of the hormones.

The chief binding protein of human serum is thyroxine-binding globulin (TBG) which carries from 1/2 to 2/3 of T_4 under normal physiological loads. Earlier results showed higher proportions of T_4 in this fraction as a result of methodological artefacts (use of barbital buffers). It migrates between the α_1- and α_2-globulins, is an acidic glycoprotein containing 32% carbohydrate including sialic acid (Seal & Doe, 1964), has an iso-electric pH $\sim$ 4·0, and is similar to, but separate from, transcortin. It has a very high affinity for T_4 and rather less for T_3, the exact value being uncertain (Robbins & Rall, 1967). The various properties are listed in Table 12.2.

TABLE 12.2
Properties of Thyroxine-Binding Proteins

	TBG	TBPA	Albumin
$S_{w.20}$	$\sim$ 3·5	$\sim$ 4·6	$\sim$ 4·3
MW(10^3)	50–60	70	67
K_{T_4}	4×10^{10}	$\sim 1 \times 10^9$(1)*	$1·6 \times 10^6$(1)*
K_{T_3}	2–10×10^9	low	2–3×10^5
Specificity	$T_4 > T_3$	$T_4 >> T_3$ Tetrac	$T_4 > T_3$
T_4 Capacity (μg./100 ml.)	20	250	

* K = affinity constant (moles^{-1}); (number of sites).

The second transport protein, carrying normally 15–25 % of the T_4 and no T_3, is thyroxine-binding prealbumin (TBPA) which is the faster of the two prealbumins in starch gel electrophoresis. Carboxylic acid side chain analogues are the preferred substrates. The protein has been purified (Seal & Doe, 1964; Oppenheimer, Surks, Smith & Squef, 1965; Purdy, Woeber, Holloway & Ingbar, 1965), has one binding site per mole of undetermined affinity. The carbohydrate content is less than in TBG and there is no sialic acid (see Table 12.2).

Albumin binds T_4 with one site of a moderate affinity constant as well as numerous other sites of low affinity (Table 12.2).

The total normal serum capacity is $\sim$ 20 μg. T_4/100 ml. on TBG, and approximately 250 μg./100 ml. on TBPA. The affinity constants and capacities are such that the distribution of T_4 amongst the proteins is approximately as shown in Fig. 12.3. Under these conditions about 75% of the TBG sites and 99% of the TBPA sites are unoccupied.

In addition, γ-globulin may bind T_4 when it contains antithyroglobulin antibodies (Premachandra, Ray, Hirata & Blumenthal, 1965), and Hoch, Sinnett, Miller & Mahady (1965) have described a dialysable substance that binds T_4. Furthermore, there is marked species variation in

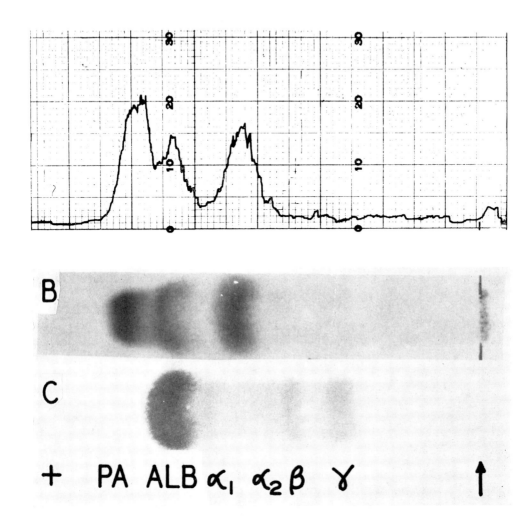

Fig. 12.3. Thyroxine binding to human serum proteins. 0·5 μg. of radioactive T_4 per ml. serum. Buffer = Tris-maleate pH 8·6. A. Scan with end-window β-counter of ^{131}I-thyroxine on electrophoretic paper strip. Ordinate: intensity of radiation in arbitrary units. B. Radioautograph of same electrophoretic strip. C. Same strip stained for protein with PA = prealbumin zone, ALB = albumin, α_1, α_2, β and γ indicate corresponding globulin fraction. ↑ indicates point of application of serum and + the anodal pole. The origins of all three figures coincide. The distribution is slightly low for TBG since a moderately high load of T_4 was used. I am indebted to Dr. M. Andreoli for this figure.

[To face p. 392.

thyroxine binding (see review by Rall *et al.*, 1964) and the results discussed above apply only to man. Some thyroxine-binding proteins have access to extravascular spaces but not to all, e.g. the cerebrospinal fluid, where the total T_4 concentration is low but the free-T_4 may be high.

The *in vivo* significance of thyroxine-binding has been clarified by studies in a variety of clinical states. An increase in available thyroxine-binding sites of TBG has been found:

(1) In pregnancy.

(2) After oestrogen therapy (both in men and women, as well as in athyreotic subjects).

(3) In certain normal families with elevated PBI levels.

(4) In the acute phase of infectious hepatitis.

(5) In hypothyroidism (slight).

(6) In carcinoma of the breast.

(7) In acute intermittent porphyria.

A decrease has been found:

(1) In the nephrotic syndrome.

(2) Following methyl testosterone, cortisol, and anabolic steroids.

(3) In the presence of diphenylhydantoin.

(4) In apparently normal patients.

(5) In hyperthyroidism (slight decrease).

(6) In acromegaly.

(For references see reviews by Rall *et al.*, 1964; Robbins & Rall, 1967).

TBPA capacity also shows fluctuations in various disease states, sometimes quite rapidly. Decreases have been shown to occur in acute and chronic illnesses and appear to play a major role when PBI changes are seen. Surgical stress may cause decreases in TBPA (Surks & Oppenheimer, 1964). Decreases found after parturition are discussed below. Dinitrophenol, salicylate and certain of its analogues and barbital displace T_4 from TBPA (Wolff, *et al.*, 1961; Woeber & Ingbar, 1964). TBPA capacity may be increased in acromegaly. It should be pointed out that T_4 displacement will reduce the number of binding sites on TBG for both T_4 and T_3, even though T_3 is not bound to TBPA.

In most of the above mentioned alterations in thyroxine-binding there is a parallel change in the PBI. In contrast, a case of analbuminaemia had a normal PBI suggesting that this protein is *not* of major importance in the control of the PBI. The cases of pregnancy, of steroid therapy, of nephrosis, and of congenital alterations in TBG, have highly abnormal PBI levels but are nevertheless euthyroid. These findings, as well as mass law considerations, led to the proposal that the unbound or free form of the hormone was the

biologically active form. Methods for determining this value depend on dialysis and are sensitive to dilution, temperature, buffer, etc. Nevertheless, approximate values for the free T_4 concentration range from 3 to 6×10^{-11}M, and for free $T_3 \sim 2 \cdot 3 \times 10^{-11}$M (see Robbins & Rall, 1967). In the case of T_4 this represents $< 0 \cdot 05 \%$ of the total T_4, whereas this fraction is about 10 times higher for T_3.

Thyroxine disposal from the circulation is best described as a function of the free T_4 concentration or, conversely, as an inverse function of the unoccupied binding sites (Rall *et al.*, 1964). The same is true, in a rough, clinical way for the thyroid status, where PBI changes are often anomalous. This in no way implies that the reactions leading to T_4 disposal are "required" for the action of the hormone. There is currently no evidence that requires such an interpretation (Wolff & Wolff, 1964; Tata, 1964a; Barker & Shimada, 1964). Furthermore, effects of bound T_4 and T_3 have not been entirely ruled out and should be considered possible, especially in effects located at the cell membrane.

DISTRIBUTION AND EXCRETION

Injected labelled thyroxine is "distributed" over a volume of 11 to 27% of the body weight in man with mean values varying from 9 to 11·2 l. per 70 Kg. (Sterling & Chodos, 1956; Berson, 1956; Gregerman, Gaffney & Shock, 1962). The tri-iodothyronine space is much larger (Sterling, Lashoff & Man, 1954; Berson & Yalow, 1954), probably because tissue T_3 concentrations are relatively much greater than in blood as suggested by equilibrium labelling experiments in rats (Albright *et al.*, 1965). The rapid formation of conjugates, e.g. the sulphate ester, makes exact values difficult to obtain. The hormones show some early concentration in the liver, kidney and stomach, whereas most of the remaining tissues accumulate the label more slowly. The pituitaries of a number of species (including man), especially the posterior lobe, concentrate radioactivity after injection of ^{131}I-labelled thyroxine (reviewed by Pitt-Rivers & Tata, 1959). Other tissues accumulate T_4 more gradually but because of their bulk (e.g. muscle) account for a substantial fraction of the total activity. The low levels of labelled T_4 for brain (Tata, 1964a) are rate-determined since equilibrium-labelled rats contain about the same T_4 and T_3 concentrations as e.g. muscle (Albright *et al.*, 1965).

The subcellular distribution of T_4 shows no particular concentration in organelles (Tata, 1964a) but these studies are made difficult by redistribution during tissue preparation and non-specific binding by organelles of added T_4. In addition a variety of cellular thyroxine-binding proteins are known to exist. They are of rather low capacity and affinity and may not, by themselves, adequately explain the concentrations of iodothyronines present (Salvatore, 1964; Lissitzky, 1960; Tata, 1964a; Hamada, Torizuka & Miyake, 1966).

Inspection of the structural formula of thyroxine or tri-iodothyronine (Fig. 12.2) reveals a number of functional groups which might be expected to undergo metabolic changes in the periphery:

(1) The amino-acid side chain.
(2) the phenolic OH.
(3) the *ortho*-iodine atoms.
(4) the diphenyl ether linkage.

All these groups can be attacked in biological systems although there is marked tissue and species variation. The literature is too voluminous for any detail here and only indications of the possible pathways will be given (Pitt-Rivers & Tata, 1959; Tata, 1964).

(1) The alanine side chain of the thyronine nucleus can be metabolized to the acetic acid analogue, apparently via the α-oxoacid. The oxoacid and lactic acids have been identified in various animals and also in human bile (Myant, 1956; Roche, Michel & Gregorio, 1961). The oxoacid stage may apparently be attained by both of the two usual routes. Tomita and coworkers have prepared a soluble DPN-linked enzyme system which leads to the formation of the acetic acid analogues (Albright, Tomita & Larson, 1959). On the other hand, a mitochondrial α-oxoglutaric transaminase system has been reported by Yamamoto, Ishikawa and Shimizu (1960).

(2) The thyroid hormones can undergo the usual "detoxification" reactions that are common to phenols. (a) Exogenous or endogenous thyroxine appears in the bile both free and as the β-glucuronide (Taurog, Tong & Chaikoff, 1951; Taurog, Briggs & Chaikoff, 1952; Briggs, Brauer, Taurog & Chaikoff, 1953). The formation of the conjugate occurs in microsome preparations of mammalian liver, and appears to require uridine diphosphate glucuronic acid (UDPGA) as a glucuronide donor (Isselbacher & Axelrod, 1955). Tri-iodothyronine appears to undergo the same fate (Roche, Michel & Tata, 1953). In the rat the ability to conjugate is limited and non-physiological doses are conjugated with decreasing efficiency. The glucuronide is hydrolysed in the bowel, and part of the liberated thyroxine is reabsorbed to complete the entero-hepatic circulation of thyroxine. The significance of this pathway for thyroxine excretion shows tremendous species variation. It is of considerable importance in the rat, while in man biliary excretion of thyroxine seems quantitatively less important (Johnson & Beierwaltes,

1953). (b) Studies with both ^{131}I and $^{35}SO_4{}^-$ have shown that the sulphate ester is another important conjugate. So far as is known this pathway is more important for tri-iodothyronine than thyroxine (Roche, Michel, Closon & Michel, 1959). The nature of the sulphate-transferring system is not yet known. Michel and co-workers have shown that o-methylation of thyroxine can occur in the rat (Roche et al., 1961). Whether or not the usual type of o-methyl transferase is involved is not yet known.

(3) In man the major pathway for thyroxine degradation is de-iodination. Most tissues can carry out this reaction and the most important quantitative consideration appears to be the relative abundance of serum and tissue thyroxine-binding proteins which compete with the enzymes for the hormone. Several systems are capable of carrying out the dehalogenation, some being heat-stable, others requiring Fe^{++} and flavines or light. There is also evidence for the participation of peroxidases (Saunders & Stark, 1958; Galton & Ingbar, 1963). Since simple Fe^{2+} chelates and H_2O_2 can accomplish T_4 de-iodination, attempts to identify de-iodinases in crude systems cannot, at present, be interpreted (Reinwein & Rall, 1966). Some laboratories have reported tri-iodothyronine formation from thyroxine in kidney tissue, as well as certain inactive products de-iodinated in the "inner" ring (Flock et al., 1961). In in vitro systems there has been some disagreement about preferential de-iodination of the "inner" ring or the phenolic ring (Barker & Shimada, 1964) but no partially iodinated thyronines appear as intermediates, although the completely de-iodinated thyronine has been demonstrated (Lissitzky, Benevent, Roques & Roche, 1958). There is no convincing proof in man that injected, labelled thyroxine can be converted to detectable levels of tri-iodothyronine (e.g. in the athyreotic subject) (Lassiter & Stanbury, 1958). Since, however, tissues concentrate T_3 relative to T_4 as seen in plasma, this problem should be re-investigated by tissue analysis.

(4) The rupture of the diphenyl ether linkage used to be considered a difficult chemical feat but is actually quite readily accomplished. The enzymic cleavage of this bond has been accomplished by Lissitzky & Bouchilloux (1957). Plaskett (1961) has obtained a product that is readily converted to di-iodotyrosine and contains the iodine atoms of the inner ring of thyroxine. Nothing is known of the importance of this step in the intact subject. However, 2,6,di-iodohydroquinone, which is a product of this reaction, has been found in the urine after administration of labelled T_4 (Wynn & Gibbs, 1964).

Summary

The evidence for the pathway of iodine metabolism in the thyroid gland to date is consonant with the following scheme (Fig. 12.4).

It can be divided into a number of steps. The first is the active accumulation of iodide (independent of its further fate) in concentrations considerably above those of plasma. This iodide is

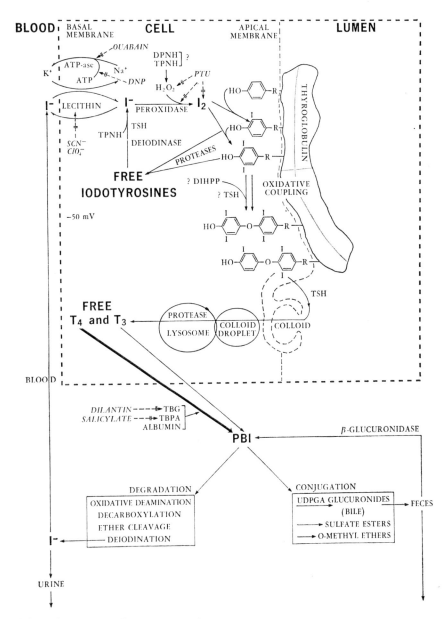

FIG. 12.4. Schematic summary of the pathway of iodine metabolism. Steps probably stimulated by TSH are indicated; inhibitors are printed in italics and their loci of action shown by - -‖- →

Abbreviations are:
PTU = 6 n-propylthiouracil
TSH = thyrotropin
DNP = 2,4-dinitrophenol
DPNH = diphosphopyridine nucleotide

TPNH = triphosphopyridine nucleotide
TBG = thyroxine-binding globulin
TBPA = thyroxine-binding prealbumin
UDPGA = uridine diphosphoglucuronic acid

oxidized, and then reacts with tyrosyl residues of thyroglobulin to form first mono-, and then di-iodotyrosine. These are coupled to form thyroxine and tri-iodothyronine probably while still in the thyroglobulin molecule. This protein is then hydrolysed by non-specific tissue proteases to yield the free iodinated amino-acids. Mono- and di-iodotyrosine are de-iodinated, and the liberated iodide re-enters the thyroid iodide or general pool. The most important factor influencing these mechanisms is the level of TSH which can independently activate both the release mechanism and, later, the iodide-concentrating mechanism. Free thyroxine (and tri-iodothyronine) is not de-iodinated to any extent, builds up a concentration gradient, and enters the circulation. Here the hormones are bound to two major binding proteins, thyroxine-binding globulin and pre-albumin. The hormones are distributed and metabolized as functions of their "free" levels. The major metabolic pathways are de-iodination, conjugation, and changes in the amino-acid side chain.

DIAGNOSTIC TESTS

There are two general classes of tests: those that measure the function of the thyroid gland *per se*, and those that measure the effects of the hormones in the periphery (BMR, cholesterol, creatine, enzyme levels, reaction time, etc.). While these often agree, there are many cases of dissociation between them, i.e. non-thyroidal factors tend to influence tests of one class without causing corresponding changes in the other.

The Basal Metabolic Rate

The basal metabolic rate (BMR) has, with the advent of other techniques, fallen into undeserved disrepute. In careful hands, and with adequate precautions to ensure basal conditions, reproducible results can be obtained. There are occasional conditions, such as the presence of large quantities of iodide or organic iodine compounds or agents that displace T_4 from binding proteins, when the BMR is one of the few readily available tests of moderate reliability. It is probably not safe to diagnose hyper- or hypometabolism on the basis of BMRs within the range of $+ 15$ to $- 15$, and exact limits vary in different geographical locations. In England the standards of Aub and Dubois appear to be somewhat high especially for the diagnosis of borderline thyrotoxicosis (Crooks, Murray & Wayne, 1958). On the other hand, since technical errors lead most often to falsely high BMR values, the Aub–DuBois standards give increased accuracy in

non-toxic disorders. Nevertheless, occasional patients with unquestioned thyroid disease (both hypo- and hyper-) are seen whose BMR lies in the "normal" range (Hendrick, 1938; Bartels, 1950; Werner & Hamilton, 1951).

Hyperthyroidism may show BMRs up to $+ 80$, but values in these high ranges are often complicated by fever and tremors, etc. BMR determinations of less than $- 45$, even in the severest case of myxoedema, are rarely found. In Table 12.3 are listed a number of conditions other than

TABLE 12.3

Changes in the BMR in conditions other than primary thyroid disease[1]

Low BMR

1. Sleep, narcolepsy.
2. Sedation (barbiturates, morphine, etc.).
3. Hypothermia (without shivering).
4. Excess body-water, e.g. in nephrosis, where there may be up to 20 kg. of non-metabolizing weight.
5. Extreme obesity, since adipose tissue has low O_2 consumption and tables are difficult to correct for this.
6. Malnutrition.
7. Anorexia nervosa and certain other mental disorders.
8. Addison's disease.
9. Simmond's or Sheehan's syndrome, i.e. secondary hypothyroidism.
10. Eunuchism (may be corrected by androgen therapy).
11. Fröhlich's syndrome.

High BMR

1. Patient is not basal (recent food or alcohol intake, restlessness or anxiety, Parkinsonism or other tremors, spastic torticollis, lack of sleep).
2. Perforated ear drum or other oxygen leaks.
3. Pregnancy.
4. Dyspnoea (cardiac, primary pulmonary disease, airway obstruction or anxiety).
5. Excess cardiac work (hypertension, severe anaemia, aortic stenosis, coarctation of the aorta, aortic regurgitation, Paget's disease).
6. Fever (subtract 10 to 13% per °C).
7. Leukaemias, lymphomas and polycythaemia.
8. Certain myopathies.
9. Acromegaly.
10. Cushing's syndrome (primary adrenal or pituitary origin).
11. Phaeochromocytoma.
12. Diabetes insipidus.
13. Drugs (dinitrophenol, salicylates, amphetamine, adrenaline, caffeine, smoking).

[1] Most of the conditions listed need not *necessarily* show an altered metabolic rate.

primary thyroid disease in which an altered BMR may be encountered on occasion. The test is most useful in confirmatory and follow-up studies, especially in therapy of hypothyroidism. In certain cases of hypermetabolism suspected of being due to anxiety it may be useful to measure the BMR under sedation or pentothal anaesthesia, during which such factitious hypermetabolism is abolished (Bartels, 1949).

Cholesterol

In hyperthyroidism serum cholesterol values tend to be low or low normal (normal range 150 to 250 mg./100 ml.), while in hypothyroidism values are often elevated. The test is more frequently abnormal in the hypothyroid states (Peters & Man, 1950; Bartels, 1950) but is perhaps most useful in following replacement therapy. The blood level is also influenced by the cholesterol content of the diet, diseases associated with poor fat absorption, some hepatobiliary diseases, nephrosis and certain other lipaemic states, xanthomatoses, etc. Cholesterol is a particularly unreliable index in untreated cretins where the level is often normal or low. Serum alkaline phosphatase levels, which are generally low, are much more valuable here. However, if such patients have once been treated and therapy is then withdrawn, the cholesterol levels rise to the hypothyroid range.

Creatine and Creatine Kinase

The creatine excretion depends on a non-specific determination of chromogens, and as a result the test is not used very often, although some feel it to be very helpful in Graves' disease (Griffiths, 1951). Since thyrotoxicosis is much more common in women, and since they also exhibit a physiological creatinuria, the test must depend on the quantity of creatine excreted (>100 mg./24 hr.) rather than on the mere appearance of creatine in the urine. In addition, the *creatine tolerance test* has been used to establish the diagnosis of Graves' disease. Normally, when 1·32 g. of creatine (equiv. to 1 g. of creatinine) are ingested, while the patient is on a low-creatine diet, less than 30% appears in the urine. In hyperthyroidism excess creatine appears in the urine ($<70\%$ retention) and the serum creatine will often exceed 0·5 mg./100 ml. (Richardson & Shorr, 1935; Tierney & Peters, 1943).

Creatine excretion and decreased creatine tolerance appear to be, in part, related to loss of muscle mass, but may appear before this is clinically demonstrable. However, other diseases involving muscle wasting, both primary, such as amyotonia congenita, pseudohypertrophic muscular dystrophy, myotonia atrophica, myasthenia gravis, etc., and beri-beri, as well as those secondary to neural lesions such as poliomyelitis, amyotrophic lateral sclerosis, etc., may show creatinuria. In addition creatinuria may be encountered during therapy with methylated androgens (Foss & Simpson, 1959).

It has been found that serum creatine kinase shows responses to variation in thyroid status not unlike that of cholesterol. It is elevated markedly in hypothyroidism and mildly depressed in thyrotoxicosis (Graig & Smith, 1965). Although not used extensively yet, it correlates well with thyroid status and the PBI. Normal values are 2·0 μmoles/ml./hr., hyperthyroid 0·7 and hypothyroid 13·2.

Measurement of serum alkaline phosphatase is occasionally useful in the diagnosis of hypothyroidism in children and is more useful for following the response to replacement therapy. Alkaline phosphatase levels may be elevated in hyperthyroidism.

Hydroxyproline

Another test of peripheral thyroid effect is urinary hydroxyproline excretion. Again it is fairly non-specific and obscured by growth and other skeletal variables yet it correlates well with thyroid status and will prove to be useful in problem cases and in follow up (Kivirikko, Laitinen & Lambeg, 1965). In general, total hydroxyproline is determined and no attempts are made to separate the small amounts of free amino acid from that present in peptides. Values are: normal: 16 to 41 mg./24 hr. in females (males slightly higher), hypothyroid: 8 to 15 mg./24 hr, hyperthyroid: 36 to 260 mg./24 hr. The normal range in children varies with the age.

Circulating Organic Iodine

Efforts to assess thyroid status by direct measure of the performance of the thyroid gland have dealt largely with two aspects of iodine metabolism: the uptake of iodine and the output and level of organic iodine. The last-named will be discussed first.

Organic iodine of the serum is to a large extent thyroxine ($\sim 85\%$), about 3% tri-iodothyronine, with traces of the iodotyrosines and up to 15% iodoprotein. A great many new methods have been developed recently for measuring these components since they may vary independently and thus give spurious results when measured as the total organic iodine, roughly equivalent to the protein-bound iodine (PBI). Nevertheless, the PBI will remain a standard first test for some time to come.

Protein-Bound Iodine (PBI)

Although T_4 and T_3 are not peptide-linked, they co-precipitate with the serum proteins, hence the name. The method is exceedingly prone to error by contamination, since 0·05 μg. amounts are generally determined; this contamination may be from iodine present in the serum or from glassware in the handling of the serum. The technical problems have been detailed (Sunderman, 1963; Davis, 1966; Robbins & Rall, 1967). Venous occlusion may raise the PBI, whereas extensive haemolysis is said to lower it.

The normal range of PBI is usually listed as 3·5 to 8·0 μg. of I/100 ml. of serum or plasma. However, the distribution curve is skewed, hence a statistical range about the mean (5·33 in males and 5·67 in females) is to be taken cautiously. Although commercial laboratories assume this normal range it has often not been tested against the clinical diagnosis. In our experience certain laboratories were consistently lower than others. This leads to a good deal of unnecessary blood letting. The width of the normal range may be partly due to differences in T_4-binding capacity since the free-T_4 appears to be the better index of peripheral thyroid status. Any diurnal, seasonal and other biological variation is apt to be < 1·0 μg./100 ml. A list of conditions influencing the PBI is given in Table 12.4. In addition high environmental temperature (summer) may decrease the PBI (Du Ruisseau, 1965).

In thyrotoxicosis the level is almost always elevated, values as high as 25 μg./100 ml. being occasionally encountered. Higher figures should arouse suspicion of contamination. Contamination can be checked by a total urine iodine determination (Fraser, Hobson, Arnott & Emery, 1953) or by one of the newer methods (see below). Contamination by iodine-containing drugs raises the PBI for highly variable periods (see Table 12.4). The specific hormone methods can avoid some but not all of these difficulties. The displacement method of Murphy et al. (1966) will likely prove the most useful for this purpose. The use of iodine compounds in floor washes, swimming pool disinfectants, as salts of various unrelated drugs, and of iodate in bread baking should be kept in mind. A list of drugs is given by Wayne et al. (1964).

Contamination by contrast media is clearly related to the function investigated. Dyes for urography are short-lived, while those for myelography or bronchography lead to contamination for many years (Table 12.4) Teridax crosses the placenta in sufficient quantity to be found in children six years after delivery from mothers exposed to this dye (Man, 1960; Shapiro, 1961; Ching & Karamourtjounis, 1960). When the organ investigated is diseased, excretion (and elevated PBI) may be prolonged. It is clear that where such studies cannot be avoided, the thyroid status should be investigated before radiography is carried out.

Other drugs will displace T_4 from binding proteins (Wolff et al., 1961) and thus lower the PBI since the free-T_4 can be maintained normal with a lowered PBI (the initial rise in free-T_4 is expected to last only a brief period—see previous section). In summary, it has been estimated that drug contamination accounts for 13% of false PBI values (Murphy et al., 1966).

An important problem in the diagnostic use of the PBI is the extensive use of oral contraceptive preparations. These may lead to an elevation of the PBI within 14 to 20 days after onset of therapy which can persist for as long as 4 to 12 weeks after cessation of medication (Williams et al., 1966). Thyroid gland function tends to be normal but the PBI is likely to be of little use in such women (see Table 12.5).

Butanol-Extractable Iodine (BEI)

Since repeated washing of serum precipitates is not useful in removing many iodine contaminants, extraction methods using butanol have been employed (Man et al., 1954). These methods removed contaminating iodoprotein, bromsulphthalein, and often, although not invariably, iodide. However, many contrast media contaminate the BEI as they do the PBI (Table 12.4). The normal range is 2·9 to 6·4 μg.I/100 ml.

Column Thyroxine

Chromatography is an obvious and effective way of removing non-hormonal iodine. Various supporting media have been used, but contamination is often not negligible and clinical analyses are usually carried out on Dowex 1 (see Robbins & Rall, 1967). Iodotyrosines and iodoproteins are readily removed when present (Pileggi, Segal & Golub, 1964) as are vast concentrations of iodide (Wolff et al., 1964). Contrast media such as Cholografin, Neo-iopax, Organidin, Priodax, Salpix and Skiodan are separated, but Hippuran, Miokon, Orabilex, Telepaque and Teridax contaminate (Pileggi, Lee, Golub & Henry, 1961; Davis, 1966). The normal range is 2·9 to 6·4 μg.I/100 ml.

Binding Displacement Method

Recently, a method has been developed in which extracted thyroxine (and T_3) is used to displace labelled T_4 from TBG and TBPA (serum). Free and bound T_4 are then separated on Sephadex or anion exchangers and counted (Murphy et al., 1966). While this method is relatively unaffected by iodine contaminants, etc., it suffers from rather poor recoveries of T_4 (77%) and may be sensitive to various dis-

TABLE 12.4

Effect of certain drugs on the ^{131}I uptake and protein-bound iodine level

Substance	^{131}I uptake	Duration[1] after cessation	PBI	Duration[1] after cessation
"Antithyroid Drugs"[2]				
KClO$_4$	decrease	days	decrease	days to weeks
Thiocarbamides	decrease	days to months	decrease	days to months
Aromatic Compounds				
p-aminosalicylic acid	decrease	days	decrease	weeks
Thiosemicarbazones[3]	decrease	days	decrease	days to weeks
p-aminobenzoic acid (PABA)	decrease	days	decrease	days to weeks
Carbutamide	decrease	?	?	?
Amphenone	decrease	< 1 day	decrease	?
Resorcinol ointment	decrease	days	decrease	weeks
Promizole	decrease	?	decrease	?
Phenylbutazone	decrease	days [5]	decrease	days
Phenylindandione	decrease	days?		
Aminoglutethimide			decrease	?
Germicides				
Betadine	decrease	days	increase	days
Parasiticides				
Floraquin	decrease	weeks	increase	weeks
Diodoquin, Vioform	decrease	weeks	increase	weeks
Iodine preparations	decrease	days to weeks	increase[4]	days to weeks
(Lugol's solution, KI syrup HI)				
Contrast Media				
Diodrast	decrease	1–4 weeks	increase	1–14 days
Hypaque	decrease	1–4 weeks	decrease	1–4 days
Salpix			increase	days
Orabilex			increase	4–9 weeks
Telepaque		2 months	increase	6–12 weeks
Cholografin		3 months	increase	3–4 months
Priodax	decrease	4–6 weeks	increase	3–4 months
Pantopaque			increase	3–12 months
Lipiodol	decrease	years	increase	years
Teridax	decrease	years	increase	many years
Displacing Drugs				
Salicylate	decrease	weeks	decrease	weeks
Diphenylhydantoin	O		decrease	?
Miscellaneous				
Mercurials	O		decrease	6–48 hours
Bromsulphthalein	O		increase	During period of retention
Thyroxine	decrease	11 weeks	increase	
Tri-iodothyronine	decrease		decrease	?
Corticosteroids	decrease	?	decrease	?
Vitamin A	decrease			
Meprobamate	decrease	?		
Low serum chloride	increase			
Erythrosin (Red Dye)			increase	2–3 weeks
2,3-Dimercaptopropanol (BAL)	decrease	hours	?	?
Disulfiram	decrease	?	decrease	?
Cobalt (CoCl$_2$)	decrease	days to weeks	decrease	weeks

Data taken from Chapman & Maloof, 1955; Grayson, 1960; Davis, 1966; Robbins & Rall, 1967.

[1] Figures for duration are highly variable.

[2] Most of these agents tend to depress the uptake while the patient is under treatment but, following cessation of therapy, they may lead to increased uptakes for varying periods because they are goitrogenic.

[3] Isoniazid, etc.

[4] In hyperthyroidism, iodine preparations may yield lower PBI measurements if special care is taken to wash out contaminating iodide.

[5] Temporary even if drug continued.

placing agents (e.g. diphenylhydantoin and probably salicylate). It is perhaps for this reason that the normal range is 4·0 to 9·8 μg. T_4/100 ml. or 2·9 to 6·4 μg. I/100 ml. and the diagnostic accuracy is somewhat less than for the PBI. Nevertheless, when contamination is a problem, this may prove to be the most useful method. A summary of blood hormone changes seen under various pathological conditions is given in Table 12.5.

TABLE 12.5

Changes in Circulating Hormones Levels in Thyroid and Other Diseases

Elevated PBI, BEI, T_4	Lowered PBI, BEI, T_4
Hyperthyroidism	Hypothyroidism (Primary, Secondary or in Hashimoto's)
Hereditary increase in TBG or (TBPA)	Hereditary decrease in TBG (or TBPA)
Subacute Thyroiditis (Acute phase)	Subacute Thyroiditis (Third stage)
Oestrogens (Ovulation suppressants)	Androgens, anabolic steroids, corticoids
Hydatidiform Mole	
Choriocarcinoma	
Embryomal Carcinoma of Testis	
Pregnancy	
T_4 Therapy	T_3 Therapy
	Nephrosis
? High Iodine Diet	Low Iodine Diet (Kempner Rice Diet)
	Malnutrition and Fasting
	Chronic Illness
Acute Intermittent Porphyria	
Acute phase of Hepatitis	
	Acromegaly (Decreased TBG)
New-born	
Contaminating drugs (see Table 12.4)	Displacing drugs (see Table 12.4)

Free Thyroxine

As mentioned earlier peripheral thyroid function correlates best with the level of free-T_4 in the blood. Changes in the PBI or total T_4 resulting from changes in the concentration of available binding sites (e.g. pregnancy or salicylates) can be better interpreted by an estimate of the dialysable fraction obtained by one of several methods under somewhat artificial conditions. This fraction is then multiplied by the total T_4, usually the PBI but preferably the column T_4. Values so obtained depend on the method and are from 0·026 to 0·050% dialysable (free) and 2·1 to 4·2

nanograms T_4/100 ml. of serum with the same method. The euthyroid range for any one method is narrower than in measurements of total T_4. Hyper- and hypothyroidism give the expected changes, whereas various euthyroid conditions with altered binding capacity have normal free-T_4 (Oppenheimer & Surks, 1964; Ingbar et al., 1965; Sterling & Brenner, 1966; Schussler & Plager, 1967). The considerable spread with different methods represent technical problems such as unpredictable effects of dilution, membrane binding of T_4, dialysable radioactive contaminants, and marked temperature sensitivity.

Tri-iodothyronine

Tri-iodothyronine determinations depend on the scrupulous removal, by chromatography, of the much more abundant T_4 as well as other contaminants. Although not yet available at a routine clinical level, the increasing realization that T_3 accounts for an important fraction of total hormone response, will soon lead to acceptance of this sort of measurement. Studies by Nauman et al., 1967 (using thin-layer chromatography for separation, followed by a displacement method) have given a total T_3 concentration of 0·33 μg./ 100 ml. with a free-T_3 fraction of 0·46%, and therefore a mean free-T_3 concentration of 1·5 nanograms T_3/100 ml. These values are similar to those from an earlier study by Pind (1957). These methods, as well as gas chromatographic analysis, have already shown that some cases of hyperthyroidism with normal PBI values may be due to excessive T_3 output.

Thyroxine-Binding Capacity

When the PBI or column T_4 measurements yield results contradicting other assessments of the thyroid status, alterations in the concentration of binding proteins or displacement of T_4 from these should be considered. Electrophoretic distribution of labelled T_4 (see Fig. 12.3) will give a rough indication of changes from the norm. Saturation of TBG and TBPA requires different optimal conditions (discussed by Ingbar & Braverman, 1965). In practice, T_4 is added to serum until the TBG is saturated (shown by electropherogram). The fraction bound to TBG multiplied by the total concentration (added plus that initially present) constitutes the capacity. Mass law considerations have been reviewed by Robbins & Rall (1967). Values for TBG capacity are 10 to 26 μg. T_4/100 ml.

An indirect test of the number of unoccupied binding sites, making no differentiation between TBG and TBPA, measures the transfer of a "tracer" dose of labelled T_3 to some adsorber. T_3

is used because its lower affinity for TBG facilitates measurement. The test is useful in cases of iodine contamination and as a rough estimate of anomalies in TBG or TBPA. Originally, washed erythrocytes were used to adsorb T_3 (Hamolsky et al., 1959). A variety of resins serve as well and give a more reproducible matrix, but each resin will have its own normal range depending on the nature of the resin and the ratio of resin to protein (see Robbins & Rall, 1967). The normal range with red cells is 11 to 19%. Values outside this range will be attained either by changes in T_4 supply or by changes in the concentration of sites.

Thyroid Function Tests Involving Radioactive Isotopes

Several isotopes emitting γ-radiation are currently in use for the evaluation of thyroid gland function. Of the 22 radioactive isotopes of iodine, three have found clinical use because of certain advantages depending on their half-lives and energies as listed in Table 12.6.

^{131}I has been and probably will be the most

tering, and directionality is therefore good (Myers & Vanderleeden, 1960); thyroid scans show better resolution than with ^{131}I (Riccabona, 1965). Tracer and scan doses can usually be less than for ^{131}I, cutting down the radiation by a factor of 10 (Porath, Hochman & Gross, 1966). However, these calculations have not included energy absorbed from the low energy Auger and internal conversion electrons and this may be quite considerable at short range. What fraction of this low energy radiation can reach the nucleus from the colloid is still uncertain. The isotope has not been widely used in routine clinical work in contrast to its great usefulness in the following:

(1) Equilibrium labelling of experimental animals (because of long half-life);
(2) labelling of synthetic compounds (because of long half-life);
(3) double isotope work (easily differentiated from ^{131}I);
(4) radioautography (because of very short range Auger and conversion electrons which give a high resolution image).

A disadvantage is the high absorption of radiation especially in media of high density and atomic number (Bakhle, Prusoff & McCrea, 1964).

TABLE 12.6

Properties of gamma-emitting isotopes used in thyroid function studies

Isotope	Chemical Form in which Used	Half-life	Principal γ-Radiation Kev	Thyroid Dose* rads/μc	Comments
^{125}I	I$^-$	60 d	27·4 (x-ray)	$\sim$ 110	Auger and Internal Conversion Electrons ^{125}Te daughter
^{131}I	I$^-$	8·05 d	364	118	β = 607 Kev, ^{131}Xe daughter
^{132}I	I$^-$	2.33 h	670, 760	4	^{132}Te parent ^{132}Xe daughter
^{99m}Tc	TcO$_4$$^-$	6.00 h	140	$\sim$ 0.32	^{99}Mo parent, ^{99}Tc daughter ($t_{1/2}$ = 2.1 · 10^{5}y)
^{186}Re	ReO$_4$$^-$	$\sim$90 h	137		Contaminated with 17 h ^{188}Re

* For complete decay, based on a 50-day biological half-life. The μc dose used for ^{99}TcO$_4$$^-$ is generally greater than for iodine isotopes so the differential factor is not as great as indicated. The effective half-life ($t_{1/2(eff.)}$) may be estimated as follows:

$$t_{1/2(eff.)} = \frac{t_{1/2} \cdot t_{1/2(biol.)}}{t_{1/2} + t_{1/2(biol.)}}$$

where $t_{1/2}$ is the physical half-life and $t_{1/2(biol.)}$ is the biological half-life in the thyroid.

extensively used isotope for biochemical, diagnostic and therapeutic purposes. It is the standard of comparison and will not be specifically discussed.

^{125}I emits a 27·4 Kev X-ray. The radiation absorbed for complete decay of a dose of equal initial disintegrations gives about 0·5 to 0·9 the energy absorbed by the thyroid after ^{131}I. There is less Compton scat-

^{132}I has two main advantages. The major one is a marked reduction in the thyroid irradiation. This amounts to about 0·03 to 0·04 of the ^{131}I dose per μc in a gland with a long biological half-life. Although the β and γ energies, as well as the dose rate are high, the very short half-life accounts for this difference (Hanbury, Heslin, Stang, Tucker & Rall, 1954; Halnan & Pochin, 1958; Goolden, 1964). The radiation dose per μc *administered* will be even less since the time to maximum uptake usually exceeds the half-life of ^{132}I. The general advantage, due primarily to the 2·3 h. half-life, but also the low radiation dose, is that repeated measurements can be made. As expected, the biological behaviour of this isotope does not differ from ^{131}I. However, short uptake times are required and this means, among other things, consideration of absorption. For this reason some groups have used intravenous injections for one hour uptakes. However, three or four hour uptakes are quite feasible and the oral route will usually be safe at these time intervals. In paediatric cases the higher radiation dose per μc should be kept in mind (because of the small gland), but size factors, etc. do not significantly change the ratio of radiation received from the three isotopes (Seltzer, Kereiakes & Saenger, 1964).

Pertechnetate (^{99}TcO$_4$$^-$) has recently become very popular because of its ideal energy characteristics which allow excellent collimation and localization (140 Kev. gamma radiation). In addition, the 6-hr. half-life and the absence of particle radiation lead to very low energy absorption in the thyroid (see Table 12.6). As shown above pertechnetate behaves to a large extent like iodide and is concentrated by all tissues that have the iodide trap, such as salivary glands, stomach, choroid plexus (which excludes it from the CSF) (Wolff & Maurey, 1962; Wolff, 1964; Andros, Harper, Lathrop & McCardle, 1965; Harden et al., 1967). Although a recent report states that as much as 50% of the anion is metabolized in the rat thyroid (Socolow & Ingbar, 1967), this is much less in beef thyroid slices (3 to 13%, mean 7%, Wolff unpublished), and in man, as shown by the nearly complete discharge obtained with perchlorate (Andros et al., 1965; Harden et al., 1967). The chief use will therefore be for scanning of the thyroid area and as a reasonably good measure of the anion trap.

The urinary ^{131}I excretion was once widely used (Skanse, 1949) but because of the problem of 24 hr. urine collections and the ease of neck counting it has been largely abandoned. The thyroid and kidney compete for circulating iodide, and hence, when the gland takes up more, less is available for urinary excretion, etc. The ranges for the 24 hr. urinary excretion of a tracer dose of radio-iodine are 40 to 70% in normals, 5 to 40% in hyperthyroids and > 70% in hypothyroid patients. The test is better for the diagnosis of hyperthyroidism since there is more overlap of the values in myxoedematous patients. Earlier intervals are more sensitive for detecting slight variations in thyroid function (Keating, Power, Berkson & Haines, 1947; Fraser et al., 1953). Extending measurements beyond 24 hr. is generally unnecessary.

In addition it is important to remember that urinary ^{127}I is readily determined and offers a clue to iodine deficiency. Due to wide regional variations in iodine intake the mean for a particular area must be known. Contamination is, of course, easily detected.

Thyroidal Uptake of Radioactivity

Two classes of problems should be kept in mind in studying thyroidal radio-iodine accumulation: (1) Technical problems in obtaining a true estimate of thyroid radioactivity. Thus early determinations show high background counts from extrathyroidal neck tissue and are corrected by subtracting the count over the thigh from that of the neck. Since the thigh contains less blood than an equivalent volume of neck tissue, such a correction will be too low. Other corrections for neck background as used, e.g. in clearance studies, have been mentioned. (2) Various physiological parameters which influence uptake. These are all influenced by factors which effect changes in thyroid activity (thyroid disease, thyroid size, TSH supply, use of drugs, etc.) and distribution of iodide (route of administration, renal clearance, volume of distribution, e.g. congestive failure). They are thus complex functions of many variables; the earlier in the pathway of iodine metabolism the fewer the variables.

The 24 hr. ^{131}I Uptake

The word "uptake" is a misnomer, since single counts measure only the radiation over the thyroid at these times and neglect that fraction of the radioactivity that has already left either as iodide or as hormonal iodine. An easy time for counting is 24 hr. after ^{131}I. Little advantage accrues from a 48 hr. count and, in addition, it occasionally misses an early peak and fall. The precise value for the normal range will depend on the "correction factor" applied for back scatter, adequacy of the phantom, on the diet and climate of the particular locality, etc. (e.g. Cassidy & Vanderlaan 1958). A normal range of 15 to 45% of the administered dose is frequently quoted, but in our own laboratory we have recently discovered that the normal range was lower than the standards we had been using (normal range 10 to 31%) hence a recheck may be necessary every 5 to 10 years. Many extraneous factors influence the uptake (see Table 12.4 and reviews by Grayson, 1960, and Sisson, 1965). In addition to those listed one should remember that thyroid depression with T$_4$ or T$_3$ may last a few weeks, sometimes longer, and that this may be followed by a brief period of rebound hyperactivity of the thyroid gland. Iodide-containing preparations (including bromides which may be contaminated with I$^-$) can influence ^{131}I$^-$ uptake in two ways: (a) by decreasing the specific activity of the tracer, and (b) by increasing the thyroidal iodide pool and organic iodine pool. Iodide given for long periods usually suppresses uptake for quite unpredictable times (except in iodide goitre) and may, of course, induce "permanent" effects in Graves' disease.

Conditions of compensatory hyperactivity such as endemic and congenital goitre (Stanbury *et al.*, 1954) or, rarely, post-thyroidectomy hyperplasia may give high uptakes in the absence of hyperthyroidism. Why this should persist in the latter is not clear—one would have to suppose either a lower than normal serum iodide level or the production of a metabolically less active secretion since thyroidal stores cannot accumulate indefinitely. Rebound hypofunction may occur after large doses of TSH (Perlmutter, Weisenfeld, Slater & Wallace, 1952). The ^{131}I uptake may be decreased in hot climates during the summer (Lewitus, Hasenfratz, Toor, Massry & Rabinowitch, 1964).

Short Term Uptakes of Radio-iodine

Unfortunately some overlap between normal and hyperthyroid uptakes does exist, and short term uptake studies with various isotopes (at present particularly ^{132}I and $^{99m}TcO_4{}^-$) were at first thought to give more satisfactory differentiation (Morton, Ottoman & Peterson, 1951; McConahey, Owen & Keating, 1956; Wayne *et al.*, 1964). While it is not clear whether these early tests are more discriminatory, they *are* more convenient, and the use of ^{132}I reduces radiation to the gland. The same is true for $^{99m}TcO_4{}^-$. Again there is wide regional variation in the normal ranges, e.g. in Glasgow the 2·5 hr. uptake is 10 to 35% and the 4 hr. uptake is 15 to 45% (Wayne *et al.*, 1964) whereas in our laboratory the normal 4 hr. range is 5 to 16%.

Thyroid clearances of ^{131}I during the early intervals after ^{131}I administration have been widely used (Keating *et al.*, 1949; Myant, Pochin & Goldie, 1949; Goodwin, Macgregor, Miller & Wayne, 1951; Berson, Yalow, Sorrentino & Roswit, 1952). These are measured by comparing changes in the neck count with either blood ^{131}I levels or with the thigh count (which is assumed to be a function of the blood level) (Foote & MacLagan, 1951; Berson *et al.*, 1952). With the latter technique, clearances are 3·7 to 41 ml./min./1·73 m² for euthyroid subjects (mean ∼ 18 ml./min.), 75 to 512 ml./min.1·73 m² for hyperthyroid patients, and 0 to 4·1 ml./min./1·73 m² in myxoedema. The neck: thigh ratio of counts serves as yet another index of thyroid status (Myant *et al.*, 1950). At two hours, using ^{132}I, the value was found to 2·7 to 6·6 in euthyroid

patients and 13 to 112 in untreated hyperthyroidism (Burkle & Lund, 1963).

Since ^{131}I uptakes do not, *per se*, measure the *amount* of iodine available to the gland for hormone biosynthesis, the use of plasma inorganic iodide (PII) has been developed (by the Glasgow group in particular). Assuming the specific activities of urine and plasma iodide to be the same, the PII is determined by measurement of urine specific activity after a tracer of labelled iodide and then determining the average plasma iodide from plasma iodide radioactivity (Wayne *et al.*, 1964). A method based on creatinine excretion yields similar results but seems less convenient (Boyle, Sloss, MacDonald & Gray, 1965). Values vary considerably, presumably mostly as a function of the diet, and range from mean values of 0·19 ± 0·04 to 0·63 ± 0·08 μg./100 ml. in different regions. The normal range within a group is, however, also very wide.

There is disagreement, at present, as to whether or not the PII is inversely related to the iodide clearance (Alexander *et al.*, 1964a; Rosen *et al.*, 1967; Oddie, Meade & Fisher, 1967). The product of the clearance and the PII is the absolute iodine uptake (AIU). These values are said to be more constant than the PII, ranging from 1 to 5·9 μg./hr. With iodide supplements the AIU will increase at least temporarily because PII rises exceed the fall in clearances. The fact that renal clearances of I^- show diurnal variation (Fisher *et al.*, 1965), and the fact that PII values vary with relation to meals, makes a 24 hr. thyroidal iodine intake difficult to estimate accurately. There are cases, however, where the AIU exceeds the output of hormone iodine. Although this may indicate a positive iodine balance in some cases, it probably attests to the fact that significant amounts of iodide may be lost from the gland (Fisher *et al.*, 1965).

The Conversion Ratio $\left(\dfrac{Protein\text{-}bound\ {}^{131}I}{Total\ {}^{131}I}\right)$ in Plasma or Serum

The rate of conversion of administered ^{131}I to plasma organic (protein-bound) ^{131}I was first suggested as a clinical test by Chaikoff, Taurog & Reinhardt (1947). Hyperthyroid patients show 45% or more of the total plasma ^{131}I in the organic fraction at 24 hr., euthyroid cases vary between 10 and 45%, and values less than 10% are suggestive of hypothyroidism (Clark, Moe & Adams, 1949; Freedberg, Ureles & Hertz, 1949; van Middlesworth, Nurnberger & Lipscomb, 1954). Some overlap into the normal range occurs from both sides, which can be reduced by employing the modification of Thode, Jaimet & Kirkwood (1954), who compare plasma protein-bound ^{131}I to salivary ^{131}I at 24 hr.

Riggs (1952) has demonstrated that the ratio is a function of at least eight variables. The calculated conversion ratio at 24 hr. forms a steep sigmoid curve when plotted against PB^{127}I over the concentration range of 4 to 12 μg./100 ml. and is useful for this reason alone. At earlier intervals the curve shifts to the right where it becomes more specific for hyperthyroidism, and at times greater than 24 hr. the test becomes useful for suspected hypothyroidism. Timing is thus important, and quantitative interpretation of this test should be cautious. For this reason the test is not used much at present.

The Tri-iodothyronine Suppression Test

^{131}I uptake in the normal thyroid gland can be suppressed by T$_3$ or dessicated thyroid and failure to obtain such suppression is characteristic of Graves' disease. Occasionally, rather large doses of hormone are required and for longer periods (usually 75 to 150 μg. of T$_3$/d. for eight days). Confusion has arisen at times because of a failure to take this into account (Greer & Smith, 1954; Werner & Spooner, 1955; Oddie, Rundle, Thomas, Hales & Catt, 1960; Burke, 1967). The test is, however, positive (no suppression) also in some cases of non-toxic nodular goitre. The exact criteria for the % suppression are debated and are not entirely independent of the pre-treatment uptake or the ability to measure small differences in rather low uptakes. In euthyroids uptake suppression is usually >20% of the pre-T$_3$ level. It is < 20% in most hyperthyroid patients but overlap will occur. Euthyroid patients with exophthalmos but suppressible thyroids tend not to develop hyperthyroidism (Burke, 1967). Suppressibility returns in many cases following successful management of hyperthyroidism. As a group the hyperfunctioning nodules fall between the normal and hyperthyroid mean percent suppression. Therefore, a neck "scan" is necessary.

In addition to the use of ^{131}I for quantitative measurement, it is extremely useful for localization studies. By the use of directional counting it is possible to localize areas of different ^{131}I concentration, and thereby (1) localize distant metastases in the rare cases when these are functioning, and (2) map the thyroid area in order to determine the functional status of thyroid nodules. In "hot nodules" (functioning adenomas) the surrounding thyroid tissue is often depressed in activity and "cold nodules" (malignancy, solitary nodules, cysts, etc.) may give counts less than or equal to the surrounding tissue (Cope, Rawson & McArthur, 1947; Dobyns, Skanse & Maloof, 1949; Allen, Kelly & Greene, 1952). For the reasons already mentioned, it is likely that the ^{99m}TcO$_4$$^-$ scan will replace ^{131}I and has already done so in some clinics. The relatively greater prominence of the salivary glands in ^{99m}TcO$_4$$^-$ scans must be kept in mind.

Measurement of TSH, LATS, the TSH reserve test, TSH responsiveness, and perchlorate discharge tests have been discussed elsewhere in this chapter.

ENDEMIC GOITRE

Endemic goitre is the most common of the thyroid disorders, its greatest prevalence coinciding in general with mountainous regions and underdeveloped areas. Endemics exist on all continents, with major areas in Northern India and the Himalayas, the Alps and Pyrenees, Burma and Southwest China, and the Andes. Other foci are found in Southern Brazil, the Northern U.S., the southwestern part of Great Britain, New Zealand, Australia and in numerous areas in Africa. While cretinism is more common in goitrous areas, the majority of patients are clinically euthyroid.

Endemics have often been correlated with areas of iodine lack, but evidence for this has, until recently, been unreliable. Iodine analyses of foods and water in goitre belts have yielded subnormal values, but, as Greenwald (1946) and Ucko (1947) have pointed out, older methods were unsatisfactory and did not necessarily support the conclusions. Many other aetiological factors have been invoked, especially foods and virus infections (reviewed by Greer, 1950). The diet may interfere with iodine metabolism, and the studies of Greer & Astwood (1948) have established that a variety of foods contain antithyroid materials. They isolated 5-vinylthio-oxazolidone (from rutabaga) which proved to be a potent antithyroid agent in man and rats. In the plant the material exists as a thioglycoside of 2-hydroxy-3-butenyl isothiocyanate which, upon hydrolysis by the plant enzyme myrosin, or by similar enzymes in the body, cyclizes to the active product (Greer & Deeney, 1959).

Studies in Tasmania and Australia (Clements & Wishart, 1956; Clements, 1957) have shown that goitre may be caused by goitrogenic agents. An increase in goitre incidence coincided with the introduction of a free milk scheme in the schools as well as to changes in the pattern of fodder crops. It was shown that the milk from cows fed chou moellier, etc. suppressed thyroidal ^{131}I accumulation in some cases. Unfortunately, the results of these ^{131}I studies were ambiguous. Children from the same area fed powdered milk instead of local milk had no goitre. A similar endemic, possibly resulting from milk goitrogens, has been reported from Finland (Peltola, 1960). In certain areas goitrogenic agents derive from cruciferous weeds such as *Rapistrum rugosum* and others. Bachelard & Trikojus (1960) have isolated the isothiocyanate cheiroline from this weed and find that it may

Progoitrin

((-)-5-vinylthio-oxazolidone)

Goitrin

be further altered in the rumen of the cow. Furthermore, benzyl isothiocyanate has been identified as a cause of taint in milk, in this case from cows feeding on the cruciferous weed "lesser swine cress" (*Coronopus didymis*) (Forss, 1951). The role of these in endemic goitre is not yet proven.

A new thioglycoside was recently isolated from a *Brassica* plant which can, upon hydrolysis by myrosin, yield SCN$^-$ ion (Virtanen, 1961).

Glucobrassicin

As yet it has not been possible to show that enough SCN$^-$ is released into cows' milk to make the latter goitrogenic. The thioglycosides and isothiocyanate are widely distributed and it is very likely that others will be identified as possible causative agents of endemic goitre. Some of the outbursts of goitre have occurred despite iodine prophylaxis, whereas in neighbouring districts iodine prophylaxis seemed to be effective over the same period, suggesting, though not proving, that iodine deficiency may have played an additional role. It is also possible that in the latter case the responsible goitrogen was of the SCN$^-$ type, i.e. these cases *should* show a better response to iodine prophylaxis. It has been pointed out that the presence of a number of positive goitrogens in the same diet, each ineffective alone, might together be responsible for goitre formation (Langer, 1966).

The best documented case for an endemic due to a positive goitrogen comes from Hokkaido (Suzuki, Higuchi, Sawa, Ohtaki & Horiuchi, 1965). The responsible agent is present in seaweed (Kombu), which is consumed in considerable quantity, and ironically, is presumably iodide. The picture is one of a block in organic iodine formation leading to diffuse goitre etc., which is relieved simply by deleting seaweed from the diet. This endemic is discussed further under "Iodide Goitre".

Many modern studies on endemic goitre have followed the now classical work of Stanbury *et al.* (1954) in Argentina. Although positive goitrogens have not been ruled out, iodine lack is directly involved in the endemics of Argentina, the Congo, and New Guinea. Evidence for this is the very low iodine intake (De Visscher, Beckers, van den Schrieck, de Smet, Ermans, Galperin & Bastenie, 1961), low urinary iodine excretion ($< 5 \mu g./day$) (Choufoer, van Rhijn, Kassenaar & Querido, 1963; Stanbury *et al.*, 1954), and the low level of circulating inorganic iodide. In an attempt to compensate, ^{131}I uptakes are very high, as are thyroid clearances. These are inversely proportional to the urinary ^{127}I output (Stanbury *et al.*, 1954; De Visscher *et al.*, 1961; Choufoer, van Rhijn & Querido, 1965).

Thyroid glands from such patients show the high MIT/DIT ratios expected for iodine deficiency (Ermans *et al.*, 1963). In some cases surprisingly little radioactivity is found in the T_4 fraction. These cases are considered to be a group with a homogeneous, slow turnover pool. Other thyroids release very high specific activity thyroxine indicating considerable heterogeneity even in such active thyroids. It is of interest that despite iodine deficiency iodide escapes from the thyroid in sizeable amounts, presumably from rapid intrathyroidal de-iodination (Ermans *et al.*, 1963).

When the patients in Argentina received supplements of iodide, their ^{131}I uptakes fell to normal very gradually. The rate at which the theoretical "equilibrium" was reached was not influenced markedly by the dose of administered iodide, although the net positive iodine balance was proportional to the dose (Stanbury *et al.*, 1954). Treatment with 200 mg./day of desiccated thyroid led to a more rapid fall in the ^{131}I uptake than did iodide therapy. After six weeks of thyroid therapy the uptake in a number of the thyroid-treated cases dropped below the normal for non-goitrous glands. Only one of the patients showed a significant decrease in goitre size, which is similar to experience in adult populations in Switzerland; hence thyroid therapy is not often employed.

HYPOTHYROIDISM

Cretinism

Deficiency of thyroid hormone produces effects of varying permanence depending on the age at which it occurs. Starting in the adult, almost all the effects are reversible. But if the deficiency occurs during the period of early growth, permanent changes may result, leading to cretinism. The constitutional defects are the result of thyroid hormone lack occurring at any time from foetal life to the end of the growth period. This may be followed in later life by any state of thyroid activity. There are a number of types of cretinism. The most common type occurs in areas of endemic goitre, especially in families where goitre has been present for several generations. Whether or not the thyroid status of the parents is a contributing cause to cretinism in the offspring has not been fully established, thus e.g. two areas of equal prevalence of endemic goitre may have a widely varying incidence of cretinism. Consanguinity in the parents of some endemic cretins suggests that genetic factors will have to be considered (*Bull. World Health Org.* Vol. 18, 1958). Such cases show thyroid enlargement with areas of hyperplasia and involution with an increased avidity for iodide unless degeneration supervenes. Besides the clinical features which define the entity, these patients may demonstrate any or most of the signs of adult hypothyroidism. The PBI is often low and there may be iodoprotein in the serum. The cholesterol level is not usually elevated. Although these patients are from endemics it is surprising how many of them do *not* have goitre or even palpable thyroid glands (Bastenie, Ermans, Thys, Beckers, van den Schrieck & De Visscher, 1962; Choufoer *et al.*, 1965). In the Congo this was associated with inadequate compensation in the ^{131}I uptake despite an apparently normal pattern of ^{131}I metabolism. They responded poorly to TSH, apparently due to existing maximal stimulation. The sellae were enlarged. Antithyroid antibodies were not present. It was concluded that cretinism ensues in those cases that do not compensate adequately to iodine deficiency (Dumont, Ermans & Bastenie, 1963). However, in other areas uptake was markedly increased (Stanbury *et al.*, 1954; Choufoer *et al.*, 1965).

The goitrous cretin in endemics may no longer show hypothyroidism when examined later in life. Thus Stanbury *et al.* (1954) encountered about 50 persons who met the criteria for cretinism, but were euthyroid by clinical standards as well as by PBI (3·4 to 6 μg./100 ml. with a mean of 4·6; two patients had PBI levels in the toxic range). The uptake of ^{131}I by such patients has been reported to be low-normal (Vogliazzo, Viole, Scorta & Marchis, 1952). Hence, at some time during early growth, the thyroids of these cretins could not supply "adequate" quantities of the hormone, and this had led to permanent damage. Today their glands show enough function to maintain them euthyroid. In other cases "exhaustion atrophy" leads to permanent hypothyroidism, while yet others may actually become thyrotoxic (Bartels, 1945; Sexton & Mack, 1954). The iodine supply of the moment may well determine the thyroid status of the cretin possessing a thyroid.

Some goitre endemics are associated with a high prevalence of deaf-mutism. While cretinism in these areas is common, and is often co-existent with deaf mutism and various motor disorders (Choufoer *et al.*, 1965), it is uncertain whether the associated defects are the result of early hypothyroidism since athyreotic cretins show no such prevalence of deaf-mutism. In other endemics these increases in deafness have been absent. From a review of the complex literature in this field Trotter (1960) tends to the view that the aetiology is related in some way to environmental rather than genetic factors, but no satisfactory explanation exists at present.

The most common cause of cretinism in areas of adequate iodine supply is due to thyroid aplasia (sporadic cretinism), sometimes defined as having a 24 hr. ^{131}I uptake of $< 10\%$. However, a sizeable fraction of these may have small remnants of functioning ectopic thyroid tissue that can be detected by careful scanning. These rests do little to diminish the hypothyroidism, but have suggested maldescent of the thyroid as an aetiological factor in athyreotic cretinism (Little, Meador, Cunningham & Pittman, 1965). In some cases ectopic tissue is found at the base of the tongue and is then called *lingual thyroid*. It may or may not be accompanied by hypothyroidism and, in some cases, a defect in organification as demonstrated by the $KClO_4$ discharge test (Ferrini & Biassoni, 1966). From a correlation between cretinism and the increased incidence of circulating antithyroid antibodies in these children (see section on thyroiditis), it has been suggested that some cases of athyreotic cretinism may result from the cytotoxic effect of placentally transferred antibodies, but there is currently no evidence to support this (Chandler, Blizzard, Hung & Kyle, 1962; Forbes, Roitt, Doniach & Johnson, 1962). An abnormally high proportion of non-tasters of phenylthiocarbamide has been reported in athyreotic cretins and their parents (Fraser, 1961).

Whether this has any aetiological significance is unknown.

Several findings in cretins are of special interest. The retarded bone age is characterized by epiphyseal dysgenesis—a widespread defect of endochondrial ossification of those centres, and only those, whose appearance is delayed by the hypothyroidism. The typical picture shows multiple irregular foci of ossification which enlarge and finally coalesce to form irregular spongy masses (Wilkins, 1941). The marked elevation of serum alkaline phosphatase expected during normal bone growth does not occur. Even before there is detectable bone growth the alkaline phosphatase level appears to be a good index of response to hormone therapy.

The most important consideration for all cretins, no matter what the aetiology, is the uncertain prognosis for mental development. The severity of the deficit depends on the onset, duration and severity of thyroid deficiency. At any period during the myelination and rapid growth of the brain thyroid deficiency may lead to permanent mental deficiency (Eayrs, 1964; Money & Lewis, 1964). Prognosis depends on early diagnosis and the time of onset and adequacy of the replacement therapy. The fraction of severe cretins who attain an IQ > 90 falls rapidly during the first year and is negligible thereafter (Wilkins, 1965). Hypothyroidism developing after the second to third year of life is not usually attended by irreversible mental deficiency.

Congenital Goitre

There are several other types of cretins whose disorders, though rare, shed considerable light on the physiology of the human gland. These patients all have goitres and the term congenital goitre is often used to classify them. Any of the identifiable steps of thyroxine biosynthesis may be deranged separately and the defects are listed here in the order of passage of iodine through the thyroid gland.

(1) An *iodide transport defect* characterizes the first group for which only five cases have, so far, been reported (Stanbury & Chapman, 1960; Wolff *et al.*, 1964). The thyroid gland is unable to concentrate iodide and has to depend on diffusion of the anion into the gland. This proves to be inadequate for hormone requirements and goitre and hypothyroidism ensue. Other iodide-concentrating tissues such as the salivary gland, gastric mucosa and choroid plexus are also unable to concentrate iodide. This widespread I^- concentrating deficit does not occur in other forms of congenital goitre or in sporadic cre-

tinism. The hypothyroidism and goitre can be entirely alleviated by "diffusing" enough iodide into the gland with large doses of KI, suggesting that no other defect occurred in the biosynthetic apparatus. In a single gland from such a patient (kindly supplied by Dr. Henry Hawkins, University of Minnesota), we have found ample Na^+-K^+-dependent ATPase, but an absence of the iodide-binding phospholipid. This suggests that the defect probably lies with the hypothetical iodide carrier.

(2) The second type of congenital goitre is characterized by *defective organification* with high ^{131}I uptakes and rapid peaking of thyroidal ^{131}I often seen in very active and/or blocked glands. Most of this activity can be almost immediately discharged by KSCN (Fig. 12.6), or $KClO_4$, indicating that these glands lack the necessary systems for the conversion of inorganic to organic iodine. Such glands are therefore low in iodine (^{127}I) and most of this is in the inorganic form (Stanbury & Hedge, 1950), whereas most of the iodine in normal glands is organic. The enzymic defect may be in the iodide peroxidase (Haddad & Sidbury, 1959) but this is, as yet, uncertain. The pituitary glands of these and other cretins have long been known to be enlarged (Niépce, 1851), and it seems most probable that there is adequate or excessive thyrotropic stimulation in these cases. The size of these goitres often decreases when such patients are treated with desiccated thyroid. About 40 such cases have been studied, but genetic interpretation is as yet uncertain (Leszynsky, 1964; Stanbury, 1966). A similar defect occurs in a transplantable rat thyroid tumour (Wolff, Robbins & Rall, 1959), a human thyroid carcinoma (Valenta, 1966), and in some cases of ectopic (lingual) thyroid tissue (Ferrini & Biassoni, 1966).

An interesting variant of this defect exists in patients with sporadic goitre and deaf-mutism (Pendred's syndrome). These cases, first studied in detail by Brain (1927), are familial and are inherited as a simple recessive. The hearing defect is of the perceptive type with greater loss for high than low tones. Vestibular function may also be impaired. The thyroidal defect is one of reduced capacity to form organic iodine from iodide as in the above cases, so that part of the accumulated ^{131}I (at early intervals) can be discharged by $KClO_4$. The "discharge" phenomenon with SCN^- or ClO_4^- resembles that from glands in which organic iodine formation was artificially blocked with antithyroid agents (Fig. 12.5). The defect is partial since most subjects affected with Pendred's syndrome are

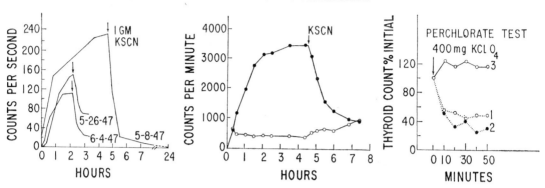

FIG. 12.5. The discharge of ^{131}I from the thyroid gland by SCN^- or ClO_4^-. *Left*—Patient with thyrotoxicosis on treatment with mercaptoimidazole (5/8/47 and 6/4/47) or propylthiouracil (5/26/47). KSCN was given orally. Note the differences in the degree of organic binding of ^{131}I on the three different dates, i.e., anti-thyroid therapy was nearly completely effective on 5/8/47—over 95% of the ^{131}I being discharged by SCN^-. In contrast only 55% of the radioactivity could be discharged on 5/26/47 indicating incomplete blocking of hormone biosynthesis (from Stanley & Astwood, 1948). *Centre*—Accumulation and discharge of ^{131}I from the goitre of a congenital cretin unable to synthesize significant quantities of organic iodine. Two grams of KSCN were given orally as indicated. Note that rise in body background (light circles) after SCN^- administration (from Stanbury & Hedge, 1950). *Right*—Discharge of accumulated ^{131}I from the thyroid glands of two patients with Pendred's Syndrome (Cases 1 and 2) and a normal sibling of the same family (Case 3). $KClO_4$ was given orally one hour after a tracer dose of [131]I. (Redrawn from Fraser, Morgans & Trotter, 1960).

euthyroid. Over 100 such cases have been described in a relatively short period and the syndrome appears to be more common than that in which deafness is absent (Fraser, Morgans & Trotter, 1960; Thould & Scowen, 1964; Nilsson, Borgfors, Gamstorp, Holst & Liden, 1964; Bax, 1966).

(3) *Partial failure in the coupling of two halogenated tyrosyl residues* to form thyroid hormone has been suggested in a few cases (reviewed by Stanbury, 1966). Claims have been made that Pendred's syndrome may also show this coupling defect, but more work is needed to establish this (Hollander, Prout, Rienhoff, Ruben & Asper, 1964; Shane, Jones & Flink, 1965).

Uptake of ^{131}I is high, retention is prolonged, and ^{131}I is not discharged by SCN^- or ClO_4^-. After [131]I^- administration, little thyroxine or tri-iodothyronine can be demonstrated in the gland despite abundant quantities of labelled mono- and di-iodotyrosines. It is thus not likely to be merely a type of iodine deficiency although to prove this defect it would be necessary to test thyroxine synthesis under conditions of iodide loading. Although the PBI is low, there is early appearance of labelled thyroxine in the circulation suggesting that coupling can occur either in a very small thyroxine pool or with considerable heterogeneity of the organic iodide. Since the thyroglobulin molecule appears to

supply conformational properties that favour the coupling reaction (Van Zyl & Edelhoch, 1967), it may be that certain changes in the tertiary structure of the protein are responsible. No evidence for this exists as yet (Stanbury, 1967).

It has often been found that thyroglobulin is absent and that the iodinated proteins are largely albumin-like or other smaller proteins (Tubiana, Mozziconacci, Attal, L'Hirondel & Girad, 1965; Lizarralde, Jones, Seal & Jones, 1966). [131]I uptake is high, as is the release rate of ^{131}I from the gland. It is not clear whether failure to find the thyroglobulin proves a defect in its synthesis. Only in congenitally goitrous sheep has there been evidence of decreased amino-acid incorporation into thyroglobulin (Falconer, 1966). Only two cases of an abnormal thyroglobulin have been demonstrated (Robbins, *et al.*, 1966; De Nayer *et al.*, 1967). In summary, a coupling defect has not been established entirely satisfactorily.

(4) Congenital goitre with inadequate thyroidal and peripheral de-iodination of the iodinated tyrosines has been described (Stanbury, 1966). In the normal thyroid, free iodotyrosine is de-iodinated locally and the liberated iodide is re-utilized. In the absence of the thyroidal de-iodinase this amino acid enters the blood. If peripheral de-iodination were intact the body could still hold on to that portion of the iodide not cleared by the kidneys. In the absence of this

second de-iodinase, the iodine leaves via the kidneys as iodotyrosine, thus creating a relative deficiency of iodine despite a normal intake. Exogenously administered labelled iodotyrosines are almost quantitatively excreted in the urine.

Although a de-iodinase like that of the thyroid exists peripherally it has recently become clear that de-iodination is much more complex (Reinwein & Rall, 1966) and may occur under many conditions. Peroxidase and other haem proteins similarly de-iodinate iodophenols (Saunders & Stark, 1958). However, when the de-iodinating defect is restricted to the thyroid, the patients are euthyroid (Kusakabe & Miyake, 1964). This suggests that failure of *peripheral* de-iodination is the determining event, and whatever the mechanism, the association of a de-iodinating defect with cretinism or hypothyroidism is established. Low PBI, high ^{131}I uptake with rapid discharge from the gland, and circulating iodotyrosines are characteristic. If this is the sole defect resulting in hypothyroidism ultimately due to iodine deficiency, then a sufficient iodide supplement *alone* should correct the hypothyroidism. This appears indeed to be the case in the few patients where this has been tried (Lissitsky, Comar, Rivière & Codaccioni, 1965; Harden, Hilditch, Kennedy, Mason, Papadopoulos & Alexander, 1967). An extensive family tree has shown that these cases are homozygous, behaving as a simple autosomal recessive trait (Hutchinson & McGirr, 1956) although di-iodotyrosine has actually been demonstrated in only a few cases.

(5) The secretion from the thyroid gland of metabolically inactive iodinated materials other than di-iodotyrosine has also been reported in congenital goitre. These compounds are not butanol-extractable and are polypeptides or proteins which become labelled with ^{131}I (De-Groot & Stanbury, 1959; Stanbury, 1966). On hydrolysis of sera containing these compounds nearly all of the radioactivity becomes butanol-extractable consisting, in addition to the iodothyronines, of mono- and di-iodotyrosine. Thyroid glands from such patients may show, in addition to thyroglobulin, an increased amount of an iodinated protein with a sedimentation coefficient of $S_{20,w} = 4S$. This material may be the precursor of the abnormal circulating substance and resembles the compound first described by Robbins in patients with cancer of the thyroid. In at least some instances this is iodinated serum protein. It is not clear why loss of part of the thyroid iodine as an "unutilizable" protein should cause hormone deficiency, and it should be pointed out that the majority of patients with such compounds are either less severely hypothyroid or euthyroid.

In summary then, cretinism can occur in patients:

(1) without thyroids (athyreotic cretins), or with ectopic tissue,

(2) from endemics, whose thyroids supplied inadequate hormone during the growth period but who may be hypothyroid, euthyroid or hyperthyroid when seen,

(3) lacking an iodide-concentrating mechanism,

(4) lacking an oxidizing system for I$^-$,

(5) with defective thyroidal iodothyronine formation from iodotyrosines (not firmly established),

(6) whose thyroids have little thyroglobulin or with abnormal thyroglobulin (not firmly established),

(7) with inadequate de-iodination of iodotyrosines,

(8) whose thyroids release an abnormal and inactive product.

Whatever the cause of cretinism, the prognosis is poor especially with regard to mental achievement, and early recognition and vigorous treatment are of the utmost importance.

Adult Hypothyroidism and Myxoedema

The aetiology of myxoedema is unknown in most cases except when it follows surgery, radioiodine, or antithyroid therapy (the hypothyroidism following such treatments may be transient). Subacute thyroiditis can, in very rare cases, be established as an antecedent event, and, more frequently, hypothyroidism may follow documented Hashimoto's thyroiditis. It has been repeatedly pointed out that the age and sex distribution, incidence of pre-existing thyrotoxicosis, level of antibodies to thyroid antigens (especially the complement-fixing type), and the histology of the thyroid, in thyroiditis and hypothyroidism are similar (Buchanan & Harden, 1965). It has been reported that hypothyroidism follows thyroidectomy for thyrotoxicosis more often when the surgical specimen reveals marked lymphocytic infiltration. Although antibody titres and tests of iodine metabolism show greater activity in thyroiditis than in myxoedema, the findings suggest that the two disorders may result from the same pathological process. Thus, hyperactivity if the gland in thyroiditis may be thought of as an attempt at compensation, which, if it fails, eventually leads to hypothyroidism. The correlation between primary myxoedema and antibody titres is so high that this test may be of aid in distinguishing primary from secondary hypothyroidism. (Vallotton, Pretell & Forbes, 1967). Other infiltrative disease rarely causes hypothyroidism. Lastly, the possibility that hypothyroidism may occur in rare patients with functioning thyroids, but who do not respond to their own or to exogenously administered hormone, presumably because of peripheral (end-organ) unresponsiveness, should be kept in mind (Reiss & Haigh, 1954; Refetoff, DeWind & DeGroot, 1967). The latter group may respond to very large doses of hormone (DeGroot, personal communication).

Foremost among the manifestations of hypothyroidism is a generalized decrease in activity in nearly all organ systems; this may lead to such signs as fatigue, weakness, sensitivity to cold, decreased sweating, constipation and decreased peristalsis, bradycardia, decrease in the voltage of the ECG complexes and increased P-R interval, and slow relaxation of the ankle jerks. Finally, puffiness, dryness and coarsening of the skin and hair, loss of hair and change in voice are observed. An estimate of the relative diagnostic usefulness of the various signs and symptoms of myxoedema (and of hyperthyroidism) has been made by Wayne (1960).

The metabolic rate is decreased and BMR values below −15 must be considered significant when other causes of hypometabolism have been ruled out (see Table 12.3). In a small group of myxoedematous patients, however, the BMR lies in the normal range (Hurxthal, 1934). The decrease in BMR is reflected in the metabolic rate of isolated tissues. Oxygen consumption (Qo_2) studies in rat tissues (Gordon & Hemming, 1944; Barker & Klitgaard, 1952; and many others) have revealed that nearly all tissues participate in the drop in O_2 consumption in hypothyroidism with the exception of adult brain, spleen and testis.

The patient who has developed myxoedema as an adult expresses herself slowly, but cerebration often appears otherwise intact and she may even seem witty. Cerebellar symptoms may be marked and respond readily to therapy (Jellinek & Kelly 1960). Psychosis apparently due to unrecognized myxoedema has been discovered in mental institutions—the so-called "myxoedema madness". Dramatic improvement often follows thyroid replacement therapy in such cases (Asher, 1949; Calvert, Smith & Andrews, 1954). Myxoedema occurring prior to brain maturation (cretinism) may lead to almost any degree of mental deficiency. The EEG yields a slow pattern and alpha waves may be absent and are a good guide to the progress of therapy.

The most serious consequence of adult myxoedema is myxoedema coma. An outstanding characteristic is a severe hypothermia which may reach temperatures of 24°C. Onset of coma is often in winter. This is often accompanied by hypotension, shallow respirations and CO_2 narcosis. Grand mal seizures may occur but otherwise the EEG may show very little cerebral activity. Hyponatraemia may occur, but evidence for adrenal insufficiency is only occasionally found. There may be gastro-intestinal bleeding (Nickel & Frame, 1961; Holvey, Goodner, Nicoloff & Dowling, 1964). The onset may be gradual but can be precipitated by trauma, infection, etc., or occasionally by the administration of drugs such as chlorpromazine. The high incidence reported from Britain may be due, in part, to the national preference for low room temperatures. The mortality rate has been very high (up to 80%). Myxoedema coma requires vigorous treatment. This includes: intravenous tri-iodothyronine or thyroxine in large initial doses (up to 100 μg. and 500 μg., respectively). assisted respiration in some cases, and perhaps adrenal steroids. The use of pressor agents, though occasionally useful, may be dangerous in conjunction with T_3 or T_4 administration (Holvey et al., 1964; Perlmutter & Cohn, 1964). Warming of the patient should probably be gradual if done at all, although the question is not settled.

Cardiac complaints occur frequently and may constitute the only presenting symptom in myxoedema. The weakness and fatigue may, in part, be related to the heart. Repeated claims are made that myxoedema predisposes to coronary arteriosclerosis (Bartels & Bell, 1939), and that angina pectoris occurs with increased frequency (Peel, 1943; and many others), but the evidence is not convincing (Hamolsky, Kurland & Freedberg, 1961). That more angina is not encountered is probably due to the decrease in the BMR, and thyroid therapy often initiates cardiac pain even before the BMR has approached normal values Hence one is wise to undertake thyroid therapy by small increments. Nevertheless, myxoedematous patients are encountered whose angina is improved by small doses of desiccated thyroid (Peel, 1943).

The decreased load on the heart resulting from a lowered BMR, and the decreased sensitivity to adrenaline, has led a number of cardiac clinics to treat intractable angina or congestive failure by induction of hypothyroidism with surgery, antithyroid medication, and more recently by ^{131}I irradiation (Blumgart, Freedberg & Kurland, 1950). Small doses of desiccated thyroid are given until the patient's maximum level of comfort is attained. Patients with angina respond more favourably than do those with congestive failure. However, this form of therapy has not been widely used.

Myxoedema heart is not common. It occurs usually in cases of full-blown myxoedema, and is characterized by diffuse dilatation (which may also occur in cretins), and/or pericardial effusion, slow and poor contractions, and decreased voltage on the ECG with or without prolongation of the P-R interval (Hamolsky et al., 1961; Kern, Soloff, Snape & Bello, 1949). At autopsy non-specific oedematous infiltration of the myocardium has been reported, occasionally accompanied by a mucinous, PAS-positive material. There is no cardiac hypertrophy.

Most of the circulatory functions are decreased As a result of the slowing of the circulation (arm to tongue circulation time 20 to 30 sec.) the A-V oxygen differences may be increased (Stewart, Deitrick & Crane, 1938; Sokoloff, Wechsler, Mangold, Balls & Kety, 1953). Consequently the cardiac output can decrease beyond that expected for the reduction in O_2 consumption, and the heart in myxoedema or hypothyroidism might thus be considered to be more efficient. Additional economy may derive from a higher mechanical efficiency (25%), claimed by Briard, McClintock & Baldridge (1935), in the conversion of calories to kilogram metres.

The general decrease in energy metabolism may be partly responsible for the increased sensitivity to cold and the decrease in sweating. However, in addition, the blood flow to the skin is reduced from an approximate normal of 4% of the total cardiac output to about 1·3% in myxoedema, where cardiac output is already diminished (Stewart & Evans, 1941, 1942). There is also an increase in capillary permeability (Lange, 1944), and it is possible that the myxoedematous infiltration of the skin and the occasional anasarca are in part related to this phenomenon, as both disappear upon treatment. No constant alterations in blood pressure are observed; the pulse pressure is sometimes decreased.

The hypodynamic peripheral circulation probably also accounts for the decreases in renal blood flow, glomerular filtration rate, filtration fraction, tubular secretory capacity or clearances and the ability to excrete a water load (Papper & Lancastremere, 1961). Albuminuria occurs not infrequently, but cells are uncommon. Pathological evidence for primary kidney disease is seldom found. Clearance of iodide decreases in myxoedema (Riggs, 1952; Hlad & Bricker, 1954).

The endocrine organs are often depressed in myxoedema and, since the pituitary may also be involved, the problem of deciding whether target organs are primarily or secondarily affected becomes a formidable one. On the other hand the pituitary increases TSH production and there may be enlargement of the sella, especially in endemic cretins. Myxoedema may be accompanied by hypo-adrenalism, or may be the apparent cause of it (Schmidt's syndrome) (Bloodworth, Kirkendall & Carr, 1954; Paul & Phillips, 1954; Genant et al., 1967). A summary of the pertinent findings relating to the adrenals in myxoedema follows: (1) Serum cortisol levels are normal although the cortisol-binding capacity may be increased. Turnover of injected cortisol is decreased (Petersen, 1958; Farese & Plager, 1962). Formation of 11-OH steroids is favoured over 11-oxosteroids (Hellman, Bradlow, Zumoff & Gallagher, 1961). (2) Urinary 17-OH and 17-oxosteroids are decreased in myxoedema. The ability to conjugate steroids is stated to be normal whereas reduction is decreased both because of reduced TPNH and 5 α-reductase (Brown, Englert & Wallach, 1958; Tomkins & McGuire, 1960). (3) The response to exogenous ACTH may be sluggish (Felber, Reddy, Selenkow & Thorn, 1959). The changes are readily reversed by thyroid therapy. It is prudent to use small initial doses of thyroid (15 mg. increments) when treating such patients, as is done for proven panhypopituitarism, in order to avoid possible adrenal crisis.

Gonadotropic function and androgen and oestrogen metabolism are discussed below.

Secondary or pituitary myxoedema used to be thought of as that form of panhypopituitarism in which the thyroid is the most prominently affected. However, pure, isolated TSH deficiency has now been documented as a result of better TSH assays (Sawin & McHugh, 1966). The signs and symptoms may be the same as those of full-blown myxoedema (Lerman & Stebbins, 1942; Cluxton, Bennett & Kepler, 1948), but often such cases do not show all the typical changes in the skin, hair or voice; the blood cholesterol and protein may be normal.

The differentiation from primary myxoedema, though often easy on clinical grounds, is most often carried out by administering TSH and then measuring the response of the ^{131}I uptake or the PBI. Recently, a one-dose test (10 units) has been most favoured. The precise criteria vary with each laboratory, but may be as low as a 10% increase in the 24 hr. ^{131}I uptake or an increase of > 1·5 mg./100 ml. in the PBI (Fore & Wynn, 1966). Thyroidal unresponsiveness in secondary hypothyroidism appears to be rarer than thought initially. In addition, there may be poor response to TSH in borderline hypothyroidism presumably due to parenchymal damage, the so-called "low thyroid reserve". Other attempts to differentiate primary from secondary myxoedema have been the demonstration of antibodies characteristic of primary disease (Vallotton *et al.*, 1967), or the high turnover rate of thyroidal ^{131}I in primary myxoedema presumed to result from maximal endogenous TSH stimulation (Greenberg, 1966). The latter test presents technical problems because of the very low initial ^{131}I uptakes.

The yellowish skin pigmentation, sometimes seen in myxoedema, has been attributed to the existence of high levels of circulating carotene. At the same time vitamin A levels may be depressed. Because of these findings as well as the skin changes seen in myxoedema, it has been held that there is a defect in the conversion of carotene to vitamin A. However, experimental evidence regarding this defect is conflicting (Drill & Truant, 1947; Kelley & Day, 1948; Arnrich & Morgan, 1954).

The majority of metabolic processes are depressed in hypothyroidism. However, depending on the relative decreases in rates of synthesis and rates of utilization, the levels of various metabolites (e.g. in the blood) may be elevated or depressed. Hence cholesterol, which is frequently though not always elevated (above levels of 280 mg./100 ml.), seems to accumulate because the rate of synthesis is not decreased as much as is the rate of utilization (Leroy, 1956). Conversely, in thyrotoxicosis, utilization outstrips an accelerated rate of synthesis until a new level is reached (Kurland, Lucas & Freedberg, 1961; Myant, (1964). The precise mechanism is difficult to ascertain because of changes in the size of precursor pools. In cholesterol synthesis thyroid hormone appears to act at a step before mevalonate, possibly by changing the ATP levels (Myant, 1964). A T_4 effect on bile acid hydroxylation may play a role in cholesterol turnover. Neutral lipid and phospholipid levels may also be increased. The response of the free fatty acids to various stimuli is diminished but whether or not this is a result of insensitivity to adrenaline is not clear at present.

Hypothyroid patients show a decreased creatine excretion and a concomitant increase in creatinine excretion when subjected to a creatine tolerance test (Wilkins & Fleischmann, 1946). It is difficult to relate this to the increased muscle creatine or creatine phosphate content in experimental animals (Wang, 1946; Kuhlbäck, 1957). The level of creatine kinase is high

(>2.0 μmoles/ml./hr.) and falls more rapidly than the cholesterol level upon treatment (Graig & Smith, 1965).

Hyperuricaemia has been reported in males and post-menopausal women with myxoedema. As this is accompanied by decreased urinary urate excretion and a moderately increased blood urea level the effect is probably of renal origin (Leeper, Benua, Breuer & Rawson, 1960). It is of interest that there seems to be a high correlation between gout and hypothyroidism (Kuzell, Schaffarzich, Naugler, Koets, Mankle, Brown & Champlin, 1955).

Absence of thyroid hormone has a profound effect on protein synthesis (see p. 420). The fact that the protein of blood and spinal fluid is at times increased in myxoedema may, perhaps, be explained by rate differences in synthesis and degradation. There is an increase in the total exchangeable albumin confined to the extravascular space, and increased transcapillary transport of albumin. There is a decrease in the rate of synthesis and breakdown of albumin, hence the half-life is increased. This is corrected by replacement therapy (Schwartz, 1955; Lewallen, Rall & Berman, 1959). There is storage of mucoproteins in many tissues and the "myxoedema fluid" is high in protein. Replacement therapy leads to excretion of excess nitrogen (negative nitrogen balance), and a moderate decrease in the size of the miscible albumin pool. This urinary N loss is accompanied by loss of Na^+, emphasizing the extracellular origin of this N (Byrom, 1934; Munro, Renschler & Wilson, 1958).

Anaemia is frequently associated with myxoedema and the total red cell mass is often reduced. Anaemia may be either normocytic or macrocytic. The former may occasionally be due to blood loss from menorrhagia or due to poor iron absorption associated with achlorhydria. Some patients with normochromic, normocytic anaemias respond to thyroid replacement alone (Tudhope & Wilson, 1960). Macrocytic anaemias are also seen in myxoedema. Until recently it was thought to be clearly differentiated from pernicious anaemia in its response to thyroid replacement therapy. However, this distinction has become blurred by recent findings. While some patients lose the requirements for parenteral vitamin B_{12} with T_4 replacement therapy, there is a high incidence of true Addisonian pernicious anaemia in myxoedema. Achlorhydria may occur in as many as half the patients with myxoedema. It does not always respond to histamine. The achlorhydria is in turn associated with poor absorption of vitamin B_{12} and is frequently associated with low serum B_{12}

levels. Of these, a number may have true pernicious anaemia (10% or more). Tudhope & Wilson (1962) found this group to have impaired intrinsic factor activity which progressed despite treatment of the hypothyroidism. Such problems are rare in induced hypothyroidism and an autoimmune process has been suggested. Anti-intrinsic factor antibodies have been found in some cases of thyroid disease and antithyroid antibodies are common in pernicious anaemia (Ardeman, Chanarin, Krafchick & Singer, 1966). These authors also point out the frequency of pernicious anaemia in hyperthyroidism. The high incidence of thyroid disease in pernicious anaemia has also been reported.

Calcium excretion is below normal, and the bone may be radiologically denser than normal (Aub, Bauer, Heath & Ropes, 1929), although serum calcium and phosphate are normal. The size of the calcium pool, and the rate of labelling of bone with ^{45}Ca, is markedly diminished but returns to normal on thyroid therapy (Krane, Stanbury & Brownell, 1956). There may be a reduced tolerance to oral calcium. Collagen turnover is diminished as shown by decreased urinary excretion of hydroxyproline (largely peptide-

bound in the urine). Hypothyroid patients all excreted less than the 16 to 25 mg./24 hr./m². In hypothyroid children the values are below the respective normal values for the age concerned (740 mg./24 hr./m²) (Kivirikko et al., 1965). Serum alkaline phosphatase may be low, a deficiency that is particularly marked in cretins. In hypothyroid rats the synthesis and breakdown of chondroitin sulphate and hyaluronic acid are decreased. Thyroxine restores these to normal (Dziewiatkowski, 1964).

The role of deficient thyrocalcitonin in athyreotic individuals is yet to be evaluated. On the other hand hypoparathyroidism must always be considered in iatrogenic hypothyroidism. Hypoparathyroidism appears to be rare after irradiation with ^{131}I, but diminished "parathyroid reserve" may occur (Harden, Harrison & Alexander, 1963).

Iodine metabolism in hypothyroidism depends on the amount of residual functioning thyroid tissue. In athyroid states a dose of ^{131}I is nearly completely excreted in three days, even though renal clearance of iodide may be reduced to about half (Riggs, 1952). The count over the neck is that due to extrathyroidal tissues. If small amounts of functioning tissue remain, the amount of ^{131}I may

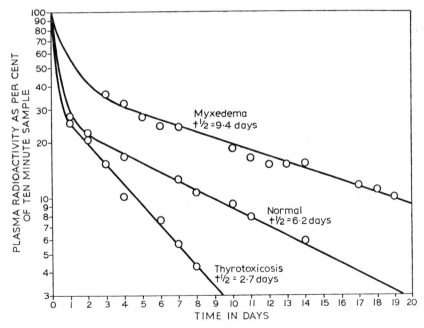

FIG. 12.6. Radiothyroxine disappearance curves in patients with altered thyroid function. Semilogarithmic plot of the plasma radioactivity as a fraction of the ten minute (initial) count. All samples are counted at the same time, thus the need for ^{131}I decay corrections is obviated and the $t_{1/2}$ values represent the true biological half-life. Reutilisation of ^{131}I⁻ from thyroxine deiodination is generally important only in patients with thyrotoxicosis and in these subjects is minimized by the administration of Lugol's solution (from Sterling & Chodos, 1956).

still be small or below the discrimination of the detecting instrument. It is claimed that such fragments can sometimes deliver organic iodine to the blood to give high conversion ratios even in full-blown myxoedema (Blom & Terpstra, 1953), indicating that the latter test may be misleading. With increasing amounts of tissue the neck count will approach normal values and the urinary ^{131}I excretion will vary inversely. Protein-bound iodine values, likewise, will range from 0 to near normal values depending on the degree of hypothyroidism. Values below 3 to $3 \cdot 5 \mu g./100$ ml. serum are considered evidence of hypothyroidism unless tri-iodothyronine has recently been administered. The corresponding value for the butanol-extractable iodine (BEI) or T_4 by column is $2 \cdot 9 \mu g./100$ ml. The extrathyroidal thyroxine pool is similarly depressed. Despite the great faith some have in the laboratory tests, there is a great deal of overlap in the tests between mild hypothyroidism and the euthyroid state. The PBI or column T_4 tests are generally more reliable than ^{131}I tests. The TSH stimulation test may elevate test values into the normal range in patients with thyroids that are not already maximally stimulated by endogenous thyrotropin.

Hypothyroid sera generally show a slight increase in thyroxine-binding capacity of TBG (Robbins & Rall, 1957; 1967). Since the PBI is low, the free thyroxine level will be decreased below that expected from the PBI alone. The results of resin tri-iodothyronine uptake are in agreement. Also in agreement with this interpretation is the decreased rate of disappearance of ^{131}-labelled thyroxine from the circulation of myxoedematous subjects (Fig. 12.6).

Mild forms of hypothyroidism are common and are often difficult to diagnose both on clinical grounds and by laboratory tests. The use of oral contraceptive preparations have recently made this diagnosis even more difficult and a high index of suspicion should be maintained.

Replacement Therapy

The initial administration of thyroid hormone (desiccated thyroid, thyroxine, tri-iodothyronine) must be undertaken with caution in profound myxoedema, since the adrenal and cardiac reserves are unknown; i.e. these systems are apt not to tolerate a large sudden increase in load. Muscle cramps are also reported with large initial doses. 15 to 30 mg. of desiccated thyroid, 25 to 50 $\mu g.$ thyroxine or 5 to 10 $\mu g.$ of tri-iodothyronine would appear to be safe initial doses in profound myxoedema, except in myxoedema coma where large initial daily doses of tri-iodothyronine or thyroxine are currently preferred. Since it is now clear that desiccated thyroid contains sizeable but variable fractions of tri-iodothyronine, the synthetic compounds are better when accurate control is desired.

The various hormone preparations have somewhat different time courses of action. Tri-iodothyronine has the most rapid calorigenic action with an onset as early as 4 to 6 hr., peak effect from a single dose (in myxoedema) at 48 to 72 hr., and an offset in the metabolic response with a half-life of seven days (Table 12.7). L-thyroxine does not cause a significant rise in the BMR until 24 to 48 hr. after a single intravenous administration, has a peak at 6 to 12 days, and the effect may still be discernible after 4 to 6 weeks. Assays in animals and man show that tri-iodothyronine is several times more active than thyroxine, 3-fold being a frequently used ratio. The response to oral desiccated thyroid is somewhat more gradual but more like thyroxine. There are reports of discernible effects 60 to 80 days after cessation of therapy.

Rapidity in response is useful in myxoedema coma and particularly when morphine has been given accidentally to a myxoedematous patient. In these cases intravenous tri-iodothyronine (or T_4) may prevent a catastrophe.

The order of response in symptomatology is variable. Changes in alertness, temperature sensitivity and pulse may be soon followed by changes in bowel habits. Chemical changes are slower although an occasional rapid drop in the serum cholesterol is reported. The improvement in these parameters may occur without changes in the BMR as shown by Lerman & Pitt-Rivers (1955) in two patients treated with tri-iodothyroacetic acid. The response in the protein-

TABLE 12.7

The calorigenic response to thyromimetic agents in myxoedema[1]

Agent	Dosage[2] and route	Time to onset	Peak	1/2 decay time	Time to offset
Desiccated thyroid	Daily p.o.	2 days	3–5 weeks	—	30–80 days
Thyroxine	Daily p.o.	2 days	3–5 weeks	—	30–80 days
Thyroxine	Single i.v.	1 day	6–13 days	12 days	4–6 weeks
Tri-iodothyronine	Single i.v.	4–6 hr.	2–3 days	7 days	10–18 days

[1] Ranges of values composed from various reports in the literature which are only roughly comparable.

[2] The effects are, to a certain extent, dosage-dependent. Values given here represent adequate or larger doses.

bound iodine is variable but in general shows a pattern similar to the BMR when thyroxine or desiccated thyroid is used. Some follow the return of the ECG toward normal during thyroid therapy.

Many attempts have been made to lower the blood cholesterol of euthyroid subjects on the assumption that this will be beneficial in arteriosclerosis (see Myant, 1964). While the dosage of many thyromimetic drugs can be so adjusted as to lead to cholesterol lowering without marked changes in the BMR, the dissociation is only temporary and appears to reflect the earlier response of cholesterol.

HYPERTHYROIDISM

Hyperthyroidism occurs in two main forms: Graves' disease (or hyperthyroidism with ophthalmopathy), also called diffuse toxic goitre, and toxic nodular goitre. The latter generally occurs in older patients, tends to be less severe, and is less often accompanied by eye signs. Solitary nodules may occasionally lead to thyrotoxicosis (Plummer's disease). Except where noted we shall treat the terms Graves' disease, hyperthyroidism and thyrotoxicosis as synonymous.

Aetiology

The aetiology of hyperthyroidism remains a mystery. Dependent personality, fright, frustrations in the attainment of too difficult goals and other emotional stresses have been blamed. Dietary regimens and war (in some countries) have been claimed to antecede the disease or an increase in its prevalence, but such evidence is difficult to evaluate and offers few other clues. There appears to be a familial pre-disposition. Relatives of patients with Graves' disease show an increased incidence both of this disease and of other thyroid disorders (Martin & Fisher, 1951). Excessive anterior pituitary activity (possibly mediated via the hypothalamus) was frequently implicated, partly because of the occasional "cure" in Graves' disease produced by irradiation of the pituitary, partly because of the occasional occurrence of thyrotoxicosis in acromegaly and partly because TSH can reproduce a number of the signs of hyperthyroidism. However, serum TSH levels are "low" or undetectable in Graves' disease (Odell, Wilber & Paul, 1965; Utiger, 1965).

Adams (1958) first showed that certain patients with hyperthyroidism have a factor in their sera which gives a much later peak effect on ^{131}I release from the thyroids of pre-labelled assay animals than does pituitary thyrotropic hormone. This factor has come to be known as the "long-acting thyroid stimulator" or LATS. Present evidence suggests that:

(1) It is not a pituitary hormone.

(2) It is a 7S γ-globulin, probably an antibody (IgG), containing no TSH or immunological cross reactivity with TSH even after partial proteolytic digestion, and having a temperature sensitivity different from TSH. The antigen for it may derive from the thyroid but this is not certain since thyrotoxic sera are reported to contain a globulin that neutralizes thyroid extracts independent of the LATS content (Adams & Kennedy, 1967). LATS is reported to be increased in some patients after radio-iodine therapy and decreased in others after subtotal thyroidectomy. Any relation to the elevated complement-fixing antibodies of Graves' disease has yet to be proven.

(3) It may be made in lymphoid tissue and serum levels are suppressed by corticosteroid therapy (McKenzie, 1965; Kriss, Pleshakov & Chien, 1964; Kirkham, 1967; McKenzie, 1967).

LATS is found in 50 to 80% of patients with Graves' disease and this high correlation has led numerous investigators to state that LATS "causes" the hyperthyroidism. This is supported by findings in the short-lived episodes of neonatal hyperthyroidism in infants of thyrotoxic mothers. The disease and its disappearance correlates well with the LATS level believed to have been transferred across the placenta. The half-life of LATS in the new-born is rather shorter than for typical γ-globulin (McKenzie, 1964; Sunshine, Kusumoto & Kriss, 1965).

On the other hand LATS is absent in a sizeable fraction of Graves' patients and efforts to explain this away as due to methodological inadequacy seem unsatisfactory. Also, by no means all children born of thyrotoxic mothers (untreated) have themselves been toxic. Contrariwise, occasional normal subjects with measurable LATS levels have been reported. In any case, there is no relation to the degree of toxicity, size of goitre, indices of thyroid function (except perhaps the rate of $PB^{131}I$ formation), and it remains to be determined whether there are several types of hyperthyroidism, only one of which is caused by LATS or whether the correlation is not aetiological (Kirkham, 1967; McKenzie, 1967). Certainly, toxic nodules appear to be autonomous, being accompanied neither by TSH or LATS (McKenzie, 1965). There are several examples of a temporal relation of a LATS rise with the onset of pretibial myxoedema and proptosis (Kriss, Pleshakov, Rosenblum, Holderness, Sharp & Utiger, 1967), but the causative role of LATS in ophthalmopathy or pretibial myxoedema is uncertain (McKenzie, 1965 and 1967; Kirkham, 1967).

LATS may fall rapidly with persistence of the eye signs, and proptosis may occur without changes in the LATS level (Kriss *et al.*, 1967).

Despite the chemical differences of the two substances, the mechanism of action of LATS is strikingly similar to TSH in such assays as glucose oxidation, phospholipid synthesis, ^{131}I uptake or release, and colloid droplet formation in the thyroid (McKenzie, 1967). This is perhaps less surprising since Larsen & Wolff (1967) have detected yet another activity (from *Cl. perfringens*) that stimulates thyroid phospholipid synthesis. This protein has since been purified by Macchia, Bates & Pastan (1967) and found to stimulate many of the other processes listed above. Whether or not these stimulating actions all operate through one or more of the components of the cyclic-AMP system, as has been repeatedly suggested, remains to be proven.

Less clear-cut evidence for the existence of an exophthalmotropic factor in the pituitary or in blood of Graves' patients with eye signs has been published (Dobyns, Wright & Wilson, 1961).

The incidence of thyrotoxicosis occasionally appears to increase shortly after iodized-salt therapy is instituted—the so-called "Jod-Base-dow" type. Whether this iodine supplies the raw material for a "potentially toxic gland" or works by other mechanisms is not known. In rare cases toxicity is caused by ingestion of excess desiccated thyroid and is then called "thyrotoxicosis factitia".

The *signs and symptoms* of Graves' disease are, with the exception of some of the ocular manifestations and localized myxoedema, largely due to the effects of excess hormone. This leads to an increased activity of most organ systems, metabolic pathways, and other biological functions of the body, and is characterized by an increase in O_2 consumption and energy production. Some tissues such as heart, liver and muscle, for example, respond more actively than the body as a whole (see p. 418).

Thyroid-catecholamine Relationships. Because of the resemblance between sympathetic over-activity and hyperthyroidism the relation between catecholamines and the thyroid gland has received much attention but no simple picture has emerged from these studies. The problem is conveniently divided into several parts: (*a*) the effect of cate-cholamines on thyroid hormone synthesis; (*b*) the role of catecholamines in the peripheral effects of the thyroid hormones; and (*c*) thyroid hormone effects on catecholamine metabolism.

The vascular bed of the thyroid is very sensitive to catecholamines and the confusing results of thyroid response probably stem from dose and time differences. Small doses of catecholamines dilate and large doses constrict thyroid blood vessels. This is reflected in the data on ^{131}I uptake and/or clearances. Most investigators find decreases in these parameters, although some find increases (Harrison, 1964; Hays, 1965). There may be a late and transient rebound increase in these measurements after cessation of adrenaline administration. Comparable effects occur in the release of ^{131}I from the thyroid. Vasoconstriction is accompanied by an increased *concentration* of ^{131}I in thyroid venous blood but the total *amount* per unit time is not altered (Harrison, 1964). Effects of adrenaline on the hypothalamus and/or pituitary gland have also been suggested. It is likely, however, that all these alterations are of a transient nature since patients with phaeochromocytomas perform normally in thyroid function tests (Gifford, Kvale, Maher, Roth & Priestley, 1964). Increases in thyroxine de-iodination produced by adrenaline, although observed in some situations, must be interpreted cautiously in view of the complicated nature of the de-iodination reaction (see p. 394).

The catecholamines and thyroid hormones share many physiological effects (increased oxygen consumption, haemodynamic effects, changes in cardiac irritability, etc.) and it is generally held that hyperthyroidism leads to exaggerated responses to catecholamines (glycogenolysis, fatty acid release, pressor response, cardiac excitability, etc.), while the reverse is true in hypothyroidism (Waldstein, 1966). For this reason it is often proposed that the catecholamines play a permissive role in these responses or, conversely, that the thyroid hormones do. It is very difficult however, to differentiate additive effects from synergism and the question can not be resolved at present. It is clear that the catecholamines are not required for thyroid hormone effects (e.g. Wollenberger, 1964), and the thyroid status profoundly affects the intrinsic contractile properties of isolated cardiac muscle independently of noradrenaline (and independently of the energy stores, creatine phosphate and ATP) (Buccino *et al.* 1967). Whether or not the response to nervous stimuli, and of the conducting system of the intact heart, is altered seems less certain. The localization of tri-iodothyronine in the bundle of His is of interest in this regard (Tommaselli, Gravina & Roche, 1965).

On the other hand, there can be no doubt that some catecholamine effects require the presence of the thyroid hormone for full expression and the excess response in hyperthyroidism certainly appears to be more than additive. In an effort to find differential effects, Bray (1966) has found that thyroidectomy has no effect on α-adrenergic responses but did influence the response of certain β-receptors mediating cardiac glycogenolysis and lipolysis. Also, it is now well known that the thyrotoxic patient shows an exaggerated increase in plasma free fatty acids to an injection of adrenaline or noradrenaline (Harlan *et al.*, 1963). It is of interest that, in the rat, stimulation of lipolysis is a very early effect of T_3 preceding any change in oxygen consumption (Bray & Goodman, 1965). Tri-iodothyronine can also sensitize the fat pad to adrenaline *in vitro* (Vaughan, 1967).

Despite the uncertain relationship between the catecholamines and thyroid hormones there is ample evidence that reduction of the body stores of catecholamines by reserpine or guanethedine, or β-adrenergic blockade, improves the signs and symptoms of thyrotoxicity. Palpitation, tachycardia, increased cardiac output, heat intolerance and sweating tremor are reduced though not usually to the normal level (Waldstein, 1966; Howitt & Rowlands, 1967; Vinik *et al.*, 1968). The response is sufficiently rapid to make this method of treatment useful in thyroid storm. Although rather large doses of guanethidine are tolerated, postural hypotension must be watched for. Thyroid function tests, the PBI or cholesterol levels, and the BMR are not significantly altered by these blocking agents.

The confusion regarding levels of catecholamines in blood and urine as a function of thyroid status probably results from technical difficulties with earlier methods. The best evidence currently available suggests normal serum and urinary levels of adrenaline and noradrenaline in hyperthyroid subjects. Diminished adrenaline excretion has been reported in response to insulin hypoglycaemia, whereas it is increased in response to CO_2 and other stimuli (Harrison, 1964). There is no agreement on the tissue content of catecholamines, nor of the changes in monoamine oxidase levels as affected by thyroid status (Harrison, 1964). What *is* clear is that the catechol-O-methyltransferase activity, which carries the major burden of catechol metabolism, seems to be little influenced by changes in thyroid status. It is probable, therefore, that whatever fraction of the hyperthyroid picture is due to adrenergic responses, this is not based on major changes in catecholamine levels or metabolism.

Muscle

While myasthenia gravis is occasionally associated with Graves' disease, and much literature is devoted to establishing a more than coincidental relation, the frequency has not been proved greater than could be statistically expected. The two diseases aggravate each other and thymic enlargement may be present in both (in Graves' disease

this is part of a general lymphatic hypertrophy in which the spleen may also be involved). There is, however, no evidence at present to suggest that the muscular weakness of the two diseases is pathogenetically related. Furthermore, weakness in thyrotoxicosis persists unchanged with rest and is usually unaffected by prostigmine. Wasting, tremor, loss of power, and, occasionally, fasciculations may be present, although not all of these need occur in the same case. The muscular weakness may be the first symptom of hyperthyroidism and may be of acute onset. The distribution tends to be centripetal (Grob, 1963; Danowski, Sarver & Bonessi, 1963). Electromyography differentiates the lesion from neuropathies. Although light microscopy of such muscles has shown only non-specific changes if anything, electron microscopic studies reveal abnormal mitochondria and focal dilatations of the transverse tubular system (Engel, 1966). In experimental hyperthyroidism in the rat, the most striking muscle finding was an increase in the size and number of mitochondria, and the number of cristae per mitochondrion without the changes seen in myopathy (Gustafsson, Tata, Lindberg & Ernster, 1965). External ophthalmoplegia is not well correlated with the general muscle weakness and the latter shows a more consistent response to therapy (Gimlette, 1959).

In the dog the oxygen consumption of thyrotoxic muscle is increased more than that of the body as a whole. This is accompanied by a proportional increase in muscle blood flow but without an increase in the A-V oxygen differences. Increasing the rate of isometric contractions leads to greater increases in the thyrotoxic than in normal muscle (Frey, 1967).

In thyrotoxic myopathy there is marked alteration in creatine metabolism. These changes are non-specific, being encountered in most diseases of muscular wasting. Normal male and female adults excrete only small amounts of creatine. Creatinuria (greater than 100 mg./24 hr.) occurs very frequently in thyrotoxicosis, with a concomitant decrease in urine creatinine, although not in equivalent amount. With treatment this disappears rather early.

Early estimates of muscle phosphocreatine and ATP content are probably unreliable and recent ones are not available. It is of interest, however, that cardiac muscle concentrations of these two substances were not significantly altered in thyrotoxic cats (Buccino *et al.*, 1967). The normal level of serum creatine kinase activity is 1·7 to 2·0 μmoles/ml./hr. This was found to be reduced in thyrotoxicosis (all patients presumably *without* significant myopathy) to 0·7 and increased in hypothyroidism to 13 μmoles/ml./hr.

Tocopherol deficiency leads to muscle and metabolic changes not unlike those of hyperthyroidism. Nevertheless, Postel (1956) found no correlation between the degree of depression of serum tocopherols and clinical estimates of the severity of muscle disease in thyrotoxicosis.

Over 200 cases of thyrotoxic periodic paralysis have been reported, mostly from Japan and China and mostly in males. It is not familial. The disorder responds well to antithyroid therapy and is exacerbated by thyroid medication (see Engel, 1961; McFadzean & Yeung, 1967). Attacks are less frequent but resemble the primary type in being accompanied by hypokalaemia, muscle inexcitability, oliguria and electrolyte retention. The only pathological change is a dilation of the sarcoplasmic reticulum (Engel, 1966).

Heart

As mentioned above, the heart can respond to thyroid status independently of neural or other hormonal factors. To what extent such effects as palpitation, and the increased pulse rate and minute volume in Graves' disease are mediated by the cardiac nerves is not known. The sleeping pulse is generally more than 80 and the great frequency with which auricular fibrillation is seen in Graves' disease has not been satisfactorily explained. There is a surprisingly low incidence of myocardial infarction during active hyperthyroidism which has not been explained (Littman, Jeffers & Rose, 1957). Hyperthyroidism in cats leads to decreased shortening time in isotonic contraction and increases the rate of tension development, but influences overall force production much less. These effects occur also after depletion of catecholamine stores (Buccino et al., 1967). On the other hand, treatment with guanethidine, etc. causes marked reduction of tachycardia, cardiac output, etc. in thyrotoxic patients.

In the presence of excess thyroid hormone the myocardium of laboratory animals shows an increased O_2 consumption and decreased glycogen content. Although this occurs early, recent results show little change in creatine phosphate or ATP concentrations (Buccino et al., 1967).

The reduced rate and inotropic responses to cardiac glycosides often seen in thyrotoxicosis may be due in part to the lower serum levels attained per unit dose despite normal turnover (Doherty & Perkins, 1966), and partly to the fact that the thyrotoxic heart is already working nearer its maximum tension while refractory

period prolongation is less (Morrow, Gaffney & Braunwald, 1963; Frye & Braunwald, 1961).

Some of the cardiac difficulties result from peripheral circulatory effects. The increased total O_2 consumption "requires" a high output, and the increased heat production "leads" to vasodilation. Cutaneous blood flow is increased to 6% of the cardiac output instead of normal of 3 to 4% (Stewart & Evans, 1941, 1942). The venous return is increased. Hypervolaemia may occur and with it some increase in the total red cell mass and a corresponding increase in active bone marrow. Part of the latter may be due to a shorter erythrocyte life span (McClellan, Donegan, Thorup & Leavell, 1958). Blood flow is accelerated (decreased circulation time, arm to tongue, less than 16 sec.). The pulse pressure may be wide.

Thyrotoxicosis may be evident almost entirely as cardiac failure. This probably can occur in the absence of pre-existing heart disease and is termed "thyrotoxic heart disease". The anaemia that occasionally occurs in thyrotoxicosis may contribute to the failure, but is seldom sufficiently severe. In those cases in which the aetiology of congestive failure is obscure the thyroid should always be considered, and the laboratory procedures are particularly useful here. The recognition of thyroid excess as a cause of heart disease is of tremendous importance, since nearly all such patients can return to a normal cardiac status upon treatment of the thyrotoxicosis, unless pre-existing heart disease was present. Supraventricular tachycardias without associated heart disease may be accompanied by increased free T_4 levels or T_3 uptake into red cells in the presence of a normal PBI. This is due presumably to decreased pre-albumin thyroxine-binding capacity (Schatz, 1967). Whether this causes the tachycardias is uncertain since elevated free T_4 in other illnesses is not accompanied by cardiac arrhythmias.

Gastro-intestinal Tract

Gastro-intestinal motility is characteristically increased in thyrotoxicosis, and this not infrequently leads to diarrhoea, although this is not as common as is generally stated. Very little is certain about transport across the mucosa in thyrotoxicosis. In animals, both increases and decreases have been reported for sugars and amino acids. Decreased transport in hyperthyroidism, or increases in hypothyroidism, predominate in the recent literature (Bronk & Parsons, 1966; London & Segal, 1967). The rapid rise and fall in oral glucose and galactose tolerance curves may well result from an effect at a site other than the gut (MacLagan, Rundle, Collard & Mills, 1940;

Lozner, Winkler, Taylor & Peters, 1941). Achlorhydria is not uncommon and may be accompanied by pernicious anaemia (see hypothyroidism).

Concomitant with the general increase in energy metabolism there appears to be an accelerated turnover of the three major food constitutents as well as of most of the vitamins. While many attempts have been made to implicate specific vitamin deficiencies, particularly of the B group, it is generally felt that in man any vitamin deficiencies that occur are probably non-specific, depending largely on the one most nearly marginal in the particular diet.

Hepatic lesions ranging from loss of glycogen and fatty infiltration to a special type of cirrhosis of the cardiac variety may be seen. The latter changes occur largely in the interlobular septa and mostly in the subcapsular zone (reviewed by Moschcowitz, 1946). Unfortunately, most of such pathological material has come from autopsies, and recent biopsy studies (Movitt, Gerstl & Davis, 1953) indicate that, in most cases of thyrotoxicosis, histopathological study of the liver does not reveal significant impairment. Occasionally, flocculation and van den Bergh tests are abnormal. The continued increase in carbohydrate load places an unusual demand on the islets for insulin, so that diabetes mellitus may be the end-result of longstanding thyrotoxicosis (reviewed by Houssay, 1945).[1] This is partially or completely reversible depending on the duration of overloading, as has been demonstrated experimentally by Houssay (1944). It is also said that thyrotoxicosis brings out latent diabetes. Whether this mechanism differs from the above is a moot point. Moreover, there may be an increased rate of destruction of insulin in thyrotoxicosis (Elgee & Williams, 1955) which further increases the demand on the islets.

Metabolism

It has long been recognized that thyrotoxicosis is accompanied by increased protein catabolism and excretion (Hoberman, 1950; Lewallen *et al.*, 1959). Nitrogen excretion is increased; the negative balance can, however, usually be abolished with adequate caloric and protein intake. A "tendency" to hypo-albuminaemia is sometimes reported (Adams *et al.*, 1967). Although blood α-amino nitrogen is high in the thyrotoxic rat (Friedberg & Greenberg, 1947) this is not the case in thyrotoxic patients. There is, however, an elevated level of tyrosine, and only of tyrosine, both in sponta-

---

[1] 2 to 4% of thyrotoxic patients have diabetes and 1 to 2·5% of diabetics have thyrotoxicosis.

neous and induced hyperthyroidism (Melmon, Rivlin, Oates & Sjoerdsma, 1964). There is also a decreased tolerance to a tyrosine load not seen with tryptophan or phenylalanine. The mechanism is unknown. It should be pointed out that urinary hydroxyproline output is markedly increased in hyperthyroidism and, in fact, shows a direct, though not linear, relation to the PBI (Kivirikko *et al.*, 1965).

Depot fat tends to disappear in the cachexia of thyrotoxicosis; this can be demonstrated by analysis of carcass fat in experimental animals. Nevertheless, the rate of synthesis of fatty acids and sterols is increased (Dayton, Dayton, Drimmer & Kendall, 1960; Myant, 1964). Many other studies dealing with this problem *in vivo* cannot be interpreted because changes in precursor pools have not been taken into account. The serum concentrations of the various lipids are decreased (cholesterol, phospholipid, carotenes, neutral lipids), as are the concentrations of both high-density and low-density lipoproteins. Lipoprotein lipase is increased in thyrotoxic rats (Alousi & Mallow, 1964). Thyrotoxicosis also increases the turnover of the low-density lipoproteins—a change readily reversed by treatment (Walton, Campbell & Tonks, 1965). In general, lipid changes, though significant, are smaller in hyperthyroidism than in myxoedema and for this reason are less useful diagnostic tools as well. A notable exception are the levels of free fatty acids which increase from 0·4 to 0·6 μEq./ml. to 0·8 to 1·0 μEq./ml. The turnover of free fatty acid is increased from 360 μEq./min. to 1670 μEq./min. In the dog uptake of free fatty acid in muscle is, to a large extent, determined by muscle blood flow but does not correlate well with the oxygen consumption (Frey, 1967). Palmitate incorporation into triglyceride is decreased and Sandhofer, Sailer & Braunsteiner (1966) suggest this may be responsible for the decreased triglyceride levels. The thyrotoxic patient responds well to the free fatty acid-lowering activity of nicotinate and shows an exaggerated increase after adrenaline or noradrenaline (Harlan *et al.*, 1963; Eaton, Steinberg & Thompson, 1965).

Thyroid hormone stimulates both the synthesis and the degradation of cholesterol. The mechanism for the former has been discussed extensively (Myant, 1964) but is still poorly understood. Degradation is increased to a large extent by increases in oxidation to bile acids. There is an increased pool as well as increased faecal excretion (Strand, 1963). The site of the thyroxine effect may be both on the 12-hydroxylase and on side chain oxidation (Mitropoulos & Myant, 1965; Berséus,

1965) with the end result of a marked shift to chenodeoxycholate excretion.

The cholesterol-lowering action of thyroxine and a large assortment of analogues has been amply reviewed and is beyond the scope of the present work (see Boyd & Oliver, 1960; Sachs, 1960; Steinberg, 1962; Myant, 1964).

Mechanism of Effect on Protein Synthesis

The more interesting aspects of thyroid hormone effects on protein metabolism deal with the stimulation of protein synthesis induced by the hormone. This has been reflected mostly in the levels of tissue enzyme activities, most of which are increased, some unchanged, and some decreased. Since co-factor concentrations, etc. could also be increased it is important to prove that the concentrations of enzyme protein are actually increased. This has been accomplished in only a few cases: various cytochromes, catalase, carbamyl phosphate synthetase in induced metomorphosis of the tadpole, and α-glycerophosphate dehydrogenase. Particularly large changes occur in cytochrome c and mitochondrial a-glycerophosphate dehydrogenase concentrations. In human hyperthyroidism, serum malic dehydrogenase and ribonuclease are elevated, while creatine kinase is decreased (Lieberthal, Benson & Klitgaard et al., 1963; Leeper, 1963; Graig & Smith, 1965). The role of synthesis and/or degradation is not, however, known. Attempts to implicate changes in enzyme levels as the primary hormone effect have not been very successful (see reviews by Wolff & Wolff, 1964; Tata, 1964b, 1966).

Attempts to localize the site of the thyroxine effect on protein synthesis have led to divergent results. Tata (1966), using the approach of time sequence of effects after a single dose of T_3 given to thyroidectomized rats in vivo, initially believed the site to be at the transcription level or RNA polymerase. Thereafter, the importance of the synthesis of ribosomal RNA and/or its attachment to membranes has been appreciated and suggested as a regulatory site. Most recently, interest has been displayed in the histone-DNA interaction but the importance of this is, as yet, obscure (Kim & Cohen, 1966). However, certain hormone responses in vivo appear to precede any seen in the above system (Gries, Matschinsky & Wieland, 1962; Bronk, 1966).

An entirely different mechanism has been proposed by Sokoloff, Kaufman, Campbell, Francis & Gelboin (1963). The thyroid hormones act on the mitochondria to release a substance, as yet unidentified, that subsequently stimulates ribosomal protein synthesis somewhere beyond the stage of amino-acid attachment to tRNA. There is also an early effect of T_3 on mitochondrial protein synthesis (Bronk, 1966).

Several laboratories have sought to prove the primacy of the protein synthetic effect in the response to thyroid hormone by experiments in which hormone effects are abolished by poisons that interfere with protein synthesis. However, these agents cannot be proved sufficiently specific to permit unequivocal interpretations. It is nevertheless established that one of the most important early effects of the thyroid hormones in mammals is on RNA and protein synthesis and many effects seen are regulated through this mechanism. Whether all effects are is uncertain, as is the obligatory role of the hormones in early mammalian differentiation (see p. 430).

Mineral Metabolism

Among the body constituents that undergo a rapid turnover, calcium is prominent. The first case of clinically demonstrable osteomalacia occurring in Basedow's disease was described by von Recklinghausen in 1891, and Revilliod called attention to augmented phosphaturia in 1895 (Sattler, 1952). Aub et al. (1929), and many others since, have demonstrated marked augmentation of both urinary and faecal calcium excretion. A negative Ca^{++} balance is a frequent finding but this may sometimes be corrected by increased Ca^{++} intake. Data on intestinal absorption are conflicting: decreases are often reported but some recent cases have shown increased Ca^{++} absorption (Adams et al., 1967). It is of interest that active transport of Ca^{++} across the gut is inhibited by thyroid hormone (Schachter, 1963). There is increased osteoblastic and osteoclastic activity. The severity of the demineralization depends on the duration of the disease, and may be so severe as to resemble hyperparathyroidism radiologically. Nevertheless, pathological fractures are very rare. The alkaline phosphatase level of serum may be elevated, but available data are inconsistent and liver disease has not always been ruled out. Changes in hydroxyproline excretion have been discussed above. In children, bone growth and maturation may be accelerated by hyperthyroidism.

Despite large increases in calcium mobilization, the serum calcium and phosphorus levels generally remain in the normal range and metastatic calcification or other renal damage is rare. Cases with elevated serum calcium levels have, however, been reported. The increased tubular resorption of phosphate may, or may not, be a consequence of the very small increases in serum Ca^{++} and consequent parathyroid suppression but no definite information is yet available (Adams, Jowsey, Kelly, Riggs, Kinney & Jones, 1967). The response to a given dose of parathormone is said to be greater in thyrotoxicosis than in the euthyroid subject (Harrison, Harden & Alexander, 1964). To what extent, if any, a deficiency of thyrocalcitonin plays a role in this picture is quite unknown.

Krane et al. (1956) have shown with ^{45}Ca that the "calcium pool" (calculated from the degree of dilution of an injected labelled dose) is vastly increased in human thyrotoxicosis, approaching values found in hyperparathyroidism. The pool shrinks to normal size upon treatment of the disease.

The serum concentration of Mg^{++} (normal range 1·7 to 2·3 mEq./l.) is slightly decreased in hyperthyroidism. The rate of urinary excretion of labelled Mg^{++} is increased although total and intracellular Mg^{++} pools are normal. The converse is true in hypothyroidism except that there is also a decrease in Mg^{++} pools (Rizek, Dimich & Wallach, 1965; Jones, Desper, Shane & Flink, 1966). The mechanism for these changes is not clear. In some reports Mg^{++} has been credited with reducing the toxicity of exogenous thyroxine. Although Mg^{++} forms insoluble complexes with the hormone, the solubility products are too high to account for these effects (see Wolff & Wolff, 1964).

A rare condition sometimes seen in thyrotoxicosis is *thyroid acropachy* which consists of clubbing of the fingers and toes, distal periosteal bone formation and soft tissue swelling especially over the affected bones. It is nearly always associated with pretibial myxoedema and exophthalmos (Gimlette, 1960).

Iodine Metabolism

The main alterations in iodine metabolism occurring in thyrotoxicosis are quantitative. However, many of the methods will not readily differentiate shifts, e.g. to increased synthesis of T_3. Since it is gradually becoming apparent that T_3, because of its greater potency, may contribute a sizeable fraction of the total metabolic response to thyroid hormone, this is an important consideration. Labelled tri-iodothyronine is more easily detected in the blood of Graves' patients treated with ^{131}I than in patients receiving radioactive iodine for other thyroid disease (Benua & Dobyns, 1955; Arons & Hydovitz, 1959). Eight cases have been reported in whom the serum ratio of *labelled* T_3/T_4 was $> 1·0$ as compared with the usual values of $< 0·2$. Some of these patients were mildly thyrotoxic but had normal PBI values (as would be expected if T_3 contributed significantly to the hyperthyroidism) (Shimaoka, 1963). It is of interest that a similar shift occurs in most tissues of "equilibrium labelled" rats made "hyperthyroid" by prolonged cold exposure (Albright *et al.*, 1965). Traces of labelled iodotyrosines are sometimes reported in blood from patients with Graves' disease (Farran *et al.*, 1959).

The quantitative changes in iodine metabolism of Graves' disease are largely those to be expected from a general increase in thyroidal iodine turnover. The extrathyroidal volume of distribution of $^{131}I^-$ may be slightly elevated in Graves' disease for reasons not well understood (Myant *et al.*, 1950). The total uptake, rate of uptake, thyroidal clearance of iodide, accumulation gradient, etc., are, with rare exceptions, all above normal in hyperthyroidism. This is true not only because of the increased amount of thyroid tissue usually present, but also because the accumulation of iodide may be greater per gram of tissue. The ratio of thyroidal iodide to plasma iodide (T/S ratio) is considerably above normal. The plasma inorganic iodide concentration (PII) may be low but clearances are sufficiently increased to yield elevated absolute iodine uptake values (AIU) (Aboul-Khair & Crooks, 1965). It should be pointed out that some of this iodine will leave the gland again as iodide but whether or not the fraction is different in thyrotoxicosis is a matter of controversy. As discussed below, the thyroid gland in Graves' disease is unusually sensitive to the inhibitory action of excess iodide. Despite the high absolute iodide uptake the toxic thyroid may be iodine-deficient (Gutman, Benedict, Baxter & Palmer, 1932). This contributes to the rapid labelling of the serum thyronines (high conversion ratio) and may contribute to the relatively greater abundance of T_3 in the serum. Occasionally ^{131}I turnover is so rapid that the peak uptake is reached well before 24 hr. and an uptake at this time may be misleading. A short term uptake (e.g. 4 hr.) will indicate this.

The half-life of thyroidal iodine shows tremendous variations. When calculated as a function of secretion rate of ^{131}I, it is somewhere between 80 and 120 days in the euthyroid patient on a good iodine intake. In hyperthyroidism the gland may be so depleted of hormone, and the turnover may (even without marked thyroidal iodine depletion) be so great, that the half-life may be reduced to less than a week (Riggs, 1952). In some patients an albumin-like protein becomes labelled and appears in plasma (Stanbury & Janssen, 1962). With rare exceptions, all methods of measuring circulating hormone levels show increases in patients with Graves' disease (PBI, BEI, column T_4, displacement of labelled T_4 from resin, fraction of binding sites occupied in binding proteins). There is a small decrease in the thyroxine-binding capacity of TBG, and possibly in TBPA (see review by Robbins & Rall, 1960). Even in the absence of these changes, the higher PBI will be accompanied by an elevated level of free T_4. Methods for this determination have not yet standardized but the mean value in normal sera is ~ 4 ng./100 ml. whereas toxic sera average ~ 20 ng./100 ml. (Ingbar *et al.*, 1965; Sterling & Brenner, 1966). This is probably an important factor, but not necessarily the only one, in the accelerated peripheral thyroxine turnover seen in thyrotoxicosis (Fig. 12.6). The claim that this increased thyroxine disappearance persists after satisfactory therapy, or is present in family members of patients with hyperthyroidism, has not been confirmed (Ingbar & Freinkel, 1958*b*; Sterling, 1958).

Chemical determination of the T_3 level (Nauman *et al.*, 1967) has given normal values of 0·26 to 0·33 μg. % (as T_3, not T_3 iodine), about 5% of the circulating thyronines (Pind, 1957; Nauman *et al.*, 1967). This value is increased in thyrotoxicosis to 0·71μg. %. More importantly, the free T_3 averages 1·5 nanograms/100 ml. (0·46% of the total as opposed to 0·046% in the case of T_4). This increases to 5·0 nanograms/100 ml. in thyrotoxicosis. The ratio free T_3/free T_4 is about 1 to 3 in normal sera. Whether it necessarily changes in thyrotoxicosis is not known.

A diagnostically useful, and mechanistically interesting, phenomenon is the fact that the ^{131}I uptake or similar measurements are not suppressed by large doses of exogenous thyroxine or tri-iodothyronine (Greer & Smith, 1954; Werner *et al.*, 1955; Burke, 1967). A response to TSH can still be shown in such glands. This can now be most easily explained in terms of LATS which is not in a feedback relation with the thyroid hormones (see p. 415).

Therapy

Excess Iodide. Iodide, or compound solution of iodine (Lugol's solution), is used widely in combination with thiocarbamides with the intent of "reducing the vascularity of the gland" at surgery. It is customarily stated that 6 mg./day of I^- will suffice to control thyrotoxicosis, but recent evidence from Glasgow suggests that larger doses are desirable (Harden, Koutras, Alexander & Wayne, 1964). The effects (e.g. on the PBI) are not prolonged and long-term control of hyperthyroidism with KI is sometimes possible but is difficult and is not generally attempted.

The mechanism of action of pharmacological doses of iodide is not understood. There are two types of effects: (*a*) inhibition of release of hormone from the gland and (*b*) inhibition of synthesis of organic iodine. There is no peripheral effect on the action of the hormone (DeGroot, 1966). Generally, it is the effect on hormone release which is the clinically useful one since Lugol's solution will reduce the level of circulating thyroid hormone (Riggs, Lavietes & Man,

1942; Harden *et al.*, 1964). This is not surprising since the absolute iodine uptake (AIU) is not decreased after two weeks of iodide therapy. Although the positive perchlorate test (i.e. discharge) which is seen in treated patients might be interpreted as faulty hormone synthesis (Harden *et al.*, 1964; Stewart & Murray, 1967), it seems more likely to us that this merely reflects a shift in the rate-limiting step from iodide trapping to organification.

The release of previously accumulated ^{131}I is abruptly decreased by KI in patients with toxic goitre. This effect may be reversed by TSH (Goldsmith & Eisele, 1956; Solomon, 1956; Greer & DeGroot, 1956). Although it is clear that excess iodide blocks hormone release from the thyroid as shown by a decrease in the PBI and is accompanied by accumulation of organic iodine in the gland, this occurs only in hyperthyroidism in man (Mercer *et al.*, 1960) and under special conditions in the experimental animal (Nakayama, 1962; Yamada *et al.*, 1963). Some evidence has been presented by these authors that this effect is not simply one of decreased specific activity of the iodine pool to be released.

The second effect of excess I^- consists of an interference in hormone production (Wolff & Chaikoff, 1948*a,b,c,d*; Stanley, 1949). It is discussed under the section on Iodide Goitre.

Inactivation of thyroid protease has also been offered as an explanation of the iodide effect (DeRobertis & Nowinsky, 1946). While I_2 inhibits the human protease (Lundblad *et al.*, 1965), there is no information on iodide and present evidence for this mechanism is inconclusive.

It is possible also that one effect of excess iodide is increased thyroxine formation at the expense of tri-iodothyronine. This type of suggestion was first made 40 years ago by Plummer. Although the difference in calorigenic activities of the two hormones would make this concept an attractive one, the decrease in the PBI that occurs after I^- therapy (Riggs *et al.*, 1942; Harden *et al.*, 1964) would seem to rule this out as a major effect. It should be pointed out that iodide, by filling the thyroid with organic iodine, may hasten the relapse in thyrotoxic patients treated with antithyroid agents of the thiourylene type.

Thiocarbamides. The other antithyroid drugs consist of two main groups: the thiocarbamides and ClO_4^-. The substituted aromatic compounds are not used clinically for thyroid disease, although their use in other disorders occasionally leads to goitres (e.g. resorcinol, *p*-aminosalicylic acid) (Bull & Fraser, 1950; MacGregor & Somner, 1954). The thiocarbamides, which include thiouracil and mercaptoimidazole derivatives, require the thiocarbamyl group:

$$> N \diagdown C = S \diagup$$

The most potent members of this class possess the thiourylene group

$$> N \diagdown C = S \diagup > N$$

characteristic of the thiouracils and mercapto-imidazoles:

HN—C—R
S=C CH
HN—C=O

HC=CH
N N—CH$_3$
C
S—R

(1) R=H in 2-thiouracil
(2) R=CH$_3$ in 6-methyl-2-thiouracil
(3) R=CH$_2$—CH$_2$—CH$_3$ in 6-n-propyl-2-thiouracil

(1) R=H in "Tapazole" or "Methimazole" (1-methyl-2-mercaptoimidazole)
(2) R= COOC$_2$H$_5$ in Carbimazole (1-methyl-2-carbethoxy-mercaptoimidazole)

These compounds act by interfering with the organification of thyroidal iodine, thereby depleting the gland of hormone. This eventually leads to hypothyroidism, resulting in TSH stimulation and finally goitre formation. The goitrogenic effect does not occur in the absence of the adenohypophysis.

The thiocarbamides are reducing agents and react with I$_2$ *in vitro* to form I$^-$ and the appropriate dithio compound (Miller, Roblin & Astwood, 1945). In this way they can interfere with various *in vitro* iodinations and presumably such an effect occurs also in the thyroid (Astwood, 1949). They could react equally well with the agent responsible for iodide oxidation rather than I$_2$ or, perhaps, act as competitive substrates for peroxidase (Randall, 1946; Rosenberg, 1952). Why many of the reducing agents present in the blood are not good antithyroid agents has not been explained. It is generally assumed that the thiocarbamides tautomerize to thiols but the equilibrium strongly favours the thione form. This probably stabilizes them in the circulation. Although the dissociated thiol form may be the reactive species, this is not necessary since tetramethyl thiourea, which cannot tautomerize, reduces I$_2$ (Wolff, unpublished). Nucleophilic sulphur may suffice to reduce I$_2$. The presence of *two* electron donating groups, as in the thiourylene or thio-oxazolidone compounds makes these very active antithyroid agents. In fact, sulphur is not necessary and any strongly nucleophilic centre will do, as shown for the case of 1,1,3-tricyano-aminopropene (Morris & Hager, 1966).

The mechanism of action of the aromatic antithyroid compounds is also not understood. Taurog, Chaikoff & Franklin (1945) considered their activity to be related to their redox potential, and Pitt-Rivers (1950) also suggested reducing power and reactivity with iodine as the mode of action. However, *meta*-substituted isomers are more active antithyroid agents whereas the *ortho*- and *para*-isomers are generally stronger reducing agents (Arnott & Doniach, 1952; Rosenberg, 1952). A number of these compounds are non-competitive inhibitors of peroxidase. Fawcett & Kirkwood (1953) have suggested that these compounds act by forming molecular compounds with iodine, or by undergoing substitution reactions. However, Wollman & Scow (1955) have presented evidence that the substitution reactions do not play a major role, and there is evidence that some addition compounds of I$_2$ may be even more active iodinating agents than the free molecule (Kleinberg & Davidson, 1948).

Although the use of the antithyroid drugs (now principally methyl- or propylthiouracil, methyl-mercaptoimidazole or carbimazole) has greatly aided in the pre-operative management of thyrotoxicosis (Astwood, 1943, 1945, 1949), prolonged medical therapy with these agents has not always been rewarding. There are few cases of hyperthyroidism that cannot be completely controlled with these agents (although "failures" or "resistant cases" appear in many series). Lahey (1953) noted no failures in over 2500 cases, and by frequent dosage all "resistant" cases could be controlled. However, the percentage of sustained remissions following discontinuation of the drug is not impressively high. Although variation is great in the published reports, roughly 50 to 60% remissions is a reasonable figure. The recurrences usually occur within 15 months; the likelihood of escape after a remission of 36 months is slight (Goodwin, Steinberg & Wilson, 1954). Optimal results seem to occur after uninterrupted therapy of over a year. Analysis of factors which might seem to influence remission (i.e. sex, age, size of goitres, change in goitre size during therapy, type of goitre, duration of disease, rapidity of response to treatment, presence of complications, Lugolization) has not yielded very satisfactory results; but an initially small, diffuse gland which decreases in size is probably a good prognostic sign. The hyperplasia initially present may regress under treatment except in those cases where doses leading to hypothyroidism have been employed (Solomon, Beck, Vanderlaan & Astwood, 1953).

Thiouracil derivatives, but not methimazole, decrease the rate of thyroxine de-iodination with a consequent greater faecal excretion. The mechanism is unknown (Jones & Van Middlesworth, 1960; Morreale de Escobar & Escobar del Rey, 1967). A similar effect appears to occur with both T_4 and T_3 degradation in man.

The chief toxic reactions to the thiocarbamides are granulocytopenia and rarely agranulocytosis ($\sim 0.5\%$), as well as drug rashes, fever, arthritis, and occasionally gastro-intestinal disturbances and jaundice (Vanderlaan & Storrie, 1955; Trotter, 1962). Aplastic anaemia is quite uncommon. In evaluating the effect on the leucocyte count it must be remembered that hyperthyroid patients may show leucopenia with a relative granulocytopenia before treatment is started. An initial count is therefore of great value. The thiocarbamides are especially useful in patients refusing surgery, and in patients who are high surgical risks. Medical therapy (either drugs or radio-iodine) is the overwhelming choice in recurrent hyperthyroidism.

Anions. Of the competitive anions only perchlorate has received extensive use. In some centres it was, until recently, the drug of choice (Crooks & Wayne, 1960). The doses used are 600 to 1000 mg./day in divided doses. Although rapidly excreted in the rat (Eichler & Hackenthal, 1962), the evidence in man regarding a "blocking" effect longer than one day is controversial (Goolden & Mallard, 1958; Halnan & Pochin, 1958; Alexander et al., 1964b). When $KClO_4$ is used it is important to remember that it is counteracted by iodide, hence Lugol's solution or KI are contraindicated. Not only will iodine metabolism no longer be blocked, but the iodine-depleted gland may avidly accumulate much of this abundant raw material so suddenly made available (Raben, 1949). This may lead to a catastrophic exacerbation of the thyrotoxicity or, at best, to replenishment of unwanted hormone stores. It also limits its usefulness in the preparation of the patient for surgery since $KClO_4$ alone does little to reduce the vascularity of the gland. The drug appears otherwise to be as effective as the organic agents and toxic reactions do not differ markedly. Reactions appear to be a good deal more frequent with daily doses > 1200 mg./day (Trotter, 1962). In 1961 five cases of aplastic anaemia were reported and as a result the drug has fallen somewhat in repute. Other anions have not been used. KSCN, which inhibits iodide transport *and* probably organic iodine formation, is no longer used. It may be that perrhenate (ReO_4^-) may prove to be useful but there have been no clinical

trials to date (Alexander & Wolff, 1966). Extreme iodine deficiency of the thyroid gland may result from antithyroid therapy either with $KClO_4$ or the thiocarbamides. There is, in addition, an iodide deficiency pattern after cessation of therapy—high thyroid I⁻ clearance, normal PBI and a low concentration of plasma iodide (< 0.08 μg./100 ml.) (Alexander et al., 1964b; Harden, Alexander, Koutras, Harrison & Wayne, 1966). This may persist for 2 years. In the rat this rebound is characterized by a burst of T_3 synthesis (Studer & Greer, 1967). It has been suggested that this iodine deficiency may delay recurrence of thyrotoxic symptoms.

Reserpine, guanethidine, propanolol, etc. have been found to cause marked amelioration of many of the signs and symptoms of hyperthyriodism without changing the underlying disease process, tissue hypermetabolism and the diagnostic tests related to iodine metabolism (Canary, Shaaf, Duffy & Kyle, 1957; Lee, Bronsky & Waldstein, 1962; Waldstein, 1966; Howitt & Rowlands, 1967; Vinik et al., 1968). The increase in cardiac glycoside requirement, characteristic of hyperthyroidism, is also reduced (Frye & Braunwald, 1961). Generally, doses required are larger than tolerated by euthyroid individuals, hence e.g. guanethidine should be used only in severe toxicity. The drug has been recommended as being especially useful in thyroid storm.

The mechanism of the guanethidine effect is credited to depletion of catecholamine stores and hence these drug effects are frequently used as proof of an interrelation between the two hormones. Interpretation should be guarded, however, since the relation of thyroid hormone effects to catecholamines is complicated and controversial.

Radioactive Iodine. Most of the effective radiation of ¹³¹I results from the β-emissions, the γ-radiation passing through the thyroid tissue before causing many ionizations. The other isotopes of iodine are poorer therapeutic agents for some of the same reasons that make them better diagnostic agents.

The remarkable similarity in the clinical results from various centres using ¹³¹I attests to the latitude that exists in the size of the administered dose. The greatest difficulty in determining dosage is the factor of thyroid weight estimation (Blomfield, Eckert, Fisher, Miller, Munro & Wilson, 1959). Scintillation scanning in the frontal and lateral planes to determine thyroid volume probably has not increased the accuracy of this estimate. In addition to gland size, it is necessary to know, as a minimum, the expected uptake of the therapy dose and this is most conveniently done by a pre-treatment tracer dose of ^{131}I. With this figure a rough estimate of the dose to be administered is:

$$\frac{\text{weight (g.)} \times \mu c\ ^{131}\text{I/g. to be delivered}}{\text{fraction of tracer taken up (24 or 48 hr.)}}$$

The dose has varied in several clinics from 100 to 140 μc./g. From what has been said about the conversion ratio it is not surprising that the more rapid appearance of hormone in the blood, measured in thyrotoxic patients roughly as the total radioactivity at 48 hr. after a tracer dose, makes possible a therapy dose calculation that includes the turnover of ^{131}I in the gland. The empirical formula derived by Rall, Sonenberg, Robbins, Lazerson & Rawson, (1953) is:

$$D = \frac{100\ (110 + 27B) \times G}{U}$$

where D is the dose to be given in μc.
   G is the gland weight in g.
   U is the 48 hr. tracer uptake (%) and
   B is the whole blood ^{131}I concentration at 48 hr. (in percent. per litre).

Remission occurs in 60 to 80 % of the cases after a single dose of ^{131}I depending on the dose. The 60 % figure usually can be brought up by repeated treatment. The fraction of patients requiring a second (or even a third) dose of ^{131}I varies from 10 to 20 % in different series. Recurrent hyperthyroidism responds well to ^{131}I (Beling & Einhorn, 1961). This is of considerable importance in view of the hazard attending a second surgical intervention in such cases. Patients with nodular goitres may show poorer responses, but rarely develop myxoedema after ^{131}I treatment—larger doses are often required and surgery is preferred in many clinics. Most patients respond in about 2–3 months, but myxoedema, if it is going to occur, generally does not appear before 4–6 months.

A complication of ^{131}I therapy that was first pointed out by the report of Beling & Einhorn (1961) is the continually rising incidence of hypothyroidism at a rate of 2 to 3 % (5 % in one report) of the treated population per year. This occurs in addition to the 8 to 12 % of patients who become hypothyroid during the first year after ^{131}I therapy. This finding came as a great blow to thyroid clinics but thorough follow-up has led to ample confirmation (Green & Wilson, 1964; Dunn & Chapman, 1964; Nofal, Beierwaltes & Patno, 1966). The incidence is related to dose,

being least in large goitres, greater in hyperthyroidism without goitre and greatest in postsurgical recurrence. In most series, "cure" by a single dose of ^{131}I produced a higher incidence of hypothyroidism than occurred after multiple doses. It should be pointed out that in some surgical series there is also a progressive increase in the incidence of hypothyroidism with a rate as high as 1·7 %/year (Nofal et al., 1966). A myxoedema incidence of 38 % after sub-total thyroidectomy for hyperthyroidism in children has been reported (Hayes, Chaves-Carballo & McConahey, 1967). In a prospective study, Smith & Wilson (1967) have compared doses delivering $\sim$ 7000 rads to the thyroid with a group of patients receiving only $\sim$ 3500 rads. Although the "cure" rate was slower in the latter (and this was easily controlled by anti-thyroid drugs), the fraction euthyroid was the same at three years. The incidence of hypothyroidism was 29 % in five years after 7000 rads compared to 7 % after half that dose. More experience of this sort is badly needed.

In addition to numerous acute disturbances in iodine metabolism resulting from ^{131}I treatment (e.g. positive perchlorate discharge), some sort of failure of the thyroid cell to multiply is currently thought to explain this progressive loss of thyroid function. Radiation is known to inhibit growth stimulation induced by a goitrogen (for references see Greig, Crooks & MacGregor, 1966). Although there is a temporary rise in cytoplasmic antibody titres after ^{131}I therapy, current evidence does not support an auto-immune mechanism for this form of hypothyroidism (Einhorn, Fagraeus & Jonsson, 1965). Pre-treatment with methylthiouracil or ClO_4^- seems to render the gland radio-resistant to a certain extent (Buchanan, Koutras, Crooks & Harden, 1965b).

Of the other untoward effects of ^{131}I, induction of thyroid neoplasms must be considered (see section on neoplasms). This is readily demonstrated in the experimental animal but has been rare with therapeutic doses in man. Nuclear changes, which appear similar to some pre-malignant lesions seen elsewhere in the body, have been noted by several investigators (Maloof, 1955; Dailey, Lindsay & Miller, 1953; Freedberg, Chamowitz & Kurland, 1952), but their significance remains obscure. Sheline, Lindsay, McCormack & Galante (1962) have found adenomas in eight thyroids 5 to 14 years after ^{131}I therapy. Frequency was highest in younger patients. They suggest that if ^{131}I therapy cannot be avoided in children, ablative doses should be used. Other reports of this complication are rare (Kogut,

Kaplan, Collipp, Tiamsic & Boyle, 1965). It is of interest that doses as low as 6 rad may produce increases in aberrant nuclear patterns of hamster thyroid cells (Moore & Colvin, 1966).

Parathyroid function is generally believed to remain unimpaired in patients treated with [131]I. However, several reports of "diminished parathyroid reserve" suggest caution in this area as well (Harden et al., 1963; Adams & Chalmers, 1965). With the doses used in the treatment of toxic goitre other untoward effects are uncommon, aside from occasional "radiation thyroiditis" during the first week.

Persistent chromosomal aberrations in the chromosomes of leucocytes have been noted after therapeutic doses of [131]I (Nofal & Beierwaltes, 1964). Such changes are, however, also seen after diagnostic X-ray procedures (Bloom & Tjio, 1964).

Although 18 cases of leukaemia are known to have occurred after ^{131}I therapy for thyrotoxicosis (through 1959), this number is not in excess of the natural leukaemia rate for a population equivalent to the nearly 60,000 cases treated (Pochin, 1960). If it can be clearly determined that thyroid cancer will be an insignificant complication of the therapy of thyrotoxicosis, it is very likely that radio-iodine will become the dominant form of treatment. At present it is already the treatment of choice in patients who present a considerable surgical risk or toxic reactions to antithyroid drugs, who are over 40–45 years of age without a very large goitre, who refuse operation, or who show persistent or recurrent (post-operative) toxicity. It is also used in selected euthyroid cardiac patients with intractable angina or failure.

Surgery. Although the operative mortality of sub-total thyroidectomy for diffuse toxic goitre is essentially zero in the major thyroid centres, the incidence of serious complications such as laryngeal nerve palsy or hypoparathyroidism is far from zero. Precise values depend on the fraction of thyroid tissue removed, etc. The same uncertainty applies to recurrence and myxoedema, the incidences of which are inversely related. The long-term incidence of post-operative hypothyroidism may well be of the progressively increasing type as seen after [131]I. The rate is less but few data are available and it may be as high as 1·7%/year (Nofal et al., 1966). While figures vary, the mortality and morbidity in hospitals not specializing in thyroid surgery is considerably higher than the above and this factor, above all, should be kept in mind when considering surgery.

IODIDE GOITRE

Excess iodide exerts its antithyroid effect not only in Graves' disease but also on the euthyroid gland. Some 150 such cases have now been reported. Goitre (usually diffuse) and hypothyroidism both occur but either may exist without the other. The majority of these patients suffer from chronic lung disease but this is not a necessary condition. Lugol's solution, KI, or HI are the usual sources of the excess iodide but organic sources such as "Iodopyrine", lipiodol and even di-iodotyrosine have also been implicated. Therapy with these agents is usually massive (720 mg. I/day) and of long duration, but small doses and treatment for only three months have been followed by goitre or myxoedema. References are too numerous to list here but representative studies will be found in: Turner & Howard, 1956; Oppenheimer & McPherson, 1961; Begg & Hall, 1963; Frey, 1964; Hadden, Montgomery & Weaver, 1965; Wolff, 1969.

A few cases of foetal iodide goitre leading to serious obstetrical complications have been recorded in women being treated with iodopyrine or KI for asthma during pregnancy (Martin & Rento, 1962; Anderson & Bird, 1961).

Recently, an endemic of iodide goitre has been described in northern Japan. This is the first series of non-iatrogenic iodide goitre, and more importantly, is the first documented goitre endemic due to a positive goitrogen, presumably iodide (Suzuki et al., 1965). The source of the iodide is the seaweed "Kombu", a species of *Laminaria*, which yields an iodine intake of ∼ 50 mg./day. These patients exhibit the criteria listed below as requirements for the syndrome but are not generally hypothyroid. Proof for the role of seaweed comes from the disappearance of the goitre if "kombu" is deleted from the diet. Proof that iodide is involved is shown by the fact that either kombu or KI will cause a return of the goitre. Why so many of these people get goitre when others who have equal iodine intakes do not, has not been explained. The presence of a compound in the diet which is synergistic with iodide, or of genetic factors, would appear to warrant further study.

The typical picture is one of goitre and hypothyroidism with all the features of a block in organic iodine formation: (1) low PBI, BEI or T_4 (these measurements require special handling because of massive iodide contamination). (2) High serum cholesterol, low BMR, etc. (3) Thyroidal [131]I^- uptake is rapid and falls rapidly. Uptakes are often substantial despite the high plasma iodide levels. Most cases are suppressed by T₃ (Harrison, Alexander & Harden, 1963). Accumulated ¹³¹I can be discharged with ClO₄⁻. (Data are confusing since the relation to the last dose of KI is not usually stated.) (4) There may be a brief rebound hyperactivity of the thyroid after iodide levels have fallen. (5) There is currently some controversy regarding the histological findings—both colloid goitre and hyperplasia have been reported. The time relation between biopsy and iodide withdrawal has not always been stated.

inhibited before trapping is saturated. This, in turn, increases the concentration of trapped iodide (Wolff & Chaikoff, 1948a,b,c,d). Acute iodide inhibition occurs also in man (Stanley, 1949; Childs, Keating, Rall, Williams & Power, 1950) and varies with the nature of the gland (Reinwein & Klein, 1962). Inhibition ensues at plasma iodide levels >20 to 35 μg./100 ml. in the rat and > 6 to 12 μg./100 ml. in normal man (Wolff & Chaikoff, 1948a,b; Stanley, 1949). (See

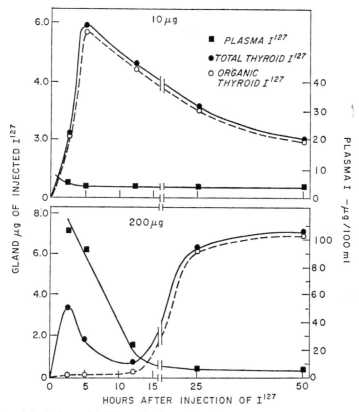

FIG. 12.7. The effect of single doses of iodide on the formation of organic iodine in the rat thyroid (from Wolff & Chaikoff, 1948).

(6) A *sine qua non* for the diagnosis is the return of the euthyroid state upon withdrawal of excess iodide alone without hormone replacement. (7) In only a few cases has a familial factor been demonstrated. Why so few patients get iodide goitre in view of the prodigal use of iodide by clinicians remains a puzzle.

The ability to concentrate iodide actively appears to be necessary in order to attain inhibitory intrathyroidal I⁻ concentration *in vivo*. With moderately large iodide loads organification is

Fig. 12.7). If iodide concentration is decreased by a partial discharge with SCN⁻, more organic iodine is formed despite the antithyroid properties of this anion (Raben, 1949). Attempts to induce hypothyroidism with KI in a patient lacking the iodide trap were unsuccessful (Wolff, Thompson & Robbins, 1964). It may be that diffused I⁻ enjoys a different cellular location than that actively transported.

In rats inhibition of organic iodine formation by excess I⁻ is short-lived (Wolff, Chaikoff,

Goldberg & Meier, 1949). In part, this is due to an "adaptive" loss in the ability to concentrate iodide following prolonged exposure to this halide (Braverman & Ingbar, 1963). The mechanism of this loss is unknown. Acute iodide block and the subsequent escape phenomenon can be demonstrated in thyroids of hypophysectomized rats suggesting that TSH changes are not involved. There is no change in thyroid K^+ levels (Lee & Ingbar, 1965).

The mechanism of iodide inhibition is entirely unknown. It has been suggested that iodide might inhibit by promoting I_3^- formation in the equilibrium: $I^- + I_2 \rightleftharpoons I_3^-$ (Fawcett & Kirkwood, 1953). However, Wollman & Scow (1954) pointed out that under the conditions of I^- concentration in the thyroid much of the I_2 would be free. Nevertheless, the complete rate expression for iodination contains a $1/[I^-]^2$ term, the second reciprocal iodide term representing the addition step to the *ortho* position (Mayberry *et al.*, 1964; Berliner, 1966). Hence this strictly chemical mode of iodide inhibition deserves further attention.

The possibility that iodide has some effect on an energy producing reaction in the thyroid has been considered. Iodide both stimulates and inhibits various Krebs cycle oxidations depending on the concentration (Green, 1966). Both levels, however, inhibit iodinations and this seems, therefore, an inadequate explanation. Inhibition due to the formation of some iodinated peptide or other inhibitor has been suggested (Halmi, 1961) but fails to account for the escape phenomenon.

Any explanation offered will have to accommodate the temporary nature of the effect. Our present view is that, for unexplained reasons, escape fails to occur in some patients and these will in time develop iodide goitre. For details the reader is referred to the review by Wolff (1969).

SEX AND THE THYROID GLAND

A reciprocal interplay of the gonads and the thyroid gland has been repeatedly demonstrated. The profound effect of oestrogenic and androgenic steroids on thyroxine-binding in serum have been discussed above. Equally profound effects are induced by the thyroid hormones on the metabolism of both oestrogens and androgens. Clinically the more important deviations from normal occur in hypothyroidism. However, what there is known of the mechanisms involved has been investigated as a function of both excessive and deficient thyroid hormone levels.

Oestrogens

The products of oestradiol-^{14}C metabolism change from oestriol in the hypothyroid state to the 2-hydroxylated products, 2-hydroxyoestrone and 2-methoxyoestrone, during hyperthyroidism. The fractions appearing as oestrone or oestradiol are not significantly changed. Thus, in the competition for C-2 and C-16 hydroxylation the thyroid hormone favours the former (Fishman, Hellman, Zumoff & Gallagher, 1965). It is of interest that thyroid control of steroid hydroxylation is seen also in the bile acids where the C-12 hydroxylation is inhibited by thyroid hormone, leading to increased proportion of chenodeoxycholic acid excretion in rat bile (Eriksson, 1957; Berséus, 1965). Furthermore, high levels of thyroid hormone lead to a higher fraction of adrenal steroid appearing in the urine as 11-ketosteroids (Hellman *et al.*, 1961).

A great deal of work has failed to shed light on the precise influence of the thyroid hormones on ovarian function both in animals (Young & Corner, 1961; Maqsood, 1952) and in man (Rogers, 1958). Much of this results from inadequate assays for gonadotropins and blood steroid determinations. The following are, however, probably correct statements. In general an optimum level of thyroid hormone is required for optimal gonadal function, but hypothyroidism causes more severe dysfunction. Infertility and delayed puberty often accompany hypothyroidism, but pregnancy is known to occur in untreated cretinism or myxoedema (Parkin & Green, 1943; Lister & Ashe, 1955). There appears, however, to be little support for the common practice of treating infertility with thyroid hormone. Thyrotoxic women are apparently normally fertile. Hyperthyroidism is frequently accompanied by oligomenorrhoea (with regular cycles), whereas severe menorrhagia may occur in myxoedema together with anovulatory cycles and low pregnanediol levels (Goldsmith, Sturgis, Lerman & Stanbury 1952; Ross, Scholz, Lamberg & Geraci, 1958). While the hypothyroid animal is unusually sensitive to exogenous gonadotropins (Janes, 1954; Mandl, 1957; Thorsøe, 1962) it is uncertain whether this occurs also in women (see below). Gonadotropin contents of hypothyroid animal pituitaries are reported to be low whereas normal urine levels are often reported in human myxoedema (Statland & Lerman, 1950; Beierwaltes & Bishop, 1954). These findings need to be reinvestigated with immune assay methods.

An interesting syndrome of precocious sexual development with menstruation and galactorrhoea in primary juvenile hypothyroidism has been reported by Van Wyk & Grumbach (1960). In addition to the above signs the sella turcica is enlarged, and there is no pubic hair. Two of three girls probably had Hashimoto's thyroiditis. All the signs of precocity disappeared upon replacement therapy with thyroid hormone and the pituitary fossa decreased in size. A related but different syndrome of primary hypothyroidism, amenorrhoea and galactorrhoea of post-partum women has been reported (Ross & Nusynowitz, 1968). A similar syndrome in the male is characterized by precocious testicular maturation (Franks & Stempfel, 1963). Although it was postulated (and supported by indirect evidence) that these were cases of inappropriate secretion of various pituitary hormones due to thyroid hormone lack, urinary gonadotropins were not elevated. Ovarian stimulation occurs in animals with pituitary tumours due to hypothyroidism (Furth & Clifton, 1958) but increased sensitivity to gonadotropins may also be involved (Janes, 1954; Mandl, 1957).

A curious and unexplained association between gonadal dysgenesis and thyroiditis has been reported (Williams, Engel & Forbes, 1964). Goitre or clinical thyroiditis was present only in chromatin-positive patients (Grumbach & Morishima, 1964), whereas antibody titres were high in both chromatin-negative and chromatin-positive cases. There appears to be a high association with X-chromosome abnormalities especially the X-iso-X type (Milet, Plunkett & Carr, 1967).

Androgens

Gallagher, Hellman Bradlow, Zumoff & Fukushima (1960) have shown a marked shift in androgen metabolites, whether of endogenous or exogenous origin, with changes in thyroid status. The normal proportion of urinary androsterone (5α) to aetiocholanolone (5β) is about 40:60. In myxoedema this ratio becomes about 15:85 while in Graves' disease ratios as high as 75:25 may occur. The authors point out that androsterone will by itself lower serum cholesterol in man (though not in animals) and suggest a possible role for this metabolite in the cholesterol-lowering effect of the thyroid hormones.

Patients with myxoedema usually have decreased urinary 17-oxosteroid excretions that return to normal upon replacement therapy (Beierwaltes & Bishop, 1954). Excess thyroid hormone leads to increased levels only in exceptional cases. Hypothyroidism of pre-pubertal onset leads to delayed maturation of the Leydig cells and tubular fibrosis associated with decreased urinary excretion of pituitary gonadotrophins and 17-oxosteroids (De La Balze et al., 1962). Hypothyroidism appearing after puberty leads to less severe Leydig cell changes.

An association between decreased thyroid gland function and Klinefelter's syndrome has come to light in recent years. It has been attributed to extra X-chromosome function. Most such patients are clinically euthyroid but may have goitre. Hypothyroidism may occur in some cases. The thyroidal iodine uptake is low, particularly in the chromatin-positive cases and there may be a poor response to exogenous TSH in some cases (Carr, Barr, Plunkett, Grumbach, Morshima & Chu, 1961; Davis, Canfield, Herman & Goter, 1963; Grand, Rosen, Di Sant'Agnese & Kirkham, 1966).

PREGNANCY

Puberty and pregnancy appear to place an increased load on the thyroid, as evidenced by the increased incidence of goitre during these two periods (Crooks, Aboul-Khair, Turnbull & Hytten, 1964). It has been suggested that these changes may, in part, be due to increased renal clearance of iodide with a consequent decrease in the plasma iodide concentration (Baschieri et al., 1959; Aboul-Khair, Crooks, Turnbull & Hytten, 1964). Since the thyroidal iodide clearance is increased after the twelfth week, the calculated amount of iodine entering the gland is likely to be normal (Myant, 1964). Placental TSH may also play a rôle.

It is well known that the BMR increases gradually to values of $+ 20$ to 25 in the third trimester of pregnancy. About three-quarters of this rise is due to the uterus and its contents, the remainder resulting from increased cardiac and respiratory work (see Freedberg, Hamolsky & Freedberg, 1957 for references).

The PBI rises during the first trimester to $6-10\mu g./100$ ml. or more (Heinemann, Johnson & Man, 1948). Dowling, Freinkel & Ingbar (1956) and Robbins & Nelson (1958) have shown that the thyroxine-binding capacity, in this case the concentration of thyroxine-binding globulin (TBG), was increased in pregnancy as early as the second month and persisted for some weeks post partum. There appears to be no rise in thyroxine-binding pre-albumin (Ingbar, 1960). As the mass-law calculations indicate, there need thus be no comparable rise in the free thyroxine of the serum (Robbins & Rall, 1967); in fact it is somewhat lower than the mean normal value. It is of interest that women with hydatidiform mole show similar blood changes as well as greatly increased thyroidal ^{131}I uptakes (see Freedberg et al., 1957).

In a small series of pregnancies, a correlation was noted between the tendency to abort and failure of the PBI to rise above values of 6 $\mu g./$

100 ml. (Man, Heinemann, Johnson, Leary & Peters, 1951; Russel, 1953), and the expected increase in thyroxine-binding globulin failed to occur in some cases of habitual abortion (Dowling et al., 1956). Although there are recurrent reports that the outcome of pregnancies is poor for women whose PBI or BEI fails to increase with pregnancy (Greenman, Gabrielson, Flanders & Wessel, 1962), not all investigators agree that there is a causal relation. Furthermore, the treatment of habitual abortion with thyroid on the basis of the above has led to no clear-cut results.

During the puerperium the BMR and serum PBI return to normal or low values, the latter at a more rapid rate (Danowski, Huff, Nirvos, Writh, George & Mateer, 1953). Trapping of iodine is also decreased following delivery (Pochin, 1952), and it would appear from these results as well as from occasional clinical observations, that mild hypothyroidism may follow delivery for a short period.

Differentiation of mild Graves' disease from the physiological changes of pregnancy is very difficult. Pregnant women tolerate moderate degrees of thyrotoxicosis remarkably well, and it is best to err on the side of under- rather than over-treatment. Diagnostic procedures with ^{131}I are contraindicated, since Chapman, Corner, Robinson & Evans (1948) have shown that human foetal thyroids accumulate ^{131}I after the 14th week. Small amounts of radio-iodine have been shown experimentally to be deleterious to the thyroid gland of the foetus (Speert, Quimby & Werner, 1951). However, the supposed increased sensitivity of the foetal thyroid is a debated subject (Skanse, 1948; Goldberg & Chaikoff, 1949; Doniach, 1957). Nevertheless, in the absence of definitive information, it would be prudent to have the pregnant or lactating mother avoid exposure to ^{131}I or material likely to be contaminated with radioactive fall-out (Beierwaltes et al., 1960).

When toxicity is severe foetal loss may be high (Bell, 1950) and the patient's condition itself may require therapy during the pregnancy. In such cases Lahey (1953) and Werner (1954a,b) favour surgery early in pregnancy and antithyroid drugs in the last trimester. However, antithyroid drugs cross the placenta and may cause goitre, etc. (Elphinstone, 1953). Although it is uncertain whether the foetal gland enlarges as a result of maternal or foetal TSH, it is probably the latter (Myant, 1964). Astwood (1951) has treated pregnant women with combinations of propylthiouracil and thyroid hormones to guard against induction of hypothyroidism. While this is useful for

the mother, the degree to which the foetus is protected depends on the rate of placental transfer of the hormones. The use of minimal doses of antithyroid drugs is safer.

The choice of therapy therefore depends on the ability to suppress these reactions, i.e. is there adequate placental transfer of T_4 and T_3? The PBI of early foetuses is very low (Osorio & Myant, 1962) whereas cord blood of full term foetuses is in the normal adult range or may be slightly increased. Although the human thyroid begins to function at about 14 weeks, it is not known how much hormone it releases. On the other hand, placental transfer of T_4 or T_3 to the foetus seems to be governed by the level of specific binding proteins. These increase with gestation leading to both increased foetal PBI levels and to increased transfer of hormone across the placenta (Myant, 1964). It is important, therefore, not to be complacent about "covering" an antithyroid agent with a few grains of desiccated thyroid.

It is quite clear that the thyroid hormone is not necessary for early foetal development or differentiation. The low PBI of young foetuses may mean only that whatever hormones get across the placenta immediately enter the tissues. However, foetuses differentiate in completely myxoedematous mothers (before the foetal thyroid makes its own hormone) (Parkin & Greene, 1943; Hodges, Hamilton & Keettel, 1952; Lister & Ashe, 1955; Myant, 1964), suggesting that thyroid hormones are not required. Precisely when the need for hormone arises is thus not clear but it seems to occur sometimes in utero, since athyroid new-born infants show defective brain development and delayed bone and tooth development (Anderson, 1961; Wilkins, 1965). Protection of the foetus is thus a complicated matter which has not been satisfactorily accomplished. The most important consideration is that, in the treatment of hyperthyroidism during pregnancy, care must be taken to avoid hypothyroidism, and a BMR around 25 and a PBI of 6 to 10 μg./100 ml. should be aimed for. Following delivery and lactation, the treatment of thyrotoxicosis is governed by the same considerations as obtain under other circumstances.

The cord blood of the new-born infant tends to reflect the maternal changes in thyroxine-binding proteins with similar PBI and T_3-uptake values (Hirschfeld & Söderberg, 1960; Michener, Tauxe & Hayles, 1962; Lindergen & Starr, 1966; Marks & Man, 1965). Premature infants show the same changes although very light foetuses will have lower PBI values. The early neonatal period is characterized by very high radio-iodine uptakes, maximal within 72 hours and decreasing rapidly thereafter. Premature infants tend to have lower 24 hr. [131]I uptakes or related parameters (Fisher, Oddie & Burroughs, 1962). Reports that radio-iodine uptakes are not elevated are probably due to the late interval after birth chosen for the test (Ogborn, Waggener & Van Hove, 1960). During the same first two days of life there is a marked rise in the PBI *not* accompanied by changes in TBP but occurring simultaneously with a drop in TBPA (Perry, Hodgman & Starr, 1965). Fisher & Oddie (1964) have attributed this to the fall in body temperature after birth, for if this is pre-vented the PBI changes are much less marked.

THYROIDITIS

We shall be concerned here with two major types of thyroiditis: (1) subacute thyroiditis (DeQuervain's thyroiditis; giant-cell, pseudo-tuberculous or granulomatous thyroiditis, and sometimes acute thyroiditis), and (2) Hashimoto's thyroiditis (struma lymphomatosa, lymphadenoid goitre, lymphocytic thyroiditis). A third, and rare type, called Riedel's struma or thyroiditis will not be discussed here except to say that it is probably *not* an end-result of either of the other two types. In addition, transient thyroiditis may be encoun-tered after ^{131}I therapy and, rarely, after injection of TSH.

Subacute Thyroiditis

The incidence of subacute thyroiditis is un-known, but mild cases may be missed if complica-ted by pharyngitis or mumps. It is defined as a self-limited inflammation of the thyroid gland that may involve one or both lobes. The disease may present as nodules which "migrate" with progression of time. The occasional confusion with solitary "cold" nodules can be resolved by the reappearance of ^{131}I uptake in the nodule (Ham-burger, Kadian & Rossin, 1965). Clinically there is local pain, sometimes radiating to the ears, often exquisite tenderness so that palpation is impossible. This is usually rather sharply confined to the area of the gland. There may be a sore throat and/or dysphagia, a marked systemic reaction including fever, sometimes with chills, sweats and malaise. There may be no symptoms other than the presence of the goitre which tends to be very firm and slightly irregular to palpation.

The aetiology of subacute thyroiditis is believed to be viral, largely on the basis of the clinical course. Virus identification has been infrequent. In 10 of 11 patients with the disease there were significantly positive complement fixation titres for mumps and the virus was isolated in two of these (Eylan, Zmucky & Sheba, 1957). Another case

with positive mumps and haemagglutination tests has also been described (Felix-Davies, 1958). Mild cases have also been observed in the adults of families where the children had mumps. A case of cat scratch thyroiditis has been reported (Shumway & Davis, 1954), as have correlations with adenovirus (Swann, 1964) and Coxsackie virus antibody titres (Volpe, Row & Ezrin, 1966). An epidemic of 44 cases of subacute thyroiditis following "colds" also supports the infectious aetiology (Hintze, Fortelius & Railo, 1964). It may be that the clinical picture is characteristic of a variety of viral infections rather than one.

The changes in iodine metabolism seen in sub-acute thyroiditis are those that would be expected from sudden destruction of the parenchyma with gradual recovery. In the acute stage of severe cases there is a period of probable hyperthy-roidism which passes through a brief euthyroid phase, to the second or hypothyroid stage. This is followed by gradual recovery. The thyrotoxic phase may show PBI values as high as 16 μg./ 100 ml. It would be expected that some of this would be thyroglobulin and the BEI values in two cases were 11–12 when the PBI was 16 μg./100 ml. (Ingbar & Freinkel, 1958a). There is probably both iodoprotein and a true elevation of the blood hormone levels. As many as two-thirds of the patients may have antibodies to thyroglobulin in their sera. The titres fall more rapidly than in Hashimoto's thyroiditis (see p. 432) (Roitt & Doniach, 1958). However, no antibody elevation has been reported in other series (Higgins, Bayley & Diosy, 1963; Hintze et al., 1964).

The ^{131}I uptake is low, often zero, and related tests, e.g. urinary ^{131}I output or conversion ratios, agree with this. It has been suggested that part of the thyroid depression is a result of the high PBI, but some patients respond poorly to exogenous TSH suggesting, not surprisingly, an element of "low thyroid reserve" (Lamberg, Hintze, Jussila & Berlin, 1960). In any case the rate of hormone synthesis is markedly reduced and the "thyro-toxicosis", when present, is produced by hormone made before the onset of the disease. The duration of this stage may thus be considered a function of the size of the thyroidal hormone pool present at the onset. The BMR may be + 40 but, as there is often considerable fever, the exact meaning of the increase is not clear. Both absolute and relative leucocytosis and lymphocytosis have been reported. The erythrocyte sedimentation rate is elevated and there may be an elevated level of plasma α_2-globulin and fibrinogen (Skillern & Lewis, 1958). In an epidemic of subacute thy-roiditis, the β-globulin remained elevated longer than the other globulin fractions (Hintze *et al.*, 1964). This toxic phase may last three weeks to three months in severe cases and can be considerably ameliorated by radiotherapy or corticosteroid therapy (Volpe, Johnston & Huber, 1958; Lamberg *et al.*, 1960). In mild cases the toxic period may be brief or absent. Since the gland is still damaged when the hormone stores are exhausted, the patient passes through a brief euthyroid period (1–2 weeks) and may then become hypothyroid both clinically and by PBI or BMR. The ^{131}I uptake is initially still low but begins to climb toward normal generally before the PBI reaches normal values. This presumably corresponds to the period of regeneration of the thyroid parenchyma. The recovery phase may show a transient rebound increase in the ^{131}I uptake. Some patients never go through a frank hypothyroid phase. Permanent myxoedema is rare after subacute thyroiditis. A few cases of true hyperthyroidism have been encountered (Volpe *et al.*, 1958; Czerniak & Harell-Steinberg, 1957). The significance of this is not yet clear. Although treatment with X-irradiation shortens the acute phase, the corticosteroids would seem to be the agents of choice. On the basis of an exacerbation of the disease with exogenous TSH, thyroid suppression with T_3 has been tried and found to be effective in about 60% of cases (Higgins *et al.*, 1963).

Hashimoto's Thyroiditis

Classically, Hashimoto's thyroiditis was a histological diagnosis characterized by diffuse lymphocytic and plasma cell infiltration of the thyroid gland sometimes developing into true germinal centres. There are also large, eosinophilic Askanazy (or Hürthle) cells. Considerable follicular damage occurs with loss of colloid, and cell masses may be found in the lumina when these are still recognizable. The later stages show fibrosis but never in the amount seen in Riedel's struma. Sufficient variability exists to make strict histological criteria difficult. Furthermore, lymphocytic infiltration is not uncommon in other thyroid diseases such as thyrotoxicosis. Variability within a single gland and lymphocytic infiltration in other goitres have limited the usefulness of needle biopsies. With the discovery of antibodies to thyroid tissue (see below) much hope was entertained that immunological tests would allow accurate diagnosis of this disorder. Unfortunately, they do not, although they are very helpful (Fig. 12.8).

The nature of the initiating insult to the thyroid is unknown. It was originally suggested that auto-immunity leads to the gradual destruction of gland, the typical histological features and finally hypothyroidism (see Roitt & Doniach, 1960). This hypothesis is based on the studies of Rose & Witebsky (1956) who produced similar lesions in rabbits by immunization with homologous thyroid extracts. However, Hashimoto sera *do not* produce the lesions in monkeys, although a cytotoxic factor for thyroid tissue culture has been demonstrated (Pulvertaft, Doniach, Roitt & Hudson, 1959). It appears to be a 7S γ-globulin requiring complement, and correlates reasonably well with the titre of the complement-fixing antibody (Irvine, 1962; Forbes *et al.*, 1962; Anderson *et al.*, 1967). It has, however, been pointed out that the appearance and decrease of the cytotoxic factor seems too rapid to explain the course of Hashimoto's thyroiditis. Even when such a factor is demonstrated for the *in situ* production of Hashimoto lesions the initial cause will still have to be demonstrated. We know that leakage of thyroglobulin does not invariably cause permanent thyroid damage, as demonstrated in cases of subacute thyroiditis, and by the fact that thyroglobulin appears to be a normal constituent of blood (Daniel *et al.*, 1967). On the other hand the reaction between thyroid antigen and antibody can produce local tissue damage of the Arthus type. It is of interest that sera of many patients with Sjögren's syndrome show antithyroid antibodies. Some of these patients have goitres and in a few cases where thyroid tissue has been available the histological picture has been consistent with Hashimoto's thyroiditis (Bunim, 1961; Anderson *et al.*, 1967). Despite the relation to this and other auto-immune diseases, and the report of a high incidence of thyroiditis in families (Thier, Black, Williams & Robbins, 1965; Anderson *et al.*, 1967), the pathogenesis of Hashimoto's thyroiditis remains obscure.

Clinical and pathological descriptions have been given by many authors (Lindsay, Dailey, Friedlander, Yee & Soley, 1952; Skillern, Nelson & Crile, 1956; Masi, 1965). The disease, though typically occurring in middle-aged women, may occur at any age and also in males. The onset is usually insidious but may be subacute which complicates differentiation from subacute thyroiditis. Goitres are diffuse to lobular and usually firm. Since the disease often progresses to rather extensive fibrosis but represents at the same time a compensatory process, various degrees of hypothyroidism may be encountered. These are reflected in the standard laboratory tests. The BMR may be low and response to desiccated thyroid occurs at dose levels typical of hypothyroidism. The serum cholesterol may be elevated. The PBI may range from below to slightly above normal. A marked discrepancy occurs with the BEI which is due to circulating iodoprotein (Gribetz, Talbot & Crawford, 1954; Skillern et al., 1956).

The ^{131}I uptakes are usually in the normal range but may sometimes be below or above normal. This is true especially in measurements made at early intervals after the isotope is given (Buchanan, Koutras, Alexander, Crooks, Richmond & Wayne, 1961). The high uptakes presumably reflect the compensatory process that is also responsible for the goitre. This explanation is supported by the fact that exogenous TSH will not generally increase the ^{131}I uptake, whereas triiodothyronine, etc. will depress it. Paradoxically, circulating TSH was found to be low (by a bioassay) in those cases with suppressible high uptakes (El Kabir, Doniach & Turner-Warwick, 1963). On the other hand, the TSH-stimulated *discharge* of PB[131]I from the gland may be elicited more frequently. The rise in serum PB[131]I is, however, usually less than in normal patients (Buchanan et al., 1961). A few cases have been observed in which the high uptakes of ^{131}I persist into the hypothyroid stage, i.e. with low BMR measurements (Skillern et al., 1956). The ^{131}I uptake is a good test to differentiate those cases of Hashimoto's thyroiditis which are symptomatic from subacute thyroiditis.

Although the ^{131}I uptakes and the absolute iodine uptakes (calculated from the plasma iodide levels) are frequently normal, a considerable number of patients cannot convert the iodide to organic forms at the normal rate. In these, a portion of the accumulated radioactivity can be discharged by ClO_4^-. This defect resembles, but is less severe than, that seen after antithyroid therapy or in certain congenital cretins. These findings may also explain the early peaks in ^{131}I uptakes (Buchanan et al., 1961; Nilsson & Berne, 1964). The same defect in organification may occur when complement fixation tests are positive in the absence of clinical thyroid disease (Buchanan, Harden, Koutras & Gray, 1965a).

In addition to the changes in iodine metabolism there are marked changes in the serum proteins. The γ-globulins are both relatively and absolutely increased and the following flocculation tests are abnormal: thymol turbidity, zinc sulphate, colloidal gold. Cephalin flocculation tests are positive less often (Skillern et al., 1956; Doniach & Vaughan-Hudson, 1957; Beare, 1958). There is no elevation of the α_2-globulins or fibrinogen as occurs in subacute thyroiditis. A marked elevation

of the erythrocyte sedimentation rate is generally found and may be helpful to differentiate simple goitre.

An association of histological thyroiditis with carcinoma of the thyroid is not infrequently pointed out from surgical material (Leboeuf & Bongiovanni, 1964). The true incidence is unknown but is probably low since many patients with thyroiditis receive no biopsy and do not go to surgery (see also Lindsay, 1964).

In addition to the cytotoxic factor mentioned above, which is a γ-globulin requiring complement, and which is found in various thyroid disorders, two classes of antigens are involved in the auto-immunity of Hashimoto's thyroiditis (see Table 12.8) (from Roitt & Doniach, 1960).

Antibodies against thyroglobulin are usually of the 7S, but occasionally also of the 19S, type. In most studies the thyroglobulin used has not been pure and in Ouchterlony plates some sera have given two precipitation lines. This may mean that

TABLE 12.8

Immune reactions in Hashimoto's thyroiditis

Antigen	Method of Detection of Auto-antibodies
Thyroglobulin	Precipitin Reaction
	Tanned Red Cell Agglutination
	Radioactive Co-precipitation
	Passive Cutaneous Anaphylaxis
Microsomes	Complement Fixation
	Fluorescent Antibody Technique on unfixed Sections
	Cytotoxic Factor

thyroglobulin fragments were used as antigens (Metzger, Sharp & Edelhoch, 1962). Small fragments, of average molecular weight 700, caused partial inhibition of the precipitin test, whereas with fractions of average molecular weight 8000 the inhibition was complete. Metzger & Edelhoch (1962) have prepared an essentially pure human auto-antibody to thyroglobulin and found material with a sedimentation coefficient $(S_{20, w})$ of 7·2S. Rabbit antibodies cross-reacted with beef, human and hog antigens, while the auto-antibody did not cross-react. It is also possible that a second soluble or colloid antigen exists in some patients who are negative for the other factors (Balfour, Doniach, Roitt & Couchman, 1961). The characteristics of these antigen-antibody interactions have been reviewed by Anderson et al. (1967).

The precipitin test is relatively insensitive and thereby seems to gain a great deal of specificity for Hashimoto's thyroiditis and myxoedema (Fig.

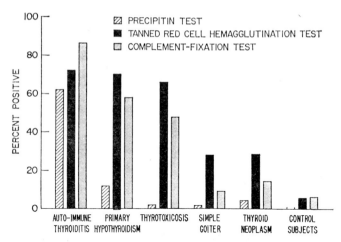

FIG. 12.8. Cumulative experience of thyroid auto-antibodies in thyroid disease (from Auto-Immune Thyroid-itis by W. Watson Buchanan in 'Disease-a-Month'. Copyright 1962, Year Book Medical Publishers, Inc. Reproduced by permission.)

12.8). The high titres present in these two diseases have been used as evidence to establish a causal relationship between them. Titres may be so high that γ-globulin levels are increased. It has also been noted that there is an increased incidence of antithyroglobulin antibodies in those patients treated with ^{131}I for thyrotoxicosis who later developed myxoedema (Blagg, 1960). The titres were rather low and will require confirmation before an auto-immune mechanism can be postulated for the genesis of this form of myxoedema. What fraction of Hashimoto's cases finally end up with myxoedema, and conversely, what fraction of the myxoedema population have lost their functional thyroid tissue as a result of thyroiditis is not known.

The tanned red cell agglutination test is very sensitive but shows positive results also in a high percentage of cases with thyrotoxicosis, simple foitre and in carcinoma of the thyroid (Fig. 12.8). Some non-thyroid disorders also show positive tests. Nevertheless, titres of Hashimoto's or myxoedema sera are generally much higher than of sera with other thyroid disorders. Polystyrene particles can be agglutinated in the same basic reaction but there seems to be no significant advantage to this method. Titres seem to be rather lower in children with thyroiditis but are at the same time more diagnostic for this disease. Fluorescent antibody methods are particularly useful.

Reaction to the microsomal antigen (complement fixation) is common both in thyrotoxicosis and Hashimoto's thyroiditis and in sera from patients with simple goitre and some sera of patients with other diseases. The most abundant source of antigen is in thyrotoxic glands, and it is of interest that in thyrotoxicosis, the positive complement-fixation test correlates with the degree of lymphocytic infiltration and the incidence of post-operative hypothyroidism (Anderson et al., 1967).

It should be clear, therefore, that these immunological tests are far from pathognomonic for Hashimoto's thyroiditis. At the same time their helpfulness cannot be denied, and the presence of positive precipitin reaction or a combination of high titres in both tanned red cell and complement-fixation tests is rare in other thyroid disorders (Anderson, McConahey, Segovia, Enslander & Wakim, 1967).

THYROID NEOPLASMS

Adenomas

Benign thyroid neoplasms readily fall into two major groups, the follicular (non-papillary) and papillary forms (Warren & Meissner, 1953). Included within the follicular group are the embryonal, foetal, simple, colloid and Hürthle cell structural patterns. Papillary adenomas are commonly cystic in contrast to the follicular variety. Moreover, papillary tumours are usually less well encapsulated; their clinical course, however, is quite similar. In marked contrast to their malignant counterparts, this is the less frequent type of benign thyroid neoplasm; it constituted but 5% of the benign lesions in the series of 500 cases reported by Meissner & McManus (1952).

It has been known since 1916 (Graham) that thyroid neoplasms contain very little thyroid hormone, and Leblond, Puppel, Riley, Radike & Curtis (1946) found that thyroid adenomas were generally less active than the surrounding tissue, as judged by iodine content, ^{131}I concentrating ability and turnover. However, nodules may be of similar or greater activity than the surrounding thyroid tissue (Dobyns & Lennon, 1951), and some thyroid nodules are "hot", i.e. are highly active in the production of hormone, which may lead to thyrotoxicosis. Scans of these nodules with ^{131}I show radio-iodine collection well in excess of the surrounding "normal" tissue, which usually shows very low background radioactivity presumably because of pituitary suppression by the "hot" nodule. One must guard against artefactual nodules resulting from differences in the amount of tissue being scanned. Exogenous TSH will stimulate this suppressed tissue. On the other hand thyroxine or tri-iodothyronine will not suppress ^{131}I accumulation in the nodule. It is considered to be independent of TSH, and the serum LATS concentration tends not to be increased (McKenzie, 1965). The appearance of such adenomas has been reported in hypophysectomized patients (Sheline & McCormack, 1960). Although a few toxic nodules have been shown to deliver a high proportion of T_3 to the circulation (Shimaoka, 1963), iodine metabolism tends not to be qualitatively abnormal in most of these. Clinically the disease (Plummer's disease) differs from Graves' disease in the rarity of exophthalmos, lack of family history of thyroid disorders, greater age, poor response to medical therapy, etc. Functional changes in other types of adenomas are on the whole similar (though often less marked) to malignant tumours and will be discussed there.

Carcinomas

Warren & Meissner (1953) have divided malignant tumours into the differentiated and nondifferentiated classes (in addition to which there are the rare non-parenchymal malignant lesions). The follicular and papillary varieties of the differentiated class correspond morphologically to their benign prototypes, but provide evidence of malignancy by metastasis or by invasion of blood or lymph vessels or capsule. The tissue diagnosis of certain thyroid tumours is difficult if not impossible, (Horn, 1960) and some feel that appropriate criteria have not been devised. Some papillary carcinomas are said to shrink or disappear on thyroid therapy while others have been observed unchanged for more than 20 years. In general they do neither but grow slowly and metastasize in time. Papillary carcinomas constitute the most frequent thyroid malignancy (especially in young persons), and are chiefly invaders of the lymphatic system in contrast to the follicular variety. The 5-yr. survival is roughly 75%, with many "cures" of 20 or more years. The follicular adenocarcinomas have a poorer prognosis (40 to 50% 5-yr. survival). In the low grade localized "carcinoma in follicular adenoma", the cure rate is approximately 90% with adequate excision. Many of the differentiated cancers show both papillary and follicular elements.

Ectopic thyroid tissue is not uncommon and may be found anywhere along the development path of the median or lateral thyroid anlagen. The tissue may exist near the gland without apparent connection or in neighbouring lymph nodes (hence called "lateral aberrant thyroid"). Although many of these have not shown cytological evidence of malignancy, they were considered to be metastases until quite recently. Some of these are now considered innocuous, and recognition of this fact will prevent unnecessary radical surgery (Klinck, 1964; Hathaway, 1965). Thyroid follicles may be found between perithyroid muscle bundles and in lymph nodes. Furthermore, ectopic thyroid tissue may be largely replaced by lymphocytic invasion. Some clues for differentiating these from true differentiated metastatic tissue have been listed by Klinck (1964). Ectopic tissue at the base of the tongue is similarly benign (lingual thyroid).

An unusual form is the medullary carcinoma of the thyroid. One form is familial and is frequently associated with *bilateral* phaeochromocytoma (up to two-thirds of cases are bilateral whereas $< 10\%$ of other phaeochromocytomas are bilateral). There is a high correlation with mucosal neuromas and with diarrhoea. The latter cases do not correlate with the presence of significant amounts of 5-hydroxytryptamine. The cells look like parafollicular cell tumours of rats and are believed to be related to these and there is abundant amyloid in the stroma (Sapira, Altman, Vandyk & Shapiro, 1965; Schimke & Hartmann, 1965; Williams, 1965; 1967). Despite this relation to parafollicular cells no functional abnormalities related to thyrocalcitonin have been detected (Freeman & Lindsay, 1965; Williams, 1965). In another group of patients with medullary carcinoma association with phaeochromocytoma is much less common, suggesting the existence of a second clinical form of this tumour. Mean postoperative survival is from 6 to 20 years.

The undifferentiated carcinomas comprise the

small and large cell carcinomas, which are highly malignant. These invade both the lymphatic and vascular system in addition to vigorous local extension; the prognosis is invariably poor.

Aetiology

There is now little doubt that irradiation is an important aetiological agent in thyroid carcinoma, at least in childhood. Duffy & Fitzgerald (1950) first pointed to such a correlation. Carcinomas are most often of the papillary type. Nodules are more common and lesions more extensive in X-irradiated infants and young children than in a comparable non-irradiated group. It has been calculated that the risk for nodule formation is about 30% and that for carcinoma 4·3% after neck irradiation (Pincus, Reichlin & Hempelman, 1967). Nine cases (seven carcinomas and two adenomas) reported by Wilson, Kilpatrick, Eckert, Curran, Jepson, Blomfield & Miller (1958) had received from 130 to 2700 r. for superficial lesions (six for naevi). The latent period for tumour detection was from 5 to 18 years. Winship & Rosvoll (1961) reported on 562 cases of childhood cancer. Of 277 cases where a history for radiation was sought, 221 gave a positive history —an incidence of about 80% with a mean latency for tumour formation of about nine years (see also Lindsay & Chaikoff, 1964). Since new series keep being reported (Hagler, Rosenblum & Rosenblum, 1966), the burden of proof that X-ray treatment is not more hazardous than the condition being treated rests with those who would use this form of therapy in children.

Tumours may also appear in children after endogenous irradiation from therapeutic doses of ^{131}I. Sheline and co-workers (1962) found thyroid nodules in 18 patients treated under the age of 20, two in the age group 21–30, and none in 186 older patients. Thus partial thyroid ablation with ^{131}I in the young must be carefully watched and is probably not indicated. There is also clear evidence that the fall-out from a hydrogen bomb exploded on Bikini has led to hypothyroidism, one case of thyroid cancer and almost a score of adenomas in children in the neighbouring islands of the Marshall group (Conard, Rall & Sutow, 1966). A symposium on fall-out and radiation problems, under the auspices of the Atomic Energy Commission, may be found in Health Physics, vol. 9 (1963).

Although the young thyroid gland appears to be more sensitive to radiation, thyroid carcinoma may perhaps also be induced in the adult by external radiation (Morris & Hardin, 1964) and victims near the epicentre in Hiroshima and Nagasaki have an increased incidence of thyroid carcinoma, although exposed as adults (Socolow, Hashizume, Neriishi & Niitani, 1963).

Chronic overstimulation of the thyroid by endogenous TSH following partial thyroidectomy, antithyroid drugs or iodine deficiency, can alone cause neoplasms (Purves, Griesbach & Kennedy, 1951; Doniach & Williams, 1962; Schaller & Stevenson, 1966; Goldberg, Lindsay, Nichols & Chaikoff, 1964; Lindsay & Chaikoff, 1964). Furthermore, adenomas and carcinomas can be induced in experimental animals with rather low doses of ^{131}I (see review by Goldberg et al., 1964), and overstimulated glands may be more sensitive to irradiation. However, in man, iodine deficiency or simple goitre correlate poorly, on the whole, with the incidence of thyroid cancer. The supposed rarity of thyroid cancer in thyrotoxicosis has been called into question (Olen & Klinck, 1965).

Solitary Nodules

The problem of the significance and therapy of solitary nodules is debated endlessly in surgical and medical clinics. Much of this controversy stems from conflicting notions regarding the prevalence of thyroid cancer. In unselected autopsy material it is quite rare (25 per million) and the mortality rate from thyroid cancer is one-third to one-fifth the incidence, reflecting, presumably, the benign course of many of these (Sokal, 1953; Mustacchi & Cutler, 1956). However, in a hospital population, and especially in centres with thyroid clinics, the sample is highly selected; this accounts, in part, for the fact that the incidence of cancer in patients presenting with single nodules is reported to be between 5 and 24%. The incidence is lower in multinodular goitre, probably of the order of 5 to 10% or less (in non-endemic areas). About half the solitary nodules diagnosed clinically turn out to be multiple at surgery. Malignant degeneration in benign nodules is probably a rare event (Sokal, 1960). The occurrence of endemic goitre in the area works in the opposite direction as does the presence of thyrotoxicity. In a recent study (Tellern, Stohl & Meranze, 1961) various selection factors were analysed. The overall incidence of cancer in clinically solitary nodules was 13%. If the group with highly suspicious lesions was selected the incidence rose to 64% whereas the remainder had a 9% incidence of malignancy. Similarly, age selection more than doubled the incidence. If scintiscanning was used as a selecting factor there was a 28% incidence of cancer in areas of decreased collection of radioactivity.

Astwood, Cassidy & Aurbach (1960) treated

nodular goitre with full doses of thyroid for many years and have achieved notable reduction in thyroid size in many cases. In our opinion some time limit, e.g. 4–6 months, should be chosen, after which failure to produce an unequivocal reduction in nodule size is considered an indication for more active therapy, especially in the young, or with a history of recent growth of the nodule, change in voice, pressure symptoms, change in consistency (hardness and fixation) and enlargement of lymph nodes, etc.

Iodine Metabolism

Many thyroid tumours do not metabolize significant amounts of iodine. Those that do usually, but not invariably, show elements of the normal architecture. Despite this the activity per gram of tissue is nearly always less than in normal tissue; thus the iodide clearance of tumour is about 0·1 ml./g./min. and the uptake $< 0·5\%$ of the dose/g. compared to a normal clearance of 0·9 ml. or an uptake of 1·5%/g. (Tata & Pochin, 1964). This may not necessarily be so in rat thyroid tumours (Wollman, 1963). An analysis of 100 cases of malignant thyroid tumours (Fitzgerald, Foote & Hill, 1950) revealed that papillary carcinomas rarely concentrate significant quantities of ^{131}I, whereas 74% of the alveolar and follicular types showed some ^{131}I concentration. There was a marked correlation of concentration with the degree of follicular differentiation and colloid content. About one-half of the solid tumours, a third of the Hürthle cell carcinomas (insignificant extent) and none of the small cell, large cell or anaplastic carcinomas concentrated ^{131}I. Primary and metastatic thyroid lesions reveal somewhat similar function as far as radio-iodine concentration is concerned. However, pleomorphism may be encountered in which the primary and metastatic sites show histological and functional differences. The concentrations are often so slight as to be therapeutically insignificant.

The turnover of ^{131}I is more rapid than in normal thyroid glands. The reason is not known but may be related to a small iodine pool of tumours. Discharge from tumours is complicated, being composed of several exponential rates. The slower components tend to be lost first after irradiation of the tumour and it is a commonplace to end up with a shorter biological half-life with the treatment dose than with the tracer (Tata & Pochin, 1964).

Defects of the individual steps of thyroxine

biosynthesis, as seen in congenital cretins, have not been very well characterized in human thyroid malignancy. Valenta (1966) has, however, reported on the function of a metastasis of a clear-cell tumour which apparently was unable to oxidize accumulated iodide. Characteristic features were rapid uptake and rapid loss, discharge by ClO_4^-, no suppression by T_3 although growth was stimulated by TSH. A similar defect had previously been reported in a transplantable rat thyroid carcinoma (Wolff et al., 1959).

Thyroglobulin is present in functioning thyroid tumours and usually behaves as expected for that protein but may, occasionally, show slightly altered electrophoretic mobility (Robbins, 1966). The MIT/DIT ratio of ^{131}I in the tumour is greater than in normal tissue. It is uncertain whether this is due to a relative iodine deficiency or is the result of the iodination of proteins other than thyroglobulin. A relatively large proportion of injected ^{131}I may appear as particulate protein but this is not specific to malignant tissue. Its role as precursor to thyroglobulin is uncertain (Robbins, 1966).

Soluble iodoproteins are readily labelled in human tumour tissue and appear rapidly in the circulation. The most abundant of these (up to 16% of thyroid iodine) appears to be serum albumin, presumably iodinated on its passage through the tumour. The substance is called both compound X or S-1 iodoprotein. It is found in other thyroid disorders and even in normal thyroid tissue but is usually associated with some degree of thyroid hyperplasia. Heterologous albumin can become iodinated as can the other normal serum proteins, though to a lesser extent (Robbins, 1966). Similar iodoproteins have been demonstrated in experimental thyroid carcinomas (Robbins, Wolff & Rall, 1959).

Labelled T_3 and T_4 are readily demonstrated in the circulation of many patients with functioning thyroid tumours. Several thyroidectomized patients with functioning metastases have been studied in whom an abnormally large fraction of the circulating ^{131}I was chromatographically identical with tri-iodothyronine (Mack, Hart, Druet & Bauer, 1961). That some metastases can maintain the euthyroid state in the absence of the thyroid and hyperthyroidism has been known to occur. In most cases metastases function less well and when they cannot be localized by scanning, it is useful to look for the formation of organic iodine provided thyroid remnants can be ruled out (Tata & Pochin, 1964).

References

ABOUL-KHAIR, S. A. & CROOKS, J. (1965). *Acta Endocrin.*, **48**, 14.

ABOUL-KHAIR, S. A., CROOKS, J., TURNBULL, A. L. & HYTTEN, F. (1964). *Clin. Sci.*, **27**, 195.

ACKERMAN, N. B., SMITH, R. W. & MILLER, J. M. (1961). *Metabolism*, **10**, 27.

ADAMS, D. D. (1958). *J. clin. Endocrin.*, **18**, 699.

ADAMS, D. D. & KENNEDY, T. H. (1967). *J. clin. Endocrin.*, **27**, 173.

ADAMS, P. H. & CHALMERS, T. M. (1965). *Clin. Sci.*, **29**, 391.

ADAMS, P. H., JOWSEY, J., KELLY, P. J., RIGGS, B. L., KINNEY, V. R. & JONES, J. D. (1967). *Quart. J. Med.*, **36**, 1.

ALBRIGHT, E. C., HENINGER, R. W. & LARSON, F. C. (1965). In "Current Topics in Thyroid Research". Eds. Cassano, C. & Andreoli, M., 346, Academic Press, N.Y.

ALBRIGHT, E. C., TOMITA, K. & LARSON, F. C. (1959). *Endocrinology*, **64**, 288.

ALEXANDER, N. M. (1959). *J. biol. Chem.*, **234**, 1530.

ALEXANDER, N. M. & CORCORAN, B. J. (1962). *J. biol. Chem.*, **237**, 243.

ALEXANDER, W. D., GUDMUNDSSON, T. V., BLUHM, M. M. & HARDEN, R. M. (1964a). *Acta Endocrin.*, **46**, 679.

ALEXANDER, W. D., HARDEN, R. M., KOUTRAS, D. A. & WAYNE, E. (1965). *Lancet*, **2**, 866.

ALEXANDER, W. D., KOUTRAS, D. A., HARDEN, H. M. & HARRISON, M. T. (1964b). *Lancet*, **2**, 558.

ALEXANDER, W. D. & WOLFF, J. (1964). *Arch. Biochem.*, **106**, 525.

ALEXANDER, W. D. & WOLFF, J. (1966). *Endocrinology*, **78**, 581.

ALLEN, H. C., KELLY, F. J. & GREENE, J. A. (1952). *J. clin. Endocrin.*, **12**, 1356.

ALOUSI, A. A. & MALLOW, S., (1964). *Amer. J. Physiol.*, **206**, 603.

ALPERS, J. B., ROBBINS, J. & RALL, J. E. (1955). *Endocrinology*, **56**, 110.

ANDERSEN, H. J. (1961). *Acta Paediat. Suppl.*, **125**.

ANDERSON, G. S. & BIRD, T. (1961). *Lancet*, **2**, 742.

ANDERSON, J., GOUDIE, R. & BUCHANAN, W. W. (1967). In "Auto-immunity Clinical and Experimental". Thomas, Charles C., Ft. Lauderdale.

ANDROS, G., HARPER, P. V., LATHROP, K. A. & McCARDLE, R. J. (1965). *J. clin. Endocrin.*, **25**, 1067.

ANDROS, G. & WOLLMAN, S. H. (1967). *Amer. J. Physiol.*, **213**, 198.

ARDEMAN, S., CHANARIN, I., KRAFCHICK, B. & SINGER, W. (1966). *Quart. J. Med.*, **35**, 421.

ARNOTT, D. G. & DONIACH, I. (1952). *Biochem. J.*, **50**, 473.

ARNRICH, L. & MORGAN, A. F. (1954). *J. Nutrit.*, **54**, 107.

ARONS, W. L. & HYDOVITZ, J. D. (1959). *J. clin. Endocrin.*, **19**, 548.

ASHER, R. (1949). *Brit. med. J.*, **2**, 555.

ASTWOOD, E. B. (1943). *J. Pharmacol.*, **78**, 79.

ASTWOOD, E. B. (1945). *Harvey Lect.*, **40**, 195.

ASTWOOD, E. B. (1949). *Ann. N.Y.Acad. Sci.*, **50**, 419.

ASTWOOD, E. B. (1951). *J. clin. Endocrin.*, **11**, 1045.

ASTWOOD, E. B., CASSIDY, C. E. & AURBACH, G. D. (1960). *J. Amer. med. Assoc.*, **174**, 459.

AUB, J. C., BAUER, W. B., HEATH, C. & ROPES, M. (1929). *J. clin. Invest.*, **7**, 97.

AUSTEN, F. K., MERONEY, W. H., RUBIN, M. E. & WOLFF, J. (1958). *J. clin. Invest.*, **37**, 1131.

BACHELARD, H. S. & TRIKOJUS, V. M. (1960). *Nature*, **185**, 80.

BAKHLE, Y. S., PRUSOFF, W. H. & McCREA, J. F. (1964). *Science*, **143**, 799.

BALASUBRAMANIAM, K. & DEISS, W. P. (1965). *Biochim. biophys. Acta*, **110**, 564.

BALFOUR, B., DONIACH, D., ROITT, I. M. & COUCHMAN, K. G. (1961). *Brit. J. exp. Path.*, **42**, 307.

BARKER, S. B. & KLITGAARD, H. M. (1952). *Amer. J. Physiol.*, **170**, 81.

BARKER, S. B. & SHIMADA, M. (1964). *Proc. Mayo Clin.*, **39**, 609.

BARTELS, E. C. (1945). *Surg. Clin. N. Amer.*, **25**, 676.

BARTELS, E. C. (1949). *J. clin. Endocrin.*, **9**, 1190.

BARTELS, E. C. (1950). *J. clin. Endocrin.*, **10**, 1126.

BARTELS, E. C. & BELL, G. (1939). *Trans. Amer. Goiter Assoc.*

BASCHIERI, L., ANDREANI, D., ANDREOLI, M., NEGRI, M. & CASSANO, C. (1959). *Folia Endocrin.*, **12**, 325.

BASTENIE, P. A., ERMANS, A. M., THYS, O., BECKERS, C., VAN DEN SCHRIECK, H. G. & DE VISSCHER, M. (1962). *J. clin. Endocrin.*, **23**, 137.

BASTOMSKY, C. H., ROSENFELD, P. S. & ROSENBERG, I. N. (1966). *Endocrinology*, **78**, 401; **79**, 505.

BATES, R. W. & CONDLIFFE, P. G. (1966). In "The Pituitary Gland". Eds. Harris, G. W. and Donovan, B. T., London, Butterworth's.

BAX, G. M. (1966). *Acta Endocrin.*, **53**, 264.

BEARE, R. L. B. (1958). *Brit. med. J.*, **1**, 480.

BECKER, D. V., RALL, J. E., PEACOCK, W. E. & RAWSON, R. W. (1953). *J. clin. Invest.*, **32**, 149.

BEGG, T. B. & HALL, R. (1963). *Quart. J. Med.*, **32**, 351.

BEIERWALTES, W. H. & BISHOP, R. C. (1954). *J. clin. Endocrin.*, **14**, 928.

BEIERWALTES, W. H., CRANE, H. R., WEGST, A., SPAFFORD, N. R. & CARR, E. A. (1960). *J. Amer. med. Ass.*, **173**, 1895.

BELING, U. & EINHORN, J. (1961). *Acta Radiol.*, **56**, 275.

BELL, G. O. (1950). *J. Amer. med. Ass.*, **144**, 1243.

BENABDELJLIL, C., MICHEL-BECHET, M. & LISSITZKY, S. (1967). *Biochem. biophys. Res. Comm.*, **27**, 74.

BENUA, R. S. & DOBYNS, B. M. (1955). *J. clin. Endocrin.*, **15**, 118.

BERLINER, E. (1966). *J. chem. Ed.*, **43**, 124.

BERMAN, M., HOFF, E., BARANDES, M., BECKER, D. V., SONENBERG, M., BENUA, R. & KOUTRAS, D. A. (1968). *J. clin. Endocrin.*, **28**, 1.

BERSÉUS, O. (1965). *Acta chem. Scand.*, **19**, 2131.

BERSON, S. A. (1956). *Amer. J. Med.*, **20**, 653.

BERSON, S. A. & YALOW, R. S. (1954). *J. clin. Invest.*, **33**, 1533.

BERSON, S. A., YALOW, R. S., SORRENTINO, J. & ROSWIT, R. (1952). *J. clin. Invest.*, **31**, 141.

BISMUTH, J., ROLLAND, M. & LISSITZKY, S. (1966). *Acta Endocrin.*, **53**, 297.

BLAGG, C. R. (1960). *Lancet*, **2**, 1364.

BLOCK, R. J., WERNER, S. C., MANDL, R. H., ROW, V. V. & RADICHEVICH, I. (1960). *Arch. biochem. biophys.*, **88**, 98.

BLOM, P. S. & TERPSTRA, J. (1953). *J. clin. Endocrin.*, **13**, 989.

BLOMFIELD, G. W., ECKERT, H., FISHER, M., MILLER, H., MUNRO, D. S. & WILSON, G. M. (1959). *Brit. med. J.*, **1**, 63.

BLOODWORTH, J. M., KIRKENDALL, W. M. & CARR, T. L. (1954). *J. clin. Endocrin.*, **14**, 540.

BLOOM, A. D. & TJIO, J. H. (1964). *New Engl. J. Med.*, **270**, 1341.

BLUMGART, H. L., FREEDBERG, A. S. & KURLAND, G. S. (1950). *Circulation*, **1**, 1105.

BOYD, G. S. & OLIVER, M. F. (1960). *Brit. med. Bull.*, **16**, 138.

BOYLE, J. H., SLOSS, A., MACDONALD, E. & GRAY, M. (1965). *J. clin. Endocrin.*, **25**, 1035.

BRAIN, W. R. (1927). *Quart. J. Med.*, **20**, 303.

BRAVERMAN, L. E. & INGBAR, S. H. (1963). *J. clin. Invest.*, **42**, 1216.

BRAY, G. A. (1966). *Endocrinology*, **79**, 554.

BRAY, G. A. & GOODMAN, H. M. (1965). *Endocrinology*, **76**, 323.

BRIARD, S. P., McCLINTOCK, T. H. & BALDRIDGE, C. W. (1935). *Arch. intern. Med.*, **56**, 30.

BRICKER, N. S. & HLAD, C. J. (1955). *J. clin. Invest.*, **34**, 1057.

BRIGGS, F. N., BRAUER, R. W., TAUROG, A. & CHAIKOFF, I. L. (1953). *Amer. J. Physiol.*, **172**, 561.

BRONK, J. R. (1966). *Science*, **153**, 638.

BRONK, J. R. & PARSONS, D. S. (1966). *J. Physiol.*, **184**, 942.

BROWN, H., ENGLERT, E. & WALLACH, S. (1958). *J. clin. Endocrin.*, **18**, 167.

BROWN-GRANT, K. (1961). *Physiol. Rev.*, **41**, 187.

BROWN-GRANT, K. (1966). *J. Physiol.*, **184**, 418.

BROWN-GRANT, K., VON EULER, C., HARRIS, G. W. & REICHLIN, S. (1954). *J. Physiol.*, **126**, 1, 29, 41.

BUCCINO, R. A., SPANN, J. F. Jr., POOL, P. E., SONNENBLICK, E. H. & BRAUNWALD, E. (1967). *J. clin. Invest.*, **46**, 1669.

BUCHANAN, W. W. (1962). *J. Endocrin.*, **24**, 115.

BUCHANAN, W. W. & HARDEN, R. McG. (1965). *Arch. Int. Med.*, **115**, 411.

BUCHANAN, W. W., HARDEN, R. McG., KOUTRAS, D. A. & GRAY, K. G. (1965*a*). *J. clin. Endocrin.*, **25**, 301.

BUCHANAN, W. W., KOUTRAS, D. A., ALEXANDER, W. D., CROOKS, J., RICHMOND, M. H. & WAYNE, E. J. (1961). *J. clin. Endocrin.*, **21**, 806.

BUCHANAN, W. W., KOUTRAS, D. A., CROOKS, J. & HARDEN, R. M. (1965*b*). *Brit. J. Radiol.*, **38**, 536.

BULL, G. M. & FRASER, R. (1950). *Lancet*, **1**, 851.

BUNIM, J. J. (1961). *Ann. Rheum. Dis.*, **20**, 1.

BURKE, G. (1967). *Amer. J. Med.*, **42**, 600.

BURKLE, J. S. & LUND, R. (1963). In "Evaluation of Thyroid and Parathyroid Functions". Eds. Sunderman, F. W. & Sunderman, F. W. Jnr., Lippincott, J. B., Philadelphia.

BYROM, F. B. (1934). *Clin. Sci.*, **1**, 273.

CALVERT, R. J., SMITH, E. & ANDREWS, L. G. (1954). *Brit. med. J.*, **2**, 891.

CANARY, J. J., SCHAAF, M., DUFFY, G. J. & KYLE, L. M. (1957). *New Engl. J. Med.*, **257**, 435.

CARR, D. H., BARR, M. L., PLUNKETT, E. R., GRUMBACH, M. M., MORISHIMA, A. & CHU, E. H. Y. (1961). *J. clin. Endocrin.*, **21**, 491.

CASSANO, C., BASCHIERI, L. & ANDREANI, D. (1959). *Presse Méd.*, **67**, 631.

CASSIDY, C. E. & VANDERLAAN, W. P. (1958). *New Engl. J. Med.*, **258**, 828.

CHAIKOFF, I. L., TAUROG, A. & REINHARDT, W. O. (1947). *Endocrinology*, **40**, 47.

CHANDLER, R. W., BLIZZARD, R. M., HUNG, W. & KYLE, M. (1962). *New Engl. J. Med.*, **267**, 376.

CHAPMAN, E. M., CORNER, G. W., ROBINSON, D. & EVANS, R. D. (1948). *J. clin. Endocrin.*, **8**, 717.

CHAPMAN, E. M. & MALOOF, F. (1955). *Medicine*, **34**, 261.

CHILDS, D. S., KEATING, F. R., RALL, J. E., WILLIAMS, M. M. D. & POWER, M. H. (1950). *J. clin. Invest.*, **29**, 726.

CHING, TSENG TENG & KARAMOURTJOUNIS, J. (1960). *Amer. J. Roent.*, **83**, 491.

CHOUFOER, J. C., VAN RHIJN, M., KASSENAAR, A. A. H. & QUERIDO, A. (1963). *J. clin. Endocrin.*, **23**, 1203.

CHOUFOER, J. C., VAN RHIJN, M. & QUERIDO, A. (1965). *J. clin. Endocrin.*, **25**, 385.

CLARK, D. E., MOE, R. H. & ADAMS, E. E. (1949). *Surgery*, **26**, 331.

CLEMENTS, F. W. (1957). *Med. J. Aust.*, **2**, 645.

CLEMENTS, F. W. & WISHART, J. W. (1956). *Metabolism*, **5**, 623.

CLUXTON, H. E., BENNETT, W. A. & KEPLER, E. J. (1948). *Ann. intern. Med.*, **29**, 732.

CONARD, R. A., RALL, J. E. & SUTOW, W. W. (1966). *New Engl. J. Med.*, **274**, 1392.

COPE, O., RAWSON, R. W. & McARTHUR, J. W. (1947). *Surg. Gynec. Obstet.*, **84**, 415.

COURRIER, R., HOREAU, A., MAROIS, M. & MOREL, F. (1951). *C. R. Acad. Sci.*, **232**, 776.

COVELLI, I. & WOLFF, J. (1966). *J. biol. Chem.*, **241**, 4444.

COVELLI, I. & WOLFF, J. (1967). *J. biol. Chem.*, **242**, 881.

CROOKS, J., ABOUL-KHAIR, S. A., TURNBULL, A. C. & HYTTEN, F. E. (1964). *Lancet*, **2**, 334.

CROOKS, J., MURRAY, I. P. C. & WAYNE, E. J. (1958). *Lancet*, **1**, 604.

CROOKS, J. & WAYNE, E. J. (1960). *Lancet*, **1**, 407.

CUNNINGHAM, L. W. (1964). *Biochemistry*, **3**, 1629.

CZERNIAK, P. & HARELL-STEINBERG, A. (1957). *J. clin. Endocrin.*, **17**, 1448.

DAILEY, M. E., LINDSAY, S. & MILLER, E. R. (1953). *J. clin. Endocrin.*, **13**, 1513.

DANIEL, P. M., PRATT, D. E., ROITT, I. M. & TORRI-GIANI, G. (1967). *Immunology*, **12**, 489.

DANOWSKI, T. S., HUFF, S. J., NIRVOS, D., WRITH, D., GEORGE, R. S. & MATEER, F. M. (1953). *Amer. J. Obstet. Gynec.*, **65**, 77.

DANOWSKI, T. S., SARVER, M. & BONESSI, J. V. (1963). *Metabolism*, **12**, 473.

DAVIS, P. J. (1966). *Amer. J. Med.*, **40**, 718.

DAVIS, T. E., CANFIELD, C. J., HERMAN, R. H. & GOLER, D. (1963). *New Engl. J. Med.*, **268**, 178.

DAYTON, S., DAYTON, J., DRIMMER, F. & KENDALL, F. E. (1960). *Amer. J. Physiol.*, **199**, 71.

DEDUVE, C. & BAUDHUIN, P. (1966). *Physiol. Rev.*, **46**, 323.

DEGROOT, L. J. (1966). *J. clin. Endocrin.*, **26**, 778.

DEGROOT, L. J. & DAVIS, A. M. (1961, 1962). *J. biol. Chem.*, **236**, 2009; *Endocrinology*, **70**, 492.

DEGROOT, L. J. & STANBURY, J. B. (1959). *Amer. J. Med.*, **27**, 586.

DEISS, C. P., BALASUBRAMANIAM, K., PEAKE, R. L., STARRETT, J. A. & POWELL, R. C. (1966), *Endocrinology*, **79**, 19.

DEISS, W. P., O'SHAUGHNESSY, P. J. & WYNN, J. O. (1959). *J. clin. Invest.*, **38**, 334.

DE LA BALZE, F. A., ARRILAGA, F., MANCINI, R. E., JONCHES, M., DAVISON, O. W. & GURTMAN, A. I. (1962). *J. clin. Endocrin.*, **22**, 212.

DEMPSEY, E. W. (1944). *Endocrinology*, **34**, 27.

DEMPSEY, E. W. & ASTWOOD, E. B. (1943). *Endocrinology*, **32**, 509.

DE NAYER, P., WEATHERS, B. & ROBBINS, J. (1967). *Endocrinology*. **81**, 118.

DEROBERTIS, E. & GRASSO, R. (1946). *Endocrinology*, **38**, 137.

DEROBERTIS, E. & NOWINSKI, W. W. (1946). *J. clin. Endocrin.*, **6**, 235.

DE VISSCHER, M., BECKERS, C., VAN DEN SCHRIECK, H. G., DE SMET, M., ERMANS, A. M., GALPERIN, H. & BASTENIE, P. A. (1961). *J. clin. Endocrin.*, **21**, 175.

DEVLIN, W. F. & WATANABE, H. (1966). *J. Pharmaceut. Sci.*, **55**, 390.

DOBYNS, B. M. & LENNON, B. (1951). *J. clin. Endocrin.*, **9**, 1171.

DOBYNS, B. M., SKANSE, B. & MALOOF, F. (1949). *J. clin. Endocrin.*, **9**, 1171.

DOBYNS, B. M., WRIGHT, A. & WILSON, L. (1961). *J. clin. Endocrin.*, **21**, 648.

DOHERTY, J. E. & PERKINS, W. H. (1966). *Ann. intern. Med.*, **64**, 489.

DONIACH, D. & VAUGHAN-HUDSON, R. (1957). *Brit. med. J.*, **1**, 672.

DONIACH, I. (1957). *Brit. med. J.*, **2**, 253.

DONACH, I. & WILLIAMS, E. I. (1962). *Brit. J. Cancer*, **16**, 222.

DOWLING, J. T., FREINKEL, N. & INGBAR, S. H. (1956). *J. clin. Endocrin.*, **16**, 280, 1491; (1956). *J. clin. Invest.*, **35**, 1263.

DRILL, V. A. & TRUANT, A. P. (1947). *Endocrinology*, **40**, 259.

DUFFY, B. J. & FITZGERALD, P. J. (1950). *J. clin. Endocrin.*, **10**, 1296.

DUMONT, J. E. (1965). *Ann. Soc. Roy. Sci. Med. Nat. Brux.*, **18**, 106.

DUMONT, J. E., ERMANS, A. M. & BASTENIE, P. A. (1963). *J. clin. Endocrin.*, **23**, 847.

DUNN, J. T. & CHAPMAN, E. M. (1964). *New Engl. J. Med.*, **271**, 1037.

DU RUISSEAU, J. P. (1965). *J. clin. Endocrin.*, **25**, 1513.

DZIEWIATKOWSKI, D. D. (1964). *Biophys. J.*, suppl. 215.

EATON, R. S., STEINBERG, D. & THOMPSON, R. H. (1965). *J. clin. Invest.*, **44**, 247.

EAYRS, J. T. (1964). In "Brain-Thyroid Relationships". Ciba Found. Study Group, No. 18, p. 60, Boston, Little Brown & Co.

EDELHOCH, H. (1962). *J. biol. Chem.*, **237**, 2778.

EDELHOCH, H. (1965). *Rec. Prog. Horm. Res.*, **21**, 11.

EICHLER, O. & HACKENTHAL, E. (1962). *Arch. exp. Path. & Pharm.*, **243**, 554.

EINHORN, J., FAGRAEUS, A. & JONSSON, J. (1965). *J. clin. Endocrin.*, **25**, 1218.

EINHORN, J. & LARSSON, L. G. (1959). *J. clin. Endocrin.*, **19**, 28.

ELGEE, N. J. & WILLIAMS, R. H. (1955). *Amer. J. Physiol.*, **180**, 13.

EL KABIR, D. J., DONIACH, D. & TURNER-WARWICK, R. (1963). *J. clin. Endocrin.*, **23**, 510.

ELPHINSTONE, N. (1953). *Lancet*, **1**, 1281.

ENGEL, A. G. (1961). *Amer. J. Med.*, **30**, 327.

ENGEL, A. G. (1966). *Mayo Clin. Proc.*, **41**, 785.

ERIKSSON, S. (1957). *Proc. Soc. exp. Biol. Med.*, **94**, 582.

ERMANS, A. M., DUMONT, J. E. & BASTENIE, P. A. (1963). *J. clin. Endocrin.*, **23**, 539, 550.

EYLAN, E., ZMUCKY, R. & SHEBA, C. (1957). *Lancet*, **1**, 1062.

FALCONER, I. R. (1966). *Biochem. J.*, **100**, 190, 197.

FARESE, R. U. & PLAGER, J. E. (1962). *J. clin. Invest.*, **41**, 53.

FARRAN, H. E. A., LEA, A. J., GOOLDEN, A. W. G. & ABBATT, J. E. (1959). *Lancet*, **1**, 793.

FAWCETT, D. M. & KIRKWOOD, S. (1953). *J. biol. Chem.*, **204**, 787; **205**, 795.

FAWCETT, D. M. & KIRKWOOD, S. (1954). *J. biol. Chem.*, **209**, 249.

FELBER, J. P., REDDY, W. J., SELENKOW, H. A. & THORN, G. W. (1959). *J. clin. Endocrin.*, **19**, 895.

FELIX-DAVIES, D. (1958). *Lancet*, **1**, 880.

FERRINI, O. & BIASSONI, P. (1966). *Folia Endocrin.*, **19**, 313.

FEUER, G. (1959). *Biochem. J.*, **73**, 349.

FISHER, D. A. & ODDIE, T. H. (1964). *Amer. J. Dis. Child.*, **107**, 574.

FISHER, D. A., ODDIE, T. H. & BURROUGHS, J. C. (1962). *Amer. J. Dis. Child.*, **103**, 738.

FISHER, D. A., ODDIE, T. H. & EPPERSON, D. (1965). *J. clin. Endocrin.*, **25**, 1353, 1580.

FISHMAN, J., HELLMAN, L., ZUMOFF, B. & GALLAGHER, F. F. (1965). *J. clin. Endocrin.*, **25**, 365.

FITZGERALD, P. J., FOOTE, F. W. & HILL, R. F. (1950). *Cancer*, **3**, 86.

FLOCK, E. U., BOLLMAN, J. L., GRINDLAY, J. H. & STOBIE, G. H. (1961). *Endocrinology*, **69**, 626.

FOOTE, J. B. & MacLAGAN, N. F. (1951). *Lancet*, **1**, 868.

FORBES, I. J., ROITT, I. M., DONIACH, D. & JOHNSON, I. L. (1962). *J. clin. Invest.*, **41**, 996.

FORD, D. H. & GROSS, J. (1958). *Endocrinology*, **62**, 416.

FORE, W. & WYNN, J. (1966). *Amer. J. Med.*, **40**, 90.

FORSS, D. A. (1951). *Aust. J. appl. Sci.*, **2**, 397.

FOSS, G. L. & SIMPSON, S. L. (1959). *Brit. med. J.*, **1**, 259.

FRANKLIN, A. L., CHAIKOFF, I. L. & LERNER, S. (1944). *J. biol. Chem.*, **153**, 151.

FRANKS, R. C. & STEMPFEL, R. S. (1963). *J. clin. Endocrin.*, **23**, 805.

FRASER, G. R. (1961). *Lancet*, **1**, 964.

FRASER, G. R., MORGANS, M. E. & TROTTER, W. R. (1960). *Quart. J. Med.*, **29**, 279.

FRASER, R., HOBSON, Q. J. G., ARNOTT, D. G. & EMERY, E. W. (1953). *Quart. J. Med.*, **22**, n.a. 99.

FREEDBERG, A. A., CHAMOWITZ, D. L. & KURLAND, G. S. (1952). *Metabolism*, **1**, 26, 36.

FREEDBERG, A. S., URELES, A. & HERTZ, S. (1949). *Proc. Soc. exp. Biol.*, **70**, 679.

FREEDBERG, I. M., HAMOLSKY, M. W. & FREEDBERG, A. S. (1957). *New Engl. J. Med.*, **256**, 505, 551.

FREEMAN, D. & LINDSAY, S. L. (1965). *Arch. Path.*, **80**, 575.

FREINKEL, N. (1964). In "The Thyroid Gland". Eds. Pitt-Rivers, R. & Trotter, W. R., vol. 1, p. 131, Washington, Butterworth's.

FREY, H. (1964). *Acta Endocrin.*, **47**, 105.

FREY, H. M. M. (1967). *Scand. J. Clin. Lab. Invest.*, **19**, 4, 15.

FRIEDBERG, F. & GREENBERG, D. M. (1947). *J. biol. Chem.*, **168**, 405.

FRYE, R. L. & BRAUNWALD, E. (1961). *Circulation*, **23**, 376.

FURTH, J. & CLIFTON, K. H. (1958). *Ciba Coll. Endocrin.*, Na. 12, 3.

GALLAGHER, T. F., HELLMAN, L., BRADLOW, H. L., ZUMOFF, B. & FUKUSHIMA, D. K. (1960). *Ann. N.Y. Acad. Sci.*, **86**, 605.

GALTON, U. A. & INGBAR, S. H. (1963). *Endocrinology*, **73**, 596.

GENANT, G., HOAGLAND, H. C. & RANDALL, R. U. (1967). *Metabolism*, **16**, 187.

GIFFORD, R. W., KVALE, W. F., MAHER, F. T., ROTH, G. M. & PRIESTLEY, J. T. (1964). *Proc. Staff. Meet. Mayo Clin.*, **39**, 281.

GIMLETTE, T. M. D. (1959). *Lancet*, **2**, 1143.

GIMLETTE, T. M. D. (1960). *Lancet*, **1**, 22.

GOLDBERG, R. C. & CHAIKOFF, I. L. (1949). *Endocrinology*, **45**, 64.

GOLDBERG, R. C. & CHAIKOFF, I. L. (1951). *Endocrinology*, **49**, 613.

GOLDBERG, R. C., LINDSAY, S., NICHOLS, C. W., Jr. & CHAIKOFF, I. L. (1964). *Cancer Res.*, **24**, 35.

GOLDBERG, R. C., NAY, L. & GREEP, R. O. (1953). *Proc. Soc. exp. Biol. Med.*, **84**, 621.

GOLDBERG, R. C., WOLFF, J. & GREEP, R. O. (1957). *Endocrinology*, **60**, 38.

GOLDSMITH, R. E. & EISELE, M. L. (1956). *J. clin. Endocrin.*, **16**, 130.

GOLDSMITH, R. E., STANBURY, J. B. & BROWNELL, G. L. (1951). *J. clin. Endocrin.*, **11**, 1079.

GOLDSMITH, R. E., STURGIS, S. H., LERMAN, J. & STANBURY, J. B. (1952). *J. clin. Endocrin.*, **12**, 846.

GOOD, B. F., HETZEL, B. S. & HOGG, B. (1965). *Endocrinology*, **77**, 674.

GOODWIN, J. F., MacGREGOR, A. G., MILLER, H. & WAYNE, E. (1951). *Quart. J. Med.*, **20**, 353.

GOODWIN, J. F., STEINBERG, H. & WILSON, A. (1954). *Brit. med. J.*, **1**, 422.

GOOLDEN, A. W. G. (1964). In "The Thyroid Gland". Eds. Pitt-Rivers, R. & Trotter, W. R., Washington, Butterworths.

GOOLDEN, A. W. G. & MALLARD, J. R. (1958). *Brit. J. Radiol.*, **31**, 589.

GORDON, E. C. & HEMMING, A. E. (1944). *Endocrinology*, **34**, 353.

GRAHAM, A. (1916). *J. exp. Med.*, **24**, 345.

GRAIG, F. A. & SMITH, J. C. (1965). *J. clin. Endocrin.*, **25**, 723.

GRAND, R. J., ROSEN, S. W., DI SANT'AGNESE, P. A. & KIRKHAM, W. R. (1966). *Amer. J. Med.*, **41**, 478.

GRAYSON, R. R. (1960). *Amer. J. Med.*, **28**, 397.

GREEN, M. & WILSON, M. (1964). *Brit. med. J.*, **1**, 1005.

GREEN, W. L. (1966). *Endocrinology*, **79**, 1.

GREENBERG, W. U. (1966). *J. clin. Endocrin.*, **26**, 559.

GREENMAN, G. W., GABRIELSON, M. O., FLANDERS, J. H. & WESSEL, M. A. (1962). *New Engl. J. Med.*, **267**, 426.

GREENWALD, I. (1946). *J. clin. Endocrin.*, **6**, 708.

GREER, M. A. (1950). *Physiol. Rev.*, **30**, 513.

GREER, M. A. & ASTWOOD, E. B. (1948). *Endocrinology*, **43**, 105.

GREER, M. A. & DEENEY, J. A. (1959). *J. clin. Invest.*, **38**, 1465.

GREER, M. A. & DeGROOT, L. J. (1956). *Metabolism*, **5**, 682.

GREER, M. A. & SMITH, G. E. (1954). *J. clin. Endocrin.*, **14**, 1374.

GREGERMAN, R. I., GAFFNEY, G. W. & SHOCK, N. W. (1962). *J. clin. Invest.*, **41**, 2065.

GREIG, W. R., CROOKS, J. & MacGREGOR, A. G. (1966). *Proc. Roy. Soc. Med.*, **59**, 599.

GRIBETZ, D., TALBOT, N. B. & CRAWFORD, J. D. (1954). *New Engl. J. Med.*, **250**, 555.

GRIES, F. A., MATSCHINSKY, F. & WIELAND, O. (1962). *Biochim. biophys. Acta*, **56**, 615.

GRIESBACH, W. E. & PURVES, H. D. (1945). *Brit. J. exp. Path.*, **26**, 13, 18.

GRIFFITHS, W. J. (1951). *Lancet*, **2**, 467.

GROB, D. (1963). *Ann. Rev. Med.*, **14**, 151.

GROSS, J. & LEBLOND, C. P. (1951). *Endocrinology*, **48**, 714.

GRUMBACH, M. M. & MORISHIMA, A. (1964). *J. Pediat.*, **65**, 1087.

GUILLEMIN, R., YAMAZAKI, E., GARD, D. A., JUTISZ, M. & SAKIZ, E. (1963). *Endocrinology*, **73**, 564.

GUSTAFSSON, R., TATA, J. R., LINDBERG, O. & ERNUSTER, L. (1965). *J. Cell. Biol.*, **26**, 555.

GUTMAN, A. B., BENEDICT, E. M., BAXTER, B. & PALMER, W. W. (1932). *J. biol. Chem.*, **97**, 303.

HADDAD, H. M. & RALL, J. E. (1960). *Endocrinology*, **67**, 413.

HADDAD, H. M. & SIDBURY, J. B. (1959). *J. clin. Endocrin.*, **19**, 1446.

HADDEN, D. R., MONTGOMERY, D. A. D. & WEAVER, J. A. (1965). In "Current Topics in Thyroid Research". Eds. Cassano, C. & Andreoli, M., p. 933, London, Academic Press.

HAGLER, S., ROSENBLUM, P. & ROSEMBLUM, A. (1966). *Pediatrics*, **38**, 77.

HALMI, N. S. (1954). *Endocrinology*, **54**, 97, 216.

HALMI, N. S. (1961). *Vitamins and Hormones*, **19**, 133.

HALMI, N. S. & PITT-RIVERS, R. U. (1962). *Endocrinology*, **70**, 660.

HALMI, N. S., SPIRTOS, B. N., BOGDANOVE, E. M. & LIPNER, H. J. (1953). *Endocrinology*, **52**, 19.

HALNAN, K. E. & POCHIN, E. E. (1958). *Brit. J. Radiol.*, **31**, 581.

HAMADA, S., TORIZUKA, K. & MIYAKE, T. (1966). *Gunma Symp. Endocrin.*, **3**, 153.

HAMBURGER, J. I., KADIAN, G. & ROSSIN, H. W. (1965). *J. Nucl. Med.*, **6**, 560.

HAMILTON, J. G., ASLING, C. W., GARRISON, W. M. & SCOTT, K. G. (1953). *Univ. of Calif. Publ. Pharm.*, **2**, 283.

HAMOLSKY, M. W., GOLODETZ, A. & FREEDBERG, A. S. (1959). *J. clin. Endocrin.*, **19**, 103.

HAMOLSKY, M. W., KURLAND, G. W. & FREEDBERG, A. S. (1961). *J. chron. Dis.*, **14**, 558.

HANBURY, E. M., HESLIN, J., STANG, L. G., TUCKER, W. D. & RALL, J. E. (1954). *J. clin. Endocrin.*, **14**, 1530.

HARDEN, R. M. & ADAMS, J. F. (1964). *Metabolism*, **13**, 843.

HARDEN, R. M., ALEXANDER, W. D., KOUTRAS, D. A., HARRISON, M. T. & WAYNE, E. (1966). *J. clin. Endocrin.*, **26**, 397.

HARDEN, R. M., ALEXANDER, W. D., PAPADOPOULOS, S., HARRISON, M. T. & MACFARLANE, S. (1967). *Acta Endocrin.*, **55**, 361.

HARDEN, R. M., HARRISON, M. T. & ALEXANDER, W. D. (1963). *Clin. Sci.*, **25**, 27.

HARDEN, R. M., HILDITCH, T. E., KENNEDY, I., MASON, D. K., PAPADOPOULOS, S. & ALEXANDER, W. D. (1967). *Clin. Sci.*, **32**, 49.

HARDEN, R. M., KOUTRAS, D. A., ALEXANDER, W. D. & WAYNE, E. J. (1964). *Clin. Sci.*, **27**, 399.

HARDEN, R. M., MASON, D. K. & BUCHANAN, W. W. (1965). *J. clin. Endocrin.*, **25**, 957.

HARINGTON, C. R. (1926). *Biochem. J.*, **20**, 300.

HARINGTON, C. R. & PITT-RIVERS, R. V. (1945). *Biochem. J.*, **39**, 157.

HARLAN, W. R., LASSLO, J., BOGDONOFF, M. D. & ESTES, E. H. (1963). *J. clin. Endocrin.*, **23**, 33.

HARRISON, M. T., ALEXANDER, W. D. & HARDEN, R. M. (1963). *Lancet*, **1**, 1238.

HARRISON, M. T., HARDEN, R. M. & ALEXANDER, W. D. (1964). *J. clin. Endocrin.*, **24**, 214.

HARRISON, T. S. (1964). *Physiol. Rev.*, **44**, 161.

HATHAWAY, B. H. (1965). *Arch. Surg.*, **90**, 222.

HAYLES, A. B., CHAVES-CARBALLO, E. & McCONA-HEY, W. M. (1967). *Mayo Clin. Proc.*, **42**, 218.

HAYS, M. T. (1965). *J. clin. Endocrin.*, **25**, 465.

HAYS, M. T. & SOLOMON, D. H. (1965). *J. clin. Invest.*, **44**, 117.

HEINEMANN, M., JOHNSON, C. E. & MAN, E. G. (1948). *J. clin. Invest.*, **27**, 91.

HELLMAN, L., BRADLOW, H. L., ZUMOFF, B. & GALLAGHER, T. F. (1961). *J. clin. Endocrin.*, **21**, 1231.

HENDRICK, J. W. (1938). *Trans. Amer. Goiter Assoc.*, 518.

HERVEG, J. P., BECKERS, C. & DE VISSCHER, M. (1966). *Biochem. J.*, **100**, 540.

HIGGINS, H. P., BAYLEY, T. A. & DIOSY, A. (1963). *J. clin. Endocrin.*, **23**, 235.

HILLMANN, G. (1956). *Z. Naturforsch.*, **11b**, 424.

HINTZE, G., FORTELIUS, P. & RAILO, J. (1964). *Acta Endocrin.*, **45**, 381.

HIRSCHFELD, J. & SÖDERBERG, U. (1960). *Acta Obst. Gynec. Scand.*, **39**, 645.

HLAD, C. J. & BRICKER, N. S. (1954). *J. clin. Endocrin.*, **14**, 1539.

HOBERMAN, H. D. (1950). *Yale J. biol. Med.*, **22**, 341; (1950). **23**, 194.

HOCH, H., SINNETT, S. L., MILLER, P. O. & MAHADY, I. B. (1965). *Biochemistry*, **4**, 931.

HODGES, R. E., HAMILTON, H. E. & KEETTEL, W. C. (1952). *Arch. intern. Med.*, **90**, 863.

HOLLANDER, C. S., PROUT, T. E., RIENHOFF, M., RUBEN, R. J. & ASPER, S. P. (1964). *Amer. J. Med.*, **37**, 630.

HOLVEY, D. N., GOODNER, C. J., NICOLOFF, J. T. & DOWLING, J. T. (1964). *Arch. intern. Med.*, **113**, 89.

HORN, R. C. (1960). *Arch. Pathol.*, **69**, 481.

HOSOYA, T. & MORRISON, M. (1967). *Biochemistry*, **6**, 1021.

HOWITT, G. & ROWLANDS, D. J. (1967). *Amer. Heart J.*, **73**, 282.

HOUSSAY, B. A. (1944). *Endocrinology*, **35**, 158.

HOUSSAY, B. A. (1945). "Accion de la tiroide sobre el metabolismo de los hidratos de carbono y en la diabetes". El Ateneo, Buenos Aires.

HURXTHAL, L. M. (1934). *Arch. intern Med.*, **53**, 762.

HUTCHINSON, J. H. & McGIRR, E. M. (1956). *Lancet*, **1**, 1035.

IFF, H. W. & WILBRANDT, W. (1963). *Biochim. biophys. Acta*, **78**, 711.

INGBAR, S. H. (1960). *Rec. Prog. Horm. Res.*, **16**, 353.

INGBAR, S. H. & BRAVERMAN, L. E. (1965). In "Endocrinologia Experimentalis". Ed. Stolc, V., p. 285, Bratislava, Slovak Academy of Sciences.

INGBAR, S. H., BRAVERMAN, L. E., DAWBER, N. A. & LEE, G. Y. (1965). *J. clin. Invest.*, **44**, 1679.

INGBAR, S. H. & FREINKEL, N. (1955). *J. clin. Invest.*, **35**, 1375.

INGBAR, S. H. & FREINKEL, N. (1957). *Endocrinology*, **61**, 398.

INGBAR, S. H. & FREINKEL, N. (1958a). *Arch. intern. Med.*, **101**, 339.

INGBAR, S. H. & FREINKEL, N. (1958b). *J. clin. Invest.*, **37**, 1603.

IRVINE, W. J. (1962). *Brit. med. J.*, **1**, 1444.

ISLER, H. (1959). *Endocrinology*, **64**, 769.

ISLER, H., LEBLOND, C. P. & AXELROD, A. A. (1958). *Endocrinology*, **62**, 159.

ISSELBACHER, K. J. & AXELROD, J. (1955). *J. Amer. chem. Soc.*, **77**, 1070.

JANES, R. G. (1954). *Endocrinology*, **54**, 464.

JELLINEK, E. H. & KELLY, R. E. (1960). *Lancet*, **2**, 225.

JENSEN, J. M. & CLARK, D. E. (1951). *J. Lab. clin. Med.*, **38**, 663.

JOHNSON, P. C. & BEIERWALTES, W. H. (1953). *J. Lab. clin. Med.*, **41**, 676.

JONES, J. E., DESPER, P. C., SHANE, S. R. & FLINK, E. B. (1966). *J. clin. Invest.*, **45**, 891.

JONES, S. L. & VAN MIDDLESWORTH, L. (1960). *Endocrinology*, **67**, 855.

KEATING, F. R., POWER, M. H., BERKSON, J. & HAINES, S. F. (1947). *J. clin. Invest.*, **26**, 1138.

KEATING, F. R., WONG, J. C., LUELLEN, T. J., WILLIAMS, M. M. D., POWER, M. H. & McCONAHEY, W. M. (1949). *J. clin. Invest.*, **28**, 191, 217, 207.

KELLEY, B. & DAY, H. G. (1948). *J. biol. Chem.*, **175**, 863.

KERN, R. A., SOLOFF, L. A., SNAPE, W. J. & BELLO, C. T. (1949). *Amer. J. med. Sci.*, **217**, 609.

KIM, K. H. & COHEN, P. P. (1966). *Proc. Natl. Acad. Sci.*, **55**, 1251.

KIRKHAM, K. E. (1967). *Vitamins and Hormones*, **24**, 173.

KIVIRIKKO, K. I., LAITINEN, O. & LAMBERG, B. A. (1965). *J. clin. Endocrin.*, **25**, 1347.

KLEBANOFF, S. J., YIP, D. & KESSLER, D. (1962). *Biochim. biophys. Acta*, **58**, 563.

KLEINBERG, J. & DAVIDSON, A. (1948). *Chem. Rev.*, **42**, 601.

KLINCK, G. H. (1964). In "The Thyroid". Ed. Hazard, J. B., p. 1, Baltimore, Williams & Wilkins.

KOGUT, M. D., KAPLAN, S. A., COLLIPP, P. J., TIAMSIC, T. & BOYLE, D. (1965). *New Engl. J. Med.*, **272**, 217.

KONDO, Y. (1961). *J. Biochem.*, **50**, 210.

KRANE, S. M., STANBURY, J. B. & BROWNELL, G. (1956). *J. clin. Invest.*, **35**, 874.

KRESS, L. F., PEANASKY, R. J. & KLITGAARD, H. M. (1966). *Biochim. biophys. Acta*, **113**, 375.

KRISS, J. P., PLESHAKOV, B. & CHIEN, J. R. (1964). *J. clin. Endocrin.*, **24**, 1005.

KRISS, J. P., PLESHAKOV, V., ROSENBLUM, A. L., HOLDERNESS, M., SHARP, G. & UTIGER, R. (1967). *J. clin. Endocrin.*, **27**, 582.

KUHLBÄCK, B. (1957). *Acta med. Scand.*, suppl. 331.

KURLAND, G. S., LUCAS, J. L. & FREEDBERG, A. S. (1961). *J. Lab. & clin. Med.*, **57**, 574.

KUSAKABE, T. & MIYAKE, T. (1964). *J. clin. Endocrin.*, **24**, 456.

KUZELL, W., SCHAFFARZICH, R. W., NAUGLER, E. W., KOETS, P., MANKLE, E. A., BROWN, B. & CHAMPLIN, B. (1955). *J. chron. Dis.*, **2**, 645.

LAHEY, F. C. (1953). *Trans. Amer. Goiter Assoc.*, 234.

LAMBERG, B. A., HINTZE, G., JUSSILA, R. & BERLIN, M. (1960). *Acta Endocrin.*, **33**, 457.

LANGE, K. (1944). *Amer. J. med. Sci.*, **208**, 5.

LANGER, P. (1966). *Endocrinology*, **79**, 1117.

LARSEN, P. R. & WOLFF, J. (1967). *Science*, **155**, 335.

LASSITER, W. B. & STANBURY, J. B. (1958). *J. clin. Endocrin.*, **18**, 903.

LAWSON, J. B. (1958). *New Engl. J. Med.*, **259**, 761.

LEBLOND, C. P. & GROSS, J. (1949). *J. clin. Endocrin.*, **9**, 149.

LEBLOND, C. P., PUPPEL, I. D., RILEY, E., RADIKE, M. & CURTIS, G. M. (1946). *J. biol. Chem.*, **162**, 275.

LEBOEUF, G. & BONGIOVANNI, A. M. (1964). *Adv. Pediat.*, **13**, 183.

LEE, G. Y. & INGBAR, S. H. (1965). *Endocrinology*, **77**, 940.

LEE, W. Y., BRONSKY, D. & WALDSTEIN, S. S. (1962). *J. clin. Endocrin.*, **22**, 879.

LEEPER, R. D. (1963). *J. clin. Endocrin.*, **23**, 426.

LEEPER, R. D., BENUA, R. S., BREUER, J. L. & RAWSON, R. W. (1960). *J. clin. Endocrin.*, **20**, 1457.

LELOUP, J. & LACHIVER, F. (1955). *C.R. Acad. Sci. Paris*, **241**, 509, 573.

LERMAN, J. & PITT-RIVERS, R. V. (1955). *J. clin. Endocrin.*, **15**, 653.

LERMAN, J. & STEBBINS, H. D. (1942). *J. Amer. med. Ass.*, **119**, 391.

LEROY, G. V. (1956). *Ann. intern. Med.*, **44**, 524.

LESZYNSKY, H. E. (1964). *Acta Endocrin.*, **46**, 103.

LEWALLEN, C. G. & GODWIN, J. T. (1962). *Radiology.*

LEWALLEN, C. G., RALL, J. E. & BERMAN, M. (1959). *J. clin. Invest.*, **38**, 88.

LEWITUS, Z., HASENFRATZ, J., TOOR, M., MASSRY, S. & RABINOWITCH, E. (1964). *J. clin. Endocrin.*, **24**, 1084.

LIEBERTHAL, A. S., BENSON, S. G. & KLITGAARD, H. M. (1963). *J. clin. Endocrin.*, **23**, 211.

LINDEGREN, L. & STARR, P. S. (1966). *Acta Endocrin.*, **51**, 77.

LINDSAY, S. (1964). In "The Thyroid Gland". Eds. Pitt-Rivers, R. & Trotter, W. R., vol. 2, p. 253, Washington, Butterworth's.

LINDSAY, S. & CHAIKOFF, I. L. (1964). *Cancer Res.*, **24**, 1099.

LINDSAY, S., DAILEY, M. E., FRIEDLANDER, J., YEE, G. & SOLEY, M. H. (1952). *J. clin. Endocrin.*, **12**, 1578.

LISSITZKY, S. (1960). *Bull. Soc. Chim. Biol.*, **42**, 1187.

LISSITZKY, S., BENEVENT, M. T., ROQUES, M. & ROCHE, J. (1958). *C.R. Soc. Biol.*, **152**, 1490.

LISSITZKY, S. & BOUCHILLOUX, S. (1957). *Bull. Soc. chim. biol. Paris*, **39**, 133.

LISSITZKY, S., COMAR, D., RIVIÈRE, R. & CODACCIONI, J. L. (1965). *Rev. Franc. Et. clin. Biol.*, **10**, 631.

LISTER, L. M. & ASHE, J. R. (1955). *Obst. & Gynec.*, **6**, 436.

LITTLE, G., MEADOR, C. K., CUNNINGHAM, R. & PITTMAN, J. A. (1965). *J. clin. Endocrin.*, **25**, 1529.

LITTMAN, D. S., JEFFERS, W. A. & ROSE, E. (1957). *Amer. J. med. Sci.*, **233**, 10.

LIZARRALDE, G., JONES, B., SEAL, V. & JONES, J. E. (1966). *J. clin. Endocrin.*, **26**, 1227.

LONDON, D. R. & SEGAL, S. (1967). *Endocrinology*, **80**, 623.

LOUGHLIN, R. E., McQUILLAN, M. T. & TRIKOJUS, V. M. (1960). *Endocrinology*, **68**, 773.

LOZNER, E. L., WINKLER, A. W., TAYLOR, F. H. L. & PETERS, J. P. (1941). *J. clin. Invest.*, **20**, 507.

LUNDBLAD, G., BERNBÄCK, M. L. & WIDEMANN, D. (1965). *Acta Chem. Scand.*, **20**, 675.

MAAYAN, M. L. & ROSENBERG, I. N. (1963). *Endocrinology*, **73**, 38.

MACCHIA, V., BATES, R. W. & PASTAN, I. (1967). *J. biol. Chem.*, **242**, 3726.

MACGREGOR, A. G. & SOMNER, A. R. (1954). *Lancet*, **2**, 931.

MACK, R. E., HART, K. I., DRUET, D. & BAUER, M. A. (1961). *Amer. J. Med.*, **30**, 323.

MacLAGAN, N. F., RUNDLE, F. F., COLLARD, H. B. & MILLS, F. H. (1940). *Quart. J. Med.*, **9**, n.s., 215.

MALOOF, F. (1955). *Endocrinology*, **56**, 209.

MALOOF, F. & SOODAK, M. (1964). *J. biol. Chem.*, **239**, 1995.

MAN, E. B. (1960). *Amer. J. Roent.*, **83**, 497.

MAN, E. B., BONDY, P. K., WEEKS, E. A. & PETERS, J. P. (1954). *Yale J. Biol. Med.*, **27**, 90.

MAN, E. B., HEINEMANN, M., JOHNSON, C. E., LEARY, D. C. & PETERS, J. P. (1951). *J. clin. Invest.*, **30**, 137.

MANDL, A. M. (1957). *J. Endocrin.*, **15**, 448.

MAQSOOD, P. (1952). *Biol. Rev. Cambridge Phil. Soc.*, **27**, 281.

MARKS, A. N. & MAN, E. B. (1965). *Pediatrics*, **35**, 753.

MARTIN, L. & FISHER, R. A. (1951). *Quart. J. Med.*, **20**, 293.

MARTIN, M. M. & RENTO, R. D. (1962). *J. Pediat.*, **61**, 94.

MASI, A. T. (1965). *J. Chron. Dis.*, **18**, 35.

MAYBERRY, W. E., RALL, J. E. & BERTOLI, D. (1964). *J. Amer. Chem. Soc.*, **86**, 5302; (1965). *J. Org. Chem.* **30**, 2029.

McCLELLAN, J. E., DONEGAN, C., THORUP, O. A. & LEAVELL, B. S. (1958). *J. Lab. clin. Med.*, **51**, 91.

McCONAHEY, W. M., OWEN, C. A. & KEATING, F. R. (1956). *J. clin. Endocrinol.*, **16**, 724.

McFADZEAN, A. J. S. & YEUNG, R. (1967). *Brit. med. J.*, **451**, 451.

McKENZIE, J. M. (1964). *J. clin. Endocrin.*, **24**, 660.

McKENZIE, J. M. (1965). *J. clin. Endocrin.*, **25**, 424.

McKENZIE, J. M. (1967). *Rec. Prog. Horm. Res.*, **23**, 1.

MEISSNER, W. A. & McMANUS, R. (1952). *J. clin. Endocrin.*, **12**, 1474.

MELMON, K. L., RIVLIN, R., OATES, J. A. & SJOERDSMA, A. (1964). *J. clin. Endocrin.*, **24**, 691.

MELTZER, R. I. & STANABACK, R. J. (1961). *J. Org. Chem.*, **26**, 1977.

MERCER, C. J., SHARARD, A., WESTERINK, C. J. M., ADAMS, D. D. (1960). *Lancet*, **2**, 19.

METZGER, H. & EDELHOCH, H. (1962). *Nature*, **193**, 275.

METZGER, H., SHARP, G. & EDELHOCH, H. (1962). *Biochemistry*, **1**, 205.

MICHEL, R. & PITT-RIVERS, R. V. (1948). *Biochim. biophys. Acta*, **2**, 223.

MICHENER, W. M., TAUXE, N. & HAYLES, A. B. (1962). *Pediatrics*, **29**, 369.

VAN MIDDLESWORTH, L. (1963). *Health Physics*, **9**, 1197.

VAN MIDDLESWORTH, L. C., NURNBERGER, C. E. & LIPSCOMB, A. (1954). *J. clin. Endocrin.*, **14**, 1056.

MILET, R. G., PLUNKETT, E. R. & CARR, D. H. (1967). *Acta Endocrin.*, **54**, 609.

MILLER, W. H., ROBLIN, R. O. & ASTWOOD, E. B. (1945). *J. Amer. chem. Soc.*, **67**, 2201.

MITROPOULOS, K. A. & MYANT, N. B. (1965). *Biochem. J.*, **94**, 594.

MONEY, J. & LEWIS, V. (1964). In "Brain-Thyroid Relationships", Ciba Found. Study Group, No. 18, p. 75, Boston, Little Brown & Co.

MOORE, W. & COLVIN, M. (1966). *Int. J. Rad. Biol.*, **10**, 391.

MORREALE DE ESCOBAR, G. & ESCOBAR DEL REY, F. (1967). *Rec. Adv. Horm. Res.*, **23**, 87.

MORRIS, D. R. & HAGER, L. P. (1966). *J. biol. Chem.*, **241**, 3582.

MORRIS, J. H. & HARDIN, C. A. (1964). *Arch. intern. Med.*, **113**, 97.

MORROW, D. H., GAFFNEY, T. E. & BRAUNWALD, E. (1963). *J. Pharm. exp. Therap.*, **140**, 324.

MORTON, M. E., OTTOMAN, R. E. & PETERSON, R. E. (1951). *J. clin. Endocrin.*, **11**, 1572.

MOSCHCOWITZ, E. (1946). *Arch. intern. Med.*, **78**, 497.

MOURIZ, J., MORREALE DE ESCOBAR, G. & ESCOBAR DEL REY, F. (1966). *Endocrinology*, **79**, 248.

MOVITT, E. R., GERSTL, B. & DAVIS, A. E. (1953). *Arch. intern. Med.*, **91**, 729.

MUNRO, D. S., RENSCHLER, H. & WILSON, G. M. (1958). *Metabolism*, **7**, 124.

MURPHY, B. N. S., PATTEE, C. J. & GOLD, A. (1966). *J. clin. Endocrin.*, **26**, 274.

MUSTACCHI, P. & CUTLER, S. J. (1956). *New Engl. J. Med.*, **255**, 889.

VON MUTZENBECHER, P. (1939). *Hoppe. Seyl. Z.*, **261**, 253.

MYANT, N. B. (1956). *Clin. Sci.*, **15**, 551.

MYANT, N. B. (1964). In "Medicinal Chemistry". Ed. R. Paoletti, vol. 2, p. 299, New York, Academic Press.

MYANT, N. B. (1964). In "The Thyroid Gland". Eds. Pitt-Rivers, R. & Trotter, W. R., vol. 1, p. 203, Washington, Butterworths.

MYANT, N. B., CORBETT, B. D., HONOUR, A. J. & POCHIN, E. E. (1950). *Clin. Sci.*, **9**, 405.

MYANT, N. B., POCHIN, E. E. & GOLDIE, E. A. G. (1949). *Clin. Sci.*, **8**, 109.

MYERS, W. G. & VANDERLEEDEN, J. C. (1960). *J. Nucl. Med.*, **1**, 149.

NADLER, N. J., SARKAR, S. K. & LEBLOND, C. P. (1962). *Endocrinology*, **71**, 120.

NAGATAKI, S. & INGBAR, S. N. (1963). *Endocrinology*, **72**, 480.

NAGATAKI, S., SHIZUME, K. & OKINAKA, S. (1961). *Endocrinology*, **69**, 199.

NAKAYAMA, K. (1962). *Endocrin. Japon.*, **9**, 131.

NAUMAN, J., NAUMAN, A. & WERNER, J. C. (1967). *J. clin. Invest.*, **46**, 1346.

NICKEL, S. N. & FRAME, B. (1961). *J. chron. Dis.*, **14**, 570.

NIÉPCE, B. (1851.) *Traité du goitre du crétinisme*, Paris, Baillière.

NILSSON, L. R. & BERNE, E. (1964). *Acta Endocrin.*, **47**, 133.

NILSSON, L. R., BORGFORS, N., GAMSTORP, I., HOLST, H. E. & LIDEN, G. (1964). *Acta Pediat.*, **53**, 117.

NISHINAGA, A., CAHNMANN, H. J., KON, H. & MATSUURA, T. (1968) *Biochemistry*, **7**, 388.

NOFAL, M. & BEIERWALTES, W. H. (1964). *J. Nucl. Med.*, **5**, 840.

NOFAL, M. & BEIERWALTES, W. H. & PATNO, M. E. (1966). *J. Amer. Med. Ass.*, **197**, 605.

NUNEZ, J., JACQUEMIN, C., BRUN, D. & ROCHE, J. (1965). *Biochim. biophys. Acta*, **107**, 441, 454.

NUNEZ, J., MAUCHAMP, J., MACCHIA, V. & ROCHE, J. (1965). *Biochim. biophys. Acta*, **107**, 241.

NUNEZ, J., POMMIER, J., EL HILALI, M. & ROCHE, J. (1965). *J. labelled Compds.*, **1**, 128.

ODDIE, T. H., MEADE, J. H. & FISHER, D. A. (1967). *J. clin. Endocrin.*, **27**, 722.

ODDIE, T. H., RUNDLE, F. F., THOMAS, I. O., HALES, I. & CATT, B. (1960). *J. Clin. Endocrin.*, **20**, 1146.

ODELL, W. D., WILBER, J. F. & PAUL, W. E. (1965). *J. clin. Endocrin.*, **25**, 1179.

OGBORN, R. E., WAGGENER, R. E. & VAN HOVE, E. (1960). *Pediatrics*, **26**, 771.

OLEN, E. & KLINCK, G. H. (1965). In "Current Topics in Thyroid Research". Eds. Cassano, C. & Andreoli, M., p. 1023, New York, Academic Press.

OPPENHEIMER, J. H. & MCPHERSON, H. T. (1961). *Amer. J. Med.*, **30**, 281.

OPPENHEIMER, J. H. & SURKS, M. I. (1964). *J. clin. Endocrin.*, **24**, 785.

OPPENHEIMER, J. H., SURKS, M. I., SMITH, J. C. & SQUEF, R. (1965). *J. biol. Chem.*, **240**, 173.

OSORIO, C. & MYANT, N. B. (1962). *Clin. Sci.*, **23**, 277.

OWEN, C. A. & POWER, M. M. (1953). *J. biol. Chem.*, **200**, 11.

PAPPER, S. & LANCASTREMERE, R. G. (1961). *J. chron. Dis.*, **14**, 495.

PARKIN, G. & GREEN, J. A. (1943). *J. clin. Endocrin.*, **3**, 466.

PASTAN, I. (1957). *Endocrinology*, **61**, 93.

PASTAN, I. (1966). *Ann. Rev. Biochem.*, **35**, Part I, 369.

PASTAN, I. & KATZEN, R. (1967). *Biochem. biophys. Res. Commun.* **29**, 792.

PAUL, A. M. & PHILLIPS, R. W. (1954). *J. clin. Endocrin.*, **14**, 554.

PEEL, A. A. F. (1943). *Brit. Heart J.*, **5**, 89.

PELTOLA, P. (1960). *Acta Endocrin.*, **34**, 121.

PERLMUTTER, M. & COHN, H. (1964). *Amer. J. Med.*, **36**, 883.

PERLMUTTER, M., WEISENFELD, S., SLATER, S. & WALLACE, E. Z. (1952). *J. clin. Endocrin.*, **12**, 208.

PERRY, R. E., HODGMAN, J. E. & STARR, P. (1965). *Pediatrics*, **35**, 759.

PETERS, J. P. & MAN, E. B. (1950). *J. clin. Invest.*, **29**, 1.

PETERSEN, R. E. (1958). *J. clin. Invest.*, **37**, 736.

PILEGGI, V. J., GOLUB, O. J. & LEE, N. D. (1965). *J. clin. Endocrin.*, **25**, 949.

PILEGGI, V. J., LEE, N. D., GOLUB, O. J. & HENRY, R. J. (1961). *J. clin. Endocrin.*, **21**, 1272.

PILEGGI, V. J., SEGAL, H. A. & GOLUB, O. J. (1964). *J. clin. Endocrin.*, **24**, 273.

PINCUS, R. A., REICHLIN, S. & HEMPELMAN, L. H. (1967). *Ann. Int. Med.*, **66**, 1154.

PIND, K. (1957). *Acta Endocrin.*, **26**, 263.

PITT-RIVERS, R. V. (1948). *Biochem. J.*, **43**, 223.

PITT-RIVERS, R. V. (1950). *Physiol. Rev.*, **30**, 195.

PITT-RIVERS, R. V. (1962). *Biochem. J.*, **82**, 108.

PITT-RIVERS, R. V. (1963). *Biochem. J.*, **87**, 340.

PITT-RIVERS, R. V. (1966). *J. Endocrin.*, **36**, 203.

PITT-RIVERS, R. & CAVALIERI, R. R. (1964). In "The Thyroid Gland". Eds. Pitt-Rivers, R. & Trotter, W. R., vol. I, p. 87, Washington, Butterworths.

PITT-RIVERS, R. V. & JAMES, A. T. (1958). *Biochem. J.*, **70**, 173.

PITT-RIVERS, R. V. & RALL, J. E. (1961). *Endocrinology*, **68**, 309.

PITT-RIVERS, R. V. & TATA, J. R. (1959). "The Thyroid Hormones". London, Permanon Press.

PLASKETT, L. G. (1961). *Biochem. J.*, **78**, 657, 649.

POCHIN, E. E. (1952). *Clin. Sci.*, **11**, 13.

POCHIN, E. E. (1960). *Brit. med. J.*, **2**, 1545.

PORATH, M. B., HOCHMAN, A. & GROSS, J. (1966). *J. Nucl. Med.*, **7**, 88, 99.

POSTEL, S. (1956). *J. clin. Invest.*, **25**, 1345.

POTTER, G. D., LINDSAY, S. & CHAIKOFF, I. L. (1960). *Arch. Path.*, **69**, 257.

POTTER, G. D., TONG, W. & CHAIKOFF, I. L. (1959). *J. biol. Chem.*, **234**, 350.

PREMACHANDRA, B. N., RAY, A. K., HIRATA, Y. & BLUMENTHAL, H. T. (1965). *Endocrinology*, **73**, 135.

PULVERTAFT, R. J. V., DONIACH, D., ROITT, I. M. & HUDSON, R. V. (1959). *Lancet*, **2**, 214.

PURDY, R. H., WOEBER, K. A., HOLLOWAY, M. T. & INGBAR, S. H. (1965). *Biochemistry*, **4**, 1888.

PURVES, H. D., GRIESBACH, W. E. & KENNEDY, T. H. (1951). *Brit. J. Cancer*, **5**, 30.

RABEN, M. S. (1949). *Endocrinology*, **45**, 296.

RALL, J. E. & CONARD, R. A. (1966). *Amer. J. Med.*, **40**, 883.

RALL, J. E., SONENBERG, M. S., ROBBINS, J., LAZERSON, R. & RAWSON, R. W. (1953). *J. clin. Endocrin.*, **13**, 1369.

RALL, J. E., ROBBINS, J. & LEWALLEN, C. G. (1964). In "The Hormones". Eds. Pincus, G. & Thimann, K. V., vol. 5, p. 159, New York, Academic Press.

RANDALL, L. O. (1946). J. biol. Chem., 164, 521.

REFETOFF, S., DeWIND, L. T. & DeGROOT, L. S. (1967). J. clin. Endocrin., 27, 279.

REICHLIN, S., VOLPERT, E. M. & WERNER, S. C. (1966). Endocrinology, 78, 302.

REICHLIN, S. (1963). New Engl. J. Med., 269, 1296.

REINWEIN, D. & KLEIN, E. (1962). Acta Endocrin., 39, 328.

REINWEIN, D. & RALL, J. E. (1966). J. biol. Chem., 241, 1636.

REISS, M. & HAIGH, C. P. (1954). Proc. R. Soc. Med., 47, 889.

RICCABONA, G. (1965). New Engl. J. Med., 273, 126.

RICHARDSON, H. B. & SHORR, E. (1935). Trans. Ass. Amer. Phys., 50, 156.

RIGGS, D. S. (1952). Pharm. Rev., 4, 284.

RIGGS, D. S., LAVIETES, P. H. & MAN, E. B. (1942). J. biol. Chem., 143, 363.

RIZEK, J. E., DIMICH, A. & WALLACH, S. (1965). J. clin. Endocrin., 25, 350.

ROBBINS, J. (1966). In "Tumors of the Thyroid Gland". Ed. Appaic, A., p. 250, Basel, S. Karger.

ROBBINS, J. & NELSON, J. H. (1958). J. clin. Invest., 37, 153.

ROBBINS, J. & RALL, J. E. (1957). Rec. Prog. Horm. Res., 13, 161.

ROBBINS, J. & RALL, J. E. (1960). Physiol. Rev., 40, 415.

ROBBINS, J. & RALL, J. E. (1967). In "Hormones in Blood". Ed. Gray, C. H., 2nd ed., London, Academic Press.

ROBBINS, J., SALVATORE, G., VECCHIO, G. & UI, N. (1966). Biochim. biophys. Acta, 127, 101.

ROBBINS, J. R., VAN ZYL, A. & VAN DER WALT, K. (1966). Endocrinology, 78, 1213.

ROBBINS, J., WOLFF, J. & RALL, J. E. (1959). Endocrinology, 64, 12, 37.

ROCHE, J., LISSITZKY, S. & MICHEL, R. (1952b). C.R. Soc. Biol., Paris, 146, 1474.

ROCHE, J., LISSITZKY, S., MICHEL, O. & MICHEL, R. (1951). Biochim. biophys. Acta, 7, 439.

ROCHE, J. & MICHEL, R. (1954). Ann. Rev. Biochem., 23, 481.

ROCHE, J., MICHEL, R., CLOSON, J. & MICHEL, O. (1959). Biochim. biophys. Acta, 33, 469.

ROCHE, J., MICHEL, R. & GREGORIO, P. (1961). Biochim. biophys. Acta, 47, 398.

ROCHE, J., MICHEL. R., MICHEL, O. & LISSITZKY, S. (1952a). Biochim. biophys. Acta, 9, 161.

ROCHE, J., MICHEL, R. & TATA, J. (1953). Biochim. biophys. Acta, 11, 543.

ROCHE, J., MICHEL, R. & WOLF, W. (1954). C.R. Acad. Sci., 239, 597.

ROCHE, J., MICHEL, R., WOLF, W. & NUNEZ, J. (1956). Biochim. biophys. Acta, 19, 308.

ROGERS, J. (1958). New Engl. J. Med., 259, 676, 721, 770.

ROITT I. M. & DONIACH, D. (1958). Lancet, 2, 1027.

ROITT, I. M. & DONIACH, D. (1960). Brit. med. Bull., 16, 152.

ROLLAND, M., BISMUTH, J., FONDARAI, J. & LISSITSKY, S. (1966). Acta Endocrin., 53, 286.

ROSE, N. R. & WITEBSKY, E. (1956). J. Immunol., 76, 408, 417.

ROSEN, F., EZRIN, C. & VOLPÉ, R. (1967). Acta Endocrin., 54, 604.

ROSENBERG, I. N. (1952). Science, 116, 503.

ROSENBERG, I. N., ATHANS, J. C. & BEHAR, A. (1960). Endocrinology, 66, 185.

ROSENBERG, I. N., ATHANS, J. C. & ISAACS, G. H. (1965). Rec. Prog. Horm. Res., 25, 33.

ROSENBERG, L. L., GOLDMAN, M., LaROCHE, G. & DIMICK, M. K. (1964). Endocrinology, 74, 212.

ROSS, F. & NUSYNOWITZ, M. L. (1968). J. clin. Endocrin, 28, 591.

ROSS, G. T., SCHOLZ, D. A., LAMBERG, E. H. & GERACI, J. E. (1958). J. clin. Endocrin., 18, 492.

RUSSEL, K. P. (1953). Surg. Gynec. & Obst., 96, 577.

SACHS, M. L. (1960). "Derivatives and Isomers of the Thyroid Hormones". Univ. of Penna., Philadelphia.

SALVATORE, G. (1964). Exp. Ann. Biochim. Med., 25, 99.

SALVATORE, G., SALVATORE, M. & WOLFF, J. (1966). Biochim. biophys. Acta, 120, 387.

SALVATORE, G., VECCHIO, G., SALVATORE, M., CAHNMANN, H. J. & ROBBINS, J. (1965). J. biol. Chem., 240, 2935.

SAMEL, M. (1958). Arch. intern. Pharm., 117, 151.

SANDHOFER, F., SAILER, S. & BRAUNSTEINER, H. (1966). Klin. Wchschr., 44, 1389.

SAPIRA, J. D., ALTMAN, M., VAN DYK, K. & SHAPIRO, A. P. (1965). New Engl. J. Med., 273, 140.

SATTLER, H. (1952). "Basedow's Disease". N.Y., Grune & Stratton.

SAUNDERS, B. C. & STARK, B. P. (1958). Tetrahedron, 4, 169.

SAWIN, C. T. & McHUGH, J. E. (1966). J. clin. Endocrin., 26, 955.

SCHACHTER, D. (1963). In "Transfer of Ca++ and Sr++ Across Biological Membranes". Ed. Wasserman, R. H., p. 206, Academic Press, N.Y.

SCHALLER, R. T. & STEVENSON, J. K. (1966). Cancer, 19, 1063.

SCHALLY, A. V., BOWERS, C. Y. & REDDING, T. W. (1966). Endocrinology, 78, 726; 79, 229.

SCHATZ, D. L. (1967). J. clin. Endocrin., 27, 165.

SCHIMKE, R. N. & HARTMANN, W. H. (1965). Ann. intern. Med., 63, 1027.

SCHNEIDER, P. B. (1964). Endocrinology, 74, 973.

SCHNEIDER, P. B. & WOLFF, J. (1965). Biochim. biophys. Acta, 94, 115.

SCHUSSLER, G. C. & PLAGER, J. E. (1967). J. clin. Endocrin., 27, 242.

SCHWARTZ, E. (1955). J. Lab. clin. Med., 45, 340.

SEAL, U. S. & DOE, R. P. (1964). Proc. Second Int. Congr. Endocrin., p. 83.

SEED, R. W. & GOLDBERG, I. H. (1965). J. biol. Chem., 240, 764.

SELA, M. & SARID, S. (1956). Nature, 178, 540.

SELLIN, H. G. & GOLDBERG, I. H. (1965). *J. biol. Chem.*, **240**, 774.

SELTZER, R. A., KEREIAKES, J. G. & SAENGER, E. L. (1964). *New Engl. J. Med.*, **271**, 84.

SEXTON, D. L. & MACK, R. (1954). *J. clin. Endocrin.*, **14**, 747.

SHANE, S. R., JONES, J. E. & FLINK, E. B. (1965). *J. clin. Endocrin.*, **25**, 1085.

SHAPIRO, R. (1961). *New Engl. J. Med.*, **284**, 378.

SHAPLAND, C. G. (1964). *J. med. Lab. Tech.*, **21**, 1.

SHELINE, G. E., LINDSAY, S., McCORMACK, K. R. & GALANTE, M. (1962). *J. clin. Endocrin.*, **22**, 8.

SHELINE, G. E. & McCORMACK, K. (1960). *J. clin. Endocrin.*, **20**, 1401.

SHIBA, T. & CAHNMANN, T. (1962). *J. Org. Chem.*, **27**, 1773.

SHIMAOKA, K. (1963). *Acta Endocrin.*, **43**, 285.

SHUMWAY, M. & DAVIS, P. L. (1954). *J. clin. Endocrin.*, **14**, 742.

SIMON, C. (1963). *Biochim. biophys. Acta*, **74**, 565.

SIMON, C. & LISSITZKY, S. (1964). *Biochim. biophys. Acta*, **93**, 494.

SISSON, J. C. (1965). *J. Nucl. Med.*, **6**, 853.

SKANSE, B. (1948). *J. clin. Endocrin.*, **8**, 707.

SKANSE, B. (1949). *Acta med. Scand. Suppl.*, 235.

SKILLERN, P. G. & LEWIS, L. A. (1958). *J. clin. Endocrin.*, **18**, 1407.

SKILLERN, P. G., NELSON, H. E. & CRILE, G., Jnr. (1956). *J. clin. Endocrin.*, **16**, 1422.

SMALL, M. D., BEZMAN, A., LONGARINI, A. E., FENNELL, A. & ZAMCHECK, N. (1961). *Proc. Soc. exp. biol. Med.*, **106**, 450.

SMITH, R. N. & WILSON, G. M. (1967). *Brit. med. J.*, **1**, 129.

SOCOLOW, E. L., HASHIZUME, A., NERIISHI, S. & NIITANI, R. (1963). *New Engl. J. Med.*, **268**, 406.

SOCOLOW, E. L. & INGBAR, S. H. (1967). *Endocrinology*, **80**, 337.

SÖDERBERG, U. (1958). *Acta Physiol. Scand.*, **42**, suppl. 147, p. 1–113.

SOKAL, J. E. (1953). *New Engl. J. Med.*, **249**, 393.

SOKAL, J. E. (1960). In "Clinical Endocrinology". Ed. Astwood, E. B., vol. 1, p. 160, N.Y. Grune Stratton.

SOKOLOFF, L., KAUFMAN, S., CAMPBELL, P. L., FRANCIS, C. M. & GELBOIN, H. V. (1963). *J. biol. Chem.*, **238**, 1432; (1964). *Proc. Natl. Acad. Sci.*, **52**, 728.

SOKOLOFF, L., WECHSLER, R. L., MANGOLD, R., BALLS, K. & KETY, S. S. (1953). *J. clin. Invest.*, **32**, 202.

SOLOMON, D. H. (1956). *Metabolism*, **5**, 667.

SOLOMON, D. H., BECK, J. L., VANDERLAAN, W. P. & ASTWOOD, E. B. (1953). *J. Amer. med. Ass.*, **152**, 201.

SPEERT, H., QUIMBY, E. H. & WERNER, S. C. (1951). *Surg. Gynec. Obstet.*, **93**, 230.

SPIRO, R. G. & SPIRO, M. J. (1965). *J. biol. Chem.*, **240**, 997, 1603.

SPIRO, R. G. & SPIRO, M. J. (1966). *J. biol. Chem.*, **41**, 1271.

STANBURY, J. B. (1966). In "The Metabolic Basis of Inherited Disease". Eds. Stanbury, J. B., Wyngaarden, J. B. & Frederickson, D. S., p. 215, N.Y., McGrew-Hill, Inc.

STANBURY, J. B. (1967). "Endocrine Genetics". Ed. Spickett, S. G., p. 107, Cambridge Univ. Press, Cambridge.

STANBURY, J. B., BROWNELL, G. L., RIGGS, D. S., PERINETTI, H., ITOIZ, S. & DEL CASTILLO, E. D. (1954). "Endemic Goiter". Harvard Univ. Press, Cambridge, Mass.

STANBURY, J. B. & CHAPMAN, E. M. (1960). *Lancet*, **1**, 1162.

STANBURY, J. B. & HEDGE, A. N. (1950). *J. clin. Endocrin.*, **10**, 1471.

STANBURY, J. B. & JANSSEN, M. A. (1962). *J. clin. Endocrin.*, **22**, 978.

STANBURY, J. B. & MORRIS, M. L. (1958). *J. biol. Chem.*, **233**, 106.

STANLEY, M. M. (1949). *J. clin. Endocrin.*, **9**, 941.

STANLEY, M. M. & ASTWOOD, E. B. (1948). *Endocrinology*, **41**, 66.

STATLAND, H. & LERMAN, J. (1950). *J. clin. Endocrin.*, **10**, 1401.

STEIN, O. & GROSS, J. (1964). *Endocrinology*, **75**, 787.

STEINBERG, D. (1962). *Adv. in Pharm.*, **1**, 59.

STERLING, K. (1958). *J. clin. Invest.*, **37**, 1342.

STERLING, K. & BRENNER, M. A. (1966). *J. clin. Invest.*, **45**, 153.

STERLING, K. & CHODOS, R. B. (1956). *J. clin. Invest.*, **35**, 806.

STERLING, K., LASHOFF, J. C. & MAN, E. B. (1954). *J. clin. Invest.*, **33**, 1031.

STEWART, H. J., DEITRICK, J. E. & CRANE, N. F. (1938). *J. clin. Invest.*, **17**, 237.

STEWART, H. J. & EVANS, W. F. (1941). *Trans. Ass. Amer. Phys.*, **56**, 233.

STEWART, H. J. & EVANS, W. F. (1942). *Amer. Heart J.*, **23**, 175.

STEWART, R. D. H. & MURRAY, I. P. C. (1967). *J. clin. Endocrin.*, **27**, 500.

STRAND, O. (1963). *J. Lip. Res.*, **4**, 305.

STUDER, H. & GREER, M. A. (1967). *Endocrinology*, **80**, 52.

SUNDERMAN, F. W. (1963). In "Evaluation of Thyroid and Parathyroid Function". pp. 53, 73, Philadelphia. J. B. Lippincott Co.

SUNSHINE, P., KUSUMOTO, H. & KRISS, J. P. (1965). *Pediatrics*, **36**, 869.

SURKS, M. I. & OPPENHEIMER, J. H. (1964). *J. clin. Endocrin.*, **24**, 794.

SUZUKI, H., HIGUCHI, T., SAWA, K., OHTAKI, S. & HORIUCHI, Y. (1965). *Acta Endocrin.*, **50**, 161.

SWANN, N. H. (1964). *Metabolism*, **13**, 908.

TATA, J. R. (1964a). In "The Thyroid". Eds. Pitt-Rivers, R. & Trotter, W. R., vol. 1, p. 163, Washington, Butterworths.

TATA, J. R. (1964b). In "Actions of Hormones on Molecular Processes". Eds. Litwack, G. & Kritchevsky, D., p. 58, New York, Wiley & Sons.

TATA, J. R. (1966). *Prog. Nucleic Acid Res.*, **5**, 191; (1966). *Biochem. J.*, **98**, 604.

TATA, J. R. & POCHIN, E. E. (1964). In "The Thyroid Gland". Eds. Pitt-Rivers, R. & Trotter, W. R., vol. 2, Washington, Butterworths.

TAUROG, A., BRIGGS, F. N. & CHAIKOFF, I. L. (1952). *J. biol. Chem.*, **194**, 29, 655.

TAUROG, A., CHAIKOFF, I. L. & FRANKLIN, A. L. (1945). *J. biol. Chem.*, **161**, 537.

TAUROG, A. & HOWELLS, E. M. (1966). *J. biol. Chem.*, **241**, 1329.

TAUROG, A., POTTER, G. D. & CHAIKOFF, I. L. (1955). *J. biol. Chem.*, **213**, 119.

TAUROG, A., TONG, W. & CHAIKOFF, I. L. (1950). *J. biol. Chem.*, **184**, 83.

TAUROG, A., TONG, W. & CHAIKOFF, I. L. (1951). *J. biol. Chem.*, **191**, 677.

TELLERN, M., STOHL, T. & MERANZE, D. R. (1961). *Cancer*, **14**, 67.

THIER, S. O., BLACK, P., WILLIAMS, H. E. & ROBBINS, J. (1965). *J. clin. Endocrin.*, **25**, 65.

THODE, H. G., JAIMET, C. H. & KIRKWOOD, S. (1954). *New Engl. J. Med.*, **251**, 129.

THORSØE, H. (1962). *Acta Endocrin.*, **40**, 161.

THOULD, A. K. & SCOWEN, E. F. (1964). *J. Endocrin.*, **30**, 69.

TIERNEY, N. A. & PETERS, J. P. (1943). *J. clin. Invest.*, **22**, 595.

TOI, K., SALVATORE, G. & CAHNMANN, H. J. (1965). *Biochim. biophys. Acta*, **97**, 523.

TOMMASELLI, A., GRAVINA, E. & ROCHE, J. (1965). In "Current Topics in Thyroid Research". Eds. Cassano, C. & Andreoli, M., p. 382, N.Y. Academic Press.

TOMKINS, G. & McGUIRE, J. M. (1960). *Ann. N.Y. Acad. Sci.*, **86**, 600.

TONG, W. (1964). *Endocrinology*, **75**, 527.

TONG, W., KERKHOF, P. & CHAIKOFF, I. L. (1962). *Biochim. biophys. Acta*, **60**, 1.

TONG, W., TAUROG, A. & CHAIKOFF, I. L. (1951). *J. biol. Chem.*, **191**, 665.

TONG, W., TAUROG, A. & CHAIKOFF, I. L. (1954). *J. biol. Chem.*, **207**, 59.

TRIANTAPHYLLIDIS, E. (1958). *Arch. Sci. Physiol.*, **12**, 191, 245.

TROTTER, W. R. (1960). *Brit. med. Bull.*, **16**, 92.

TROTTER, W. R. (1962). *J. New Drugs*, **2**, 333.

TUBIANA, M., MOZZICONACCI, P., ATTAL, C., L'HIRONDEL, J. & GIRARD, F. (1965). *Ann. d'Endocrin.*, **26**, 109.

TUDHOPE, G. R. & WILSON, G. M. (1960). *Quart. J. Med.*, **29**, 513.

TUDHOPE, G. R. & WILSON, G. M. (1962). *Lancet*, **1**, 703.

TURNER, H. H. & HOWARD, R. B. (1956). *J. clin. Endocrin.*, **16**, 141.

UCKO, H. (1947). *J. clin. Endocrin.*, **7**, 820.

UTIGER, R. D. (1965). In "Current Topics in Thyroid Research", Eds. Cassano, C. & Andreoli, M. New York, Academic Press.

VALENTA, L. (1966). *J. clin. Endocrin.*, **26**, 1317.

VALLOTTON, M. B., PRETELL, J. Y. & FORBES, A. P. (1967). *J. clin. Endocrin.*, **27**, 1.

VANDERLAAN, W. P. & CAPLAN, R. (1954). *Endocrinology*, **54**, 427.

VANDERLAAN, W. P. & GREER, M. A. (1950). *Endocrinology*, **47**, 36.

VANDERLAAN, W. P. & STORRIE, V. M. (1955). *Pharm. Rev.*, **7**, 301.

VAN WYK, J. J. & GRUMBACH, M. M. (1960). *J. Pediat.*, **57**, 119, 416.

VAN ZYL, A. & EDELHOCH, H. (1967). *J. biol. Chem.*, **242**, 2423.

VAUGHAN, M. (1967). *J. clin. Invest.*, **46**, 1482.

VECCHIO, G., EDELHOCH, H., ROBBINS, J. & WEATHERS, B. (1966). *Biochemistry*, **5**, 2617.

VILKKI, P. (1962). *Arch. Biochem.*, **97**, 425.

VILKKI, P. & JAAKONMÄKI, I. (1966). *Endocrinology*, **78**, 453.

VINIK, A. I., PIMSTONE, B. L. & HOFFENBERG, R. (1968). *J. clin. Endocrin.*, **28**, 725.

VIRTANEN, A. I. (1961). *Experientia*, **17**, 241.

VOGLIAZZO, U., VIOLE, G., SCORTA, A. & MARCHIS, E. (1952). *Rassegna clin. Sci.*, **28**, 3.

VOLPE, R., JOHNSTON, M. W. & HUBER, N. (1958). *J. clin. Endocrin.*, **18**, 65; (1957). *Can. med. Ass. J.*, **77**, 297.

VOLPE, R., ROW, V. U. & EZRIN, C. (1966). Program American Thyroid Association Meeting, p. 48.

WALDSTEIN, S. S. (1966). *Ann. Rev. Med.*, **17**, 123.

WALSER, M. & RAHILL, W. J. (1965). *J. clin. Invest.*, **44**, 1371.

WALTON, K. W., CAMPBELL, D. A. & TONKS, E. L. (1965). *Clin. Sci.*, **29**, 199, 217.

WANG, E. (1946). *Acta med. scand. Suppl.*, **169**.

WARREN, S. & MEISSNER, W. A. (1953). "Atlas of Tumour Pathology". Section IV, Fascicle 14, Washington, D.C. AFIP.

WAYNE, E. J. (1960). *Brit. med. J.*, **1**, 78.

WAYNE, E. J., KOUTRAS, D. A. & ALEXANDER, W. D. (1964). "Clinical Aspects of Iodine Metabolism". Oxford. Blackwell Scientific Publications.

WERNER, S. C. (1954a). In "Glandular Physiol. & Therapy". 5th Ed., Chicago, Lippincott.

WERNER, S. C. (1954b). *J. clin. Endocrin.*, **14**, 1260.

WERNER, S. C. & HAMILTON, H. E. (1951). *J. Amer. med. Ass.*, **146**, 450.

WERNER, S. C. & SPOONER, M. A. (1955). *Bull. N.Y. Acad. Med.*, **31**, 137.

WESTERFELD, W. W. & LOWE, C. (1942). *J. biol. Chem.*, **145**, 463.

WETZEL, B. K., SPICER, S. S. & WOLLMAN, S. H. (1965). *J. Cell. Biol.*, **25**, 593.

WHITEHEAD, J. K. & BEALE, D. (1959). *Clin. Chim. Acta*, **4**, 710; (1960). **5**, 150.

WIBERG, G. S., DEVLIN, W. F., STEPHENSON, N. R., CARTER, J. R. & BAYNE, A. J. (1962). *J. Pharm. Pharmol.*, **14**, 777.

WILKINS, L. (1941). *Amer. J. Dis. Child.*, **61**, 13.

WILKINS, L. (1965). "Endocrine Disorders in Childhood and Adolescence". 3rd Ed., Springfield, C. C. Thomas.

WILKINS, L. & FLEISCHMANN, W. (1946). *J. clin. Invest.*, **25**, 360.

WILLIAMS, D. W., DENARDO, G. L. & ZELENIK, J. S. (1966). *Obst. Gynec.*, **27**, 232.

WILLIAMS, E. D. (1965). *J. clin. Path.*, **18**, 288.

WILLIAMS, E. D. (1967). Symposium on Thyroid Neoplasia, Imperial Cancer Res. Fund.

WILLIAMS, E. D., ENGEL, C. & FORBES, A. P. (1964). *New Engl. J. Med.*, **270**, 805.

WILSON, G. M., KILPATRICK, R., ECKERT, H., CURRAN, R. C., JEPSON, R. P., BLOMFIELD, G. W. & MILLER, H. (1958). *Brit. med. J.*, **2**, 929.

WINSHIP, T. & ROSVOLL, R. V. (1961). *Cancer*, **14**, 734.

WISSIG, S. L. (1964). In "The Thyroid". Eds. Pitt-Rivers, R. & Trotter, W. R., vol. I, p. 32, Washington, Butterworths.

WOEBER, K. A. & INGBAR, S. H. (1964). *J. clin. Invest.*, **43**, 931.

WOLF, O. & GREEP, R. O. (1937). *Proc. Soc. exp. Biol.*, *N.Y.*, **36**, 856.

WOLFF, E. C. & WOLFF, J. (1964). In "The Thyroid Gland". Eds. Pitt-Rivers, R. & Trotter, W. R., vol. I, p. 237, Washington, Butterworths.

WOLFF, J. (1951). *Endocrinology*, **48**, 284.

WOLFF, J. (1960). *Biochim. biophys. Acta*, **38**, 316.

WOLFF, J. (1964). *Physiol. Rev.*, **44**, 45.

WOLFF, J. (1969). *Am. J. Med.* (in press).

WOLFF, J. & AUSTEN, F. K. (1958). *J. clin. Invest.*, **37**, 1144.

WOLFF, J. & CHAIKOFF, I. L. (1947). *Endocrinology*, **41**, 295.

WOLFF, J. & CHAIKOFF, I. L. (1948*a,b*). *J. biol. Chem.*, **172**, 855; **174**, 555.

WOLFF, J. & CHAIKOFF, I. L. (1948*c,d*). *Endocrinology*, **42**, 468; **43**, 174.

WOLFF, J., CHAIKOFF, I. L., GOLDBERG, R. C. & MEIER, J. R. (1949). *Endocrinology*, **45**, 504.

WOLFF, J., CHAIKOFF, I. L., TAUROG, A. & RUBIN, L. (1946). *Endocrinology*, **39**, 140.

WOLFF, J. & COVELLI, I. (1966). *Biochemistry*, **5**, 867.

WOLFF, J. & HALMI, N. S. (1963). *J. biol. Chem.*, **238**, 847.

WOLFF, J. & MAUREY, J. R. (1962). *Biochim. biophys. Acta*, **57**, 422.

WOLFF, J. & MAUREY, J. R. (1963). *Biochim. biophys. Acta*, **69**, 58.

WOLFF, J., ROBBINS, J. & RALL, J. E. (1959). *Endocrinology*, **64**, 1.

WOLFF, J., RUBIN, L. & CHAIKOFF, I. L. (1950). *J. Pharm. Exp. Therap.*, **98**, 45.

WOLFF, J., STANDAERT, M. E. & RALL, J. E. (1961). *J. clin. Invest.*, **40**, 1373.

WOLFF, J., THOMPSON, R. H. & ROBBINS, J. (1964). *J. clin. Endocrin.*, **24**, 699.

WOLLENBERGER, A. (1964). *Arch. exp. Path. Pharm.*, **249**, 288.

WOLLMAN, S. H. (1963). *Rec. Prog. Horm. Res.*, **19**, 579.

WOLLMAN, S. H. (1965). In "Current Topics in Thyroid Research". Eds. Cassano, C. & Andreoli, M., New York, Academic Press.

WOLLMAN, S. H. & REED, F. E. (1962). *Amer. J. Physiol.*, **202**, 182.

WOLLMAN, S. H. & SCOW, R. O. (1954). *Endocrinology*, **55**, 828, 837.

WOLLMAN, S. H. & SCOW, R. O. (1955). *Endocrinology*, **56**, 448, 445.

WOLLMAN, S. H., SCOW, R. O., WAGNER, B. & MORRIS, H. P. (1953). *J. Nat. Canc. Inst.*, **13**, 785, 807.

WOODBURY, D. M. & WOODBURY, J. W. (1963). *J. Physiol.*, London, **169**, 553.

WYNN, J. (1960). *Arch. Biochem. Biophys.*, **87**, 120.

WYNN, J. & GIBBS, R. (1964). *J. biol. Chem.*, **239**, 527.

YAGI, Y., MICHEL, R. & ROCHE, J. (1953). *Bull. Soc. Chim. Biol.*, **35**, 289.

YAMADA, T., IINO, S. & SHICHIJO, K. (1963). *Endocrinology*, **72**, 83.

YAMAMOTO, K., ISHIKAWA, I. & SHIMIZU, S. (1960). *Jap. J. Physiol.*, **10**, 221.

YOUNG, W. C. & CORNER, G. W. (1961). In "Sex and Internal Secretions", vol. 1, p. 478, Baltimore, Williams & Wilkins Co.

Chapter 13

DISEASES OF THE NERVOUS SYSTEM

by

R. H. S. Thompson and J. N. Cumings

Courtauld Institute of Biochemistry, Middlesex Hospital Medical School, and
Institute of Neurology, London

IT is many years since the conception was first introduced that certain of the diseases of the nervous system might be explained in terms of some underlying chemical disorder. Thudichum's monograph on the chemical constitution of the brain, which appeared in 1884, described practical investigations carried out nearly a century ago with this end in view, and his studies of the structure of brain lipids have provided a notable and lasting background for subsequent work. The more modern conception of disordered cell metabolism underlying and leading up to visible tissue damage, a conception aptly summarized in the term "biochemical lesion", had, however, to wait upon the growth of more detailed knowledge of metabolic biochemistry, and is still in its early stages as regards its application to neurological disease.

It might indeed be expected that a tissue showing such specialized features, both anatomical and functional, as exist within the nervous system would also exhibit some specialized aspects of metabolism, derangements of which might readily occur, and such indeed is the case.

But this complexity of structure is one of the major difficulties in the way of advance, and our knowledge of the biochemistry of localized areas of the central nervous system, or of the different types of neurone or glial cell, is still limited. Information in this field is, however, now beginning to accumulate, as can be seen, for example, from the studies on the relative rates of oxidative metabolism of neurones and neuroglia described by Pope (1958) and Hess (1961). Numerous other examples of regional differences in various aspects of brain metabolism have been presented in the Proceedings of the Fourth International Neurochemical Symposium (Kety & Elkes, 1961).

Certain aspects of the normal chemical structure and of metabolism which are peculiar either quantitatively or qualitatively to the nervous system, were reviewed in the last edition of this book (Thompson & Cumings, 1964).

ALTERATIONS IN THE LEVEL OF NERVOUS ACTIVITY

Before embarking on a consideration of "organic" nervous disorders it is proposed to describe briefly the changes in brain metabolism that have been shown to accompany alterations in the level of nervous activity. Such changes may be exhibited in physiological variations in the state of cerebral activity, as, for example, between sleep and excitement. From the point of view of the pathologist, the wider problems of narcosis and anaesthesia, on the one hand, and convulsive states including both epilepsy and artificially induced convulsions, on the other hand, are of more immediate interest, and, as may be expected, changes in metabolism that are only slight in sleep or excitement may reveal themselves more obviously in these more extreme, unphysiological alterations of function.

Narcosis and Anaesthesia

One of the earlier observations pointing the way to a relationship between drug action and enzyme inhibition was provided by Quastel & Wheatley (1932), who showed that various barbiturates are capable of inhibiting the O_2 consumption of brain preparations *in vitro*. This inhibitory action is selective and is centred round the main stream of energy-yielding reactions in brain; thus, while the oxidations of glucose, lactate and pyruvate are powerfully depressed, glutamate oxidation is affected to a lesser extent, and succinate is oxidized normally. It was also shown that concentrations of the barbiturate, estimated to be of the same order as those required to produce narcosis in the living body, were able to bring about a small but definite inhibition (15 to 32%) of the respiration of brain slices *in vitro* (Jowett & Quastel, 1937; Jowett, 1938).

The question arises then as to whether the narcotic effect of these drugs (barbiturates, chloretone) is the direct outcome of a slowing-down of the oxidative metabolism of the neurones in the brain, or whether this fall in respiration is merely the result of a lowering of the level of cerebral activity brought about by the drug by means of some other action affecting excitation, conduction or synaptic transmission.

The *in vitro* findings of Quastel and his colleagues have been confirmed *in vivo*; in the monkey, Schmidt, Kety & Pennes (1945) have shown that the O_2 consumption of the brain varies with the state of cerebral activity, and is more profoundly depressed in deep than in light anaesthesia; and in man, Himwich and his group have demonstrated that during anaesthesia induced by intravenous thiopental the cerebral metabolic rate, calculated from measurements of A-V oxygen differences and cerebral blood flow, fell from a mean normal level of 2·5 ml. O_2/100 g. tissue/min. to a level of 1·6, i.e. a reduction of approximately 35% (see Himwich, 1951).

The extension of these observations to the intact brain does not, however, fully answer the above question. But if the primary action of narcotics is to inhibit brain oxidations it might be expected, as Richter (1952) has pointed out, that the energy-rich phosphates would be depleted in narcotized brain; experiment has shown, however, that the levels of phosphocreatine, ATP and acetylcholine are well maintained, while the lactic acid, inorganic phosphate and NH_3 levels are low. These findings would seem to be more consistent with a state of economy, of non-utilization of energy, rather than with a block in the energy-yielding mechanism of the cells. Also, it has been reported that in the narcotized superior cervical ganglion, transmission is depressed before any fall in O_2 consumption occurs (Larrabee, Ramos

& Bulbring, 1950). In the face of this evidence against the view that narcotic action is due to a suppression of oxidations, it must be remembered that cell respiration involves a complex chain of reactions, and it is still possible that an action at some point in this chain may affect function before any measurable effect on overall respiration can be detected.

There is also experimental evidence indicating that alcohol, ether and cyclopropane depress cerebral metabolism *in vivo*. It has been estimated that ether anaesthesia can cause a 10 to 40% decrease in the O_2 utilization of the brain.

In view of the dependence of the brain on carbohydrate oxidation, lack of glucose, as in an insulin-induced hypoglycaemia, will clearly depress cerebral metabolism and consequently affect function; these effects are reversible provided that the hypoglycaemia is short-lived and not excessive, but permanent damage and death have been recorded following prolonged hypoglycaemia.

Epilepsy and Other Convulsive States

In convulsive states the metabolic changes in the brain are in general the opposite of those seen in narcosis, and indicate a very rapid utilization of energy-rich phosphates, glucose and O_2, necessary for the maintenance of the high level of nervous activity underlying the convulsions. The O_2 consumption of the brain is increased, and there is a rise in the levels in the brain of lactic acid, inorganic phosphate, ADP and NH_3; at the same time the levels of glycogen, glucose, phosphocreatine, ATP and acetylcholine fall (Gurdjian, Stone & Webster, 1944; Stone, Webster & Gurdjian, 1945; Klein & Olsen, 1947; Olsen & Klein, 1947; Richter & Dawson, 1948 *a,b*; Richter & Crossland, 1949; Dawson & Richter, 1950).

Useful new techniques for the study of the effects of electrical stimulation *in vitro* on the metabolism of separated portions of the central nervous system have been worked out by McIlwain and his colleagues. They have provided further information on the effects of activity on the levels of a number of phosphate and nucleotide components, and have studied the action of various drugs (atropine, cocaine, ergotoxine, mescaline, dibenamine) on the metabolic response to electrical stimulation; concentrations of these drugs which have no effect on the metabolism of the unstimulated tissue were found to inhibit the extra respiration produced by stimulation (see McIlwain, 1952; Lewis & McIlwain, 1954).

Much less information is available concerning metabolism in epilepsy than in the case of artificially induced convulsions. In idiopathic epilepsy it has been reported that the cerebral metabolic rate is high during the seizure, which is to be expected in view of the greatly increased nervous activity, although it is normal between the attacks. Elliot & Penfield (1948) have examined the respiratory and glycolytic activity of focal epileptogenic tissue from patients, but have been unable to find any defect in these mechanisms.

Since the epileptic convulsion appears to consist essentially of an uncontrolled discharge of cortical neurones it is natural that the part played by acetylcholine should have been explored in this connection. Miller (1937), Miller, Stavraky & Woonton (1940), Williams & Ritchie Russell (1941), Brenner & Merritt (1942) and Forster (1945) have all brought forward evidence suggesting that the convulsions may be associated with an abnormality of acetylcholine metabolism. Further, it has been shown that the injection of DFP (di*iso*propyl fluorophosphonate) results in electroencephalographic changes resembling those seen in epilepsy (Grob, Harvey, Langworthy & Lilienthal, 1947; Freedman, Bales, Willis & Himwich, 1949).

Acetylcholine metabolism in epilepsy has been studied intensively by a group of workers at the Montreal Neurological Institute. Their approach to the problem has been based on the hypothesis that there must exist "a biochemical lesion which represents, so to speak, a common denominator through which the many and diverse causative, predisposing and precipitating factors concerned in epilepsy can be finally resolved into the seizure discharge" (Tower, 1952); they have also stressed the view that this lesion must represent some *chronic* biochemical defect in epileptogenic brain tissue, which, by virtue of its chronicity, might account for the liability to seizures. Their study *in vitro* of epileptogenic cortical tissue, removed at operation from patients with focal cortical seizures, has brought to light two such biochemical abnormalities: first, a small increase in the level of cholinesterase activity in epileptogenic tissue (Pope, Morris, Jasper, Elliott & Penfield, 1947; Tower & Elliott, 1952), and, secondly, a failure to form bound acetylcholine when slices of epileptogenic cortex are incubated in bicarbonate-Ringer solution containing glucose and eserine (see Table 13.1). Tower & Elliott (1952) have suggested that the increased cholinesterase activity may be an adaptive response to an increased tendency to release acetylcholine, resulting from this partial failure to bind it. There is as yet no evidence that these abnormalities are responsible for the attacks, but, from what is now known about the central effects of acetylcholine, these findings in excised epileptogenic tissue, taken together, represent a chronic lesion which is certainly compatible with a state of excitatory instability in the focal area.

Tower & McEachern (1949) have also shown that the cerebrospinal fluid from epileptic patients contains detectable amounts of acetylcholine, whereas none is usually to be found in the cerebrospinal fluid from non-epileptic persons.

sulphoximine, and of normal cortex maintained under conditions of partial anoxia, to form normal amounts of bound acetylcholine. It is too early to assess the relevance of these observations to the aetiology and control of human epilepsy, but it is noteworthy that this defect in the binding of acetylcholine by epileptogenic tissue would appear to be yet another example of a reversible lesion.

Methionine sulphoximine has been shown to inhibit the enzyme glutamine synthetase both *in*

TABLE 13.1

Cholinesterase levels and ability to bind acetylcholine in normal and epileptogenic cerebral cortex.
(Nos. in parentheses = No. of determinations)

Type of sample[1]	Cholinesterase (μl.CO_2/g./hr.)	Change in bound acetylcholine (μg.ACh./g./hr.)
Normal area	950 (5)	1.15 (4)
Non-focal abnormal area	1050 (10)	0·65 (8)
Epileptogenic focus	1250 (10)	0·3 (13)

[1] Normal area = sample not far distant from site of epileptogenic activity.
Non-focal abnormal area = samples showing scarring or atrophy on gross inspection, abnormal electrocorticographically, but having no signs of being the focus of epileptic activity.

(Taken from Tower & Elliott (1952))

A failure to form bound acetylcholine has also been demonstrated in slices of cerebral cortex taken from animals poisoned with methionine sulphoximine (Tower & Elliott, 1953); this toxic agent was isolated from "agenized" flour and produces fits in animals very closely resembling human epilepsy (Mellanby, 1946, 1947; Bentley, McDermott, Pace, Whitehead & Moran, 1950). Exposure of slices of normal cerebral cortex to partial anoxia *in vitro* also results in a failure to form bound acetylcholine. Tower & Elliott (1953) have made some interesting observations on the control and reversal of this defect in acetylcholine-binding; they have demonstrated that the addition of glutamine or asparagine (but not glutamic acid) to the incubating medium restores the power of human focal epileptogenic tissue, of cerebral cortex from animals treated with methionine

vitro and *in vivo* (Gershenovich, Krichevskaya & Kolousek, 1963; Sellinger & Weiler, 1963; Lamar & Sellinger, 1965). If therefore glutamate is concerned with excitatory processes inside the central nervous system, it is possible that methionine sulphoximine may in part act by inhibiting processes concerned with the extracellular destruction of this substance.

The discovery of relatively large amounts of γ-aminobutyric acid (GABA) in brain tissue, and the subsequent study of the actions of this compound on the central nervous system and of the various factors that influence its level in the brain (see Elliott, 1959; Roberts & Baxter, 1959), provide a new approach to the study of certain types of central convulsant disorders. GABA can be formed from glutamic acid by a decarboxylase enzyme which is present in brain:

$$COOH . CH(NH_2) . CH_2CH_2COOH \rightarrow H_2N . CH_2CH_2CH_2COOH + CO_2$$
$$\text{Glutamic acid} \qquad\qquad \gamma\text{-Aminobutyric acid}$$

This decarboxylase requires pyridoxal phosphate, a derivative of vitamin B_6 (pyridoxine), as a co-enzyme.

The effect that GABA is capable of exerting on the state of neuronal activity in the central nervous system has been shown in a number of ways. In the first place, it has been demonstrated that when applied locally to the exposed cerebral cortex GABA produces changes in the electrical activity of that tissue (Purpura, Girado & Grundfest, 1957; Iwama & Jasper, 1957). Secondly, evidence has been produced suggesting that diminished levels of GABA in the brain, or an inhibition of the decarboxylase responsible for its formation, may be associated with the development of epileptiform convulsant states. Thus, epileptiform seizures are known to be a part of the syndrome of vitamin B_6 deficiency both in experimental animals and in human infants (Maloney & Parmelee, 1954; Hunt, Stokes, McCorry & Stroud, 1954), and the occurrence of these seizures in animals has been correlated with lowered levels of GABA in the brain.

It has indeed been suggested that GABA may act by exerting a tonic inhibitory or moderating effect on neuronal activity in the CNS, but the precise nature or significance of its action is at present undecided. The part, if any, that alterations in the level of GABA may play in the production of convulsant states is, therefore, also at present undecided.

MIGRAINE

Considerable attention is now being focused on the pathogenesis of migraine, and in particular on the possible role that abnormalities of tyramine or catecholamine metabolism may play in the production of certain types of migrainous attacks.

The development of headaches and hypertensive crises in certain individuals under therapy with monoamine oxidase inhibitors following the eating of cheese has been described by Blackwell in 1963. Blackwell & Marley (1964) later concluded that the inhibition of monoamine oxidase in the intestine and liver must allow the absorption of some constituent of cheese which is capable of influencing peripheral adrenergic receptors, but which in the normal subject is inactivated by the action of this enzyme. Certain cheeses are known to contain tyramine and phenylethylamine, and pharmacological and chemical evidence suggests that tyramine may be the constituent responsible for these attacks.

The mechanism underlying the development of the migraine headache has been studied by Wolff and his collaborators (Graham & Wolff, 1937;

Wolff & Sutherland, 1938; Schumacher & Wolff, 1941). It is believed that a period of vasoconstriction of cerebral blood vessels occurs during the stage of the premonitory symptoms, and that vasodilatation subsequently occurs accompanying the pain (Greene, 1959). The blood vessels concerned are thought to be mainly the branches of the external carotid artery.

It has been estimated that in about 5% of migraine patients the onset of the attack appears to be associated with certain dietary factors, the consumption of chocolate, cheese or citrus fruits being most frequently incriminated. Hanington (1967) therefore studied the effect of administering tyramine orally to a group of migraine patients who had observed this association with dietary factors, and was able to show that tyramine hydrochloride, in oral doses of 100 mg., regularly precipitated typical attacks of migraine headache in these sufferers. She has suggested therefore that patients with migraine associated with dietary factors may exhibit an inborn defect in the metabolism of tyramine and related compounds, including possibly the catecholamines, (see also Hanington & Harper, 1968).

The sequence of events underlying the development of the migraine headache in the majority of sufferers from this disease who are unable to relate the onset of the attacks to the consumption of certain dietary constituents is at present unknown.

Reserpine is known to produce attacks of migraine in susceptible subjects; recently it has been shown that plasma serotonin levels fall following reserpine, and that the headache is relieved by intravenous injection of serotonin (Anthony, Hinterberger & Lance, 1967).

NERVE DEGENERATION

It has been known for over a hundred years that when a nerve is cut characteristic degenerative changes (Wallerian degeneration) take place peripheral to the point of section. Very similar changes are also found in spinal tracts and peripheral nerves in a number of conditions associated with metabolic lesions of nerve cells, for example in thiamine deficiency in man and in pigeons (Pekelharing & Winkler, 1887; Swank & Prados, 1942) and in subacute combined degeneration of the cord (Greenfield & Carmichael, 1935).

Histological examination of degenerating nerve has shown that there is destruction of myelin, and specific staining methods have been employed in an attempt to demonstrate the nature of the end-products of such degeneration. Chemical studies on degenerating nerves were also early carried out. Noll (1899) described a decrease in "protagon", which is now assumed to have been a fraction composed largely of cerebroside. Mott & Halli-burton (1901 *a,b*) reported an increase in wet weight and also a loss of phosphorus from degene-rating nerve. May (1930) also found a loss of total phosphorus. More recently, modern micro-chemi-cal methods have been applied to this problem, and the group led by Rossiter in Canada has been foremost in this field.

The myelin sheath consists principally of the "myelin lipids", which are composed mainly of cerebroside, free cholesterol and sphingomyelin, together with protein, and the changes found in these after nerve section will be described in some detail. Changes in other components of the de-generating nerve, for example in nucleoprotein content or in the activity of certain enzymes, also take place due to the multiplication of Schwann cells and macrophages (Young, 1942) or to the disintegration of the axon, both of which processes are taking place at the same time as the break-up of the myelin.

Water

There is an increase of about 30% in the wet weight of the peripheral part of the cut nerve four days after section. No further increase in water content occurs after that time, but there is a slow reduction in weight, until after about 60 days it is no longer heavier than a control, uncut nerve (Johnson, McNabb & Rossiter, 1949).

Lipids

The total lipids of degenerating nerve decrease steadily over at least 96 days (Johnson *et al.* 1949; Brante, 1949; Bodian & Dziewiatkowski, 1950). The neutral fat fraction decreases rapidly up to 4 to 8 days, but returns to normal by about 32 days; this loss of neutral fat may in part be due to loss from the cut axon or from the perineurium, rather than a result of damage to the myelin itself.

Sphingomyelin and cerebroside decrease more slowly during the first eight days, but thereafter there is a much more rapid drop, so that by 96 days only about 7% of the normal sphingomyelin content remains, while at this time cerebrosides can no longer be detected (Johnson *et al.* 1949; Brante, 1949). Total cholesterol also changes little during the first eight days, but by 96 days only about 24% remains; between 8 and 32 days there is, however, a rapid fall in the amount of free cholesterol and an increase in esterified cholesterol, so that by the end of 16 days choles-terol esters, which are normally virtually absent

from nerve, may be found in appreciable amounts (Johnson *et al.* 1949). There is also a release of choline, assumed to be derived from sphingomye-lin, in the early stages of degeneration (Brante, 1949). A rapid hydrolysis of cephalin and some hydrolysis of lecithin also occur; both of these constituents are probably in large part derived from the degenerating axons.

Proteins and Nucleoproteins

At the same time that this loss of lipids is taking place there is a loss of non-extractable N from the nerve (Abercrombie & Johnson, 1946), which may indicate a breakdown of the so-called "neuro-keratin" (Block, 1937), probably a component of the sheath.

Other changes are found in the levels of nucleic acids in degenerating nerve. There is an increase over the first 16 days in these acids, but thereafter they fall towards normal (Logan, Mannell & Rossiter, 1952; Samuels, Boyarsky, Gerard, Libet & Brust, 1951). This increase seems to parallel the rapid rise in the number of Schwann cells and infiltrating leucocytes. The ribonucleic acid increases more rapidly, and to a greater extent, than the deoxyribonucleic acid. The increase in nucleic acid concentration is already detectable on the second day after nerve section, and is well established before any significant decrease in lipid P can be detected. This would seem to indicate that cell proliferation commences before the chemical break-up of the myelin lipids.

The phosphoprotein content of nerve also falls throughout the course of the degeneration in cut nerve; in nerve-crush injuries, where re-innerva-tion of the distal degenerating segment eventually takes place, the phosphoproteins gradually rise again after 96 days, reaching the normal level by about 250 days (Logan *et al.* 1952).

According to studies with polarized light and by X-ray diffraction (Schmitt & Bear, 1939; Schmitt, Bear & Palmer, 1941) there is evidence that the myelin sheath is made up of co-axial concentric sheets of orientated lipid molecules alternating with thin layers of protein, so that changes in the above-mentioned protein components are to be expected to accompany the lipid changes.

Enzymes

Detailed studies have been made of the changes in the activity of a number of enzymes in nerve during Wallerian degeneration. Early studies on *cholinesterase* in degenerating nerve were made by Couteaux & Nachmansohn (1938) and Hellauer & Umrath (1939). Sawyer in 1946 examined the levels of both acetyl-and butyrylcholinesterases, and reported that while the level of acetyl-cholinesterase fell following nerve section, butyrylcholinesterase was unaffected. More recently, Cavanagh, Thompson & Webster (1954) have re-investigated these enzymes in degenerating chicken sciatic nerve; they found that acetylcholinesterase activity falls to zero by about 8 to 10 days after nerve section. Butyryl-cholinesterase activity, on the other hand, showed a striking increase, reaching a value of more than double the pre-operative level by about seven days after section, and thereafter slowly declining to the normal level. These results are consistent with the view that while acetylcholinesterase is wholly neuronal in its location in peripheral nerve, butyrylcholinesterase is associated with the sheath, probably with the Schwann cells whose multiplication after nerve section would seem to be concerned with the observed increase in enzyme activity.

The *choline acetylase* system has also been shown to undergo a rapid fall in activity following nerve section (Feldberg, 1943; Nachmansohn, John & Berman, 1946; Banister & Scrase, 1950), and von Muralt & von Schulthess (1944) have described a fall in the acetylcholine content of degenerating nerve.

As in the case of butyrylcholinesterase, *acid phosphatase* also increases during Wallerian degeneration (Bodian, 1947; Heinzen, 1947; Hollinger, Rossiter & Upmalis, 1952). The last-named workers have shown that this increase and subsequent fall follow very closely the changes in deoxyribonucleic acid in degenerating nerve, suggesting that this enzyme too is probably a Schwann sheath component.

Alkaline phosphatase activity in degenerating nerve has been studied by Hollinger et al. (1952) using standard biochemical techniques; they found a rapid decrease in activity, so that by 32 days only about 20 to 25% of the normal amount was present. If the nerve had been cut, activity remained at this low level for the 96 days over which the experiment was conducted, but after nerve crush this initial fall was followed by a gradual return to values considerably greater than in the controls. These workers concluded that alkaline phosphatase, like acetylcholinesterase, is probably associated with the axon rather than with the sheath, and that the delayed increase in activity after nerve crush is concerned with nerve regeneration. Rossiter has commented on the fact that chemical and histochemical methods of study of phosphatases in degenerating nerve have yielded conflicting results. As has been indicated, chemical studies have shown that acid phosphatase in-

creases and alkaline phosphatase decreases during Wallerian degeneration; using histochemical methods, however, Lassek & Bueker (1947) and Smith (1948) have reported a decrease in acid phosphatase, while Marchant (1949) has described an increase in alkaline phosphatase which she concluded was mostly in the cytoplasm of the Schwann cells.

5′-Nucleotidase activity also increases after either nerve section or nerve crush; *adenosine-triphosphatase* was found to increase only after nerve crush (Hollinger et al. 1952).

In addition to the cholinesterases, nervous tissue exhibits *ali-esterase* activity and rapidly splits simple aliphatic esters such as methyl butyrate or tributyrin. Lumsden (1952) has described a fall in the ability to hydrolyse methyl butyrate in degenerating nerve, followed by a striking increase apparently associated with re-innervation. Cavanagh & Webster (1955), on the other hand, using tributyrin as substrate, found an early increase (4 to 9 days) followed by a second increase showing a maximum at about 25 to 30 days after section, which they have interpreted as being probably due to Schwann cell and macrophage activity respectively.

β-Glucuronidase, which is believed to be concerned with cell proliferation (Levvy, Kerr & Campbell, 1948; Kerr, Campbell & Levvy, 1949, 1950), is present in peripheral nerve, and has been shown by Hollinger & Rossiter (1952) to undergo a striking increase after either nerve section or nerve crush.

More recently, use has been made of isotopic phosphorus (^{32}P), and it has been suggested that the enzymes which catalyse the exchange between inorganic phosphorus and the phosphorus of the phospholipids are present in the Schwann cells and macrophages (Magee & Rossiter, 1954).

Using normal nerve and portions of nerve obtained at varying times after transection, Magee, Berry, Magee & Rossiter (1959) found an incorporation of ^{32}P into phospholipids during the period 8 to 32 days following section. This increase was related to the phosphatidylcholine and phosphatidylethanolamine fractions of the phospholipids. Pritchard & Rossiter (1959) obtained very similar results with ^{14}C, increased labelling being observed in both myelin and non-myelin lipids, suggesting that the increased incorporation of radioactive substances into the various compounds is related not only to changes in the myelin lipids, but also to the increased proliferation of Schwann cells.

On the basis of this evidence obtained from experimental studies in animals it is now possible to form a picture, albeit rough and incomplete of, some of the chemical and biochemical changes that occur during nerve degeneration and break-up of the myelin sheath. Thus, while the acetyl-cholinesterase, choline acetylase and alkaline phosphatase activity each decrease following nerve section, butyrylcholinesterase, acid phosphatase, 5-nucleotidase, tributyrinase and β-glucuronidase all show an increase. The observed losses of lipid and of protein from the sheath, together with the decline in the activity of some enzymes and the increase of others, are providing some of the essential preliminary information not only for an understanding of the processes underlying one of the important reactions of the nervous system to disease, but also in connection with the wider problems of the functions of the Schwann cells and the biochemistry of the axis cylinders, whose distal ends are so often situated so remotely from the nucleus of their cell.

VITAMIN DEFICIENCY DISORDERS

The high rate of metabolism of the brain and its dependence on glucose as a source of fuel, together with the part played by various components of the vitamin B complex in the reactions involved in glucose utilization, render the nervous system particularly sensitive to deficiency of a number of the water-soluble vitamins.

Thiamine Deficiency

The manifestations of severe and acute thiamine deficiency as they occur among rice-eating peoples in many countries of the East are present as part of the symptom-complex of beri-beri. Three forms of the disease are known: (1) wet beri-beri, characterized by generalized oedema with a liability to heart failure and sudden death, (2) dry beri-beri, which is a chronic nutritional polyneuropathy associated with degenerative changes in the peripheral nerves leading to muscle wasting, and (3) infantile beri-beri, a chronic marasmus often associated with a sudden heart failure.

Wernicke's encephalopathy, a condition that may be seen in chronic alcoholics or in patients suffering from chronic cachexia secondary to carcinoma of the stomach or other debilitating disease, can respond promptly to thiamine therapy, and can possibly be regarded as yet another type of manifestation of thiamine deficiency, a cerebral beri-beri. It is characterized by nystagmus, often associated with various ocular palsies, mental changes, disorientation and hallucinations, leading, if untreated, to complete loss of consciousness and death. A similar condition was described

among British prisoners of war in the Far East by de Wardener & Lennox (1947).

The less severe degrees of thiamine deficiency are characterized more by the development of a chronic polyneuritis, and because of the problems of differential diagnosis from other forms of peripheral neuritis, and the relationship of thiamine deficiency to alcoholic polyneuritis, this question will be considered later under the heading of Polyneuritis.

Largely owing, however, to the difficulties in gauging the response to therapy of long-standing chronic diseases of the nervous system, there has been, and still is, considerable uncertainty as to the part played by thiamine deficiency in chronic peripheral neuritis. Because of this, a number of studies of experimentally induced thiamine deficiency under controlled conditions in volunteers have been carried out, and it will be helpful at this point to consider the main points that have emerged from these experiments (Elsom, 1935; Elsom, Lukens, Montgomery & Jonas, 1940; O'Shea, Elsom & Higbe, 1942; Jolliffe, Goodhart, Gennis & Cline, 1939; Williams, Mason, Wilder & Smith, 1940; Williams, Mason, Power & Wilder, 1943).

These various studies have together shown that under carefully controlled conditions experimental thiamine deficiency in man leads to well-marked mental symptoms, such as depression, irritability, defective memory and failure of concentration, but can also cause both subjective and objective changes in the peripheral nerves of the lower limbs; tenderness of the calf muscles, impairment of superficial sensation, weakness of the feet and legs, hyperaesthesiae and paraesthesiae and reduced or absent tendon reflexes have all been recorded. While some of the changes, notably the mental symptoms, improved rapidly with thiamine therapy, the symptoms and signs of peripheral nervous disorders did not in every case respond promptly, suggesting that irreversible or only slowly reversible structural changes in the nerves had taken place. A reduction or even an abolition of secretion of gastric hydrochloric acid was observed in some of the volunteers while on the deficient diet.

The blood pyruvate level was found to be raised in these studies; the significance of this finding will be discussed later in connection with the changes found in other types of polyneuritis.

Subacute Combined Degeneration of the Spinal Cord

Although not usually due to any dietary deficiency, subacute combined degeneration of the cord results from a deficiency of vitamin B_{12} consequent on a failure of secretion of Castle's "intrinsic factor" by the gastric mucosa. The biochemistry of vitamin B_{12} and its relationship to the intrinsic and extrinsic factors and to the anti-pernicious anaemia principle have been described elsewhere in this volume.

The relationship existing between subacute combined degeneration of the cord and pernicious anaemia is obscure. Neurological involvement very frequently occurs early in the development of the anaemia, and may even precede it. The severity of the neurological symptoms does not parallel the degree of anaemia, and subacute combined degeneration of the cord does not occur in other macrocytic anaemias such as tropical nutritional macrocytic anaemia or the anaemia accompanying sprue. The neurological lesions are not, therefore, simply the result of the anaemia on the cells of the central nervous system, but are to be regarded as due to an abnormal metabolism of the nerve cells resulting directly from the deficiency of vitamin B_{12}.

In both subacute combined degeneration of the cord and pernicious anaemia, gastric achlorhydria is invariably present.

Unfortunately, when compared with most of the other members of the vitamin-B complex, our knowledge of the biochemical function of vitamin B_{12} is still obscure. It is known to exist in the body in a variety of forms—hydroxocobalamin, cyanocobalamin, methylcobalamin and in the form of a co-enzyme, cobamide co-enzyme. The cobamide co-enzyme is known to participate in a variety of reactions including the methylation of homocysteine to form methionine, and in the methylation of uridine to thymidine.

The work of Dubnoff (1950, 1952), Ling & Chow (1953, 1954), Register (1954) and others suggests that vitamin B_{12} is also intimately concerned with the reduction of disulphide compounds to the —SH form. Thus, the glutathione (GSH) content of rat blood falls during a deficiency of the vitamin and rises again on its reinclusion in the diet. The same changes have been described in pernicious anaemia. It has been claimed that the reduction of co-enzyme A to the —SH form may be interfered with in vitamin B_{12} deficiency, thereby inhibiting the normal metabolic path of both carbohydrates and fats. Consistent with this view, Ling & Chow (1954) have described disturbances of carbohydrate and fat metabolism (hyperglycaemia and impaired glucose tolerance) in vitamin B_{12}-deficient rats.

Earl, El Hawary, Thompson & Webster (1953) have described high blood pyruvate levels in three untreated cases of subacute combined degeneration of the cord, and have shown that treatment, limited to the parenteral administration of vitamin B_{12}, led to a rapid return to normal of these levels. These findings have been confirmed by Hornabrook & Marks (1960) and by Buckle (1967). The latter worker measured pyruvate and α-oxoglutarate levels in 33 patients with vitamin B_{12} deficiency; in contrast to the abnormally high levels of pyruvate he found that the level of α-oxoglutarate was abnormally low. He too found that treatment with vitamin B_{12} led to a return to normal of the pyruvate level, the improvement being noticeable after 2 to 3 days' treatment and maximal improvement being obtained in 5 to 7 days. Scheinberg (1951) has demonstrated that the O_2 consumption of the brain is low in pernicious anaemia and subacute combined degeneration of the cord, the degree of diminution in the latter condition appearing to be related to the severity of the neurological involvement.

The relationship of vitamin B_{12} to cyanide metabolism is discussed on p. 465.

Nutritional Neuropathies of Obscure Origin

In addition to the well-defined neurological manifestations that can accompany thiamine or vitamin B_{12} deficiency, a number of nutritional neuropathies have been described, the underlying mechanism of which remains obscure.

The occurrence of nervous lesions in pellagra, particularly in severe and long-standing cases, is well known. They may be present in acute or chronic forms, and may be primarily cerebral, spinal or peripheral. How far lack of nicotinic acid can be held responsible *per se* for the mental and other neurological changes in pellagra is not certain. There is, however, good evidence that the peripheral nervous lesions in pellagrins are due in large part to an accompanying deficiency of thiamine, and it seems likely that the final syndrome represents the outcome of a multiple deficiency state.

Although animal experiments have shown that nerve lesions can develop in certain species in the course of riboflavin, pyridoxine or pantothenic acid deficiencies, the importance of these vitamins in connection with nutritional neuropathies in man is not yet known.

The "burning feet" syndrome, retrobulbar neuritis, nerve deafness, sensory ataxia and other syndromes seen in the tropics and in the prisoner-of-war camps during the last war have been described by Spillane (1947) and Cruickshank (1952). Suggestions, based on therapeutic response to various vitamins, have from time to time been put forward as to their aetiology, but it must be admitted that at present we have no clear understanding of the nature of the deficiency in these syndromes.

Apart from dietary deficiencies it is now clear that nutritional deficiency states can not infrequently arise as a result of some abnormality of the gastro-intestinal tract. Thus, it is well known that a failure to absorb adequate amounts of essential food factors can occur in chronic diarrhoeas. It is known also that several members of the vitamin-B complex are synthesized by micro-organisms in the gut, and there is good evidence that the vitamins so synthesized are available for absorption. Disturbances of gastric acidity or other factors that may upset the populations and types of intestinal micro-organisms may therefore affect the amounts of certain vitamins available for absorption. The relatively frequent association of achlorhydria with certain forms of peripheral neuritis may be relevant in this connection, and it has been suggested that this may allow bacterial multiplication at abnormally high levels in the intestine and so upset the balance between synthesis and utilization of vitamins by the intestinal micro-organisms. For in addition to the synthesis of vitamins by these micro-organisms (see Najjar & Barrett, 1945), it is also possible that vitamins ingested with the food or synthesized by other species may remain stored in the cells of certain bacterial species and so be rendered unavailable for absorption by the host (Alexander & Landwehr, 1945; Citron & Knox, 1954).

POLYNEURITIS

As its name implies, polyneuritis manifests itself as an impairment of function of many peripheral nerves, and may therefore present a clinical picture showing a relatively widespread disturbance of the nervous system, not infrequently involving the central nervous system as well as the peripheral nerves. Because of this tendency to widespread lesions it is not surprising that the condition can in some cases be traced to factors affecting the body as a whole, such as, for example, certain vitamin deficiency disorders, a variety of intoxications by both inorganic and organic chemical compounds and generalized metabolic disorders such as diabetes mellitus.

The principal causes and types of polyneuritis are listed below:

(1) *Deficiency disorders.* Beri-beri, pellagra, sprue, subacute combined degeneration of the cord, and chronic alcoholism.

(2) *Chemical intoxications.* Compounds of arsenic, antimony, bismuth, mercury, copper and lead; carbon monoxide; a wide range of organic compounds including carbon disulphide, dinitrobenzene, aniline.

(3) *Metabolic disorders.* Diabetes mellitus, porphyria, amyloidosis, and in association with carcinoma of the lung and of the stomach.

(4) *Acute infective polyneuritis* (Guillain-Barré syndrome).

(5) *Bacterial infections.* Polyneuritis can occur as a complication of many bacterial infections, both acute and chronic.

(6) *Unknown origin.* Chronic progressive peripheral neuritis of unknown origin.

An increasing number of chemical compounds in use in industry or therapeutically are being found liable to produce polyneuritic manifestations; an interesting example that has recently come to light is the simple vinyl monomer, acrylamide ($CH_2 = CHCONH_2$), which is now being used extensively in industry as the basis of flocculators used for aiding the separation of suspended solids from aqueous systems in various processes such as mining, soil stabilization and the disposal of industrial wastes. Fullerton & Barnes (1966) have made a detailed histological and physiological study of the peripheral neuropathy which can be produced in rats by the chronic administration of acrylamide, but little is at present known about the biochemical basis of the lesions.

From the standpoint of the chemical pathologist, the polyneuritis of thiamine deficiency occupies the central position of this group of conditions, since it was from the work of Peters and his colleagues on avian polyneuritis in rice-fed pigeons that our present knowledge of the biochemical lesion underlying thiamine deficiency stemmed (see Peters, 1936). With this came also a widening of the conception that other biochemical derangements, either related or of a fundamentally different type, may underlie other types of polyneuritis. As a result of this work it became known that the outstanding defect in thiamine deficiency is an impairment in the normal metabolism of pyruvate which results in a rise in the blood pyruvate level (Thompson & Johnson, 1935; Platt & Lu, 1939). Pyruvate metabolism has therefore been studied in a variety of different types of polyneuritis. Since this work is relevant to several of the causes of polyneuritis, and since blood pyruvate determinations are of some value in differential diagnosis, the outcome of these studies will be summarized before proceeding to describe separately the biochemical characteristics of some of the different polyneuritides.

Pyruvate Metabolism in Peripheral Neuritis

In the studies in man made by Platt & Lu in 1939 in Shanghai, it was found that although very considerable elevations in the blood pyruvate level occurred in the acute, advanced type of beri-beri, in the more subacute or chronic types the values were usually within normal limits or only very slightly raised. Shortly afterwards Bueding, Wortis & Stern (1942) also reported that while elevated fasting values were found in "acute peripheral neuropathy" the levels were normal in the chronic forms, and in further studies both in America and in England it has been repeatedly found that the degrees of thiamine deficiency occurring in these countries are not usually associated with any obvious elevation of the fasting pyruvate level.

To reveal these less severe degrees of thiamine depletion it is necessary to determine blood pyruvate levels after a loading dose of glucose, that is to say, after the tissues have been subjected to an abnormal load of pyruvate formed from the absorbed glucose. This was first demonstrated in induced thiamine deficiency by Elsom, Lukens, Montgomery & Jonas (1940), and in Wernicke's syndrome and in peripheral neuropathy associated with chronic alcoholism by Bueding, Stein & Wortis (1941).

Williams, Mason, Power & Wilder (1943) carried out an extensive study on normal and experimentally induced thiamine-deficient subjects fasting and at rest in bed; after withdrawing a fasting blood specimen they gave 50 g. of glucose by mouth followed 30 min. later by a second dose of 50 g., further blood specimens being taken at 30, 60 and 90 min. after the first dose. With this procedure they found that while normal subjects showed only a slight rise in the blood pyruvate level, the maximum value at any of the times never exceeding 1·4 mg. pyruvic acid/100 ml., the thiamine-deficient subjects showed a significantly greater rise, many of them giving values of well over 2 mg./100 ml.

This "pyruvate tolerance test" was later used by Joiner, McArdle & Thompson (1950) in a study of 40 cases of polyneuritis of various types, together with a group of 50 control subjects. Just over half of the cases of polyneuritis studied showed high values at either 60 or 90 min. after the first dose of glucose (see Fig. 13.1), but only three gave high fasting values. The cases studied by these workers were completely unselected, except that their symptoms were sufficiently severe to warrant admission to hospital, and it would seem unlikely that nearly half of these cases, occurring in this country, were due to, or were associated with, a deficiency of thiamine. Also it is known clinically

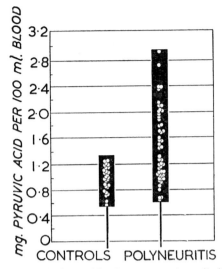

FIG. 13.1. Maximum blood pyruvate values obtained after administration of glucose in unselected cases of polyneuritis.

that thiamine therapy, even when given parenterally in large doses, is only of value in a relatively small proportion of cases of peripheral neuritis.

The system of enzymes responsible for pyruvate oxidation can of course be inhibited in a number of ways other than by a lack of the essential co-enzyme thiamine pyrophosphate. This enzyme system contains highly reactive essential SH groups in at least one of its components, and it is now known that a number of toxic agents can inhibit pyruvate oxidation and lead to the development of high blood pyruvate levels by interaction with these SH groups. For example, many compounds of arsenic (Peters, Sinclair & Thompson, 1946), antimony, gold and mercury (Thompson & Whittaker, 1947) act in this way. In this connection it is interesting that many points of clinical resemblance have long been recognized between arsenical neuritis and the neuritis of dry beri-beri (Ross & Reynolds, 1901). In addition to these metal poisons certain organic compounds are also known to inhibit pyruvate oxidation. For example, the toxic alkaloid sanguinarine, obtained from argemone oil, has been shown to be a potent inhibitor of this enzyme system (Sarkar, 1948). Intoxication with this compound, present as a natural contaminant in certain oriental cooking oils, is believed to be the cause of the epidemic dropsy occurring in parts of India. This condition is very similar to wet beri-beri, and it was shown as long ago as 1937 by Wilson & Ghosh that a rise in the bisulphitebinding capacity of the blood (and presumably therefore of the blood pyruvate) occurs in cases of epidemic dropsy. All of these toxic agents inhibit pyruvate oxidation by reaction with essential SH groups and not by any interference with the action of thiamine, so that we have reason for thinking that a block in pyruvate metabolism, detected by the presence of abnormally high blood pyruvate levels, might be due to causes other than a deficiency of thiamine.

In the hope of differentiating between those cases with high pyruvate levels due to a deficiency of thiamine and those due to some other cause, Joiner *et al.* (1950) studied the effect of massive therapy (100 mg. vitamin B_1/day) given parenterally for 14 days. At the end of this time they carried out a second pyruvate test on those patients in their group of polyneuritics who had shown high blood pyruvate levels before treatment. If the high levels found originally had been due to lack of thiamine it was felt that it might reasonably be expected that they would have been restored to normal by 14 days of such treatment. It was found (Fig. 13.2) that in some of the cases studied thiamine

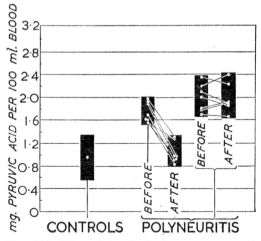

FIG. 13.2. Effect of vitamin B_1 therapy on cases of polyneuritis with raised blood pyruvate levels (after glucose load).

therapy caused the originally high pyruvate levels to return to well within the normal range, whereas in other cases the blood levels were entirely unaffected by this treatment, and remained so even when thiamine therapy was carried out for longer periods.

It was concluded from this work that from the biochemical point of view cases of polyneuritis occurring in this country fall into three groups:

(1) Patients in whom no abnormality of pyruvate metabolism can be detected. Such cases appeared to correspond to about half of the total number of patients studied. Judged by this test there would seem to be no reason to suspect a significant degree of thiamine deficiency in this group.

(2) Patients showing impaired pyruvate metabolism, but in whom the blood pyruvate level falls to normal after intramuscular thiamine therapy for 14 days. The polyneuritis in these patients is presumably due to, or is associated with, thiamine deficiency.

(3) Patients showing impaired pyruvate metabolism in whom this biochemical disturbance remains unaffected by massive and prolonged thiamine therapy. In these patients it would appear that the polyneuritis is not associated with a simple deficiency of thiamine, but must be due to some other cause, possibly some interference with essential SH groups.

The value to the clinician of blood pyruvate determinations in cases of polyneuritis of unknown origin is that even in cases due to simple thiamine lack in the diet, the clinical response following treatment with thiamine is often slow and incomplete, as indeed is to be expected when the nature of the neuronal lesion is taken into account. A pyruvate metabolism test carried out after 14 days of intensive parenteral therapy may therefore give a much more rapid indication of the value of such therapy than would be obtained by basing conclusions solely on clinical criteria.

With patients falling into the third of the above biochemical types, and particularly if any history can be obtained of exposure to arsenic or heavy metals, it would seem logical to try treatment with dimercaprol (BAL) (see Stocken & Thompson, 1946; Thompson, 1948). Furmanski (1948) has reported the successful treatment of four cases of "toxic" polyneuritis with BAL, but blood pyruvate levels in these cases were not reported.

Blood Transketolase Levels

A further biochemical test that has attracted attention in recent years as a possible aid in the diagnosis of thiamine deficiency is the determination of the level of erythrocyte transketolase activity. This enzyme is known to require thiamine pyrophosphate as a co-factor (Horecker & Smyrniotis, 1953; Racker, De la Haba & Leder, 1953). It is present in red blood cells, and satisfactory methods for its estimation have been worked out. The clinical applications of blood transketolase determinations have been described by Dreyfus (1962, 1967).

Alcoholic Polyneuritis

The symptomatology of this condition bears a very striking resemblance to that of dry beri-beri, and it has for long been thought that it may be due to a thiamine deficiency brought about by the unbalanced, deficient diet of the chronic alcoholic, together with the chronic gastritis and the associated disturbances of gastro-intestinal function.

Minot, Strauss & Cobb (1933) carried out a dietary survey in a group of patients with alcoholic polyneuritis, and showed that in the great majority of these the diet was inadequate; they also reported on the high incidence (well over 50%) of achlorhydria and hypochlorhydria in these patients. That this condition is primarily dietary in origin and not due to any direct toxic action of alcohol, as had earlier been suggested despite the contrary evidence that polyneuritis does not follow bouts of acute alcoholism, was indicated by the observations of Spies & de Wolf (1933), Blankenhorn & Spies (1935), Strauss (1935) and Jolliffe, Colbert & Joffe (1936), who showed that the continued intake of alcohol did not prevent the improvement of the condition which can be brought about by an adequate diet rich in thiamine.

The existence of a thiamine deficiency in patients suffering from alcoholic polyneuritis is supported by the finding of raised blood pyruvate levels (Bueding & Wortis, 1940) and low levels of vitamin B_1 (Sinclair, 1939) and of co-carboxylase (Goodhart & Sinclair, 1939).

Polyneuritis due to Organo-phosphorus Compounds

The neurotoxic action of tri-o-cresyl phosphate (TOCP) has been widely recognized as a result of an outbreak of severe motor neuritis in the United States in 1930. The paralysis affecting these patients was shown to follow the drinking of a beverage, one constituent of which was an extract of Jamaica ginger subsequently shown to contain TOCP (Smith & Elvove, 1930; Smith, Elvove & Frazier, 1930). For this reason this type of neuritis has been called "ginger paralysis". Numerous other instances of poisoning by TOCP have since come to light. Lorot in 1899 described the occurrence of polyneuritis in patients with pulmonary tuberculosis treated with preparations of "phosphocreosote" shown to contain TOCP. More recently outbreaks have occurred as a result of its presence in apiol (Ter Braak, 1931; Germon, 1932), in cooking oils (Sampson, 1938; Staehelin, 1941; Humpe, 1942; Wlathard, 1946; Hotston, 1946), and of its use in the plastics industry (Hunter, Perry & Evans, 1944).

Degenerative lesions affecting both the axis cylinders and the myelin sheaths are found in the peripheral nerves and the long tracts of the spinal cord. Experimentally it has been shown that paralysis and nerve lesions can be produced by TOCP in certain animals, notably the hen, although the rat appears to be resistant. A striking characteristic of the experimental condition in the hen is the latent period of 10 to 14 days prior to the onset of the paralysis, during which time the bird appears healthy except for some loss of appetite.

In a study in cats intoxicated by subcutaneous injections of TOCP, Cavanagh & MacDermot (1961) have demonstrated the considerable damage that takes place in the sensory terminals of muscle spindles and tendon organs, in contrast to the relatively minor changes found in motor endings; they have further shown, by means of fibre diameter measurements, that it is the nerve fibres of large diameter that are selectively damaged.

As TOCP is a stable substance it has been thought for some time that it is probably converted inside the body into a more reactive compound which then produces the toxic effects, and Aldridge in 1954 first obtained direct evidence in support of this view by showing that, following incubation with rat liver slices, the inhibitory action of TOCP on horse serum cholinesterase is markedly increased. This conversion to a more toxic compound has now been studied in detail, and it has been shown (Casida, Eto & Baron 1961) that a major pathway of the metabolism of TOCP involves hydroxylation of a methyl group with subsequent cyclization:

TOCP

Cyclic metabolite

This cyclic metabolite is a potent esterase inhibitor, and also produces a neurotoxic syndrome at dose levels as low as 4 mg./kg. (Baron, Bennett & Casida, 1962).

The biochemical effect of TOCP which has been studied most extensively is its inhibitory effect on cholinesterase and tributyrinase activity (Bloch, 1941; Hottinger & Bloch, 1943; Mendel & Rudney, 1944). Earl & Thompson (1952a) showed that it is a selective inhibitor of human butyrylcholinesterase in nervous tissue and in plasma, the acetylcholinesterase of nervous tissue, muscle and red blood cells being unaffected. It was also found that in hens poisoned by a single oral dose of TOCP the butyrylcholinesterase activity in the brain and spinal cord is very nearly abolished, the acetylcholinesterase being again almost unaffected (Earl & Thompson, 1952b). Tributyrinase activity in the cords of poisoned hens is also inhibited; no defect could be demonstrated in glucose or pyruvate metabolism (Earl, Thompson & Webster, 1953).

More recently, a fall in erythrocyte acetylcholinesterase has been reported by Piccoli, Ferrari & Daniele (1962); Hern (1967) has found a significant reduction of both red cell and muscle acetylcholinesterase following the administration of TOCP to baboons.

A very similar motor paralysis has also been reported following intoxication by certain of the new organo-phosphorus anti-cholinesterase insecticides. In 1951 Petry described the onset of paralysis in a man who three months earlier had been exposed to parathion (diethyl-p-nitrophenyl thiophosphate). Two years later a full report appeared of two cases of paralysis following poisoning by mipafox, bis-(monoisopropylamino)-fluorophosphine oxide (Bidstrup, Bonnell & Beckett, 1953); in each of these cases the levels of both plasma and erythrocyte cholinesterases were markedly lowered. Barnes & Denz (1953) have succeeded in producing paralysis in hens with mipafox and DFP (diisopropyl fluorophosphonate) as well as with TOCP, and have described the pathology of the lesions (see also Cavanagh, 1954).

It is to be noted that each of these "paralysing" compounds is an ester of a phosphorus-containing acid, and that each is an inhibitor, or is converted into an inhibitor, of certain esterases. Other organophosphorus compounds, however, which are also selective inhibitors of these esterases, do not cause paralysis or degenerative lesions of the nerves, even although they may be capable of producing an extensive degree of inhibition of pseudocholinesterase activity in the spinal cord after administration to animals (Davison, 1953; Thompson, 1954). It is clear therefore that if inhibition of this enzyme is playing any part in the production of these lesions in the nervous system other factors must also be concerned. On present evidence it would certainly be premature to conclude that butyrylcholinesterase inhibition is causally concerned with this type of paralysis. Present ideas concerning the mechanism of the delayed neurotoxicity caused by these various organo-phosphorus compounds have been discussed by Aldridge, Barnes & Johnson (1969).

Diabetic Neuropathy

Symptoms of peripheral neuropathy have been found in both severe and controlled diabetics, with or without arteriosclerotic lesions. The clinical manifestations are usually sensory (Epstein, 1951), but may be purely motor (Garland & Taverner, 1953; Garland, 1955).

Considerable differences of opinion have existed as to the aetiological factor or factors involved, and the three main hypotheses have been those of degenerative vascular disease, thiamine deficiency and the disordered metabolism of diabetes mellitus. Martin (1953) does not consider that peripheral vascular disease plays any part in this condition. The observations of Epstein (1951) and Hirson, Feinmann & Wade (1953) do not support the theory of thiamine deficiency, although previous workers had claimed good results with thiamine therapy.

Bueding, Wortis & Fein (1942) demonstrated that diabetic subjects show little or no rise in the blood pyruvate level following glucose administration, although a significant rise occurs when insulin is given as well. Martin (1953) has, however, reported on pyruvate tolerance tests in diabetic subjects following the intravenous injection of pyruvate, and has concluded that pyruvate metabolism is normal in cases of diabetic neuropathy. Thompson, Butterfield & Kelsey Fry (1960) have reported on the blood pyruvate levels in glucose-insulin tests carried out on a series of diabetic subjects with and without neuropathy. The fasting and the 60 min. pyruvate levels were distinctly higher in the diabetic group taken as a whole than in healthy control subjects, but there was no evidence that the levels were any higher in the patients with neuropathy than in the other diabetics. Goodhart & Sinclair (1940) found normal levels of blood co-carboxylase in four out of five patients with diabetic neuropathy, the fifth patient, in whom a low level was found, being also an alcohol addict.

In an investigation of 150 cases of diabetic neuropathy Martin (1953) found that the condition occurred more commonly in those patients who had neglected their diabetic control, or in whom the condition had not been recognized.

However, there appears to be no direct connection between the blood sugar level and the neuritis (Bonkalo, 1950; Hirson, Feinmann & Wade, 1953). In 1950 Handelsman, in a review of carbohydrate metabolism in diabetes, concluded that the mechanism of the nervous changes was unknown, and this is still true.

Neurological symptoms occur not infrequently in patients with insulinomas. Attacks not typically epileptic, altered states of consciousness and even degrees of mental deterioration may be present unassociated with food intake (Marks, Marrack & Rose, 1961). The diagnosis can usually be confirmed by the finding of low blood glucose concentrations (obtained on more than one occasion) following fasting. The glucagon (Cochrane, Payne, Simpkins & Woolf, 1956) and intravenous tolbutamide tests (Fajans & Conn, 1959) are valuable aids in diagnosis (Marrack, Rose & Marks, 1961).

Polyneuritis of Acute Porphyria

Nervous symptoms are frequently associated with the acute type of porphyria occurring usually but not exclusively in adults. The derangement of porphyrin metabolism in this condition is described in Chapter 8. The nervous symptoms, apart from the mental abnormalities, consist of some form of paralysis, most frequently of the extremities, although an ascending paralysis of the Landry type may be found. The patient is usually passing excessive amounts of porphyrin in the urine, but this is not invariable and the colourless precursor porphobilinogen may be found alone.

The cause of the nervous lesions in this condition is still obscure. Denny-Brown & Sciarra (1945) have described two cases, with histological examination of the nervous system; they suggested that some vaso-constrictor substance acting locally might be the factor involved. Perrault, Klotz, Canivet & Caroit (1953) examined the nervous system of autopsy, but could find no evidence of any deposit of porphyrin. Klüver (1944) has stated that microscopic granules exhibiting a red fluorescence in ultra-violet light can be found in the normal central nervous system, and Rimington & Gray (1947) have concluded that on present evidence porphyrin cannot be regarded as neurotoxic and that there is no evidence that the nerve lesions found in this condition are the result of the formation of porphyrins.

ACTH was not shown to be of any therapeutic benefit (Goldberg, Macdonald & Rimington, 1952) even though marked changes in electrolyte levels had been found earlier by Linder (1947).

Cyanide Neuropathy

The role that chronic cyanide intoxication may play in the production of degenerative neurological disease has recently become of interest as a result of a study of Leber's hereditary optic atrophy carried out by Wilson (1965).

Leber's optic atrophy is a rare inherited disorder characterized by visual failure and in some patients by more widespread evidence of central nervous system damage. The hereditary nature of the condition suggests that it may be the outcome of some inborn metabolic error which becomes revealed because of some exogenous factor; the development of the disease appears often to be related to smoking, and it has been suggested that some toxic agent in tobacco smoke may be such a factor (Wilson, 1963).

Tobacco smoke is known to contain hydrogen cyanide, which in the normal person is rapidly converted to less toxic compounds. One important detoxication pathway involves its conversion to thiocyanate by the enzyme thiusulphate : cyanide sulphurtransferase (also known as rhodanese):

Thiosulphate + cyanide →
Sulphite + thiocyanate

Wilson (1965) therefore investigated the levels of cyanide and thiocyanate in the plasma and urine of healthy smokers and non-smokers and of patients with Leber's optic atrophy who were also smokers. He found that the mean plasma concentration and urinary excretion of thiocyanate was significantly higher in the control smokers than in the control non-smokers, a fact which he interpreted as indicating absorption of cyanide by the smokers, and its conversion to thiocyanate. Smokers who also suffered from Leber's disease failed, however, to show this increment in mean thiocyanate levels. These findings are certainly consistent with the possibility that patients with this condition have an inborn error of metabolism as a result of which they are unable to detoxicate cyanide to thiocyanate in the normal way, while the diffuse damage to the central nervous system in these patients is also consistent with the known neurotoxic effects that have been produced experimentally by repeated exposure to cyanide.

More recently Monekosso & Wilson (1966) have commenced an epidemiological and laboratory study of a degenerative neuropathy, often associated with the so-called tropical amblyopia, which is common in certain parts of Nigeria. They have found that patients with this neurological disorder have very much higher levels of plasma thiocyanate than either healthy controls or "hospital controls", i.e. patients suffering from a variety of non-neurological disorders. Since cassava, which is known to be rich in cyanogenic gluco-sides, is the staple diet of a large number of Nigerians, work is now in progress in the hope of correlating more closely the incidence of this tropical neuropathy with cassava consumption, and hence with cyanide intake.

The possibility that vitamin B_{12} may also have a physiological role to play in connection with cyanide metabolism is also receiving increasing attention. It is known that cyanide combines readily with various forms of vitamin B_{12} to form cyanocobalamin, and it has been suggested by Wokes (1955, 1958) and by Smith (1961) that vitamin B_{12} takes part in the detoxication of exogenous cyanide; it has also been claimed that cyanide administered chronically to animals depletes liver B_{12} (Braekkan, Njaa & Utne, 1957).

Wilson & Matthews (1966) have studied the metabolic inter-relationships of cyanide and vitamin B_{12}. They obtained evidence of a recipro-cal relationship between cyanide (or thiocyanate) and vitamin B_{12} concentrations in the plasma, and they have suggested that at low serum B_{12} levels plasma cyanide concentration might be sufficiently elevated to produce neurotoxic effects.

DEMYELINATING DISEASES

The "demyelinating diseases" of the nervous system comprise an important and relatively com-mon group of disorders whose aetiology is in most cases unknown, but which are characterized by the presence of scattered, sharply localized areas of myelin break-down and gliosis, mainly restric-ted to the white matter of the brain, spinal cord and optic nerves. Wilson (1940) has pointed out that the manifestations of reaction of the nervous system to injury or disease, as with other tissues of the body, are strictly limited, so that the same end-result may ensue from very different primary causes. Destruction of the myelin sheath repre-sents one of these standard reactions to a wide variety of injuries, and, as has been pointed out already, is therefore commonly found in diseases of both the central and peripheral nervous sys-tems. In many conditions the demyelination appears to be a secondary reaction to neuronal damage, but in the group of conditions known as the demyelinating diseases damage to the myelin sheath is the outstanding change, and would appear to precede damage to the axis-cylinders.

The demyelinating diseases include multiple sclerosis (or disseminated sclerosis), neuromyelitis optica, the various forms of diffuse sclerosis, in-cluding Schilder's encephalitis periaxialis diffusa, and such allied conditions as the acute dissemi-nated encephalomyelitis that occurs as a rare complication of vaccination and of certain of the acute infections of childhood such as measles, German measles, mumps, chicken pox and small-pox. Somewhat similar demyelinating lesions have been described in association with hepatic disease, uraemia, eclampsia and porphyria.

Although the incidence of multiple sclerosis appears to show striking variations in different parts of the world, in many countries of northern Europe and in North America it is one of the commonest organic diseases of the nervous system. For this reason the pathology of multiple sclerosis has been more studied than that of the other demyelinating diseases, and this account of the chemical pathology of this group of diseases will therefore centre round multiple sclerosis.

MULTIPLE SCLEROSIS
Pathology of Multiple Sclerosis

The distribution of the plaques of demyelina-tion and glial sclerosis, which occur scattered throughout the central nervous system, and the macroscopic and minute pathology of these lesions have brought to light a number of observations that have had a distinct bearing on the views con-cerning the aetiology of the condition and the nature of the disease process. Some of these facts will therefore be briefly summarized before pro-ceeding to describe the more chemical observa-tions that have been made.

The lesions in multiple sclerosis appear to be restricted to the central nervous system; although a few cases have been reported of lesions in the nerve roots it would seem that these have been extensions from plaques situated in the adjoining brain-stem or spinal cord. The occurrence of characteristic lesions in peripheral nerves has not been established.

The plaques vary much in size, some being microscopic and others 1 or 2 cm. in diameter or even larger, but are characterized by the much greater degree of myelin break-down than of damage to the axon. The earlier lesions, in which the demyelination is only partial are known as "shadow plaques". It has been stated that the degenerating myelin sheath in some instances gives an appearance suggesting that the myelin is undergoing a process of erosion or lysis from without, the more external part of the sheath suffering before the more central parts imme-diately surrounding the axon (McAlpine, Comp-ston & Lumsden, 1955); the possible significance of this observation in connection with the aetio-logy of the condition will be discussed later. If this suggestion of an initial marginal lysis of the myelin is correct, it would seem that the process must differ fundamentally from the demyelination accompanying thiamine deficiency, where the whole thickness of the myelin sheath is affected, presumably as a result of primary changes in the axon.

The contours of the plaques are sharply demarcated, giving rise to their "punched-out" appearance. In the plaque itself there is a disappearance both of myelin and, to some extent, of the oligodendrocytes. A full account of the pathology and cytology of these lesions has been given by Lumsden (see McAlpine *et al.* 1955).

It is of interest to note in this connection that Luse & McDougal (1960) have reported that in the acute stages of allergic encephalomyelitis, induced in rabbits by the injection of white matter from bovine brain together with adjuvants, one of the early changes observed was a striking swelling of the mitochondria of the oligodendrocytes, although the mitochondria of adjacent axons and cells remained morphologically unaffected.

There is a tendency for the plaques to be distributed symmetrically, and the question of their relation to blood vessels has received much attention. Putnam (1936, 1937) indeed suggested that the lesions of multiple sclerosis might be in large part the result of local anoxia resulting from thrombotic occlusion of small blood vessels. Although this view has been contested by various workers (see, for example, Dow & Berglund, 1942) it has been pointed out that "plaques are *sometimes* centred round veins and venules, particularly in the acute lesions, in such a way as to suggest a more than fortuitous relationship" (Lumsden, 1951).

Plasma Protein Levels in Multiple Sclerosis

Although changes in the levels of the cerebrospinal fluid proteins are well recognized as occurring frequently in multiple sclerosis, the plasma protein levels do not appear to be much affected, except perhaps for some lowering of the plasma albumin. The claims that have been made are conflicting, and seem to depend on the criteria of significance adopted by the investigators.

The association, if any exists, of multiple sclerosis with any characteristic alteration in plasma protein levels, or with any significant degree of liver dysfunction, has therefore yet to be proved.

CSF Protein Levels in Multiple Sclerosis

While it is true to say that there are certainly no changes in the cerebrospinal fluid that can be

regarded as diagnostic of the condition, it has been known for many years that the total protein level, and even more frequently the globulin fraction, is not uncommonly raised. Thus, it has been estimated that a positive Pandy or Nonne-Apelt reaction is given by the cerebrospinal fluid of about 30% of cases (Freedman & Merritt, 1950). Over a nine-year period the following results have been obtained at the National Hospital for Nervous Diseases, London:

Total number of specimens examined	438
Positive Nonne-Apelt reaction	94 (21%)
Positive Pandy reaction	178 (41%)
Positive Lange test	189 (43%)
Protein 50 mg./100 ml. or more	215 (49%)

Immunological and electrophoretic techniques have shown that it is the γ-globulin fraction which is increased (Kabat, Freedman, Murray & Knaub, 1950; Field, 1954). Yahr, Goldensohn & Kabat (1954) have studied the cerebrospinal fluid in 681 patients with neurological disease; they found raised γ-globulin levels in 67% of patients with multiple sclerosis, in 74% of patients with neurosyphilis, and in 6% of patients having other diseases of the nervous system.

Immunoelectrophoresis has recently been applied to the study of CSF proteins, and by these means Gavrilescu has identified the presence of an abnormal globulin in some cases of multiple sclerosis (see McMenemey, 1961).

Lipid Metabolism in Multiple Sclerosis

Lipid metabolism has also been extensively studied in multiple sclerosis. As regards the levels of blood lipids, contradictory claims are again to be found. The blood cholesterol level has been stated to be normal by Fog (1951), Wilmot & Swank (1952) and Chiavacci & Sperry (1952). On the other hand, Frisch (1937), Altmann & Goldhammer (1937), Pichler & Reisner (1938), Jones, Jones & Bunch (1950) and Dobin & Switzer (1954) have claimed that the levels of both total and esterified cholesterol in the blood are high.

Conflicting reports have also appeared concerning the levels of phospholipids in the blood of patients with multiple sclerosis. Thus, to quote only from more recent statements, Sercl, Kovarik & Jicka (1961) reported low levels of total phospholipids in this disease, although Plum & Fog (1959) found no significant change.

More recently, Baker, Thompson & Zilkha (1964, 1966) have carried out a study of the fatty acid composition of the total lipid extract of serum taken from patients with multiple sclerosis.

Using gas chromatographic methods they found that the level of linoleic acid (18:2) was significantly reduced in patients in the active, advanced stages of the disease (Table 13.2). The levels of the

TABLE 13.2

Mean levels of linoleate
(free and esterified) in serum from patients with multiple sclerosis

	Clinical evidence of deterioration within preceding month	No. of subjects	μmoles/ml. $\pm$ S.E.M.
Controls	—	20	3·68 ± 0·09
Multiple Sclerosis	Nil or slight	7	3·74 ± 0·18
Multiple Sclerosis	Moderate	8	3·06 ± 0·20
Multiple Sclerosis	Extensive	11	2·79 ± 0·16

other fatty acids did not appear to be affected in any of the patients studied. Since the cholesteryl ester fraction of the serum lipids contains more linoleate than either the triglyceride or phospholipid fractions, the concentration of cholesteryl linoleate in the serum was measured after separation by thin-layer chromatography (Baker, Sanders, Thompson & Zilkha, 1965); these measurements showed that the mean cholesteryl linoleate

fraction was strikingly reduced in the group of patients with active multiple sclerosis.

Montfoort, Baker, Thompson & Zilkha (1966) also studied the levels of plasma phospholipids in 27 patients with multiple sclerosis and in 17 controls, and found reduced levels only in patients in the active phases of the disease; the proportions of the different fatty acids, however, showed no change in this fraction even in the active phases.

When we turn to the examination of the brain the findings are more consistent and the changes more pronounced. As might be expected in a condition where it is known from histological studies that there is a loss of myelin, chemical estimations show that the brain phospholipids are decreased in amount in the plaques of multiple sclerosis (Weil, 1948). Cumings (1953, 1955) has made a detailed study of the various lipid fractions in the brain from patients with multiple sclerosis and diffuse sclerosis. He has shown that there is a profound loss of lecithin, cephalin, sphingomyelin, cholesterol and cerebroside from the demyelinated areas. He also described the interesting finding of the presence of cholesterol esters, which are not normally present in appreciable amounts in human brain; this finding is of particular interest in view of the appearance of esterified cholesterol in peripheral nerve undergoing Wallerian degeneraton following transection. It is also noteworthy in connection

TABLE 13.3

Lipid content of cerebral white matter from normal human brain and from the brains of two cases of multiple sclerosis and one of diffuse sclerosis

(Expressed as g./100 g. wet weight of brain)

	Total phospholipid	Sphingomyelin	Lecithin	Cephalin	Cholesterol Total	Cholesterol Free	Cerebroside
Normal brain	6·0	2·3	1·2	2·5	4·83	4·83	5·5
Case 1. Demyelinated area	2·7	0·8	0·46	1·04	2·84	1·17	1·2
Case 2. Demyelinated area	1·82	0·49	0·34	0·99	2·84	1·08	0·58
Case 3. Early demyelination	2·34	0·8	0·78	0·76	3·3	1·74	1·2
Case 3. Late demyelination	1·8	0·54	0·53	0·73	3·0	1·2	1·03
Case 1. Normal area	4·8	2·04	1·7	1·06	2·8	2·8	3·5
Case 2. Normal area	5·78	2·40	0·93	2·46	4·06	3·81	4·23
Case 3. Normal area	4·9	1·9	1·0	2·0	3·9	3·8	2·3

Cases 1 and 2—multiple sclerosis
Case 3—diffuse sclerosis

with the pathogenesis of the condition that areas of histologically normal cerebral white matter from the brains of these cases, and also the cortex overlying the plaques, were found to show a similar though less marked reduction in lipid, although cholesterol esters were not found in these areas. The results of these analytical studies in the brain from these demyelinating conditions are summarized in Table 13.3.

A study has also been reported of the fatty acid composition of the lecithin fraction extracted from the white matter of the brains of six persons dying from non-neurological causes and from nine patients with multiple sclerosis (Baker, Thompson & Zilkha, 1963). In the brains from the patients with multiple sclerosis samples were taken for analysis only from areas of white matter which appeared normal on visual inspection. The analytical results showed that there is a change in the proportions of saturated and unsaturated fatty

TABLE 13.4

Proportions of fatty acids in the lecithins of apparently normal white matter in multiple sclerosis brains

(Mean values, expressed as eq. individual fatty acids/100 eq. total fatty acids)

Fatty acid	Normals (6)	Multiple Sclerosis (9)
Palmitic (P)	24·6	33·6
Palmitoleic (PO)	4·9	2·3
Stearic (S)	13·3	10·4
Oleic (O)	51·1	44·4
Arachidonic (A)	3·3	1·7
Total saturated acids (P + S)	37·9	44·0
Total unsaturated acids (PO + O + A)	59·3	48·4

(Number of brains studied indicated in brackets)

acids in the lecithin fraction from patients with this disease. It will be seen from Table 13.4, which shows the proportions of the five most plentiful fatty acids present in this fraction, that there is a shift towards a degree of greater saturation of the fatty acids in the lecithins from the diseased brains.

These changes in the levels of lipids in the demyelinated areas appear to be, to some extent, reflected by changes in the CSF. Poser & Curran (1958) for example, have studied the cholesterol and cholesterol ester levels in the CSF of patients with multiple sclerosis, and have found an increase in the level of total cholesterol, associated with the appearance of free cholesterol (Table 13.5). Green, Papadopoulos, Cevallos, Foster & Hess (1959) and Plum & Fog (1959) have also reported raised cholesterol levels in the CSF in multiple sclerosis.

Phospholipid levels in the CSF in various demyelinating conditions have recently been reported on by McArdle & Zilkha (1962). Not only is the total phospholipid level raised in these conditions, but the relative proportions of different phospholipids are altogether different from that of normal CSF; in diseases associated with demyelination, as opposed to inflammatory conditions of the central nervous system, the percentage distribution of the individual phospholipids shows a striking similarity to that in nervous tissue, the cephalin content in particular being markedly raised.

Cumings (1955) has also examined the neuraminic acid content of the cerebral cortex in five cases of multiple sclerosis, and in four of them found levels considerably above the range found in the normal brain.

Carbohydrate Metabolism in Multiple Sclerosis

It has been claimed that patients with multiple sclerosis present certain biochemical features suggesting an abnormality of glucose metabolism.

TABLE 13.5

Levels of total and free cholesterol in the CSF (mg./100 ml.) in multiple sclerosis

Condition	No. of subjects	Cholesterol	
		Total	Free
Normal controls	25	0·11	0·03
M.S.[1] ("inactive")	17	0.17	0·01
M.S. ("questionably active")	14	0·28	0·04
M.S. ("active")	19	0·33	0·13
Amyotrophic lateral sclerosis	8	0·37	0·11

[1] M.S. = multiple sclerosis.

(Taken from Poser & Curran, 1958)

Although no change in the fasting blood sugar level has been recorded, Jones, Jones & Bunch in 1950 described a lowered glucose tolerance, and confirmed an earlier report (Weil & Bradburne 1948) of a low fasting level of serum inorganic P. This group of workers also reported that the fasting blood pyruvate level was high in patients with multiple sclerosis, and that there was an extra accumulation of pyruvate in the blood following the oral administration of glucose.

Henneman, Altschule, Goncz & Alexander (1954) have examined keto-acid metabolism in this condition in greater detail, using a chromatographic method for the separate estimation of pyruvic and α-ketoglutaric acids, and have also studied the blood lactate and citrate levels. They were unable to confirm the findings, mentioned above, of high fasting blood pyruvate levels, although there was a suggestion that slightly high levels might be found after the ingestion of glucose. They did, however, detect abnormally high levels of α-ketoglutarate and citrate.

Both Jeanes & Cumings (1958) and McArdle, Mackenzie & Webster (1960) have also reported an abnormal rise in the blood pyruvate level after ingestion of glucose in approximately 50% of cases; and the latter authors also found that the α-ketoglutarate level was not infrequently raised. The cerebrospinal fluid level, however, was found to be normal in the 12 patients studied.

From the work of McArdle et al. (1960), however, it now seems likely that high levels of pyruvate, when present, are due more to the presence of spasticity in the patient than to any intrinsic abnormality of pyruvate metabolism connected directly with the disease process, an association that had indeed been suggested earlier by Bauer (1956). It is well known that muscular activity can cause an elevation of the blood pyruvate level, so that it is certainly to be expected that spasticity might be responsible for abnormalities in the pyruvate tolerance test.

Aetiology of Multiple Sclerosis

The biochemical findings described above give little lead to an understanding of the pathogenesis of the plaques of multiple sclerosis. As is to be expected, a number of hypotheses have been put forward and some experimental work has been carried out. Some further facts relating to the formation of myelin have been obtained from the study of a naturally occurring demyelinating disease of lambs. In order to give some indications of the lines along which present-day biochemical research is proceeding in connection with the problem of multiple sclerosis, the question of its aetiology will be considered under the following headings.

(1) *Cerebral anoxia*. It has been demonstrated experimentally in monkeys, cats, dogs and rats that, under suitable conditions, demyelination of areas in the central nervous system can be brought about by various respiratory poisons such as cyanide, azide or carbon monoxide. Both Ferraro (1933 a, b) and Weston Hurst (1940, 1941, 1942) have produced such disseminated lesions with cyanide. Weston Hurst demonstrated that the size of the dose of cyanide was important, and that repeated small doses were most suitable for the production of scattered focal lesions in the white matter. Although both myelin sheaths and axis cylinders are affected there is a tendency for the latter to show less damage (Lumsden, 1950), so that in this respect the lesions show a resemblance to those of multiple sclerosis. For this reason it has been thought that the production by some means of cerebral anoxia, possibly of a localized nature, may be the underlying change responsible for the development of the plaques of multiple sclerosis. As has been mentioned earlier (p. 467), localized thrombotic occlusion of blood vessels was suggested by Putnam as the cause, but this theory has been largely abandoned, chiefly owing to a failure to demonstrate such thromboses as regular occurrences early in the development of the plaques. It should also be pointed out that, even in the experimental cyanide lesions, Wyndham (1941) was unable to demonstrate any overall diminution in the oxidative processes of the brain, so that it is not yet established that the lesions are due to a direct poisoning of the respiratory processes in the white matter by the cyanide.

(2) *Trace metal deficiency*. The possibility of a trace metal deficiency playing a part in the pathogenesis of multiple sclerosis has also been considered, and indeed it has been clearly established that a naturally occurring demyelinating disease of young lambs is due to a deficiency of copper (Cu).

Enzootic ataxia, the name given to this disease in Australia, occurs in areas where the pasture is deficient in copper (Bennetts & Beck, 1942); ewes grazing these pastures have low levels of Cu in the blood and in their milk, and the Cu content of the livers of affected lambs is also low (Bennetts & Chapman, 1937). The administration of Cu to the lambs arrests the progress of the ataxia, while if it is given to the ewes the condition in the lambs is prevented.

Swayback is a clinically similar ataxic disease occurring in lambs in various parts of Great Britain. It would seem that in this condition the

Cu in the pasture is not assimilated normally, since although the Cu content of the pasture is normal the levels of Cu are low in the tissues of the pregnant ewes and ataxic lambs (Innes & Shearer, 1940). Here also Cu therapy by mouth is effective (Dunlop & Wells, 1938; Dunlop, Innes, Shearer & Wells, 1939).

In the lamb, therefore, Cu is necessary for the normal laying down of myelin, although its precise role in this complex process is not known. As yet, however, there are no clear reasons for associating Cu deficiency with the development of multiple sclerosis in man. Mandelbrote, Stanier, Thompson & Thruston (1948) studied the blood and urine Cu levels in a series of 26 patients with multiple sclerosis, but were unable to find any conclusive abnormality of Cu metabolism. Plum & Fog (1959) have confirmed these findings, by also showing that there is no reduction of the serum copper level in this disease.

It has also been suggested, on the other hand, that the ingestion of excessive amounts of certain minerals present in the soil or in the water may play a part in the causation of multiple sclerosis. Thus, Campbell, Herdan, Tatlow & Whittle (1950) have claimed that the disease is associated with a high intake of lead (Pb), possibly due to a high Pb content in the soil, and in support of this they have stated that the Pb content of the teeth in patients with multiple sclerosis is higher than that of teeth from normal persons. Butler (1952), however, has measured the concentration of Pb in urine, blood, cerebrospinal fluid, bone, teeth and various soft tissues from patients with multiple sclerosis, but has found that the values are all within normal limits, and has concluded that his studies do not support the view that Pb plays any part in the aetiology of this disease.

(3) *"Allergic" demyelination.* The possibility of the lesions of multiple sclerosis arising as a result of an allergic response in the central nervous system has also been envisaged, and the association of a demyelinating encephalomyelitis with vaccinia and with the acute infections of childhood might be taken to support such a hypothesis.

Furthermore, it is now well established that an "allergic" encephalomyelitis can be produced experimentally by the subcutaneous injection of sterile extracts of brain, either homologous or heterologous, together with an "adjuvant" of a preparation obtained from killed tubercle bacilli (Rivers & Schwentker, 1935; Ferraro & Jervis, 1940; Kabat, Wolf & Bezer, 1947; Morgan, 1947; Lumsden, 1949 *a, b*). This experimental disease appears to resemble fairly closely the acute encephalomyelitis complicating vaccinia or the infec-

tions of childhood, but it differs in a number of important ways from multiple sclerosis, and on present evidence there is insufficient cause to conclude with any certainty that an allergic mechanism is involved in this latter condition.

A great deal of work by Lumsden, Kies, Roboz, Field and others has been put into the isolation and characterization of this encephalitogenic factor in brain.

Active protein preparations have been obtained from white matter, grey matter, brain mitochondria and myelinated axon fragments. Laatsch, Kies, Gordon & Alvord (1962) described a preparation derived from guinea pig brain myelin, and showed that the encephalitogenic activity of myelin was higher than that of whole brain; they also isolated from the myelin fraction a basic protein of high encephalitogenic activity. At about the same time Robertson, Blight & Lumsden (1962) isolated an active dialysable peptide from bovine spinal cord, and Field and his colleagues (Caspary & Field, 1963; Field, Caspary & Ball, 1963) obtained a preparation from human brain of a protein fraction with a molecular weight of 20,000 to 50,000, 1 μg. of which regularly caused encephalomyelitis when injected into guinea pigs. More recently, Lumsden, Robertson & Blight (1966) have described a dialysable, basic, small molecular weight peptide with encephalitogenic activity, which they claim is responsible for the encephalogenicity of all the various active preparations that have been obtained from cerebral tissue. However, the relevance of this experimental "allergic" condition to the changes in multiple sclerosis has still to be defined.

(4) *"Myelinolysis."* The possibility that the plaques of multiple sclerosis might be due to an enzymic "lysis" of myelin was suggested as long ago as 1906 by Marburg. This view was taken up later by Brickner, who claimed that plasma from patients with multiple sclerosis was capable of producing a greater degree of "myelinolysis" of segments of rat spinal cord *in vitro* than that which was produced by normal plasma (Brickner, 1930). A series of reports then appeared claiming to establish the presence of abnormal amounts of a lipase in the plasma in multiple sclerosis. The titrimetric methods used for estimating lipase activity, however, were inexact and involved prolonged incubation with the substrate, so that much of this earlier work is difficult to assess. Weil & Cleveland (1932), however, confirmed some of Brickner's claims, but considered that the results were too slight to be considered important aetiologically. Crandall & Cherry (1932) also reported high lipase activity in the serum in multiple sclerosis,

but as they found equally high values in patients with liver disease they interpreted their results as indicating an associated hepatic disturbance. Brickner (1935) next reported that this serum lipase or esterase was high only during the inactive phases of the disease, normal values being found during relapses. Swan & Myers (1937), on the other hand, found no evidence of abnormal lipolytic activity. Using more exact manometric methods of assay Richards & Wolff (1940) were also unable to detect any increase in serum esterase activity in patients with multiple sclerosis. More recently still, however, Lesny & Polacek (1951) have again reported the finding of high lipolytic activity in the serum, the levels rising during exacerbations and falling during remissions. The finding by Jones, Jones, Howard & Bunch (1954) of high serum cholinesterase levels in cases of the "progressive" type has already been mentioned.

In view of these conflicting claims it would clearly be premature to conclude that myelinolysis is taking place because of the presence of excess circulating lipase, and indeed from the nature of the lesions there are reasons for thinking more in terms of some local disturbance rather than of a systemic disorder involving changes in the blood level of an active enzyme.

The possibility of a local disturbance causing the release or activation of a myelinolytic mechanism, and thereby being responsible for initiating the actual breakdown of the myelin sheaths in the plaques of multiple sclerosis, would be strengthened if it were known whether "myelin" exhibited any metabolic turnover, i.e. whether it is continually being broken down and resynthesized. If this were so, then demyelination might take place either as a result of a failure of resynthesis or of increased rates of breakdown induced by a local process of myelinolysis. If, on the other hand, myelin is a "stable" substance which, when once laid down, shows no appreciable rate of turnover, its disintegration in multiple sclerosis by a failure of resynthesis would be less likely, and it would seem at any rate reasonable to look for some myelinolytic agent or process.

Payling Wright and his colleagues attempted to answer this question by long-term studies involving the injection of radioactive cholesterol, serine (a precursor of sphingosine) and inorganic phosphate into young animals at a time when myelination is proceeding rapidly; they then killed the animals at intervals of up to 200 days and longer following the injection, and measured the amount of radioactivity still remaining in the lipids of the central nervous system. They showed that a large proportion of the labelled cholesterol, for example, persists in the brain for as long as a year after its administration, whereas in tissues such as liver, kidney or heart, it disappears relatively rapidly (Davison, Dobbing, Morgan and Payling Wright, 1958, 1959). Radioactive serine (Davison, Morgan, Wajda & Payling Wright, 1959) and phosphate (Davison & Dobbing, 1958) have also been shown to persist for long periods of time when once incorporated into brain lipids. From this and other work they have concluded that when once myelin is laid down it persists with relatively little evidence of turnover for long periods of time (see Payling Wright, 1961). If this is so, and there is now considerable evidence in support of this view, it could be argued that the demyelination occurring in the plaques is therefore more likely to be due to a simple lysis by some locally released agent of the metabolically stable and inert proteolipid layers of the myelin sheath. At the same time, it must be realized that such an agent might be released from, say, the neighbouring oligodendrocytes as a result of some process affecting the energy-yielding reactions in these cells.

As regards the nature of this postulated lytic substance, Morrison & Zamecnik (1950), and Birkmayer & Neumayer (1957), have shown experimentally that both lysolecithin and phospholipase A, the enzyme that forms lysolecithin from lecithin, can cause demyelinating changes in isolated segments of central nervous tissue under *in vitro* conditions, and they have suggested (see also Debuch, 1957) that lysolecithin or some other lysophosphatide may be the agent concerned in the production of the plaques of demyelination in multiple sclerosis. It is of interest therefore that small amounts of lysolecithin have now been identified as a normal component of brain tissue (Thompson, Niemiro & Webster, 1960; Papadopoulos, Cevallos & Hess, 1960; Blomstrand & Nakayama, 1961; Webster & Thompson, 1962). Moreover, both phospholipase A, an enzyme capable of forming lysophosphatides, and phospholipase B, an enzyme that breaks down lysolecithin to glycerylphosphorylcholine and free fatty acid, are also both present in brain tissue (Gallai-Hatchard, Magee, Thompson & Webster, 1962; Marples & Thompson, 1960).

While these observations may eventually throw light on processes concerned in myelin metabolism, it is not possible at present to relate these findings in any direct way to the problem of the aetiology of multiple sclerosis.

(5) *Viral infection.* It will be apparent from the variety of different aetiological possibilities which have from time to time been considered that no

agreement has yet been reached regarding the pathogenesis of multiple sclerosis. It is clear, however, that whatever view is finally adopted it must take into account the striking variations in geographical distribution of the disease. A theoretically possible explanation of these regional variations might be that the disease is due primarily to an infective agent such as a virus. However, repeated attempts to demonstrate an infective agent have been unsuccessful, and the pathology of the lesions does not obviously support the conception of a reaction to such an infective agent.

The detailed discussion of this approach is outside the scope of this book, but the analogy of certain naturally occurring diseases of sheep, together with recent work on circulating viral antibodies, is sufficient to indicate that the possibility of infection with a virus cannot be ruled out as a causative agency.

(6) *Dietary causes.* Variations in nutritional habits might be expected to be another environmental factor that might operate to different extents in different parts of the world. Dietary customs are known to vary with climate and latitude, and the view has been put forward that the high prevalence of multiple sclerosis in certain parts of the world may be related to the high intake of animal fats (Swank & Backer, 1950; Swank, Lerstad, Strom & Backer, 1952; Swank, 1961).

Sinclair (1956), however, has stressed the possible importance of a deficiency of unsaturated fatty acids rather than an excess of saturated animal fats, and it is of interest that, as mentioned earlier (see p. 468) low levels of plasma linoleate are found in patients in the active phases of the disease (Baker *et al.*, 1964, 1965, 1966).

The relationship between these changes in plasma linoleate and the development of the demyelinated plaques in the central nervous system is obscure, but Clausen & Moller (1967) have recently shown that rats raised on a diet deficient in polyunsaturated fatty acids exhibit an increased susceptibility to the development of allergic encephalomyelitis induced by the subcutaneous injection of guinea-pig brain homogenate. There is, furthermore, evidence suggesting that saturated and polyunsaturated fatty acids differ strikingly in the effects which they exert on blood platelet aggregation and stability (Kerr, MacAulay, Pirie & Bronte-Stewart, 1965; Shore & Alpers, 1963), and it has also been established by several groups of workers that platelet adhesiveness is increased in patients with multiple sclerosis (Nathanson & Savitsky, 1954; Fog,

Kristensen & Helweg-Larsen, 1955; Caspary, Prineas, Miller & Field, 1965; Wright, Thompson & Zilkha, 1965; Millar, Merrett & Dalby, 1966).

It is not possible on present evidence to formulate any clear-cut aetiological hypothesis embodying these various findings, although Thompson (1966) has discussed them more fully in relation both to the nutritional possibilities mentioned above and to Putnam's platelet microthrombi (see p. 467).

More recently, Millac (1967*a*) has claimed that there is a significant correlation between the extent of the disease, as evidenced by clinical disability, and the increase in adhesiveness. He has, however, also found increased platelet adhesiveness in patients with invasive intracerebral tumours (Millac, 1967*b*) and has suggested that the platelet changes are due to acute degradation of neural tissue.

Diffuse Sclerosis

A number of disorders, occurring infrequently, have been grouped together under the term diffuse sclerosis, in only some of which is there acute demyelination. Attempts at classification, such as that of Greenfield (1950), are all open to some criticism. It is probably advantageous to exclude all cases involving abnormalities of sphingolipid metabolism and to include these and the cases of amaurotic family idiocy together under the general term of the sphingolipidoses (see below).

The *sudanophil* variety, seen in both children and adults, shows widespread demyelination, but with sparing of the U fibres. There is a severe loss of myelin in the white matter with the presence of esterified cholesterol in varying amounts dependent upon the stage of the disease process. There are raised total and water-soluble hexosamine levels in the white matter, but the cerebral cortex shows little variation from the normal (Cumings, 1953, 1962).

The *Pelizaeus-Merzbacher* type occurs in rather older children, and some areas of perivascular myelination still persist. Here there is a diminution of cerebral lipids in the white matter; in the cerebral cortex there is only a slight loss of lipids, but with the presence of cholesterol esters (Blackwood & Cumings, 1954).

The *spongy* (Canavan) type, which is a very rare condition commencing in early infancy and inherited in a recessive manner, has been shown to be associated with a very low level of phospholipids, cerebroside and cholesterol (i.e. of the myelin lipids) in the brain (Blackwood & Cumings, 1954). It was thought by these authors that maturation of myelin did not take place, and van

Bogaert & Bertrand (1949) from histological studies concluded that the condition was a degenerative one, possibly abiotrophic in nature.

SPHINGOLIPIDOSES

A number of disorders are now known to occur in which a sphingolipid is predominently involved, and in some of which an enzymic abnormality is now known to be present. These conditions include Gaucher's disease, Niemann-Pick's disease, Tay-Sachs' disease, other forms of amaurotic family idiocy, metachromatic leucodystrophy and the Krabbe or globoid body type of diffuse sclerosis.

Cerebral changes are only rarely encountered in *Gaucher's* disease and *Niemann-Pick's* disease, and few biochemical studies have been made. The few cases of *Gaucher's* disease studied have shown a slight increase in cerebral cerebrosides which on further study were shown to contain both glucose and galactose (Maloney & Cumings, 1960), whereas normal brain cerebrosides contain only the latter hexose. The finding of the presence of glucose agrees with the analysis of the splenic cerebrosides in this disease for these contain large amounts of glucose.

In *Niemann-Pick's* disease there is some increase of sphingomyelin in the brain, together with a raised level of cholesterol. The most striking feature is, however, an increase of ganglioside in both white matter and cerebral cortex, and on examination by thin-layer chromatography (TLC) two fast moving bands (G_{M3} and G_{M4}) are present (Booth, Goodwin & Cumings, 1966). A similar ganglioside pattern is seen on TLC in lipid extracts of the liver and spleen. In both this condition and in Gaucher's disease there is a widespread distribution of the lipid disorder so that they can be regarded as examples of generalized sphingolipidoses.

Originally, the form of cerebral lipidosis occurring most commonly went under the title of *Amaurotic family idiocy* (AFI), but in recent years more exact biochemical and electron microscopic studies have resulted in a more definite terminology than one relying upon age or the existence of a cherry-red macula.

Tay-Sachs' Disease

This condition, occurring in very young infants, frequently of Jewish origin, and with a relatively high level of multiple sibship affection, is inherited in an autosomal recessive manner.

The examination of the level of aldolase (Aronson, Perle, Saifer & Volk, 1962) showed an almost complete absence, whereas in other forms of AFI the enzyme is not significantly reduced. The parents of the patient also showed a reduction in the level of the enzyme.

Klenk, examining cerebral tissue from subjects with this disease (Klenk, 1939–40; Klenk & Langerbeins, 1941), found raised levels of ganglioside, using neuraminic acid as an index of its increase. This finding has been confirmed by many authors since, but the white matter did not appear at first to show any significant abnormality relating to gangliosides. However, with the introduction of thin-layer chromatography an absolutely diagnostic feature has been demonstrated. Müldner, Wherrett & Cumings (1962) and Svennerholm (1962) showed that there is a very considerable increase of a monosialoganglioside (G_{M2}), in which there are two moles of hexose instead of the normal three to each mole of sphingosine present in the ganglioside. Wherrett & Cumings (1963) showed that some 85% of the total N-acetylneuraminic acid is present in this specific band. This abnormality has not been detected in any other lipid disorder. It is of interest that one of us (J.N.C.) has demonstrated this abnormality in the cerebral white matter, in the liver and in peripheral nerve. Gangliosides are present only in the microsomal fraction of brain extracts (Thompson, Goodwin & Cumings, 1967) and this is true also of the Tay-Sachs' G_{M2} fraction.

There is a varying loss of phospholipid in the brain in this condition (Klenk, 1939–40; Thannhauser, 1950; Cumings, 1965a).

It would appear probable that there is an enzymic defect involving a defective galactose-transferring enzyme, which results in an accumulation of G_{M2}. There are other possibilities but all suggest an abnormality in carbohydrate metabolism.

Other Forms of Amaurotic Family Idiocy

Patients with AFI may be of any age, for although most are children some are adults. There is in all a generalized loss of cerebral lipids with no special increase in ganglioside content. However the level of gangliosides is not depressed in proportion to the lipid level; in fact it may be normal (Cumings, 1953, 1965a).

There are now a number of case records of a more generalized lipid disorder, usually termed generalized gangliosidosis (O'Brien, Stern, Landing, O'Brien & Donnell, 1965). There is in this condition a deposition of a ganglioside in the liver, kidney and spleen, which these authors have shown by thin-layer chromatography to be a monosialoganglioside (G_{M1}). Other cases have been seen in which a disialoganglioside was the dominant ganglioside present and this too may be present in the organs (Cumings—personal observation).

The conditions so far described are all due to an enzymic defect, which has been postulated and in some instances verified. In Gaucher's disease there is a very considerable lack of glucocerebrosidase, while in Niemann-Pick's disease sphingomyelinase is grossly reduced. These changes can be demonstrated by an examination of the leucocytes of the patient's blood (Brady, 1967). It is suggested that a reduction in galactosyl transferase may result in the accumulation of G_{M2} in Tay-Sachs' disease, while a somewhat similar enzyme defect at a later stage in the metabolic cycle would result in a relative accumulation of the G_{M1} ganglioside.

Metachromatic Leucodystrophy

This condition, although most commonly affecting children, may also occur in later life. Males are more frequently affected, more than one member of the family may suffer from the condition, and inheritance is by a recessive gene.

The condition was regarded by Poser (1961) as dysmyelinitic in nature for there is a reduction in the normal myelin lipids, but without a significant amount of cholesterol ester. An increase in hexosamine was found originally (Edgar, 1957; Cumings, 1957), but more recently it has been demonstrated that there is a marked increase in sulphatides with a corresponding severe reduction in cerebrosides (Austin, 1959; Black & Cumings, 1961; Mossakowski, Mathieson & Cumings, 1961).

It has been known for some time that the results of the metabolic abnormality can be seen in various parts of the body. The nerves show a reduction in conduction velocity (Fullerton, 1964), and Austin (1957) found that the urine contains intracellular metachromatic material. Abnormal amounts of urinary sulphatide have also been observed (Cumings, 1965b). In 1963 Austin and his colleagues found a reduced amount of the enzyme arylsulphatase in the urine, while further details of the methods employed and results obtained were published by Austin, Armstrong, Shearer & McAfee (1966) in which a deficiency of sulphatase A was found.

Edgar (1957) originally suggested that the condition was an inborn error of metabolism and it was later suggested that it was a genetically determined metabolic defect of enzymic origin (Cumings, 1960). These suggestions have been fully confirmed by Austin and his co-workers and by Jatzkewitz and Mehl. The former group

(Austin, McAfee, Armstrong, O'Rourke, Shearer & Bachhawat, 1964; Austin, McAfee & Shearer, 1965) demonstrated a deficiency in arylsulphatase A in the brain, kidney and liver, while in some cases arylsulphatases B and C were also reduced. Mehl & Jatzkewitz (1965) claimed from their experiments that only one enzyme, cerebrosidesulphatase was deficient, and the same authors have shown arylsulphatase A to be part of cerebrosidesulphatase.

One further abnormality has been described by O'Brien (1964), who found a defect in synthesis of cerebrosides containing long-chain fatty acids.

Recent experimental work on myelin prepared from the white matter of cases of metachromatic leucodystrophy has shown a very much greater amount of sulphatide relative to cerebroside (20:1 as sphingosine) compared with examination of normal myelin when the ratio is 1 : 4. It is also of interest that a small amount of ganglioside is also present in myelin whereas normal myelin does not contain any (Cumings, Thompson & Goodwin, 1968).

Krabbe or Globoid Body Disease

This condition occurs in very young children who usually die by the age of 3 years; there is a peculiar and characteristic histological appearance of globoid cells or bodies staining positively with PAS, which suggested to Hallervorden (1950) that they were composed of kerasin. The cerebrospinal fluid almost invariably contains more than 100 mg. of protein per 100 ml.

There is a general loss of phospholipids and cholesterol but without esterified cholesterol being present. Cerebrosides and sulphatides are reduced although not to the same extent as the phospholipids, with a raised cerebroside to sulphatide ratio in the white matter (Austin, 1963; Menkes, Duncan & Moossy, 1966). Menkes et al. have also shown an increase in ceramide di- and trihexoside in the white matter and Cumings et al. (1968) have also found raised levels of ceramide dihexoside.

Austin, Armstrong & Shearer (1965) found that levels of β-galactosidase and of soluble sulphatases were well maintained in the brain, while more recently Bachhawat, Austin & Armstrong (1967) found that cerebroside sulphotransferase was considerably reduced in the white matter from cases of this disease.

It is of interest that the ganglioside pattern of a lipid extract of the cerebral cortex is similar to that seen in Niemann-Pick's disease with the presence of bands G_{M3} and G_{M4} (Booth et al. 1966).

Austin (1962), by injecting cerebroside into normal rat brain, obtained bodies, containing PAS positive material, which were very similar to typical globoid bodies.

REFSUM'S DISEASE

Refsum (1945, 1946) described a condition, inherited by a rare recessive gene, which he named heredopathia atactica polyneuritiformis, but which in recent literature usually bears his name. Parental consanguinity and affection of more than one sib of normal parents is not uncommon. The striking clinical features are a retinitis pigmentosa, polyneuritis and a raised protein in the cerebrospinal fluid. Cammermeyer (1956) supported the view of Refsum (1946) that the condition was akin to the lipidoses.

Until 1963 the only biochemical abnormality found was the raised CSF protein, but in that year it was reported that phytanic acid (3,7,11,15-tetramethylhexadecanoic acid) was present in excess in the liver, kidney and blood serum of patients (Klenk & Kahlke, 1963; Richterich, Kahlke, van Mechelen & Rossi, 1963; Kahlke, 1963). Since that date a number of other workers have reviewed cases and have reported similar findings (Nevin, Cumings & McKeown, 1967). Phytanic acid has also been found in excess in muscle, fat and nerve as well as in the liver, although no increase has been detected in the brain (Cumings, personal observations).

The cause of the abnormalities would appear to be an inborn defect in the degradation pathway concerned with branched chain fatty acids. Eldjarn (1965) suggested a defect in omega oxidation of fatty acids, but later it was reported that a pathway involving a CO_2-fixation mechanism is lacking in subjects with Refsum's disease (Eldjarn, Try & Stokke, 1966a).

An attempt has been made to alter the abnormal metabolism by means of a dietary restriction of precursors of phytanic acid (Eldjarn, Try, Stokke, Munthe-Kaas, Refsum, Steinberg, Avigan & Mize, 1966b). Foods containing chlorophyll and other substances known to have a high content of phytol were omitted from the diet. Two patients were treated on this type of regime and serum phytanic acid levels followed. One patient showed a considerable fall, and the other a lesser fall in the level of this acid, but clinical improvement was not so marked. Remissions and relapses are well known in this condition so that evaluation of such findings are very difficult to assess accurately. Others have tried a similar dietary restriction but without significant success.

Many other biochemical estimations have been made, such as serum copper, caeruloplasmin, phosphocreatine kinase and proteins but none has yielded any consistent abnormalities.

HEPATOLENTICULAR DEGENERATION

In 1912 Kinnier Wilson described a clinical entity, often called after him, exhibiting muscular rigidity, tremor and incoordination, and involving damage to both the basal ganglia and the liver. It was later found that many patients suffering from this condition also show the presence of a zone of golden-brown pigmentation in the cornea, now known as the Kayser-Fleischer ring. There have been many speculations as to the chemical nature of this pigment, and it has been suggested at different times that deposits of iron, silver or copper are responsible for its appearance.

The condition mainly occurs in adolescents and young adults, but older adults in the third to fifth decades may also be affected. There is also another group of adult patients who show involuntary movements but no Kayser-Fleischer ring and none of the abnormal biochemical features that have so far been found, and which are discussed below; these cases should not be regarded as examples of hepatolenticular degeneration.

Wilson's disease is now known to be a metabolic disorder, and one in which, as shown by Bearn (1953), there is a strong suggestion that it is inherited in an autosomal recessive manner. The underlying metabolic characteristic of the disease appears to be an accumulation of copper in the tissues.

Brain and Liver Copper

Most organs of the body contain copper usually combined with a protein. Porter & Folch (1957a, b) have described three different Cu protein compounds; the major portion of the Cu in the brain is present in the fraction named cerebrocuprein I. Similarly in the liver there is at least one related protein, but with certain different characteristics to those of cerebrocuprein (Morell, Shapiro & Scheinberg, 1961).

Porter, Sweeney & Porter (1964) have isolated a mitochondrocuprein in neonatal liver which contains 10 times the copper content of other liver copper complexes. The level of this copper compound is rapidly lowered in the first weeks of life.

The distribution of the metal within the brain is widespread as shown originally by Tingey (1937) and Cumings (1948). Warren, Earl & Thompson (1960) have made a more extensive survey and report that the cerebral cortex throughout has a higher Cu content than the white matter. They also found very high concentrations of Cu in the substantia nigra and the locus caeruleus, areas not previously examined in any detail.

Rumpel (1913) and Haurowitz (1930) were among the first to show that the livers and brains of patients suffering from Wilson's disease contain excess Cu. This finding has since been amply confirmed by Luthy (1932), Glazebrook (1945), Cumings (1948, 1954), Spillane, Keyser & Parker (1952) and Cartwright, Hodges, Gubler, Mahoney, Daum, Wintrobe & Bean (1954). The last-named workers have also given figures for some other organs. Table 13.6 shows the range of values obtained. This increased Cu content is present in

TABLE 13.6

Copper content of tissues in normal subjects and in patients with hepatolenticular degeneration

(All figures in mg./100 g. dry tissue)

Tissue	Normal	Hepato-lenticular degeneration
Brain frontal cortex	1–8	4–45
Brain frontal white	1–8	10–25
Brain globus pallidus	10–18	10–40
Brain putamen	6–12	30–70
Brain thalamus	3–12	20–60
Brain caudate nucleus	3–9	10–32
Brain stem	1·0	24
Spinal cord	1·0	10
Liver	5–17	30–160
Kidney	1	4–28

almost all areas of the brain so far examined, including the medulla and the cerebral cortex as well as the basal ganglia, which may be strikingly affected to naked eye examination and which may contain a 10-fold excess of Cu.

Porter (1961) has reviewed the distribution of the cerebral Cu proteins in Wilson's disease, and he has shown that cerebrocuprein I, although containing the major part of the Cu, does not have identical properties with normal cerebrocuprein I. It is more labile and some of the Cu appears to be bound to different brain proteins, since electrophoretically these proteins have mobilities similar to those of plasma β-globulins.

Urinary Copper

The first report of increased excretion of Cu in the urine in Wilson's disease arose from a chance observation made by Mandelbrote, Stanier, Thompson & Thruston in 1948, and it is now established that in this condition an increased urinary excretion of Cu is present in all advanced cases (Cumings, 1951, 1954; Denny-Brown & Porter, 1951; Matthews, Milne & Bell, 1952; Spillane *et al.* 1952; Warnock & Neill, 1954). Copper excretion may rise from the normal level, which has been variously estimated as from 10 to 100 μg. Cu/day, to values of 400 to 600 μg./day or higher, although one *early* case has been reported in which Cu excretion was not excessive (Cumings, 1951).

Amino-aciduria

An amino-aciduria is also present in this disease (Uzman & Denny-Brown, 1948), although two cases have been recorded in which the only urinary abnormality to be found was the increased Cu excretion (Cumings, 1951; Cartwright *et al.* 1954). There is usually an increase in the excretion of all the amino acids normally found in urine, up to a total of as much as 300 to 800 mg./day. In some cases proline and citrulline may also be present (Dent & Harris, 1951; Stein, Bearn & Moore, 1954). Conditions showing involuntary movements, but which are not examples of hepatolenticular degeneration, do not exhibit either amino-aciduria or increased copper excretion. A fuller account of the amino-aciduria in this condition is given on p. 598.

Blood Copper

Plasma normally contains about 80 to 130 μg. Cu/100 ml.; most of this Cu is firmly bound to protein (Mann & Keilin, 1938) and the action of acids is needed to liberate it. A very small amount of the plasma Cu, less than 5% of the total, is more loosely bound to protein, and is capable of reacting directly with Na diethyldithiocarbamate, the reagent commonly used for Cu estimations; most of the Cu present in the cerebrospinal fluid is in the direct-reacting form (Cartwright *et al.* 1954).

In Wilson's disease the total plasma Cu level is reduced to values of about 40 to 60 μg. Cu/100 ml. (Bearn, 1953; Lahey, Gubler, Cartwright & Wintrobe, 1953; Bearn & Kunkel, 1954a).

It was found both by Bearn & Kunkel (1954a) and by Cumings, Goodwin & Earl (1955) that only about 40 to 60% of the total blood Cu is attached to the globulins. Cartwright *et al.* (1954) have, in addition, shown that there is an increase in the amount of direct-reacting Cu in the plasma, which presumably corresponds to this fraction loosely bound to albumin, so that the reduction in the firmly bound indirect-reacting fraction is even more marked than is indicated by the reduced total plasma Cu level.

Copper Proteins

Copper is present in the body combined with a number of proteins and some but not all possess enzymic properties. These copper protein complexes include caeruloplasmin, cerebrocuprein, hepatocuprein and tyrosinase.

Caeruloplasmin

Holmberg & Laurell in 1948 isolated from both pig and human blood a blue Cu protein with a molecular weight of about 150,000, the Cu being combined with an α_2-globulin. They named this compound caeruloplasmin, and showed later, using p-phenylenediamine as substrate, that it can act as an oxidase (Holmberg & Laurell, 1951). Scheinberg & Gitlin (1952), using immunological as well as chemical methods, showed that there was a lowered caeruloplasmin level in the blood in Wilson's disease, accompanied by an absence of oxidase activity. This latter finding has been confirmed by Bearn & Kunkel (1954a) and Cumings et al. (1955).

Recent work on caeruloplasmin has been mainly related either to the preparation of pure caeruloplasmin (Sanders, Miller & Richard, 1959; Curzon & Vallet, 1960; Deutsch, 1960) or to a study of its properties. It has been found from chromatographic studies of purified caeruloplasmin that, although in the adult there is one main component, there may be up to three minor fractions (Broman, 1958; Morell & Scheinberg, 1960). Although caeruloplasmin has oxidase properties *in vitro*, there is no proof that it acts in this way *in vivo*. Another remarkable characteristic is the effect of EDTA (Curzon, 1961a), probably related to the sensitivity to iron (Curzon, 1961b). In the presence of iron a coupled Fe-caeruloplasmin oxidation system is formed. It has been suggested that of the eight Cu atoms in caeruloplasmin four are in a more active and available state (Scheinberg & Sternlieb, 1960b). Further studies indicate a highly complex arrangement of its Cu atoms, but one possible arrangement of four valence-changing copper atoms of reduced caeruloplasmin would make possible an explanation for inhibition by a single azide group (Curzon & Cumings, 1966). Cyanide has also been shown to be an inhibitor as powerful as azide even if its mode of action is not identical. It has recently been suggested that there may be only seven Cu atoms (Morell, van den Hamer & Scheinberg, 1966) but further work is necessary before this view can be accepted.

Treatment

In view of the accumulation of Cu in the brain, liver and other tissues, numerous attempts have been made to treat Wilson's disease with dimercaprol (BAL) since both McCance & Widdowson (1946) and Mandelbrote et al. (1948) had shown that this compound can produce an increased urinary excretion of Cu in man. The earliest reports on the effects of this treatment came from Cumings (1951) and Denny-Brown & Porter (1951). The dosage suggested at the present time is 2·5 mg./kg. twice daily for 5 days, these courses being repeated at intervals of 10 days. Clinically it has been concluded that definite improvement results, particularly in patients of the young adult or older age groups.

Versene has not proved so useful a therapeutic tool as had at first been hoped, but potassium sulphide, given by mouth, can play a valuable part in diminishing Cu absorption.

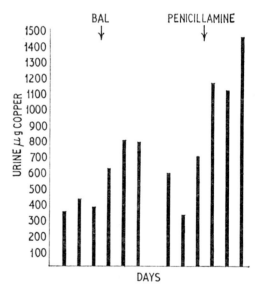

FIG. 13.3. Effect on the urinary excretion of copper by patients with Wilson's disease of treatment with British Anti-Lewisite (BAL) or penicillamine. (By permission of the Editor, *Proceedings of the Nutritional Society*.)

In 1956 Walshe introduced penicillamine ($\beta\beta'$-dimethylcysteine) as a therapeutic tool. The value of this substance, which is given orally and very rarely produces any toxic changes, has been proved by very many workers (Fister, Boulding & Baker, 1958; Osborn & Walshe, 1958; Scheinberg & Sternlieb, 1960a). The effect of BAL and penicillamine on the urinary Cu excretion of patients with Wilson's disease is shown in Fig. 13.3.

There are now a number of patients who have responded very well to therapy and who have survived for 10 years or more (Cumings, 1968). Neurological abnormalities are minimal but in most if not all, evidence of cirrhosis of the liver persists. The Kayser-Fleischer ring, while still present, often diminishes in intensity of colour indicating a reduction of copper content.

Variation from the Normal Picture

There are now many records of young children whose first symptom was jaundice and who showed no abnormal neurological signs (Chalmers, Iber & Uzman, 1957; Sass-Kortsak, Glatt, Cherniak & Cederlund, 1961). These children show a post-necrotic cirrhosis on histological examination of the liver, a raised liver copper (Cumings, 1968) and sometimes blood and urine copper levels consistent with Wilson's disease. These children respond well to penicillamine.

Recently McIntyre, Clink, Levi, Cumings & Sherlock (1967) have described three patients in whom Wilson's disease presented with evidence of acute haemolytic episodes. They record similar cases from the literature and suggest that the possible explanation may be the sudden release of copper from the tissues into the blood which results in red cell haemolysis. Some of these patients also improve with penicillamine therapy.

The Nature of the Biochemical Lesion

Most of the recent work on this disease has been directed to elucidating the reasons for these rather remarkable biochemical findings; one in particular has caused much thought, namely, how is it that on the one hand there is excessive urinary excretion of Cu associated with low levels of Cu and caeruloplasmin in the blood, while on the other hand more Cu is retained in the tissues in this disease? Some light has been thrown on this question by means of studies with radioactive copper (^{64}Cu) carried out by Earl, Moulton & Selverstone (1954) and by Bearn & Kunkel (1954b). These workers found that in normal subjects the administered ^{64}Cu first became attached to the plasma albumin fraction, but after 24 hr. it became transferred to the globulin fraction which normally contains the caeruloplasmin. In the patients with Wilson's disease this transfer to the globulin fraction was either very slow or did not take place. It has been suggested therefore that the underlying fault in this condi-

tion may be a failure to synthesize caeruloplasmin at the normal rate. This would be consistent with the decrease in the amount of indirect-reacting globulin-bound Cu in the plasma of these patients. As a result of this failure, most of the absorbed Cu remains "unattached" and free to combine in other ways, such as with the proteins of the brain and liver, or to be excreted by the kidney. If this is so, however, the accumulation of Cu in the tissues, coupled with the increased urinary excretion, must imply that the lowered caeruloplasmin levels result also in increased absorption of dietary Cu. Zimdahl, Hyman & Cook (1953), in a balance experiment, found that there was increased absorption of Cu from the gut, and this was the basis for the use of potassium sulphide therapeutically. Using radioactive Cu Matthews (1954) found a higher percentage of administered ^{64}Cu in the faeces of control subjects than in those of patients with hepatolenticular degeneration, while the urine of these patients contained relatively more of the isotopic Cu than in normal subjects. Cartwright et al. (1954) have shown the presence of a positive Cu balance in four of their patients with Wilson's disease.

Uzman & Hood (1952) and Uzman (1953), examining the urine of patients with this disease, have obtained a polypeptide to which the Cu is linked, and have suggested that such peptides may also be present in the blood. However, one of us (J.N.C.) has been unable to locate Cu in the blood apart from the albumin or globulin fractions.

The nature of the Kayser-Fleischer ring is still somewhat obscure. It has been suggested that Cu is deposited in the cornea where it forms the characteristic zone of granules (Gerlach & Rohrschneider, 1934; Brand & Takáts, 1951; Denny-Brown & Porter, 1951).

Our knowledge of the full metabolic abnormality in this disease is still incomplete, but it may be useful even at this stage to summarize the known facts and to state the working hypothesis that has emerged from them. First, it appears possible that there is an increased absorption of Cu from the gut, but whether or not this is a secondary phenomenon is not known. There is also a failure in the synthesis of caeruloplasmin resulting from a failure to transfer the absorbed Cu from albumin to the appropriate globulin. However, the actual function of caeruloplasmin in this disease is still uncertain and no final decision as to its role can yet be reached. It is nevertheless certain that the Cu attached to the albumin, being more labile, is readily bound to the tissue proteins and is also excreted in the urine in excess of normal, being chelated by amino acids and peptides. The deposits of Cu in the brain and liver cause the characteristic functional and pathological changes in these organs, while its accumulation in the kidney causes a functional impairment in the reabsorption of amino acids and peptides which are accordingly excreted in greater amounts than normal.

PARKINSON'S DISEASE

It is only in the last decade, that biochemical studies in this condition have yielded results which may eventually prove of value. Most of these are related to catecholamine metabolism, but there are also some concerned with nucleic acid, especially ribonucleic acid.

Amines

Three compounds, dopamine, noradrenaline and 5-hydroxytryptamine have specially interested investigators. Dopa is synthesized from tyrosine by hydroxylation by means of tyrosine hydroxylase, and this in turn is decarboxylated to dopamine. Noradrenaline is derived from dopamine, as is homovanillic acid, the latter through a final step involving monoamine oxidase.

All three compounds are found in normal cerebral tissues in varying quantities. The basal ganglia, especially the putamen and globus pallidus, contain relatively large amounts of dopamine, but are relatively low in noradrenaline, while the red nucleus and the hypothalamus contain more adrenaline than dopamine (Bertler, 1961; Sano, Gamo, Karimoto, Taniguchi, Takesada & Nishinuma, 1959). It has also been shown by elegant fluorescent techniques (Carlsson, Falck & Hillarp, 1962; Falck, 1962) that all three compounds are present in terminal parts of axons forming synaptic contacts.

There has been found to be a variation from the normal distribution in Parkinson's disease, for when the corpus striatum has been examined in this disease low levels of dopamine and of noradrenaline have been found (Ehringer & Hornykiewicz, 1960). This was true whether the condition was post-encephalitic in origin or was idiopathic in nature. Barolin, Bernheimer & Hornykiewicz (1964) examined one patient affected unilaterally with a corresponding reduction in amine levels in the appropriate basal ganglia as compared with the normal side.

Some experimental work has been performed in animals relating to this problem. Electrocoagula-

tion of the substantia nigra of the monkey results in a fall in dopamine and noradrenaline in the striatum (Poirier & Sourkes, 1965), while in rats a similar reduction in dopamine is found (Andén, Carlsson, Dahlström, Fuxe, Hillarp & Larsson, 1964). These workers (1965a,b) have shown that the catecholamine terminals are in spinal neurones with cell bodies in the lower brain stem.

Reserpine, which depletes the brain of catecholamines, produces a parkinson-like condition in rabbits, and this can be reversed by dopa (Carlsson, 1959). The caudate nucleus is rich in dopa decarboxylase (Kuntsman, Shore, Bogdanski & Brodie, 1961) as well as containing dopamine β-oxidase (Udenfriend & Creveling, 1959) but the distribution of the enzymes does not parallel that of the various catecholamines.

The urinary excretion of various catecholamine metabolites has been studied frequently, but without success. Urinary dopamine has been estimated in various forms of basal ganglia disorder (Sourkes, Murphy, Sankoff, Wiseman-Distler & Saint Cyr, 1963; Barbeau, 1960) and higher figures than normal were found in Wilson's disease but even so the level was very variable. Greer and Williams (1963) also determined homovanillic acid excretion but found no abnormality in Parkinson's disease. Numerous workers have also estimated 5-hydroxyindole acetic acid (O'Reilly, Loncin & Cooksey, 1965; Barbeau, Jasmin & Duchastel, 1963) but the results have usually indicated that there is no variation from the normal.

Some patients who had been treated surgically by pallidotomy have not shown abnormal urinary levels of catecholamines (Nashold & Kirshner, 1963), while others have demonstrated raised urinary levels of dopamine (Westlake & Tew, 1966).

Nucleic Acid

Hydén has employed a number of elegant techniques to study quantitatively the amounts of ribonucleic acid (RNA) and of adenine, guanine, cytosine and uracil in isolated single nerve cells. Gomirato & Hydén (1963) have applied these techniques to cases of Parkinson's disease. They found that in cerebral biopsy material from the basal ganglia there were increased amounts of RNA in both glial cells and neurones in disease. The glial RNA base composition showed an increased amount of adenine with a reduced uracil and guanine, but the composition of the neuronal RNA was not altered.

References

ABERCROMBIE, M. & JOHNSON, M. L. (1946). *J. Neurol. Neurosurg. Psychiat.*, **9**, 113.

ALDRIDGE, W. N. (1954). *Biochem. J.*, **56**, 185.

ALDRIDGE, W. N., BARNES, J. M. & JOHNSON, M. K. (1969). *Proc. N.Y. Acad. Sci.*, in press

ALEXANDER, B. & LANDWEHR, G. (1945). *Science*, **101**, 229.

ALTMANN, O. & GOLDHAMMER, H. (1937). *Klin. Wschr.*, **16**, 1017.

ANDÉN, N-E., CARLSSON, A., DAHLSTRÖM, A., FUXE, K., HILLARP, N-Å. & LARSSON, K. (1964). *Life Sciences*, **3**, 523.

ANDÉN, N-E., DAHLSTRÖM, A., FUXE, K. & LARSSON, K. (1965a). *Amer. J. Anat.*, **116**, 329.

ANDÉN, N-E., DAHLSTRÖM, A., FUXE, K. & LARSSON, K. (1965b). *Life Sciences*, **4**, 1275.

ANTHONY, M., HINTERBERGER, H. & LANCE, J. W. (1967). *Arch. Neurol.* (Chicago), **16**, 544.

ARONSON, S. M., PERLE, G., SAIFER, A. & VOLK, B. W. (1962). *Proc. Soc. exp. Biol. N.Y.*, **111**, 664.

AUSTIN, J. H. (1957). *Neurology* (Minneap.), **7**, 716.

AUSTIN, J. H. (1959). *Proc. Soc. exp. Biol. N.Y.*, **100**, 361.

AUSTIN, J. H. (1962). In "Proceeding of IV International Congress of Neuropathology", Volume 1, p. 35. Ed. Jacob, H. Stuttgart, Georg Thieme Verlag.

AUSTIN, J. H. (1963). *Arch. Neurol.* (Chicago), **9**, 207.

AUSTIN, J., ARMSTRONG, D. & SHEARER, L. (1965). *Arch. Neurol.* (Chicago), **13**, 593.

AUSTIN, J., ARMSTRONG, D., SHEARER, L. & MCAFEE, D. (1966). *Arch. Neurol.* (Chicago), **14**, 259.

AUSTIN, J. H., BALASUBRAMANIAN, A. S., PATTABIRAMAN, T. N., SARASWATHI, S., BASU, D. K. & BACHHAWAT, B. K. (1963). *J. Neurochem.*, **10**, 805.

AUSTIN, J., MCAFEE, D., ARMSTRONG, D., O'ROURKE, M., SHEARER, L. & BACHHAWAT, B. (1964). *Biochem. J.*, **93**, 15C.

AUSTIN, J., MCAFEE, D. & SHEARER, L. (1965). *Arch. Neurol.* (Chicago), **12**, 447.

BACHHAWAT, B. K., AUSTIN, J. & ARMSTRONG, D. (1967). *Biochem. J.*, **104**, 15C.

BAKER, R. W. R., SANDERS, H., THOMPSON, R. H. S. & ZILKHA, K. J. (1965). *J. Neurol. Neurosurg. Psychiat.*, **28**, 212.

BAKER, R. W. R., THOMPSON, R. H. S. & ZILKHA, K. J. (1963). *Lancet*, **1**, 26.

BAKER, R. W. R., THOMPSON, R. H. S. & ZILKHA, K. J. (1964). *J. Neurol. Neurosurg. Psychiat.*, **27**, 408.

BAKER, R. W. R., THOMPSON, R. H. S. & ZILKHA, K. J. (1966). *J. Neurol. Neurosurg. Psychiat.*, **29**, 95.

BANISTER, J. & SCRASE, M. (1950). *J. Physiol.*, **111**, 437.

BARBEAU, A. (1960). *Neurology* (Minneap.), **10**, 446.

BARBEAU, A., JASMIN, G. & DUCHASTEL, Y. (1963). *Neurology* (Minneap.), **13**, 56.

BARNES, J. M. & DENZ, F. A. (1953). *J. Path. Bact.*, **65**, 597.

BAROLIN, G. S., BERNHEIMER, H. & HORNYKIEWICZ, O. (1964). *Schweiz. Arch. Neurol. Psychiat.*, **94**, 241.

BARON, R. L., BENNETT, D. R. & CASIDA, J. E. (1962). *Brit. J. Pharmacol.*, **18**, 465.

BAUER, H. (1956). *Biochem. Z.*, **327**, 491.

BEARN, A. G. (1953). *Amer. J. Med.*, **15**, 442.

BEARN, A. G. & KUNKEL, H. G. (1954a). *J. clin. Invest.*, **33**, 400.

BEARN, A. G. & KUNKEL, H. G. (1954b). *Proc. Soc. exp. Biol.*, (N.Y.), **85**, 44.

BENNETTS, H. W. & BECK, A. B. (1942). *Bull. Coun. Sci. Industr. Res. Aust.*, No. 147.

BENNETTS, H. W. & CHAPMAN, F. E. (1937). *Aust. vet. J.*, **13**, 138.

BENTLEY, H. R., MCDERMOTT, E. E., PACE, J., WHITEHEAD, J. K. & MORAN, T. (1950). *Nature*, (Lond.), **165**, 150.

BERTLER, A. (1961). *Acta physiol. Scand.*, **51**, 97.

BIDSTRUP, P. L., BONNELL, J. A. & BECKETT, A. G. (1953). *Brit. med. J.*, i, 1068.

BIRKMAYER, W. & NEUMAYER, E. (1957). *Deutsch. Z. f. Nervenheilk*, **177**, 117.

BLACK, J. W. & CUMINGS, J. N. (1961). *J. Neurol. Neurosurg. Psychiat.*, **24**, 233.

BLACKWELL, B. (1963). *Lancet*, **2**, 849.

BLACKWELL, B. & MARLEY, E. (1964). *Lancet*, **1**, 530.

BLACKWOOD, W. & CUMINGS, J. N. (1954). *J. Neurol. Neurosurg. Psychiat.*, **17**, 33.

BLANKENHORN, M. A. & SPIES, T. D. (1935). *Trans. Ass. Amer. Phys.*, **50**, 164.

BLOCH, H. (1941). *Helv. med. Acta.*, **8**, Suppl. 7, 15.

BLOCK, R. J. (1937). *Yale J. Biol. Med.*, **9**, 445.

BLOMSTRAND, R. & NAKAYAMA, F. (1961). *J. Neurochem.*, **8**, 230.

BODIAN, D. (1947). *Symp. Soc. exp. Biol.*, **1**, 163.

BODIAN, D. & DZIEWIATKOWSKI, D. (1950). *J. cell. comp. Physiol.*, **35**, 155.

BONKALO, A. (1950). *Arch. intern. Med.*, **85**, 944.

BOOTH, D. A., GOODWIN, H. & CUMINGS, J. N. (1966). *J. Lipid. Res.*, **7**, 337.

BRADY, R. O. (1967). *Clin. Chem.*, **13**, 565.

BRAEKKAN, O., NJAA, L. R. & UTNE, F. (1957). *Acta pharmacol.* (Kbh), **13**, 228.

BRAND, I. & TAKÁTS, I. (1951). *v. Graefes Arch. Ophth.*, **151**, 391.

BRANTE, G. (1959). *Acta physiol. Scand.*, **18**, 1 (Suppl. No. 63).

BRENNER, C. & MERRITT, H. H. (1942). *Arch. Neurol. Psychiat.* (Chicago), **48**, 382.

BRICKNER, R. M. (1930). *Arch. Neurol. Psychiat.* (Chicago), **23**, 715.

BRICKNER, R. M. (1935). *Arch. Neurol. Psychiat.* (Chicago), **34**, 466.

BROMAN, L. (1958). *Nature* (Lond.), **182**, 1655.

BUCKLE, R. M. (1967). *Proc. Roy. Soc. Med.*, **60**, 48.

BUEDING, E., STEIN, M. H. & WORTIS, H. (1941). *J. biol. Chem.*, **140**, 697.

BUEDING, E. & WORTIS, H. (1940). *Proc. Soc. exp. Biol.* (N.Y.), **44**, 245.

BUEDING, E., WORTIS, H. & FEIN, H. D. (1942). *Amer. J. med. Sci.*, **204**, 838.

BUEDING, E., WORTIS, H. & STERN, M. (1942). *J. clin. Invest.*, **21**, 85.

BUTLER, E. J. (1952). *J. Neurol. Neurosurg. Psychiat.*, **15**, 119.

CAMMERMEYER, J. (1956). *J. Neuropath. exp. Neurol.*, **15**, 340.

CAMPBELL, A. M. G., HERDAN, G., TATLOW, W. E. T. & WHITTLE, E. G. (1950). *Brain*, **73**, 52.

CARLSSON, A. (1959). *Pharmacol. Rev.*, **11**, 490.

CARLSSON, A., FALCK, B. & HILLARP, N-Å. (1962). *Acta physiol. Scand.*, **56**, Suppl. 196.

CARTWRIGHT, G. E., HODGES, R. E., GUBLER, C. J., MAHONEY, J. P., DAUM, K., WINTROBE, M. M. & BEAN, W. B. (1954). *J. clin. Invest.*, **33**, 1487.

CASIDA, J. E., ETO, M. & BARON, R. L. (1961). *Nature* (Lond.), **191**, 1396.

CASPARY, E. A. & FIELD, E. J. (1963). *Nature* (Lond.), **197**, 1218.

CASPARY, E. A., PRINEAS, J., MILLER, H. & FIELD, E. J. (1965). *Lancet*, **2**, 1108.

CAVANAGH, J. B. (1954). *J. Neurol. Neurosurg. Psychiat.*, **17**, 163.

CAVANAGH, J. B. & MACDERMOT, V. (1961). *Lancet*, **2**, 583.

CAVANAGH, J. B., THOMPSON, R. H. S. & WEBSTER, G. R. (1954). *Quart. J. exp. Physiol.*, **39**, 185.

CAVANAGH, J. B. & WEBSTER, G. R. (1955). *Quart. J. exp. Physiol.*, **40**, 12.

CHALMERS, T. C., IBER, F. L. & UZMAN, L. L. (1957). *New Engl. J. Med.*, **256**, 235.

CHIAVACCI, L. V. & SPERRY, W. M. (1952). *Arch. Neurol. Psychiat.* (Chicago), **68**, 37.

CITRON, K. M. & KNOX, R. (1954). *J. gen. Microbiol.*, **10**, 482.

CLAUSEN, J. & MØLLER, J. (1967). *Acta Neurol. Scand.*, **43**, 375.

COCHRANE, N. A., PAYNE, W. W., SIMPKINS, M. J. & WOOLF, L. I. (1956). *J. clin. Invest.*, **35**, 411.

COUTEAUX, R. & NACHMANSOHN, D. (1938). *Nature* (Lond.), **142**, 481.

CRANDALL, L. A. & CHERRY, D. A. (1932). *Arch. Neurol. Psychiat.* (Chicago), **27**, 367.

CRUICKSHANK, E. K. (1952). *Vitam. & Horm.*, **10**, 1.

CUMINGS, J. N. (1948). *Brain*, **71**, 410.

CUMINGS, J. N. (1951). *Brain*, **74**, 10.

CUMINGS, J. N. (1953). *Brain*, **76**, 551.

CUMINGS, J. N. (1954). *Proc. R. Soc. Med.*, **47**, 152.

CUMINGS, J. N. (1955). *Brain*, **78**, 554.

CUMINGS, J. N. (1957). In "Cerebral Lipidoses". Eds. van Bogaert, L. Cumings, J. N. & Lowenthal, A. Blackwell, Oxford, p. 112.

CUMINGS, J. N. (1960). "In Modern Scientific Aspects of Neurology". Ed. Cumings, J. N. p. 330, London, Arnold.

CUMINGS, J. N. (1962). *J. Kansas med. Soc.*, **63**, 377.

CUMINGS, J. N. (1965a). *Proc. Roy. Soc. Med.*, **58**, 21.

CUMINGS, J. N. (1965b). In "Biochemical Aspects of Neurological Disorders", Second Series. Eds. Cumings, J. N. & Kremer, M. Oxford, Blackwell Scientific Publication, p. 229.

CUMINGS, J. N. (1968). *J. clin Path.*, **21**, 1.

CUMINGS, J. N., GOODWIN, H. J. & EARL, C. J. (1955). *J. clin. Path.*, **8**, 60.

CUMINGS, J. N., THOMPSON, E. J. & GOODWIN, H. (1968). *J. Neurochem.*, **15**, 243.

CURZON, G. (1961a) In "Wilson's Disease: Some Current Concepts". Eds. Walshe, J. M. & Cumings, J. N. Oxford, Blackwell.

CURZON, G. (1961b). *Biochem. J.*, **79**, 656.

CURZON, G. & CUMINGS, J. N. (1966). In "The Biochemistry of Copper". Eds. Peisach, J., Aisen, P. & Blumberg, W. E., Academic Press, New York & London, p. 545.

CURZON, G. & VALLET, L. (1960). *Biochem. J.*, **74**, 279.

DAVISON, A. N. (1953). *Brit. J. Pharmacol.*, **8**, 212.

DAVISON, A. N. & DOBBING, J. (1958). *Lancet*, **2**, 1158.

DAVISON, A. N., DOBBING, J., MORGAN, R. S. & PAYLING WRIGHT, G. (1958). *J. Neurochem.*, **3**, 89.

DAVISON, A. N., DOBBING, J., MORGAN, R. S. & PAYLING WRIGHT, G. (1959). *Lancet*, **1**, 658.

DAVISON, A. N., MORGAN, R. S., WAJDA, M. & PAYLING WRIGHT, G. (1959). *J. Neurochem.*, **4**, 360.

DAWSON, R. M. C. & RICHTER, D. (1950). *Amer. J. Physiol.*, **160**, 203.

DEBUCH, H. (1957). "Cerebral Lipidoses". Ed. Cumings, J. N., p. 203, Oxford, Blackwell.

DENNY-BROWN, D. & PORTER, H. (1951). *New Engl. J. Med.*, **245**, 917.

DENNY-BROWN, D. & SCIARRA, D. (1945). *Brain*, **68**, 1.

DENT, C. E. & HARRIS, H. (1951). *Ann. Eugen.*, (*Camb.*), **16**, 60.

DEUTSCH, H. F. (1960). *Arch. Biochem. Biophys.*, **89**, 225.

DOBIN, N. B. & SWITZER, J. L. (1954). *Arch. Neurol. Psychiat.* (Chicago), **71**, 405.

DOW, R. S. & BERGLUND, G. (1942). *Arch. Neurol. Psychiat.* (Chicago), **47**, 1.

DREYFUS, P. M. (1962). *New Engl. J. Med.*, **267**, 596.

DREYFUS, P. M. (1967). In "Thiamine Deficiency". Eds. Wolstenholme, G. E. W. & O'Connor, M., London, J. & A. Churchill Ltd.

DUBNOFF, J. W. (1950). *Arch. Biochem.*, **27**, 466.

DUBNOFF, J. W. (1952). *Arch. Biochem.*, **37**, 37.

DUNLOP, G., INNES, J. R. M., SHEARER, G. D. & WELLS, H. E. (1939). *J. comp. Path.*, **52**, 259.

DUNLOP, G. & WELLS, H. E. (1938). *Vet. Rec.*, **50**, 1175.

EARL, C. J., EL HAWARY, M. F. S., THOMPSON, R. H. S. & WEBSTER, G. R. (1953). *Lancet*, **1**, 115.

EARL, C. J., MOULTON, M. J. & SELVERSTONE, B. (1954). *Amer. J. Med.*, **17**, 205.

EARL, C. J. & THOMPSON, R. H. S. (1952a). *Brit. J. Pharmacol.*, **7**, 261.

EARL, C. J. & THOMPSON, R. H. S. (1952b). *Brit. J. Pharmacol.*, **7**, 685.

EARL, C. J., THOMPSON, R. H. S. & WEBSTER, G. R. (1953). *Brit. J. Pharmacol.*, **8**, 110.

EDGAR, G. W. F. (1957). In "Cerebral Lipidoses". Eds. Bogaert, L., Cumings, J. N. & Lowenthal, A. Blackwell, Oxford, p. 186.

EHRINGER, H. & HORNYKIEWICZ, O. (1960). *Klin. Wschr.*, **38**, 1236.

ELDJARN, L. (1965). *Scand. J. clin. Lab. Invest.*, **17**, 178.

ELDJARN, L., TRY, K. & STOKKE, O. (1966*a*). *Biochim. Biophys. Acta.*, **116**, 395.

ELDJARN, L., TRY, K., STOKKE, O., MUNTHE-KAAS, A. W., REFSUM, S., STEINBERG, D., AVIGAN, J. & MIZE, C. (1966*b*). *Lancet*, **1**, 691.

ELLIOTT, K. A. C. (1959). "Proc. IV Int. Congr. Biochem.", p. 251. London, Pergamon Press.

ELLIOTT, K. A. C. & PENFIELD, W. (1948). *J, Neurophysiol.*, **11**, 485.

ELSOM, K. O. (1935). *J. clin. Invest.*, **14**, 40.

ELSOM, K. O., LUKENS, F. D. W., MONTGOMERY, E. H. & JONAS, L. (1940). *J. clin. Invest.*, **19**, 153.

EPSTEIN, S. H. (1951). *Neurology*, (Minneap.), **1**, 228.

FAJANS, S. S. & CONN, J. W. (1959). *J. Lab, clin. Med.*, **45**, 811.

FALCK, B. (1962). *Acta physiol. Scand.*, **56**, Suppl. 197.

FELDBERG, W. (1943). *J. Physiol.*, **101**, 432.

FERRARO, A. (1933*a*). *Psychiat. Quart.*, **7**, 267.

FERRARO, A. (1933*b*). *Arch. Neurol. Psychiat.* (Chicago), **29**, 1364.

FERRARO, A. & JERVIS, G. A. (1940). *Arch. Neurol. Psychiat.* (Chicago), **43**, 195.

FIELD, E. J., CASPARY, E. A. & BALL, E. J. (1963). *Lancet*, **2**, 11.

FIELD, E. J. (1954). *J. Neurol. Neurosurg. Psychiat.*, **17**, 228.

FISTER, W. P., BOULDING, J. E. & BAKER, R. A. (1958). *Canad. Med. Ass. J.*, **78**, 79.

FOG, M. (1951). *Acta Psychiat.* (Kbh.), Suppl. **74**, 22.

FOG, T., KRISTENSEN, I. & HELWEG-LARSEN, H. F. (1955). *Arch. Neurol.* (Chicago), **73**, 267.

FORSTER, F. M. (1945). *Arch. Neurol. Psychiat.* (Chicago), **54**, 391.

FREEDMAN, A. M., BALES, P. D., WILLIS, A. & HIMWICH, H. E. (1949). *Amer. J. Physiol.*, **156**, 117.

FREEDMAN, D. A. & MERRITT, H. H. (1950). *Res. Publ. Ass. Nerv. Ment. Dis.*, **28**, 428.

FRISCH, C. (1937). *Wien. klin. Wschr.*, **50**, 596.

FULLERTON, P. M. (1964). *J. Neurol. Neurosurg. Psychiat.*, **27**, 100.

FULLERTON, P. M. & BARNES, J. M. (1966). *Brit. J. Industr. Med.*, **23**, 210.

FURMANSKI, A. R. (1948). *Arch. Neurol. Psychiat.* (Chicago), **60**, 270.

GALLAI-HATCHARD, J., MAGEE, W. L., THOMPSON, R. H. S. & WEBSTER, G. R. (1962). *J. Neurochem.*, **9**, 545.

GARLAND, H. (1955). *Brit. med. J.*, **2**, 1287.

GARLAND, H. & TAVENER, D. (1953). *Brit. med. J.*, **i**, 1405.

GERLACH, W. & ROHRSCHNEIDER, W. (1934). *Klin. Wschr.*, **13**, 48.

GERMON, G. (1932). "Intoxication mortelle par l'Apiol". Thèse de Paris. Quoted by Hunter, D. (1944). "Industrial Toxicology", Oxford Univ. Press.

GERSHENOVICH, Z. S., KRICHEVSKAYA, A. A. & KOLOUSEK, J. (1963). *J. Neurochem.*, **10**, 79.

GJESSING, R. (1932). *Arch. Psychiat. Nervenkrank*, **96**, 319.

GJESSING, R. (1939). *Arch. Psychiat. Nervenkrank*, **109**, 525.

GLAZEBROOK, A. J. (1945). *Edinburgh med. J.*, **52**, 83.

GOLDBERG, A., MACDONALD, A. C. & RIMINGTON, C. (1952). *Brit. med. J.*, **ii**, 1174.

GOMIRATO, G. & HYDÉN, H. (1963). *Brain*, **86**, 773.

GOODHART, R. & SINCLAIR, H. M. (1939). "C.R. IIIme Congress. Neurol. Internat. Copenhagen", p. 891.

GOODHART, R. & SINCLAIR, H. M. (1940). *J. biol. Chem.*, **132**, 11.

GRAHAM, J. R. & WOLFF, H. G. (1937). *Trans. Amer. Neurol. Assoc.*, **63**, 164.

GREEN, J. B., PAPADOPOULOS, N. M., CEVALLOS, W., FOSTER, F. M. & HESS, W. C. (1959). *J. Neurol. Neurosurg. Psychiat.*, **22**, 117.

GREENE, R. (1959). *Brit. med. J.*, **i**, 574.

GREENFIELD, J. G. (1950). *Folia Psychiat.* (Amst.), **53**, 255.

GREENFIELD, J. G. & CARMICHAEL, E. A. (1935). *Brain*, **59**, 483.

GREER, M. & WILLIAMS, C. M. (1963). *Neurology* (Minneap.), **13**, 73.

GROB, D., HARVEY, A. M., LANGWORTHY, O. R. & LILIENTHAL, J. L. (1947). *Bull. Johns Hopk. Hosp.*, **81**, 257.

GURDJIAN, E. S., STONE, W. E. & WEBSTER, J. E. (1944). *Arch. Neurol. Psychiat.* (Chicago), **51**, 472.

HALLERVORDEN, J. (1950). *Verh. dtsch. Ges. path.*, **32**, 96.

HANDELSMAN, M. B. (1950). *Bull. N.Y. Acad. Med.*, **26**, 611.

HANINGTON, E. (1967). *Brit. med. J.*, **2**, 550.

HANINGTON, E. & Harper, A. M. (1968). *Headache*, **8**, 84.

HAUROWITZ, F. (1930). *Hoppe-Seyl. Z.*, **190**, 72.

HEINZEN, B. (1947). *Anat. Rec.*, **98**, 193.

HELLAUER, H. & UMRATH, K. (1939). *Z. Biol.*, **99**, 624.

HENNEMAN, D. H., ALTSCHULE, M. D., GONCZ, R. M. & ALEXANDER, L. (1954). *Arch. Neurol. Psychiat.* (Chicago), **72**, 688.

HERN, J. E. C. (1967). *Nature*, **215**, 963.

HESS, H. H. (1961). "Regional Neurochemistry". Eds. Kety, S. S. & Elkes, J., p. 200. Oxford, Pergamon Press.

HIMWICH, H. E. (1951). "Brain metabolism and cerebral disorders". Baltimore, Williams & Wilkins.

HIRSON, C., FEINMANN, E. L. & WADE, H. J. (1953). *Brit. med. J.*, **i**, 1408.

HOLLINGER, D. M. & ROSSITER, R. J. (1952). *Biochem. J.*, **52**, 659.

HOLLINGER, D. M., ROSSITER, R. J. & UPMALIS, H. (1952). *Biochem. J.*, **52**, 652.

HOLMBERG, C. G. & LAURELL, C-B. (1948). *Acta chem. Scand.*, **2**, 550.

HOLMBERG, C. G. & LAURELL, C-B. (1951). *Scand. J. clin. Lab. Invest.*, **3**, 103.

HORECKER, B. L. & SMYRNIOTIS, P. Z. (1953). *J. Amer. Chem. Soc.*, **75**, 1009.

HORNABROOK, R. W. & MARKS, V. (1960). *Lancet*, **2**, 893.

HOTSTON, R. D. (1946). *Lancet*, **1**, 207.

HOTTINGER, A. & BLOCH, H. (1943). *Helv. chim. Acta*, **26**, 142.

HUMPE, F. (1942). *Münch. med. Wschr.*, **89**, 448.

HUNT, A. D., STOKES, J., MCCORRY, W. W. & STROUD, H. H. (1954). *Pediatrics*, **13**, 140.

HUNTER, D., PERRY, K. M. A. & EVANS, R. B. (1944). *Brit. J. indust. Med.*, **1**, 227.

INNES, J. R. M. & SHEARER, G. D. (1940). *J. comp. Path.*, **53**, 1.

IWAMA, K. & JASPER, H. H. (1957). *J. Physiol.*, **138**, 365.

JEANES, A. L. & CUMINGS, J. N. (1958). *Confin. neurol.*, **18**, 397.

JOHNSON, A. C., MCNABB, A. R. & ROSSITER, R. J. (1949). *Biochem. J.*, **45**, 500.

JOINER, C. L., MCARDLE, B. & THOMPSON, R. H. S. (1950). *Brain*, **73**, 431.

JOLLIFFE, N., COLBERT, C. N. & JOFFE, P. M. (1936). *Amer. J. med. Sci.*, **191**, 515.

JOLLIFFE, N., GOODHART, R., GENNIS, J. & CLINE, J. K. (1939). *Amer. J. med. Sci.*, **198**, 198.

JONES, H. H., JONES, H. H. & BUNCH, L. D. (1950). *Ann. intern. Med.*, **33**, 831.

JONES, H. H., JONES, H. H., HOWARD, R. R. & BUNCH, L. D. (1954). *Ann. N.Y. Acad. Sci.*, **58**, 656.

JOWETT, M. (1938). *J. Physiol.*, **92**, 322.

JOWETT, M. & QUASTEL, J. H. (1937). *Biochem. J.*, **31**, 565.

KABAT, E. A., FREEDMAN, D. A., MURRAY, J. P. & KNAUB, V. (1950). *Amer. J. med. Sci.*, **219**, 55.

KABAT, E. A., WOLF, A. & BEZER, A. E. (1947). *J. exp. Med.*, **85**, 117.

KAHLKE, W. (1963). *Klin. Wschr.*, **41**, 783.

KERR, J. W., MACAULAY, I., PIRIE, R. & BRONTE-STEWART, B. (1965). *Lancet*, **1**, 1296.

KERR, L. M. H., CAMPBELL, J. G. & LEVVY, G. A. (1949). *Biochem. J.*, **44**, 487.

KERR, L. M. H., CAMPBELL, J. G. & LEVVY, G. A. (1950). *Biochem. J,*, **46**, 278.

KETY, S. S. & ELKES, J. (1961). "Regional Neurochemistry", Oxford, Pergamon Press.

KLEIN, J. R. & OLSEN, N. S. (1947). *J. biol. Chem.*, **167**, 747.

KLENK, E. (1939/40). *Hoppe-Seyl. Z.*, **262**, 128.

KLENK, E. & KAHLKE, W. (1963). *Hoppe-Seyl. Z.*, **333**, 133.

KLENK, E. & LANGERBEINS, H. (1941). *Hoppe-Seyl. Z.*, **270**, 185.

KLÜVER, H. (1944). *Science*, **99**, 482.

KUNTZMAN, R., SHORE, P. A., BOGDANSKI, D. & BRODIE, B. B. (1961). *J. Neurochem.*, **6**, 226.

LAATSCH, R. H., KIES, M. W., GORDON, S. & ALVORD, E. C. (1962). *J. exp. Med.*, **115**, 777.

LAHEY, M. E., GUBLER, C. J., CARTWRIGHT, G. E. & WINTROBE, M. M. (1953). *J. clin. Invest.*, **32**, 329.

LAMAR, C. & SELLINGER, O. Z. (1965). *Biochem. Pharmacol.*, **14**, 489.

LARRABEE, M. G., RAMOS, J. G. & BULBRING, E. (1950). *Fed. Proc.*, **9**, 75.

LASSEK, A. M. & BUEKER, E. D. (1947). *Anat. Rec.*, **97**, 395.

LESNY, I. & POLACEK, L. (1951). *Acta neurol. psychiat. belg.*, **51**, 601.

LEVVY, G. A., KERR, L. M. H. & CAMPBELL, J. G. (1948). *Biochem. J.*, **42**, 462.

LEWIS, J. L. & MCILWAIN, H. (1954). *Biochem. J.*, **57**, 680.

LINDER, G. C. (1947). *Lancet*, **2**, 649.

LING, C. T. & CHOW, B. F. (1953). *J. biol. Chem.*, **202**, 445.

LING, C. T. & CHOW, B. F. (1954). *J. biol. Chem.*, **205**, 797.

LOGAN, J. E., MANNELL, W. A. & ROSSITER, R. J. (1952). *Biochem. J.*, **51**, 482.

LOROT, C. (1899). "Les Combinaisons de la Creosote dans le Traitement de la Tuberculose Pulmonaire". Thèse de Paris. Quoted by Hunter, D. (1944). "Industrial Toxicology". London, Oxford Univ. Press.

LUMSDEN, C. E. (1949a). *Brain*, **72**, 198.

LUMSDEN, C. E. (1949b). *Brain*, **72**, 517.

LUMSDEN, C. E. (1950). *J. Neurol. Neurosurg. Psychiat.*, **13**, 1.

LUMSDEN, C. E. (1951). *Brit. med. J.*, **i**, 1035.

LUMSDEN, C. E. (1952). *Quart. J. exp. Physiol.*, **37**, 45.

LUMSDEN, C. E., ROBERTSON, D. M. & BLIGHT, R. (1966). *J. Neurochem.*, **13**, 127.

LUSE, S. A. & MCDOUGAL, D. B. (1960). *J. exp. Med.*, **112**, 735.

LUTHY, P. (1932). *Dtsch. Z. Nervenheilk*, **123**, 101.

MCALPINE, D., COMPSTON, N. D. & LUMSDEN, C. E. (1955). "Multiple Sclerosis". Edinbrugh, E. & S. Livingstone.

MCARDLE, B., MACKENZIE, I. C. K. & WEBSTER, G. R. (1960). *J. Neurol. Neurosurg. Psychiat.*, **23**, 127.

MCARDLE, B. & ZILKHA, K. J. (1962). *Brain*, **85**, 389.

MCCANCE, R. A. & WIDDOWSON, E. M. (1946). *Nature* (Lond.), **157**, 837.

MCILWAIN, H. (1951). *J. ment. Sci.*, **97**, 674.

MCILWAIN, H. (1952). *Biochem. Soc. Symp.*, **8**, 27.

MCMENEMEY, W. H. (1961). *Proc. R. Soc. Med.*, **54**, 127.

MCINTYRE, N., CLINK, H. M., LEVI, A. J., CUMINGS, J. N. & SHERLOCK, S. (1967). *New Engl. J. Med.*, **276**, 439.

MAGEE, W. L., BERRY, J. F., MAGEE, M. & ROSSITER, R. J. (1959). *J. Neurochem.*, **3**, 333.

MAGEE, W. L. & ROSSITER, R. J. (1954). *Biochem. J.*, **58**, 243.

MALONEY, A. F. J. & CUMINGS, J. N. (1960). *J. Neurol. Neurosurg. Psychiat.*, **23**, 207.

MALONEY, C. J. & PARMELEE, A. H. (1954). *J. Amer. Med. Ass.*, **154**, 405.

MANDELBROTE, B. M., STANIER, M. W., THOMPSON, R. H. S. & THRUSTON, M. N. (1948). *Brain*, **71**, 212.

MANN, T. & KEILIN, D. (1938). *Proc. roy. Soc. B.*, **126**, 303.

MARBURG, O. (1906). *Jg. Psychiat. Neurol.*, **27**, 213.

MARCHANT, J. (1949). *J. Anat.* (Lond.), **83**, 227.

MARKS, V., MARRACK, D. & ROSE, F. C. (1961). *Proc. R. Soc. Med.*, **54**, 747.

MARPLES, E. A. & THOMPSON, R. H. S. (1960). *Biochem. J.*, **74**, 123.

MARRACK, D., ROSE, F. C. & MARKS, V. (1961). *Proc. R. Soc. Med.*, **54**, 749.

MARTIN, M. M. (1953). *Brain*, **76**, 594.

MATTHEWS, W. B. (1954). *J. Neurol. Neurosurg. Psychiat.*, **17**, 242.

MATTHEWS, W. B., MILNE, M. D. & BELL, M. (1952). *Quart. J. Med.*, **21**, 425.

MAY, R. M. (1930). *Bull. Soc. Chim. biol.*, **12**, 934.

MEHL, E. & JATZKEWITZ, H. (1965). *Biochem, biophys. Res. Commun.*, **19**, 407.

MELLANBY, E. (1946). *Brit. med. J.*, **2**, 885.

MELLANBY, E. (1947). *Brit. med. J.*, **2**, 288.

MENDEL, B. & RUDNEY, H. (1944). *Science*, **100**, 499.

MENKES, J. H., DUNCAN, C. & MOOSSY, J. (1966). *Neurology* (Minneap.), **16**, 581.

MILLAC, P. (1967a). *Deutsch. Z. f. Nervenheilk.*, **191**. 74.

MILLAC, P. (1967b). *Brit. med. J.*, **2**, 25.

MILLAR, J. H. D., MERRETT, J. D. & DALBY, A. M. (1966). *J. Neurol. Neurosurg. Psychiat.*, **29**, 187.

MILLER, F. R. (1937). *J. Physiol.*, **91**, 212.

MILLER, F. R., STAVRAKY, G. W. & WOONTON, G. A. (1940). *J. Neurophysiol.*, **3**, 131.

MINOT, G. R., STRAUSS, M. B. & COBB, S. (1933). *New Engl. J. Med.*, **208**, 1244.

MONEKOSSO, G. L. & WILSON, J. (1966). *Lancet*, **1**, 1062.

MONTFOORT, A., BAKER, R. W. R., THOMPSON, R. H. S. & ZILKHA, K. J. (1966). *J. Neurol. Neurosurg. Psychiat.*, **29**, 99.

MORRELL, A. G. & SCHEINBERG, I. H. (1960). *Science*, **131**, 930.

MORELL, A. G., SHAPIRO, J. R. & SCHEINBERG, I. H. (1961). In "Wilson's Disease: Some Current Concepts", p. 36. Eds. Walshe, J. M. & Cumings, J. N. Oxford, Blackwell.

MORELL, A. G., VAN DEN HAMER, C. J. A. & SCHEINBERG, I. H. (1966). *J. biol. Chem.*, **241**, 3745.

MORGAN, I. M. (1947). *J. exp. Med.*, **85**, 131.

MORRISON, L. R. & ZAMECNIK, P. C. (1950). *Arch. Neurol. Psychiat.* (Chicago), **63**, 367.

MOSSAKOWSKI, M., MATHIESON, G. & CUMINGS, J. N. (1961). *Brain*, **84**, 585.

MOTT, F. W. & HALLIBURTON, W. D. (1901a). *Phil. Trans. B.*, **194**, 437.

MOTT, F. W. & HALLIBURTON, W. D. (1901b). *Lancet*, **1**, 1077.

MÜLDNER, H. G., WHERRETT, J. R. & CUMINGS, J. N. (1962). *J. Neurochem.*, **9**, 607.

MURALT, A. VON & SCHULTHESS, G. VON (1944). *Helv. physiol. pharmacol. Acta*, **2**, 435.

NACHMANSOHN, D., JOHN, H. M. & BERMAN, M. (1946). *J. biol. Chem.*, **163**, 475.

NAJJAR, V. A. & BARRETT, R. (1945). *Vitam. & Horm.*, **3**, 23.

NASHOLD, B. S. & KIRSHNER, N. (1963). *Neurology*, (Minneap.), **13**, 753.

NATHANSON, M. & SAVITSKY, J. P. (1954). *Bull. N.Y. Acad. Med.*, **28**, 462.

NEVIN, N. C., CUMINGS, J. N. & MCKEOWN, F. (1967). *Brain*, **90**, 419.

NOLL, A. (1899). *Hoppe-Seyl. Z.*, **27**, 370.

O'BRIEN, J. S. (1964). *Biochem. biophys. Res. Commun.*, **15**, 484.

O'BRIEN, J. S., STERN, M. D., LANDING, B. H., O'BRIEN, J. K. & DONNELL, G. N. (1965). *Amer. J. Dis. Child.*, **109**, 338.

OLSEN, N. S. & KLEIN, J. R. (1947). *J. biol. Chem.*, **167**, 739.

O'REILLY, S., LONCIN, M. & COOKSEY, B. (1965). *Neurology* (Minneap.), **15**, 980.

OSBORN, S. B. & WALSHE, J. M. (1958). *Lancet*, **1**, 70.

O'SHEA, H. E., ELSOM, K. O. & HIGBE, R. V. (1942). *Amer. J. med. sci.*, **203**, 388.

PAPADOPOULOS, N. M., CEVALLOS, W. & HESS, W. C. (1960). *A.M.A. Arch. Neurol.*, **3**, 677.

PAYLING WRIGHT, G. (1961). *Proc. R. Soc. Med.*, **54**, 26.

PEKELHARING, C. A. & WINKLER, C. (1887). *Dtsch. med. Wschr.*, **13**, 845.

PERRAULT, M., KLOTZ, B., CANIVET, J. & CAROIT, M. (1953). *Bull. Soc. med. Hôp.* (Paris), **69**, 1048.

PETERS, R. A. (1936). *Lancet*, **1**, 1161.

PETERS, R. A., SINCLAIR, H. M. & THOMPSON, R. H. S. (1946). *Biochem. J.*, **40**, 516.

PETRY, H. (1951). *Zbl. Arbeitsmed. Arbeitsschütz*, **1**, 86.

PICCOLI, P., FERRARI, M. & DANIELE, E. (1962). *Folia Med. Napoli*, **45**, 342.

PICHLER, E. & REISNER, H. (1938). *Wien. klin. Wschr.*, **51**, 1304.

PLATT, B. S. & LU, G. D. (1939). *Biochem. J.*, **33**, 1525.

PLUM, C. M. & FOG, T. (1959). *Acta psychiat. Scand.*, **34**, Suppl. 128.

POIRIER, L. J. & SOURKES, T. L. (1965). *Brain*, **88**, 181.

POPE, A. (1958). "Biology of the Neuroglia". Ed. Windle, W. F., p. 211. Springfield, Illinois, C. C. Thomas.

POPE, A., MORRIS, A. A., JASPER, M. H., ELLIOTT, K. A. C. & PENFIELD, W. (1947). *Res. Publ. Ass. Nerv. Ment. Dis.*, **26**, 218.

PORTER, H. (1961). In "Wilson's Disease: Some Current Concepts". Ed.s Walshe, J. M. & Cumings, J. N. Oxford, Blackwell.

PORTER, H. & FOLCH, J. (1957a). *Arch. Neurol. Psychiat.* (Chicago), **77**, 8.

PORTER, H. & FOLCH, J. (1957b). *J. Neurochem.*, **1**, 260.

PORTER, H., SWEENEY, M. & PORTER, E. M. (1964). *Arch. Biochem. Biophys.*, **104**, 97.

POSER, C. M. (1961). *A.M.A. Arch. Neurol.*, **4**, 323.

POSER, C. M. & CURRAN, G. L. (1958). *Arch. Neurol. Psychiat.* (Chicago), **80**, 304.

PRITCHARD, E. T. & ROSSITER, R. J. (1959). *J. Neurochem.*, **3**, 341.

PURPURA, D. P., GIRADO, M. & GRUNDFEST, H. (1957). *Science*, **125**, 1200.

PUTMAN, T. J. (1936). *Ann. intern. Med.*, **9**, 854.

PUTNAM, T. J. (1937). *Arch. Neurol. Psychiat.* (Chicago), **37**, 1298.

QUASTEL, J. H. & WALES, W. T. (1940). *Lancet*, **1**, 402.

QUASTEL, J. H. & WHEATLEY, A. H. M. (1932). *Proc. roy. Soc. B.*, **112**, 60.

RACKER, E., DE LA HABA, G. & LEDER, I. G. (1953). *J. Amer. Chem. Soc.*, **75**, 1010.

REFSUM, S. (1945). *Nord. Med.*, **28**, 2682.

REFSUM, S. (1946). *Acta psychiat. neurol. Scand.*, Suppl. **38**, 1.

REGISTER, U. D. (1954). *J. biol. Chem.*, **206**, 705.

RICHARDS, C. H. & WOLFF, H. G. (1940). *Arch. Neurol. Psychiat.* (Chicago), **43**, 59.

RICHTER, D. (1952). *Biochem. Soc. Symp.*, **8**, 62.

RICHTER, D. & CROSSLAND, J. (1949). *Amer. J. Physiol.*, **159**, 247.

RICHTER, D. & DAWSON, R. M. C. (1948a). *J. biol. Chem.*, **176**, 1199.

RICHTER, D. & DAWSON, R. M. C. (1948b). *Amer. J. Physiol.*, **154**, 173.

RICHTERICH, R., KAHLKE, W., VAN MECHELEN, P. & ROSSI, E. (1963). *Klin. Wschr.*, **41**, 800.

RIMINGTON, C. & GRAY, C. H. (1947). *Brit. med. J.*, ii, 629.

RIVERS, T. M. & SCHWENTKER, F. F. (1935). *J. exp. Med.*, **61**, 689.

ROBERTS, E. & BAXTER, C. F. (1959). "Proc. IV Int. Congr. Biochem.", p. 268. London, Pergamon Press.

ROBERTSON, D. M., BLIGHT, R. & LUMSDEN, C. E. (1962). *Nature* (Lond.), **196**, 1005.

ROSS, R. & REYNOLDS, E. S. (1901). *Brit. med. J.*, ii, 979.

RUMPEL, A. (1913). *Dtsch. Z. Nervenheilk*, **49**, 54.

SAMPSON, B. F. (1938). *Bull. Off. int. Hyg. publ.*, **30**, 2601.

SAMUELS, A. J., BOYARSKY, L. L., GERARD, R. W., LIBET, B. & BRUST, M. (1951). *Amer. J. Physiol.*, **164**, 1.

SANDERS, B. E., MILLER, O. P. & RICHARD, M. N. (1959). *Arch. Biochem. Biophys.*, **84**, 60.

SANO, L., GAMO, T., KARIMOTO, Y., TANIGUCHI, K., TAKESADA, M. & NISHINUMA, K. (1959). *Biochim. Biophys. Acta*, **32**, 586.

SARKAR, S. N. (1948). *Nature* (Lond.), **162**, 265.

SASS-KORTSAK, A., GLATT, B. S., CHERNIAK, M. & CEDERLUND, I. (1961). In "Wilson's Disease: Some Current Concepts". Eds. Walshe, J. M. & Cumings, J. N. p. 151. Oxford, Blackwell.

SAWYER, C. H. (1946). *Amer. J. Physiol.*, **146**, 246.

SCHEINBERG, I. H. & GITLIN, D. (1952). *Science*, **116**, 484.

SCHEINBERG, I. H. & STERNLIEB, I. (1960a). *Amer. J. Med.*, **29**, 316.

SCHEINBERG, I. H. & STERNLIEB, I. (1960b). *Pharmacol. Rev.*, **12**, 355.

SCHEINBERG, P. (1951). *Blood*, **6**, 213.

SCHMIDT, C. F., KETY, S. S. & PENNES, H. H. (1945). *Amer. J. Physiol.*, **143**, 33.

SCHMITT, F. O. & BEAR, R. S. (1939). *Biol. Rev.*, **14**, 27.

SCHMITT, F. O., BEAR, R. S. & PALMER, K. L. (1941). *J. cell. comp. Physiol.*, **18**, 31.

SCHUMACHER, G. A. & WOLFF, H. G. (1941). *Arch. Neurol. Psychiat.*, **45**, 199.

SELLINGER, O. Z. & WEILAR, P. (1963). *Biochem. Pharmacol.*, **12**, 989.

SERCL, M., KOVARIK, J. & JUCHA, J. (1961). *Acta neurol. Scand.*, **37**, 317.

SHORE, P. A. & ALPERS, H. S. (1963). *Nature* (Lond.), **199**, 495.

SINCLAIR, H. M. (1939). "C.R. IIIme Congres. Neurol. Internat. Copenhagen", p. 885.

SINCLAIR, H. M. (1956). *Lancet*, **1**, 381.

SMITH, A. D. M. (1961). *Lancet*, **1**, 1001.

SMITH, M. I. & ELVOVE, E. (1930). *Publ. Hlth. Rep.* (Wash.), **45**, 1703.

SMITH, M. I., ELVOVE, E. & FRAZIER, W. H. (1930). *Publ. Hlth. Rep.* (Wash.), **45**, 2509.

SMITH, W. K. (1948). *Anat. Rec.*, **102**, 523.

SOURKES, T. L., MURPHY, G. F., SANKOFF, L., WISEMAN-DISTLER, M. H. & SAINT CYR, S. (1963). *J. Neurochem.*, **10**, 947.

SPIES, T. D. & DE WOLF, H. F. (1933). *Amer. J. med. Sci.*, **186**, 521.

SPILLANE, J. D. (1947). "Nutritional Disorders of the Nervous System". Eeinburgh, E. & S. Livingstone.

SPILLANE, J. D., KEYSER, J. W. & PARKER, R. A. (1952). *J. clin. Path.*, **5**, 16.

STAEHELIN, R. (1941). *Schweiz. med. Wschr.*, **71**, 1.

STEIN, W. H., BEARN, A. G. & MOORE, S. (1954). *J. clin. Invest.*, **33**, 410.

STOCKEN, L. A. & THOMPSON, R. H. S. (1946). *Biochem. J.*, **40**, 535.

STONE, W. E., WEBSTER, J. E. & GURDJIAN, E. S. (1945). *J. Neurophysiol.*, **8**, 233.

STRAUSS, M. B. (1935). *Amer. J. med. Sci.*, **189**, 378.

SVENNERHOLM, L. (1962). *Biochem. biophys. Res. Commun.*, **9**, 436.

SWAN, K. C. & MYERS, H. B. (1937). *Arch. Neurol. Psychiat.* (Chicago), **38**, 288.

SWANK, R. L. (1950). *Amer. J. med. Sci.*, **220**, 421.

SWANK, R. L. (1953). *Arch. Neurol. Psychiat.* (Chicago), **69**, 281.

SWANK, R. L. (1961). "A Biochemical Approach to Multiple Sclerosis". Springfield, Ill.

SWANK, R. L. & BACKER, J. (1950). *Trans. Amer. Neurol. Ass.*, **75**, 274.

SWANK, R. L., LERSTAD, O., STROM, A. & BACKER, J. (1952). *New Engl. J. Med.*, **246**, 721.

SWANK, R. L. & PRADOS, M. (1942). *Arch. Neurol. Psychiat.* (Chicago), **47**, 97.

TER BRAAK, J. W. G. (1931). *Ned. Tijdschr. Geneesk.*, **75**, 2329.

THANNHAUSER, S. H. (1950). "Lipidoses", 2nd Ed., New York, Oxford University Press.

THOMPSON, E. J., Goodwin, H. & CUMINGS, J. N. (1967). *Nature* (Lond.), **215**, 168.

THOMPSON, R. H. S. (1948). *Brit. med. Bull.*, **5**, 319.

THOMPSON, R. H. S. (1954). "Chem. & Ind. (Rev.), p. 749.

THOMPSON, R. H. S. (1966). *Proc. R. Soc. Med.*, **59**, 269.

THOMPSON, R. H. S., BUTTERFIELD, W. J. H. & KELSEY FRY, I. (1960). *Proc. R. Soc. Med.*, **53**, 143.

THOMPSON, R. H. S. & CUMINGS, J. N. (1964). "Biochemical Disorders in Human Disease", 2nd Ed., London, J. & A. Churchill.

THOMPSON, R. H. S. & JOHNSON, R. E. (1935). *Biochem. J.*, **29**, 694.

THOMPSON, R. H. S., NIEMIRO, R. & WEBSTER, G. R. (1960). *Biochim. Biophys. Acta*, **43**, 142.

THOMPSON, R. H. S. & WHITTAKER, V. P. (1947). *Biochem. J.*, **41**, 342.

THUDICHUM, J. L. W. (1884). "A Treatise on the Chemical Constitution of the Brain". London, Bailliere, Tindall & Cox.

TINGEY, A. H. (1937). *J. Ment. Sci.*, **83**, 452.

TOWER, D. B. (1952). "Montreal Neurological Institute". Reprint No. 414.

TOWER, D. B. & ELLIOTT, K. A. C. (1952). *J. appl. Physiol.*, **4**, 669.

TOWER, D. B. & ELLIOTT, K. A. C. (1953). *J. appl. Physiol.*, **5**, 375.

TOWER, D. B. & MCEACHERN, D. (1949). *Canad. J. Res.*, **27**, Sect. E, 120.

UDENFRIEND, S. & CREVELING, C. R. (1959). *J. Neurochem.*, **4**, 350.

UZMAN, L. L. (1953). *Amer. J. med. Sci.*, **226**, 645.

UZMAN, L. L. & DENNY-BROWN, D. (1948). *Amer. J. Med. Sci.*, **215**, 599.

UZMAN, L. L. & HOOD, B. (1952). *Amer. J. med. Sci.*, **223**, 392.

VAN BOGAERT, L. & BERTRAND, I. (1949). *Acta neurol. Psychiat. belg.*, **49**, 572.

WALLER, A. (1850). *Phil. Trans.*, **140**, 423.

WALSHE, J. M. (1956). *Lancet*, **1**, 25.

WALTHARD, K. M. (1946). *Schweiz. Arch. Neurol. Psychiat.*, **58**, 189.

DE WARDENER, H. E. & LENNOX, B. (1947). *Lancet*, **1**, 11.

WARNOCK, C. G. & NEILL, D. W. (1954). *J. Neurol. Neurosurg. Psychiat.*, **17**, 70.

WARREN, P. J., EARL, C. J. & THOMPSON, R. H. S. (1960). *Brain*, **83**, 709.

WEBSTER, G. R. & THOMPSON, R. H. S. (1962). *Biochim. Biophys. Acta*, **63**, 38.

WEIL, A. (1948). *J. Neuropath. exp. Neurol.*, **7**, 453.

WEIL, A. & BRADBURNE, G. (1948). *J. Neuropath. exp. Neurol.*, **7**, 447.

WEIL, A. & CLEVELAND, D. A. (1932). *Arch. Neurol. Psychiat.* (Chicago), **27**, 375.

WESTLAKE, R. J. & TEW, J. M. (1966). *Neurology*, (Minneap.), **16**, 619.

WESTON HURST, E. (1940). *Aust. J. exp. Biol. Med. Sci.*, **18**, 201.

WESTON HURST, E. (1941). *Med. J. Aust.*, **ii**, 661.

WESTON HURST, E. (1942). *Aust. J. exp. Biol. Med. Sci.*, **20**, 297.

WHERRETT, J. R. & CUMINGS, J. N. (1963). *Trans. Amer. Neurol. Ass.*, **88**, 108.

WILLIAMS, R. D., MASON, H. L., POWER, M. H. & WILDER, R. M. (1943). *Arch. intern. Med.*, **71**, 38.

WILLIAMS, R. D., MASON, H. L., WILDER, R. M. & SMITH, B. F. (1940). *Arch. intern. Med.*, **66**, 785.

WILLIAMS, D. & RITCHIE RUSSELL, W. (1941). *Lancet*, **1**, 476.

WILMOT, V. A. & SWANK, R. L. (1952). *Amer. J. med. Sci.*, **223**, 25.

WILSON, H. E. C. & GHOSH, B. L. (1937). *Indian med. Gaz.*, **72**, 147.

WILSON, J. (1963). *Brain*, **86**, 347.

WILSON, J. (1965). *Clin. Sci.*, **29**, 505.

WILSON, J. & MATTHEWS, D. M. (1966). *Clin. Sci.*, **31**, 1.

WILSON, S. A. K. (1912). *Brain*, **34**, 295.

WILSON, S. A. K. (1940). "Neurology", vol. 1, Ed. Bruce, A. N. London, Arnold.

WOKES, F. (1955). *Amer. J. clin. Nutr.*, **3**, 383.

WOKES, F. (1958). *Lancet*, **2**, 526.

WOLFF, H. G. & SUTHERLAND, A. M. (1938). *Trans. Amer. Neurol. Assoc.*, **64**, 103.

WRIGHT, H. P., THOMPSON, R. H. S. & ZILKHA, K. J. (1965). *Lancet*, **2**, 1109.

WYNDHAM, R. A. (1941). *Aust. J. exp. Biol. med. Sci.*, **19**, 243.

YAHR, M. D., GOLDENSOHN, S. S. & KABAT, E. A. (1954). *Ann. N.Y. Acad. Sci.*, **58**, 613.

YOUNG, J. Z. (1942). *Physiol. Rev.*, **22**, 318.

ZIMDAHL, W. T., HYMAN, I. & COOK, E. D. (1953). *Neurology* (Minneap.), **3**, 569.

Chapter 14

DISEASES OF MUSCLE

by

KENNETH L. ZIERLER

The Johns Hopkins University, Baltimore

IN man, cross-striated muscle constitutes more than two-fifths of total body weight and over one-half of the weight of soft tissues. It is the function of this huge mass of tissue to contract, and, in so doing, to produce movement of bone about a joint, movement of the eye, a change in volume (as that produced in the thorax by the diaphragm), or fixation as when agonist and antagonist act together. Disease of cross-striated muscle threatens life when muscles of respiration are involved. Because metabolism and function of cross-striated muscle are related closely, but not completely, to those of heart muscle, myopathy and myocardiopathy have much in common, and myocardiopathy may be life-threatening. But for the most part, muscle disease is disabling and alters the quality of life, but does not directly end it.

Muscle disease occurs secondarily to disorders of nerve and to disturbed blood supply. It occurs as part of systemic infectious disease and as part of endocrinopathy for which skeletal muscle is the largest, if not the most dramatic, target tissue. Muscle is involved in hyperimmune states, alone or with other tissues. Muscle may share in body-wide metabolic and nutritional disorders. Finally, there is a group of diseases, often heritable, which seem to be largely, if not entirely, limited to muscle.

There have been rapid advances in descriptive detail of muscle anatomy, thanks to electron microscopy, and in comprehension of mechanisms by which motor nerve signals are translated to produce contraction of muscle. There is better awareness of the contractile process and of the energetics underlying it. But there is a chasm of ignorance between the mountain of information concerning morphology, physiology, and biochemistry of muscle, normal or diseased, and the garden of genuine understanding of the molecular mechanism of disease. Reasons for failure to bridge this gap are that many studies of natural disease cannot distinguish among observed phenomena between results of the disease and its causes, and that despite the impressive accumulation of basic knowledge, we still do not understand enough about normal muscle, particularly in the realm of structure, function, and reactions of fibre membranes.

Because appreciation of muscle disease depends on comprehension of function and chemistry of normal muscle, we begin by summarizing current knowledge of muscle physiology and chemistry.

CHEMICAL ANATOMY
AND PHYSIOLOGICAL CHEMISTRY
Morphology

A muscle is an orderly assembly of muscle fibres. Each muscle fibre is a cell, roughly cylindrical, ending in fibrous extensions that fuse to form, for example, tendons. There are no regular, well-defined, cross-wise connections between fibres, but rather there is more or less loose connective tissue linking a fibre with its neighbours throughout its length. A capillary net clothes each fibre, the richness of blood supply varying greatly.

Muscle fibres vary in length, in diameter, and in colour. Darker fibres, called red muscle, tend to be narrower. Lighter fibres, called white muscle, tend to be larger. Most human muscle contains mixed red and white fibres, often in no obvious pattern. Blood capillary supply tends to be more lush about red fibres. Red muscle fibres have more mitochondria, more lipid, more oxidative phosphorylation activity, and less glycogen than white fibres.

Every muscle fibre is encased in several layers of membranes, collectively called sarcolemma. Outermost is a dense collagen mesh. Beneath this is an amorphous layer, often called the basement membrane, composed largely of mucoprotein, perhaps 500 to 1000Å thick, and conceivably the analogue of the bacterial cell wall. Innermost is the plasma membrane, about 100Å thick, thought by many, but not all, to be made of two protein layers separated by lipid.

Muscle fibres are made up of repeating cylindrical units, sarcomeres, in series. Sarcomeres are bounded by Z lines. Each Z line bisects a band sotropic to polarized light, the I band. Between I bands is a band anisotropic to polarized light, the A band. A relatively isotropic mid-zone in the A band is called the H zone. The alternation of A and I bands give cross-striated muscle its name. A bands are about 1·5 μ long, and their length is invariant at rest or during contraction of muscle.

When a muscle shortens, the Z lines move closer together. A sarcomere at rest is about 2·1 μ long. Its maximum shortening is to about 1·5 μ. It can be stretched reversibly to about 3·5 μ. These changes in length occur at the expense of the I band.

Electron microscopy reveals the instruments of these changes in sarcomere length. Every sarcomere is filled with an orderly array of long rods, the fibrils. Fibrils are themselves orderly bundles of filaments. There are no membranes around fibrils. Fibrils are separated from one another by cytoplasm through which courses an endoplasmic reticulum, the longitudinal components of the sarcoplasmic reticulum.

Fibrils contain two types of filaments. Thin filaments, anchored to the Z line, about 1 μ long, and, in the centre of the sarcomere, parallel thick filaments, about 1·5 μ long. I bands contain only thin filaments. A bands contain only thick filaments in their centre and overlapping thin and thick filaments at their edges toward the I bands. Thin filaments are aggregates of actin, and perhaps also of tropomyosin. Thick filaments are aggregates of myosin. In the zone of overlap there are cross-bridges between thick and thin filaments (Hanson & Huxley, 1953; Huxley, 1957).

The length of thick and thin filaments is approximately invariant. When a sarcomere shortens, each thick filament slides between a hexagonal array of thin filaments.

Myosin, actin, and tropomyosin are the contractile proteins. Their chemistry is considered in a separate section of this chapter.

To continue with the anatomy of the skeletal muscle fibre, the sarcolemma has regular invaginations. In mammalian muscle these invaginations occur at every Z line. The invaginations are in fact tubular structures dipping perpendicularly into fibres, dividing to form an annulus about the Z line of every fibril. This system, open to outside interstitial fluid, lined with a plasma membrane and probably with an amorphous mucoprotein membrane, is the transverse tubular, or T, system of the sarcoplasmic reticulum. Each annulus of the T system, encircling a fibril, is connected, probably by a tight junction, to dilated terminal cisterns of the longitudinal tubules of the sarcoplasmic recitulum. The longitudinal tubules are walled by the plasma membrane. On longitudinal section of muscle one sees about the Z line of every fibril a triad of which the central member is a fragment of the T system and the lateral members are terminal cisterns of the longitudinal system (Porter & Palade, 1957).

The entire membrane system—sarcolemma, T system, and longitudinal reticulum—is essential for the spread of excitation, initiation of contraction, and, probably, termination of contraction.

A specialized area, or areas, of sarcolemma on every mammalian muscle fibre is the motor end-plate. The end-plate is a hollow ball-like structure into which fits a terminal bud of a motor nerve. The assembly, nerve bud and motor end-plate, constitutes the myoneural junction. Usually one efferent nerve fibre supplies a number of muscle fibres, perhaps as many as 1000 in man.

Mitochondria tend to be concentrated in the vicinity of the triads at the Z lines. In mature mammalian skeletal muscle, numbers of nuclei lie just beneath the sarcolemma.

Contractile Proteins

About two-thirds of the total protein of skeletal muscle is in filaments of myofibrils. Of the myofibrillar protein about 54% is myosin, 21% actin, 15% tropomyosin B, and 10% unidentified.

Myosin accounts for 95% or more of the thick filaments. Actin and tropomyosin make up nearly all the protein of the thin filaments. Filaments that form the Z line may be tropomyosin B.

Myosin is a fibrous protein of uncertain molecular weight, 470,000 or 600,000. A myosin molecule is a rod, about 1500Å long and 15 to 20Å thick, with a club at one end at right angles to the long axis. The club is about 200Å long and 40Å thick. It is about the size of the cross-bridges between thick and thin filaments.

Trypsin or chymotrypsin can split myosin into two fragments, one about twice the weight of the other. The heavy fragment, heavy meromyosin, is 600 to 900Å long and contains the clubbed end. The lighter fragment, light meromyosin, is a straight rod, about 600Å long.

Myosin and heavy meromyosin, but not light meromyosin, aggregate with actin, a reaction that may be fundamental to muscle contraction.

Myosin forms a remarkable polymer. It first forms an end-to-end dimer with the clubs at both ends. Further polymerization proceeds by side-to-side aggregation with the club away from the centre. The clubs are displaced from one another by about 400Å and seem to be arranged in a spiral. Polymerization continues until the macromolecule is about 100Å thick and about 1·5 to 2 μ long; that is, about the size of a thick filament.

(Rice, 1961; Zobel & Carlson, 1963; Huxley, 1963).

Myosin, as well as heavy meromyosin, but not light meromyosin, is an ATPase. This suggests that the ATPase may be in the club end. Since the club end looks like the cross-bridges, and has the proper spacing, it may be that ATPase plays a role in connecting thick to thin filaments in contracted muscle.

There are two forms of actin. A monomer, globular or G-actin, molecular weight 60,000 to 70,000, contains bound ATP. G-actin dimerizes. In the presence of salts the dimer of G-actin polymerizes to a large fibrous form, F-actin. During polymerization the bound ATP is dephosphorylated to ADP, but actin itself is not an ATPase.

F-actin is made of two strands twisted about each other. The basic unit is a sphere, about 55Å in diameter, and perhaps it is G-actin, or something close to it. There are 13 globular units per complete turn of the helix (Hanson & Lowy, 1963).

Tropomyosin B, or soluble tropomyosin, molecular weight about 50,000, forms a substantial portion of thin filaments. It has been suggested that tropomyosin B and actin are coiled together to form the thin filaments of the I band.

Actin and myosin, and actin and heavy meromyosin, spontaneously complex. Actin-heavy meromysin complexes are filaments with a strong axial periodicity and amazing structural polarity. What appear to be arrowheads all point in the same direction along the whole length of the filament, suggesting that F-actin is itself polarized.

Chemistry of the Contractile Process

ATP is dephosphorylated during muscle contraction. Ordinarily there is such a large supply of phosphocreatine (PC) that ADP is re-phosphorylated rapidly to ATP. In excised muscle, repeated stimulation reduces PC concentration (Carlson & Siger, 1959; Mommaerts et al., 1962). The reactions are

$$ATP \rightarrow ADP + P_1$$
$$PC + ADP \rightarrow ATP + Creatine,$$

the latter reaction involving creatine phosphoryltransferase. When creatine phosphoryltransferase is inhibited by 2,4-dinitrofluorobenzene, muscle ATP content decreases during contraction (Davies et al., 1964).

Although the present evidence is not as quantitative as one hopes to get eventually, owing to great technical difficulties, within considerable experimental error the energy from splitting

ATP or PC accounts quantitatively for the total energy of contraction work plus initial heat (Carlson, Hardy & Wilkie, 1963). It is likely, but not yet proven, that ATP is split early in contraction, and not during relaxation.

Excitation

Acetylcholine is packaged in packets in the terminal buds of motor nerves (Fatt & Katz, 1952). When a motor nerve fibre is stimulated the impulse arriving at nerve-endings releases acetylcholine from many points over the broad nerve-ending into a wide, shallow hemispheric trough that separates the nerve-ending from the motor end-plate. Acetylcholine diffuses rapidly over the short distance, arriving at many specific receptor sites on the end-plate. Permeability of the end-plate to monovalent cations is increased by the interaction of acetylcholine with its receptors. The increased permeability leads to net influx of Na^+, as a result of which the end-plate is depolarized. The consequent end-plate potential spreads only by electrotonus; i.e., it is not propagated. However, if it is sufficiently large it will depolarize immediately adjacent areas of the muscle fibre, and the impulse from these areas can then be propagated.

A propagated impulse occurs as follows. The initial electrotonic end-plate potential alters the permeability of an adjacent sarcolemmal surface. This permeability change is a rather specific increase in permeability to Na^+. Because the electrochemical potential gradient for Na^+ across the sarcolemma is large and in the direction of driving Na^+ from extracellular fluid into sarcoplasm, there is inward movement of Na^+. This inward movement of Na^+ depolarizes the muscle membrane locally. The electric field alters permeability of an adjacent area of sarcolemma so as to increase permeability to Na^+. Na^+ flows into muscle at this spot, depolarizing this area, altering permeability over an adjacent area, and so on. Though permeability is increased some 500-fold over that of membrane permeability to Na^+ at rest, the actual flux of Na^+ is still only hundreds of picamoles per second per cm^2 of sarcolemma (Hodgkin, 1951; Hodgkin & Huxley, 1952).

Excitation-contraction Coupling

As a result of microinjection of Ca^{++} into muscle fibres (Niedergerke, 1955) and studies of effects of Ca^{++} solutions applied locally to muscles stripped of sarcolemma (Podolsky & Constantin, 1964) and, as a result of many studies of an ATP-linked Ca^{++} pump in microsomal fractions of skeletal muscle (Frank, 1961;

Hasselbach & Makinose, 1961), it is now held that the action potential, as it depolarizes the transverse tubular membrane, stimulates release of Ca^{++} from the wall of the longitudinal reticulum, and that Ca^{++} diffuses probably to sites of potential cross-bridges between thick and thin filaments, activating myosin ATPase. Contraction results. Relaxation occurs, or at least the active state ceases, when Ca^{++} is pumped back into, or on the wall of, the longitudinal reticulum.

Distribution of Water

In organs and tissues in general, one tends to consider that there is a volume of water not included in blood and excluded from cells, so-called interstitial water, and a volume of water inside cells. In skeletal muscle the distribution of water is complicated by the fact that the sarcoplasmic reticulum is open to interstitial fluid. The volume of water in sarcoplasmic reticulum is, in a sense, outside the fibre, perhaps to the extent that intestinal juices are outside the body. Water content and distribution of water in organs and tissues are determined ordinarily by a series of measurements in which (a) total water is determined by drying the tissue to constant weight, and (b) the tissue content at equilibrium of a reference substance, presumably excluded from cells but distributed at uniform concentration in interstitial fluid, is divided by the extracellular concentration of the reference substance. The volume determined by the latter analysis is designated extracellular volume. Difference between total water and extracellular volume is considered cell water.

There are problems in determination of cell water, or more pertinently, sarcoplasmic or fibre water in muscle. One problem is that it is not clear that various extracellular reference substances diffuse freely throughout all interstitial space. It is conceivable that the tightly woven collagen mesh about fibres may serve as a molecular seive, although it is not likely to exclude a molecule even as large as inulin, a standard polyfructose reference substance. It is more conceivable that various carbohydrate reference substances, such as inulin and sucrose, may associate with the amorphous mucoprotein basement membrane, so that their concentration is not uniform. However, the fraction of total reference carbohydrate so associated may be negligible. The second problem has to do with the volume of endoplasmic reticulum and with access of the reference substance to it. It is likely that all commonly used reference substances find their way into the T-system because even proteins can be demonstrated in at least portions of the T-system. However, the

T-system is, in volume, the lesser component of the sarcoplasmic reticulum. Peachey (1965), on the basis of electron microscopy of frog sartorius muscle, has estimated that the T-system is but 0·3 % of fibre volume. On the other hand, it is likely that some reference substances enter longitudinal reticulum and others do not, and that, of those that enter, the concentration of reference substance in the longitudinal reticulum may be quite different from that in the interstitial fluid. The volume of the longitudinal reticulum is not negligible; it is probably of the same order as the volume of fluid between muscle fibres, based on Peachey's estimates by electron microscopy of frog muscle, and on our estimates (Rogus & Zierler, 1968) based on analysis of radio-sodium flux from rat skeletal muscle.

Total water in mammalian skeletal muscle varies with age and among different muscles. It is usually between 750 and 800 g./kg. fresh weight of muscle. Inulin space, a measure of interstitial water, probably including the T-system, has been estimated variously at from 120 to 250 g./kg. fresh weight. The longitudinal reticulum may have a water content of 140 to 170 g./kg. fresh weight. The difference between total water and the sum of interstitial and reticular water is sarcoplasmic water, which is about 500 g./kg. fresh weight.

There is a difference of opinion about the structure of sarcoplasmic water. There is general agreement that it is structured to a certain extent. By this is meant that individual water molecules do not have the complete freedom of movement they enjoy in the liquid state in bulk dilute solutions in the macroscopic world. There are hydration shells about proteins and ions. There is an electric field that may orientate polarized substances. It is not at all understood to what extent sarcoplasmic water is organized. Some hold that it is totally structured. In any event, the implication is that laws of dilute aqueous solutions from the macroscopic world may not apply. Furthermore, changes in muscle proteins may be associated with changes in the structure of water, as a result of which there may be secondary effects on muscle metabolism and function. This is, of course, quite speculative at this stage.

Movement, Distribution, and Rôle of Monovalent Ions, Na+, K+, Cl−

Mammalian skeletal muscle contains more K+ and less Na+ and Cl− per unit wet weight, or fresh weight, than does plasma, plasma water, or extracellular fluid. To determine their concentrations in muscle fibre water one needs to know the volume of muscle fibre water and whether or not the ion is distributed at uniform concentration within that volume. Neither of these is known accurately.

From analyses of radio-sodium efflux from rat skeletal muscle, Rogus & Zierler (1968) estimated that about 95 % of muscle fibre Na+ is in sarcoplasmic reticulum. True sarcoplasmic Na+, then, is at a concentration of about 2 millimoles/kg. of sarcoplasmic water. Sarcoplasmic K+ is at a concentration of 150 to 160 millimoles/kg. of sarcoplasmic water. There is great uncertainty about the Cl− concentration. Sarcoplasmic Cl− concentration is much smaller than that in extracellular fluid, but an exact measurement of the concentration has been impossible owing to uncertainties in measurement of water distribution. A small error in the estimate of inulin space can even lead to the ridiculous estimate that intracellular Cl− concentration is negative.

It is often assumed that Cl− flux in both directions across the sarcolemma is completely passive; that is, that Cl− is driven only by its electrochemical potential gradient. If this is true, then

$$E_R = E_{Cl} = \frac{RT}{F} \ln \frac{(Cl^-)_o}{(Cl^-)_i}$$

where E_R is the observed electrical potential difference across the sarcolemma with the muscle at rest, E_{Cl} is the Cl− equilibrium electrical potential difference, R, T, and F are constants, and $(Cl^-)_o$ and $(Cl^-)_i$ are chloride concentrations in water outside and inside the cell, respectively. For mammalian muscle, E_R is probably about −75 mV. This predicts that $(Cl^-)_i$ should be about 6 millimoles/kg. of sarcoplasmic water.

The equilibrium electrical potential difference for K+,

$$E_K = \frac{RT}{F} \ln \frac{(K^+)_i}{(K^+)_o}$$

is about −95 mV. Since the observed resting electrical potential difference, E_R, is much less for mammalian muscle, the electrical potential gradient, tending to drive K+ into muscle, is less than the chemical potential gradient, tending to drive K+ out of muscle.

In the steady state, influx and efflux of K+ must be equal. If the fluxes of K+ in both directions were passive (i.e., driven only by electrochemical potentials), efflux would exceed influx. There must therefore be an active transport system at least for inward K+ movement.

The reverse is true with respect to Na+. The Na+ equilibrium potential difference, E_{Na}, is about +120 mV, of sign opposite that of the observed electrical potential difference. This means that more than 99% of outward Na^+ flux is against an electrochemical potential gradient.

An ATPase system, activated by Na^+, K^+, and Mg^{++}, and inhibited by ouabain, has been found in a number of tissues. Skou (1965) and others have proposed that this is the energy source and the carrier for outward pumping of Na^+, with simultaneous, or coupled, inward pumping of K^+, usually in a 1 : 1 ratio. In mammalian skeletal muscle, this enzyme system is limited to a fraction, obtained by centrifugation, that appears on electron microscopy to contain only fragments of sarcoplasmic reticulum. This seems to imply that the $Na^+ - K^+$ pump is not in the sarcolemma, but in the membrane of the sarcoplasmic reticulum.

From measurements of membrane resistance to passage of electric currents in controlled extracellular ionic environments, Adrian & Freygang (1962) deduced that the sarcolemma is mainly permeable to Cl^- and the reticular system is mainly permeable to K^+, with the muscle at rest. The various muscle membranes, at rest, are quite poorly permeable to all ions, compared to the case in which there is no membrane (e.g., diffusion of aqueous solution). The apparent diffusibility of K^+ is several hundred million times greater in aqueous solution than it is from muscle; that is, the resistance to diffusion is enormous across muscle membranes. At rest, permeability to Na^+ is only a few percent of permeability to K^+.

When muscle is excited to contract, its permeability to Na^+ is increased specifically by perhaps two orders of magnitude. The electrical potential difference across the membrane moves toward the equilibrium potential for Na^+, but usually reaches only +30 to +50 mV. The rise from resting potential to the peak at +30 to +50 mV and the subsequent return to the resting value constitute the action potential. The actual net influx of Na^+ and net efflux of K^+ during the action potential is only at a rate of about 10^{-10} Eq/sec./cm² of cell surface, too small to measure by flame photometry. Restitution of original concentrations may occur by means of a $Na^+ - K^+$ coupled pump, but neither the time course of restitution nor its exact mechanism is known.

The magnitude of the steady electrical potential depends on the gradients of monovalent ions across the membrane and on the permeability of the membrane ot these ions. This is described by the Goldman-Hodgkin-Katz equation,

$$\psi = \frac{RT}{F} \ln \frac{P_K(K^+)_i + P_{Na}(Na^+)_i + P_{Cl}(Cl^-)_o}{P_K(K^+)_o + P_{Na}(Na^+)_o + P_{Cl}(Cl^-)_i}$$

where P is the permeability coefficient to the particular ion. P has dimensions of velocity, length per time, and at a given temperature varies only with some intrinsic property of the membrane. The resting potential can be modified by alterations in the gradient in K^+ concentration, but not very much by altered gradient in Na^+. In practice this usually means that changes in serum K^+ concentration alter the resting potential. Intracellular K^+ concentration does not vary widely in life. The amplitude of the action potential depends on the Na^+ concentration gradient, but extracellular Na^+ rarely varies over a sufficiently wide range in life to make an important difference in the height of the action potential.

Many of the symptoms and signs of hypokalaemia and hyperkalaemia can be attributed to changes in the resting membrane potential. Hypokalaemia would be expected to increase the resting membrane potential. Increased (more negative) membrane potential is called hyperpolarization. It is more difficult to depolarize a hyperpolarized membrane; that is, it is more difficult to initiate a propagated action potential.

On the other hand, hyperkalaemia would be expected to decrease the membrane potential, or to depolarize the membrane. Such a membrane might conceivably be more easily depolarized further to lead to a propagated action potential; it might be unstable. More likely, however, associated with the clinical states that produce hyperkalaemia there are other derangements. Among them is the possibility that ionic recovery processes function poorly, since the $Na^+ - K^+$ pump depends on energy coupled with cell metabolism. It is conceivable, therefore, that some of the disturbances of the neuromuscular apparatus, associated clinically with hyperkalaemia, may be due to impaired recovery processes.

There are probably functions for intracellular Na^+ and K^+ other than those concerned directly with transmembrane electrical potential differences. The sum of Na^+ and K^+ concentrations may play a rôle in the physical state of contractile proteins. Myosin is precipitated from aqueous solutions at K^+ concentrations not much less than those which occur normally inside cells; and for this purpose K^+ and Na^+ are virtually interchangeable.

K^+ may be required in a certain concentration for optimum activity of several enzyme systems. Positive nitrogen balance in the whole body, with increase in clinically-observable muscle mass, does not occur in patients in whom there is K deficit.

Metabolic Fuels

It was noted earlier that there are at least two types of muscle fibres, with respect to metabolic characteristics, and that in man muscles tend to contain mixtures of the two types. In general, there are small diameter, red, mitochondrial-rich fibres, and large diameter, pale, mitochondrial-poor fibres. The mitochondrial-rich fibres of course have active oxidative phosphorylation. They have a relatively low glycogen content, they stain for lipid, and they metabolize fatty acids. Such fibres are predominant in human muscle. The large, pale fibres have little oxidative phosphorylation, are rich in glycogen and poor in lipid. Their major metabolic route is probably by way of the Embden-Meyerhof pathway. Skeletal muscle contains little TPN, so that the pentose phosphate shunt is not very active. Such large, pale fibres are typical of frog sartorius muscle, from which so much information about muscle has been gained, but they are of far less importance in man.

It is possible to consider metabolism of muscle at rest as separate from metabolism occurring during contraction and recovery.

Resting metabolism is spent in cellular house-keeping, keeping the muscle in readiness for contraction. Presumably it involves such things as maintenance of energy-coupled transport systems, such as a Na^+ pump, as well as continuing syntheses.

In man, evidence for the nature of the metabolic mixture comes from studies of metabolism of forearm muscles *in situ*. Blood flow to forearm muscles, multiplied by arterio-venous concentration differences across forearm muscles under steady-state conditions, gives a measure of uptake (quantity per time) or release of various metabolites. From such studies it has been concluded that only 15% of forearm muscle oxygen consumption can be accounted for by oxidation of glucose extracted from arterial blood, and that the rest of the oxygen consumption is spent in oxidation of free fatty acids (FFA) extracted from plasma (Zierler, Maseri, Klassen, Rabinowitz & Burgess, 1968). This quantitative result is supported by the respiratory quotient of forearm muscles, which is about 0·74.

The major substrates are the most abundant free fatty acids, oleic acid, which constitutes about 45% of arterial plasma FFA, and palmitic acid, which constitutes 25–30% of the total. Both of these fatty acids are extracted by muscle from arterial plasma to about the same proportion, so that about 45% of forearm oxygen consumption at rest is accounted for by oxidation of oleic acid, and about 25% by oxidation of palmitic acid.

The contribution of metabolism of ketone bodies to oxygen consumption is negligible except during periods of prolonged fasting.

To what extent skeletal muscle suffers anaerobic metabolism at rest is unknown. There are no reliable measurements of the very small amount of heat released from resting muscle. If there were, one could calculate whether or not the heat equivalent of the observed oxygen consumption equalled the measured heat. There is a suggestion that in man there may be substantial anaerobic metabolism at rest. Specifically, lactic acid concentration in venous blood draining forearm muscles exceeds that in arterial blood, even at rest. Indeed, lactate production by forearm muscles at rest can account for about half the observed glucose uptake from arterial blood by forearm muscles (Baltzan, Andres, Cader & Zierler, 1962). This observation has been interpreted as evidence that there is anaerobic metabolism at rest. It is possible that although a substantial fraction of skeletal muscle fibres may metabolize anaerobically at any instant, no muscle fibre remains at the extremely low oxygen tension needed for anaerobic metabolism for very long. Blood flow to skeletal muscle at rest is relatively small. It is conceivable that this small blood flow is rationed so that while some fibres are perfused adequately, others are not, and that this small blood flow is redistributed among fibres so that no fibre remains poorly perfused for a period long enough to produce irreversible damage.

When a skeletal muscle contracts there is increased evolution of heat. This heat occurs with initiation of contraction and is maintained during the course of contraction. It is possible, during steady, maintained muscle contraction in man, to obliterate arterial pulsations. In experimental preparations, although blood flow is not likely to be reduced, an increase in blood flow is limited during contraction, depending on the force of contraction. When contraction ceases, if the load on the muscle or the force of contraction has been sufficiently great to restrict blood flow, there is immediate post-contraction hyperaemia, much like hyperaemia following release of arterial occlusion. At peak hyperaemia, blood flow to skeletal muscle may be 20–50 times resting blood flow. Blood flow returns to normal over a period of 5–20 minutes. During this hyperaemic period there is a large increase in oxygen consumption.

The questions concerning metabolic fuels are: What are the substrates during contraction? What are the substrates during recovery? Has the composition of muscle returned to its resting values by the time blood flow, oxygen consumption and heat production have returned to resting values?

Some of these questions have not been answered adequately in man, or in any preparation.

During contraction, as indicated earlier in this chapter, ATP is hydrolysed. ATP is resynthesized from the pool of creatine phosphate. Most, if not all, of the initial heat (that produced during the mechanical response, in excess of that produced a rest) can be accounted for by the heat of hydrolysis of creatine phosphate. Eventually, there must be regeneration of creatine phosphate. This can be accomplished anaerobically or, more effectively, aerobically, and there are reasons for believing that both processes proceed in man.

If exercise is sufficiently strenuous, lactic acid production by forearm muscles, measured as the product of blood flow and arterio-venous difference in lactic acid concentration, can exceed the lactate equivalent of glucose uptake (defined as two moles of lactate produced per mole of glucose uptake). This means not only that there is anaerobic metabolism, but also that the glycogen content of muscle must decrease. It is not known yet how long is needed to replenish muscle glycogen in man, but in experimental preparations many hours, up to 18 or more, can be required to mend the loss incurred during seconds or minutes of muscle stimulation (Cori & Cori, 1933; Sacks & Sacks, 1933; Hines & Knowlton, 1935; Flock & Bollman, 1940).

There is abundant evidence that oxidation of fatty acids is the major pathway for oxygen consumption during exercise.

Earliest evidence that lipids are used during exercise was provided by Lafon (1913), who found a higher arterial than venous lipid concentration at rest, and an increase in the difference during exercise (chewing) in blood to and from the levator of the upper lip in the intact horse, and by Palazzolo (1913), who discovered that electrical stimulation decreased fatty acid content of isolated gastrocnemius from winter frogs and from fasted summer frogs and of the hind limb of the hibernating hedgehog. Some years later Ochoa (1930) and Gemmill (1932) found that glycogen-poor frog muscle could develop isometric tension at least as great as normal muscle, and that glycogenolysis under these conditions was only in small part the source of energy for contraction. However, Buchwald & Cori (1931) could detect no significant decrease in lipid content of rat gastrocnemius stimulated *in situ*, although in poorly-nourished frogs repeated stimulation of one sciatic nerve decreased lipid in the stimulated

leg. George and his colleagues (1958) demonstrated histochemically that, in birds and flying mammals, exercise decreases glycogen in glycogen-rich fibres and decreases lipid in lipid-rich fibres. But Neptune, Foreman & Reisch (1960) failed to find decreased endogenous fatty acids in electrically stimulated excised rat diaphragm and Masoro, Rowell, MacDonald & Steiert (1966) found no change in intracellular lipid ester content in contracting skeletal muscle.

Despite uncertainty about the use of lipid already present inside muscle fibres, there is little doubt that during exercise muscle extracts more free fatty acids from plasma than at rest, and that oxidation of this free fatty acid can account for most of the oxygen consumed. Fritz et al. (1958) observed that FFA removal from the bathing solution (or its appearance as labelled CO_2) increased compared to that at rest and accounted for much of the increased O_2 consumption by electrically stimulated, excised rat muscle.

Friedberg, Sher, Bodgonoff & Estes (1963) and Havel, Pernow & Jones (1967) estimated, from infusion of labelled palmitic acid into man, that there is increased FFA uptake by exercising muscle and increased oxidation of FFA during exercise. Hagenfeldt & Wahren (1966) and Zierler et al. (1968) have quantitated FFA uptake by forearm muscles during forearm exercise and found it increased. Zierler et al. (1968) found that the RQ of forearm muscles remained at about 0·7 during mild exercise, indicating continuing preferential lipid oxidation, and that the oxidation-equivalent of FFA abstracted from blood during forearm exercise was about five times that of glucose.

The question of whether or not there is a store of muscle lipid used in part during exercise remains unsettled. Earlier experiments in a number of preparations, cited above, gave equivocal results. The more recent studies of Havel et al. (1967) and of Zierler et al. (1968) suggest that in man there may be oxidation of muscle lipid stores. Techniques used in these experiments may be more sensitive for this purpose than direct analysis of chemical content of muscle samples, since it has not been possible to obtain skeletal muscle samples free of adipose tissue.

In summary, in man skeletal muscles at rest can oxidize lipid and carbohydrate. All the O_2 consumed by muscle at rest can be accounted for by oxidation of FFA and of glucose abstracted from arterial blood, and, under standard conditions, 85% or more is attributed to oxidation of FFA. During exercise uptake of FFA and of glucose from blood is increased, and the ratio of uptakes remains about the same as at rest. Whether all O_2 consumption during exercise can be accounted for by oxidation of substrates abstracted from blood or whether some of it is spent in oxidation of stored lipid and carbohydrate is not yet determined clearly, but most signs suggest that the latter occurs.

CHEMICAL PATHOLOGY

Atrophy

There are few biological puzzles more mysterious than the delicate trophic relationship which exists between a striated muscle fibre and its motor nerve. When the nerve is severed there follows within several days a series of events which, if permitted to continue without re-innervation, lead over months to the virtual disappearance of the muscle fibre (Tower, 1939; Sunderland & Ray, 1950; Adams, Denny-Brown & Pearson, 1953). This reaction to denervation, with its progressive wasting of muscle bulk, is unique in the appearance of two distinct phenomena: the development of random, spontaneous discharges in single fibres, fibrillation (Denny-Brown & Pennybacker, 1938; Jarcho, Berman, Dowben & Lilienthal, 1954), and of exquisite sensitivity to various stimulating agents, especially acetylcholine (Cannon & Rosenblueth, 1949). The progressive loss of bulk is an accompaniment common to simple disuse, inanition, immobilization, ischaemia, tenotomy and local injection of tetanus toxin (Davenport, Ranson & Stevens, 1929) as well as denervation, and in all forms there is a marked loss in contractile strength of remaining muscle fibres. The loss in bulk of muscle fibre follows the familiar exponential curve which appears so frequently to describe processes of both growth and decay in biological systems (Sutfin, Thomson & Hines, 1954). In the muscles they studied, the rate of weight loss, in terms of residual weight, was remarkably constant, similar to the findings by Bowden in monkeys (1951); nevertheless, there seems reason to believe that in some specialized muscles the rate of loss may vary appreciably (Adams et al., 1953) and that species differences may be very large indeed. Lest it be inferred that denervation releases some inexorable catabolic process, attention should be directed to the findings of Dreyfus and the Schapiras (1949) that in growing rabbits the total weight of the denervated muscle continues to rise, albeit at a much slower rate than its contralateral control. Experiments on diaphragm from adult rats show that in certain cases the denervated muscle may in fact gain weight during the week following denervation (Sola & Martin

1953), a gain which has been attributed simply to local retention of water (Thomson, Morgan & Brodish, 1951). In any event, it is plain that although contractile strength decreases in atrophying muscle in rough proportion to the loss of muscle fibre bulk, nevertheless, there may occur significant discrepancies.

With respect to the time course of weight-loss accompanying various forms of atrophy, a number of factors have been observed to play a modifying rôle. Virtually every observer has reported that daily brief periods of direct electrical stimulation of denervated muscle will retard the rate of atrophy (Hines, 1952), although contractile strength per unit mass of muscle is not preserved to the same degree (Fischer, 1939). It would seem that the work performed by the atrophying muscle, which is stimulated electrically, is related closely to the prevention of weight loss, because stimulation is more effective in the partially stretched muscle and of little or no effect in the tenotomized muscle which shortens against very little resistance (Wehrmacher, Thomson & Hines, 1945). Those factors which share a capacity to accelerate body metabolism (e.g. thyroxine) increase rate of atrophy slightly, while those which depress such processes (e.g., thiourea) have the reverse effect (Diaz-Guerrero, Thomson & Hines, 1947; Huf & Fischer, 1949). Although it has been known since Langley & Itagaki's (1917) original observation that the resting rate of O_2 consumption is accelerated in atrophying muscle, Slack (1954), who measured the rate of incorporation of labelled glycine into the residual proteins of atrophying muscle, could not detect any difference from the rate of protein "synthesis" proceeding in the control muscles. Once regeneration begins, rate of weight gain is rapid at first and decreases progressively (Hines, Thomson & Lazere, 1942).

Extensive changes in composition occur in muscle undergoing atrophy, but there still is some uncertainty as to the absolute degree of some of these changes. This uncertainty arises from the fact that the available pool of data is made up of observations on various species, and of measurements which vary in the account taken of the difficult problem of reference base, discussed elsewhere.

There appears to be a slight increase in water content approximating 1% (Humoller, Griswold & McIntyre, 1950a), although there are peculiar instances of considerably greater gain exemplified by the findings of Thomson (1955) in rat diaphragm.

It has been known for decades (Audova, 1923)

that lipid increases in atrophic muscle, but there are no quantitative data on the extent to which this increase may lie within muscle fibres.

The question of ionic composition is confused. In the denervated muscle of the rat Humoller *et al.* (1950*b*) found a sharp increase in Na and Ca content and a slight fall in K, expressed in terms of wet weight of muscle. On the other hand Baldwin, Robinson, Zierler & Lilienthal (1952), who examined atrophic muscle in man, could discover no significant change in either K or Mg content when the amounts were referred to the non-collagenous N content of the muscle, although there were apparent losses when these cations were referred to wet weight of muscle. There is evidence that the normal rates of flux and of penetrability of Cl^- (Fischer, 1952) and of K^+ (Harris & Nicholls, 1954) are altered appreciably by atrophy, and the slowed conduction of fibrillary potentials in denervated muscle is consistent with a significant decrease in the concentration of reactants of the fibre (Jarcho *et al.*, 1954). Perhaps the best that can be said at this time is that no overall characteristic alteration in ionic composition has been disclosed, although there is much to suggest that changes do occur.

Among the few constant components is an Fe fraction, called non-haemin Fe by Schapira & Dreyfus (1959) who first characterized it. The concentration of this Fe increases in denervated muscle in proportion to the loss of muscle weight; that is, the total amount of Fe per muscle is unchanged and might therefore serve as a reference base. Also constant, per muscle but increasing per muscle wet weight, is deoxyribonucleic acid (Clavert, Mandel & Jacob, 1949; Schmidt & Schlief, 1956).

There are undoubtedly remarkable changes in muscle proteins, although it is not clear what they are. There is certainly an increase in collagen. Fischer (1952), Fischer & Ramsey (1946), Stewart (1955) and Schapira & Dreyfus (1959) and their colleagues have studied alterations in contractile proteins characterizing atrophy owing to various causes. Most remarkable is an apparent reduction in the particle size of myosin, determined by its flow birefringence, remarkable because it is demonstrable within a few minutes following denervation (Dreyfus, Joly, Schapira & Raeber, 1953), a fact that its discoverers suggest may be secondary to a rapid change in internal ionic environment. Late in atrophy the ATPase activity of the remaining myosin is decreased (Fischer, 1955). It has also been reported that myosin from denervated muscle is immunochemically distinct from normal (Samuels, 1957). Quantification of

myosin and actin content is treacherous and their concentration is uncertain. There seems little doubt, however, that their rate of synthesis is decreased, an observation first made in the laboratories of Schapira & Dreyfus (1959) and evident after the first day following denervation.

A curious situation arises with regard to other proteins, collagen excepted. No definite persistent increase in enzymic content of atrophic muscle has appeared; indeed, most measurements show decreases. Yet the O_2 consumption of residual muscle is accelerated, and there is the intriguing observation that after many weeks there is an increase in muscle ribonucleic acid, hinting at a possible increase in synthesis of some undetected protein, as Schapira & Dreyfus (1959) have pointed out. The accelerated O_2 consumption is not obviously due to the uncoupling of oxidative phosphorylation, although direct measurement is lacking, but at least there is no great change in ATP content of residual muscle.

One of the things atrophying muscle may be oxidizing is itself. Its glycogen content decreases. There is evidence of autolysis. Certain amino acids, particularly glutamic acid, increase (Yudaev, Smirnov, Razina & Dorbert, 1953). There are alterations in di- and tri-peptides. Carnosine content decreases steadily (Yudaev *et al.*, 1953), but glutathione doubles (Okuda, 1930).

In short, we are faced with a plethora of observations on isolated biochemical events during the process of atrophy, but we have no clear image of how they tie together. Gutmann (1959) suggests that denervation leads to a reduction in synthetic processes.

The supersensitivity of denervated muscle, specifically to acetylcholine, recalls the foetal state. Acetylcholine depolarizes not only the end plate, as it does in normal muscle, but many spots along the denervated muscle fibre (Thesleff, 1960).

The phenomenon of fibrillation which characterizes denervation has certain aspects which link it to metabolic activity in general (Feinstein, Pattle & Weddell, 1945). Although there is substantial evidence that atrophy is not an exhaustion effect of fibrillation (Solandt & Magladery, 1940) yet the two processes are accelerated and delayed by the same sort of metabolic modulators.

Ischaemic injury to muscle effects a storm of disorganization that erases recognizable chemical patterns and obliterates the structure of the fibre (Green & Stoner, 1952).

Muscular Dystrophies
Experimentally produced muscular dystrophies.
In a variety of laboratory animals there has been

produced by any one of several means—vitamin E deficiency (Pappenheimer, 1948) and large doses of cortisone (Ellis, 1952), in particular—a disorder of skeletal muscle characterized grossly by weakness and histologically by architectural changes reminiscent of those occurring spontaneously in naturally occurring progressive muscular dystrophy in man. Although the variety of exciting agents, which produce similar lesions in muscle, suggests that muscle may be capable only of a stereotyped response, this does not rule out the possibility that the primary mechanism for this response may be shared by several agents. For example, cortisone accelerates urinary excretion of several vitamins, thus producing a vitamin deficiency state. There are no data concerning the effect of cortisone on vitamin E disposal, and it remains possible that the myopathy produced by cortisone may be in fact due to deficiency of vitamin E.

Most thoroughly studied of the experimental dystrophies is that which follows dietary lack of vitamin E, sometimes called nutritional muscular dystrophy, described first by Pappenheimer & Goettsch (1931), Morgulis & Spencer (1936) and Mackenzie & McCollum (1940). Since it is not established that examples of vitamin E deficient dystrophy have appeared in man, only a brief summary of the rôle of vitamin E will be considered here. Further information will be found in reports of an International Conference on Vitamin E (Mason, 1949), in a review (Mackenzie, 1953), and in the Annotated Bibliography of Vitamin E (Harris & Kuzawski, 1950, 1952, 1955).

How deficiency of vitamin E, or tocopherol, produces muscular dystrophy remains unsolved. It was appreciated early in the study of nutritional muscular dystrophy that dystrophic animals (Kaunitz & Pappenheimer, 1943) and their isolated skeletal muscle (Victor, 1934) consumed much more O_2 than did normal animals or their isolated skeletal muscle. This effect is obliterated by administration of therapeutic doses of vitamin E (Friedman & Mattill, 1941; Kaunitz & Pappenheimer, 1943) and reversed by excessive doses (Zierler, Folk, Eyzaguirre, Jarcho, Grob & Lilienthal, 1949a).

Assays of various enzyme systems in muscle from animals with nutritional muscular dystrophy have demonstrated a number of defects. It is difficult to see how these defects, in which enzyme activity is reduced, can explain the accelerated O_2 consumption observed in total muscle, unless they imply a shift of energetic processes to as yet unidentified systems in which O_2 is consumed less efficiently. In some cases, the decrease in enzyme

activity may be more apparent than real, reflecting only a gross loss of cellular substance in dystrophic muscle.

In contrast to these observations there is accelerated ribonuclease activity in muscles from vitamin E deficient rabbits with increased turnover of nucleic acids (Dinning, 1955). Whether this is an immediate result of vitamin E deficiency (i.e. whether vitamin E normally checks ribonuclease activity), or whether this is to be expected when there is necrosis of tissue from a number of causes, is undetermined. Also accelerated in vitamin E deficient muscle are the activities of certain proteolytic (Weinstock, Goldrich & Milhorat, 1955; Koszalka, Mason & Krol, 1961) and autolytic enzymes (Koszalka et al., 1961), which are restored to or toward normal when the animal is treated with vitamin E. The meaning of these observations in terms of underlying mechanism is obscure.

There are several bits of evidence linking vitamin E to muscle glycolysis (Zierler, Levy & Lilienthal, 1953; Gray & DeLuca, 1954), which suggest that the use of energy stored as carbohydrate within muscle may be faulty in the presence of excess or insufficiency of vitamin E. Zierler et al. (1953) reported that the phosphoglucomutase system, among the enzymes of the Embden-Meyerhof chain, was inhibited specifically by administration of a tocopherol, an observation confirmed in vitro by more modern methods by Rosenkrantz & Laferte (1961). In contrast, assay of white muscle, but not of red muscle, from E-deficient chicks yielded reduced phosphoglucomutase activity (Hazzard & Leonard, 1961). In any case, whatever vitamin E or its lack may appear to do to carbohydrate metabolism, this rôle seems inadequate to explain the devastation overtaking skeletal muscle deprived of this vitamin.

However, the biological role so far assigned to vitamin E is intellectually dissatisfying, in that it makes no use of what is perhaps the most striking chemical property of tocopherol, that it is a reducing agent with a potential which should be effective in living tissue (Golumbic & Mattill, 1940). It might be expected that tocopherol should participate in an electron transport system which itself is central to a number of key reactions, or, conceivably, it might simply prevent oxidation of fatty acids which are important in this regard.

A link between tocopherol and electron transport was suggested by the work of Nason and his colleagues (Donaldson, Nason & Garrett, 1958), but unfortunately the evidence that tocopherol is concerned directly is no longer substantial.

Largely from studies of bizarre disturbances among livestock it is clear that dietary deficiency of selenium or of vitamin E produces similar clinical and morphological disturbances. Zalkin & Tappel (1960) reported that, in the E-deficient rabbit, lipid peroxidation of mitochondria and microsomes could trigger metabolic alterations, and that either dietary selenium or tocopherol inhibited lipid peroxidation in tissues from the chick (Zalkin, Tappel & Jordan, 1960). The effect of neither selenium nor tocopherol may be direct. In deficiency of either there is decreased tissue ubiquinone content, restorable when either is administered. Tocopheronolactone acts with extraordinary speed to raise in minutes the ubiquinone content of heart muscle from E-deficient rats (Diplock, Edwin, Green & Bunyan, 1961). Influence on ubiquinone synthesis, or on its activation, is shared by many substances, and may be the common pathway underlying a number of nutritional and toxic myopathies. There is no evidence that any of these underlies naturally occurring progressive muscular dystrophy in man.

Hereditary myopathy of mice. Michelson, Russell & Harman (1955) discovered a myopathy in mice, inherited as an autosomal recessive, histologically reminiscent of human progressive muscular dystrophy. Although its mode of inheritance differs from those of the two commonest types of human progressive muscular dystrophy, and hence presumably it is apt to represent a different metabolic defect, mouse hereditary myopathy gave new opportunities for honing tools with which to dissect muscle disease. Many studies, previously performed in E-deficiency and in patients with muscular dystrophy, were repeated in the mice. Although the disease is now well-described in many details, its metabolic origin is not obviously nearer exposition than is that of the disease in man. In addition to the original histological description of the disease by Michelson *et al.* (1955), more recent morphological and histochemical studies (Kitivakara, 1961) show that the number of nuclei per muscle is normal, but that, owing to the presence of many narrower muscle fibres, nuclear material per unit muscle mass is increased. There was no evidence of altered DNA synthesis. Golarz & Bourne (1960), who earlier suggested, on the basis of histochemical study of human muscle, that muscular dystrophy might be primarily a disease of connective tissue and not of muscle, found no such evidence in mouse myopathy, and concluded that they could not support the hypothesis that the two were the same disease.

The following observations will be placed in perspective after we have discussed progressive muscular dystrophy in man:

In mouse dystrophy there is increased excretion of creatine in urine. There is some dispute as to whether or not urinary creatinine excretion is diminished. Muscle creatine concentration is reduced and phosphorylation of creatine may be inadequate, or at any rate muscle is unable to retain creatine normally (Fitch, Oates & Dinning, 1961).

Increases in concentrations of several serum enzymes occur as in human muscular dystrophy, and there are probably reductions in muscle content of several of these enzymes. In normal muscle at rest most of the phosphorylase is in the inactive form, phosphorylase *b*. Electrical stimulation rapidly converts more of it to the active phosphorylase *a* (Rulon, Schottelius & Schottelius, 1961). Although total phosphorylase is reduced in dystrophic mouse muscle, the fraction of it that is *a* at rest is normal and its activation with electrical stimulation is approximately normal, although it may be activated even more rapidly than normal (Rulon, Schottelius & Schottelius, 1962).

That the concentration of certain enzymes is high in serum and low in muscle suggests that dystrophic muscle is inordinately leaky. This has been demonstrated for the case of aldolase (Zierler, 1958*a*, 1961*b*). That the leak may be for many substances is suggested by the fact that both the influx (Burr & McLennan, 1961) and efflux (Zierler, 1961*b*) of K^+ is accelerated.

Prior to elucidation by electron microscopy of the details of sarcoplasmic reticulum, it had been assumed that an enzyme leak occurred across the sarcolemma. With more refined knowledge of morphology one now must include the possibility that the leak occurs from sarcoplasm across walls of longitudinal reticulum, through the tubular longitudinal reticulum, across the junction of cysternae and transverse tubules, through the transverse tubules of interstitial space.

Sreter, Ikemoto & Gergely (1967) have found morphological and functional abnormalities (reduced calcium uptake) in fragmented sarcoplasmic reticulum (microsomes) from myopathic mice. Aloisi & Margreth (1967) have deduced, from studies of parallel increases in sarcoplasmic enzyme content and growth in volume of sarcoplasmic reticulum, that most of the so-called sarcoplasm enzymes are in the longitudinal reticulum. A wide variety of factors can swell the terminal cysternae of longitudinal reticulum. If these swollen cysternae cause an increase in the permeability of the junction between cysternae and transverse tubules, then enzymes already in the longitudinal reticular system could not be prevented from leaking through the transverse system into interstitial space. Aloisi & Margreth (1967) have also shown that the sarcoplasmic reticulum is only scantily developed in new-born rats.

There is no doubt that hereditary myopathic muscles are abnormally leaky. The question is, is this leakiness of some limiting membrane the fundamental defect or is there a more primary cause acting upon the membrane? It is not yet established that the affected membrane is that of the cysterna-T system junction, or that more than one membrane is not involved. Since chloride conductance across muscle membranes is largely if not entirely across sarcolemma, an appropriate experiment would measure chloride conductance in myopathic muscle.

One of the difficulties in studying heritable disorders lies in distinguishing results of the disease from more primary defects. By the time animals or patients with these dystrophies are studied they have been ill for a long time. How long is illustrated by the report by Meier, West & Hoag (1965) that histological changes in tongue, masseter, and psoas muscles are apparent even in prenatal stages of mouse muscular dystrophy. Even though such studies are technically difficult, the greatest value of naturally occurring muscular dystrophies in animals may lie in the examination of foetal abnormalities, and first attention might be paid to those that concern development of membrane systems.

Other hereditary myopathies in animals. An autosomal recessive myopathy has been reported in chickens (Asmundsen, Kratzer & Julian, 1966) and in the Syrian hamster (Homburger, Nixon, Eppenberger & Baker, 1966). The latter is of interest because it is associated with a high incidence of cardiac necrosis, in some series including 100% of dystrophic animals. There is also an hereditary myopathy in the white Pekin duck, but its genetic transmission is unknown (Rigdon, 1966). In general, these other animal myopathies share the biochemical features of mouse myopathy insofar as they have been studied. Specifically, there are high concentrations of various enzymes in the serum and a reduced content of the same enzymes in muscle.

The disease in chickens is interesting in that red muscle is relatively spared, the white breast muscles being involved most severely. Peters (1967) has reported a decrease in content of a number of enzymes from white muscle of myopathic chickens, and noted that these enzymes have in common the capacity to shuttle reducing equivalents from $NADH_2$ into mitochondria. They are, however, enzymes of the non-particulate fractions of muscle, and, in general, are those that have been found in abnormally high concentrations in serum.

Progressive muscular dystrophies. The progressive muscular dystrophies are inherited disorders, mainly, but not necessarily only, affecting skeletal muscle. In recent years there have been several attempts to classify these diseases on the basis of patterns of inheritance and clinical features, but there is no general agreement, and it is entirely possible that much of the difference of opinion regarding classification reflects a real difference in the types of dystrophy seen in different geographical areas. Furthermore, despite classification there are patients who suffer an hereditary dystrophy not resembling any of the forms widely distributed geographically, and many others whose dystrophy appears spontaneously without family history. The subject is discussed fully in an admirable review by Walton & Nattrass (1954).

Often some phenomena in patients with progressive muscular dystrophy have suggested disturbance of the autonomic nervous system, or of one or other of the endocrine glands. Critical examination of these extramuscular factors, however, has failed to reveal dysfunction, which might be considered either primary or essential to the muscular dystrophy (Hoagland, Gilder & Shank, 1945; Tyler & Perkoff, 1951).

Interpretation of metabolic observations in patients with the muscular dystrophies is difficult, because superimposed upon the primary dystrophy there are apt to be chronic pulmonary infection, atrophy of disuse of many muscle groups and nutritional deficiencies as in many chronic debilitating diseases. For example, many patients with dystrophy have a low basal metabolic rate by normal standards. It might be suspected that subnormal O_2 consumption in such patients simply reflects the replacement of skeletal muscle by much less actively respiring fat and connective tissue. Indeed, it has been suggested that the basal metabolic rate in these patients be corrected for loss of muscle mass (estimated from the quantity of urinary creatinine), and when this is done the basal metabolic rate appears to be normal (Shank, Gilder & Hoagland, 1944).

Similar difficulties arise in interpretation of carbohydrate tolerance tests of various sorts. On the basis of such tests there have been reports that glucose tolerance in dystrophic patients is impaired (Meldolesi & Garretto, 1938) or normal (Tyler & Perkoff, 1951), or that there is hypoglycaemia (McCrudden & Sargent, 1916). Varying experience with glucose tolerance tests in dystrophy is not surprising, since patients may vary greatly with respect to the extent and severity and rate of progression of the dystrophy, and with respect to their general physical development and nutritional status. In part, impaired carbohydrate tolerance may result from the immediate dietary habits of these patients who may find eating a chore, and in part it may result from the fact that although remaining muscle may remove its share of administered glucose from blood, the total bulk of muscle is reduced and some glucose, which would in normals have moved into muscle, accumulates in blood. The so-called flat glucose tolerance curve may be the result of intestinal malabsorption. In some patients with muscular dystrophy there is oedema of the intestinal mucosa (Bevans, 1945) which, while it may or may not be a manifestation of the underlying dystrophy, resembles lesions of dietary insufficiency.

Metabolic balance studies, that is, quantitative assessment of dietary intake and excretory losses of certain elements, have sometimes shown overall losses of N, P and K. This array, classically interpreted, implies net loss of cellular substance, presumably muscle, and its presence suggests progression of the disease. Such losses are results of the disease, not causes, and occur, for example, during immobilization with its attendant atrophy (Cuthbertson, 1929; Howard, Parson & Bingham, 1944; Deitrick, Whedon & Shorr, 1948).

The concentration of creatine in serum is elevated and that of creatinine is normal or, perhaps, low (Cumings, 1953). Urine of dystrophic patients also gives evidence of continuing muscle destruction and of loss of muscle mass. The hallmark of progressive muscular dystrophy has been a reduction in the daily excretion of creatinine and excessive urinary loss of creatine (Milhorat & Wolff, 1937). These will be discussed later. In addition, there is increased urinary excretion of amino acids (Ames & Risley, 1948), though not larger than seen in association with negative N balance in a variety of states, and presumably explainable as the result of muscle destruction. A pentose, probably not ribose (Drew, 1955), also appears prominently in the urine of many patients with progressive muscular dystrophy (Minot, Frank & Dziewiatkowski, 1949). Since pentose is commonly incorporated into nucleotides, its presence in the urine can be interpreted as the result of some cellular catastrophe with subsequent degradation of nucleotides.

It is assumed generally that, if there is a metabolic defect underlying muscular dystrophy, it is primarily in the muscle fibre or its sarcolemma. However, Bourne & Golarz (1959) and Golarz, Bourne & Richardson (1961), from histochemical evidence of unusual quantities of certain hydrolytic enzymes in connective tissue in human dystrophic muscle, suggest that the primary defect may lie in the connective tissue and not in muscle proper. The study does not seem to have included examination of other states in which connective tissue proliferates, so that it may be that their observation is characteristic of connective tissue proliferation and not of muscular dystrophy.

Sibley & Lehninger (1949) reported high concentration of aldolase in the serum from muscular dystrophies, a finding confirmed by Schapira, Dreyfus & Schapira (1953) who also demonstrated that dystrophic muscle was deficient in aldolase. When muscle cells disintegrate or lose their selective permeability, their contents are swept into the blood stream. It was predictable, therefore, that serum concentrations of other enzymes would also be elevated. Schapira, Dreyfus, Schapira and their colleagues have investigated the matter most widely, but many others have confirmed the fact that not only aldolase but also glutamic oxaloacetic and pyruvic transaminases, lactic dehydrogenase, malic dehydrogenase and creatine phosphokinase all may occur in abnormally high concentration in serum. There is some evidence that some occur in greater quantities than others; in particular, Schapira et al. find creatine phosphokinase is apt to be elevated when other serum enzyme concentrations are not yet high. In general, the more extensive the dystrophy the more elevated are the serum enzyme concentrations, until rather late in the disease when their concentrations in serum fall. Nothing is known about the metabolic fate of serum enzymes, and a high serum concentration is still small compared to the concentration of these enzymes in muscle. Although there is no evidence that any reduction so far observed in muscle enzyme concentration is sufficiently great to limit metabolic events within muscle (Ronzoni, Berg & Landau, 1960), assessment of enzymic activity rests on analysis of groups of many fibres in varying states of disrepair, so that it is possible, indeed likely, that the more obviously diseased fibres suffer the greatest loss. In some of these, conceivably, enzymic losses may be sufficient to limit the rates of certain metabolic processes.

Owing to what is undoubtedly accelerated loss of these enzymes from muscle, the biological half-life of these enzymes is usually rapid. There may be some mechanism for adjusting rates of synthesis of these enzymes in order to maintain a nearly normal concentration. At least in dystrophic mice synthesis, measured by incorporation of labelled amino acid, is accelerated, though not sufficiently to meet the deficit (Kruh, Dreyfus, Schapira & Grey, 1960). A considerable portion of muscle's resting metabolism may be spent in this ultimately futile effort, although it is unknown whether it is the small degenerating dystrophic fibres that perform this extra job, or the abnormally large dystrophic fibres, or the remaining apparently normal muscle fibres, or proliferating extramuscular cells within muscle bundles.

It has been suggested that measurement of serum enzyme concentrations might lead to earlier recognition of cases of progressive muscular dystrophy, and that clinically normal carriers might be identified by demonstration of serum enzyme concentrations intermediate between those of normals and dystrophics, by analogy with other heritable disorders. Several groups have reported that, in families containing dystrophic members, serum enzyme concentrations may be high before the disease is apparent clinically (Brugsch, Brockmann-Rohne & Fromm, 1960; Pearson, Chowdhury, Fowler, Jones & Griffith, 1961), but, whenever muscle has been obtained by biopsy, there has also been histological evidence of muscular dystrophy (Pearson, 1962). Efficacy of the method for the detection of carriers is doubtful. Either there is no difference between normals and presumed carriers (Leyburn, Thomson & Walton, 1961) or there is a slight difference, most evident among mothers of boys with the Duchenne type of progressive muscular dystrophy (Chung, Morton & Peters, 1960; Schapira, Dreyfus, Schapira & Demos, 1960; Emery, 1967).

What does all this mean with regard to the cause or causes of muscular dystrophy? Because serum concentrations of enzymes are high and muscle concentrations are low, and because these enzymes are probably synthesized in muscle (Richterich, Gautier, Egli, Zuppinger & Rossi, 1961), and not blood-borne from some remote organ to muscle (in which case, high serum-low muscle concentrations would imply that entrance into muscle was difficult), it is likely that dystrophic muscle is leaky. There are many factors affecting flux of aldolase from rat and mouse muscle (Zierler, 1957, 1958a, b, c, 1961b) besides overt rupture of the membrane. In man, exercise is adequate to increase serum aldolase (Richter & Konitzer, 1960). The effectiveness of the cell membrane as a barrier to diffusion depends on the metabolism of the cell it envelops. On the other hand, inordinate leakiness must lead to altered

metabolism, even though not necessarily owing to the relatively small loss of enzyme. There is as yet no way to decide whether the presumed leakiness of human dystrophic muscle is due to a primary defect in construction of the cell membrane or is secondary to a more primary defect within the cell.

Just as there are abnormalities in the sarcoplasmic reticulum from myopathic mice, so there are similar defects in the sarcoplasmic reticulum of muscle obtained by biopsy from patients with progressive muscular dystrophy (Sugita, Okimoto, Ebashi & Okinaka, 1967).

There is no reason to believe that any chemical changes so far observed are specific. Similar enzyme leaks occur in patients with neurogenic atrophy. It is conceivable that the leak may sometimes be across the sarcolemma, sometimes through the T-system, and sometimes over both routes. It is also conceivable that morphological changes in the sarcoplasmic reticulum may be secondary to altered intracellular environment produced by a leak across the sarcolemma, and that diminished microsomal calcium uptake occurs pari passu with morphological deterioration of the sarcoplasmic reticulum. Or it is possible that there is from the beginning some error in the construction of membranes or of certain membranes. If the error is limited to skeletal muscle (or to myocardium and skeletal muscle) one might profitably inquire into what differences there are between muscle membranes and those of other cell types. Rather than being in the plasma membranes may not the difference be in mucopolysaccharide basement membranes, which may be more apt to be cell type-specific?

No one has demonstrated the fundamental defect in muscular dystrophy, and there may be as many fundamental defects as there are genetic variants of this group of diseases. So great is the devastation that it has not been possible to distinguish the results of the disease from its cause.

In the past much effort has gone into studies of creatine metabolism in muscular dystrophy, often with the assumption, at least implicit, that the creatinuria reflected a primary defect. Therapeutic attention was directed at times towards the creatinuria rather than the disease. Creatinuria will occur in any state in which there is dissolution of muscle and reduced muscle bulk in the face of continuing synthesis of creatine at normal velocity. Hoagland, Gilder & Shank (1945) concluded from the response of dystrophic patients to administration of precursors of creatine and to methyltestosterone that there was normal ability to synthesize creatine, but that there was simply inadequate muscle mass into which newly synthesized creatine might be deposited. This conclusion has been confirmed by tracer techniques (Benedict, Kalinsky, Scarrone, Wertheim & Stetten, 1955).

There have been chemical analyses of muscle, obtained by biopsy or at autopsy, from patients with progressive muscular dystrophy. As pointed out by Hoagland (1946*a*, *b*), it is particularly difficult to interpret chemical data from dystrophic muscle owing to uncertainties about the reference base. One g. wet weight of dystrophic muscle may contain a large amount of fat and connective tissue and very little muscle. If the sample is defatted and dried, there remains the dry weight of the connective tissue along with that of muscle fibres. Several expedient solutions to the problem have been offered, but many of the analyses of dystrophic muscle antedated the use of these reference bases and cannot be treated rigorously.

The earliest chemical analyses of muscle from patients with muscular dystrophy were those of Nevin (1934), who examined creatine phosphate and ATP in specimens of resting muscle, of contracted muscle and of muscle recovered from faradic stimulation. In dystrophic muscle these organic phosphates were low when expressed as a percentage of total acid-soluble phosphate, and they were split to a less extent than normal in contracted muscle. These observations were not specific for muscular dystrophy, however, insofar as they were also obtained by Nevin in muscle atrophic by reason of nerve degeneration. Somewhat similar results were reported later by Nevin (1936) for muscle from two patients with a disease which he called late progressive myopathy, which is considered by some to be not a dystrophy but a polymyositis.

A few years later Reinhold & Kingsley (1938) confirmed that the creatine concentration of dystrophic muscle was diminished (this observation is difficult to interpret owing to the lack of adequate reference base), and that phosphocreatine and ATP represented less than normal fractions of acid-soluble phosphate. Again, these observations were not specific for muscular dystrophy and were obtained, though this time to a slightly less extent, in muscle secondarily atrophied.

In muscles from dystrophic children Vignos & Lefkowitz (1959) reported that there is increased collagen, decreased myosin per unit non-collagenous N, decreased ATPase, creatine kinase and glycolysis (but these enzymic changes occur similarly in neurogenic atrophy). In adults with late onset of muscular dystrophy the enzymic changes

were not evident, but myosin was reduced to an even greater extent.

Horvath & Proctor (1960) confirmed chemically an increase in collagen and in fat and a decrease in muscle protein in muscular dystrophy, although they found that myosin may be decreased less than remaining muscle protein in some specimens. Na and Cl increased and K decreased.

Again, it is difficult to interpret these observations as other than changes secondary to destruction of muscle fibres.

Electrolytes

The participation of various electrolytes in the function of muscle is well recognized to be crucial. Accumulations or depletions of several ions result variously in inexcitability or hyperexcitability, weakness or contracture, shrinking or swelling. For many of these ions the effects of change of concentration in interstitial fluid or within the fibre are well described (Manery, 1954); the synergistic or antagonistic results of various combinations are known. But fundamental information is meagre as to how these effects are produced.

Because current methods of analysis yield knowledge mainly about the concentration of electrolytes in extracellular fluids, and less is known about either concentration or state within muscle fibre, concepts are based naturally enough on what has been discovered to occur outside the cell. In a few instances there are measurements which suggest the direction of movement of ions into or out of the cell, but they are as yet not complete or certain enough to allow much more than entertaining speculation.

In the main, distortions of electrolyte distribution follow several large categories of functional disorder: excessive or prolonged loss *via* watery secretions or dejecta; expansion or contraction of aqueous compartments; inadequate or excessive intake (dietary or absorptive) or rapid cellular dissolution; disturbances in hormonal and cerebral function; congenital or acquired faults in renal or pulmonary economy; and a group of rare inborn defects of which periodic paralysis is a paradigm (Peters, 1952).

Potassium. There is scarcely an end to the list of functions and specific biochemical processes which depend on precise regulation of K for the maintenance of normal behaviour. Concentration of K in muscle varies less than that in serum. It is not possible in the animal to increase intramuscular K by much more than 10%. In excised muscle K concentration can be raised a good deal higher simply by incubation in hypertonic sucrose solutions, but this has no quantitative counterpart in life owing to the lethal effects of severe hypertonicity. Nor can intramuscular K be reduced in the experimental animal to less than 40% of normal. In man, the most clinically serious K depletion, estimated from repletion studies, is not apt to represent loss of more than 20% of body K, although this does not indicate what the K concentration may be in muscle.

K concentration in serum need have little relation to that in muscle. K, entering plasma from muscle, may be collected by other tissues and, more likely, may be excreted in the urine. The change in mass of circulating K depends on the difference between the rate at which K enters plasma and the rate at which it leaves. It is possible, therefore, to find the serum K concentration abnormally high in the face of accelerated loss from muscle because renal excretion of K is impaired. This, of course, is a common event in diabetic ketosis. The mass of K in muscle is more than 50 times greater than that in extracellular fluid. If muscle were to dump 1% of its K into extracellular fluid, where it remained, the concentration of serum K would rise by more than 50%. Conversely, if half the extracellular K were to move into muscle it would be futile to seek the event by measuring muscle K, because muscle K concentration would rise by less than 1%.

Effects of altered K content must be the result of changes in concentration of intracellular K (because so many enzymic processes are K-requiring, and because the physical state of myosin is K-concentration-dependent) and of changes in the logarithm of the ratio of intracellular to extracellular K (because the resting membrane electrical potential difference is affected by this value), and these effects must be modulated by many changes in concentrations of other electrolytes that happen to accompany the state in which K is altered. Many clinical states are complicated by widespread distortion of electrolyte concentrations, and it is not surprising that quantitative correlation between measurements of K concentrations and some clinical phenomena is not as clear-cut as it can be under certain controlled laboratory conditions.

When K is lost from the body, as in continuing urinary losses during starvation, in vomiting, in diarrhoea, or in exaggerated urinary losses, a major symptom is weakness. In severe loss there may be absence of tendon reflexes, and muscle may not respond to direct percussion. When the myocardium or muscles of respiration are involved, life is threatened and K repletion is urgent. Transition from clinically minor to clinically severe involvement may be alarmingly abrupt. Yet it is astonishing how often neuromuscular function is maintained despite reduction in concentration of serum K to nearly half normal (Mudge & Vislocky, 1949; Tarail, Hacker & Taymer, 1952).

Muscle weakness, to which the word paralysis has been applied frequently, has been reported as due to reduction in body K, usually with hypokalaemia, secondary to urinary loss in so-called K-losing nephritis and in renal tubular acidosis, including Fanconi's syndrome, following bilateral ureterosigmoidostomy, in recovery from diabetic acidosis, associated with prolonged use of certain drugs such as chlorothiazide, p-aminosalicylic acid, adrenal corticoids and laxatives, in primary hyperaldosteronism, in hyperthyroidism and in chronic diarrhoeas.

In a separate category is a group of diseases in which paralysis occurs intermittently, usually in one or another of several well-defined clinical patterns, the *familial periodic paralyses*. Owing to the heterogeneous nature of the reported cases there must be reasonable doubt that familial periodic paralysis is a single disease.

Classical familial periodic paralysis, reviewed comprehensively by Talbott (1941) and later by Gass, Cherkasky & Savitsky (1948), McArdle (1956), Shy, Wanko, Rowley & Engel (1961) and Mollaret, Goulon & Tournilhac (1961), is characterized by episodes of weakness, increasing to paralysis, usually beginning in the middle of the night. Paralysis, with loss of tendon reflexes, often begins in the lower extremities, may extend to all extremities and the trunk and neck. It may last for hours or several days. It seldom occurs during the first few years of life, increases in frequency and severity and then often wanes and even disappears. Often the attack is heralded by an aura which patients describe so poorly that it may be attributed to a subtle decrease in muscle tone, whatever that is, that precedes objective signs of weakness. Sometimes patients find they can abort attacks by mild exercise, which, to anticipate the story, is a device for extruding K from muscle into plasma.

Observations made by many observers, since the first descriptions by Aitken, Allott, Castleden & Walker (1937) and Allott & McArdle (1938), have indicated almost uniformly a precipitate hypokalaemia which ushers in and is coincident with the paralysis. In many instances the attack is preceded and accompanied by an abrupt decrease in renal excretion of K (Ferrebee, Atchley & Loeb, 1938; Gammon, Austin, Blithe & Reid, 1939). On the basis of balance studies Danowski,

Elkinton, Burrows & Winkler (1948) concluded that there was good indirect evidence to indicate that K had entered an intracellular phase. Simultaneous measurements of the concentration of K in arterial plasma and in plasma of venous blood draining muscles of the forearm have been made during development of a spontaneous attack in a patient with classical familial periodic paralysis. When the arteriovenous difference in K concentration is multiplied by the flow of plasma through these muscles, the rate of net exchange of K between muscle and plasma is determined. During the development of an attack, in the patient so studied, K moved from plasma into muscle and the rate of movement into muscle was adequate to account for the hypokalaemia which occurred (Zierler & Andres, 1957). Measurements by others (Grob, Johns & Liljestrand, 1957; Mollaret *et al.*, 1961) of arteriovenous differences in K concentration across the forearm support this observation.

That attacks begin classically during the night is related to the diurnal variation in K movement that occurs in normals (Andres, Cader, Goldman & Zierler, 1957). During the waking hours, even in the absence of gross muscle activity, K moves in the net out of muscle into plasma. Activity probably increases this movement and postprandially it is probably reversed. During the night, synchronously with the normal decreased urinary K excretion, muscle loss of K ceases and may even reverse. In classical periodic paralysis, K movement across the muscle membrane is exaggerated. Movement of K into muscle during the night is abnormally great. During waking hours, movement of K out of muscle is extraordinarily large, serum K concentration is restored and the attack terminates. Thus, the muscle membrane in patients with periodic paralysis seems to be unusually permeable to K in both directions. There are hints that whatever impels K movement across the muscle membrane in normal man acts with less restraint in patients with familial periodic paralysis. Witness the classical methods of inducing attacks by a high carbohydrate meal, by insulin and by adrenaline, and the spontaneous attacks in response to emotional crises and during recovery from severe exercise (Ziegler & McQuarrie, 1952). That attacks do not occur nightly implies that, when nocturnal attacks do appear, superimposed on the normal diurnal fluctuation in K movement is another K-moving event, such as follows an indiscreet evening meal or recovery from a day of heavy exercise.

There are few resports of muscle K analysis in patients with classical familial periodic paralysis.

Shy *et al.* (1961) found muscle K concentration less than normal in two patients in an interval between attacks; during an attack K-poor water entered muscle so that K concentration fell, but the quantity of K per unit dry weight of muscle was, within measurement error, unchanged, as would be expected from our earlier argument that only a 1% increase in muscle K is expected. Bekény, Hasznos & Solti (1961a), on the other hand, reported normal muscle K concentration between attacks and a few per cent increase during an attack. In their patient muscle water decreased slightly, though perhaps not significantly, during an attack. In the cases reported by Conn, Fajans, Louis, Streeten & Johnson (1957), to be considered later, as intermittent aldosteronism with periodic paralysis, muscle K was subnormal, but, if there really were aldosteronism, this is to be expected. It is not surprising that muscle K may become reduced in some cases of familial periodic paralysis. We have suggested that the muscle membrane in this disease is more permeable to K in both directions. During the day, when unusual quantities of K leak from muscle, there may be consequent high urinary K loss. Reduction in total body K follows.

There have been many descriptions of morphological changes in muscle, reviewed recently by Shy *et al.* (1961) and by Bekény (1961). Most striking are vacuoles staining for glycogen or glycogen products. Electron microscopy seems to place the vacuoles within the sarcoplasmic reticulum and they appear to expand during an attack. In some cases, however, no morphological abnormality has been detected (Mollaret *et al.*, 1961), suggesting that the changes reported may be a secondary result of the disease. Because they are so reminiscent of those found in experimental K deficiency, this may be their cause.

Allott & McArdle (1938) first suggested that the unusual K movement in periodic paralysis might be only a manifestation of a more fundamental defect in carbohydrate metabolism; they suggested a lesion at a hexose phosphate stage. Since then others have noticed impaired glucose tolerance, high blood lactate and pyruvate and several miscellaneous observations along these lines (McArdle, 1956); Shy *et al.*, 1961; Bekény *et al.*, 1961a; Mollaret *et al.*, 1961), but no definitive evidence of a unique imperfection at any known step in carbohydrate metabolism has been demonstrated. It is possible that these rather non-specific findings reflect the muscle's difficulty in metabolizing in the presence of either a loss of K or of the consequent morphological changes, or that alterations in the membrane are not specific for K permeation and may influence the metabolism of the cell.

Conn *et al.* (1957) called attention to movement of Na and water in their cases. Again, opinion is divided as to whether initial inward movement of K may cause later movement of water and of other ions, or whether K movement is secondary to a primary movement of water and Na.

The cause of paralysis is still debated. Those accustomed to think in electrophysiological terms do not doubt that the great reduction in extracellular K concentration must lead to hyperpolarization of the muscle membrane, a suggestion, according to McArdle (1956), first made by Merton. It is, of course, more difficult to depolarize such a membrane, and this can account for the observed failure of the patient's muscle to propagate an impulse during paralysis. Shy *et al.* (1961) measured resting membrane potentials during an attack and found them identical with those found in the attack-free interval. However, if their remote electrode sat in an artificial solution of constant K composition, rather than in the patient's extracellular fluid, the observation is irrelevant. Mammalian muscle is hyperpolarized when bathed by a solution low in K concentration. If the patient's muscles are not hyperpolarized during an attack, when serum K is half normal or less, some unusual mechanism must operate to prevent it.

Other explanations are based on metabolic changes within the cell consequent upon distorted intracellular K concentration. There are many K-dependent reactions, but since intracellular K changes little, if at all, it is difficult to accept this sort of explanation in the classical cases of hypokalaemic familial periodic paralysis.

There are, however, other forms of this group of diseases. In some, clinically close to classical cases, there is no change in serum K during attacks (Watson, 1946; Tyler, Stephens, Gunn & Perkoff, 1951), and in Tyler's case K was administered to no avail. Clearly a different, though unknown, lesion is present.

Periodic paralysis has been reported in patients who have muscular dystrophy, and in families including members who have either periodic paralysis or a muscular dystrophy. Many of these have hypokalaemic paralysis. This implies a close genetic association but there is no assurance that the cause of periodic paralysis is the same in these patients as in the first group we discussed.

There is an unusual association between periodic paralysis and hyperthyroidism, particularly in Japan from where most of the cases have been reported (Okinaka, Shizume, Iino, Watanabe,

Irie, Noguchi, Kuma, Kuma & Ito, 1957). In some Japanese series the incidence of association is remarkable. Satoyoshi (1961) found 8% of 409 hyperthyroids, including 34% of the males, had periodic paralysis. In these cases onset of periodic paralysis is later in life, beginning with or after onset of hyperthyroidism, and periodic paralysis disappears when euthyroidism is achieved. In classical familial periodic paralysis, hyperthyroidism produced by exhibition of triiodothyronine or of thyrotropin did not exacerbate attacks (Engel, 1961). Although thyrotoxic periodic paralysis is hypokalaemic it must be regarded as a different disease.

Conn *et al.* (1957) reported two patients who had episodes of flaccid paralysis related to hypokalaemia. In them daily urinary excretion of aldosterone was rather more variable than one expects in normotensive normals, and it was suggested that when aldosterone production became sufficiently high, Na moved into muscle and somehow induced paralysis. Attacks were prevented by low Na intake. Others have confirmed and failed to confirm this report of aldosteronism as a cause of periodic paralysis, and the evidence is that aldosteronism is not the cause of classical familial periodic paralysis, although there may be cases of aldosteronism in whom paralysis appears episodically. Nevertheless, even when aldosteronism has not been found, dietary Na restriction has been salutary (Shy *et al.*, 1961), probably by modulating K movement, though not always (DeGraeff, 1961).

Gamstorp (1956) reported as *hereditary episodic adynamia* a group of cases in whom transient attacks of flaccid paralysis were associated with hyperkalaemia. These patients are distinguishable clinically from those with familial periodic paralysis by the facts that onset tends to occur earlier in life, attacks begin during the day, last usually for minutes rather than hours, though occasionally longer, are provoked by phenomena that raise serum K and are relieved by those that reduce it. Drager, Hammill & Shy (1958) discovered transient hyperkalaemia in a family suffering from paramyotonia congenita, and Van der Meulen, Gilbert & Kane (1961) demonstrated persistent contraction and percussion myotonia in a family with hyperkalaemic hereditary episodic adynamia. The disease is inherited as a single autosomal dominant with complete penetrance (Van der Meulen *et al.*, 1961; Helweg-Larsen, Hauge & Sagild, 1955). Many repetitive phenomena, including myotonia, are enhanced by K (Eyzaguirre *et al.*, 1948) and it is not surprising that myotonia should appear in this disease. The increases in serum K are seldom greater than 50%, and paralysis occurs at a K concentration that is too low to be associated with paralysis in those not afflicted with this disease. During the attack venous K in plasma from an extremity exceeds arterial K concentration (Egan & Klein, 1959; Bekény, Hasznos & Solti, 1961b; McArdle, 1962). Liljestrand (1957) found muscle K and exchangeable body K reduced in one patient, but this does not appear to be generally the case (Sagild, cited by Buchtal, Engbaek & Gamstorp, 1958; McArdle, 1962).

An electrophysiologist might guess at once that in these patients hyperkalaemia reduces resting membrane potential across muscle. Slight hypopolarization increases excitability; marked hypopolarization prevents a propagated impulse. There are bizarre, unexplained electrical abnormalities even during the attack-free periods (Buchtal et al., 1958), and the expected hypopolarization has been reported (Abbott, Creutzfeld, Fowler & Pearson, 1962).

Myotonias

Myotonia is a physical sign characterized by apparent delay in relaxation of stimulated muscle. Analysis by electrophysiological techniques has shown the basic change to be a repetitive response of muscle to a single stimulus or a short volley. The phenomenon is obliterated by repeated stimulation, either voluntary, electrical or mechanical. Whatever the cause, it is intrinsic in muscle and not in the myoneural junction or in nerve. It can be erased by quinine and not by curare.

Myotonia occurs in man in at least two diseases: myotonia congenita (Thomsen's disease) and myotonic dystrophy. It occurs also in the state known as paramyotonia, in which the phenomenon appears only on exposure to cold, but this is thought by some to be but a variant of myotonia congenita and in certain cases it is a symptom associated with hereditary episodic adynamia (see above). Clinical phenomena resembling myotonia appear with or following certain systemic diseases, for example infectious neuronitis, and in these instances the myotonia disappears eventually. Although these temporary states, called myotonia acquisita, resemble myotonia clinically, there are no electromyographic studies to confirm the identity. Much of our understanding of myotonia has come from studies of goats, in whom the disease occurs as an hereditary lesion (Brown & Harvey, 1939). Repetitive phenomena closely resembling myotonia have been produced in rats, particularly by administration of 2:4-dichloro-phenoxyacetate, a commercial weed-killer (Eyzaguirre et al., 1948).

Both myotonia congenita and myotonic dystrophy are inherited disorders, and although it has been suggested that they are fuudamentally the same disorder they differ importantly. Myotonia congenita is a benign though awkward ailment in which myotonia may be distributed among many muscles. Muscle bulk and strength are at least normal and may be supernormal, and no other organs or tissues are involved. In myotonic dystrophy, on the other hand, myotonia is apt to be limited to certain muscle groups, those of the hand and tongue, chiefly, and is not the striking aspect of the disease. These patients exhibit muscle wasting which may become universal and severe, and which early and characteristically affects the sternomastoids. Histologically, muscle in this disease resembles that in progressive muscular dystrophy, from which it can possibly be distinguished with difficulty (Wohlfart, 1951). But myotonic dystrophy is a disorder of more than muscle. Patients with this disease have a high incidence of skeletal anomalies. They tend to have a high arched palate, hyperostosis frontalis and frequent alteration of the hypophyseal fossa. They are apt to have cataracts and, indeed, early cataracts may be the only sign of the disease in some members of families in which there is frank myotonic dystrophy. Among males there is often gynaecomastia, testicular atrophy and laboratory evidence of disturbed gonadal function, low urinary excretion of 17-ketosteroids and abnormally high excretion of follicle-stimulating hormone. Goitre is found frequently and, although these patients, in common with others who have massive wasting of muscle, may have low basal metabolic rates by normal standards, they are not truly hypothyroid. Two cases of coincidental hypothyroidism and myotonic dystrophy have, however, been reported (Stanbury, Goldsmith & Gillis, 1954).

Patients with myotonic dystrophy excrete in their urine an amount of creatinine which is less than normal to a degree probably commensurate with the reduction in muscle mass. It has been noted (Thomasen, 1948; Zierler, Folk, Magladery & Lilienthal, 1949b), however, that they excrete surprisingly little creatine in contrast to most other examples of severe muscle wasting. Since creatinuria should occur whenever there is severe wasting of muscle, providing that the rate of synthesis of creatine is normal, and providing that creatine is metabolized only to creatinine and not dissimilated along other pathways not known to play a rôle in normal metabolism, explanation of the relative lack of creatinuria should lie in one or both of these provisos.

The proximate cause of creatinuria in most diseases of muscle is an elevation of serum creatine concentration beyond the renal threshold. In myotonic dystrophy, serum creatine concentration is either normal or only slightly increased (Zierler et al., 1949b). When creatine is fed to such patients, serum creatine concentration rises at a rate similar to that seen in normals, suggesting that there is no unusual alternative disposition of creatine. It is suspected, therefore, that the rate of creatine synthesis is retarded in this disease, a deduction which awaits confirmation by direct tests of that rate. The rate of synthesis of creatine can be accelerated in normal subjects, it is supposed, by administration of methyltestosterone. In a patient with myotonic dystrophy, methyltestosterone provoked a great increase in serum creatine concentration and appropriate creatinuria, as in normal persons (Zierler et al., 1949b). Thus, the rate of synthesis of creatine, presumably reduced in myotonic dystrophy, can be stimulated, indicating that the materials for synthesis of creatine are at hand and suggesting that some unknown regulator of the rate of creatine synthesis is awry in this disease.

If there is diminished synthesis of creatine in myotonic dystrophy, it is not to be considered a cause of the disease, but it may be representative of a more widespread disturbance in orderly synthesis of nitrogenous compounds which may characterize the disease.

Endocrinopathies

Although weakness and wasting occurring in the course of endocrinopathies may signal affection of skeletal muscle, knowledge of the molecular effects of hormones is often inadequate to explain rigorously the observed response of muscle, either because the rôle of the hormone in biochemical events within muscle is mapped incompletely, or because the gap between metabolism and function is bridged only by the imagination. Detailed discussion of the interplay of muscle and hormones belongs in other chapters of this volume, but some of the disturbances of muscle associated with endocrine disease will be considered briefly here.

Acromegaly. Patients with acromegaly may have weakness of certain muscle groups despite the large bulk of these muscles. In some cases this may be due to limitation of motion secondary to affection of joints, but this is not always obviously the explanation. It has been noted (Schrire, 1937; Cumings, 1953) that patients with acromegaly

have a somewhat excessive urinary output of creatinine and a moderate creatinuria, the latter associated with a slight increase in concentration of creatine in serum. Although there are no studies which would explain these observations in detail, excessive creatinuria implies that the rate of synthesis of creatine has been accelerated. Since this possibility exists, the increased serum creatine concentration and the creatinuria may possibly be explained in part in the same way.

In patients with active acromegaly, there is uptake of K by forearm muscles at rest, in contrast to the normal basal leak of K from muscle, and there is increased O_2 uptake by forearm muscle (Rabinowitz & Zierler, 1962). Glucose and K uptake by muscle in response to intra-arterial insulin is markedly reduced.

Hyperthyroidism. Following administration of thyroid substance to laboratory animals, and in patients with hyperthyroidism, there is loss of muscle mass with decreased urinary excretion of creatinine and abnormal creatinuria. Analysis of muscle of rabbits with experimental hyperthyroidism suggests that the concentration of creatine and of phosphocreatine is reduced (Wang, 1939). Serum creatine concentration is high (Tierney & Peters, 1943) and the creatinuria is not due to decreased renal tubular re-absorption of creatinine. In contrast, the creatinuria which accompanies administration of thyroid substance to myxoedematous subjects is largely the result of an alteration in renal function (Zierler et al., 1949b).

In a group of older patients myopathy may be the most prominent feature of hyperthyroidism. In these patients, in whom muscle wasting is striking, there is surprisingly little or no creatinuria, although there is the anticipated reduction in urine creatinine and in creatine tolerance (Zierler, 1951). It has been suggested that creatine synthesis may be impaired in this state, although direct evidence is lacking.

Rundle, Finlay-Jones & Noad (1953) found in malignant exophthalmos that the extra-ocular muscles enlarge some two- to five-fold and show degeneration, in contrast to thyrotoxicosis where the enlargement may be due to extra-muscular deposition of fat (Rundle & Pochin, 1944).

Satoyoshi (1961) was the first to examine chemically muscles from patients with hyperthyroidism. He found K low and Na high, creatine, phosphocreatine and ATP reduced. The concentrations of several enzymes were reduced in muscle, though not raised in serum. These, then, are the rather non-specific changes in damaged muscle we have considered earlier.

Myxoedema. Most, if not all, myxoedematous subjects are weak. Many have objective weakness of proximal muscles (Nickel & Frame, 1961). Their muscles exhibit metachromasia of sarcoplasm and surrounding connective tissue, but there are no definitive histochemical or chemical studies of this phenomenon.

Diabetes mellitus. Weakness so commonly seen in patients with diabetes mellitus remains unexplained, and indeed probably has many explanations. In experimental diabetes produced by alloxan the concentration of muscle glycogen is reduced (Lackey, Brindle, Gill & Harris, 1944). It might be suspected that reduced muscle glycogen would impair the ability of muscle to synthesize so-called high-energy phosphate compounds. This conjecture is only weakly supported by measurement of high-energy phosphate fractions in the gastrocnemius of alloxan diabetic and of depancreatized rats (Peterson, Beatty, Bocek & West, 1954). Among these animals the only difference was a lower creatine phosphate in the depancreatized rats, as compared to unoperated controls, and in alloxan diabetes there was not even this difference. In depancreatized rats acetoacetate uptake by muscle is deficient (Beatty, Marco, Peterson, Bocek & West, 1960). In diabetic patients glucose uptake by forearm muscles at rest is less than normal, and even in patients never treated with insulin the response to intra-arterial insulin, with respect to glucose and K uptake by forearm, is reduced (Andres & Zierler, 1958).

Addison's disease. Although weakness and wasting in adrenal insufficiency is complicated by circulatory disturbances (Goldstein, Ramey & Levine, 1950), there are real changes in skeletal muscle, in addition to the familiar changes in the electrolyte composition of the interstitial fluid environment of muscle cells. There is, in experimental adrenal insufficiency, an increase in muscle intracellular water, a loss of muscle Na and Cl and an increase in K (Muntwyler, Mellors, Mautz & Mangun, 1940). From consideration of the change in Cl, on the assumption that Cl is entirely extracellular even in this distorted state, it has been adduced that the gain in water is intracellular at the expense of interstitial fluid.

Cushing's syndrome. Similarly complicated is the weakness and wasting of Cushing's syndrome. In part this may be due to circulatory disturbance, to atrophy of disuse, to nutritional deficiency, to the abnormal electrolyte environment and to the familiar but incompletely understood alterations in organic metabolism. It may be noted that muscle from patients with this syndrome had less K than normal (Kepler, Sprague, Mason & Power, 1948). Closely related is the myopathy produced by adrenal cortical hormones or by ACTH, although in one study total exchangeable K in patients treated with triamcinolone was not detectably different from that of controls (Bauer, Dubois & Telfer, 1960).

Disorders of androgenic secretions. The increase in muscle mass produced by administration of androgens to castrated animals is well established. It is of interest that this increased mass is associated with an increase in total protein content and in amino acid and creatine concentration (Coffman & Koch, 1940). An interesting example of the heterogeneity of skeletal muscle may be found in the observation that the muscles of mastication suffer to a greater extent following castration than do limb muscles in the guinea-pig (Scow & Roe, 1953). In muscles from testosterone-treated castrated rats DPNH cytochrome *c* reductase activity is greater than in muscles from non-treated castrated rats (Loring, Spencer & Villee, 1961). What may be a more primary effect of testosterone, demonstrated in rat seminal vesicles but presumably applicable to muscle, is its rôle in stimulating protein synthesis by converting soluble RNA-amino-acid complexes to microsomal ribonucleoprotein (Wilson, 1962).

Miscellaneous Myopathies

Myoglobinuria. Although myoglobinuria is relatively rare it merits somewhat detailed consideration because it appears so nearly to permit correlation of a rich background of fundamental information with a clinical state. Much of the material in this section will be found in more complete reviews by Millikan (1939), Biörck (1949) and Bywaters (1950).

Myoglobin is a ferrous-porphyrin-protein complex related closely to haemoglobin but differing from the latter, according to Theorell (1934) who first crystallized it, in that it contains but one atom of Fe and has a mol. wt. of about 17,000, compared to haemoglobin's four atoms of Fe and mol. wt. of about 68,000. Myoglobin is distributed in smooth muscle, skeletal muscle and the myocardium. Its concentration may vary for any given skeletal muscle from species to species, among different skeletal muscles within the same individual, and for any given skeletal muscle in any individual depending, among other factors, upon age and accustomed activity. Red muscle is higher in myoglobin content than white. In mammals the concentration tends to be higher in muscles of locomotion. Although the variation among individual muscles is not great in adults, in the 9-week pup there may be a two-fold variation in myoglobin content among various muscles. In the adult dog, the myoglobin concentration of the muscles of the legs is 10 times that in the pup (Whipple, 1926), and about the same as that in man. According to Biörck's (1949) extensive analyses, adult human muscle contains about 700 mg. of myoglobin/100 g. wet weight, approximately 3% of total muscle protein. No information is available concerning the intracellular distribution of this substance.

Like haemoglobin, myoglobin combines rapidly and reversibly with O_2 and with CO. Its ferrous Fe is oxidized easily to yield metmyoglobin. The curve relating O_2 tension to % saturation of myoglobin is hyperbolic rather than sigmoid, as in the case of haemoglobin. Myoglobin is nearly saturated at low O_2 tension, 40 mm. Hg, and is precipitously desaturated at tensions below 20 mm. Hg. Although the rôle of myoglobin remains incompletely understood, there is general acceptance of Millikan's hypothesis that it is a reservoir supplying O_2 for brief periods when local O_2 tension falls. Myoglobin is not assigned a critical rôle in the contractile process, and there are no substantial reasons for inferring that decreased myoglobin content of muscle is the cause of paralysis seen in the myoglobinurias.

Perhaps owing to its smaller molecular weight, when myoglobin pours from muscle into plasma it is filtered rapidly through the renal glomeruli and excreted in the urine; it is not apt to accumulate in plasma in concentrations sufficient to tinge it as does haemoglobin. Myoglobinuria is consequent upon dissolution of muscle by diverse means. It occurs when there is sufficiently great necrosis of muscle secondary to ischaemia (Bywaters & Stead, 1945), trauma (Bywaters, 1945), electric shock (Fischer & Rossier, 1947) and perhaps in acute disease such as polymyositis (Günther, 1924). It has been recorded in cases resembling progressive muscular dystrophy (Louw & Nielsen, 1944; Acheson & McAlpine, 1953), where it may be again only a manifestation of loss of integrity of a large mass of muscle. In some instances outpouring of myoglobin may have been due to extraneous toxic agents, as in Haff disease (Berlin, 1948) although the agents remain unidentified. Finally, there are the paroxysmal paralytic myoglobinurias seen in horses and man.

There is little to suggest that equine and human paroxysmal myoglobinurias are closely related. The disease in the horse has been studied extensively by Carlström (1931), who described a sudden onset of paralysis in draft horses with the first heavy exercise following a few days of rest and high carbohydrate diet (see Minett (1935) for a thorough review in English of this work). During attacks the concentration of K, glucose and lactate are increased in blood, changes attributed to intense glycogenolysis in glycogen-laden tissues. It is difficult to see the relevance of these observations to either the paralysis or the change in permeability of muscle required for outflux of myoglobin.

Reported cases of idiopathic myoglobinuria in man are rare, numbering perhaps less than 50. In some of these the urinary pigment was not identified, and in others, in which the clinical descriptions suggests paroxysmal myoglobinuria, the urinary pigment was identified, presumably incorrectly, as haemoglobin. In six of the reported cases, and one case seen in this institution, there was a family history (paroxysmal paralysis with passage of dark urine related to exercise) strongly suggesting myoglobinuria. Although, in most of these patients, and in several others without patent family histories, the calves were described as large, suggesting pseudohypertrophy, there are features in the available descriptions which distinguish them from typical pseudohypertrophic muscular dystrophy. For example, none of these patients was severely dystrophic. In the family with the largest pedigree, although eight males and no females in five generations had muscle disease, suggesting a sex-linked recessive, the two men in the fourth generation had a relatively late onset of dystrophy without myoglobinuria. Furthermore, the myoglobinuric, although only 10 years old, had no creatinuria except during attacks (Louw & Nielsen, 1944). Another myoglobinuric had stigmata suggesting mild myotonic dystrophy, and a sister who, though not myoglobinuric, had rather more definite dystrophy (Acheson & McAlpine, 1953). Schmid & Mahler (1959) found myoglobinuria in their patient with McArdle's syndrome (see below). In most patients with myoglobinuria, however, the disease has appeared as an isolated phenomenon.

There are too many differences among reported cases to permit aphorism, but the myoglobinuria seems to be precipitated by heavy exercise, usually of the lower extremities. Within minutes to a few hours, the exercised muscles become weak, sometimes swollen, board-like and tender, sometimes accompanied by local skin eruptions. With this there is passage of dark urine in which the pigment is a varying mixture of myoglobin and metmyoglobin. The paresis is seldom extensive, but it may involve the muscles of respiration and thereby threaten life. There may be fever, leucocytosis, signs of shock and acute renal failure, the last being the most serious complication of the episode and the cause of death in several patients. Paresis and myoglobinuria are self-limited and subside in a matter of hours.

In the absence of reliable measurement of the quantity of myoglobin in the urine, it can only be estimated that less than a gram of myoglobin is apt to be excreted in a full-blown attack, representing less than 0·5% of total body myoglobin in the adult. Collateral evidence of release of muscle contents into blood has not always been found. Serum K has been reported to rise, to fall and to remain unchanged. In an unreported case known to me, death was due to cardiac effects of hyperkalaemia. Serum creatine has been reported high or unchanged. Creatinuria has usually, but not always, accompanied myoglobinuria. In one case certain serum enzymes were present in extraordinarily high concentrations early in the attack (Pearson, Beck & Blahd, 1957).

There are no chemical analyses of muscle from these patients. Histochemical studies have not been helpful (Reiner, Konikoff, Altschule, Dammin & Merrill, 1956; Farmer, Hammack & Frommeyer, 1961). Although Theorell & de Duve (1947) have crystallized the myoglobin from one patient and described it as normal, it is not yet certain that there may not be abnormal myoglobins just as there are abnormal haemoglobins.

Clearly, owing to its incidental occurrence in other diseases, myoglobinuria is not pathognomonic of the syndrome under discussion. Diagnosis of paroxysmal myoglobinuria or idiopathic rhabdomyolysis depends on the combination of clinical events described above and demonstration of myoglobinuria. In the past the latter was performed chiefly spectroscopically. Paper electrophoresis (Fletcher & Prankerd, 1955) appears to be a convenient and perhaps more reliable method.

It has been difficult to study metabolic disturbances which may underlie this disease. Experience has shown that the real risk of acute renal failure makes reprehensible provocation of attacks for experimental purposes. Whatever is responsible for it, necrosis of muscle seems adequate to account for the paresis. Although there are no data on the turnover rate of myoglobin in patients with myoglobinuria, the normal turnover rate of myoglobin is so slow (Helwig & Greenberg, 1952) that it is scarcely conceivable that myoglobin lost from muscle during an attack can be replaced in the brief period during which recovery occurs. This does not eliminate the possibility that other substances, not yet identified, whose rôle in muscle function is critical, may be lost in an attack and replaced rapidly. It is possible that the disruption of muscle is due to an agent, provoked by heavy exercise, which attacks the muscle membrane, but no pertinent data are available.

In certain respects idiopathic paralytic myoglobinuria resembles other syndromes in which exercise is followed by unusual muscle spasm and weakness but not by myoglobinuria. Some of these may share the same basic defects with myoglobinuria and may be but quantitative variants of that disorder.

Glycogenoses. There are 11 enzymically-determined types of glycogenosis, of which five occur primarily or prominently in skeletal muscle. These are:

(1) *Lysosomal glucosidase defect* (cardiac glycogen storage disease, Pompe's disease). An autosomal recessive trait, lysosomal α-glucosidase is absent. In those surviving the heart disease for more than a year or two symptoms mimic those of progressive muscular dystrophy (Zellweger, Brown, McCormick & Tu, 1965; Smith, Amick & Sidbury, 1966).

(2) *Debrancher enzyme defect* (limit dextrinosis). Abnormal glycogen is deposited in liver and muscle. Inheritance is uncertain, probably autosomal recessive. Larner (1964) reported a middle-aged adult with the disease whose complaints were referable primarily to muscle.

(3) *McArdle's disease* (muscle phosphorylase absence). McArdle (1951) described a myopathy attributed to a defect in muscle glycogen breakdown, and manifested by pain, weakness and stiffness of muscles provoked by moderate exercise. From measurements of changes in blood lactate and pyruvate concentrations following exercise and administration of adrenaline, it was adduced that the development of contractures in this patient was the result of inability to dissimilate glycogen to lactate, reminiscent of the effect of iodoacetate on isolated muscle. This was a remarkably prescient hypothesis, though it has proved to be not exactly correct. By the time the second and third cases of this disease turned up, sufficient information on basic metabolic processes was available to pinpoint the defect. Schmid & Mahler (1959) and, independently, Mommaerts, Illingworth, Pearson, Guillory & Seraydarian (1959)—data from the same patient were reported later *in extenso* by Pearson, Rimer & Mommaerts (1961)—demonstrated almost complete absence of muscle phosphorylase in their patients. The defect is due to a single recessive, rare, autosomal gene (Schmid & Hammaker,

1961). Engel, Eyerman & Williams (1963) described late onset of muscle phosphorylase deficiency, unique because one patient had some phosphorylase activity.

(4) *Muscle phosphofructokinase defect.* Tarui, Okuno, Ikura, Tanaka, Suda & Nishikawa (1965) discovered a family, male and female children of first cousins, with symptoms similar to those of McArdle's disease. Blood lactate concentration did not rise with anaerobic exercise. However, muscle phosphorylase content was normal. Muscle glycogen content was increased and phosphofructokinase was markedly decreased in muscle, and low in erythrocytes.

(5) *Phosphohexose isomerase deficiency.* Satoyashi & Kowa (1965) found two brothers in whom symptoms developed only after age 35. These were muscle aches produced by exercise, accompanied by dark urine. Blood lactate concentration did not rise with anaerobic exercise, but did rise if a large quantity of fructose was administered prior to exercise. Symptoms were controlled by daily administration of 50 g. of fructose. Analyses of muscle obtained by biopsy showed slightly increased glycogen, normal glycolytic enzymes except phosphofructokinase. However, normal quantities of lactate were produced with fructose-6-phosphate or fructose diphosphate as substrates, but no lactate was formed from glycogen, glucose-1-, or glucose-6-phosphate. From these observations it was deduced that muscle hexose isomerase was inhibited.

Central core disease. Shy & Magee (1956) described a non-progressive myopathy, inherited probably as a dominant, in which, among the clinically involved proximal muscles, nearly every skeletal muscle fibre was distinguished by a central core that, while approximately normally cross-striated, exhibited unusual staining characteristics. Greenfield, Cornman & Shy (1958) christened it central core disease, and Engel, Foster, Hughes, Huxley & Mahler (1961) came upon a second family whom they and Dubowitz & Pearse (1960) studied by means to which the word exhaustively might properly apply.

The transition between the core and the normal outer annulus is abrupt, but electron microscopy detects neither membrane nor space separating the two regions. Myofibrils in the core are packed more densely. Infrequently myofibrils are lost in patches. With the muscle tied at rest-length, core sarcomeres are about 10% shorter than those of the normal annulus. But perhaps most important for its biochemical implications is the almost complete absence of mitochondria. Probably in consequence of this defect oxidative enzymes are

histochemically absent from the core. This does not explain why the core also lacks phosphorylase. The outer annulus stains normally for both oxidative enzymes and phosphorylase, although the uniform distribution of the stains is unusual. Muscle from both parents was normal histologically and histochemically.

A curious discrepancy between histochemistry and gross analysis of muscle homogenates was revealed in these studies and, while the discrepancy is unexplained, it may serve as a note of caution in interpretation of this sort of study. Phosphorylase activity of muscle homogenates was completely absent, although there was ample phosphorylase in the normal annulus demonstrated histochemically. Furthermore, in the father's muscle, completely normal histochemically, there was no phosphorylase activity in the homogenate. In both patient and father, activation of phosphorylase by addition of adenosine-5-phosphate to the homogenate increased activity only slightly. The discrepancy in the patient's case was not owing to phosphorylase inhibitors, say in the core, because his muscle did not inhibit phosphorylase activity of normal muscle.

Unlike McArdle's disease, blood pyruvate and lactate rose normally in response to exercise and muscle glycogen was not elevated.

Finally, an unidentified sarcoplasmic protein was absent in the patient. The fact that it was present in the father suggests that this loss was a result of the disease.

The disease, then, seems to be an inherited error in foetal development in which hypomitochondriosis may be central.

There are several groups of disorders, not specifically muscular in origin, yet which may involve muscular function in an important fashion. These categories are exemplified by the avitaminoses (beri-beri, pellagra, scurvy), and the primary or secondary effects of some bacterial toxins (diphtheria). In each instance, the involvement of muscle is simply a reflection or counterpart of the more extensive rôle played by the agent, or lack of it, on other systems and tissues.

Neuromuscular Transmission

In terms of the oversimplified description of neuromuscular transmission given earlier there are several mechanisms which, if disturbed, might break the chain of events underlying normal neuromuscular performance. General categories of possible disturbances follow:

(1) Failure of the impulse to reach and excite the terminal nerve-endings.

(2) Failure of release of transmitter by reason of

unfavourable environment, impermeability of membrane, exhaustion of stores, or inadequate resynthesis, among others.

(3) Failure of normally released transmitter to gain functional access to a receptor site on the endplate, because of accelerated hydrolysis due to excess cholinesterase, or because of prior occupation of the receptor by some other agent (curariform).

(4) Failure of the endplate to respond to the transmitter because of continuing depolarization resulting from persistence of transmitter or its hydrolyzed products, or because of other functional changes in the reactivity of the endplate itself.

(5) Failure of a normal endplate potential to excite a propagated potential in the muscle fibre.

(6) Failure of excitation and mechanical contraction of the muscle fibre itself.

There are several physiological and pharmacological agents capable of inducing failure in one or another of the sites listed above, and several disease states produce changes that appear to interfere similarly. For some examples one may point to the observation that the amount of acetylcholine released by a community of nerve-endings is conditioned by the level of Ca in the surrounding fluids; to curariform agents which reduce the effectiveness of acetylcholine in exciting an endplate potential ("competitive block"); and to persistent depolarization of the endplate which follows in the train of excess K, excess acetylcholine, or the presence of many quaternary ammonium compounds like the methonium series (Lilienthal, 1952; Paton & Zaimis, 1952).

At this juncture it seems appropriate to emphasize some logical pitfalls that occasionally trap speculative thought concerning aetiology of diseases of neuromuscular transmission. The first of these is oversimplication from superficial resemblance of certain experimental preparations to natural disease; e.g. if excess local acetylcholine produces weakness experimentally, then the weakness of myasthenia gravis is the result of the same process. The second is analysis by exclusion on the false premise that possible mechanisms are mutually exclusive; e.g. an agent which produces neuromuscular block does so by depolarization or competition with transmitter, neglecting the possibility that both may occur (Jarcho, Berman, Eyzaguirre & Lilienthal, 1951; Thesleff, 1955). The third is neglect of possible species variations (Paton & Zaimis, 1952); e.g. the response of a hind-limb muscle in the cat to various agents is the exact counterpart of that which occurs in man or other species. Perhaps listing these errors is

as offensive as it is naïve; but the reason is that these errors have been made. The list may serve then as a partial reminder that although our store of knowledge about neuromuscular transmission is rich, the leap from it to certain understanding of the basic mechanism of disease may be very wide indeed.

Myasthenia gravis. The first definite clue that this disease was related in some fashion to the acetylcholine transmitter mechanism transpired when Walker's astute recognition of the curare-like manifestations of myasthenia led her to demonstrate the reparative effect of physostigmine, an anticholinesterase and decurarizing agent. The unfolding of knowledge about myasthenia has been built on this theme, that every observation fits the concept that the functional defect is restricted to the neuromuscular apparatus (Harvey & Masland, 1941; Harvey & Lilienthal, 1941; Grob & Harvey, 1953).

Until recently the hypothesis which fitted certain of the observed facts was based on the second category of failure listed above. In view of the reparative effect of several anticholinesterase agents, as well as others known to enhance the action of acetylcholine (e.g. ephedrine, K, guanidine), and in view of the lack of evidence that any disturbance existed in cholinesterase systems, the working hypothesis has been based on a suspicion that the normal quantum of acetylcholine released was diminished. A basis for the assumed decrease was not established, but was thought perhaps to result from inadequate synthesis or release.

Neuromuscular block appearing in myasthenia has certain characteristics which implicate the endplate itself. Churchill-Davidson & Richardson (1953) demonstrated that in the myasthenic subject, involved muscles were especially sensitive to the blocking action of decamethonium. The block which developed displayed characteristics of a "competitive" block: reversed by anticholinesterases, deepened by repetitive stimulation, absence of fasciculations, etc. On the other hand, the "normal" muscles of the myasthenic showed remarkable resistance to the blocking action of decamethonium. The generalization at which these authors arrived "suggested that the failure of neuromuscular transmission in myasthenia is derived from abnormalities in the response of the motor endplate to acetylcholine".

Grob, Johns & Harvey (1955) discovered that the intra-arterial injection of acetylcholine produced the familiar transient neuromuscular block, followed by a prolonged block lasting many minutes. In the normal subject, this later block possessed characteristics which suggest that it was the result of persistent depolarization; i.e. it was intensified by anticholinesterases and the presumed resulting persistence of acetylcholine. The possibility that this prolonged block was due to hydrolysis products of acetylcholine was tested by injecting choline, which produced a long-lasting block which exhibited characteristics of both competitive and predominantly depolarizing blocks. In the myasthenic patient, by contrast, the prolonged depression of neuromuscular transmission induced by excess acetylcholine was of the competitive sort, as was that produced by choline alone. These observations confirm the report that there is some disorder of the endplate in myasthenia; yet, on the other hand, they continue to implicate the acetylcholine mechanism by raising the possibility that choline, or some related by-product of hydrolysis, exerts the blocking effect of the endplate. On the other hand, Desmedt (1958, 1961), from studies in cats of effects of hemicholinium HC3, an inhibitor of acetylcholine synthesis in nervous tissue, has mimicked the electrophysiological evidence of myasthenia gravis, and suggests that what may appear to be an endplate disorder can be secondary to defective synthesis of acetylcholine. Desmedt suggests that there may be a circulating hemicholinium-like substance in this disease. Dahlbäck, Elmqvist, Johns, Radner & Thesleff (1961) measured miniature endplate potentials in excised muscle from myasthenic patients (though not clinically myasthenic muscle). These tiny potentials signal random spontaneous release of acetylcholine packets from nerve endings. In muscle from myasthenics, although the amplitude of miniature endplate potentials was normal, their frequency was reduced, suggesting a decrease in the number of packets produced or released by nerve endings. Coërs & Desmedt (1959) have found structural abnormalities in terminal motor nerve arborization in myasthenic muscle.

Whatever may be the defect, there are certain clinical observations which must be borne in mind when speculation is entertained about the pathogenesis of the disease. The first of these is the extraordinary similarity between myasthenia and curarization (Harvey & Lilienthal, 1941), a relationship made even more provocative by the recent demonstration of the competitive (curariform) block occurring in myasthenic muscle. The second point is the remarkable variation in the location of muscles which become overtly myasthenic. On occasions the disease may be ushered in by a sudden weakness in a single muscle, in other instances virtually every muscle may be involved; some patients exhibit myasthenia in extra-ocular muscles without any weakness elsewhere for years. The third point is the undoubted fact that a severely myasthenic mother may be delivered of a severely myasthenic child in whom the myasthenia is almost certain to wane and vanish during the first neonatal days or weeks (Grob & Harvey, 1953). Although unproved, it is difficult to explain this occurrence except in terms of transplacental transfer of some hypothetical myasthenogenic substance. The fourth point is the striking effect on myasthenia of the hormonal changes accompanying menstruation and pregnancy, as well as the unpredictable effects of hyperthyroidism and of cortical steroids (Grob & Harvey, 1952).

And finally, there is the confused issue of the thymus in relation to myasthenia. There is general agreement that the appearance of germinal centres or neoplasm is encountered almost uniformly in myasthenia gravis (Castleman & Norris, 1949). Of some interest, but as yet no help in understanding, is the frequency with which thymic enlargement is discovered in exophthalmic goitre, hypoadrenalism, acromegaly and in the rare instance of thymic hypertrophy of infants; in each of these conditions weakness of muscle may be an outstanding development. Nevertheless, the suspicion remains that some relationship exists, likely not to be directly causal, and yet tantalizing in the thin promise that illumination of the rôle played by the thymus might be a long step towards understanding pathogenesis. That the thymus is not the persistent source of the circulating myasthenic agent is certain from the fact that neonatal myasthenia has occurred despite thymectomy of the mother before pregnancy (Nilsby, 1949; Geddes & Kidd, 1951). Yet there is growing evidence that the thymus is responsible for certain immune functions, reviewed by Harvey & Johns (1962), and Strauss, Seegal, Hsu, Burkholder, Nastuk & Osserman (1960) have found a muscle-binding, complement-fixing serum globulin fraction in blood of myasthenic patients. That it is a myasthenic agent is unproven.

Botulism. The terrifying effect of botulinum toxin is made especially dramatic by its potency; the amounts involved suggest that a single molecule may disorganize a nerve-ending. It may be considered here as a model of various poisons, derived from plants, microbes, molluscs, fish and snakes, which share a dual action on erythrocytes and on neuromuscular structures. For the most part, little is known about the mechanism of action of these naturally occurring toxins. The recent crystallization of botulinum toxin provided a potent tool for investigation of its action, but a clear answer is not yet apparent. Burgen, Dickens & Zatman (1949) established that the neuromuscular block was not the result of any fault in the synthesis of acetylcholine. Their evidence showed that the block was not curariform, in that the endplate remained sensitive to acetylcholine, and Stover, Fingerman & Forester (1953) have shown in the frog that botulinum poisoning leads to the evocation of an inadequate endplate potential. The observations of these authors all supported the conclusion that interference with spread of impulse in the terminal arborizations of the motor nerve, or with normal release of acetylcholine, was the basis of botulinum block. Brooks (1954), however, localized the probable site of defect even further by showing that external stimuli evoked normal discharge of acetylcholine, and concluded that botulinum toxin blocked transmission of nerve impulses into the final presynaptic arborization, which retained the capacity to release acetylcholine but failed to receive stimulation. The block is supposed to result from some alteration in ionic permeance of hyperpolarization.

CONCLUSION

There are still great gaps in our understanding of basic processes in skeletal muscle, in our total description of chemical events in diseases of muscle, and in our ability to relate disease to basic processes.

Most diseases of muscle considered in this chapter are long-standing. By the time the physician sees the patient hosts of secondary changes have occurred, and with the exception of those disorders such as glycogenoses, in which there is total absence of an enzyme, it has not been possible to array biochemical lesions in chronological order.

In many diseases of muscle substances leak, ultimately into plasma or urine. In general, such leaks signal abnormal permeability, disorganization, or even disruption of some envelope normally responsible for limiting ebb and flow between a muscle fibre and its surroundings.

In the history of study of muscle disease, probably the first chemical finding associated with myopathies was creatinuria. Creatinuria is of course quite non-specific. It occurs during disruption of muscle, as in myoglobinuria, dermatomyo-

sitis and hyperthyroidism. It occurs in those states in which there is reduced muscle mass in the face of continuing synthesis of creatine, such as severe atrophies and muscular dystrophies, because there is no effective feedback inhibition of creatine synthesis in man. And it occurs when renal reabsorption of creatine is diminished, since filtered creatine is reabsorbed completely by renal tubules at low concentration, and partially at high concentrations, by a mechanism poorly competitive with α-amino acids.

More recently, attention has shifted from creatinuria to measurement of various enzymes in blood. High concentration of enzymes in blood is again a non-specific manifestation of leaky cells. Even though it may be possible to deduce that the enzymes in blood in high concentration came from skeletal muscle, it is not yet possible to state what disease process made the muscle fibre leaky to such large molecules. Sometimes these enzyme leaks are accompanied by leaks of myoglobin, creatine, potassium and other sarcoplasmic contents.

The fact that muscle has two cell membrane systems, sarcolemma and sarcoplasmic reticulum, may help explain features unique to skeletal muscle. Rhabdomyolysis may involve sarcolemma predominantly, with prominent myoglobinuria. There are suggestions that the more common route for leak of sarcoplasmic enzymes is through transverse tubules. It may be that myoglobin, the intracellular localization of which is undetermined, is more closely associated with sarcolemma.

Unique features of muscle membranes, distinguishing them from other cells, are less apt to lie in the plasma membrane than in the mucopolysaccharide basement membrane and in the peculiar structure of the sarcoplasmic reticulum, particularly the T-system and the junction between the T-system and the cysternae of the longitudinal reticulum. These may be the sites at which specific myopathies begin to act.

Acknowledgement

Original studies described here have been aided by grants from the National Institutes of Health, Bethesda, Md. (A-999, A-750, AM-05524) and from the Muscular Dystrophy Associations of America, Inc.

References

ABBOTT, B. C., CREUTZFELD, O., FOWLER, B. & PEARSON, C. (1962). *Fed. Proc.*, **21**, 318.

ACHESON, D. & McALPINE, D. (1953). *Lancet*, **2**, 372.

ADAMS, R. D., DENNY-BROWN, D. & PEARSON, C. M. (1953). "Diseases of Muscle. A Study in Pathology." New York, Hoeber.

ADRIAN, R. H. & FREYGANG, W. H. (1962). *J. Physiol.*, **163**, 61.

AITKEN, R. S., ALLOTT, E. N., CASTLEDEN, L. I. M. & WALKER, M. (1937). *Clin. Sci.*, **3**, 47.

ALLOTT, E. N. & McARDLE, B. (1938). *Clin. Sci.*, **3**, 229.

ALOISI, M. & MARGRETH, A. (1967). In Milhorat: "Exploratory Concepts in Muscular Dystrophy and Related Disorders." New York, Excerpta Medica Foundation.

AMES, S. R. & RISLEY, H. A. (1948). *Proc. Soc. Exp. Biol., N.Y.*, **68**, 131.

ANDRES, R., CADER, G., GOLDMAN, P. & ZIERLER, K. L. (1957). *J. Clin. Invest.*, **36**, 723.

ANDRES, R. & ZIERLER, K. L. (1958). *Clin. Res.*, **6**, 250.

ASMUNDSEN, V. S., KRATZER, F. H. & JULIAN, L. M. (1966). *Ann. N.Y. Acad. Sci.*, **138**, 49.

AUDOVA, A. (1923). *Skand. Arch. Physiol.*, **44**, 1.

BALDWIN, D., ROBINSON, P. K., ZIERLER, K. L. & LILIENTHAL, J. L., Jr. (1952). *J. clin. Invest.*, **31**, 850.

BALTZAN, M. A., ANDRES, R., CADER, G. & ZIERLER, K. L. (1962). *J. clin. Invest.*, **41**, 116.

BAUER, F. K., DUBOIS, E. L. & TELFER, N. (1960). *Proc. Soc. Exp. Biol., N.Y.*, **105**, 671.

BEATTY, C. H., MARCO, A., PETERSON, R. D., BOCEK, R. M. & WEST, E. S. (1960). *J. biol. Chem.*, **235**, 2774.

BEKÉNY, G. (1961). *Dtsch. Z. Nervenheilk.*, **182**, 119.

BEKÉNY, G., HASZNOS, T. & SOLTI, F. (1961a). *Dtsch. Z. Nervenheilk.*, **182**, 92.

BEKÉNY, G., HASZNOS, T. & SOLTI, F. (1961b). *Dtsch. Z. Nervenheilk.*, **182**, 69.

BENEDICT, J. D., KALINSKY, H. J., SCARRONE, L. A., WERTHEIM, A. R. & STETTEN, D., Jr. (1955). *J. clin. Invest.*, **34**, 141.

BERLIN, R. (1948). *Acta Med. Scand.*, **129**, 560.

BEVANS, M. (1945). *Arch. Path.*, **40**, 225.

BIÖRCK, G. (1949). *Acta Med. Scand.*, Suppl. 226.

BOURNE, G. H. & GOLARZ, M. N. (1959). *Nature*, **183**, 1741.

BOWDEN, R. E. M. (1951). *Bull. Johns Hopk. Hosp.*, **89**, 153.

BROOKS, V. B. (1954). *J. Physiol.*, **123**, 501.

BROWN, G. L. & HARVEY, A. M. (1939). *Brain*, **62**, 341.

BRUGSCH, J., BROCKMANN-ROHNE & FROMM, H. (1960). *Z. Ges. Inn. Med.*, **15**, 891.

BUCHTHAL, F., ENGBAEK, L. & GAMSTORP, I. (1958). *Neurology*, **8**, 347.

BUCHWALD, K. W. & CORI, C. F. (1931). *Proc. Soc. Exp. Biol., N.Y.*, **28**, 737.

BURGEN, A. S. V., DICKENS, F. & ZATMAN, L. J. (1949). *J. Physiol.*, **109**, 10.

BURR, L. H. & McLENNAN, H. (1961). *J. Physiol.*, **158**, 324.

BYWATERS, E. G. L. (1945). *J. Path. Bact.*, **57**, 394.

BYWATERS, E. G. L. (1950). In Schapira: "Le Muscle." Paris, L'Expansion Scientifique Francaise.

BYWATERS, E. G. L. & STEAD, J. K. (1945). *Clin. Sci.*, **5**, 195.

CANNON, W. B. & ROSENBLUETH, A. (1949). "The Supersensitivity of Denervated Structures." New York, Macmillan.

CARLSON, F. D., HARDY, D. J. & WILKIE, D. R. (1963). *J. gen. Physiol.*, **46**, 851.

CARLSON, F. D. & SIGER, A. (1959). *J. gen. Physiol.*, **43**, 301.

CARLSTRÖM, B. (1931). *Skand. Arch. Physiol.*, **61**, 161.

CASTLEMAN, B. & NORRIS, E. H. (1949). *Medicine*, **28**, 27.

CHUNG, C. S., MORTON, N. E. & PETERS, H. A. (1960). *Amer. J. Hum. Genet.*, **12**, 52.

CHURCHILL-DAVIDSON, H. C. & RICHARDSON, A. T. (1953). *J. Physiol.*, **122**, 252.

CLAVERT, J., MANDEL, P. & JACOB, M. (1949). *C.R. Soc. Biol.*, Paris, **143**, 539.

COËRS, C. & DESMEDT, J. E. (1959). *Acta Neurol. Belg.*, **59**, 539.

COFFMAN, J. R. & KOCH, F. C. (1940). *J. biol. Chem.*, **135**, 519.

CONN, J. W., FAJANS, S. S., LOUIS, L. H., STREETEN, D. H. P. & JOHNSON, R. D. (1957). *Lancet*, **1**, 802.

CORI, G. T. & CORI, C. F. (1933). *J. biol. Chem.*, **99**, 493.

CUMINGS, J. N. (1953). *Brain*, **76**, 299.

CUTHBERTSON, D. P. (1929). *Biochem. J.*, **23**, 1328.

DAHLBÄCK, O., ELMQVIST, D., JOHNS, T. R., RADNER, S. & THESLEFF, S. (1961). *J. Physiol.*, **156**, 336.

DANOWSKI, T. S., ELKINTON, J. R., BURROWS, B. A. & WINKLER, A. W. (1948). *J. clin. Invest.*, **28**, 65.

DAVENPORT, H. K., RANSON, S. W. & STEVENS, E. (1929). *Arch. Path.*, **7**, 978.

DAVIES, R. E., CAIN, D. F., INFANTE, A. A., KLAUPIKS, D. & EATON, W. A. (1964). In Gergely, J.: "Biochemistry of Muscle Contraction." Boston, Little, Brown & Co., p. 463.

DeGRAEFF, J. (1961). In Stewart & Strengers: "Water and Electrolyte Metabolism." Amsterdam, Elsevier Publishing Co.

DEITRICK, J. E., WHEDON, G. D. & SHORR, E. (1948). *Amer. J. Med.*, **4**, 3.

DENNY-BROWN, D. & PENNYBACKER, J. B. (1938). *Brain*, **61**, 311.

DESMEDT, J. E. (1958). *Nature*, **182**, 1673.

DESMEDT, J. E. (1961). In Viets: "Myasthenia Gravis." Springfield, Ill. Charles C. Thomas.

DIAZ-GUERRERO, R., THOMSON, J. D. & HINES, H. M. (1947). *Amer. J. Physiol.*, **151**, 91.

DINNING, J. S. (1955). *J. biol. Chem.*, **212**, 735.

DIPLOCK, A. T., EDWIN, E. E., GREEN, J. & BUNYAN, J. (1961). *Biochem. Biophys. Acta*, **51**, 594.

DONALDSON, K. O., NASON, A. & GARRETT, R. H. (1958). *J. biol. Chem.*, **233**, 572.

DRAGER, G. A., HAMMILL, J. F. & SHY, G. M. (1958). *Arch. Neurol. Psychiat.*, **80**, 1.

DREW, A. L. (1955). *Amer. J. Phys. Med.*, **35**, 309.

DREYFUS, J. C., JOLY, M., SCHAPIRA, G. & RAEBER, L. (1953). *C.R. Acad. Sci.*, (Paris), **236**, 2351.

DREYFUS, J. C., SCHAPIRA, G. & SCHAPIRA, F. (1949). *C.R. Soc. Biol.*, (Paris), **143**, 681.

DUBOWITZ, V. & PEARSE, A. G. E. (1960). *Histochemie*, **2**, 105.

EGAN, T. J. & KLEIN, R. (1959). *Pediatrics*, **24**, 761.

ELLIS, J. T. (1952). *Amer. J. Path.*, **28**, 542.

EMERY, A. E. H. (1967). In Milhorat: "Exploratory Concepts in Muscular Dystrophy and Related Disorders." New York, Excerpta Medica Foundation.

ENGEL, A. G. (1961). *Amer. J. Med.*, **30**, 327.

ENGEL, W. K., EYERMAN, E. L. & WILLIAMS, H. E. (1963). *New Engl. J. Med.*, **268**, 135.

ENGEL, W. K., FOSTER, J. B., HUGHES, B. P., HUXLEY, H. E. & MAHLER, R. (1961). *Brain*, **84**, 167.

EYZAGUIRRE, C., FOLK, B. P., ZIERLER, K. L. & LILIENTHAL, J. L., Jr. (1948). *Amer. J. Physiol.*, **155**, 69.

FARMER, T. A., Jr., HAMMACK, W. J. & FROMMEYER, W. B., Jr. (1961). *New Engl. J. Med.*, **264**, 60.

FATT, P. & KATZ, B. (1952). *J. Physiol.*, **117**, 109.

FEINSTEIN, B., PATTLE, R. E. & WEDDELL, G. (1945). *J. Neurol. Neurosurg. Psychiat.*, **8**, 1.

FERREBEE, J. W., ATCHLEY, D. W. & LOEB, R. F. (1938). *J. clin. Invest.*, **17**, 504.

FISCHER, E. (1939). *Amer. J. Physiol.*, **127**, 605.

FISCHER, E. (1952). In Schapira: "Le Muscle." Paris, L'Expansion Scientifique Francaise.

FISCHER, E. (1955). *Amer. J. Phys. Med.*, **36**, 212.

FISCHER, E. & RAMSEY, V. W. (1946). *Amer. J. Physiol.*, **145**, 571.

FISCHER, H. & ROSSIER, P. H. (1947). *Helv. Med. Acta*, **14**, 212.

FITCH, C. D., OATES, J. D. & DINNING, J. S. (1961). *J. clin. Invest.*, **40**, 850.

FLETCHER, W. D. & PRANKERD, T. A. J. (1955). *Lancet*, **1**, 1072.

FLOCK, E. V. & BOLLMAN, J. L. (1940). *J. biol. Chem.*, **136**, 469.

FOLLIS, R. H., Jr. (1943). *Amer. J. Physiol.*, **138**, 246.

FRANK, G. B. (1961). In Shanes: "Biophysics of Physiological and Pharmacological Actions." Washington, American Association for the Advancement of Science.

FRIEDBERG, S. J., SHER, P. B., BOGDONOFF, M. D. & ESTES, E. H., Jr. (1963). *J. Lipid Research*, **4**, 34.

FRIEDMAN, I. & MATTILL, H. A. (1941). *Amer. J. Physiol.*, **131**, 595.

FRITZ, I. B., DAVIS, D. G., HOLTROP, R. H. & DUNDEE, H. (1958). *Amer. J. Physiol.*, **194**, 370.

GAMMON, G. D., AUSTIN, J. H., BLITHE, M. D. & REID, C. G. (1939). *Amer. J. Med. Sci.*, **197**, 326.

GAMSTORP, I. (1956). *Acta paediat.* Suppl. 108.

GASS, H., CHERKASKY, M. & SAVITSKY, N. (1948). *Medicine*, **27**, 105.

GEDDES, A. K. & KIDD, H. M. (1951). *Canad. Med. Ass. J.*, **64**, 152.

GEMMILL, C. L. (1932). *Biochem. Z.*, **246**, 319.

GEORGE, J. C. & NAIK, R. M. (1958). *Nature*, **181**, 709.

GEORGE, J. C. & SCARIA, K. S. (1958). *Nature*, **181**, 783.

GOLARZ, M. N. & BOURNE, G. H. (1960). *Acta Anat,.* **43**, 13.

GOLARZ, M. N., BOURNE, G. H. & RICHARDSON, H. D. (1961). *J. Histochem. Cytochem.*, **9**, 132.

GOLDSTEIN, M. S., RAMEY, E. R. & LEVINE, R. (1950). *Amer. J. Physiol.*, **163**, 561.

GOLUMBIC, C. & MATTILL, H. A. (1940). *J. biol. Chem.*, **134**, 535.

GRAY, D. E. & DELUCA, H. A. (1954). *Canad. J. Biochem. Physiol.*, **32**, 491.

GREEN, H. N. & STONER, H. B. (1952). In Schapira: "Le Muscle." Paris, L'Expansion Scientifique Francaise.

GREENFIELD, J. G., CORNMAN, T. & SHY, G. M. (1958). *Brain*, **81**, 461.

GROB, D. & HARVEY, A. M. (1952). *Bull. Johns Hopk. Hosp.*, **91**, 124.

GROB, D. & HARVEY, A. M. (1953). *Amer. J. Med.*, **15**, 695.

GROB, D., JOHNS, R. J. & HARVEY, A. M. (1955). *Amer. J. Med.*, **19**, 684.

GROB, D., JOHNS, R. J. & LILJESTRAND, Å. (1957). *Amer. J. Med.*, **23**, 356.

GÜNTHER, H. (1924). *Virchows Arch.*, **251**, 141.

GUTMANN, E. (1959). *Amer. J. Phys. Med.*, **38**, 104.

HAGENFELDT, L. & WAHREN, J. (1966). *Life Sciences*, **5**, 357.

HANSON, J. & HUXLEY, H. E. (1953). *Nature*, **172**, 530.

HANSON, J. & LOWY, J. (1963). *J. Molecular Biol.*, **6**, 46.

HARRIS, E. J. & NICHOLLS, J. G. (1954). *J. Physiol.*, **123**, 3P.

HARRIS, P. L. & KUZAWSKI, W. (1950, 1952, 1955). "Annotated Bibliography of Vitamin E", Vols. I, II and III. New York, The National Vitamin Foundation.

HARVEY, A. M. & JOHNS, R. J. (1962). *Amer. J. Med.*, **32**, 1.

HARVEY, A. M. & MASLAND, R. L. (1941). *Bull. Johns Hopk. Hosp.*, **68**, 81.

HARVEY, A. M. & LILIENTHAL, J. L., Jr. (1941). *Bull. Johns Hopk. Hosp.*, **69**, 566.

HASSELBACH, W. & MAKINOSE, M. (1961). *Biochem. Ztschr.*, **333**, 518.

HAVEL, R. J., PERNOW, B. & JONES, N. L. (1967). *J. Appl. Physiol.*, **23**, 90.

HAZZARD, W. R. & LEONARD, S. L., (1961). *Proc. Soc. Exp. Biol.*, *N.Y.*, **106**, 839.

HELWEG, LARSEN, H. F., HAUGE, M. & SAGILD, U. (1955). *Acta Genet.*, **5**, 263.

HELWIG, H. L. & GREENBERG, D. M. (1952). *J. biol. Chem.*, **198**, 703.

HINES, H. M. (1952). In Schapira: "Le Muscle." Paris, L'Expansion Scientifique Francaise.

HINES, H. M. & KNOWLTON, G. C. (1935). *Amer. J. Physiol.*, **111**, 243.

HINES, H. M., THOMSON, J. D. & LAZERE, B. (1942). *Amer. J. Physiol.*, **137**, 527.

HOAGLAND, C. L. (1946a). *Advanc. Enzymol.*, **6**, 193.

HOAGLAND, C. L. (1946*b*). In Green: "Currents in Biochemical Research." New York, Interscience.

HOAGLAND, C. L., GILDER, H. & SHANK, R. E. (1945). *J. Exp. Med.*, **81**, 423.

HODGKIN, A. L. (1951). *Biol. Rev.*, **26**, 399.

HODGKIN, A. L. & HUXLEY, A. F. (1952). *Cold Spring Harbor Symp. Quant. Biol.*, **17**, 43.

HOMBURGER, F., NIXON, C. W., EPPENBERGER, M. & BAKER, J. R. (1966). *Ann. N.Y. Acad. Sci.*, **138**, 14.

HORVATH, B. & PROCTOR, J. B. (1960). *Res. Publ., Ass. Nerv. Ment. Dis.*, **38**, 740.

HOWARD, J. E., PARSON, W. & BIGHAM, R. S. (1944). *Bull. Johns Hopk. Hosp.*, **75**, 209.

HUF, E. G. & FISCHER, E. (1949). *Amer. J. Physiol.*, **159**, 6.

HUMOLLER, F. L., GRISWOLD, B. & MCINTYRE, A. R. (1950*a*). *Amer. J. Physiol.*, **161**, 406.

HUMOLLER, F. L., GRISWOLD, B. & MCINTYRE, A. R. (1950*b*). *J. gen. Physiol.*, **33**, 723.

HUXLEY, H. E. (1957). *J. Biophys. & Biochem. Cytol.*, **3**, 631.

HUXLEY, H. E. (1963). *J. Molecular Biol.*, **7**, 281.

JARCHO, L. W., BERMAN, B., DOWBEN, R. M. & LILIENTHAL, J. L., Jr. (1954). *Amer. J. Physiol.*, **178**, 129.

JARCHO, L. W., BERMAN, B., EYZAGUIRRE, C. & LILIENTHAL, J. L., Jr. (1951). *Ann. N.Y. Acad. Sci.*, **54**, 337.

KAUNITZ, H. & PAPPENHEIMER, A. M. (1943). *Amer. J. Physiol.*, **138**, 328.

KEPLER, E. J., SPRAGUE, R. G., MASON, H. L. & POWER, M. H. (1948). *Rec. Progr. Horm. Res.*, **2**, 345.

KITIYAKARA, A. (1961). *Arch. Path.*, **71**, 579.

KOSZALKA, T. R., MASON, K. E. & KROLL, G. (1961). *J. Nutrit.*, **73**, 78.

KRUH, J., DREYFUS, J. C., SCHAPIRA, G. & GEY, G. O., Jr. (1960). *J. clin. Invest.*, **39**, 1180.

LACKEY, R. W., BRINDLE, C. A., GILL, A. J. & HARRIS, L. C. (1944). *Proc. Soc. Exp. Biol., N.Y.*, **57**, 191.

LAFON, G. (1913). *C.R. Acad. Sci.*, (Paris), **156**, 1248.

LANGLEY, J. N. & ITAGAKI, M. (1917). *J. Physiol.*, **51**, 202.

LARNER, J. (1964). In Whelan and Cameron: "Control of Glycogen Metabolism," Ciba Foundation Symposium. London, J. and A. Churchill Ltd.

LEYBURN, P., THOMSON, W. H. S. & WALTON, J. N. (1961). *Ann. Hum. Genet.*, **25**, 41.

LILIENTHAL, J. L., Jr. (1952). "The Biology of Mental Health and Disease." (Milbank Memorial Fund Conference). New York, Paul B. Hoeber.

LILJESTRAND, Å. (1957). *Opuscula Medica* p. 183.

LORING J. SPENCER J. & VILLEE C. (1961). *Endocrinology* **68**, 501.

LOUW, A. & NIELSEN H. E. (1944). *Acta Med. Scand.* **117**, 424.

MCARDLE, B. (1951). *Clin. Sci.* **10**, 13.

MCARDLE, B. (1956). *Brit. Med. Bull.*, **12**, 226.

MCARDLE, B. (1962). *Brain*, **85**, 121.

MCCRUDDEN, R. H. & SARGENT, C. S. (1916). *Arch. Intern. Med.*, **17**, 465.

MACKENZIE, C. G. (1953). In Herriott: "Symposium on Nutrition." Baltimore, Johns Hopkins Press.

MACKENZIE, C. G. & MCCOLLUM, E. V. (1940). *J. Nutrit.*, **19**, 345.

MANERY, J. F. (1954). *Physiol. Rev.*, **34**, 334.

MASON, K. E. (1949). *Ann. N.Y. Acad. Sci.*, **52**, 63.

MASORO, E. J., ROWELL, L. B., MACDONALD, R. M. & STEIERT, B. (1966). *J. biol. Chem.*, **241**, 2626.

MEIER, H. W., WEST, W. T. & HOAG, W. G. (1965). *Arch. Pathol.*, **80**, 165.

MELDOLESI, G. & GARRETTO, U. (1938). *Policlinico (Sez. Med.)*, **45**, 1.

MICHELSON, A. M., RUSSELL, E. S. & HARMAN, P. J. (1955). *Proc. Nat. Acad. Sci.*, **41**, 1079.

MILHORAT, A. T. & WOLFF, H. G. (1937). *Arch. Neurol. Psychiat.*, **38**, 992.

MILLIKAN, G. A. (1939). *Physiol. Rev.*, **19**, 503.

MINETT, F. C. (1935). *Proc. R. Soc. Med.*, **28**, 672.

MINOT, A. S., FRANK, H. & DZIEWIATKOWSKI, D. (1949). *Arch. Biochem.*, **20**, 394.

MOLLARET, P., GOULON, M. & TOURNILHAC, M. (1961). *Sem. Hôp., Paris*, **37**, 603.

MOMMAERTS, W. F. H. M., ILLINGWORTH, B., PEARSON, C. M., GUILLORY, R. J. & SERAY-DARIAN, K. (1959). *Proc. Nat. Acad. Sci.*, **45**, 791.

MOMMAERTS, W. F. H. M., SERAYDARIAN, K. & WALLNER, A. (1962). *Biochem. et Biophys. Acta*, **63**, 75.

MORGULIS, S. & SPENCER, H. C. (1936). *J. Nutrit.*, **11**, 573.

MUDGE, G. H. & VISLOCKY, K. (1949). *J. Clin. Invest.*, **28**, 482.

MUNTWYLER, E., MELLORS, R. C., MAUTZ, F. R. & MANGUN, G. H. (1940). *J. biol. Chem.*, **134**, 367.

NEPTUNE, E. M., Jr., FOREMAN, D. R. & REISH, J. J. Jr. (1960). *Amer. J. Physiol.*, **199**, 1048.

NEVIN, S. (1934). *Brain*, **57**, 239.

NEVIN, S. (1936). *Quart. J. Med.*, **5**, n.s., 51.

NICKEL, S. N. & FRAME, B. (1961). *J, Chronic Dis.*, **14**, 570.

NIEDERGERKE, R. (1955). *J. Physiol.*, **128**, 12P.

NILSBY, I. (1949). *Acta Paediat.*, **37**, 489.

OCHOA, S. (1930). *Biochem. Z.*, **227**, 116.

OKINAKA, S., SHIZUME, K., IINO, S., WATANABE, A., IRIE, M., NOGUCHI, A., KUMA, S., KUMA, K. & ITO, T. (1957). *J. clin. Endocr.*, **17**, 1454.

OKUDA, M. (1930). *J. Biochem., Tokyo*, **11**, 183.

PALAZZOLO, G. (1913). *Arch. Fisiol.*, **11**, 558.

PAPPENHEIMER, A. M. (1948). "On Certain Aspects of Vitamin E Deficiency." Springfield, Ill., Charles C. Thomas.

PAPPENHEIMER, A. M. & GOETTSCH, M. (1931). *J. Exp. Med.*, **53**, 11.

PATON, W. D. M. & ZAIMIS, E. J. (1952). *Pharmacol. Rev.*, **4**, 219.

PEACHEY, L. D. (1965). *J. Cell. Biol.*, **25**, 209.

PEARSON, C. M. (1962). *Brain*, **85**, 109.

PEARSON, C. M., BECK, W. S. & BLAND, W. H. (1957). *Arch. Intern. Med.*, **99**, 376.

PEARSON, C. M., CHOWDHURY, S. R., FOWLER, W. M., JONES, M. H. & GRIFFITH, W. H. (1961). *Pediatrics*, **28**, 962.

PEARSON, C. M., RIMER, D. G. & MOMMAERTS, W. F. H. M. (1961). *Amer. J. Med.*, **30**, 502.

PETERS, J. P. (1952). In Duncan: "Diseases of Metabolism." Philadelphia, W. B. Saunders.

PETERS, J. B. (1967). In Milhorat: "Exploratory Concepts in Muscular Dystrophy and Related Disorders." New York, Excerpta Medica Foundation.

PETERSON, R. D., BEATTY, C. H., BOCEK, R. M. & WEST, E. S. (1954). *Amer. J. Physiol.*, **179**, 499.

PODOLSKY, R. J. & CONSTANTIN, L. L. (1964). *Fed. Proc.*, **23**, 933.

PORTER, K. R. & PALADE, G. E. (1957). *J. Biophys. & Biochem. Cytol.*, **3**, 269.

RABINOWITZ, D. & ZIERLER, K. L. (1962). *J. clin. Invest.*, **41**, 1393.

REINER, L., KONIKOFF, N., ALTSCHULE, M. D., DAMMIN, G. J. & MERRILL, J. P. (1956). *Arch. Intern. Med.*, **97**, 537.

REINHOLD, J. G. & KINGSLEY, G. R. (1938). *J. clin. Invest.*, **17**, 377.

RICE, R. V. (1961). *Biochem. Biophys. Acta*, **52**, 1961.

RICHTER, K. & KONITZER, K. (1960). *Klin. Wschr.*, **38**, 998.

RICHTERICH, R., GAUTIER, E., EGLI, W., ZUPPINGER, K. & ROSSI, E. (1961). *Klin. Wschr.*, **39**, 346.

RIGDON, R. H. (1966). *Ann. N.Y. Acad. Sci.*, **138**, 28.

ROGUS, E. & ZIERLER, K. L. (1968). *Fed. Proc.*, **27**, 702.

RONZONI, E., BERG, L. & LANDAU, W. (1960). *Res. Publ. Ass. Res. Nerv. Ment. Dis.*, **38**, 721.

ROSENKRANTZ, H. & LAFERTE, R. O. (1961). *Proc. Soc. Exp. Biol., N.Y.*, **106**, 391.

RULON, R. R., SCHOTTELIUS, D. D. & SCHOTTELIUS, B. A. (1962). *Amer. J. Physiol.*, **202**, 821.

RUNDLE, F. F., FINLAY-JONES, L. R. & NOAD, K. B. (1953). *Aust. Ann. Med.*, **2**, 128.

RUNDLE, F. F. & POCHIN, E. E. (1944). *Clin. Sci.*, **8**, 9.

SACKS, J. & SACKS, W. C. (1933). *Amer. J. Physiol.*, **105**, 151.

SAMUELS, A. (1957). *Fed. Proc.*, **16**, 399.

SATOYOSHI, E. (1961). *Clin. Neurol.*, **1**, 439.

SATOYASHI, E. & KOWA, H. (1965). *Trans. Amer. Neurol. Ass.*, **90**, 46.

SCHAPIRA, F., DREYFUS, J. C., SCHAPIRA, G. & DEMOS, J. (1960). "Revue francaise d'Etudes cliniques et biologique." **5**, 990.

SCHAPIRA, G. & DREYFUS, J. C. (1959). *Amer. J. Phys. Med.*, **38**, 207.

SCHAPIRA, G., DREYFUS, J. C. & SCHAPIRA, F. (1953). *Sem. Hôp., Paris*, **29**, 1917.

SCHMID, R. & HAMMAKER, L. (1961). *New Engl. J. Med.*, **264**, 223.

SCHMID, R. & MAHLER, R. (1959). *J. clin. Invest.*, **38**, 2044.

SCHMIDT, C. G. & SCHLIEF, H. (1956). *Z. Ges. Exp. Med.*, **127**, 53.

SCHRIRE, I. (1937). *Quart. J. Med.*, **6**, n.s., 17.

SCOW, R. O. & ROE, J. H., Jnr. (1953). *Amer. J. Physiol.*, **173**, 22.

SHANK, R. E., GILDER, H. & HOAGLAND, C. L. (1944). *Arch. Neurol. Psychiat.*, **52**, 431.

SHY, G. M. & MAGEE, K. R. (1956). *Brain*, **79**, 610.

SHY, G. M., WANKO, T., ROWLEY, P. T. & ENGEL, A. G. (1961). *Exp. Neurol.*, **3**, 53.

SIBLEY, J. A. & LEHNINGER, A. (1949). *J. Nat. Cancer Inst.*, **9**, 303.

SKOU, J. C. (1965). *Physiol. Rev.*, **45**, 596.

SLACK, H. G. B. (1954). *Clin. Sci.*, **13**, 155.

SMITH, H., AMICK, L. & SIDBURY, J. B., Jr. (1966). *Amer. J. Dis. Child.*, **111**, 475.

SOLA, O. M. & MARTIN, A. W. (1953). *Amer. J. Physiol.*, **172**, 324.

SOLANDT, D. Y. & MAGLADERY, J. W. (1940). *Brain*, **63**, 255.

SRETER, F. A., IKEMOTO, N. & GERGELY, J. (1967). In Milhorat: "Exploratory Concepts in Muscular Dystrophy and Related Disorders." New York, Excerpta Medica Foundation.

STANBURY, J. B., GOLDSMITH, R. R. & GILLIS, M. (1954). *J. clin. Endocrinol.*, **14**, 1437.

STEWART, D. M. (1955). *Biochem. J.*, **59**, 553.

STOVER, J. H., FINGERMAN, M. & FORESTER, R. H. (1953). *Proc. Soc. Exp. Biol., N.Y.*, **84**, 146.

STRAUSS, A. J., SEEGAL, B. C., HSU, J. C., BURKHOLDER, P. M., NASTUK, W. L. & OSSERMAN, K. E. (1960). *Proc. Soc. Exp. Biol., N.Y.*, **105**, 184.

SUGITA, H., OKIMOTO, K., EBASHI, S. & OKINAKA, S. (1967). In Milhorat: "Exploratory Concepts in Muscular Dystrophy and Related Disorders." New York, Excerpta Medica Foundation.

SUNDERLAND, S. & RAY, L. J. (1950). *J. Neurol. Neurosurg. Psychiat.*, **13**, 159.

SUTFIN, D. C., THOMSON, J. D. & HINES, H. M. (1954). *Amer. J. Physiol.*, **178**, 535.

TALBOTT, J. H. (1941). *Medicine*, **20**, 85.

TARAIL, R., HACKER, E. S. & TAYMOR, R. (1952). *J. clin. Invest.*, **31**, 23.

TARUI S., OKUNO, G., IKURA, Y., TANAKA, T., SUDA, M. & NISHIKAWA, M. (1965). *Biochem. Biophys. Res. Commun.*, **19**, 517.

THEORELL, H. (1934). *Biochem. Z.*, **268**, 46.

THEORELL, H. & DE DUVE, C. (1947). *Arch. Biochem.*, **12**, 113.

THESLEFF, S. (1955). *Nature*, **175**, 594.

THESLEFF, S. (1960). *Physiol. Rev.*, **40**, 734.

THOMASEN, E. (1948). Myotonia, Aarhus, Universtets Forlaget.

THOMSON, J. D. (1955). *Amer. J. Physiol.*, **180**, 202.

THOMSON, J. D., MORGAN, J. A. & BRODISH, A. (1951). *Amer. J. Physiol.*, **167**, 832.

TIERNEY, N. A. & PETERS, J. P. (1943). *J. clin. Invest.*, **22**, 595.

TOWER, S. S. (1939). *Physiol. Rev.*, **19**, 1.

TYLER, F. H. & PERKOFF, G. T. (1951). *Arch. Intern. Med.*, **88**, 175.

TYLER, F. H., STEPHENS, F. E., GUNN, F. D. & PERKOFF, G. T. (1951). *J. clin. Invest.*, **30**, 492.

VAN DER MEULEN, J. P., GILBERT, G. J. & KANE, C. A. (1961). *New Engl. J. Med.*, **264**, 1.

VICTOR, J. (1934). *Amer. J. Physiol.*, **108**, 229.

VIGNOS, P. J. & LEFKOWITZ, M. (1959). *J. Clin. Invest.*, **38**, 873.

WALTON, J. N. & NATTRASS, F. J. (1954). *Brain*, **77**, 169.

WANG, E. (1939). *Acta Med. Scand., Suppl.* **105**, 1.

WATSON, C. W. (1946). *Yale J. Biol. Med.*, **19**, 127.

WEHRMACHER, W. H., THOMSON, J. D. & HINES, H, M. (1945). *Arch. Phys. Med.*, **26**, 261.

WEINSTOCK, I. M., GOLDRICH, A. D. & MILHORAT, A. T. (1955). *Proc. Soc. Exp. Biol., N.Y.*, **88**, 257.

WHIPPLE, G. H. (1926). *Amer. J. Physiol.*, **76**, 708.

WILSON, J. D. (1962). *J. clin. Invest.*, **41**, 153.

WOHLFART, G. (1951). *J. Neuropath. Exp. Neurol.*, **10**, 109.

YUDAEV, N. A., SMIRNOV, M. I., RAZINA, P. G. & DORBERT, N. N. (1953). *Biokhimya*, **18**, 732.

ZALKIN, H. & TAPPEL, A. L. (1960). *Arch. Biochem.*, **88**, 113.

ZALKIN, H., TAPPEL, A. L. & JORDAN, J. P. (1960). *Arch. Biochem. Biophys.*, **91**, 117.

ZELLWEGER, H., BROWN, B. I., McCORMICK, W. F. & TU, J.-B. (1965). *Ann. Paediat.* (Basel), **205**, 413.

ZIEGLER, M. R. & McQIARRIE, I. (1952). *Metabolism*, **1**, 116.

ZIERLER, K. L. (1951). *Bull. Johns Hopk. Hosp.*, **89**, 263.

ZIERLER, K. L. (1957). *Amer. J. Physiol.*, **190**, 201.

ZIERLER, K. L. (1958a). *Bull. Johns Hopk. Hosp.*, **102**, 17.

ZIERLER, K. L. (1958b). *Amer. J. Physiol.*, **192**, 283.

ZIERLER, K. L. (1958c). *Amer. J. Physiol.*, **193**, 534.

ZIERLER, K. L. (1961b). *Bull. Johns Hopk. Hosp.*, **108**, 208.

ZIERLER, K. L. & ANDRES, R. (1957). *J. clin. Invest.*, **36**, 730.

ZIERLER, K. L., FOLK, B. P., EYZAGUIRRE, C., JARCHO, L. W., GROB, D. & LILIENTHAL, J. L., Jr., (1949a). *Ann. N.Y. Acad. Sci.*, **52**, 180.

ZIERLER, K. L., FOLK, B. P., MAGLADERY, J. W. & LILIENTHAL, J. L., Jr., (1949 b). *Bull. Johns Hopk. Hosp.*, **85**, 370.

ZIERLER, K. L. LEVY, R. I. & LILIENTHAL, J. L., Jr. (1953). *Bull. Johns Hopk. Hosp.*, **92**, 41.

ZIERLER, K. L., MASERI, A., KLASSEN, G. A., RABINOWITZ, D. & BURGESS, J. A. (1968). *Trans. Assoc. Am. Physicians* (in press).

ZOBEL, C. R. & CARLSON, F. D. (1963). *J. Molecular Biol.*, **7**, 78.

Chapter 15

DISORDERS OF IMMUNOGLOBULIN PRODUCTION

by

S. Cohen and N. H. Martin

Department of Chemical Pathology, Guy's Hospital Medical School, London, and
Department of Chemical Pathology, St. George's Hospital Medical School, London

ACQUIRED immunity depends essentially upon a process of lymphoid cell multiplication and differentiation which occurs in response to antigenic stimulation and leads to the production of serum immunoglobulins and probably also cell-bound antibody. The essential components of the immune response are shown diagrammatically in Fig. 15.1.

Antigens are usually large molecules in which at least part of the structure is foreign to the recipient host. The initial step in the immune response to soluble and particulate antigens involves their phagocytosis by macrophage cells (see Mitchison, 1967). This is shown for example by the fact that antigen which has circulated in one animal for some hours, so that all phagocytosable material is removed, is no longer immunogenic when tested in other recipients. Indeed, such material may induce a long-lasting state of specific immunolo-

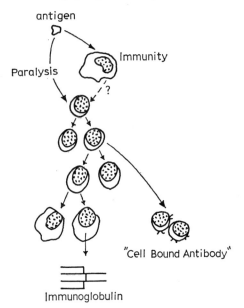

FIG. 15.1. Diagrammatic representation of the immune response. Phagocytic cells ingest antigen and liberate material which stimulates lymphoid cells to divide, differentiate and produce specific antibody (serum and cell-bound). Antigen in non-phagocytosable form may lead to specific immune paralysis, perhaps by direct interaction with lymphoid cells.

gical paralysis, possibly by direct interaction with lymphoid cells of appropriate specificity (Fig. 15.1). The way in which antigen ingested by macrophages is able to stimulate lymphocytes to produce antibody remains unknown. There is evi-

dence of close physical contact between lymphocytes and macrophages, and highly antigenic material, sometimes associated with RNA, has been extracted from macrophages after immunization. Material liberated from macrophages must interact with lymphocytes, perhaps selectively with those which carry antibody of the appropriate specificity on the cell surface. The stimulated lymphocytes undergo repeated mitotic divisions and differentiate into larger cells, some of which resemble plasma cells, and contain and secrete specific antibody. Newly formed antibody passes into the extracellular fluid and enters the venous blood-stream through lymphatic ducts. The synthesis of antibody molecules is balanced by a continual process of catabolism so that serum immunoglobulin concentrations remain within narrow limits in healthy individuals.

Certain immunological responses cannot be passively transferred with serum, but are transferable with lymphoid cell suspensions. This is true for delayed hypersensitivity responses in general, e.g. the tuberculin reaction, and applies also to specific sensitivity to grafts of organized tissue. Such immunological phenomena which appear to depend upon the direct interaction of antigen with sensitized cells, have led to the concept of "cell-bound antibody." (Fig. 15.1.) Whether such cells are passive carriers of absorbed antibody or actively synthesize the specific combining sites which are presumably carried at their surface, is at present unknown (see Coombs, 1967).

It is now established that the rejection of genetically foreign tissue grafts is fundamentally dependent upon an immunological process evoked by transplantation antigens of the graft. If these antigenic molecules are actually released from the graft, as they appear to be from certain cultured cells, then the process of immunization would be similar to that outlined above for soluble or particulate antigens. However, the time of contact required for grafts to evoke sensitization and their failure to sensitize the host when contained in cell-impermeable filter chambers suggest that tissue antigens may remain fixed to the transplanted cells. If this is so, then the afferent arc of the immune process probably involves sensitization of host lymphocytes by direct contact with foreign cells during their passage through the grafted tissue (Fig. 15.2). Such sensitized cells probably divide and differentiate in remote lymphoid tissues and liberate showers of specific effector lymphocytes (carrying cell-bound antibody) capable of invading and destroying the graft.

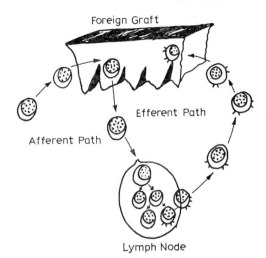

Foreign Graft

Efferent Path

Afferent Path

Lymph Node

FIG. 15.2. Diagrammatic representation of the afferent pathway for sensitisation of host lymphocytes to foreign tissue, and the efferent pathway leading to graft rejection by "cell-bound antibody".

Various disorders of immunoglobulin and specific antibody production are observed in clinical medicine. These include:

(i) Diffuse overproduction of immunoglobulin.
(ii) Diminished production of immunoglobulin.
(iii) Production of "monoclonal" immuno-globulins.
(iv) Production of autoantibodies.

Before discussing each of these phenomena, the chemical structure and some properties of normal immunoglobulins will be described.

NORMAL IMMUNOGLOBULIN

Classes and Types of Immunoglobulin

Tiselius & Kabat (1939) first demonstrated that precipitating antibodies in a strongly immunized rabbit were associated with γ-globulin. This fraction, originally defined as the component which moves most slowly during electrophoresis of serum at alkaline pH, is known to include several classes of protein associated with antibody activity. The predominant component of γ-globulin has a molecular weight of about 150,000 and is now referred to as IgG; immunoelectrophoresis has shown that protein having the antigenic specificity of IgG extends into the β- and α-globulin regions. About 5 to 10% of human γ-globulin consists of protein having a molecular weight of about 900,000 and referred to as IgM; this fraction can be identified by immuno-

electrophoresis and was previously called β_2M- or γ_1M globulin. Immunoelectrophoresis has also led to the identification of a third antigenically distinct type of γ-globulin now known as IgA (Grabar, Fauvert, Burtin & Hartmann, 1956) which is mainly of similar molecular size to IgG, but like IgM has a relatively high carbohydrate content. Two additional classes of human immunoglobulins have recently been described. IgD is present in low and variable concentration and has not been shown to carry antibody activity (Rowe & Fahey, 1965). IgE is also a trace component, but there is growing evidence that, in some subjects, this class may be associated with reaginic antibodies which mediate various immediate type hypersensitivity responses in man (Stanworth, Humphrey, Bennich & Johansson, 1967). Despite their diversity the three types of immunoglobulin have a basically similar structure and all are associated with certain common chemical and biological properties (Table 15.1) (Reviewed by Lennox & Cohn, 1967; Cohen & Milstein, 1967a,b; Schultze & Heremans, 1966).

Immunoglobulin G (IgG)

This fraction comprises about 85% of the total immunoglobulin and contains about 3% carbohydrate. IgG can be prepared free of other immunoglobulin fractions by elution of serum from diethylaminoethyl (DEAE) cellulose columns. In all species investigated molecular weight estimations have fallen within the range 140,000 to 190,000; recent studies suggest that this wide scatter arises from differences of technique and that the lower figure, which corresponds to the original estimates of Heidelberger & Pedersen (1937), is more probably correct. The heterogeneity of this protein is shown by its wide range of electrophoretic mobility and diffuse spread on ion-exchange chromatography. Most of the antibodies which have been studied in detail belong to this subfraction of the immunoglobulins. Several antigenically distinct types of human IgG have been recognized and the nomenclature used for these by different authors is shown in Table 15.2. These types of IgG are present in all normal human sera so that, in contrast to allotypic specificities (Table 15.1), they do not reflect a genetic polymorphism. There is evidence that IgG types differ in biological properties, e.g. in regard to skin fixation (Table 15.2).

Immunoglobulin M (IgM)

This fraction has an average molecular weight of about 900,000 and constitutes 5 to 10% of electrophoretically isolated γ-globulin and approxi-

TABLE 15.1

Properties of human immunoglobulins

	IgG	IgA	IgM	IgD
Biological				
Serum Conc. mg./100ml.	800–1680	140–420	50–190	0·3–40
Synthesis rate (mg./Kg./d.)	20–40	2·7–55	3·2–16·9	0·03–1·49
Catabolic rate (% I–V pool/d.)	4–7	14–34	14–25	18–60
Distribution (% in I–V pool)	48–62	40	65–100	63–86
Antibody activity	+	+	+	
Complement fixation	+	0	+	
Placental passage	+	0	0	0
Presence in cerebrospinal fluid	+	+	0	
Selective seromucous secretion*	0	+	0	
Skin sensitization				
heterologous species	+	0	0	
homologous species	0	0	0	
Immunological				
Light chain types	κ, λ	κ, λ	κ, λ	κ, λ†
Heavy chain classes	γ	a	μ	δ
types	4	2	2	
Allotypes Gm	+	0	0	0
Inv	+	+	+	
Physico-chemical				
S20W	6·5–7·0	7·0, 13, 15, 17	18–20 > 30	6·2–6·8
Ammonium sulphate precipitation	1·49–1·64M		1·64–2·05M	
Total carbohydrate %	2·9	7·5	11·8	
Hexose%	1·10	3·2	5·4	
Acetylhexosamine %	1·30	2·3	4·4	
Sialic acid %	0·30	1·8	1·3	
Fucose %	0·20	0·22	0·7	

* see text.

† Myeloma IgD's usually have λ-chains (Hobbs, Slot, Campbell, Clein, Scott, Crowther & Swan, 1966; Hansson, Laurell & Bachmann, 1966).

TABLE 15.2

Types of human IgG

Nomenclature				% Total IgG	Location of Specificity	Skin Sensitisation
(2)	(3)	(4)	(1)			(5)
We	γ2b	C	γ1	60–70%	γ chain—Fc [3]	+
Vi	γ2c	Z	γ3	< 20%	γ chain—Fd [2]	+
Ge	γ2d		γ4	< 20%		
Ne	γ2a		γ2	< 20%	γ chain—Fc [3]	0

(1) Kunkel, Fahey, Franklin, Osserman & Terry (1966).
(2) Grey & Kunkel (1964).
(3) Terry & Fahey (1964).
(4) Ballieux, Bernier, Tominaga & Putnam (1964).
(5) Terry (1964).

mately 1 % of the total protein in human serum. IgM shows a characteristic heterogeneity in the ultracentrifuge; the major component has a sedimentation constant of 19S and there are two additional components (29S and 35–40S) which are thought to be polymers of IgM (Kunkel, 1960). The electrophoretic mobility of IgM is intermediate between γ- and β-globulins and the fraction contains about 10 % carbohydrate (Table 15.1). IgM can be observed by immuno-electrophoresis and isolated in relatively pure form by preparative ultracentrifugation or by a combination of density gradient centrifugation, chromatography and gel filtration (Chaplin, Cohen & Press, 1965). Heidelberger & Pedersen (1937) first showed in their classical experiments that horse anti-pneumococcal antibody has a relatively high molecular weight. Since that time several biologically active proteins have been demonstrated in human IgM; some of these, including cold agglutinins, antibodies to the 0 antigen of salmonella and the rheumatoid factor, are almost entirely confined to this fraction, while others, such as isohaemagglutinins, anti-thyro-globulin and the antibodies mediating the Wasserman reaction, are present in both IgG and IgM (Fahey & Goodman, 1960).

Immunoglobulin A (IgA)

This fraction, which comprises about 10% of human immunoglobulin, has been isolated from normal serum by a combination of zinc sulphate and ammonium sulphate precipitation and preparative electrophoresis. Serum IgA is usually heterogeneous in the ultracentrifuge; the main component has a sedimentation constant of approximately 7S, but additional components, ranging from 9S to 15S may be present (Laurell, 1961b). IgA has a relatively high carbohydrate content, an electrophoretic mobility corresponding to γ_1-globulin, and is now known to be associated with antibody activity.

IgA is present in relatively high concentration in various seromucous secretions, including saliva, colostrum, tears and secretions of the bronchial and gastro-intestinal tracts; in these secretions IgA exists largely in polymerized form and has a sedimentation coefficient of 11S.

Immunoglobulin E (IgE)

This fraction is present in normal human serum at very low concentration (mean value 0·25 μg./ml.) and appears to be increased in about 50% of patients with allergic diseases and probably also in parasitic and helminthic infections. The association of reaginic antibody with a new class of immunoglobulin (IgE) was suggested by Ishizaka et al. 1966, 1967) who showed that skin sensitizing antibodies did not contain the class specific determinants of IgG, IgA, IgM or IgD. This view was given support by studies on a myeloma protein having similar properties (Johansson, Bennich & Wide, 1968). IgE has the general 4-chain structure common to all immunoglobulins, migrates with γ1 mobility on electrophoresis, has a molecular weight of about 200,000, does not pass from maternal to foetal circulations across the placenta, is heat-labile and able to inhibit completely passive skin sensitization by reaginic antibody (Prausnitz-Küstner reaction). The tissue attachment site is present on the Fc fragment which, in the unreduced state, has full inhibitory activity.

Peptide Chains of Immunoglobulins

The multichain structure of antibodies was established by Edelman and his collaborators (Edelman, 1959; Edelman & Poulik, 1961) who separated subunits of human and rabbit immuno-globulins after reduction in urea solution. The products obtained by this method, which splits about 15 of the 20 disulphide bonds of the molecule, were separable by chromatography, but were biologically inactive and insoluble in aqueous solutions. Fleischman, Pain & Porter (1962) subsequently isolated the constituent peptide chains in a more soluble form and with several biological activities intact by reduction of immunoglobulin in neutral aqueous solution, followed by dissociation in N-acetic or N-propionic acid and gel filtration on Sephadex columns; two classes of chains now referred to as heavy and light were separated with 100% recovery of the original protein.

The heavy chain comprises about three-quarters of the molecule and has a molecular weight of about 50,000 while the light chain has a molecular weight of about 20,000 (Pain, 1963; Small, Kehn & Lamm, 1963). The relative yields and molecular weights suggest that the molecule is made up of two heavy and two light chains and this is supported by amino-acid analyses. These facts led Porter (1962) to postulate a diagrammatic four chain structure for rabbit immunoglobulin (Fig. 15.3) and subsequent work indicates that this is characteristic of all species investigated.

Enzymic Fragments of Immunoglobulins

Ig molecules can be split not only by separation of peptide chains but also by a variety of enzymes which appear to act at slightly different sites, but all within a limited and as yet incompletely defined area of the heavy chain (Fig. 15.3). Following earlier studies on the enzymic hydrolysis of horse antibodies, Porter (1959) used papain in the presence of reducing agent to split rabbit immunoglobulin into three fragments. The largest (F_c) has a molecular weight of 48,000, carries no antibody activity, but is associated with other biological activities of the original molecule including the ability to fix complement, combine with rheumatoid factor and cross the placenta from maternal to foetal circulations. This F_c fragment is made up of portions of the heavy chain and, when proteolysis has been carried out in low concentrations of reducing agent, these are joined by a disulphide bond so that the molecular weight of the fragment is halved by reduction. The other two fragments (F_{ab}) have molecular weights of 42,000, each contains one combining site, and consists of the light chain together with a portion of the heavy chain (F_d). These observations suggest that papain cleaves the heavy chains of immunoglobulin on the N-terminal side of the inter-heavy chain disulphide bond shown in Fig. 15.3. The fact that papain splits the IgG molecule only in the presence of reducing agents suggests that enzymic cleavage occurs either at a point bridged by an intrachain disulphide bond or between two crossed interchain disulphide bonds.

Digestion of immunoglobulin with pepsin at pH 5 leaves a fragment ($F_{(ab')}2$) which has a molecular weight of 91,000 and contains both the original combining sites. $F_{(ab')}2$ is split on reduction to give univalent fragments which resemble F_{ab} but unlike the latter can be reoxidized to the

$F_{(ab')}2$ dimer. Pepsin splits the remainder of the molecule (corresponding to the F_c region) into at least three groups of fragments, two of which contain all the antigenic determinants of F_c while the third contains all the carbohydrate and none of the original antigenic determinants (Utsumi & Karush, 1965). There was no evidence for interchain disulphide bonds in any of these peptides isolated from the F_c region. These observations suggest that pepsin may split the immunoglobulin molecule on the C-terminal side of the inter-heavy chain disulphide bond as shown in Fig. 15.3.

The fact that the heavy chain is readily split by several agents at approximately the same site has led to speculation that it may, in fact, consist of two separate peptide chains. Support for this idea comes from the fact that certain biological observations can be more readily explained on the basis of a six-chain rather than a four-chain Ig molecule (see Cohen & Porter, 1964). For example, the F_c portions of heavy chains from IgG, IgA and IgM are known to be structurally distinct and yet their F_d fragments are presumably common in antibodies of the same specificity; moreover, the F_d fragment in the rabbit carries allotypic specificities controlled by a single genetic locus (A) and these are apparently common to all classes of Ig. There is, however, no chemical evidence for two separate peptide chains. Moreover, genetically controlled allotypic specificities have now been recognized on both F_c and F_d and the invariable pairing of some of these specificities on individual molecules indicates that both halves of the human γ chain are inherited as a single genetic unit; this offers no support for the view that F_c and F_d are, in fact, separate peptide chains.

Structural Relationships Between Classes of Immunoglobulins

Although the classes of Ig differ considerably in physical, chemical and biological properties (Table 15.1) all appear to have a basically similar four-chain structure (Fig. 15.3) which is polymerized in the case of higher molecular weight antibodies; thus, IgM (molecular weight 900,000) probably contains five four-chain units of molecular weight 180,000 covalently linked to one another by disulphide bonds between heavy chains. The IgA which is secreted in relatively high concentration in the parotid saliva and colostrum exists largely in polymerized form and probably consists of two four-chain units. An associated fragment (T-piece) has antigenic specificity distinct from α or light chains, but its exact relationship to IgA has not been determined.

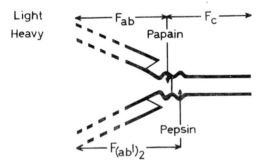

FIG. 15.3. Diagrammatic representation of IgG antibody. The molecule is made up of two heavy and two light chains linked by three inter-chain disulphide bonds. Broken lines show the highly variable portions of the molecule which contain the two antibody combining sites. The undulating portion of the heavy chain represents the area susceptible to proteolytic digestion; the enzymes papain and pepsin give rise to the fragments indicated (from Cohen & Milstein, 1967a).

A variety of observations indicate that the three classes of immunoglobulin contain light chains of closely similar structure (Cohen, 1963a). Thus the light chains from normal IgG and IgM have the same amino-acid compositions and are identical on electrophoresis at pH 3·5 and 8. The light chains from all classes of human Ig occur in two forms (κ and λ chains); these are antigenically distinct and present on different molecules, about 70% having κ and 30% having λ chains (Mannik & Kunkel, 1963a,b; Fahey, 1963a). The κ chains are associated with the allotypic specificity (Inv.) which is common to all Igs. Heavy chains from IgG, IgA and IgM, on the other hand, are structurally distinct and are referred to as γ, α and μ chains respectively. Observed differences between these three classes of heavy chains include molecular weights, amino-acid composition and carbohydrate content, electrophoretic mobilities, and antigenic and allotypic specificities (see Cohen & Milstein, 1967a).

Heterogeneity of Immunoglobulin Peptide Chains

It is apparent from the findings outlined above that the three main classes of Ig are made up from five distinct peptide chains arranged as shown in Table 15.3. Further analyses have shown that the individual chains exist in multiple, chemically distinct forms.

TABLE 15.3

Peptide chains of human immunoglobulins

		IgG	IgA	IgM
Serum	70%	$\kappa_2\gamma_2$	$\kappa_2\alpha_2$	$(\kappa_2\mu_2)_5$
	30%	$\lambda_2\gamma_2$	$\lambda_2\alpha_2$	$(\lambda_2\mu_2)_5$

Human IgG contains several types of γ chains which differ antigenically and chemically. The type specificity is localized either on the F_c or F_d portion of the γ-chain (Table 15.2). The normal human μ and α chains also appear to be heterogeneous as judged by reactions to antisera against monoclonal proteins. It seems likely that further degrees of heavy chain heterogeneity will be defined as methods of analysis become more refined.

As mentioned above the human light chain occurs in two forms (κ and λ) which are antigenically distinct and chemically different. In addition, whole human light chain is resolved into 10 components on starch gel electrophoresis at pH 7–8. These electrophoretic components are themselves heterogeneous since each contains both κ

and λ chains. The κ chain shows a further degree of heterogeneity associated with allotypic specificity (Inv); it appears on the basis of antigenic, allotoypic and electrophoretic variability, that there are at least 40 chemical variants of the human light chain. The total number of light chain variants is, however, certainly far greater, since κ-chains which are alike in regard to electrophoretic mobility and Inv specificity may differ significantly in peptide patterns and primary structure (see Cohen & Milstein, 1967a,b).

The Antibody-combining Site

The hall-mark of all immunological reactions is the specificity of combination between antigen and antibody. The most familiar example of this is seen in acquired immunity which shows specificity for the particular strain of pathogenic organism which caused the original infection. Since individual antibodies have a narrow specificity and the number of antigenic substances is very great, it follows that the body must be able to synthesize a very large number of different antibodies; the minimum number is generally regarded as being of the order of 10^5, but may be very much greater. The fact that every individual can synthesize a remarkable range of different antibodies raises a problem of fundamental interest and importance—namely, what structural features of the molecule determine combining specificity and how are these features characteristic of individual molecules accommodated within the basic four-chain peptide structure described above.

The sites on antigen and antibody which enter into direct combination are visualized as areas of similar size and complementary configuration. From the estimated size of antigenic sites, it appears that the antibody-combining site is equivalent to about 1% of the antibody surface and this would comprise 10 to 20 amino acids. In contrast to what is observed with antigens, every four-chain antibody molecule carries only two combining sites and these always have identical specificities. The number of combining sites or valency of antibody molecules is inferred from various physical measurements such as electrophoresis, ultracentrifugation and equilibrium dialysis carried out on antigen–antibody complexes formed in an excess of antigen when all antibody-combining sites are saturated. The isolation of two antibody fragments each with a single combining site (Fig. 15.3) also indicates convincingly that antibody molecules are bivalent. Non-precipitating antibodies found in certain antisera are sometimes regarded as univalent, but there is no evidence to support this assumption. Higher molecular weight antibodies appear to carry only one active combining site per four-chain unit.

Since each four-chain antibody molecule carries a maximum of two combining sites which occupy about 2% of the molecular surface, it is evident that 98% of the structure is not directly involved in combining specificity. Many attempts have been made to locate these small active sites on the macromolecular four-chain structure represented in Fig. 15.3. The enzymic fragments of the antibody molecule which carry full combining activity consist of the light chain together with the N-terminal portion of the heavy chain known as the F_d fragment (Fig. 15.3). The combining site could therefore be present on one or other of these peptide chains, but in fact most of the experimental evidence suggests that it is usually formed by portions of both chains. The structural differences which characterize antibody sites of different specificities have not been defined. Combining specificity could be determined by variations in the three-dimensional folding of a peptide chain of constant structure, but this now appears to be unlikely. More probably, the configuration characteristic of each specific antibody is determined by the sequence of amino acids in the combining site. Support for this view comes from amino-acid sequence studies of immunoglobulin chains. The C-terminal halves of chains appear to have invariant sequences in a given class of Ig. The N-terminal halves, which contain the combining sites (Fig. 15.3), show a degree of structural variation which is unique among proteins and is presumably related to differences in combining specificity.

Antibodies must therefore be visualized as large protein molecules made up of a similar basic four-chain unit. This consists of two heavy and two light polypeptide chains which occur in multiple molecular forms even in highly purified antibody preparations. Each antibody molecule carries two combining sites of identical specificity determined by variable amino-acid sequences in the N-terminal sections of chains and possibly formed jointly by portions of both heavy and light chains. Combining sites of identical specificity may occur on all three classes of antibody, but the different immunoglobulins vary in regard to several other important biological properties (Table 15.1) and also in their patterns of response in various pathological states.

Metabolism of Immunoglobulins

In all mammalian species investigated little or no synthesis of immunoglobulin occurs during pre-

natal life and the developing foetus acquires antibody by passive transfer from the maternal circulation. In the pig, horse and goat immunoglobulin is present only in trace amounts at birth and is absorbed from colostrum during the first two days of life. The human foetus, on the other hand, acquires maternal antibody during prenatal life, apparently by transfer across the placental membrane, and the immunoglobulin present in human colostrum does not appear to be absorbed.

Transmission of immunoglobulin across the foetal membranes is a highly selective process since IgG is freely transferred whereas IgA and IgM are not. Investigations using papain fragments of rabbit IgG labelled with ^{131}I have suggested that the chemical configuration essential for transmission of IgG to the foetus is located on the F_c fragment (Fig. 15.3). This explains why horse antisera used in pregnant women fail to confer passive immunity on the developing foetus; such antisera are commonly treated with pepsin during commercial preparation and, as discussed above, this destroys F_c and leaves a bivalent antibody fragment which lacks the transmission site.

At birth the level of IgG in the human infant is similar to that of the mother; the concentration falls progressively during the first few weeks of life at which time the catabolism of maternal IgG exceeds active synthesis. The lowest levels occur at 3–6 months and the concentration then increases progressively to reach adult levels between one and four years. Serum of new-born infants contains very low levels of IgM and no detectable IgA; the levels of both rise progressively after birth, the adult level of IgM being attained at about 4–6 months and IgA at about one year of age. Work in germ-free animals suggests that contact with bacteria and other antigens stimulates immunoglobulin production.

Immunoglobulin synthesis occurs in lymphoid tissue throughout the body and notably in lymph nodes, spleen and bone marrow. Experimental evidence suggests that immunoglobulin-producing stem cells may all be derived from bone marrow. The *in vitro* production of antibody by single lymph node cells indicates that a single cell can synthesize both heavy and light chains and assemble these into the complete antibody molecule. Immunofluorescent studies have confirmed the presence of heavy and light chains in the same cell and shown that individual cells have a restricted potential, being able to synthesize either κ or λ chains together with either γ, μ or α chains; cells containing α chains are especially common in the gastro-intestinal tract. In addition, it appears that individual cells synthesize peptide chains carrying only a single allelic form of allotypic specificity even in heterozygotes. Individual cells therefore have a restricted capacity for synthesizing the heavy and light chain variants of immunoglobulin molecules, but the exact number of chains which can be produced by one cell is not known.

The total IgG of the body (about 80 g.) in healthy adults is distributed equally between the circulating plasma and the interstitial fluids. Fluorescent antibody techniques have shown that extravascular γ-globulin is present in all extracellular fluids as well as in the ground substance of connective tissue. About 25% of the circulating IgG fraction passes across capillaries into the extravascular fluids each day and a similar amount is returned to the bloodstream through the main lymphatic ducts. The concentration of γ-globulin in the interstitial fluids varies considerably in different sites, being highest in the hepatic lymph (about 1 g. per 100 ml.) and relatively low (200 mg./100 ml.) in the interstitial fluids of muscle and subcutaneous tissue. The distribution of IgM differs from that of IgG in that only a small proportion of the total pool is present in extravascular tissues. IgA is present in relatively high concentration in human milk as well as in saliva and tears; it has been suggested that the antigenically distinct fragment (T-piece) found in IgA in seromucous secretions may contain a transmission site responsible for secretion into these biological fluids.

All plasma protein fractions including γ-globulin are in a state of dynamic equilibrium undergoing constant degradation and replacement by newly synthesized molecules. A homogeneous protein, such as human albumin, when labelled with ^{131}I has a constant rate of breakdown (measured by urinary excretion of label) over a period of several weeks. On the other hand, the fractional catabolic rate of ^{131}I-labelled human γ-globulin prepared by zone electrophoresis falls progressively during the first one to two weeks after injection, suggesting the presence of a mixed population of molecules having different breakdown rates. This metabolic heterogeneity is attributable to differences in the turnover rates of the immunoglobulins. Thus, human IgM isolated by ultracentrifugation and zone electrophoresis or by electrophoresis and gel filtration, has a relatively high turnover rate which is probably similar to IgA. IgG is catabolized at a slower rate (Table 15.1). Little is known about the site and mechanism of immunoglobulin catabolism. On the basis of labelled protein studies it has been suggested that

plasma cells which are known to be involved in antibody synthesis may also be responsible for immunoglobulin breakdown. However, perfusion experiments in which biologically screened proteins are used show that the normal rat liver, which is not a site of antibody synthesis, catabolizes IgG at a rate equivalent to 30% of the total breakdown in vivo. The fractional breakdown rate of IgG can be increased in the mouse by infusing large amounts of either IgG or F_c derived from it, but not by injecting IgA or IgM. The removal of circulating protein by a process such as pinocytosis cannot easily account for such selectivity, and the presence of specific mechanisms controlling immunoglobulin breakdown appears likely (Fahey & Robinson, 1963; Brambell, 1965).

Urinary Fragments of Immunoglobulins

Human urine is known to contain low molecular weight proteins antigenically related to immunoglobulin and apparently identical to free light chains. More recently, fragments of light chain have been identified in the urine of several patients with Bence-Jones proteinuria. Immunological tests have shown that these urinary fragments corresponded to either the variable or the constant portion of the light chain and it now appears likely that these fragments arise through enzymic splitting which occurs when light chain is incubated with serum, but not readily on incubation with urine.

A similar explanation probably accounts for the presence in urine of heavy chain fragments antigenically related to F_c (Fig. 15.3). In the rare syndrome originally described by Franklin, on the other hand, fragments of heavy chain having some structural features of F_c and present in serum and urine, seem to be synthesized de novo (Franklin, 1964).

Antibody activity which has frequently been reported in urine is confined mainly to IgG (Turner & Rowe, 1964). However, activity has also been found in fractions thought to have molecular weights of about 10 to 15,000. Such fragments have not been fully characterized; they appear to contain determinants of F_{ab} and their precipitating activity is lost on reduction (Merler, 1966).

ABNORMAL LEVELS OF IMMUNOGLOBULINS

Recognition that the γ-globulin fraction of serum contains several classes of immunoglobulins, has indicated the need to reappraise the clinical conditions associated with hyper- and hypo-gammaglobulinaemia, in terms of individual fractions since these have distinctive biological properties (Table 15.1) and may react independently in pathological states.

The levels of Ig classes in the normal adult are shown in Table 15.1 and changes in concentration from birth are shown in Fig. 15.4. It will be seen that serum levels and the rates of increase during early childhood vary from one Ig class to another. The new-born infant has a level of IgG approximating that of the adult and derived from the maternal circulation. The IgG concentration drops by 60% during the first three weeks after birth reaching a minimum between the third and fifth month and rising steadily thereafter to approach adult levels at about the fifth to sixth year. IgM which may be as low as 5 mg./100 ml. at birth, rises relatively rapidly reaching about 30 mg./100 ml. by the third week. IgA is absent at birth, increases to about 10 mg./100 ml. by the third week and may not reach adult concentrations until late adolescence.

Measurements of immunoglobulin concentrations in health and disease have usually been made by methods based on agar diffusion. Fahey & McKelvey (1965), comparing results obtained by this technique with inhibition methods using isotopically labelled proteins, found discrepancies between the two methods. The mean value for IgA was some 50% lower by the diffusion technique. Monoclonal IgA proteins often contain molecules with sedimentation values ranging from 8S to 14S. The use of IgA standards containing varying proportions of macromolecular species would affect the results obtained by the diffusion technique (Cwynarski, 1968) and may account in part for the wide variations in IgA observed in normal populations.

The primary antibody response to most antigenic stimuli is heralded by an increase in circulating IgM followed by a rise in IgG. An associated rise of IgA is usually observed, but this is more variable. The response varies with the physical characteristics of the antigen and its site of entry. Following intensive immunization not all the circulating immunoglobulin increment can be accounted for by specific antibody so that anti-

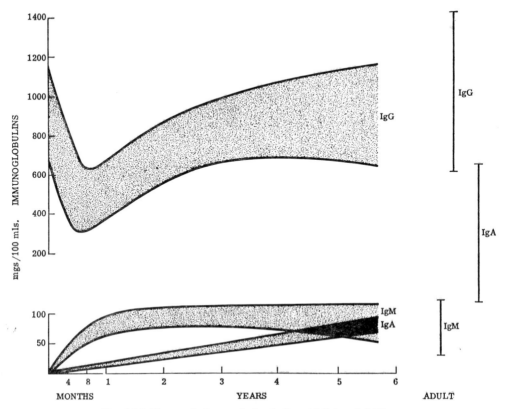

FIG. 15.4. Changes in human Ig levels from birth to adult life.

genic stimulation appears to produce a partly non-specific response.

Diffuse Hyperimmunoglobulinaemia

Hyperimmunoglobulinaemia leading to a diffuse increase in the electrophoretic γ-globulin fraction is found in a wide variety of clinical disorders. In many of these increased Ig levels appear to result from prolonged antigenic stimulation, but in others, e.g. liver disease, the cause of the hypergammaglobulinaemia is obscure. A list of such diseases, which is by no means comprehensive, appears in Table 15.4 (see also Gitlin, Gross & Janeway, 1959; Martin, 1964). At the time of writing this review comparatively few

TABLE 15.4

Conditions associated with diffuse hypergammaglobulinaemia

I. INFECTIONS
    Bacterial and mycobacterial—
        Streptococcal
        Staphylococcal
        Chronic Tuberculosis
        Lepromatous Leprosy
    Spirochaetal
        Leptospirosis
        Syphilis
    Viral
        Lymphogranuloma
        Infective Mononucleosis
        Viral Hepatitis
    Rickettsial
        Typhus
    Protozoal
        Malaria
        Trypanosomiasis
        Visceral Leishmaniases
    Helminthic
        Trichinosis

II. GRANULOMATA
    Sarcoidosis
    Chronic Beryllium poisoning

III. HYPERIMMUNIZATION

IV. LIVER PARENCHYMAL DISEASE

V. NEOPLASIA OF THE RETICULO-ENDOTHELIAL SYSTEM

VI. "CONNECTIVE TISSUE" DISEASE
    Diffuse Lupus Erythematosus
    Rheumatoid Arthritis
    Periarteritis nodosa
    Dermatomyositis

VII. "HYPERSENSITIVITY" DISEASE
    Serum sickness
    Acquired immune haemolytic anaemia
    Thyroiditis

quantitative data are available concerning the levels of individual classes of immunoglobulins in these disorders. Hyperimmunoglobulinaemia always appears to be the result of increased synthesis rather than reduced catabolism of Ig. In chronic malarial infection and hepatic cirrhosis, the rate of production of IgG (Fig. 15.5) may be up to eight times that observed in normal subjects (see Cohen, 1963b).

Bacterial Infections

The majority of hyperglobulinaemias following bacterial infection show a predominant increase in IgG with a modest increase in IgA and little or no increase in IgM (McKelvey & Fahey, 1965). Occasional sera from patients suffering from leprosy show a significant increase in IgM (Lim & Fusaro, 1967).

Viral Infections

Wollheim & Williams (1966) in studies on sera from patients suffering from infectious mononucleosis showed that levels of heterophil agglutinin titres have a linear relationship to levels of circulating IgM. IgM increases of up to 100% above normal were recorded but neither these levels nor the heterophil agglutinin titres collate with the severity of the disease.

Protozoal Infections

Infection with trypanosomes produces a significant increase in the IgM component which may reach concentrations of 700 mg./100 ml. (Mattern, Masseyeff, Michel & Peretti, 1961). In chronic malarial infection, hypergammaglobulinaemia is associated mainly with an increase of IgG, but the increment of IgM also suggests a relationship to infection; levels of IgA and IgD are not obviously related to the disease (Rowe & McGregor, 1968). Only a small proportion of the IgG in immune subjects appears to be specific malarial antibody (see Cohen, McGregor & Carrington, 1961).

Diseases of the Liver Parenchyma

Increased levels of immunoglobulin are commonly observed in hepatic parenchymal disease. The highest levels occur in the so-called "juvenile" hepatitis (Mackay & Burnet, 1963) and involve predominantly IgG (Hobbs, 1967). In primary biliary cirrhosis IgM is commonly raised while levels of IgG and IgA may be normal (McKelvey & Fahey, 1965; Hobbs, 1967; Feizi, 1968). Alcoholic cirrhosis, on the other hand, is associated with an increase mainly in IgA (Hobbs, 1967) while IgM may be disproportionately elevated in

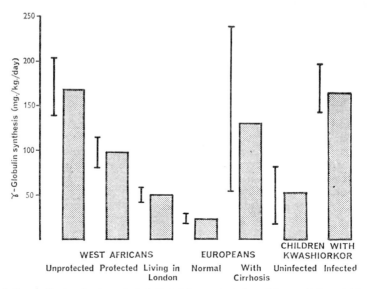

FIG. 15.5. γ-Globulin synthesis rates in malaria-infected (unprotected) and in non-infected Africans, in healthy Europeans and in Europeans with cirrhosis, and in children suffering from kwashiorkor with infection and without infection. Average rate shown by blocked area and range by vertical line (Cohen, 1963b).

cases of infectious hepatitis; however, no pattern of Ig change is specific for particular hepatic lesions.

The reason for the increase in serum immunoglobulins in liver disease is not understood. Otaki, Read, Stubbs & Sculthorpe (1960) examined the progressive changes in the globulin pattern following partial hepatectomy and noted a globulin increase from 2·8 to 4·8 g. between the first and twelfth day post-operatively. This was regarded as a reaction against necrotic parenchyma from the cut surface of the liver. Hypergammaglobulinaemia in liver disease has also been ascribed to diminished osmotic pressure due to hypoalbuminaemia, but this does not readily account for the increased antibody response to immunization reported in patients with hepatic cirrhosis (see Havens, 1959).

Lymphoreticular Neoplasms

Disturbances in the circulating immunoglobulins appear to be commonest in those lymphoreticular neoplasms in which the predominant proliferating cell is of a primitive morphological type (Rundles, Coonrad & Arends, 1954). In Hodgkin's disease levels of IgG are usually raised slightly while IgM and IgA are normal (McKelvey & Fahey, 1965) or subnormal (Goldman & Hobbs, 1967). In general, delayed hypersensitivity responses are depressed while antibody production

is normal (Aisenberg & Leskowitz, 1963). Reticuloses have been associated with the presence of so-called α_3-globulin migrating between the α_2- and β_1-globulin components (Sunderman, 1964). Goldman & Hobbs (1967) confirmed the presence of this fraction in the majority of their patients with Hodgkin's disease and other reticuloses, but found that it was also present in several other disorders; the identity of this fraction has not been established.

Diseases of Connective Tissue

About 80% of patients suffering from diffuse lupus erythematosus show an increase in circulating immunoglobulins which involves the three main classes, IgG, IgA and IgM. A smaller proportion (about 50%) of patients suffering from rheumatoid arthritis show significant increases in immunoglobulins which usually occur during the active phase of the disease. Meltzer & Franklin (1962) have noted the presence of high molecular weight complexes consisting of IgM rheumatoid factor together with IgG or IgA. In periarteritis nodosa and related vascular disorders including dermatomyositis levels of IgG, IgA or IgM show a variable response.

Stein & Fudenberg (1966) found levels of IgG, over 1900 mg./100 ml. and of IgA over 340 mg./100 ml. in a group of mongols. It is well known that mongols have an increased susceptibility to infection and a diminished immunological response to specific toxins has been reported. IgM levels are normal or subnormal in these subjects and Stein & Fudenberg, with these observations in mind, suggest the possibility that a genetic block occurs in the development of the immunological response of the mongol.

Primary Immunological Deficiency

Conditions associated with a failure to maintain adequate levels of circulating immunoglobulins have aroused interest among clinicians since Bruton in 1952 first described a sex-linked syndrome in young boys associated with a lack of serum γ-globulin (reviewed by Martin, 1964; Peterson, Cooper & Good, 1965; Janeway, Rosen, Merler & Alper, 1966). Improved methods for the clinical study of immunological deficiency diseases have led to the recognition of many related disorders at present designated by a most confused terminology. An expert Committee of W.H.O. has recently drawn up a classification of these disorders which focuses attention upon measurable cellular, immunoglobulin and functional deficiencies (Table 15.5).

As pointed out in the introduction to this Chapter, there is now growing evidence that immunological responses are mediated by two distinct kinds of antibody—the serum immunoglobulins and specifically sensitized cells usually referred to as "cell-bound" antibody (Fig. 15.1). These immunological responses appear to be mediated by two distinct populations of cells. Those responsible for cell-mediated immune responses depend upon the functional integrity of the thymus. On the other hand lymphoid cells which differentiate into plasma cells involved in immunoglobulin synthesis, are independent of the thymus gland. In birds such cells appear to differentiate in the bursa of Fabricius and there is some evidence that in mammals, the lymphoepithelial areas of the appendix and Peyer's patches, may serve a comparable function.

Among the immunological deficiency disorders which occur clinically (see Table 15.5) some involve predominantly the thymus-independent immunoglobulin-producing system, e.g. infantile recessive sex-linked agammaglobulinaemia. Such disorders are characterized by a reduction of circulating Ig, usually affecting all classes but to a variable extent. The antibody response to antigenic stimulation is diminished and susceptibility to bacterial infections is increased. Delayed hypersensitivity responses are unimpaired and resistance to viral infections and response to vaccination are normal. Although all classes of Ig are commonly affected,

several examples of partial immunoglobulin deficiency have been described. The most common are a decrease of IgA and IgG together with normal or increased amounts of IgM (Type 1 dysgammaglobulinaemia), and a decrease of IgA and IgM together with normal or near normal levels of IgG (Type 2 dysgammaglobulinaemia). A selective deficiency of IgA (Type 3 dysgammaglobulinaemia) occurs in association with ataxia telangiectasia and is seen also in subjects predisposed to infections of mucous surfaces. However, IgA has been reported absent in apparently normal subjects, so the clinical significance of this finding is sometimes obscure.

Other Ig deficiencies involve only thymus-dependent cells and cell-mediated responses, e.g. thymic aplasia. In these conditions immunoglobulin levels are normal although the antibody response to antigenic stimulation may be rather variable. Lymphocytes are deficient in tissues and blood, delayed hypersensitivity responses are absent and these infants frequently succumb to viral or fungal infections in early life. Several immunological deficiency syndromes show evidence of a developmental defect of both cell systems, e.g. ataxia telangiectasia, with corresponding deficiencies of cell-bound and serum antibodies.

Many of the diseases associated with immunological deficiency appear to have a genetic basis. Such disorders could arise from mutations of structural or regulator genes and the latter might control either synthesis of immunoglobulins or differentiation of cells involved in the immune response. Several of the defects show a sex-linked inheritance, but the role of the X-chromosome in immunoglobulin synthesis or lymphoid cell differentiation is unknown.

Secondary Ig Deficiency

Hypogammaglobulinaemia in adolescence and adult life may result from the form of primary Ig deficiency having a variable age of onset and listed in Table 15.5. This syndrome which probably includes several related disorders is equally common in males and females and there is no obvious underlying pathology. Ig deficiency at this age may however be secondary to:

(i) proliferative disorders of the lymphoid system—especially reticulum cell sarcoma, lymphosarcoma, Hodgkin's disease, chronic lymphatic leukaemia, myelomatosis and macroglobulinaemia (reviewed by Scharff & Uhr, 1965).

(ii) excessive protein loss—as in protein-losing enteropathy, exfoliative dermatitis, extensive burns, nephrotic syndrome.

TABLE 15.5.

Diseases associated with primary immunoglobulin deficiency
(From report of WHO expert Committee)

| Syndrome | CELLS | | | IMMUNOLOGICAL RESPONSE | | | Genetics | Comments |
	Thymus	Plasma cells	Others	Circulating Lympho-cytes	Main Ig Deficiency	Humoral antibody	Cellular antibody		
Transient hypogamma-globulinaemia of infancy	?	Deficient		Normal	IgG	Low or absent	Normal	Familial ? Genetic	Usually recover by two years. IgG low or normal in later life.
Primary Ig deficiency-variable onset ("acquired", "congenital", non-sex-linked a-γ)	?	Deficient but variable	Reticular hyper-plasia	Normal	All classes but variable	Variable response to antigen	Variable	? Autosomal recessive ? Multi-factorial	A heterogeneous group of disorders. Malabsorption common.
Infantile sex-linked recessive a-γ (Bruton's disease)	Normal	Absent		Normal	All classes	Absent or very low	Normal	X-linked	Recurrent infections with pyogenic organisms
Selective IgA deficiency	Normal	IgA cells absent		Normal	IgA-serum and sero-mucous	Normal, but no IgA ab	Normal	? Autosomal recessive	Bronchitis, sinusitis, exudative enteropathy. Some are healthy
A-γ with thymoma (Good's syndrome)	Thymic enlarge-ment	Absent or deficient	Eosino-phils deficient. Red cell aplasia in some	Low	All classes	Deficient to all antigens	Deficient to all antigens		

Thrombocytopenia. Immune deficiency and Eczema (T.I.E. syndrome, Wiskott-Aldrich syndrome)	Normal	Normal	Lymphocytes deficient in thymus-dependent para-cortical areas	Low	Variable. Low IgM, high IgA common	Deficient to some antigens	Deficient to some antigens	X-linked	Associated with eczema and thrombocytopenia
Ataxia telangiectasia (Louis-Bar's syndrome)	Embryonic type	Variable	Lymphocytes deficient in thymus-dependent areas	Decreased	Variable but low IgA in about 80%	Deficient to some antigens	Deficient to some antigens	Autosomal recessive	Associated with progressive cerebellar ataxia, ovarian dysgenesis, telangiectasia (may appear late)
Sex-linked recessive lymphopenic immunological deficiency (Swiss type a-γ)	Hypoplasia	Variable	Tissue lymphocytes deficient	Low but variable	Class variable	Deficient to some antigens	Deficient to some antigens	X-linked recessive	Often die of fungal or virus infections
Autosomal recessive alymphocytic a-γ	Hypoplasia	Absent	Tissue lymphocytes absent	Very low	All classes	Absent	Deficient	Autosomal recessive	Do not survive infancy
Autosomal recessive lymphopenia (Nezelof's syndrome)	Hypoplasia	Present	Tissue lymphocytes depleted	Low	Normal	Present	Decreased or absent	Autosomal recessive	
Thymic aplasia (Di George's syndrome)	Absent (failure of development 3rd, 4th pharyngeal pouch)	Present	Lymphocytes deficient in thymus-dependent areas. Parathyroid absent	Low but variable	Normal	Variable	Absent		Neonatal tetany

(iii) toxic states—especially uraemia.

Secondary immunoglobulin deficiency may also occur in early life. For example, in cases of congenital rubella IgG levels may be greatly reduced in the first year of life and IgM markedly increased (Soothill, Hayes & Dudgeon, 1966).

MONOCLONAL IMMUNOGLOBULINS

Homogeneous immunoglobulin fractions appearing as sharp peaks on electrophoresis are found characteristically in patients with multiple myelomatosis and macroglobulinaemia, but also occur in other clinical states. These conditions are generally thought to result from the proliferation of cells derived from single clones and for this reason it is becoming customary to refer to their products as monoclonal immunoglobulins (Waldenström, 1962a). These proteins have the same general configuration as normal immunoglobulins, but in contrast to the latter, their peptide chain structure is remarkably homogeneous. When considered collectively, monoclonal immunoglobulins show approximately the same distribution of antigenic and allotypic factors as the normal Ig population (see below). Some monoclonal proteins are associated with antibody-like properties including those of cold agglutinins (Harboe & Lind, 1966), rheumatoid factors (Kritzman, Kunkel, McCarthy & Mellors, 1961), capacity for cell agglutination (Ozer & Chaplin, 1963) as well as anti-streptolysin (Zetterval, Sjöquist, Waldenström & Winblad, 1966) and anti-lipoprotein activity (Beaumont, 1967). These findings suggest that monoclonal proteins can be regarded as individual species of normal Ig, and when considered in this light the elucidation of their detailed chemical structure becomes a matter of the greatest importance. Such studies are, in fact, beginning to illuminate many fundamental questions concerning the structure of antibodies (see Cohen & Milstein, 1967a,b).

Although purified myeloma proteins are homogeneous according to several criteria, some may show evidence of heterogeneity. Thus, the majority of IgA (Laurell, 1961b; Deutsch, 1962) and IgM (Kunkel, 1960) monoclonal immunoglobulins show multiple peaks in the ultracentrifuge; this phenomenon is generally ascribed to polymer formation rather than chemical heterogeneity. In addition, many IgG and IgA proteins which are homogeneous on conventional electrophoresis separate into multiple bands on starch gel electrophoresis (Creyssel & Fine, 1958; Fine, Creyssel & Morel, 1959; Engle, Woods, Castillo & Pert, 1961; Laurell, 1961a; Fahey,

1963b). This heterogeneity cannot be ascribed to polymer formation and its chemical basis has not been determined. There is evidence that monoclonal immunoglobulins present within cells are electrophoretically homogeneous and that the banding observed on starch gel electrophoresis develops either during passage through the cell or after entry into the serum. Finally, a small proportion of cases have shown two distinct monoclonal immunoglobulins which in some instances belong to different classes or antigenic types (Vaerman, Johnson, Mandy & Fudenberg, 1965; Imhof, Ballieux, Mul & Poen, 1966; Engle & Wackman, 1966).

Structure of Serum Monoclonal Proteins

Monoclonal serum immunoglobulins have a structure fundamentally similar to that of normal immunoglobulin being composed of heavy and light chains covalently linked by interchain disulphide bonds as shown in Fig. 15.3. However, as compared with normal Ig, the peptide chains of monoclonal proteins are homogeneous according to several criteria. Individual monoclonal proteins belong to one or other of the major Ig classes and the distribution of these in multiple

TABLE 15.6

Distribution of antigenic specificities on monoclonal IgG, IgA, IgM and Bence-Jones proteins

Ig Class	%Total Cases (1)	Light Chain Type (2)	
		% κ	% λ
IgG	32	61	39
IgG + B.J.	15		
IgA	14	66	34
IgA + B.J.	6		
IgM	13	60	40
IgM + B.J.	1		
B.J. only	20	57	43

(1) Osserman & Takatsuki (1963)—distribution of Ig specificities in 300 proteins from cases of multiple myelomatosis and macroglobulinaemia.

(2) Imhof, Ballieux, Mul & Poen (1966)—distribution of κ and λ chains in 242 proteins from cases of multiple myelomatosis and macroglobulinaemia.

myelomatosis and macroglobulinaemia is shown in Table 15.6. IgG myeloma proteins carry the antigenic specificity of only one of the four γ1-chain subtypes, and are associated with Gm factors which are inherited as a single genetic unit. The majority are of subtype γ1 (We) and are either Gm a+ z+ or Gm y+ f+ (Table 15.7).

Myeloma proteins and macroglobulins also carry light chains of a single antigenic type (either κ or

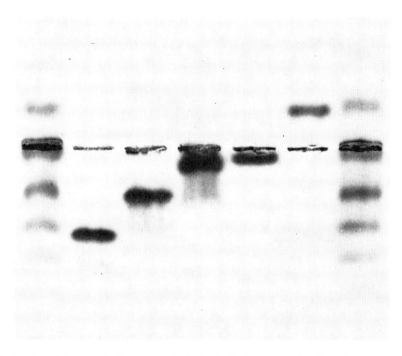

Fig. 15.6. Electrophoresis in urea-glycine starch gel of light chains from normal and myeloma immunoglobulins. (From Cohen & Porter, 1964.)

TABLE 15.7

Distribution of antigenic and allotypic specificities in IgG myeloma proteins
(Caucasians)

IgG type		Approximate % Total cases	Gm type						
			a	z	y	f	b′	b³	n
We	$\gamma 1$	65	+	+	−	−	−	−	−
(γ_{2b}, C)			−	−	+	+	−	−	−
Vi	$\gamma 3$	7	−	−	−	−	+	+	−
(γ_{2c}, Z)									
Ge	$\gamma 4$		−	−	−	−	−	−	−
(γ_{2d})									
Ne	$\gamma 2$	15	−	−	−	−	−	−	+
(γ_{2a})									

See Terry & Fahey (1964), Grey & Kunkel (1964), Mårtensson (1966), Litwin & Kunkel (1966).

λ chains); the distribution of these in 242 proteins from cases of multiple myelomatosis and macroglobulinaemia is shown in Table 15.6 (Imhof, Ballieux, Mul & Poen, 1966). In addition, myeloma light chains contain only one or two of the 10 electrophoretic components of normal light chain (Fig. 15.6) and those of type K are associated with a single allelic form of Inv specificity, even in heterozygotes.

Structure of Bence-Jones Proteins

In about 40% of patients with myelomatosis or macroglobulinaemia, the urine contains a protein antigenically related to Ig and known as Bence-Jones protein. A variety of studies (summarized by Putnam, 1957) have shown that these proteins differ from serum Ig in having a lower molecular weight (40,000), fewer antigenic determinants and usually no carbohydrate. In about 20% of all cases Bence-Jones protein occurs without an associated monoclonal serum protein (Table 15.6). Bence-Jones proteins are usually detected on the basis of their characteristic thermosolubility behaviour; some, however, give a negative result on the heating test and are demonstrated by paper electrophoresis or immunoelectrophoresis of concentrated urine. Urinary Bence-Jones proteins are now known to be composed of light chains (Edelman & Gally, 1962) present in urine in the form of dimers which may be joined by disulphide bonds or by non-covalent linkages. Bence-Jones proteins are either of type K or L and like the light chains of monoclonal Ig's are relatively homogeneous on electrophoresis. They appear to have unique chemical sequences and these have been completely determined in a few instances; this work has established the chemical basis of Inv specificity and has shown that the C-terminal

halves of κ and λ chains are relatively constant in structure while the N-terminal halves are variable (see Cohen & Milstein, 1967a,b).

Monoclonal Heavy Chains

In 1964 Franklin and co-workers described a patient having an unusual low molecular weight Ig present in serum and urine. The disorder was referred to as heavy chain disease and four other cases of this very rare syndrome were subsequently described (Osserman & Takatsuki, 1964). The abnormal protein was shown to have a molecular weight of 51,000; it was split by reduction and alkylation and from antigenic analysis appeared to correspond to the F_c fragment of the IgG molecule shown in Fig. 15.3 (Franklin, 1964). However, one such protein contains both the C- and N-terminal sequences of the γ-chain suggesting that a deletion has occurred in the mid-portion of the heavy chain (Prahl, 1967).

Metabolism of Monoclonal Serum Immunoglobulins

The distribution and turnover of serum monoclonal proteins have been investigated using radioactive iodine labelling of whole serum (Berson & Yalow, 1957) or isolated immunoglobulins (Gabuzda, 1962; Korman, Corcoran, Fine & Lipincott, 1962; Solomon, Waldmann & Fahey, 1963; Alper, Freeman & Waldenström, 1963; Birke, Liljedahl, Olhagen, Plantin & Ahlinder, 1963). Such studies have shown that the distribution of monoclonal immunoglobulins is essentially the same as that of the corresponding normal Ig. Increased levels of monoclonal immunoglobulins result from accelerated synthesis and not from reduced catabolism as was suggested by earlier studies with labelled amino acids. The rate of monoclonal protein production may be 20 times normal but varies considerably in different cases. The fractional catabolic rate of normal Ig may be increased (Alper et al., 1963; Solomon, Waldmann & Fahey, 1963) and is sometimes appreciably higher than that of the pathological globulin (Cohen, 1963b); these findings suggest that hypercatabolism may contribute towards the reduction of normal Ig frequently observed in association with monoclonal proteins.

Metabolism of Bence-Jones Protein

In the majority of cases newly synthesized Bence-Jones protein is rapidly excreted in the urine (Putnam & Hardy, 1955; Putnam, Meyer & Miyaki, 1956; Osserman, Graff, Marshall, Lawlor & Graff, 1957), the renal clearance for proteins of both type K and L being 9 to 50% of the creatinine clearance (Harrison, Blainey, Hardwicke, Rowe & Soothill, 1966). In some cases, however, Bence-Jones protein can be demonstrated in serum by either physicochemical or immunochemical techniques (Gutman, Moore, Gutman, McClellan & Kabat, 1941; Moore, Kabat & Gutman, 1943; Morton & Deutsch, 1956). Solomon & Fahey (1964) found that the level of serum Bence-Jones protein was greater than 0·3 g./100 ml. in 10% of cases of multiple myelomatosis; such Bence-Jones proteinaemia was always associated with some degree of renal insufficiency affecting both glomerular filtration and tubular function. The extent of renal damage observed morphologically did not correlate with the level of Bence-Jones protein in serum or urine. In these cases Bence-Jones protein is present in extravascular body fluids and can also be identified in the cerebrospinal fluid.

The possibility that some Bence-Jones protein may be catabolized was suggested by Meyer & Putnam (1963) who reinjected a patient with his own ^{14}C-labelled Bence-Jones protein and recovered only a fraction of the labelled protein in the urine. Similar findings were reported with ^{131}I-labelled Bence-Jones protein in human subjects (Perkins, Doherty & Towbin, 1959) and in mice (Humphrey & Fahey, 1961). Solomon, Waldmann, Fahey & McFarlane (1964) carried out turnover studies using ^{131}I-labelled Bence-Jones protein supplemented by determinations of non-protein-bound [131]I. The labelled protein was catabolized at rates equivalent to 1·8 to 42% of the intravascular pool per hour and was highest (10 to 42%) in patients with normal renal function suggesting that the kidneys play a role in the catabolism of Bence-Jones protein. From these

studies it appeared that the amount of Bence-Jones protein excreted in the urine was far less than that synthesized, being as little as 10% when the total formed was about 3 g./day and 50% with very high rates of synthesis.

It is evident that the level of Bence-Jones protein in serum and the amount excreted in urine depend upon a balance between rates of synthesis, catabolism and excretion. Bence-Jones proteinaemia is favoured by high rates of synthesis in the presence of renal insufficiency which probably reduces both catabolism and excretion.

Clinical Features of Monoclonal Protein Diseases

The clinical features of diseases associated with monoclonal protein production have been reviewed in detail (Osserman, 1959; Waldenström, 1961a,b; Osserman & Takatsuki, 1963; Osserman, 1965). These studies have drawn attention to the fact that monoclonal proteins occur in association with several distinct clinical states (Table 15.8). In about 65% of cases the monoclonal

TABLE 15.8

Clinical diagnosis in 400 cases with monoclonal proteins (Osserman & Takatsuki, 1963)

Clinical Diagnosis	No. of cases
Multiple myelomatosis	262
Macroglobulinaemia	41
H-chain disease	3
Lymphoma	23
Unrelated neoplasm	31
Idiopathic	40

protein (IgG or IgA) is associated with multiple myelomatosis; this is essentially a neoplastic disease of plasma cells characterized clinically by skeletal lesions and commonly associated with anaemia, hypercalcaemia, hyperuricaemia, renal functional impairment, defects of coagulation and increased susceptibility to infection. The disease is equally common in males and females and the peak incidence occurs in patients aged over 80 (Axelsson, Bachman & Hallén, 1966). Bence-Jones proteinuria is found in about 50% of cases of multiple myelomatosis and in about 20% constitutes the only manifestation of monoclonal protein production (Table 15.6). Deposits of amyloid material occur in the tissues in about 10% of cases and the great majority of these also have Bence-Jones proteinuria (Magnus-Levy, 1933; Osserman, Takatsuki & Talal, 1964). The diagnosis of multiple myelomatosis depends upon the demonstration of a monoclonal protein in serum or urine together with radiographic evidence of osteolytic lesions and the finding of increased numbers of plasma cells in the bone marrow. The disease usually pursues a progressive course without spontaneous remissions; the average duration of life from the onset of symptoms is about two years (Snapper, Turner & Moscovitz, 1953; Mandema, 1956; Osserman, 1959; Nordenson, 1966), but survival may be prolonged by the use of chemotherapeutic agents, such as Melphelan (Osserman, 1963; Bergsagel, Sprague, Austin & Griffith, 1962; Bernard, Seligmann & Danon, 1962).

The clinical picture of macroglobulinaemia differs from that of multiple myelomatosis, although syndromes with the features of both are observed (Waldenström, 1962a,b). The condition occurs predominantly in males usually between the ages of 50 and 70; lymphadenopathy and splenic enlargement are common; a bleeding tendency is frequently observed, while osteolytic lesions are very rare, and only about 10 to 15% of cases show Bence-Jones proteinuria (Kappeler, Krebs & Riva, 1958; Osserman & Takatsuki, 1963). The blood lymphocytes are usually increased and the bone marrow is characteristically infiltrated with small lymphocytes and may contain large numbers of mast cells (Tischendorff & Hartmann, 1950). The clinical course tends to be protracted and the drug of choice in many cases appears to be Chlorambucil (Waldenström, 1965).

The clinical features of heavy chain disease have been reviewed by Osserman & Takatsuki (1964). The five cases described were males; all showed lymphadenopathy together with fever and in four splenomegaly was present. Three patients developed an unusual oedematous swelling and erythema of the soft palate which subsided spontaneously. Lymph node and bone marrow sections showed atypical and immature plasma cells, but osteolytic lesions did not occur. Proteinuria (4–15 g./24 hr.) was present in all cases but tests for Bence-Jones protein were negative; the serum and urinary proteins appeared to be identical and by immunochemical tests were shown to be related to heavy chains. The disease runs a protracted course extending over some years; recurring bacterial infection is common and death has been associated with pneumonia or sepsis.

As a result of studies initiated by Waldenström (1942) it has become apparent that about 20 to 30% of patients having monoclonal serum proteins do not show the clinical manifestations of either multiple myelomatosis or macroglobulinaemia. About a third of these cases present with a monoclonal protein and some have been followed for as long as 10 years without developing clinical symptoms (Osserman & Takatsuki, 1963); in other instances, however, clinical and pathological evidence of multiple myelomatosis has become manifest up to 17 years after the monoclonal protein was first observed (Wallerstein, 1951; Norgaard, 1964). This asymptomatic and possibly presymptomatic state has been referred to as idiopathic monoclonal gammapathy (Waldenström, 1961a). Contrary to earlier observations the monoclonal serum Ig may be present in high concentration in these cases; however, Bence-Jones protein is not observed and its presence appears to be diagnostic of either multiple myelomatosis or macroglobulinaemia (see data of Osserman & Takatsuki, 1963). As reported by several authors, monoclonal proteins may also occur either in association with neoplasms unrelated to lymphoid tissues (Owen, Pitney & O'Dea, 1959; Waldenström, 1961a; Osserman & Takatsuki, 1963) or in cases showing the clinical and cytological features of lymphosarcoma or chronic lymphatic leukaemia (Waldenström, 1961a; Osserman & Takatsuki, 1963).

The factors which lead to the production of monoclonal proteins in several apparently diverse clinical states, are not understood. It is significant in this connection that certain inbred strains of mice show a genetic predisposition to develop spontaneous plasma cell tumours associated with the production of monoclonal proteins (Rask-Nielsen, 1956; Rask-Nielsen, Gormsen & Clausen, 1959; Dunn, 1957; Potter, Fahey & Pilgrim, 1957). Such plasma cell neoplasms appear to originate in the ileocaecal area (Dunn, 1957); this observation may prove to be of great interest since experimental evidence indicates that in mammals the lymphoid tissue of this area, like the avian bursa of Fabricius, is the site of origin or maturation of immunoglobulin-producing cells (Cooper, Perey, McKneally, Gabrielsen, Sutherland & Good, 1966). In another inbred strain of mice plasma cell neoplasms never occur spontaneously, but can be induced by the intraperitoneal administration of a variety of substances including plastic, Freund's adjuvant and mineral oil (Merwin & Algire, 1959; Potter & Robertson, 1960; Potter & Boyce, 1962). In human subjects Seligmann (1966) has obtained evidence for a genetic predisposition towards monoclonal protein production, but this is unusual in familial studies of such patients. The possible role of extrinsic factors including chronic inflammatory lesions acting upon a genetically predisposed individual has been the subject of discussion (see Osserman & Takatsuki, 1965).

Pathological Effects of Monoclonal Proteins

As mentioned above, monoclonal proteins appear to represent individual molecular species of normal immunoglobulin. They may vary considerably in physico-chemical properties such as solubility, intrinsic viscosity, tendency to polymer formation and ability to form complexes with other circulating proteins. These specific properties can, in some instances, be directly related to certain clinical and pathological manifestations.

Impairment of Renal Function

Pathological evidence of renal damage is observed in 50 to 90% of patients with multiple myelomatosis, while uraemia has been found, after pneumonia, to be the most common cause of death. Moreover, myelomatosis may present clinically as renal disease and elude diagnosis before other signs become manifest (Osserman, 1948; Sanchez & Domz, 1960). Impairment of renal function is commonly but not invariably seen in association with Bence-Jones proteinuria. In some instances this appears to result, at least in part, from the precipitation of Bence-Jones protein forming casts which may extend up the nephron to the proximal convoluted tubules (Bell, 1933; Forbes, Perlzweig, Parfentjer & Burwell, 1935; Oliver, 1944; Greenwald, Bronfin & Auerbach, 1953); in other cases the protein apparently interferes with specific tubular transport mechanisms (Sirota & Hammerman, 1954; Engle & Wallis, 1957; Dedmon, West & Schwartz, 1963). The recognition of myelomatosis in cases of renal disease is of considerable importance to the radiologist, since intravenous pyelography may lead to acute and irreversible renal failure in such patients (Bartels, Brun, Gammeltoft & Gjørup, 1954; Myhre, Brodwall & Knutsen, 1956; Kielmann, Gjørup & Thaysen, 1957; Perillie & Conn, 1958; Sanchez & Domz, 1960), although adequate hydration and use of appropriate contrast media minimize this risk (Lasser, Lang & Zawadzki, 1966).

Hyperviscosity Syndrome

Certain important clinical manifestations in patients with monoclonal proteins can be attributed to elevated serum viscosity; this occurs particularly with macroglobulinaemia but is also observed in multiple myelomatosis. The relative viscosity of solutions of IgG shows a linear increase at concentrations of 1 to 5%, whereas the viscosity of IgM solutions increases sharply at higher concentrations (Fig. 15.7). Symptoms attributable to hyperviscosity are not observed

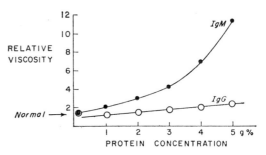

Fig. 15.7. Relative viscosity in relation to IgG and IgM concentration. (From Fahey & Solomon, 1965.)

with relative viscosity levels of below 4 (normal 1·4 to 1·8). The threshold level associated with clinical symptoms shows considerable individual variation, but in most subjects symptoms appear when the serum viscosity reaches 6 or 7 (Fahey & Solomon, 1965). The commonest clinical features associated with hyperviscosity are related to circulatory impairment and include recurrent, spontaneous bleeding, ocular disturbances and various neurological symptoms.

Cryoglobulinaemia

Severe circulatory disturbances aggravated by exposure to low temperatures are observed with those monoclonal proteins which on cooling show an increase in viscosity or precipitate either in the form of a floccular deposit or a gel. This phenomenon was first described by Wintrobe & Buell (1933) and the term "cryoglobulin" was introduced by Lerner & Watson (1947). Cryoglobulins may belong to any of the three major classes of immunoglobulin and quite commonly contain both IgG and IgM (Waller & Vaughan, 1956; Edelman, Kunkel & Franklin, 1953; Meltzer & Franklin, 1966). The temperature at which precipitation occurs varies considerably and in most instances complete re-solution occurs at 37°. On repeated warming and cooling the property of precipitation may diminish; in some instances the ability to precipitate is lost on heating the serum to 56°C, suggesting that the process is complement-dependent (Volpé, Bruce-Robertson, Fletcher & Charles, 1956; Luckey, Russ & Barr, 1951; Barnett, Curtain & Hayes, 1956). The temperature-dependent changes in viscosity and solubility observed with these proteins are influenced by pH, ionic environment and protein concentration and the interaction of these factors leads to great variation in the clinical picture associated with cryoglobulinaemia (Lerner & Watson, 1947;

Watson & Lerner, 1947; MacKay, Eriksen, Motulsky & Volwiler, 1956; Osserman, 1959).

Blood Clotting Disturbances

A variety of blood clotting disturbances have been observed in association with monoclonal proteins, but for the most part their nature is obscure. It is generally assumed that the defects arise from the interaction of the monoclonal protein with platelets or with one or more of the coagulation factors including factors V and VII, prothrombin, antihaemophilic globulin and fibrinogen (Uehlinger, 1949; Luscher & Labhart, 1949; Nilsson & Wenckert, 1953; Niléhn, 1962); however, such interactions have not been directly demonstrated. The abnormality often affects the conversion of fibrinogen to fibrin (Frick, 1955) and in one recorded instance could be overcome by the addition of Ca ions (Craddock, Adams & Figueroa, 1953). An IgA myeloma protein has been described which interfered with the first stage of clotting by inhibiting the action of antihaemophilic globulin (Glueck & Hong, 1965).

Immunological Deficiency

Infection is a frequent and often terminal event in diseases associated with the production of monoclonal proteins. In a series studied at the Clinical Centre, Bethesda, infection was found to occur in 82% of patients with multiple myelomatosis and in 56% of cases of macroglobulinaemia; in multiple myelomatosis infection was equally common in those with IgG, IgA and Bence-Jones monoclonal proteins (Fahey, Scoggins, Utz & Szwed, 1963). In these diseases there is characteristically a reduction of the normal immunoglobulin levels as shown by paper electrophoresis (Laurell, 1961a), chromatography (Fahey, 1962), immunoelectrophoresis (Grabar & Burtin, 1960; Heremans & Heremans, 1961) or by specific immunochemical methods (Fahey, Scoggins, Utz & Szwed, 1963; Cwynarski, 1968). This state of hypogammaglobulinaemia is associated with a diminished capacity to form circulating antibodies. Thus, patients with multiple myelomatosis may have progressively decreasing isohaemagglutinin levels (Lawson, Stuart, Paull, Phillips & Phillips, 1955) and show a poor antibody response to pneumococcal polysaccharides (Larson & Tomlinson, 1952; Zimmerman & Hall, 1954), typhoid-paratyphoid vaccine (Zimmerman & Hall, 1954; Fahey, Scoggins, Utz & Szwed, 1963), brucella abortus polysaccharides (Zimmerman & Hall, 1954), influenza vaccine (Heath, Fairley & Malpas, 1964), mumps vaccine and diphtheria toxoid. Patients with multiple myelomatosis show a particularly poor response to primary antigenic stimulation and an almost normal response to secondary stimulation (Fahey, Scoggins, Utz & Szwed, 1963; Cone & Uhr, 1964). Similarly, such patients show a decreased capacity to develop delayed hypersensitivity to antigens encountered after the onset of the disease. Thus, the cases investigated by Cone & Uhr (1964) all showed delayed skin reactivity to at least one of eight commonly encountered antigens, but only 50% could be sensitized with dinitrofluorobenzene. These data suggest that immunologically committed clones of cells may remain relatively unaffected in diseases leading to monoclonal protein production; the capacity of uncommitted cells to respond to primary stimulation, on the other hand, is greatly diminished. As pointed out by Scharff & Uhr (1965) this may imply that committed cells are non-dividing long-lived lymphocytes, whereas uncommitted cells may be short-lived and easily replaced by the expanding clone which produces the monoclonal protein.

The fact that infection is extremely common in multiple myelomatosis and can be correlated with hypogammaglobulinaemia and defective immunological responsiveness, suggest that γ-globulin therapy may be of value in these cases.

AUTOIMMUNE DISEASE

The Problem of Self-recognition

It has become apparent during recent years that cells of the immunological system have the capacity to respond in two alternate ways in the presence of antigen. On the one hand, antigenic stimulation may induce a cycle of cell proliferation and differentiation which culminates in antibody synthesis. Alternatively, antigen may lead to a state of immunological paralysis; this is not merely a failure to produce antibody, but represents a long-lasting inhibition of the capacity to synthesize antibodies specific for the antigen which induced paralysis. It is in terms of this phenomenon that an explanation must be sought for the remarkable ability of the immunological system to differentiate between antigens originating within the organism itself and those of genetically foreign origin—in other words to distinguish between "self" and "non-self".

This discriminatory power was for long accepted as a biological axiom and appropriately named by Ehrlich the "horror autotoxicus". An experimental analysis of this phenomenon of self-recognition grew out of observations made on cattle twins. When these are male and female, the latter is often sterile and referred to as a free-martin; it has been postulated that as the result of anastomoses between chorionic vessels of the two placentae, male hormone is present in the circulation of the female and inhibits development of sexual organs. Such anastamoses also result in the exchange of cells between developing bovine twins, and in 1945 Owen showed that after birth such cells of foreign genetic origin survived long into adult life without provoking the expected immunological reaction. A similar state of affairs was later found in a woman whose blood cells were of both group O and group A; her saliva contained H and not A substance indicating that her true blood group was O and that the A cells were derived *in utero* from a twin brother who had died 25 years before at the age of 3 months (Dunsford, Bowley, Hutchison, Thompson, Sanger & Race, 1953). On the basis of Owen's observations in cattle Burnet & Fenner (1949) postulated that antigen present during foetal life acted upon the developing immunological system and suppressed its subsequent capacity to synthesize antibodies of the corresponding specificity. Experimental confirmation of this penetrating hypothesis was provided by Billingham, Brent & Medawar (1953) who induced a state of immunological tolerance to genetically foreign grafts by injecting mice *in utero* with cells derived from the strain which was to act as the graft donor. Subsequent experiments have shown that long-lasting immunological tolerance can be induced in many different species by exposure of the foetus to a variety of antigens.

The occurrence of immunological paralysis is not confined to the period of foetal development. In adult life such specific unresponsiveness has, for example, been induced by the administration of large doses of antigen. This reaction was first noted with pneumococcal polysaccharide antigens which tend to resist intracellular destruction, but has since been observed with foreign proteins given in large doses by repeated parenteral administration. In addition, a state of immunological paralysis has been induced in some instances by administration of protein antigens from which aggregated material liable to phagocytosis has been removed either by ultracentrifugation or by preliminary circulation through a live animal. These and related experiments suggest that the immune response may be initiated by some form of "processed antigen" derived from phagocytic cells; on the other hand, antigen which by-passes phagocytic cells may, through direct interaction with lymphocytes, induce a state of immunological paralysis (Fig. 15.1).

The foetus tends to respond to antigenic material by paralysis rather than specific antibody formation and this may be attributable to some functional immaturity of developing phagocytic cells. Whatever the mechanism, contact of auto-antigens with the foetal immunological system apparently eliminates clones of cells having the capacity to form the corresponding auto-antibodies; in this way the pattern of "self-recognition" is established during prenatal development. It is evident that alterations in the structure and distribution of auto-antigens, or changes in the immunological system itself could disturb the

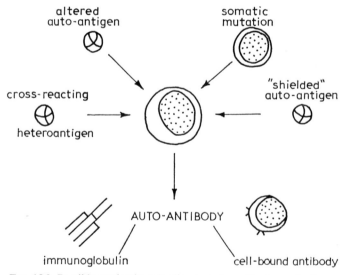

FIG. 15.8. Possible mechanisms leading to auto-antibody production.

mechanism of self-recognition and lead to the production of auto-antibodies through mechanisms such as those outlined in Fig. 15.8. For example, it has been shown that when the antigenic structure of platelets is altered by combination with the drug Sedormid, antibodies specific for the complex are formed and these destroy platelets and produce thrombocytopenic purpura (Ackroyd, 1949). Some antigens, such as thyroglobulin, are normally shielded from the immunological system; since these have never been in contact with foetal immunological cells, their release into the circulation in later life will lead to auto-antibody production. The occurrence of somatic mutations in the rapidly dividing cells which comprise the immunological system may result in the reappearance of cell lines suppressed in foetal life and capable of synthesizing auto-antibodies.

The clinical concept of autoimmune disease is based upon the identification of antibodies present in serum and having an affinity for some human tissue component. Such antibodies are being found in association with an ever-growing number of pathological states; their identity and significance have been the subject of intensive investigation in recent years and several reviews of this work have been written in which the original literature is fully documented (Doniach & Roitt, 1962; Anderson, 1963; MacKay & Burnet, 1963; Gell & Coombs, 1963; Glynn & Holborrow, 1965; Whipple, 1965; Samter, 1965). No attempt will be made here to deal comprehensively with the subject which is discussed in various other chapters of this book; the serological properties of certain relatively common auto-antibodies will be outlined and the significance of autoimmune processes in human disease will be briefly discussed.

Diseases Associated with Auto-antibodies

Rheumatoid arthritis. The rheumatoid factor (R.F.) is usually present in the IgM fraction of serum; it reacts with homologous or heterologous γ-globulin which has been denatured or is present in the form of complexes with antigen. The determinants of the γ-globulin molecule which react with the rheumatoid factor are located on part of the γ-chain contained in the F_c fragment (Fig. 15.3). Rheumatoid factors are of heterogeneous specificity since they differ in their reactivity with γ-globulins from various species and in their combination with genetically distinct types of γ-globulin. R.F. is detected by its ability to agglutinate various particles, bacteria or cells which have been coated with γ-globulin usually of human or rabbit origin.

The incidence of positive reactions in cases of rheumatoid arthritis varies with different techniques. The simplest and most widely used test which makes use of latex particles coated with normal γ-globulin, gives positive tests with serum dilutions of more than 1/20 in over 70% of cases diagnosed clinically as rheumatoid arthritis; positive tests are especially common in the presence of subcutaneous nodules. Detection of the R.F. is not diagnostic of rheumatoid arthritis. Positive tests are found in about 5% of normal subjects, occasionally in high titre, and in a higher proportion of patients with other disorders of connective tissues as well as in subjects with a variety of illnesses including pulmonary tuberculosis, syphilis and liver disease.

Systemic lupus erythematosus. This disease is characterized by the presence in the serum of a variety of anti-nuclear and anti-cytoplasmic antibodies which react *in vitro* with several different tissue constituents, but lack species or organ specificity. The most readily identifiable is the L.E. factor which is an immunoglobulin (usually IgG) reacting with deoxyribonucleohistone of the cell nucleus and responsible for the formation of L.E. cells (phagocytes containing ingested nuclei). Anti-nuclear factors which may be either IgG, IgA or IgM can also be detected by immunofluorescent methods using a fluorescein-labelled antibody to human Ig; antibodies to cytoplasmic constituents are detected by complement fixation and haemagglutination tests. The L.E. cell factor is present in about 90% of patients with clinically diagnosed systemic lupus erythematosus; positive tests have also been reported in up to 50% of patients with rheumatoid arthritis and in a significant proportion of other rheumatic diseases and occasionally in ulcerative colitis, liver disease and drug hypersensitivity, for example, to penicillin.

Sjögren's Syndrome. This syndrome consists essentially of chronic inflammation of lacrimal and salivary glands, occurring in many cases together with a "connective tissue disorder"; it is associated with a great diversity of serological reactions, many of which are similar to those of rheumatoid arthritis and systemic lupus erythematosus. The rheumatoid factor is present in more than 75% of cases, but unlike that of rheumatoid arthritis, often lacks anti-Gm activity. Anti-nuclear factor has been reported in 50 to 75% of patients, but the L.E. cell phenomenon seems to occur only in patients having clinical features of systemic lupus erythematosus or rheumatoid arthritis. The serum of patients with Sjögren's syndrome may give precipitin and complement fixation reactions with extracts of human salivary and lacrimal glands, but such reactions appear to have neither organ nor species specificity, being similar in this respect to the anti-tissue reactions observed in systemic lupus erythematosus. Antibodies reacting with thyroglobulin or thyroid microsomes have been demonstrated in up to 50% of patients with Sjögren's syndrome, frequently in the absence of detectable thyroid disease; antibody to gastric parietal cells occurs in about one quarter of patients.

Thyroid Disease

Thyroiditis. Various forms of lymphocytic thyroiditis, of which Hashimoto's disease is the commonest, are very commonly associated with serum anti-thyroid antibodies; these differ in their specificities and may interact with any of three distinct thyroid antigens. The commonest antibodies are directed against thyroglobulin; these antibodies may be either IgG or IgM and in suitable test systems give precipitin or agglutinin reactions but rarely fix complement. In a small percentage of patients the antibodies present combine with colloid giving a pattern of immunofluorescence in thyroid sections which is quite distinct from that obtained by the same technique with thyroglobulin antibodies. This second antigen of the colloid contains no iodine and its physicochemical properties are distinct from thyroglobulin. A third antigen has been localized in the microsomal fraction of thyroid homogenates; antibodies to this component are detected by immunofluorescence or complement fixation and appear to be responsible for the cytotoxic action seen when sera from patients with thyroiditis are applied to monolayer cultures of trypsinized human thyroid gland.

In Hashimoto's disease antibodies directed against all three thyroid antigens are usually present and the complete absence of anti-thyroid antibody practically excludes the diagnosis. Similar serological findings are common in primary myxoedema, but in other forms of thyroid disease including thyrotoxicosis, non-toxic colloid goitre and carcinoma of the thyroid, auto-antibodies are found in less than 60% of patients, and are present in lower titre. About 5% of hospital patients with no clinical evidence of thyroid disease give positive tests for thyroid auto-antibodies, but the incidence is much higher (about 15%) in apparently healthy women over the age of 50 years.

Thyrotoxicosis. Serum from some patients with thyrotoxicosis causes prolonged stimulation of thyroid secretion when injected into animals pretreated with radioactive iodine and with thyroid hormone to suppress the secretion of endogenous thyrotropin. In this assay pituitary thyroid-stimulating hormone (T.S.H.) causes a prompt and relatively brief increase of circulating radioactive iodine, whereas thyrotoxic serum has a long-lasting effect with a blood-iodine peak at 10 to 12 hr. after injection. This phenomenon is attributed to the presence in sera from patients with Grave's disease of a long-acting thyroid stimulator (LATS) which acts on the thyroid gland and not indirectly through the pituitary (reviewed by McKenzie, 1965).

Although the chemical identity of LATS has not been established with certainty, various fractionation procedures indicate that it is probably a 7S immunoglobulin. Moreover, its biological activity can apparently be abolished by reaction with anti-human Ig serum (Dorrington, Munro & Carneiro, 1964; Kriss, Pleshakov & Chien, 1964). A claim that its activity is localized to the heavy chain after reductive cleavage of the Ig molecule (Meek, Jones, Lewis & Vanderland, 1964) has not been confirmed (Dorrington, Munro & Carneiro, 1964). Further purification of LATS and a study of its combining specificity are required to establish whether or not it can be regarded as an auto-antibody.

LATS can be detected in the serum of about 60 to 70% of patients with Grave's disease and in a higher proportion of those with exophthalmos; its presence in individual cases may show poor correlation with the clinical state and with other tests of thyroid function.

Acquired Haemolytic Disease

Cases of acquired haemolytic disease associated with red cell auto-antibodies may be classified on the basis of the optimum temperature of interaction between antibody and erythrocyte antigen. The commoner "warm antibodies" are active at body temperature while "cold antibodies" have an optimum temperature of about 4 to 10°C.

"Warm Antibody"

In the majority of cases of acquired haemolytic disease of the warm type serum antibody can be demonstrated only when the patient is acutely ill; this is generally taken to mean that the antibody is of high affinity and is mainly bound to red blood cells. These cell-bound antibodies are present in over 80% of patients and can be detected by the Coombs test, i.e. by the agglutination of antibody-coated erythrocytes with antisera to human γ-globulin; in other cases cells react, not with anti-Ig sera, but with antisera to various components of complement. Red cell auto-antibodies can be eluted from sensitized erythrocytes by heat, mild acid or other solvents; they have the properties of IgG, but are sometimes relatively homogeneous and in this respect may resemble myeloma proteins (Leddy & Bakemeier, 1965). The eluted antibody sensitizes normal human red blood cells to the anti-globulin test and the majority appear to combine with some structural unit common to erythrocytes of several, or all, rH types (Wiener, Gordon & Gallop, 1953; Wiener & Vos, 1963). Occasionally these antibodies are of a specific anti-rH type, usually anti-e, and the red blood cells of the patient from which the eluates have been made show a corresponding specificity; in rare instances, the specificity of the antibody is different from that of the autologous red blood cells (Dacie, 1962).

"Cold Antibody"

Paroxysmal cold haemaglobinuria. The antibodies associated with this syndrome are detected by the Donath and Landsteiner test. Fresh serum from the patient is mixed with homologous or autologous erythrocytes at 4°C and the mixture is warmed to 37°; rapid haemolysis then occurs due to the attachment of antibody and complement in the cold. The antibody responsible for this reaction is a 7S immunoglobulin and frequently has a specificity within the P blood-group system (Levine, Celano & Falkowski, 1963; Worlledge, 1965).

Cold agglutinins. The auto-antibodies which cause intense haemagglutination in the cold belong to the IgM class and usually have anti-I specificity, although other specificities have been described (van Loghem, Pectoom, van der Hart, van der Veer, van der Giessen, Prins, Zucher & Engelfriel, 1963). Antibodies associated with the idiopathic forms of the disease occasionally show the property of cryoprecipitation and are unusual in that the great majority are relatively homogeneous and have light chains of type K only. The cold agglutinins which appear transiently after *Mycoplasma pneumoniae* infection are also IgM antibodies usually with anti-I specificity, but appear to carry both classes of light chains (Costea, Yakulis & Heller, 1966). Cold agglutinins may also be found in association with malignant disease of the reticulo-endothelial system.

Pernicious Anaemia and Gastritis

The primary lesion in pernicious anaemia appears to affect the gastric mucosa where atrophy is associated with a failure to secrete acid, pepsinogen and intrinsic factor. This clinical syndrome is, in some cases, associated with the presence of auto-antibodies directed against the intrinsic factor and against a microsomal component of gastric parietal (acid producing) cell cytoplasm. Using the most sensitive techniques, about 60% of patients have serum intrinsic factor antibodies (Chanarin & Ardeman, 1966) and almost 90% have antibodies directed against parietal cells (Taylor, Roitt, Doniach, Couchman & Shapland, 1962). Patients with chronic gastritis without pernicious anaemia may have parietal cell antibodies, but their sera are always negative for intrinsic factor antibodies. The incidence of parietal cell antibodies is lower in chronic gastritis than in pernicious anaemia but much higher than in healthy controls (Taylor, 1965). In addition to intrinsic factor and parietal cell antibodies, a high proportion (about 40%) of patients with pernicious anaemia have antibodies to the microsomal fraction of the thyroid gland. Conversely, gastric antibodies are unusually common in thyroiditis, thyrotoxicosis, iron deficiency anaemia and diabetes mellitus (Doniach, Roitt & Taylor, 1963); gastric antibodies are also present in about one third of the relatives of pernicious anaemia patients and in a small proportion of apparently healthy people (Doniach & Roitt, 1966).

Ulcerative Colitis

Serum antibodies which combine with antigens present in saline or phenol extracts of colonic mucosa are demonstrable in many cases of ulcerative colitis in adults and are especially frequent in children with this disease (Broberger & Perlmann, 1959; Asherson & Broberger, 1961). The reactive antigens appear to be present in normal colon as well as that from ulcerative colitis patients. The titre of anti-colon antibodies appears to be no higher in patients with active ulcerative colitis than those in remission (Harrison, 1965). An immunological basis for the disease is suggested by the finding that circulating leucocytes (mainly lymphocytes) from ulcerative colitis patients, in the presence of complement, have a cytotoxic effect on cells of the colon maintained in tissue culture (Broberger & Perlmann, 1963; Perlmann & Broberger, 1963). It has been suggested that autosensitization may result from an immune reaction against lipopolysaccharide derived from *Escherichia coli* since this material appears to have antigenic specificities in common with colonic cells (Perlmann, Hammarstrom, Lagercrantz & Gustafsson, 1965). In addition to anti-colon antibodies, patients with ulcerative colitis show a significantly higher incidence of gastric parietal cell antibody than do normal controls (Taylor, 1965); there are conflicting reports concerning the incidence of anti-nuclear antibodies in ulcerative colitis.

Liver Disease

Various circulating antibodies may be present in the serum of patients with chronic hepatitis. Anti-nuclear factors detected by the L.E. cell reaction or by immunofluorescent staining occur in about 25% of such cases. Active chronic hepatitis associated with a positive L.E. test has been designated "lupoid hepatitis", but indistinguishable forms of liver disease occur in the absence of anti-nuclear factor. Antibodies which react with cytoplasmic antigens from various human tissue homogenates giving the so-called autoimmune complement fixation (AICF) test are present in the serum of 20 to 40% of patients with chronic hepatitis. In some instances this reaction does not detect auto-antibodies since the patient's serum fails to react with autologous tissue but gives strong reactions with homologous tissue; the AICF reaction may be weakly positive in some normal subjects while strong reactions occur in several diseases including macroglobulinaemia and systemic lupus erythematosus.

Demyelinating Diseases

The evidence that demyelinating diseases in man have an immunological basis is largely indirect and has been critically reviewed by Paterson (1965). Several laboratories have reported the presence of complement-fixing anti-brain antibodies in sera of some patients with multiple sclerosis, but their incidence appears to be no greater than in control patients. In patients who develop encephalitis after receiving injections of rabies vaccine prepared from rabbit brain or spinal cord, complement-fixing anti-brain antibodies are found which are organ-specific but not species-specific; similar antibodies are frequently present in those who receive the vaccine but do not develop encephalitis. Of great interest are the findings of Bornstein (1963, 1965) who used cultures of central nervous tissue to demonstrate myelinotoxic and glial-toxic factors in the sera of some patients with multiple sclerosis; however, demyelinating activity may be present also in sera from patients with motor neurone disease while glial cells are easily damaged by serum in high concentration (Berg & Källén, 1962).

Significance of Auto-antibodies in Human Disease

The concept of autoimmune disease has been clearly established in experimental animals. A great variety of lesions, some of which closely resemble those encountered in clinical medicine, have been produced by autoimmunization. Experimental allergic encephalitis and thyroiditis produced by injecting extracts of brain or thyroid gland together with adjuvants, have been extensively studied. Such experimental autoimmune lesions are associated with the appearance of serum antibodies having the appropriate organ specificities. However, sera which contain high titres of auto-antibody, when passively transferred, fail to induce tissue damage in recipient animals. Lesions have, on the other hand, been passively transferred in some instances, by injecting leucocytes from the sensitized animal into genetically similar recipients. On the basis of these findings it has been postulated that autoimmune processes may be initiated by "cell-bound" antibody, similar to that thought to be responsible for delayed hypersensitivity. However, it is not known whether the cells passively transferred in these experiments produce tissue damage directly or through the production of serum antibody, which may have high affinity for tissue antigen and therefore be undetectable in the circulation.

Antibodies which combine with various homologous or autologous tissue components are, as outlined above, found in a wide variety of human diseases. There are several facts which throw doubt upon the role of these antibodies in the initiation of pathological lesions. In the first place, auto-antibodies may be demonstrable in only a proportion of patients who show a particular clinical syndrome; for example, no more than 60% of pernicious anaemia cases have detectable serum antibodies to intrinsic factor. Conversely, specific auto-antibodies may occur without disease of the corresponding tissue; for example, anti-thyroglobulin antibodies are found in euthyroid subjects. In addition, the presence and the level of auto-antibodies may show little correlation with the clinical state; in both acquired haemolytic anaemia and ulcerative colitis, for instance, there may be little change in the titre of auto-antibodies during exacerbations and remissions of the disease. Finally, it has not been possible to transmit autoimmune disease to human volunteers by repeated injections of serum containing high levels of auto-antibody. In this connection it is of interest that during pregnancy transfer of circulating isoantibodies from the maternal blood stream may seriously damage the foetus whereas maternal auto-antibodies seldom, if ever, lead to pathological changes in the offspring. It is clear that the role of auto-antibodies in the pathogenesis of human disease has not been clearly established. There appears to be a marked familial predisposition to form auto-antibodies (Doniach, Roitt & Taylor, 1963), presumably in response to the liberation of tissue antigens by some damaging agent or as a result of primary alteration in the lymphoid system itself. Such antibodies could lead to significant pathological complications or play no part at all in the pathogenesis of the disease. On the basis of findings in experimental animals, it has been postulated that tissue damage in human auto-immune disease is mediated by "cell-bound" antibody. This idea is of potential importance, but will be of practical value in the clinic only if techniques become available for the identification and measurement of such antibodies.

References

ACKROYD, J. F. (1949). *Clin. Sci.*, **8**, 269.

AISENBERG, A. C. & LESKOWITZ, S. (1963). *New Engl. J. Med.*, **268**, 1269.

ALPER, C. A., FREEMAN, T. & WALDENSTRÖM, J. (1963). *J. clin. Invest.*, **42**, 1858.

ANDERSON, J. B. (1963). *Brit. med. Bull.*, **19**, 251.

ASHERSON, G. & BROBERGER, O. (1961). *Brit. med. J.*, **1**, 1429.

AXELSSON, U., BACHMAN, R. & HALLÉN, J. (1966). *Acta med. Scand.*, **179**, 235.

BALLIEUX, R. E., BERNIER, G. M., TOMINAGA, K. & PUTNAM, F. W. (1964). *Science*, **145**, 168.

BARNETT, A. J., CURTAIN, C. C. & HAYES, R. A. (1956). *Australas. Ann. Med.*, **5**, 177.

BARTELS, E. D., BRUN, G. C., GAMMELTOFT, A. & GJØRUP, P. A. (1954). *Acta med. Scand.*, **150**, 297.

BEAUMONT, J. L. (1967). *Compt. rend. Acad. Sci.*, **264**, 185.

BELL, E. T. (1933). *Am. J. Path.*, **9**, 393.

BERG, O. & KÄLLÉN, B. (1962). *Lancet*, **1**, 1051.

BERGSAGEL, D. E., SPRAGUE, C. C., AUSTIN, C. & GRIFFITH, K. M. (1962). *Cancer Chemother. Rep.*, No. 21, p. 87.

BERNARD, J., SELIGMANN, M. & DANON, F. (1962). *Nouv. Rev. Franc. Hémat.*, **2**, 611.

BERSON, S. A. & YALOW, R. S. (1957). *J. Lab. clin. Med.*, **49**, 386.

BILLINGHAM, R. E., BRENT, L. & MEDAWAR, P. B. (1953). *Nature*, **172**, 603.

BIRKE, G., LILJEDAHL, S. O., OLHAGEN, B., PLANTIN, L. O. & AHLINDER, S. (1963). *Acta med. Scand.*, **173**, 589.

BORNSTEIN, M. B. (1963). *Nat. Cancer Inst. Monogr.*, **11**, 197.

BORNSTEIN, M. B. (1965). "Immunopathology IVth International Symposium". Ed. Grabar, P. & Miescher, P. A. Schwabe & Co., Basel. p. 374.

BRAMBELL, F. W. R. (1965). *Nature*, **203**, 1352.

BROBERGER, O. & PERLMANN, P. (1959). *J. exp. Med.*, **110**, 657.

BROBERGER, O. & PERLMANN, P. (1963). *J. exp. Med.*, **117**, 705.

BRUTON, O. C. (1952). *Paediatrics*, **9**, 722.

BURNET, F. M. & FENNER, F. (1949). "The production of Antibodies". 2nd edition. McMillan, Melbourne.

CHANARIN, I. & ARDEMAN, S. (1966). *Proc. R. Soc. Med.*, **59**, 690.

CHAPLIN, H., COHEN, S. & PRESS, E. M. (1965). *Biochem. J.*, **95**, 256.

COHEN, S. (1963a). *Nature*, **197**, 253.

COHEN, S. (1963b). *Brit. med. Bull.*, **19**, 202.

COHEN, S., McGREGOR, I. A. & CARRINGTON, S. (1961). *Nature*, **192**, 733.

COHEN, S. & MILSTEIN, C. (1967a). *Nature*, **214**, 449.

COHEN, S. & MILSTEIN, C. (1967b). *Adv. Immunol.*, **7**, 1.

COHEN, S. & PORTER, R. R. (1964). *Adv. Immunol.*, **5**, 287.

CONE, L. & UHR, J. W. (1964), *J. clin. Invest.*, **43**, 2241.

COOMBS, R. R. A. (1967). *Proc. R. Soc. Med.*, **60**, 594.

COOPER, M. D., PEREY, D. Y., McKNEALLY, M. F., GABRIELSEN, A. E., SUTHERLAND, D. E. R. & GOOD, R. A. (1966). *Lancet*, **1**, 1388.

COSTEA, N., YAKULIS, V. & HELLER, P. (1966). *Science*, **152**, 1520.

CRADDOCK, C. G., ADAMS, W. S., FIGUEROA, W. G. (1953). *J. Lab. clin. Med.*, **42**, 847.

CREYSSEL, R. & FINE, J. M. (1958). *Rev. Franc. Etude Clin. et Biol.*, **9**, 984.

CWYNARSKI, M. T. (1968). *Clinica chim. Acta*, **19**, 1.

DACIE, J. V. (1962). "The Haemolytic Anaemias". Part 2. Pub. Churchill.

DEDMON, R. E., WEST, J. H. & SCHWARTZ, T. B. (1963). *Med. Clin. N. Amer.*, **47**, 191.

DEUTSCH, H. F. (1962). *Fedn. Proc. Fedn. Am. Socs. exp. Biol.*, **21**, 77.

DONIACH, D. & ROITT, I. M. (1962). *A. Rev. Med.*, **13**, 213.

DONIACH, D. & ROITT, I. M. (1966). *Proc. R. Soc. Med.*, **59**, 691.

DONIACH, D., ROITT, I. M. & TAYLOR, K. B. (1963). *Brit. med. J.*, **1**, 1374.

DORRINGTON, K. J., MUNRO, D. S. & CARNEIRO, L. (1964). *Lancet*, **2**, 889.

DUNN, T. B. (1957). *J. Natn. Cancer Inst.*, **19**, 371.

DUNSFORD, I., BOWLEY, C. C., HUTCHISON, A. M., THOMPSON, J. S., SANGER, R. & RACE, R. R. (1953). *Brit. med. J.*, **ii**, 81.

EDELMAN, G. M. (1959). *J. Am. chem. Soc.*, **81**, 3155.

EDELMAN, G. M. & GALLY, J. A. (1962). *J. exp. Med.*, **116**, 207.

EDELMAN, G. M., KUNKEL, H. G. & FRANKLIN, E. C. (1953). *J. exp. Med.*, **100**, 105.

EDELMAN, G. M. & POULIK, M. D. (1961). *J. exp. Med.*, **113**, 861.

ENGLE, R. L. & WACKMAN, R. L. (1966). *Blood*, **27**, 74.

ENGLE, R. L. & WALLIS, L. A. (1957). *Am. J. Med.*, **22**, 5.

ENGLE, R. L., WOODS, K. R., CASTILLO, G. & PERT, J. H. (1961). *J. Lab. clin. Med.*, **58**, 1.

FAHEY, J. L. (1962). *J. biol. Chem.*, **237**, 440.

FAHEY, J. L. (1963*a*). *J. Immun.*, **91**, 438.

FAHEY, J. L. (1963*b*). *J. clin. Invest.*, **42**, 111.

FAHEY, J. L. & GOODMAN, H. C. (1960). *J. clin. Invest.*, **39**, 1259.

FAHEY, J. L. & MCKELVEY E. M. (1965). *J. Immun.*, **94**, 84.

FAHEY, J. L. & ROBINSON, A. G. (1963). *J. exp. Med.*, **118**, 845.

FAHEY, J. L., SCOGGINS, R., UTZ, J. P. & SZWED, F. (1963). *Am. J. Med.*, **35**, 698.

FAHEY, J. L. & SOLOMON, A. (1965). *J. Am. med. As.*, **192**, 464.

FEIZI, T. (1968). "Gut". (In press.)

FINE, J. M., CREYSSEL, R. & MOREL, P. (1959). *Rev. Haematol.*, **14**, 75.

FLEISCHMAN, J. B., PAIN, R. H. & PORTER, R. R. (1962). *Archs. Biochem. Biophys.*, Suppl. 1, 174.

FORBES, W. D., PERLZWEIG, W. A., PARFENTJER, I. A. & BURWELL, J. C. (1935). *Bull. Johns Hopkins Hosp.*, **57**, 47.

FRANKLIN, E. C. (1964). *J. exp. Med.*, **120**, 691.

FRICK, P. G. (1955). *Am. J. clin. Path.*, **25**, 1263.

GABUZDA, T. G. (1962). *J. Lab. clin. Med.*, **59**, 65.

GELL, P. G. H. & COOMBS, R. R. A. (1963). "Clinical Aspects of Immunology". Blackwell, Oxford.

GITLIN, D., GROSS, P. A. M. & JANEWAY, C. A. (1959). *New England J. Med.*, **280**, 121.

GLUECK, H. I. & HONG, R. (1965). *J. clin. Invest.*, **44**, 1866.

GLYNN, L. E. & HOLBORROW, E. J. (1965). "Auto-immunity and Disease". Blackwell, Oxford.

GOLDMAN, J. M. & HOBBS, J. R. (1967). *Immunology*, **13**, 421.

GRABAR, P. & BURTIN, P. (1960). "Analyse Immuno-electrophoretique". p. 93. Masson & Cie., Paris.

GRABAR, P., FAUVERT, R., BURTIN, P. & HARTMANN, L. (1956). *Rev. Franc. Etude Clin. et Biol.*, **1**, 175.

GREENWALD, H. P., BRONFIN, G. J. & AUERBACH, O. (1953). *Am. J. Med.'* **15**, 198.

GREY, H. M. & KUNKEL, H. G. (1964). *J. exp. Med.*, **120**, 253.

GUTMAN, A. B., MOORE, D. H., GUTMAN, E. B., MCCLELLAN, V. & KABAT, E. A. (1941). *J. clin. Invest.*, **20**, 765.

HANSSON, U.-B., LAURELL, C.-B. & BACHMANN, R. (1966). *Acta med. Scand.*, Suppl. 445, p. 89.

HARBOE, M. & LIND, K. (1966). *Scand. J. Haematol.*, **3**, 269.

HARRISON, W. J. (1965). *Lancet*, **1**, 1346.

HARRISON, J. F., BLAINEY, J. D., HARDWICKE, J., ROWE, D. S. & SOOTHILL, J. F. (1966). *Clin. Sci.*, **31**, 95.

HAVENS, W. P. (1959). *Int. Archs. Allergy appl. Immun.*, **14**, 75.

HEATH, R. B., FAIRLEY, G. H. & MALPAS, J. S. (1964). *Br. J. Haemat.*, **10**, 365.

HEIDELBERGER, M. & PEDERSEN, K. O. (1937). *J. exp. Med.*, **65**, 393.

HEREMANS, J. F. & HEREMANS, M.-Th. (1961). *Acta Med. Scand.*, Suppl. 367, p. 27.

HOBBS, J. R. (1967). *Proc. R. Soc. Med.*, **60**, 1250.

HOBBS, J. R., SLOT, G. M. J., CAMPBELL, C. H., CLEIN, G. P., SCOTT, J. T., CROWTHER, D. & SWAN, H. T. (1966). *Lancet*, **2**, 614.

HUMPHREY, J. H. & FAHEY, J. L. (1961). *J. clin. Invest.*, **40**, 1696.

IMHOF, J. W., BALLIEUX, R. E., MUL, N. A. J. & POEN, H. (1966). *Acta med. Scand.*, **179**, Suppl. 445, p. 102.

ISHIZAKA, K., ISHIZAKA, T. & HORNBROOK, M. M. (1966). *J. Immunol.* **97**, 75.

ISHIZAKA, K. & ISHIZAKA, T. (1967). *J. Immunol.* **99**, 1187.

JANEWAY, C. A., ROSEN, F. S., MERLER, E. & ALPER, C. A. (1966). "The Gammaglobulins". Churchill, London.

JOHANSSON, S. G. O., BENNICH, H. & WIDE, L. (1968). *Immunology*, **14**, 265.

KAPPELER, R., KREBS, A. & RIVA, G. (1958). *Helv. med. Acta*, **25**, 54.

KIELMANN, S., GJØRUP, S. & THAYSEN, J. H. (1957). *Acta med. Scand.*, **158**, 43.

KORMAN, S., CORCORAN, C., FINE, S. & LIPINCOTT, S. W. (1962). *J. Lab. clin. Med.*, **59**, 371.

KRISS, J. P., PLESHAKOV, V. & CHIEN, J. R. (1964). *J. clin. Endocr. Metab.*, **24**, 1005.

KRITZMAN, I. J., KUNKEL, H. G., MCCARTHY, J. & MELLORS, R. C. (1961). *J. Lab. clin. Med.*, **57**, 905.

KUNKEL, H. G. (1960). "The Plasma Proteins". **1**, 279. Ed. Putnam, F. W. Academic Press, New York,

KUNKEL, H. G., FAHEY, J. L., FRANKLIN, E. C., OSSERMAN, E. & TERRY, W. D. (1966). *Bull Wld. Hlth. Org.*, **30**, 953.

LARSON, D. L. & TOMLINSON, L. J. (1952). *J. Lab. clin. Med.*, **39**, 129.

LASSER, E. C., LANG, J. H. & ZAWADZKI, Z. A. (1966). *J. Am. Med. Ass.*, **198**, 945.

LAURELL, C.-B. (1961*a*). *Acta med, Scand.*, **170**, 17.

LAURELL, H. F. (1961*b*). *Acta med. Scand.*, Suppl. 367 **170**, 69.

LAWSON, H. A., STUART, C. A., PAULL, A. M., PHILLIPS, A. M. & PHILLIPS, R. W. (1955). *New England J. Med.*, **252**, 13.

LEDDY, J. P. & BAKEMEIER, R. F. (1965). *J. exp. Med.*, **121**, 1.

LENNOX, E. S. & COHN, M. (1967). *A. Rev. Biochem.* **36**, 365.

LERNER, A. B. & WATSON, C. J. (1947). *Am. J. med. Sci.*, **214**, 410.

LEVINE, P., CELANO, M. J. & FALKOWSKI, F. (1963). *Transfusion*, **3**, 278.

LIM, S. D. & FUSARO, R. M. (1967). *Int. J. Lepr.*, **35**, 355.

LITWIN, S. & KUNKEL, H. G. (1966). *Fedn, Proc. Fedn. Am. Socs. exp. Biol.*, **25**, 371.

LUCKEY, E. H., RUSS, E. & BARR, D. P. (1951). *J. Lab. clin. Med.*, **37**, 253.

LÜSCHER, E. & LABHART, A. (1949). *Schwiz. Med. Wschr.*, **79**, 598.

MacKay, I. R. & Burnet, F. M. (1963). "Auto-immune Disease". C. C. Thomas, Springfield, Illinois.

MacKay, I. R., Eriksen, N., Motulsky, A. G. & Volwiler, W. (1956). Am. J. Med., 20, 564.

McKelvey, E. M. & Fahey, J. L. (1965). J. clin. Invest., 44, 1778.

McKenzie, J. M. (1965). J. clin. Endocr. Metab., 25, 424.

Magnus-Levy, A. (1933). Z. Klin. Med., 126, 62.

Mandema, E. (1956). "Over het Multiple Myeloom, het Solitaire Plasmocytoom en de Macro-globulinaemie." Groninger. Dijkstra's Drukkery, N.V.

Mannik, M. & Kunkel, H. G. (1963a). J. exp. Med., 117, 213.

Mannik, M. & Kunkel, H. G. (1963b). J. exp. Med., 118, 817.

Mårtensson, L. (1966). Vox Sanguin., 11, 393, 521.

Martin, N. H. (1964). In "Biochemical Disorders in Human Disease". Eds. Thompson, R. H. S. & King, E. J. Churchill, London.

Mattern, P., Masseyeff, R., Michel, R. & Peretti, P. (1961). T. Gambieuse Ann. Institute Pasteur, 101, 302.

Meek, J. C., Jones, A. E., Lewis, V. J. & Vanderland, W. P. (1964). Proc. natn. Acad. Sci., (U.S.A.), 52, 342.

Meltzer, M. & Franklin, E. C. (1962). Arthritis Rheum., 5, 117.

Meltzer, M. & Franklin, E. C. (1966). Am. J. Med., 40, 828.

Merler, E. (1966). Immunology, 10, 249.

Merwin, R. M. & Algire, G. H. (1959). Proc. Soc. exp. Biol. Med., 101, 437.

Meyer, F. & Putnam, F. W. (1963). J. exp. Med., 117, 573.

Mitchison, N. A. (1967). In "Regulation of the Antibody Response". Ed. Cinader, B. C. C. Thomas, Springfield, Illinois.

Moore, D. H., Kabat, E. A. & Gutman, A. B. (1943). J. clin. Invest., 22, 67.

Morton, J. I. & Deutsch, H. F. (1956). Proc. Soc. exp. Biol. Med., 93, 402.

Myhre, J. R., Brodwall, E. K. & Knutsen, S. B. (1956). Acta med. Scand., 156, 263.

Niléhn, J.-E. (1962). Acta med. Scand., 171, 491.

Nilsson, I. M. & Wenckert, A. (1953). Blood, 8, 1067.

Nordenson, N. G. (1966). Acta med. Scand., 179, Suppl. 445, 178.

Norgaard, O. (1964). Acta med. Scand., 176, 137.

Oliver, J. (1944). Harvey Lect., 40, 102.

Osserman, E. F. (1948). Radiology, 71, 157.

Osserman, E. F. (1959). New England J. Med., 261, 952, 1006.

Osserman, E. F. (1963). Proc. Am. Ass. Cancer Res., 2, 50.

Osserman, E. F. (1965). In "Immunological Diseases". Ed. Samter, M. Little Brown & Co., Boston. p. 353.

Osserman, E. F., Graff, A., Marshall, M., Lawlor, D. & Graff, S. (1957). J. clin. Invest., 36, 352.

Osserman, E. F. & Takatsuki, K. (1963). Medicine, 42, 357.

Osserman, E. F. & Takatsuki, K. (1964). Am. J. Med., 37, 351.

Osserman, E. F., Takatsuki, K. & Talal, N. (1964). Seminars. Haematol., 1, 3.

Osserman, E. F. & Takatsuki, K. (1965). Series Haematol. Suppl., Scand. J. Haematol., 4, 28.

Otaki, A., Read, A. E., Stubbs, J. & Sculthorpe, H. (1960). Brit. med. J., ii, 256.

Owen, R. D. (1945). Science, 102, 400.

Owen, J. A., Pitney, W. R. & O'Dea, J. F. (1959). Br. J. clin. Path., 12, 344.

Ozer, F. J. & Chaplin, H. (1963). J. clin. Invest., 42, 1735.

Pain, R. H. (1963). Biochem. J., 88, 234.

Paterson, P. Y. (1965). In "Immunological Diseases". Ed. Samter, M. Little Brown & Co., Boston. p. 788.

Perillie, P. E. & Conn, H. O. (1958). J. Am. med. Ass., 167, 2186.

Perkins, W. H., Doherty, J. E. & Towbin, E. J. (1959). Clin. Res., 7, 133.

Perlmann, P. & Broberger, O. (1963). J. exp. Med., 117, 717.

Perlmann, P., Hammarstrom, S., Lagercrantz, R. & Gustafsson, B. E. (1965). Ann. N.Y. Acad. Sci., 124, 337.

Peterson, R. D., Cooper, M. D. & Good, R. A. (1965). Am. J. Med., 38, 579.

Porter, R. R. (1959). Biochem. J., 73, 119.

Porter, R. R. (1962). In "Basic Problems in Neo-plastic Disease". Eds. Gellhorn, A. & Hirschberg, E. Columbia University Press, New York. p. 177.

Potter, M. & Boyce, C. R. (1962). Nature, 193, 1086.

Potter, M., Fahey, J. L. & Pilgrim, I. (1957). Proc. Soc. exp. Biol. Med., 94, 327.

Potter, M. & Robertson, C. L. (1960). J. Natn. Cancer Inst., 25, 847.

Prahl, J. W. (1967). Nature, 215, 1386.

Putnam, F. W. (1957). Physiol Rev., 37, 512.

Putnam, F. W. & Hardy, S. (1955). J. biol. Chem., 212, 361.

Putnam, F. W., Meyer, F. & Miyaki, A. (1956). J. biol. Chem., 221, 517.

Rask-Nielsen, R. (1956). J. Natn. Cancer Inst., 16, 1137.

Rask-Nielsen, R. Gormsen, H. & Clausen, J. (1959). J. Natn. Cancer Inst., 22, 509.

Rowe, D. S. & Fahey, J. L. (1965). J. exp. Med., 121, 185.

Rowe, D. S. & McGregor, I. A. (1968). J. clin. exp. Immunol. (In press.)

Rundles, R. W., Coonrad, E. V. & Arends, T. (1954). Am. J. Med., 16, 842.

Samter, M. (1965). "Immunological Diseases". Little Brown, Boston.

Sanchez, L. M. & Domz, C. A. (1960). Ann. intern. Med., 52, 44.

SCHARFF, M. D. & UHR, J. W. (1965). *Seminars Haematol.*, **2**, 47.

SCHULTZE, H. E. & HEREMANS, J. F. (1966). "Molecular Biology of Human Proteins". Vol. 1. Elsevier, Amsterdam.

SELIGMANN, M. (1966). *Acta med. Scand.*, **179**, Suppl. 445, 140.

SIROTA, J. H. & HAMMERMAN, D. J. (1954). *Am. J. Med.*, **16**, 138.

SMALL, P. A., KEHN, J. E. & LAMM, M. E. (1963). *Science*, **142**, 393.

SNAPPER, I., TURNER, L. B. & MOSCOVITZ, H. L. (1953). "Multiple Myeloma". Grune & Stratton, New York.

SOLOMON, A. & FAHEY, J. L. (1964). *Am. J. Med.*, **37**, 206.

SOLOMON, A., WALDMANN, T. A. & FAHEY, J. L. (1963). *J. Lab. clin. Med.*, **62**, 1.

SOLOMON, A., WALDMANN, T. A., FAHEY, J. L. & MCFARLANE, A. S. (1964). *J. clin. Invest.*, **43**, 103.

SOOTHILL, J. F., HAYES, K. & DUDGEON, J. A. (1966). *Lancet*, **1**, 1385.

STANWORTH, D. R., HUMPHREY, J. H., BENNICH, H. & JOHANSSON, S. G. O. (1967). *Lancet*, **2**, 330.

STEIN, E. R. & FUDENBERG, H. H. (1966). *Pediatrics*, **37**, 715.

SUNDERMAN, F. W. (1964). *Am. J. clin. Path.*, **42**, 1.

TAYLOR, K. B. (1965). *Gastroenterology*, **24**, 23.

TAYLOR, K. B., ROITT, I. M., DONIACH, D., COUCHMAN, K. G. & SHAPLAND, C. (1962). *Br. med. J.*, **2**, 1347.

TERRY, W. D. (1964). *Proc. Soc. exp. Biol. Med.*, **117**, 901.

TERRY, W. D. & FAHEY, J. L. (1964). *Science*, **146**, 400.

TISCHENDORFF, W. & HARTMANN, F. (1950). *Acta Haematol.*, **4**, 374.

TISELIUS, A. & KABAT, E. A. (1939). *J. exp. Med.*, **69**, 119.

TURNER, M. W. & ROWE, D. S. (1964). *Immunology*, **7**, 639.

UEHLINGER, E. (1949). *Helvet. med. Acta*, **16**, 508.

UTSUMI, S. & KARUSH, F. (1965). *Biochemistry*, **4**, 1766.

VAERMAN, J. P., JOHNSON, L. B., MANDY, W. & FUDENBERG, H. H. (1965). *J. Lab. clin. Med.*, **65**, 18.

VAN LOGHEM, J. J., PECTOOM, E., VAN DER HART, M., VAN DER VEER, M., VAN DER GIESSEN, M., PRINS, H. K., ZUCHER, C. & ENGELFRIEL, C. P. (1963). *Vox Sanguin.*, **8**, 33.

VOLPÉ, R., BRUCE-ROBERTSON, A., FLETCHER, A. A. & CHARLES, W. B. (1956). *Am. J. Med.*, **20**, 533.

WALDENSTRÖM, J. (1942). *Acta chir. Scand.*, **87**, 365.

WALDENSTRÖM, J. (1961a). *Acta med. Scand.*, **170**, Suppl. 376, 110.

WALDENSTRÖM, J. (1961b). *Harvey Lect.*, **56**, 211.

WALDENSTRÖM, J. (1962a). *Prog. Allergy*, **6**, 320.

WALDENSTRÖM, J. (1962b). *Prog. Haematol.*, **3**, 266.

WALDENSTRÖM, J. (1965). *Adv. Metab. Dis.*, **2**, 116.

WALLER, M. V. & VAUGHAN, J. H. (1956). *Proc. Soc. exp. Biol. Med.*, **92**, 198.

WALLERSTEIN, R. S. (1951). *Am. J. Med.*, **10**, 325.

WATSON, C. J. & LERNER, A. B. (1947). *Acta med. Scand.*, **128**, Suppl. 196, p. 489.

WHIPPLE, H. E. (1965). Symposium on Autoimmunity in Disease. *Ann. N. Y. Acad. Sci.*, **124**, 1.

WIENER, A. S., GORDON, E. B. & GALLOP, C. (1953). *J. Immun.*, **71**, 58.

WIENER, W. & VOS, G. H. (1963). *Blood*, **22**, 606.

WINTROBE, M. M. & BUELL, M. V. (1933). *Bull. Johns Hopkins Hosp.*, **52**, 156.

WOLLHEIM, F. A. & WILLIAMS, R. C. (1966). *New England J. Med.*, **274**, 61.

WORLLEDGE, S. M. (1965). In "Autoimmunity". Eds. Baldwin, R. W. & Humphrey, J. H. Blackwell, Oxford, p. 52.

ZETTERVALL, O., SJÖQUIST, J., WALDENSTRÖM, J. & WINBLAD, S. (1966). *Clin. exp. Immunol.*, **1**, 213.

ZIMMERMAN, H. H. & HALL, W. H. (1954). *Ann. Int. Med.*, **41**, 1152.

Chapter 16

SOME ABNORMALITIES OF AMINO ACID METABOLISM

by

M. D. MILNE

Westminster Medical School, London

AMINO-ACIDURIA

THE term "amino-aciduria" is nowadays used in chemical pathology to describe any situation where one or more free amino acids are encountered in the urine in larger amounts than usually occur among normal individuals. Clearly the extent and significance of such conditions can only be assessed against a background knowledge of the quantities of these substances excreted by normal healthy subjects.

Amino Acids in Normal Urine

The normal adult excretes about 1·1 g. of free amino acids daily in the urine (Stein, 1953). This represents about 180 mg. of nitrogen, which is about 1·2% of the total nitrogen excreted. It corresponds to about 120 mg. of α-amino nitrogen. A further 2 g. of amino acids are excreted in conjugated form (Stein, 1953), and these are liberated after acid hydrolysis. These are only average figures, and there is much variation between individuals.

An approach to the analysis of the particular amino acids that go to make up these quantities is possible by three main methods: microbiological assay using organisms dependent for their growth on the particular amino acid to be estimated; two-dimensional partition chromatography on filter paper; elution chromatography from columns of ion-exchange resins. A few individual amino acids may also be determined in urine by specific chemical methods.

Microbiological assay is not possible for a number of the amino acids present in urine because appropriate micro-organisms are not available. Furthermore, the determination of free amino acids by this method may on occasion be equivocal, because many amino acids are present in combined forms, the microbiological availabilities of which are not known.

Two-dimensional chromatography on filter paper has the advantage of simplicity and speed. The chief disadvantage is that it is at best only semi-quantitative. This method does, however, provide a reliable approach to the detection of most of the major abnormalities of amino acid

excretion encountered in clinical medicine. It indicates qualitative disturbances in the pattern of amino acid excretion, and draws attention to any unusual amino acids which may be present in abnormal amounts.

Elution chromatography from ion-exchange resins as developed by Moore & Stein (1951, 1954) probably represents the most satisfactory analytical method yet available. Its main drawback is the elaborate nature of the system required.

For the isolation and subsequent characterization of individual amino acids from urine the method of displacement chromatography from ion-exchange resins has proved of considerable value (Westall, 1952, 1955).

Many studies in recent years using a variety of these methods have made it clear that the amino acid content of normal urine is very complex. Typical figures for the free amino acids in 24 hr. urine specimens of normal adult males are given in Table 16.1. They are largely derived from the results of Stein (1953). They were all determined by elution chromatography from the ion-exchange resin Dowex 50, with the exception of the glutamine value for which this method is unsatisfactory. Even such an analysis as this is probably incomplete, because amino acids excreted at levels below 5–10 mg./day may well not have been detected. Westall (1955), for example, has demonstrated the presence of at least seven unknown acid-stable ninhydrin-reacting amphoteric substances excreted in amounts of probably less than 10 mg./day in normal human urine. It is interesting to note that already two new amino acids, β-amino*iso*butyric acid (Crumpler, Dent, Harris & Westall, 1951), and 3-methylhistidine (Tallan, Stein & Moore, 1954), have been discovered by studies on normal human urine (Fig. 16.1).

Side by side with the average values of the urinary amino acids in Table 16.1 are given data obtained by Stein & Moore (1954), using similar methods, for the plasma levels of individual amino acids. It is evident that the relative proportions of various amino acids in the two fluids are very different. Estimates of renal

TABLE 16.1

Amino acids in normal urine and plasma
(*Based on data of Stein, 1953; Stein, Bearn & Moore, 1954; Stein & Moore, 1954;
Evered, 1954; Archibald, 1944*)

| | Urine (mg./24 hr.) | | Plasma (mg./100 ml.) |
	Range	Average value	Average value (post absorptive)
Aspartic acid	—	< 10	0·03
Asparagine	30–90	54	0·58
Glutamic acid	—	< 10	0·70
Glutamine	—	100	8·30
Glycine	70–200	132	1·54
Alanine	20–70	46	3·41
Aminobutyric acid	—	< 10	0·30
Valine	—	< 10	2·88
Leucine	10–25	14	1·69
Isoleucine	10–30	18	0·89
Serine	25–75	43	1·12
Threonine	15–50	28	1·39
Cysteine and cystine	10–20	10	1·18
Methionine	—	< 10	0·38
Taurine	85–300	156	0·55
Proline	—	< 10	2·36
Phenylalanine	10–30	18	0·84
Tyrosine	15–50	35	1·03
Tryptophan	—	—	1·11
Histidine	110–320	216	1·15
1-Methylhistidine	50–210	180	0·11
3-Methylhistidine	—	50	0·08
Ornithine	—	< 10	0·72
Lysine	10–50	19	2·72
Arginine	—	< 10	1·51
Citrulline	—	< 10	0·50
β-Aminoisobutyric acid β-Alanine	4–180	20	0·20

clearances suggest that these are of the order of 0·5–2·5 ml./min. for most amino acids.

Cusworth & Dent (1960) have reinvestigated amino acid excretion and clearance both in normal subjects and in diseases with aminoaciduria. The essential amino acids are almost completely reabsorbed from the glomerular filtrate. Glycine and histidine have relatively high renal clearances, as only 95 to 98% of the filtered glycine is reabsorbed by the tubules and 90 to 95% of histidine. Although the clearance of histidine is higher than that of glycine, normal urine contains more glycine because of higher plasma values. Some amino acids and related ninhydrin-reacting compounds are excreted at clearances approximating to that of inulin, e.g. argininosuccinnic acid, cystathionine, phosphoethanolamine, β-aminoisobutyric acid, and 1- and 3-methyl-histidines. These "non-threshold" ninhydrin-reacting substances may be regarded either as waste products of nitrogen metabolism or as metabolic intermediates which normally occur intracellularly and are only found in plasma and extracellular fluid in disease. Jagenburg (1959) has investigated the effects of diet on amino acid excretion in more detail. A high protein intake considerably increased the output both in children and adults. In infants the type of milk protein fed had no effect, but bottle-fed infants consumed more protein than those breast-fed with a corresponding rise of urinary amino acids. Adult males and females excrete the same amount of total amino acid in relation to body weight or total urinary nitrogen output. The

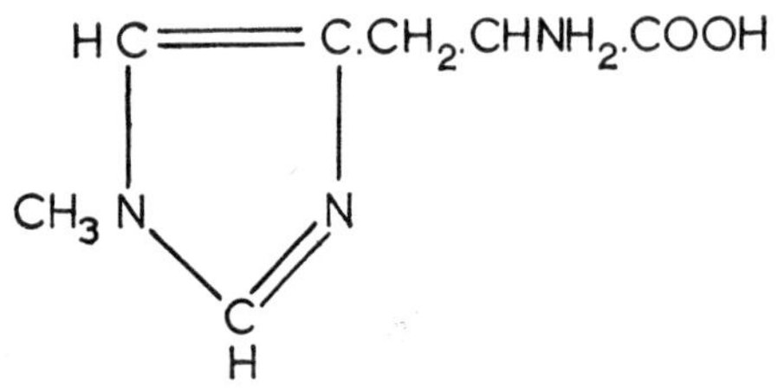

$$HC = C.CH_2.CHNH_2.COOH$$

$$CH_3 \, N \qquad\qquad N$$

$$C$$
$$H$$

3-methylhistidine

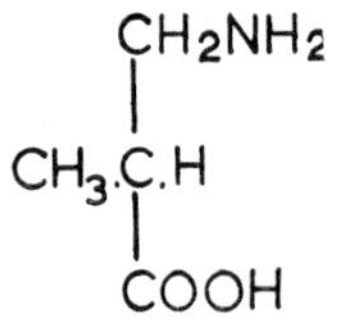

$$CH_2NH_2$$
$$CH_3.C.H$$
$$COOH$$

β-amino*iso*butyric acid

FIG. 16.1. 3-methylhistidine and β-amino*iso*butyric acid.

urinary amino-nitrogen/creatinine ratio is lower in men than in women whether creatinine alone is used as the reference compound or whether creatinine *plus* creatine is used.

After acid hydrolysis there is a considerable liberation of glycine, glutamic acid and aspartic acid from conjugates (Stein, 1953; Eckhardt & Davidson, 1949). About 70% of the extra glycine can be accounted for as coming from hippuric acid, which is excreted in quantities of 1·0–2·5 g./day (Stein, Paladini, Hirs & Moore, 1954). The source of the rest is not yet known. The increase in glutamic and aspartic acids, which are hardly present at all in the free state, cannot be accounted for in terms of the glutamine and asparagine known to be present. About 50% of the glutamic acid is, however, derived from phenylacetyl-glutamine which is normally excreted in amounts of 0·25–0·5 g./day (Stein *et al.*, 1954).

Many other amino acids are also liberated after acid hydrolysis, though in smaller amounts (Stein, 1953; Eckhardt *et al.*, 1949; Ling, 1955). The nature of the conjugated forms from which they are derived is not in general known, though Westall (1955) has demonstrated the presence of a number of small peptides in normal urine.

There are considerable variations in the amounts of particular amino acids excreted by different normal individuals, and by the same individual from day to day (Steele, Reynolds & Baumann, 1950; Berry, 1953). The causes of this variation are not entirely understood, and

evidently differ from amino acid to amino acid. It is known, however, that differences in diet, genetical differences between individual people, and physiological changes such as pregnancy may contribute to such variations.

In general, it has been found that neither the total quantity nor the distribution of the amino acids in normal urine can be correlated closely with the dietary intake of protein (Steele *et al.*, 1950; Stein, Bearn & Moore, 1954). Ten- to 15-fold increases in the dietary protein give rise in most cases to no more than a two- or three-fold increase in the excretion of individual amino acids. The one exception to this is 1-methylhistidine. The excretion of this substance is closely related to the amount of meat in the diet (Datta & Harris, 1951), and it is probable that it is largely derived from the dipeptide anserine often present in quite large quantities in muscle. However, apart from 1-methylhistidine, it is clear that the variations encountered between different individuals in amount and pattern of amino acid excretion are greater than can be accounted for in terms of dietary differences (Steele *et al.*, 1950).

The excretion of β-amino*iso*butyric acid appears under ordinary conditions to be little influenced by ordinary dietary variations, though it has been found that complete fasting for 2 to 3 days may lead to an increased excretion (Sandler & Pare, 1954). Large differences in excretion are observed between different individuals on similar diets, and these appear in the main to be genetically determined (Crumpler *et al.*, 1951; Harris, 1953). About 5 to 10% of white subjects excrete from 50 to 200 mg. of this amino acid daily, whereas most individuals excrete only trace amounts. High excretions are especially common in Polynesians and Micronesians in the Marshall Isles (Blumberg & Gartler, 1959), where an incidence of up to 80% of the population occurs. Experiments in rats, both *in vivo* and by the tissue slice technique (Fink, 1956; Fink, Cline, Henderson and Fink, 1956; Fink, McCaughy, Cline & Fink, 1956), suggest that the amino acid is derived from thymine (Fig. 16.2).

Thymine ⇌ DHT ⇌ BUIB → BAIB
where DHT = dihydrothymine,
       BUIB = β-ureido*iso*butyric acid,
       BAIB = β-amino*iso*butyric acid.

Gartler (1959) considers that thymine is the only significant source of the amino acid in man.

The difference between excretors and non-excretors is only present at low levels of thymine, dihydrothymine and β-ureido*iso*butyric acid intake. This argues against a difference in the

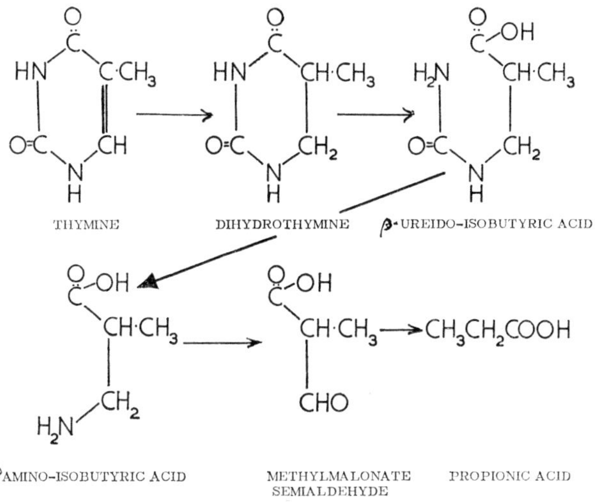

THYMINE   DIHYDROTHYMINE   β-UREIDO-ISOBUTYRIC ACID

β-AMINO-ISOBUTYRIC ACID   METHYLMALONATE SEMIALDEHYDE   PROPIONIC ACID

FIG. 16.2. Metabolic pathways in the production of β-amino*iso*butyric acid from thymine. The probable cause of the anomaly of excess excretion of β-amino*iso*butyric acid is absence or deficiency of the oxidase converting this amino acid to methylmalonate semialdehyde.

clearance of the amino acid in excretors and non-excretors. Probably there is a block in excretors in the further degradation of β-amino*iso*butyric acid to methylmalonate semialdehyde or to *iso*butyric acid itself.

During pregnancy there is an increase in the excretion of several urinary amino acids, histidine and threonine being the ones most markedly affected (Wallraff, Brodie & Borden, 1950). Threonine increases steadily throughout gestation, whereas histidine reaches a maximum at about 4 months and thereafter remains at more or less the same level till term (Ruttinger, Miller, Andrecovitz & Perdue, 1954). During lactation the excretion levels fall rapidly, often to values below those found in the non-pregnant state.

Dustan, Moore & Bigwood (1955) studied the physiological amino-aciduria of full term and premature infants. The plasma levels of amino acids were identical with those of the adult, but glycine, alanine, threonine, serine, asparagine, glutamine, cystine, glutamic acid and proline were present in excess amounts in the urine. Output of the basic amino acids was not increased. Presumably, the amino-aciduria of infants is due to incomplete maturation of transport mechanisms involved in amino acid reabsorption from the glomerular filtrate.

Amino-aciduria in Pathological States

During the last few years the widespread application of paper chromatography to the study of urinary amino acids has brought to light the occurrence of grossly abnormal amino acid excretion in certain conditions in which a disorder of amino acid metabolism had not previously been suspected. It is probable that further examples of such conditions remain to be discovered. Furthermore, abnormal amino acid excretion can only be assessed against the still incomplete background of what is known about the excretion of these compounds in normal individuals. It is likely that so far only gross deviations from the normal pattern of excretion have been detected, and that more subtle disturbances will become apparent only when a comprehensive picture of normal excretion and its variations has been obtained.

It is useful to classify amino-acidurias into two main groups: the "overflow" amino-acidurias, and the "renal" amino-acidurias (Dent, 1950, 1954*a*). The "overflow" amino-acidurias arise because there is some defect in intermediary metabolism leading to an increase in the plasma levels of one or more amino acids, to such a degree that the normal renal tubular reabsorptive mechanism is unable to deal with them adequately, and they therefore pass in increased quantities into the urine. The "renal" amino-acidurias are due to some defect in the processes of renal tubular reabsorption, so that even at normal plasma concentrations, and hence normal concentrations in the glomerular filtrate, inefficient reabsorption of one or more amino acids takes place, and so abnormal amounts are found in the urine. The particular amino acids occurring in excess in the urine will depend in the "overflow" type on the specific character of the disturbance in intermediary metabolism, and in the "renal" type on the particular way in which the renal tubules are defective. Mixed types of amino-aciduria have now been recognized (Milne, 1964). In these cases the basic abnormality is a metabolic defect causing an increase of a single amino acid, and therefore a corresponding rise in the glomerular filtrate and the tubular lumen. Increased proximal tubular reabsorption of this amino acid may saturate a transport system shared by a group of amino acids. There is thus an "overflow" amino-aciduria of the amino acid involved in the metabolic block and a "renal" amino-aciduria of the other members of the transport group.

In general, a differentiation between the types of amino-aciduria may be obtained by a consideration of the plasma concentrations of the particular amino acids excreted in excess. More precise information is, however, obtained by detailed clearance studies, preferably at different plasma amino acid concentrations (Dent, 1954b). In practice this is often difficult to achieve, but it becomes critical in cases where there is any doubt as to the mechanism involved, or where it is thought that both mechanisms are operating.

Most examples of pathological amino-aciduria are due either to hereditary disease or to the effects of nephrotoxic drugs or poisons. An hereditary disease could conceivably cause an amino-aciduria by six different mechanisms, five of which are actually known to occur (Mudge, 1958).

(1) There may be a metabolic disorder causing an increase of plasma level of one or several amino acids with an amino-aciduria of a pure "overflow" type. It is useful to subdivide this type according to the clearance of the affected amino acid, i.e. whether of the "threshold" or "non-threshold" group. Examples of the "threshold" type include phenylketonuria—phenylalanine in excess; maple-syrup urine disease—leucine, isoleucine and valine in excess; histidinuria—histidine in excess; and citrullinuria—citrulline in excess. The "non-threshold" group includes cystathioninuria—cystathionine in excess; hypophosphatasia—phosphoethanolamine in excess; and argininosuccinic aciduria—argininosuccinic acid in excess.

(2) The excess excretion of a single amino acid from increase of its plasma level could saturate a specific proximal tubular transport system, and thus cause a secondary amino-aciduria of the renal type. The best example is hereditary prolinuria (Scriber, Shafer & Efron, 1961), where

increase of plasma proline causes excess urinary proline which saturates the tubular reabsorption mechanism for proline, hydroxyproline and glycine. Thus, the urine contains abnormal amounts of all three amino acids. An analogous situation can easily be produced experimentally by intravenous infusions of proline or hydroxyproline (Scriber et al., 1961). Similarly, infusions of lysine (Robson & Rose, 1957), or of arginine (Ruszkowski, Baertl & Gabuzda, 1960), will saturate reabsorptive mechanisms for dibasic amino acids with the temporary production of an amino-aciduria of a pattern similar to that found in cystinuria. Probably, hereditary citrullinuria is strictly an example of this type of amino-aciduria, as there is also excess excretion of alanine, aspartic acid, glycine, histidine and serine, without any rise of plasma levels of these amino acids (McMurray & Mohyuddin, 1962).

(3a) There might be a specific hereditary defect of an amino acid transport system confined to the proximal renal tubules. No certain example of this type is known, and in fact it seems that amino acid transport mechanisms in the tubules are very similar to those in the jejunum.

(3b) There is a specific amino acid transport defect in the proximal renal tubules, and also elsewhere in the body. The two examples are cystinuria involving dibasic amino acids and Hartnup disease involving many mono-amino mono-carboxylic amino acids, with the notable exceptions of proline, hydroxyproline and glycine. In these diseases there is a dual transport defect in the proximal renal tubules and the jejunal cells of groups of amino acids sharing a common transport system. There is no proof that the abnormality is also present in other body organs or cells.

(4) There is a known or unknown metabolic abnormality which causes generalized and non-specific proximal tubular damage. Typical examples are the Lignac-Fanconi syndrome, adult Fanconi syndrome and Lowe's syndrome. In these conditions there are many other proximal tubular defects besides amino-aciduria, e.g. renal glycossuria, increased phosphate and uric acid clearances, reduced capacity to secrete organic acids as shown by lower Tm_{PAH}, and a mild proteinuria, especially globulinuria. This is unlike the isolated proximal tubular defects of cystinuria and Hartnup disease, where the amino-aciduria is the sole abnormality of renal function. In addition, the amino-aciduria is less specific and less constant in pattern. There are differences in detail in different patients, and amino acids thought to be reabsorbed by different transport mechanisms,

e.g. the dibasic amino acids in one group and many of the mono-amino mono-carboxylic acids in another, are excreted together in the same patient.

(5) There is a metabolic disorder resulting in overproduction of metabolites which are directly nephrotoxic. Typical examples are the amino-aciduria of galactosaemia, where excess galactose-1-phosphate within proximal tubular cells is probably the toxic substance, and hepato-lenticular degeneration where evidence is accumulating that deposits of copper within tubular cells directly interfere with transport mechanisms. In this type there is again generalized tubular damage with effects on transport of other substances besides amino acids, but the renal

lesion is not an essential part of the disease, and, as in galactosaemia, may only occur during exacerbations, or before effective therapy has been arranged.

In all these conditions the main features of the abnormality in amino acid excretion can be readily identified by means of paper chromatography. This is certainly the method of choice in routine chemical pathology for the detection of amino-aciduria. A full account of the technique as applied to urine and plasma has been given by Dent (1951).

Figs. 16.3 and 16.4 and 16.9–16.14 illustrate diagrammatically the kind of chromatograms obtained when urines from normal people and from patients with some of these disorders are

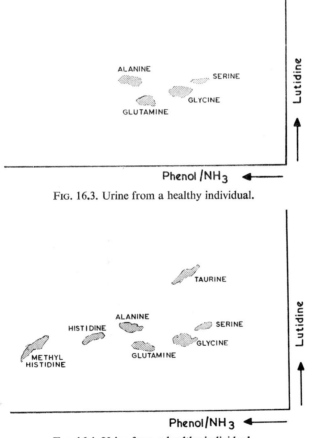

FIG. 16.3. Urine from a healthy individual.

FIG. 16.4. Urine from a healthy individual.

FIGS. 16.3 and 16.4 are diagrams of amino acid chromatograms of urine from normal individuals. In each case the equivalent of a two-second sample of urine was chromatographed and the completed chromatograms developed with ninhydrin. The urine samples had been treated with H_2O_2 in order to oxidize any S-containing amino acids present.

examined by this method. It will be seen that in certain cases the abnormality is confined to a single amino acid or to a small group of particular amino acids. Thus in phenylketonuria, phenylalanine is the only amino acid excreted abnormally, and all the many other amino acids are present in their normal amounts. Similarly, in cystinuria the defect is confined to cystine, lysine, arginine and ornithine. On the other hand, in other disorders a large number of different amino acids may be found in excess in the urine. Such a situation is often referred to as a "generalized" amino-aciduria, and is found for example in Wilson's disease, the Fanconi syndrome and lead poisoning. However, it must be borne in mind that even among these so-called "generalized" amino-acidurias specific differences may be found in the qualitative pattern of amino acid excretion from condition to condition. For example, histidine is often found in large amounts in the urine of patients with Wilson's disease, but is very much less prominent in the Fanconi syndrome, though in other respects the amino-aciduria occurring in these two disorders is very similar. The gross amino-aciduria found in the Hartnup syndrome is peculiar, in that proline excretion is quite normal, whereas in the Fanconi syndrome and in Wilson's disease large amounts of proline are frequently found in the urine. β-amino*iso*butyric acid excretion is particularly prominent in lead poisoning but not in most of the other conditions listed.

These qualitative differences in pattern can usually be detected by paper chromatography, and are likely to be of some diagnostic significance. When they can be placed on a more quantitative basis their importance in this respect is even greater.

Amino Acid Transport Mechanisms

The pattern of amino acid excretion in disease has been considerably elucidated by increased knowledge of amino acid transport. All amino acids derived from protein are actively transported by the jejunum and proximal cells, as well as by many other cells and tissues. There are obviously three alternatives:

(*a*) All amino acids could be transported as a single large group;

(*b*) Each amino acid could have its own specific transport group;

(*c*) Various groups of amino acids could share a transport system which is specific only for the particular amino acids involved.

There is now clear evidence that the last alternative is the one which actually occurs and that probably five separate transport groups exist. These are:

(1) A large group of neutral amino acids. Transport of this group is defective in Hartnup disease (Baron *et al.*, 1956);

(2) The dibasic amino acids lysine, ornithine, arginine and cystine. Transport in this group is deficient in cystinuria (Dent & Rose, 1951).

(3) The imino-glycine group consisting of proline, hydroxyproline and glycine. Transport in this group is deficient in prolinuria.

(4) The diacidic amino acids aspartic and glutamic acids. No human disease is known where transport of these amino acids is specifically altered.

(5) β-amino acids involved in the very rare condition of β-amino-aciduria (Scriver *et al.*, 1966).

GROUP I. TRUE DISORDERS OF AMINO ACID METABOLISM
AMINO ACID EXCRETION IN LIVER DISEASE

The liver plays a key role in the deamination of amino acids and in the regulation of their plasma levels. It might therefore be expected that disorders of the liver would lead to abnormal elevation of plasma amino acid levels and hence to amino-aciduria. However, the liver possesses a considerable reserve of function in this respect, and in practice gross amino-aciduria is encountered only in cases of massive liver necrosis or very advanced hepatic cirrhosis (Dent, 1946; Walshe, 1953). With less severe forms of liver damage, amino-aciduria is a much less marked finding, though it undoubtedly occurs to some extent in a proportion of the patients (Dunn, Akawaie, Yeh & Martin, 1950; Gabuzda, Eckhardt & Davidson, 1952; Walshe, 1953). Walshe (1953), who has made a detailed study by paper chromatography of urines from 119 patients with all forms of liver disease, considers that the extent of the amino-aciduria runs roughly parallel with the degree of underlying liver damage both in the same patient and from patient to patient.

In comatose patients with acute hepatic necrosis there is an appreciable increase in the plasma levels of all the amino acids normally present, and associated with this is a very generalized gross amino-aciduria. In most, but not all, cases of this sort the appearance of the gross amino-aciduria heralds a fatal outcome. In hepatic coma due to advanced progressive cirrhosis of the liver, similar findings are obtained, but in lesser degree.

In cirrhosis of the liver Walshe (1953) emphasizes the variation in pattern of amino acid excretion from patient to patient and in the same patient at different stages of the illness. Some increase in the output of most of the urinary amino acids may be detected in different cases, but cystine, β-amino*iso*butyric acid, and the amine, ethanolamine, are most frequently involved and appear to give the most sensitive indication of liver damage.

In acute infectious hepatitis about one-third of the patients show a moderate amino-aciduria in the early stages of the illness, and another third give borderline values (Hsia & Gellis, 1954). When amino-aciduria is found, the plasma *a*-amino nitrogen is raised.

No major abnormalities in amino acid excretion have been detected in patients with "inactive" cirrhosis, obstructive jaundice, secondary carcinoma of the liver, or infiltrations of the liver (Walshe, 1953).

Diseases Due to a Metabolic Block in Amino Acid Catabolism

In the second edition of this book only six examples of this class of disease were described, i.e. phenylketonuria, maple syrup urine disease, histidinaemia, cystathioninuria, citrullinuria and argininosuccinuria. In the last few years numerous other examples have been recognized. Many of these are extremely rare, but are disproportionately important in view of the specificity of a metabolic disorder produced by lack of a single enzyme. Mental deficiency is by far the most common clinical manifestation, emphasizing the susceptibility of the developing brain to major abnormalities of the biochemical environment.

DEFECTS IN METABOLISM OF AROMATIC AMINO ACIDS

These include phenylketonuria, tyrosinaemia, and alkaptonuria. Phenylketonuria is especially important as it is the most common of all the innate disorders of amino acid metabolism and is the disorder in which the greatest experience of dietary therapy has been accumulated.

PHENYLKETONURIA

Phenylketonuria was first recognized by Fölling (1934*a, b*) who demonstrated the presence of large amounts of phenylpyruvic acid in the urine of several mentally deficient patients. The presence of phenylpyruvic acid in these quantities (0·5–2 g./day) may be readily shown by the addition of a few drops of 5% $FeCl_3$ solution to the urine. A deep bluish-green colour develops which slowly fades over the next few minutes.

All individuals who have so far been found to excrete phenylpyruvic acid continuously in their urine have shown a greater or lesser degree of intellectual impairment. Generally this has been severe, amounting to idiocy or imbecility, but occasionally higher-grade feeble-minded individuals have been encountered. About 2% of untreated phenylketonurics have intelligence quotients between 60 and 100% of the average normal (Jervis, 1954; Hsia, Knox, Quinn & Paine, 1958), and therefore can be classified as dull and backward rather than as imbeciles or idiots. The addition of $FeCl_3$ is nowadays a routine procedure in urine examinations for ordinary clinical purposes, and it is likely that if phenylketonuria in the absence of mental defect occurred it would have been discovered in this way.

Neurologically, phenylketonurics show no paralysis and no increase in muscular tone, but a constant and peculiar feature is a marked accentuation of all the reflexes, both superficial and deep. There is also a slight reduction in stature and in head measurements as compared with the normal averages of the same age and sex. The other peculiar feature of this condition is a slight dilution of the hair and skin pigmentation (Fölling, Mohr & Ruud, 1945; Cowie & Penrose, 1951).

The condition accounts for about 0·5 to 1% of all patients in mental-deficiency hospitals, and has a frequency in the general population of between 1 in 25,000 and 1 in 50,000. It is inherited as a typical mendelian recessive character (Penrose, 1935; Jervis, 1937; Fölling, Mohr & Ruud, 1945). Heterozygotes though clinically normal may be detected by the phenylalanine tolerance test (Hsia, Driscoll, Troll & Knox, 1956).

Biochemical findings in phenylketonuria. (1) *The urine.* Although phenylpyruvic acid was the first abnormal metabolite to be found in the urine of these patients, and therefore became incorporated in the nomenclature, it is now known that a number of other substances are also present in abnormal quantities.

Quantitatively the most important of these are phenyllactic acid, phenylacetylglutamine and phenylalanine (Fölling, Closs & Gammes, 1938; Dann, Marples & Levine, 1943; Jervis, 1950; Woolf, 1951; Stein, Bearn & Moore, 1954). Phenyllactic acid and phenylacetylglutamine are, like phenylpyruvic acid, excreted in amounts of 0·5–2·0 g./day, while the phenylalanine excretion is about 0·2–0·4 g./day.

Appreciable quantities of *p*-hydroxyphenyl-acetic acid, *p*-hydroxyphenyllactic acid and *o*-hydroxyphenylacetic acid also occur in the urine of these patients (Boscott & Bickel, 1953).

A number of indole compounds, derived from tryptophan, are also found in increased quantities in the urine of phenylketonuric patients (Armstrong & Robinson, 1954). These include indolelactic acid, indoleacetic acid and indican (Bessman & Tada, 1960). They have been shown to be derived from excess bacterial degradation of tryptophan within the colon (Yarbro & Anderson, 1966). Increased levels of phenylalanine in body fluids acts as a competitive inhibitor of jejunal absorption of neutral amino acids, including tryptophan. A greater proportion of ingested amino acids is, therefore, unabsorbed and degraded by colonic bacteria.

(2) *The Blood.* The blood plasma shows a very high level of free phenylalanine. The normal content of phenylalanine in plasma is about 1 mg./100 ml. In phenylketonuria values ranging from 15 mg./100 ml. to 60 mg. have been reported (Jervis, Block, Bolling & Kanze, 1940; Borek, Brecher, Jervis & Waelsch, 1950; Stein, Bearn & Moore, 1954; Armstrong & Tyler, 1955).

The other amino acids present in plasma occur in normal amounts. There is also a slight increase in phenylpyruvic acid in the plasma (Jervis, 1952), but no other abnormal constituents have been found.

(3) *The cerebrospinal fluid.* Phenylalanine is present in considerably increased amounts, but other amino acids are not abnormal. The concentration of phenylalanine is of the order of 7 mg./100 ml. (Borek *et al.*, 1950), and this represents an increase over the normal values of the same order of magnitude as that observed in blood.

(4) *The tissue proteins.* No peculiarity in the tissue proteins has been found. Block, Jervis, Bolling & Webb (1940) prepared proteins from sera, erythrocytes, brain, liver and kidney of normal individuals and from phenylketonurics, and analysed them for a number of amino acids including phenylalanine, tyrosine and tryptophan. No significant differences were detected.

Thus, biochemically the outstanding feature of phenylketonuria is the high level of phenylalanine in the blood, cerebrospinal fluid, and urine of the affected individuals. This is associated with the occurrence of phenylpyruvic acid, phenyllactic acid and phenylacetylglutamine in grossly abnormal amounts in the urine, and also some phenolic acids and indole derivatives. It is evident that the disorder represents a severe disturbance of phenylalanine metabolism.

The normal metabolism o, phenylalanine. Phenylalanine is an essential amino acid. Rose, Haines, Johnson & Warner (1943) showed that in man it is an indispensable dietary constituent, and that its omission from the diet is followed by a pronounced negative nitrogen balance. The body has no capacity to synthesize the benzene ring, which is mainly supplied in the diet by the aromatic amino acids phenylalanine and tyrosine. Tyrosine, however, is not essential (Rose *et al.*, 1943), though it may become a limiting factor for growth and nutrition if the diet does not contain enough phenylalanine. This indicates that while tyrosine can be formed from phenylalanine, the formation of phenylalanine from tyrosine is not possible.

This irreversible conversion of phenylalanine to tyrosine (Fig. 16.5) is now generally believed to be the first step in the oxidation of phenylalanine, derived either from proteins taken in the diet or from the breakdown of tissue proteins. There is much evidence to indicate that this reaction has a central place in phenylalanine metabolism. Moss & Schoenheimer (1940), for example, prepared DL-deuterophenylalanine, in which most of the

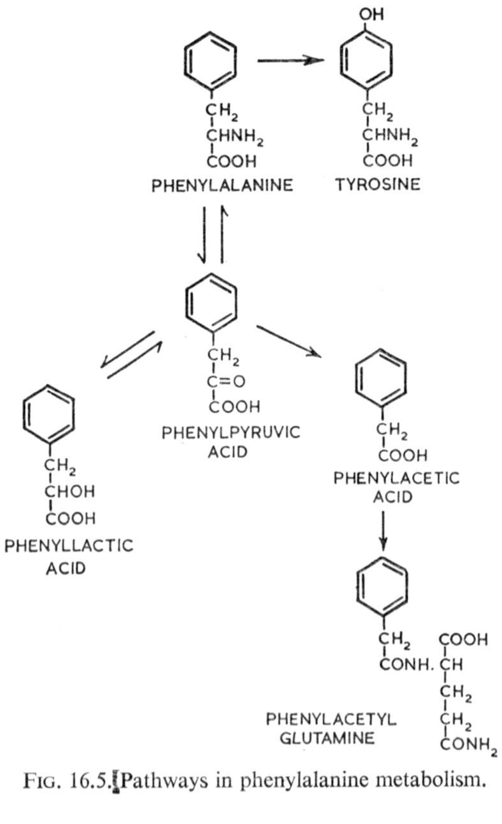

Fig. 16.5. Pathways in phenylalanine metabolism.

deuterium was present in the benzene ring. This amino acid was added to a casein stock diet and fed to growing and adult rats. Subsequently, samples of tyrosine were isolated from the proteins of these animals and the deuterium content determined. The tyrosine from the internal organs contained a concentration of deuterium, indicating that about 20 to 30 % of this tyrosine was derived from the deuterophenylalanine. In another experiment non-isotopic tyrosine in addition to the deuterophenylalanine was added to the stock diet of adult rats. Despite the abundance of tyrosine in the diet, about 13 % of the tyrosine in the internal organs was found to be derived from the deuterophenylalanine. These experiments showed that phenylalanine is rapidly converted into tyrosine, not only by growing, but also by fully grown rats of constant body weight.

Hier (1947) studied the plasma levels of various amino acids after feeding given individual amino acids to dogs. They found that after feeding phenylalanine there was a considerable rise in the tyrosine level in the plasma, but after feeding tyrosine the phenylalanine level was not raised. Levine, Dann & Marples (1943) studied a series of normal and premature infants on diets high in protein but low in vitamin C. Various amounts of extra tyrosine and phenylalanine were administered. Ingestion of phenylalanine led to the excretion of phenylalanine and tyrosine and the keto and hydroxyacids derived from them. Feeding tyrosine, however, led to no phenylalanine, phenylpyruvic or phenyllactic acid excretion, although tyrosine and its derivatives were excreted in abundant amounts. These results have been confirmed and extended by Woolf & Edmunds (1950), and similar effects have been demonstrated in vitamin C-deficient guinea-pigs (Sealock & Goodland, 1951; Sealock, Goodland, Sumerwell & Brierly, 1952).

The enzyme system catalysing the oxidation of phenylalanine to tyrosine has been studied by Udenfriend & Cooper (1952). They found that the enzyme was present in the water-soluble fractions of liver preparations from the rat, guinea-pig, rabbit, dog, chicken and man. Rat lung, kidney, brain and muscle did not contain the enzyme. The system required oxygen and pyridine nucleotide for activity. It was specific for L-phenylalanine and had no activity on N-acetylphenylalanine, the ethyl ester of phenylalanine, phenylglycine, phenylserine or phenylpyruvic acid. Mitoma & Leeper (1954) have shown that the system is complex, and that at least two enzymes may be separated by fractional precipitation. Phenylalanine hydroxylase is a labile enzyme found only in liver. It requires for activity a second more stable protein fraction (Fraction II), which is present in many animal tissues including liver. Oxygen is essential for the reaction, and the activity of Fraction II is dependent on ferrous iron, the reaction being inhibited by 1,1'-dipyridyl and restored by Fe++ (Knox, 1961).

Another series of reactions in which phenylalanine is normally concerned involves changes in the side chain (Fig. 16.5). Growth experiments have shown that phenylpyruvic acid and phenyllactic acid can replace phenylalanine in the diet (Rose, 1937; Bubl & Butts, 1949). Thus, it seems that these two acids can be converted to phenylalanine. The administration of phenylpyruvic acid by mouth will result in the excretion of some phenyllactic acid, and ingestion of phenyllactic acid results in the excretion of some phenylpyruvic acid (Kotake, Masai & Mori, 1922). Thus the conversion of phenylpyruvic acid to phenyllactic acid is presumably reversible. Furthermore, it has been found that labelled phenyllactic acid can be converted to tyrosine (Moss, 1941). Phenylpyruvic acid when fed by mouth will also give rise to phenylacetic acid (Chandler & Lewis, 1932). This reaction is, however, not reversible. The phenylacetic acid is in human beings largely conjugated with glutamine to give phenylacetylglutamine which is excreted in the urine (Thierfelder & Sherwin, 1914, 1915). The normal adult under ordinary conditions excretes phenylacetylglutamine to the extent of 250–500 mg./day (Stein, Paladini, Hirs & Moore, 1954). This is presumably derived from phenylalanine via phenylpyruvic acid.

Metabolic investigations in phenylketonuria. The biochemical findings in the blood, cerebrospinal fluid and urine of phenylketonuria patients can to a large extent be interpreted in the light of our knowledge of the normal processes concerned in phenylalanine metabolism. Phenylalanine derived from the food proteins or from the breakdown of tissue proteins tends to accumulate in the body fluids and is excreted in abnormal amounts. Phenylpyruvic acid, phenyllactic acids and phenylacetylglutamine are formed in excess. Since the renal threshold for these latter substances is very low, they are found in large amounts in the urine but hardly at all in the blood or C.S.F.

Jervis (1950) showed that the excretions of phenylalanine, phenyllactic and phenylpyruvic acids were greatly increased if a high-protein diet is fed, and diminished proportionately if the protein content of the diet was reduced. The effect of various amino acids on the excretion of these compounds was tested by determining the daily output of patients kept on a nitrogen-constant diet, following the ingestion of some pure amino acids. The following amino acids produced no change: glycine, glutamic acid, tyrosine, alanine and cystine. The ingestion of phenylalanine, however, produced a greatly increased excretion of both the keto and hydroxy acids as well as phenylalanine itself. Feeding phenylpyruvic or phenyllactic acids leads to an increase in excretion of these compounds in the

The question as to whether or not the block is complete has been investigated by Udenfriend & Bessman (1953) using labelled phenylalanine. They administered 3-^{14}C-DL-phenylalanine orally to two normal adults and two phenylketonuric children. Tyrosine and phenylalanine were subsequently isolated from the plasma proteins, and their specific activities were determined. The ratio of the activity of tyrosine to phenylalanine (T:P) was used as a rough index of the extent of conversion of phenylalanine to tyrosine (Table 16.2). The labelled phenylalanine administered to

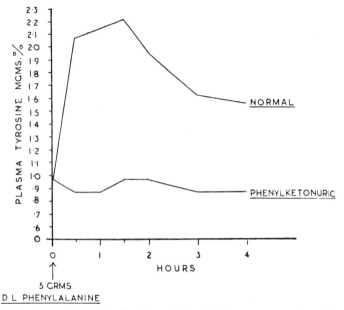

Fig. 16.6. Effect on plasma tyrosine of feeding 5 g. of phenylalanine to a normal and to a phenylketonuric individual. (After Jervis, 1947.)

urine (Penrose & Quastel, 1937; Jervis, 1938, 1950), and also a rise in phenylalanine level in the blood (Jervis et al., 1940). Thus, it seems that the metabolic disorder is primarily concerned with the hydroxylation of phenylalanine, and that in these patients, as in normal individuals, phenylpyruvic acid, phenyllactic acid and phenylalanine are interconvertible.

Jervis (1947) demonstrated that in normal individuals the feeding of phenylalanine or phenylpyruvic acid led to a rise in Millon-reacting substance (presumably tyrosine) in the blood. In phenylketonurics this did not occur (Fig. 16.6). After feeding tyrosine, however, a rise occurred both in phenylketonurics and in normals. This indicates that the conversion of phenylalanine to tyrosine is blocked in these patients.

normal subjects was rapidly incorporated into proteins, not only as phenylalanine but also as tyrosine. Values for the T:P ratio were very much lower in the phenylketonurics than in the controls. It appeared that some conversion of phenylalanine to tyrosine did take place in the phenylketonurics but to a very much diminished degree. This experiment would suggest that either the phenylalanine hydroxylase activity in the liver may be much smaller than usual, but not entirely absent; or that the phenylalanine hydroxylase may be completely absent, but a small amount of tyrosine may be formed from phenylalanine through an alternative pathway or by intestinal bacteria.

A direct attempt to discover whether any L-phenylalanine oxidase activity could be detected

TABLE 16.2

Incorporation of ^{14}C into plasma protein phenylalanine and tyrosine after the administration of $3\text{-}^{14}C\text{-}DL\text{-}phenylalanine$

(Udenfriend & Bessman, 1953)

Expt.	Time after administration (hr.)	Phenylalanine (counts/min./ μmol.)	Tyrosine (counts/ min./ μmol.)	Ratio: Tyrosine/ Phenylalanine
Control (a)	24	10·4	2·79	0·26
	48	7·84	2·24	0·29
Control (b)	24	24·6	4·90	0·20
	48	21·0	4·70	0·22
Phenylketonuric (c)	24	55·0	0·91	0·016
	48	39·0	0·89	0·023
Phenylketonuric (d)	24	46·0	0·70	0·016
	48	33·0	0·69	0·021

in the liver of phenylketonuric patients has been made by Jervis (1953). Fragments of liver obtained at autopsy from two phenylketonurics and three controls were used. Autopsy was performed within a few hours of death. Crude liver extracts were used in the test system for L-phenylalanine hydroxylase of Udenfriend & Cooper (1952). It was found that tyrosine was formed from phenylalanine under the conditions of the experiment in all the controls, but no formation of tyrosine was observed when the liver extracts of the phenylketonuric patients were used.

The later experiments of Wallace, Moldave & Meister (1957) and Mitoma, Auld & Udenfriend (1957), have conclusively proved that the primary abnormality in phenylketonuria is absence of the labile Fraction I of phenylalanine hydroxylase in the liver, whereas the amount of the more stable Fraction II is normal.

Other abnormalities of metabolism. Fig. 16.5 shows that phenylalanine can be converted to phenylpyruvic acid, which itself may reversibly be converted to phenyllactic acid and irreversibly to phenylacetic acid. The latter acid is almost quantitatively excreted as the conjugate, phenyl-acetylglutamine. Similar series of reactions occur in relation to tyrosine, o-hydroxyphenylalanine and tryptophan, and many of the corresponding metabolites are also greatly in excess in phenyl-ketonuria.

The following compounds have been shown to be excreted in excess in the disease:

(a) Derivatives of phenylalanine: phenyl-pyruvic acid, phenyllactic acid, phenylacetyl-glutamine and hippuric acid.

(b) Derivatives of tyrosine: p-hydroxyphenyl-pyruvic acid, p-hydroxyphenyllactic acid and p-hydroxyphenylacetic acid.

(c) Derivatives of o-hydroxyphenylalanine: o-hydroxyphenylacetic acid.

(d) Derivatives of typtophan: indolyl-3-pyruvic acid, indolyl-3-lactic acid and indolyl-3-acetic acid *plus* its conjugate indolylacetylglutamine. Approximate quantitative figures of their output corrected to adult male amounts as compared to normal controls is given in Table 16.3.

The excess excretion of p-hydroxyphenylalanine derivatives is mostly known from paper chromato-graphic data, and therefore no accurate figures can be given.

The excess output of these compounds indicates abnormally high transamination of phenylalanine, tyrosine, tryptophan and o-hydroxyphenyl-alanine to the corresponding keto-acids, and then to the hydroxy and substituted acetic acid derivatives. Increased transamination of phenyl-alanine is obviously due to increase of substrate, but that of the other amino acids must be due either to stimulation of transamination or to a secondary partial metabolic block in other major pathways of amino acid metabolism. Formation of o-hydroxyphenylacetic acid can probably occur both *via ortho*hydroxylation of phenylalanine and of phenylpyruvic acid. Phenylalanine in high concentration may also be degraded to benzoic acid which is excreted as the glycine conjugate, i.e.,

TABLE 16.3

Excretion of various metabolites in cases of phenylketonuria
(Amounts corrected for body size to that expected in an average adult male)

Metabolite	Phenylketonuria (mg./day)	Normal excretion (mg./day)
Phenylalanine	300–750	10–30
Phenylpyruvic acid	1700–2700	Traces
Phenyllactic acid	600–1350	Traces
Phenylacetylglutamine	300–2400	250–500
o-Hydroxyphenylacetic acid	140–560	< 1
Indolic acids	100–400	<20

hippuric acid. Grüner (1961), after feeding ^{14}C-labelled phenylalanine to phenylketonuric patients, showed that part of the labelled carbon was excreted as hippuric acid. Table 16.3 shows that phenylalanine, phenylpyruvic acid, phenyllactic acid, phenylacetylglutamine and o-hydroxy-phenylacetic acid are in especially high concentration in phenylketonuric urine. The last four compounds are organic acids excreted by the proximal tubular secretory mechanism, which is easily saturated by organic acid excess. Their excretion may therefore have important secondary effects on the output of other organic acids in phenylketonuria.

The clearance of indican, another organic acid secreted by the proximal tubules, is reduced in phenylketonuria, as after indole administration the abnormally high plasma indican is associated with a relatively low rate of urinary indican output. There is reduced output of 5-hydroxy-indolylacetic acid (Armstrong & Robinson, 1954; Ferrari, Campagnari & Guida, 1955; Pare, Sandler & Stacey, 1957). Pare *et al.* (1957) also found an abnormally low 5-hydroxytryptamine concentration in serum from phenylketonurics, and a reduced output of 5-hydroxyindolylacetic acid after ingestion of 5-hydroxytryptophan (Pare, Sandler and Stacey, 1958). These results were interpreted as due to inhibition of 5-hydroxytryptophan decarboxylase by phenylalanine and its metabolites, especially phenyllactic acid, and o- and p-hydroxyphenylacetic acids. These substances inhibit the enzyme *in vitro* (Davison & Sandler, 1958), but only at concentrations of 15–20 μmol./ml., which are much higher than could occur in body fluids in the disease. An alternative explanation (Milne, 1959) is that there is a block in excretion of 5-hydroxyindolylacetic acid due to saturation of the proximal tubular secretory mechanism for organic acids. Proximal tubular transport systems for organic acids are not, however, completely saturated in the disease, as Jervis (1952) showed that probenecid decreased the renal excretion of phenylpyruvic acid to half the original rate with corresponding increase of plasma levels of the acid.

Inhibition of p-hydroxyphenylpyruvate oxidase provides an interesting comparison. This enzyme is completely inhibited by concentrations of phenylpyruvate of only 2 μmol./ml. (Hager, Gregerman & Knox, 1957). Even this value is, however, about 50 times the amount of phenylpyruvate in phenylketonuric plasma, and in fact p-hydroxyphenylpyruvic acid is not excreted in gross excess in phenylketonuric urine even after administration of large doses of tyrosine. Thus there is in fact no significant block in the enzymic oxidation of p-hydroxyphenylpyruvic acid to homogentisic acid. Inhibition of tyrosinase by phenylalanine is of undoubted clinical importance. Miyamoto & Fitzpatrick (1957) showed that mammalian tyrosinase was competitively inhibited by phenylalanine at concentrations of 5 μmol./ml. There should be at least 15 to 30% inhibition of the enzyme at phenylalanine concentrations known to occur in the phenylketonuric patients. This probably explains the failure of melanin formation in many such patients. As the inhibition is competitive, more melanin is produced if a high tyrosine diet is given. Tashian (1961) has shown that phenylacetic acid and o-hydroxyphenylacetic acid will inhibit glutamic acid decarboxylase prepared from mammalian brain at concentrations of 7·5 μmol./ml., and considers this may be of significance in reducing formation of γ-aminobutyric acid. Again, the *in vitro* concentration is much higher than could conceivably occur *in vivo*. In summary, the only enzyme inhibition demonstrated to date which is of unequivocal clinical importance is that of mammalian tyrosinase by phenylalanine.

These results do not, therefore, explain the serious disorder of the central nervous system in phenylketonuria.

The mental defect. All individuals who have been found to excrete phenylpyruvic acid and the other abnormal metabolites continuously in their urine have shown a greater or lesser degree of intellectual impairment. There is some considerable variation in different patients with apparently the same metabolic disturbance. Most cases are severely affected and can be graded as idiots or imbeciles. Occasionally, higher-grade feeble-minded persons have been encountered.

The cause of the mental defect is not known with any certainty. One would expect that it was in some way determined by the profound metabolic disturbances which occur, and could ultimately be traced back to the primary biochemical lesion. This is known to be a failure to oxidize phenylalanine to tyrosine, due to the absence or inactivity of L-phenylalanine hydroxylase in the liver. One can, however, only speculate on what are the intervening connecting links.

One attractive hypothesis is that the mental defect results from the toxic action of one or other of the various metabolites, which occur in abnormal amounts as a result of the block in phenylalanine oxidation. Phenylalanine itself, which occurs in the blood and cerebrospinal fluid in concentrations 20–40 times those normally encountered and which presumably is found in the tissue cells in similarly increased concentrations, may well have some such action.

However, no correlation has been found between the phenylalanine concentration in the plasma and the degree of mental defect (Borek et al., 1950). Similarly, there is no direct relation between the plasma phenylpyruvic acid content and the degree of mental defect (Jervis, 1953).

Many recent papers have reported on the character of the brain damage in untreated cases and the possibilities of simulation of the disease in the experimental animal. The characteristic abnormality is widespread degeneration of the cerebral white matter with secondary gliosis. The defects seem to be chiefly due to abnormality and delay in the laying down of myelin, but gradual demyelination cannot be excluded (Crome & Pare, 1960). The water content of the brain is high and the cerebroside and cholesterol content is reduced (Crome, Tymms & Woolf, 1962). Cholesterol esters are increased, a biochemical abnormality which also occurs in demyelination from other causes. Occasionally, the lesions are more extreme with widespread degeneration and atrophy of the central white matter as in Schilder's disease (Crome, 1962). High phenylalanine diets in young animals may simulate the disease. Ammon (1961) using infantile rabbits produced profound neurological disturbances and pathological lesions of the central nervous system. Waisman, Wang, Palmer & Haslow (1960) found that in monkeys learning ability was greatly reduced, and that the animals excreted phenylpyruvic acid as well as phenylalanine.

Treatment. The results of treatment with low phenylalanine diets have been published by Woolf, Griffiths & Moncrieff (1955), Lang, Knopp & Weber (1957), Murphy (1958), Horner & Streamer (1959), Brimblecombe, Stoneman & Maliphant (1959), Gruttner, Muller & Wallis (1958), and Brimblecombe, Blainey, Stoneman & Wood (1961). Precise control of phenylalanine intake is the main difficulty as it varies with the age and rate of growth of the child. Excess will cause mental deterioration, whereas too severe limitation results in defective protein synthesis with retardation of growth and development, and skin lesions consisting of an irritative fiery rash or even exfoliative dermatitis (Woolf, 1962). The maximum requirement of phenylalanine is at about 7 months. During the age range 10–18 months there is a considerable fall in metabolic requirements, e.g. in a case recorded by Woolf, the required amount of the amino acid was 430 mg./day at 11 months, but this was seven times as much as was necessary several months earlier and later. Repeated determinations of phenylalanine in plasma, supplemented by estimations of o-hydroxyphenylacetic acid in urine give the best biochemical control. Berry et al. (1967) consider that serum phenylalanine levels should be maintained between 3–8 mg./100 ml. but Koch et al. (1967) advise lower values of 1–4 mg./100 ml. Intelligence and growth are normal if control is adequate and the diagnosis is made very early in life. Satisfactory results usually occur if treatment is started below the age of 3 months, but if later, irreversible abnormalities are always present.

Beneficial effects of therapy include amelioration of eczema, darkening of the hair, improvement in behaviour, restlessness and irritability, and increased concentration and ability to learn. There is progressive improvement in E.E.G. abnormalities and in motor performance. Fits may occur early in treatment, but not usually after efficient control has been maintained for several months. Although the treatment is difficult, expensive and time-consuming, there is now no doubt that it will save the community a life-time of institutional care and be of immeasurable benefit to the individual patient.

An undecided point is whether dietary control can be relaxed later in childhood or in adolescence. There is certainly a risk of seizures if a normal diet is resumed (Langdell, 1965). Biochemical relapse always occurs, but high plasma phenylalanine concentrations are not so serious in later childhood. Bickel & Grüter (1963) consider that if possible the diet should be continued until adolescence, but obviously discipline in older children is much more difficult than in infancy. There is no doubt that the diet should be resumed if an adult phenylketonuric patient becomes pregnant. The infant will otherwise be exposed to high phenylalanine concentrations *in utero* and will be born an imbecile even though he or she will almost certainly be genetically a heterozygote for the abnormal gene.

TYROSINAEMIA

No patient similar to the case described in the classical paper of Medes (1932) has since been described. Defects of tyrosine metabolism occur as a relatively common condition in premature infants and as a rare inborn error of metabolism usually termed tyrosinaemia.

Para-hydroxyphenylpyruvate oxidase is present in low concentration in the liver of premature infants and the enzyme requires vitamin C as co-enzyme. Tyrosine and tyrosyl metabolites may therefore often be found in the urine of premature infants, but the abnormality is usually reversed on feeding excess ascorbic acid (Huisman & Jonxis, 1957). In the rare, hereditary disease infantile tyrosinaemia, the main clinical abnormalities are a nodular cirrhosis of the liver and multiple proximal renal tubular defects causing rickets and a Fanconi syndrome (Halvorsen & Gjessing, 1964; Gentz *et al.*, 1965; Halvorsen, Parde, Loken & Gjessing, 1966). More commonly, there may be a thrombocytopenia, darkening of the skin, and sometimes slight mental impairment. Biochemically, there is hypertyrosinaemia causing a considerable output of tyrosine in the urine. Tyrosyl compounds in the urine, especially *p*-hydroxyphenylpyruvic acid, *p*-hydroxyphenyllacetic acid and *p*-hydroxyphenyllactic acid, are grossly increased. The primary defect is an absence of *p*-hydroxyphenylpyruvic acid oxidase, tyrosine transaminase and homogentisic acid oxidase activities in the liver being within normal limits. The disease may be of the acute or chronic type (Halvorsen, 1967). In the former there is vomiting, diarrhoea, failure to thrive with death from liver failure in the first seven months of life.

In the chronic type symptoms occur later in infancy and are milder, hepato-splenomegaly, growth impairment and rickets being the most prominent symptoms and signs.

Serum tyrosine may be increased to 10 mg./ 100 ml. or even more. In the early stages the prominent amino acid in the urine is tyrosine itself, but later there is a generalized amino-aciduria due to proximal renal tubular damage. In the later stages of the disease plasma methionine may also be increased (Scriver *et al.*, 1967), an abnormality ascribed to severe liver failure.

Like phenylketonuria, results of dietary treatment are better the earlier the disease is diagnosed. Early cases are recognized by a positive urinary reaction to ferric chloride during screening for phenylketonuria, and in younger sibs of a previously diagnosed patient. Restriction of both phenylalanine and tyrosine is obviously essential, the usual daily amount being 45 mg./Kg. body weight of each amino acid initially, this being gradually reduced to 25 mg./Kg. (Halvorsen, 1967). There is a rapid fall of plasma tyrosine and early improvement of the renal tubular defects as shown by a rise in serum phosphate and reduction in the degree of amino-aciduria. Improvement in established liver cirrhosis is less likely, and therefore every effort should be made to start therapy before irreversible liver damage has occurred.

ALKAPTONURIA

Alkaptonuria is a rare condition readily recognized by the characteristic changes in colour which occur in the urine. The urine when freshly passed is normal in appearance, but if left to stand it soon begins to darken. Alkalinity speeds up the change, and the urine passes through a series of shades of brown and finally appears quite black. Linen and woollen fabrics moistened with the urine become darkly stained, and as a result the condition is frequently recognized in early infancy by the characteristic staining of the napkins. On other occasions the abnormality is detected for the first time in the course of a life insurance examination, or a routine medical investigation when the urine is found to have strongly reducing properties, and then its other peculiar characteristics are noted.

These curious properties of the urine persist unchanged throughout life. In other respects the affected individuals appear quite healthy, except that as they grow older their ligaments and cartilages tend to become darkened and they are rather prone to develop osteoarthritis. These changes in pigmentation are called "ochronosis".

Biochemical findings. The urinary changes in colour are due to the presence of large quantities of homogentisic acid.

HO—OH

CH₂ . COOH

This is itself colourless, but it is readily oxidized to a series of brown and black pigments. Homogentisic acid was first isolated from the urine of these patients by Wolkow & Baumann (1891). Alkaptonurics excrete several grams of this substance daily. The amount excreted varies somewhat with the diet and is larger as the protein intake is increased. Consequently, the output of homogentisic acid in these patients is highly correlated with the total nitrogen output, and the ratio of homogentisic acid to total nitrogen excretion has often been used as a convenient index in the study of this condition. Given a constant diet this ratio is probably much the same in all alkaptonuric patients (Garrod, 1923).

Apart from homogentisic acid, no other substance has been reported as occurring in abnormal amounts. In particular, Neuberger, Rimington & Wilson (1947), in a search for other aromatic compounds, failed to find any abnormal quantities of tyrosine, *p*-hydroxyphenyllactic acid, *p*-hydroxyphenylpyruvic acid or phenylpyruvic acid. The reducing properties of the urine could be attributed entirely to the homogentisic acid present.

The exact concentration of homogentisic acid in the blood plasma of alkaptonurics is still somewhat uncertain. Katsch & Metz (1927), Lanyar & Lieb (1931), and Neuberger *et al.* (1947) all obtained values of the order of 3 mg./100 ml. Such concentrations are so low as to be near the lower limits of the applicability of the methods used, and, moreover, minute amounts of other reducing substances reacting like homogentisic acid are present even in the plasma extracts obtained from non-alkaptonuric individuals, so that the plasma levels reported cannot be considered as very accurate (Neuberger *et al.*, 1947). No other abnormal constituents have been reported in the blood of these patients.

Metabolic investigations. Homogentisic acid is believed to be an intermediate in normal metabolism. Normal individuals, after taking by mouth amounts of the substance of the order of 5 g., appear to metabolize it completely and no homogentisic acid appears in the urine (Falta,

1904; Leaf & Neuberger, 1948). Embden (1893) did, in fact, succeed in producing a slight transitory alkaptonuria by giving as much as 8 g. of the acid, but he found that smaller doses had no such effect. In sharp contrast with these findings in the normal, homogentisic acid when fed to alkaptonurics is excreted almost quantitatively, in addition to that already being put out by these patients (Embden, 1893). It appears therefore that the alkaptonuric is completely incapable of metabolizing this substance.

The simplest interpretation of the metabolic disorder in alkaptonuria is that the further oxidation of homogentisic acid, a normal intermediate in the breakdown of phenylalanine and tyrosine, is completely blocked, and that consequently homogentisic acid accumulates and is excreted in large amounts in the urine. Apparently the failure lies essentially in the body's inability to break down the benzene ring with hydroxyl groups in the 2 : 5 position. It has been shown that liver preparations can enzymically oxidize homogentisic acid to fumarylacetoacetic acid, and this in the presence of a second enzyme is hydrolysed to fumaric and acetoacetic acids (Ravdin & Crandall, 1951).

Homogentisic acid is an intermediate on the main, though not the only, metabolic pathway in the degradation of the two aromatic amino acids phenylalanine and tyrosine. Some 70 to 90% of these amino acids present in the diet are converted to homogentisic acid by the alkaptonuric. A similar conversion rate is obtained when either L-phenylalanine or L-tyrosine are fed alone. Other pathways not leading through homogentisic acid do exist, though they are probably quantitatively limited. Thus, phenylacetylglutamine is found in normal urine, and is presumably derived from phenylalanine. Adrenaline, noradrenaline, 3:4-dihydroxyphenylalanine (dopa), melanin, diiodotyrosine, thyroxine and triiodothyronine are also derived from tyrosine in the body.

Taking the view that homogentisic acid is a normal intermediary metabolite, the results of administering various aromatic acids to alkaptonurics might be expected to throw light on the intermediate metabolic steps which precede the formation of this compound. A substance which represents a link in the chain should be destroyed in the normal organism, and should increase the output of homogentisic acid in the alkaptonuric. With this in mind, many substances have been fed to alkaptonurics, and the earlier literature is fully reviewed by Garrod (1923) and Neubauer (1928).

Both phenylalanine and tyrosine, when fed to these subjects, greatly increase the excretion of homogentisic acid in the urine and there seems no doubt that these are the parent substances from which it is derived. Phenylpyruvic acid, phenyllactic acid, and p-hydroxyphenylpyruvic acid, likewise give rise to an increased elimination of homogentisic acid in alkaptonuric patients (Neubauer & Falta, 1904; Grutterinck & van den Bergh, 1907). On the other hand, o-tyrosine and m-tyrosine do not increase the excretion of homogentisic acid (Blum, 1908), and neither do the o- nor m-hydroxyphenylpyruvic acids. Thus, it seems that the presence of the hydroxyl group in the *para* position, as in tyrosine, is not only no hindrance to the change to homogentisic acid, but is probably essential, and the transformation occurs not by removal of the hydroxyl group in the *para* position but by a shifting of the side chain.

Modern views (Edwards, Hsai & Knox, 1955; La Du & Zannoni, 1955) of the conversion of phenylalanine and tyrosine to homogentisic acid, and the subsequent degradation of this intermediate to fumaric and acetoacetic acids are given in Fig. 16.7.

La Du, Zannoni, Laster & Seegmiller (1958) showed that homogentisic acid oxidase activity was completely absent in a sample of liver from an alkaptonuric patient, and also proved that the defect was due to the actual absence of the enzyme rather than to the presence of an inhibitor or to lack of a co-factor. Zannoni, Seegmiller & La Du (1962) were later able to prove that there was a similar enzymic defect in kidney tissue in a necropsy specimen from an alkaptonuric. The enzymes maleylacetoacetic acid isomerase and fumarylacetoacetic acid hydrolase were present in normal amounts, even though they had presumably never been in contact with their substrate until the moment of the *in vitro* reaction.

The renal threshold of homogentisic acid. It is probable that both in normal subjects and in alkaptonurics the renal threshold for homogentisic acid is extremely low. Leaf & Neuberger (1948) were able, by intravenous injection of quantities of the order of 0·3 g., to produce a transient alkaptonuria in normal individuals. On the

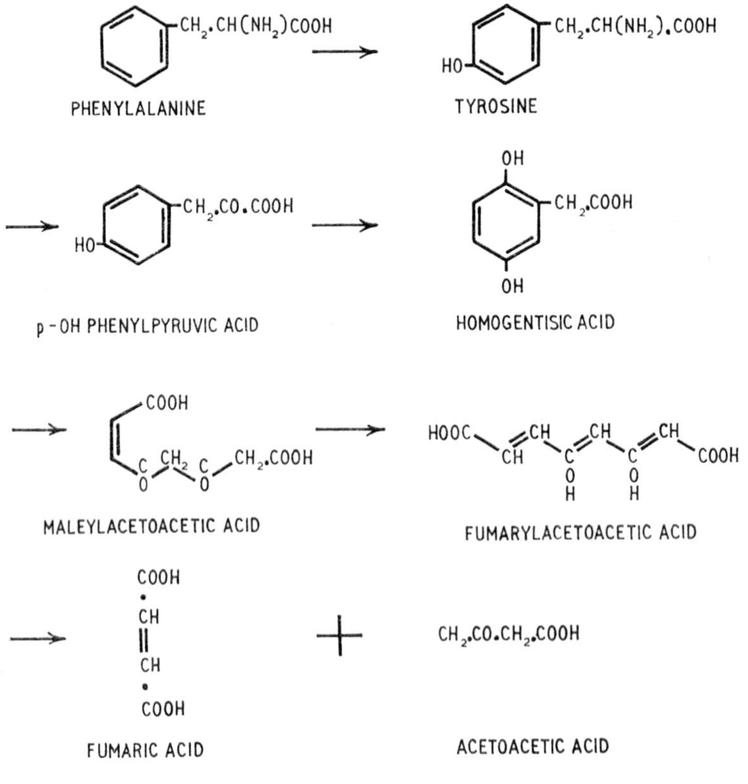

PHENYLALANINE

TYROSINE

p-OH PHENYLPYRUVIC ACID

HOMOGENTISIC ACID

MALEYLACETOACETIC ACID

FUMARYLACETOACETIC ACID

FUMARIC ACID

ACETOACETIC ACID

FIG. 16.7. The formation and breakdown of homogentisic acid.

average about one-third of the dose administered appeared in the urine. The concentration in the plasma was of the order of 1·5–3·5 mg./100 ml., and they concluded that the renal threshold for this substance must be well below 4·0 mg./100 ml. In normal subjects alkaptonuria cannot be produced by feeding tyrosine or phenylalanine, and it must be assumed that homogentisic acid, if it is formed as an intermediate, never appears in the blood in appreciable quantities, and it may well be rapidly oxidized in the organ where it is first formed. The alkaptonuric probably has the same low renal threshold for this substance as does the normal, and this could account for the high urine concentration, and the low concentration in the plasma, which is observed.

However, the values for the renal clearance of homogentisic acid in alkaptonuria actually obtained by Neuberger et al. (1947) in one patient were remarkably high, about 400–500 ml./min. This was much more than could be readily accounted for by filtration alone, as a substance which was filtered by the glomeruli and not at all absorbed by the tubules might have been expected to show a clearance of about 100 ml./min. in this patient.

Seegmiller, Zannoni, Laster & La Du (1961) have developed a specific spectrofluorimetric enzymic method for homogentisic acid, and confirm that the concentration in alkaptonuric plasma is less than 3 mg./100 ml. and that the renal clearance is considerably above the glomerular filtration rate. Like many other organic acids, homogentisic acid is presumably secreted by the proximal renal tubules despite considerable binding to plasma albumin.

Ochronosis. Apart from the excretion of homogentisic acid in the urine, the most notable clinical feature of alkaptonuria is the development of the condition known as ochronosis. This does not generally become apparent till middle or later life, and is due to the development of a dark pigmentation of the cartilages, tendons and ligaments, and of the sclerotics of the eyes. The earliest signs are bluish discoloration of the ears, and the appearance of triangular brown patches in the sclerotics with their bases towards the corneae. Later, owing to the staining of the underlying tendons, the nose may appear bluish and a blue tint may appear on the knuckles. The post-mortem appearances are very striking. The cartilages and fibro-cartilages are deeply pigmented, the staining of the tracheal rings and of the interstitial discs being particularly noticeable. Pigmentation in the tendons, sclerotics and in advanced cases in the bones may be observed, and patches of pigment in the endocardium and intima of the arteries have also been described. (For detailed description see Garrod, 1923; Lichtenstein & Kaplan, 1954.) These patients are particularly prone to develop arthritic changes. The changes are prominent in the spine and may lead to rigidity and kyphosis. Typical X-ray appearances have been described by Pomeranz, Friedman & Tunick (1941), the main features of which are an extensive calcification in tendon sheaths, bursal sacs, synovial membranes and in the intervertebral discs.

After injection homogentisic acid is bound both by connective tissue and by plasma albumin. The distribution pattern closely resembles that previously described for gentisic acid in rats (Roof & Turner, 1955). Milch (1961) and Milch & Murray (1961) showed that the acid was irreversibly bound to connective tissue elements by a tanning-like reaction requiring preliminary oxidation to benzoquinone-acetic acid (Fig. 16.8). This subsequently polymerizes with formation of a melanin-like pigment, explaining the ochronosis of the disease. The mechanism leading to the

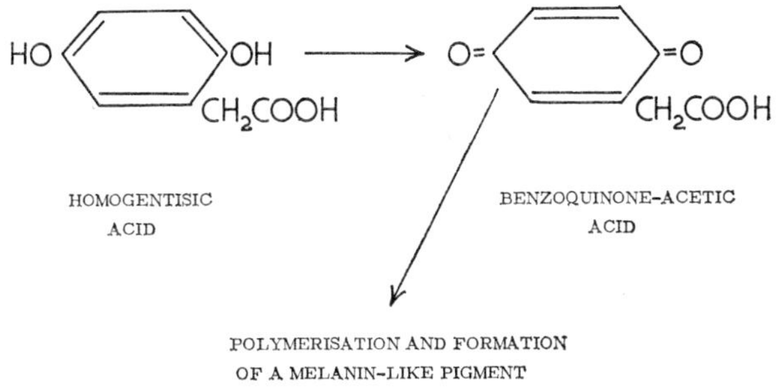

HOMOGENTISIC
ACID

BENZOQUINONE-ACETIC
ACID

POLYMERISATION AND FORMATION
OF A MELANIN-LIKE PIGMENT

FIG. 16.8. A minor pathway of the metabolism of homogentisic acid. In alkaptonuria there is absence of the enzyme homogentisic acid oxidase. This results in accumulation of homogentisic acid in body fluids with especial deposition in cartilage and connective tissue. Ochronosis is due to excess formation of benzoquinone-acetic acid and melanin-like pigments produced by its polymerization.

arthritis is still unknown. Greiburg (1957) has shown that hyaluronidase is inhibited by oxidation products of homogentisic acid, but not by the acid itself.

Genetics. Garrod (1902) was the first to point out that alkaptonuria had a characteristic familial distribution. It occurred frequently among the brothers and sisters of affected relatives, but rarely among their parents, children or more distant relatives. Furthermore, he pointed out that there was an unusually high incidence of parental consanguinity. He concluded that this must imply that the condition is genetically determined, and that it is in fact inherited in the manner of a typical mendelian recessive character. The affected individuals would thus be homozygous for the rare abnormal gene involved. These conclusions have been largely confirmed by further work (Hogben, Worrall & Zieve, 1932), and there is little doubt that the majority of cases of alkaptonuria are determined in this way.

DEFECTS IN TRYPTOPHAN METABOLISM

These are rare metabolic blocks in the main pathway of tryptophan metabolism via kynurenine and its derivatives. Investigations of this important metabolic pathway require rather sophisticated biochemical methods and it is probable that the disorders of metabolism described will prove to be more common than is suggested by present reports.

HYPERTRYPTOPHANAEMIA

Tada *et al.* (1963) reported a 9-year old mentally deficient patient who was undersized and had additional symptoms and signs suggestive of Hartnup disease, i.e. a photosensitive pellagrous rash and cerebellar ataxia. There was

excess plasma and urinary tryptophan, but no generalized amino-aciduria and no excess output of indolic metabolites in the urine. Oral tryptophan caused a greater rise of plasma and urinary tryptophan as compared to controls, but only a slight rise of urinary kynurenine. The basic defect was claimed to be a deficiency of tryptophan pyrrolase, but no absolute proof of this was possible.

DEFECTS IN KYNURENINE METABOLISM

Three hereditary defects of the kynurenine-nicotinamide pathway have been described. Hydroxykynureninuria (Komrower *et al.*, 1964; Komrower & Westall, 1967) is associated with growth-retardation, bony abnormalities, mental retardation and symptoms of pellagra. There is excessive urinary output of hydroxykynurenine and some increase of kynurenine, kynurenic acid and xanthurenic acid. The primary defect was assumed to be a deficiency of the enzyme kynureninase. Some clinical improvement occurred on pyridoxine and nicotinamide therapy, but the abnormal biochemistry persisted.

In the families described by Knapp (1960) there was an undue incidence of asthma, urticaria, varicose ulcers, anaemia and diabetes. An abnormal output of kynurenine, hydroxykynurenine and xanthurenic acid was present. Although there was no pyridoxine deficiency, clinical and biochemical improvement occurred on high doses of the vitamin. The condition apparently resembles cystathioninuria in that there is an inherited abnormality of the apo-enzyme, kynureninase, such that it can only function in the presence of abnormally high concentrations of the co-enzyme, pyridoxal.

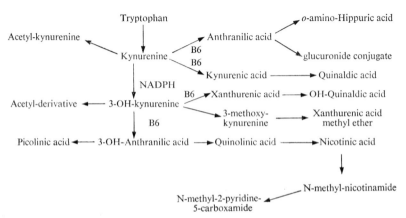

FIG. 16.9. Tryptophan-kynurenine-nicotinic acid pathway.

Kynureninuria (Price *et al.*, 1967) is a further defect in that kynurenine was the major urinary metabolite, although the outputs of *o*-amino-hippurate, kynurenic acid and acetylkynurenine were also abnormally high. The propositus had an unusual form of scleroderma with a predominantly unilateral distribution, but the biochemical abnormality was found in many of her relatives. Pyridoxal therapy proved ineffective, and it was thought that the defect was a partial deficiency of kynurenine hydroxylase.

DEFECTS IN METABOLISM OF BRANCHED-CHAIN AMINO ACIDS

These are of considerable theoretical importance with regard to the specificity of human enzymes. Knowledge of these diseases suggests that the amino acid transaminases are specific to each amino acid, the three oxo-acids are further metabolized by a single common enzyme, and the resultant carboxylic acids are further degraded by separate specific oxidative enzymes. Dietary treatment of maple syrup urine disease is more difficult than that of phenylketonuria, and available evidence suggests that control will need to be continued much longer, and possibly throughout adult life.

HYPERVALINAEMIA

This condition was reported in a Japanese infant (Wada *et al.*, 1963) with failure to thrive,

inability to suck, nystagmus and vomiting. There was increase of plasma and urinary valine, but not of leucine or isoleucine. There was no accumulation of oxo-acids, and no maple-syrup odour in the urine. Plasma valine was five times the normal value, but was reduced to normal levels by a low valine diet. With dietary treatment there was weight gain and vomiting was less severe. Intravenous valine or milk feeding caused a rapid relapse and electro-encephalographic deterioration. Although not fully proven, the basic defect is probably a deficiency of valine transaminase.

MAPLE SYRUP URINE DISEASE

This condition was first described by Menkes, Hurst & Craig (1954) in four siblings dying early in infancy. There was vomiting with feeding difficulties, hypertonicity of muscle, and a peculiar characteristic maple syrup odour of the urine. Westall, Dancis & Miller (1957) reported a similar finding in a mentally deficient boy aged 20 months. The branched-chain amino acids valine, leucine and isoleucine were found in excess in plasma and urine, and they also recorded excess methionine in the plasma. Later investigations have proved that the condition is due to a metabolic block in a pathway shared by the three branched-chain amino acids (Mackensie & Woolf, 1959; Menkes, 1959; Dancis, Levitz, Miller & Westall, 1959).

Amino acids	*a*-oxo acids	*a*-hydroxy acids
Valine	*a*-oxo*iso*valeric acid	*a*-hydroxy*iso*valeric acid
Leucine	*a*-oxo*iso*caproic acid	*a*-hydroxy*iso*caproic acid
Isoleucine	*a*-oxo-*β*-methylvaleric acid	*a*-hydroxy-*β*-methylvaleric acid

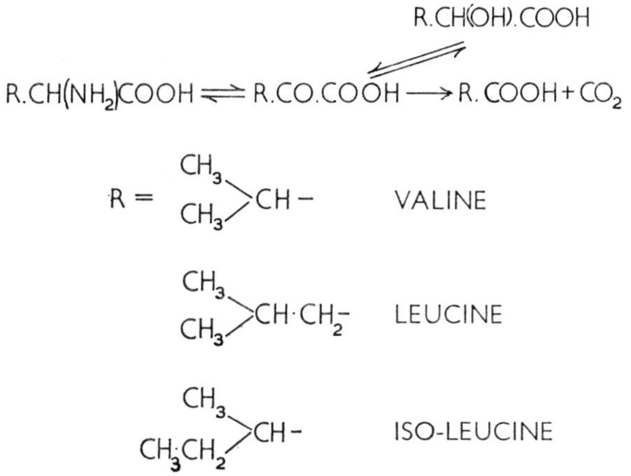

$$R.CH(OH).COOH$$
$$R.CH(NH_2)COOH \rightleftharpoons R.CO.COOH \longrightarrow R.COOH + CO_2$$

$$R = \quad \genfrac{}{}{0pt}{}{CH_3}{CH_3}\!\!>CH- \qquad VALINE$$

$$\genfrac{}{}{0pt}{}{CH_3}{CH_3}\!\!>CH\cdot CH_2- \qquad LEUCINE$$

$$\genfrac{}{}{0pt}{}{CH_3}{CH_3CH_2}\!\!>CH- \qquad ISO\text{-}LEUCINE$$

FIG. 16.10. Metabolic pathways of the branched chain amino acids. The defect in maple syrup urine disease is an absence of an enzyme involved in the oxidative decarboxylation of the oxo-acid to the corresponding aliphatic acid.

Metabolism of the branched-chain amino acids. As shown in Fig. 16.10 these amino acids are first transaminated to the corresponding α-oxo-acid, pyridoxal phosphate acting as co-enzyme. The α-oxo-acids may be reversibly reduced to the corresponding hydroxy acids, or degraded by irreversible oxidative decarboxylation. Thiamine pyrophosphate, lipoic acid, co-enzyme A, diphosphopyridine nucleotide, and flavinadenine dinucleotide are co-factors in the complex process of oxidative decarboxylation (Coon, Robinson & Backawat, 1955; Kinnory, Takeda & Greenberg, 1955; Block, 1944; Coon & Abrahamsen, 1952).

Biochemical abnormalities. As the block in maple syrup urine disease is at the stage of oxidative decarboxylation, nine organic acids accumulate in blood and urine (Fig. 16.10).

Westall, Dancis & Miller (1957) found an increase of the three branched-chain amino acids up to 10 times the normal value in plasma. Mackensie & Woolf (1959) reported a similar excess concentration in cerebrospinal fluid as well as in plasma and urine. The oxo- and hydroxy-acids are easily demonstrable in urine, but are in less concentration in other body fluids. In the case described by Dent & Westall (1961) plasma levels of oxo-acids averaged 10 mg./100 ml. and urinary oxo-acids 50–60 mg./100 ml. *Iso*butyric, *iso*valeric and α-methylbutyric acids produced by oxidative decarboxylation have not been detected, as the block prevents their formation. Transaminases in tissues, from cases of the disease obtained at necropsy, have been shown to be active in transfer of the amino group of the branched-chain amino acids to α-oxoglutarate. Dancis, Hutzler & Levitz (1960) found that leucocytes obtained from affected patients failed to produce $^{14}CO_2$ labelled valine, leucine and isoleucine, due to failure of decarboxylation. The defect therefore seems to affect many, if not all, body cells.

The apparent increase in plasma methionine first reported by Westall *et al.* (1957) was an anomalous feature, as its presence could not easily be reconciled with the known enzymic defect. Dent & Westall (1961) reported that plasma methionine fell on a synthetic diet containing a low content of branched-chain amino acids, but inexplicably rose to over twice the original value after oral ingestion of isoleucine. This anomaly has now been partly explained by Norton, Roitman, Luyderman & Holt (1962) who found that the peak on Moore and Stein column separation, previously considered to be methionine, was, in fact, one-tenth methionine, and nine-tenths another amino acid provisionally identified

as *allo*-isoleucine. Isoleucine, like threonine, hydroxylysine and hydroxyproline, is a diastereo-isomeric amino acid with two dissimilar asymmetric C atoms. The source of *allo*-isoleucine in maple syrup urine disease remains unexplained, but could possibly be derived from transamination of α-oxo-β-methylvaleric acid. Both L-isoleucine and D-*allo*-isoleucine produce the L-form of this α-oxo-acid by transamination. Reversal of the usual direction of the transamination reaction can certainly occur in the rat as α-oxo-β-methyl-valeric acid can completely replace isoleucine in a synthetic diet (Wood & Cooley, 1954). An abnormally low blood glucose may often occur (Dancis, Levitz & Westall, 1960), probably due to a mechanism similar to that of leucine-induced hypoglycaemia (Cochrane, Payne, Simpkiss & Woolf, 1956). There is excess excretion of indolyl-3-acetic and indolyllactic acids (Mackensie & Woolf, 1959), comparable to the finding in phenylketonuria, possibly secondary to increased transamination of tryptophan.

Clinical aspects and pathology. Maple syrup urine disease is in many ways comparable to phenylketonuria, but, because three essential amino acids are involved rather than one, is an even more serious disorder of metabolism. Mental retardation and histopathological lesions of the central nervous system are more extreme, and cause obvious disability at an earlier age. The affected babies are often apparently normal for the first week after birth, but after this there are feeding difficulties and failure to thrive. There is hypertonicity of muscle, with frequent jerking movements, and attacks of opisthotonus. As in phenylketonuria, there is often some flexural eczema. Progressive deterioration with death in infancy occurs unless dietary treatment is given. Pathological abnormalities in the central nervous system are more severe than in phenylketonuria. The main changes are gross status spongiosus of the central nervous system with defective myelinization and gliosis of the white matter (Crome, Dutton & Ross, 1961).

Treatment. Dietary management of maple syrup urine disease is much more difficult than of phenylketonuria, as there is no easy method of removing branched-chain amino acids from protein hydrolysates. Suitable commercial diets are available for phenylketonurics, but corresponding diets in maple syrup urine disease have to be laboriously prepared by clinicians and biochemists. Dent & Westall (1961) used a basis of gelatin to which was added synthetic amino acids. In some cases DL-amino acids were the only ones available in sufficient quantity, e.g.

phenylalanine. This causes certain biochemical complications, as the only route of metabolism of D-phenylalanine is oxidation by D-amino acid oxidase to phenylpyruvic acid, which, together with its derivatives, phenyllactic acid and phenylacetyl-glutamine, is excreted in the urine. Dent & Westall (1961) reported considerable biochemical improvement, with fall in plasma and urine concentrations of branched-chain amino acids and their keto and hydroxy acid derivatives. The smell of maple syrup in the urine, which is possibly due to α-hydroxy-acids, disappeared on treatment. Addition of any one of the branched-chain amino acids caused the expected biochemical relapse. Addition of leucine produced the most severe biochemical and clinical deterioration, and in particular was the only amino acid which resulted in gross increase of oxo-acid excretion, in this case almost entirely α-oxoisocaproic acid. Isoleucine caused an increased plasma level both of isoleucine itself and of another amino acid, which can now be interpreted as a rise of D-alloisoleucine, either by reversed transamination of α-oxo-β-methylvaleric acid, or possibly indicative of impurity of the isoleucine given. Commercial samples of this amino acid usually contain appreciable amounts of alloisoleucine.

Studies on the cerebrospinal fluid were of particular interest and importance. Abnormally high concentrations of branched-chain amino acids were present in the CSF, and in fact were in higher concentration than glutamine, the amino acid most prominent in chromatograms of normal CSF. Treatment reduced the levels of leucine and isoleucine, but valine was less well controlled both in plasma and CSF. Concentrations of oxo-acids in CSF also fell, but again α-oxoisovaleric acid derived from valine was still present despite attempts at dietary control.

Snyderman (1967) reports that normal growth can be expected with adequate dietary therapy. There is improvement in the hypertonicity of muscle and the increased tendon reflexes characteristic of the untreated patient. Cessation of fits and improvement in the electroencephalogram almost always occur. Improvement in the mental state is related to the age at which therapy is started. A patient in whom therapy was commenced at the age of 10 days had normal intelligence at the age of three. Present evidence suggests that dietary control may well have to be lifelong, unlike phenylketonuria when restrictions become less important in adolescence and adult life. When a patient with maple syrup urine disease is allowed to try a normal diet there is rapid deterioration with early return of seizures.

ISOVALERIC ACIDAEMIA

This condition was described by Tawaka, Budd, Efron & Isselbacher (1966) in two affected sibs, and a further case has been reported by Newman, Wilson, Callaghan & Young (1967). There are recurrent attacks of vomiting, acidosis and lethargy and coma. Death may occur in early infancy from severe metabolic acidosis. The diagnosis is made by the characteristic odour of short-chain fatty acids in sweat and urine; this has been compared to the odour of sweaty feet. Isovaleric acid is in high concentration in body fluids, the plasma level being about 100 mg./100 ml., or 1,500 times the normal value. There is no increase of amino or oxo-acids in plasma or urine. The condition is due to absence of the acyl dehydrogenase converting isovaleryl-Co-A to β-methyl crotonyl-Co-A. Oxidation of ^{14}C-labelled isovaleric acid by isolated white cells from the patients is markedly depressed as compared to controls (Budd et al., 1967; Efron, 1967). The only similar clinical condition is one with comparable depression of oxidation of n-butyric and n-hexanoic acids (Sidbury et al., 1967). This is due to a deficiency of the acyl dehydrogenase specific for oxidation of 4-carbon and 6-carbon fatty acids (Steyn-Parve & Beinert, 1958), but is a disorder of fatty acid metabolism. No simple screening tests are available in the diagnosis of these conditions, and therefore familiarity with the characteristic odour is of crucial importance in their early diagnosis. It would obviously be useful to try either a low leucine diet or general protein restriction in the control of isovaleric acidaemia, but no information on the effects of this is currently available. Exacerbations with temporary severe acidosis should be controllable by complete protein restriction and glucose infusions.

DEFECTS IN METABOLISM OF SULPHUR-CONTAINING AMINO ACIDS

Homocystinuria is the second most common disorder of amino acid metabolism, being second in frequency to phenylketonuria. Many cases having been described in the last five years. The metabolic defects afford supportive evidence for the metabolic pathway of sulphur-containing amino acids first elucidated in a case of cystinuria by du Vigneau et al. (1944).

HYPERMETHIONAEMIA

Perry, Hardwick, Dixon, Dolman & Hansen (1965) described three sibs, each of whom died during the third month of life after an illness associated with a peculiar odour of the urine, expired air and sweat. There was irritability and increasing somnolence, and terminally hypoglycaemia with a haemorrhagic diathesis. At necropsy, hepatic cirrhosis, renal tubular degeneration and dilatation, and pancreatic islet hypertrophy were found in each infant. Detailed biochemical studies were only possible in the third infant where there was a considerable elevation of plasma and urinary methionine, plasma methionine being elevated to 30–100 times normal values. In addition, there was a generalized amino-aciduria of a "renal" type. The peculiar odour was probably due to accumulation of α-oxo-γ-methiolbutyric acid in body fluids including plasma, sweat and urine. This acid is formed from methionine by transamination and is subsequently degraded to methyl mercaptan

Although only recently described (Carson & Niell, 1962; Gerritsen, Vaughn & Waisman, 1962) the condition appears fairly common, being second in frequency only to phenylketonuria in hereditary disorders of amino acid metabolism.

Clinically, in addition to mental deficiency in the majority of cases, there is dislocation of the lens of the eye, fine sparse hair, and skeletal deformities, often with knock-knee and a shuffling gait. Thrombo-embolic complications due to an abnormality of platelet stickiness are often seen and may prove fatal. There is often a superficial resemblance to cases of arachnodactyly (Marfan's syndrome), but the two conditions are quite distinct biochemically.

There is a positive urinary cyanide-nitroprusside test due to excretion of homocystine. This can easily be distinguished from cystine

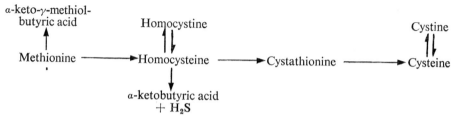

FIG. 16.11. Metabolism of sulphur-containing amino acids.

(Canellakis & Tarver, 1953). There was a normal content of cystathionine in the brain, making it likely that the main pathway of methionine metabolism was intact (Fig. 16.11). It was suggested that the basic metabolic defect was an enzymic block in the further breakdown of α-oxo-γ-methiolbutyric acid. If this is true, the defect is comparable to that present in maple syrup urine disease, where there is a block in the metabolism of the three oxo-acids produced from the branched-chain amino acids by transamination. There was no opportunity to try the effect of a low methionine diet.

HOMOCYSTINURIA

This is an autosomal recessive disease now proved to be due to lack of cystathionine synthetase (Mudd, Finkelstein, Irreverre & Laster, 1964). This primarily causes accumulation of homocystine in body fluids, but there is often some increase of methionine, as conversion of this amino acid to homocystine is impeded by the high concentration of the latter compound. Brain damage and intellectual impairment are variable, about 40% of the cases being of normal intelligence (McKusick, Arang & Pollack, 1965).

either by paper or column chromatographic techniques. Homocystine can be detected with greater difficulty in plasma and in the more severe cases there is hypermethioninaemia in addition. Increased platelet stickiness has been shown to occur by in vitro addition of homocystine to blood (McDonald, Bray, Field, Love, & Davies, 1964). As there is complete lack of cystathionine synthetase, cystathionine and cystine are not formed from dietary methionine. This causes a reduced cerebral content of cystathionine, and cystine becomes an essential amino acid in homocystinuric patients.

Treatment consists of giving a low methionine and cystine-enriched diet as soon as the diagnosis has been made. This causes a rapid biochemical improvement with fall of plasma and urinary homocystine levels. Improvement in the clinical abnormalities and particularly the mental retardation were not striking in a case where treatment was commenced at 5 years of age (Carson, 1967), but very satisfactory in a child diagnosed within a few days of birth (Komrower, 1967). It might be theoretically advantageous to give cystathionine as this metabolite is abnormally low in the brains of affected patients.

This compound is, however, extremely expensive and is rapidly excreted by the kidney (Waisman, 1967).

CYSTATHIONINURIA

Harris, Penrose & Thomas (1959) reported the finding of excess cystathionine excretion in an imbecile female aged 64. Subsequent necropsy showed no significant abnormality except a very small thyroid. The patient excreted about 0·5 g. of the amino acid/day, but cystathionine could not be detected in blood plasma by paper chromatography. Administration of 5 g. DL-methionine by mouth increased cystathionine output two-and-a half times. Excess cystathionine was found at necropsy in the patient's liver and kidney, whereas the amino acid could not be detected in similar tissue from controls. The content in the patient's brain was probably greater than in controls, although this was not certain. Normal concentrations of cystathionine in these tissues are: brain, 22·5–56·6 mg./100 g. wet weight, and less than 1 mg./100 g. wet weight in liver and kidney (Tallan, Moore & Stein, 1958).

Two of the patient's blood relations excreted cystathionine, but in only one-tenth the amount of the patient, and were thought to be heterozygotes. The primary abnormality was considered to be a block in the cleavage of cystathionine to cysteine and homoserine. As cystathionine could not be detected in plasma this amino acid, like β-amino-*iso*butyric acid, phosphoethanolamine and argininosuccinic acid, must have a high urinary clearance, with little if any tubular reabsorpton from the glomerular filtrate (Cusworth & Dent 1960).

Unlike most diseases of amino acid metabolism this condition does not cause a uniformly recognizable clinical syndrome. Three of the cases described were mentally retarded (Harris *et al.*, 1959; Frimpter, Haymoritz & Horwith, 1963; Berlow, 1966), but the other patient was normally intelligent (Mongeau, Hilgartner, Worthen & Frimpter, 1966). In adult cases, from 500–1300 mg. of cystationine are excreted in the urine daily, with considerable increase after methionine loading. The condition is of especial interest because of the beneficial effects of therapy with large doses of pyridoxine. There is however no evidence of generalized pyridoxal deficiency. In two patients samples of homogenized liver were assayed for cystathionase activity with and without the presence of excess pyridoxal phosphate (Frimpter, 1965). Cystine was produced only when excess pyridoxal was present. The results suggest that the apo-enzyme

is abnormal in the disease, possibly with a defect in the binding of the co-enzyme. Heterozygotes can be recognized by excretion of cystathionine after methionine loads.

HISTIDINURIA

Fig. 16.12 gives the metabolic pathways of histidine in normal subjects and in cases of histidinuria. Ghadimi, Partington & Hunter (1961) described elevated plasma and urinary levels of histidine in two sisters. The urine gave a reaction with ferric chloride similar to that found in phenylketonuria. Auerbach *et al.* (1961), investigating a third case of the condition, identified imidazolepyruvic, imidazolelactic and imidazoleacetic acids in the urine, the first acid giving a positive ferric chloride test similar to phenylpyruvic acid. Urocanic acid, given intravenously, was found to be metabolized normally via formiminoglutamic acid, showing that urocanase and enzymes involved in the subsequent pathways of histidine metabolism were normal. They suggested that the primary abnormality was lack of histidase, which catalyses the conversion of histidine to urocanic acid. La Du, Howell & Jacoby (1962) have investigated two further cases of the same disease in two siblings. Histidase was found to be completely absent from the epithelium of the patients, although normally there are considerable amounts of the enzyme in the epidermis, and in fact about half as much as in the liver.

Skin tissue was ideal both from the points of view of accessibility and because it contains no urocanase, which would have further degraded the enzymic reaction product. The presence of an inhibitor was excluded by performing experiments in which homogenates of skin from the cases were mixed with similar homogenates from controls. An apparently normal sibling and the father had a reduced but not absent skin content of histidase, and were presumably heterozygotes.

Plasma histidine in the cases was 13·4 and 17·3 mg./100 ml. as compared to normal levels of less than 2 mg./100 ml. The sweat of the affected children contained no urocanic acid, whereas it can always be detected in normal sweat.

The similarities to the metabolic disorders of phenylketonuria and maple syrup urine disease are obvious, but none of the first five cases of histidinuria described showed any mental deficiency or signs of organic disease. It is, however, a strange coincidence that three of the five were reported to have a speech defect.

At least 20 cases have since been described (Ghadimi & Partington, 1967). Of the 17 patients

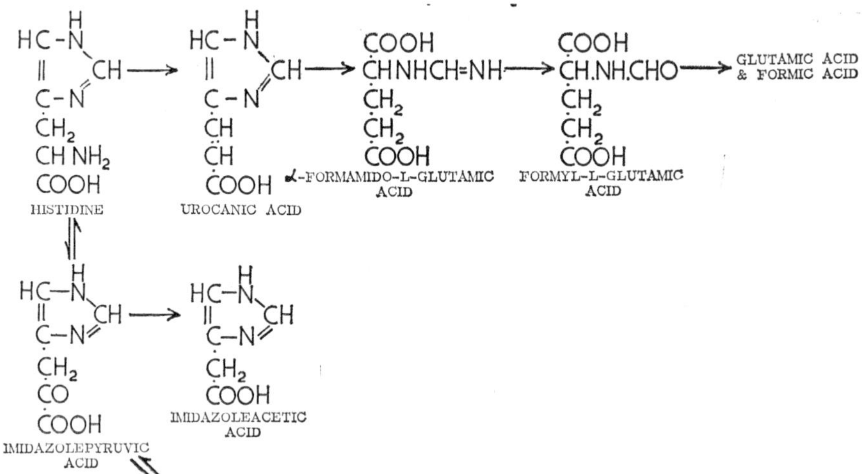

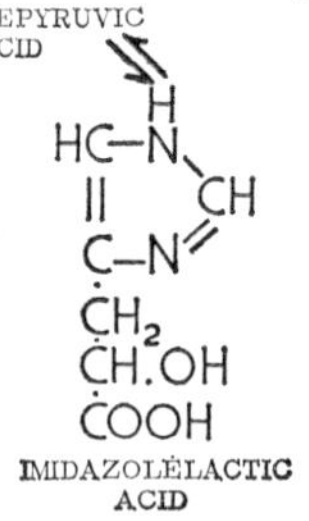

HISTIDINE → UROCANIC ACID → α-FORMAMIDO-L-GLUTAMIC ACID → FORMYL-L-GLUTAMIC ACID → GLUTAMIC ACID & FORMIC ACID

IMIDAZOLEPYRUVIC ACID → IMIDAZOLEACETIC ACID

IMIDAZOLELACTIC ACID

FIG. 16.12. Metabolic pathways of histidine. In histidinuria there is absence of the enzyme histidase converting histidine to urocanic acid. This results in accumulation of histidine, and imidazolepyruvic, imidazolelactic and imidazoleacetic acids in body fluids.

over 1 year of age, 13 had speech defects. Mental ability is very variable as 4 of the 17 were normal, 6 were very retarded with I.Q.s of about 50, and the remainder were backward with I.Q.s between 65 and 85. Histidine is a non-essential amino acid and therapy with reduced histidine intake causes only slight falls in plasma histidine levels, and probably no clinical improvement (Waisman, 1967).

Imidazole-amino-aciduria in cerebromacular degeneration. Bessman & Baldwin (1962) have described another disorder of histidine metabolism. Three families were studied in which there were five patients with late cerebromacular degeneration (juvenile Tay-Sachs disease). The biochemical abnormality was present in all the patients, but also in many apparently normal relatives. Cerebromacular degeneration is inherited as a recessive disorder, whereas the biochemical defect appeared to be dominant. The authors suggest that the metabolic defect alone is the heterozygous manifestation of an abnormal gene, whereas in homozygotes both the metabolic defect and the central nervous system defect are found. The severity of the metabolic abnormality was not, however, correlated with that of the neurological disease.

Carnosine and anserine, peptides containing histidine, were present in urine in amounts of from 20 to 100 mg./day, whereas in normals the amount excreted is 2–3 mg. of the former peptide and 5–7 mg. of the latter (Westall, 1955).

There was also an increased urinary output of histidine and 1-methylhistidine and other unidentified compounds reacting both with ninhydrin and Pauly's reagent. Imidazole-aciduria was also probably present as in histidinuria. No biochemical abnormalities were found in the plasma, suggesting that the urinary abnormalities were at least in part due to a renal tubular defect.

The association of these biochemical abnormalities with the juvenile form of Tay-Sachs disease has since been fully confirmed by Levenson *et al.* (1964).

Hypercarnosinaemia is a further allied metabolic disorder involving carnosine metabolism. The condition was described in two sibs presenting with fits and mental deficiency (Perry, Hansen, Tischler, Bunting & Berry, 1967). There was excess of the dipeptide carnosine (β-alanyl histidine) in fasting plasma and urine, and similarly of the methylated derivative anserine after eating large amounts of meat. The condition is probably due to deficiency of the dipeptidase, carnosinase. This enzyme also splits homocarnosine, a peptide in high concentration in the brain, to γ-aminobutyric acid and histidine (Abraham, Risano & Udenfriend, 1962). Carnosinase deficiency could reduce formation of cerebral γ-aminobutyric acid and thus explain the fits which were a major feature of the disease.

DEFECTS IN AMINO ACIDS METABOLISM AFFECTING THE ORNITHINE-UREA CYCLE

Five hereditary disorders are known in which a metabolic block of the Krebs-Henseleit cycle of urea formation results in a high blood ammonia level. These are hyperlysinaemia, citrullinuria, arginino-succinuria, and two types of hyper-ammonaemia.

HYPERLYSINAEMIA

Three unrelated patients have been described with persistent hyperlysinaemia (Ghadimi, Binnington & Pecora, 1965; Woody, Hutzler & Dancis, 1966). There was considerable physical and mental retardation, hypotonia and weakness of muscle, and electro-encephalographic abnormalities. Plasma concentrations of lysine ranged from 3·5–8·5 mg./100 ml., which is about twice the normal value. There was also excess lysine in urine and CSF. Lysine loading caused higher plasma peaks than controls, and the return to basal levels was considerably delayed. The precise block in lysine metabolism in these patients has not been elucidated as yet. After administration of ^{14}C-labelled lysine less of the

radio-activity was recovered as CO_2 in the expired air in one patient as compared to controls (Woods et al., 1966). No information is as yet available of the value of possible therapy with a low lysine diet.

It is uncertain whether these patients are identical with the condition described as "lysine intolerance with periodic ammonia intoxication" (Colombo, Richterich, Donath, Spahr & Rossi, 1964). The patient was an infant who had suffered from vomiting fits, episodes of coma, and variable muscle tonicity from birth. On a low protein diet of 1·5 g./Kg. body weight/day, the infant was improved clinically, blood ammonia was only slightly increased (2·4 μg./ml.) and plasma lysine and arginine were normal. On a normal protein intake, at this age 3 g./Kg. body weight/day, there was rapid deterioration, blood ammonia rose to 5·6 μg./ml., lysine was increased to 6·8 mg./100 ml. and arginine to 6·2 mg./100 ml., about three times the normal value, but plasma ornithine remained normal. There was no associated amino-aciduria. Lysine loads were toxic, whereas excess arginine, leucine, or glycine had no unusual effects. Some improvement occurred on a low lysine diet. Buergi, Ritchterick & Colombo (1966) have claimed that there is deficiency of L-lysine dehydrogenase in a liver biopsy. It was postulated that the high lysine content of body fluids results in competitive inhibition of arginase. This would account for a normal plasma level of ornithine, an amino acid which is usually

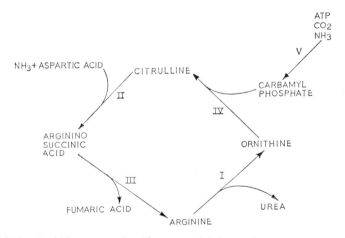

Fig 16.13. Ornithine-urea cycle. Absence or deficiency of enzymes occurs as follows:
I. Arginase in hyperlysinaemia.
II. Argininosuccinic acid synthetase in citrullinaemia.
III. Argininosuccinic acid lyase in argininosuccinic aciduria.
IV. Ornithine transcarboxylase in hyperammonaemia (type 1).
V. Carbamyl phosphate synthetase in hyperammonaemia (type 2).

produced in excess if plasma arginine levels are raised.

ARGININOSUCCINIC ACIDURIA

Allan, Cusworth, Dent & Wilson (1958) described two mentally deficient siblings, who were children of a non-consanguineous marriage. There was very severe mental deficiency in both cases with major fits in one child, and electro-encephalography showed a grossly abnormal tracing. There was a characteristic abnormality of the hair, which was irregular, matted and friable. A systolic murmur suggestive of ventricular septal defect was present in both patients. An abnormal amino acid was found in CSF, plasma and urine. The clearance of the amino acid was approximately equal to the glomerular filtration rate. The concentration in CSF was 2·5–3 times that in the plasma.

The substance was identified by Westall (1960) as argininosuccinic acid, and each patient excreted about 3 g./day. The excretion was little affected by protein restriction or by adding arginine to the diet, but was increased by feeding ornithine and citrulline. Urea formation was normal, indicating that there was no abnormality of the Krebs-Henseleit cycle. The high concentration of argininosuccinic acid in the CSF suggests that the source of the abnormal amino acid may be in the brain.

Levin, Mackay & Oberholzer (1961) have described a third case of the disease. There was a severe illness in the first week of life with abdominal distension, gross hepatomegaly, blood-stained vomiting, and periods of unconsciousness. Later there was severe retardation of mental and physical development, persistent liver enlargement, and changes in the hair similar to the two previous cases. Microscopy showed the hair defect was typical of trichorrexis nodosa, and it was suggested that the abnormality was due to reduced incorporation of arginine into keratin. In this case, protein restriction reduced argininosuccinic acid output, whilst addition of arginine increased its excretion.

The primary biochemical disorder is absence of argininosuccinic acid lyase (Levin, 1967). Other enzymes of the urea cycle are normal. It now seems probable that the clinical effects are more due to post-prandial rises of blood ammonia, similar to those of citrullinuria, rather than to a high level of argininosuccinic acid in body fluids. Similar difficulties in control of post-prandial blood ammonia occur to those in the management of citrullinuria. Reduction of protein in infancy may be of value in both conditions, and

the feeds should be small and frequent to reduce dangerous elevations of blood ammonia as far as is possible.

CITRULLINURIA

McMurray, Mohyuddin, Rossiter, Rathbun, Valentine, Koegler & Zarfas (1962) reported the excretion of citrulline averaging 1·41 g./day in a mentally retarded child of 18 months born of a consanguinous marriage. There was increased citrulline concentration both in the plasma (20–30 mg./100 ml.; normal 0·38–0·57 mg./100 ml.) and the cerebrospinal fluid (6 mg./100 ml.; normal < 0·1 mg./100 ml.). The urea excretion was normal, suggesting that there was no abnormality of the Krebs-Henseleit cycle.

Citrulline output was proportionate to the intake of protein, was increased by oral citrulline or ornithine (McMurray, Mohyuddin, Rossiter, Rathbun & Zarfas, 1962), but was unaffected by administration of a broad-spectrum antibiotic. There was also some increase of urinary alanine, aspartate, glycine, histidine and serine, although the plasma concentrations of these amino acids were normal (McMurray & Mohyuddin, 1962) suggesting partial saturation of an amino acid transport system in the proximal renal tubules by the high concentration of citrulline in the glomerular filtrate.

An important feature of the condition is a high blood ammonia concentration, particularly after protein ingestion. The metabolic defect appears to be a partial deficiency of the enzyme argininosuccinic acid synthetase. The patient is capable of maintaining normal amounts of arginine and urea in plasma, but is less efficient than the normal subject in rapid conversion of ammonia arising from deamination of ingested amino acids to urea. Neomycin therapy causes reduction of ammonia 4 hr. after protein ingestion, but does not affect the values at 2 hr. which are due to endogenous metabolism of amino acids (Mohyuddin et al., 1967). The greatest increases of blood ammonia occurred after glutamine ingestion. A low-protein diet causes little if any improvement. No effective therapy for this disease is known to date.

HYPERAMMONAEMIA

This disease was described in identical twins and their cousin (Russell, Levin, Oberholzer & Sinclair, 1962). In one affected infant there was early development of vomiting, screaming fits, and agitation, followed by stupor and coma. One of the twins appeared normal in physique and mentality until the age of 9 years, when she developed headache, malaise and lethargy.

Amino acid excretion is normal or at the most only marginally high, with some increase of glutamine output. The main biochemical abnormality is increase of blood and cerebrospinal fluid ammonia, the rise being less fluctuant than in citrullinuria and argininosuccinic aciduria. The primary defect has been shown to be absence of ornithine transcarbamylase in the liver.

An allied but probably distinct disorder has been described by Freeman Nicholson, Masland, Rowland & Carter (1964). Here there was also elevation of plasma glycine as well as of ammonia, and a liver biopsy showed deficiency of carbamyl phosphate synthetase, and not of ornithine transcarbamylase.

DEFECTS IN GLYCINE AND SARCOSINE METABOLISM
HYPERGLYCINAEMIA

Ketotic type. This disease causes mental and growth retardation, attacks of ketosis with vomiting, weakness, stupor, fits, thrombocytopenia and neutropenia. This disease and Type I glycogenosis are almost the only conditions where ketones are found in neonatal urine. Most cases of the disease have proved fatal within the first year (Nyhan, 1967). There are often signs of both pyramidal and extra-pyramidal damage in the central nervous system. Exacerbations were found to be produced by ingestion of excess protein, and it has since been shown that the responsible amino acids are leucine, isoleucine, valine, threonine and methionine (Childs & Nyhan, 1964). Menkes (1966) showed that the ketosis in the condition was unlike more common types in that neutral ketones were not exclusively composed of acetone. In fact, the acetone content was little more than 50% of the total, the rest being chiefly 2 : butanone (methyl ethyl ketone) with lesser amounts of 2 : pentanone, 3 : pentanone, acetaldehyde and a hexanone, probably 2 : hexanone. The source of these unusual ketones remains unknown, but possibly 2 : butanone is produced by decarboxylation of *a*-methylacetoacetyl coenzyme A, a compound formed during catabolism of *iso*leucine. There is, in addition, reduced urinary output of *a*-oxoglutarate, but possibly this may be a non-specific effect of the systemic acidosis of the condition. A low-protein diet or the administration of large doses of sodium benzoate, by sequestrating glycine as hippuric acid, reduces the plasma and urinary glycine content, and the size of the expanded body pool of glycine. Simultaneously, there is a rise of polymorphonuclear leucocytes in the blood, showing that the neutropenia of the disease is due to the high content of glycine in body fluids. Sodium benzoate has, however, no effect on the ketosis, this being only improved by dietary restriction of branched-chain amino acids, threonine, and methionine. Dietary treatment consists of a low protein diet of about 0·5 g./Kg. body weight, with or without supplementation of the amino acids which do not produce ketosis or elevate plasma glycine. A positive test for ketones in the urine is an indication for a period on a protein-free regime with glucose infusions. Patients diagnosed early in life appear to improve considerably on this regime. The precise enzymatic defect has not been defined. The conversion of glycine to serine was slower than that of normal subjects, but this could be caused by the increased glycine pool in the patient's metabolism of glycine to δ-amino-laevulinic acid. Conjugation with benzoic and salicylic acids, and creatinine and oxalate formation are all normal. Metabolism of glycine to CO_2 and incorporation of glycine into tissue proteins are either normal or not grossly defective.

Non-ketotic type. This metabolic defect is associated with failure to thrive, fits and mental deficiency (Gerritsen, Kaveggia & Waisman, 1965). Plasma glycine ranged from 7–9·5 g./ 100 ml. and urinary glycine 1·5–2·0 g./day, values about four times the normal. Other similar cases have been described by Mabry (1963), and Schreier (1964). There was no ketosis and a leucine load failed to produce a positive reaction for urinary ketones. Oxalate excretion is almost zero, but glyoxylic acid is oxidized to oxalate in normal amount. This probably indicates deficiency of glycine oxidase, with reduced or absent conversion of glycine to glyoxylate. Theoretically, a low-protein diet might be beneficial in a case diagnosed early in life, but trials have not yet been reported.

HYPERSARCOSINAEMIA

Sarcosine, although closely related to glycine, is not a constituent of body protein and is not normally detectable in either plasma or urine. Gerritsen & Waisman (1966) have described a mentally retarded infant with hypersarcosinaemia. There was, in addition, failure to thrive, dysphagia, hypertonia, tremor and marked muscle weakness. An older sib was also affected but the clinical symptoms, although causing mental retardation, were less severe. Heterozygotes showed slight but abnormal sarcosinuria.

It was thought probable that the patient was defective in sarcosine dehydrogenase, which catalyses oxidative demethylation of the amino acid to glycine. Ethanolamine was in increased concentration in plasma, this being formed by a minor pathway of sarcosine metabolism. No dietary or other effective therapy is known to date.

DEFECTS OF IMINO-ACID METABOLISM
HYPERPROLINAEMIA

Several different clinical syndromes appear to be associated with hyperprolinaemia and in many cases there is a relationship to hereditary nephritis which remains completely unexplained.

Hyperprolinaemia due to deficiency of proline oxidase has been reported in two separate families associated with congenital renal defects and haematuria (Schafer, Scriver & Efron, 1962; Efron, 1965). In both families some of the affected members were mentally retarded, and in one there was nerve deafness and major fits. The renal disease was, however, found in several generations and was, therefore, presumably due to dominant heredity, whereas the biochemical disorder was only found in a single sibship and was therefore thought to be recessive. Two other families, however, have been recorded (Kopelman, Asatoor & Milne, 1964; Fuhrmann, 1963) in which hyperprolinaemia was found in two generations of families afflicted with hereditary nephritis. Unfortunately, enzyme studies were not possible in these families, although presumably proline oxidase could not be absent in heterozygotes. In all reported cases there has been an "overflow" amino-aciduria of proline and a "renal" leak of hydroxyproline and glycine which share a common renal transport system with proline. Plasma proline concentrations have been of the order of 1–2 μmole/ml., a value about ten times the normal.

A second type of hyperprolinaemia (Efron, 1967) has been reported in two unrelated patients with mental retardation and fits but no renal disease. The condition was shown to be due to deficiency of the enzyme Δ^1-pyrroline-5-carboxylic acid oxidase and therefore both proline and its oxidized derivative Δ^1-pyrroline-5-carboxylate are present in excess in plasma and urine. The latter gives a characteristic reaction with o-aminobenzaldehyde. Although it would reasonably be expected that plasma proline should be higher in cases due to proline oxidase, the reverse seems to be the case. Efron (1967) reports plasma proline concentrations up to 40 mg./100 ml. As proline is a non-essential amino acid, dietary measures are unlikely to lower plasma proline concentrations, nor is it certain that such a reduction would necessarily produce any therapeutic benefit.

HYDROXYPROLINAEMIA

Only a single case of this condition has been recorded to date (Efron, Bixby, Pallata & Pryles, 1962). It is therefore uncertain whether the excess plasma concentration of the amino acid was the cause of the patient's severe mental deficiency. Plasma hydroxyproline values were reported as 0·2–0·4 μmole/ml. as compared to the normal value of 0·01 μmole/ml. Although excess free hydroxyproline was excreted in urine, the imino-glycine transport system remained unsaturated and there was no excess urinary loss of proline or glycine. The condition was shown to be due to lack of hydroxyproline oxidase. Like prolinaemia, dietary control of the biochemical defect is unlikely to be effective.

DEFECTS OF β-AMINO ACID METABOLISM
HYPER-β-ALANINAEMIA

Scriver, Pueschel & Davies (1966) have described an infant suffering from somnolence and major fits in which there was found an increased plasma concentration of β-alanine. The primary defect appeared to be a deficiency of β-alanine-α-oxoglutarate transaminase. The urinary transport system for β-amino acids was saturated by the excess β-alanine transport, with consequent increased urinary output of β-amino-isobutyric acid and taurine. In addition, there was a high concentration of γ-aminobutyric acid in plasma, CSF and urine. This was thought to be due to an increased leak from the central nervous system due to high plasma concentrations of β-alanine. The fits were probably due to low concentration of the central nervous inhibitor γ-aminobutyric acid, within cerebral tissue.

GROUP II. DISEASE CAUSED BY A SPECIFIC AMINO ACID TRANSPORT DEFECT IN THE RENAL TUBULES AND THE SMALL INTESTINE

There are three conditions in this group each affecting a separate amino acid transport group, i.e. cystinuria involving the dibasic amino acids, Hartnup disease involving a large group of neutral amino acids and prolinuria, the imino-glycine group. In each disorder there is a similar transport defect in the proximal renal tubules and the jejunum. The defect is highly specific, transport of all other substances being within normal limits.

CYSTINURIA

In 1812 Wollaston described a urinary calculus of unusual composition. During the following 100 years many further examples of the same kind of stone were recognized, and it was found that they were composed almost entirely of the amino acid cystine. Furthermore, patients who showed a tendency to form such stones were observed to be excreting continuously in their urine large amounts of cystine. The disorder was frequently familial and it was concluded that it was genetically determined.

recurrent calculus formation, first described by Wollaston, and now known to involve specifically the abnormal excretion not only of cystine but also of lysine, arginine and ornithine.

The loss of these four amino acids even in these considerable amounts does not lead to any nutritional disturbances in the patients on an ordinary diet. All the clinical features of the disease can in fact be attributed to the formation of stones in the renal tract.

Cystine is one of the least soluble amino acids. In urine of between pH 5 and 7 it is soluble only

TABLE 16.4

Excretion of cystine, lysine, arginine and ornithine in five patients with cystinuria
(Stein, 1951)

| Amino acid | Excretion in g./day | | | | |
	Case 1	Case 2	Case 3	Case 4	Case 5
Ornithine	0·42	0·18	0·36	0·50	0·42
Cystine	0·97	0·42	0·82	0·74	0·70
Arginine	1·24	0·55	0·92	0·77	0·67
Lysine	2·30	1·00	1·98	2·38	1·35

Despite considerable interest in the condition, little progress was made until it became possible to apply modern biochemical techniques, notably chromatography (Dent & Rose, 1951; Stein, 1951) to the problem. It then emerged that patients who form cystine calculi in the renal tract excrete in their urine not only cystine but also the basic amino acids lysine, arginine and ornithine in grossly increased amounts. The quantities involved are remarkable (Table 16.4). On the average, 0·73 g. of cystine, 1·8 g. of lysine, 0·83 g. of arginine and 0·37 g. of ornithine are excreted each day (Stein, 1951), and this is continuous and probably persists unchanged throughout their lives. Furthermore, the abnormality is highly specific for these four amino acids.

Cystine may also be excreted in unusual amounts in a number of other genetically determined conditions, notably in the Fanconi syndrome and in Wilson's disease; in the past the Fanconi syndrome was certainly confused with the type of cystinuria described above. It is now clear, however, that these disorders may be sharply differentiated on clinical, biochemical and genetical grounds (Dent & Harris, 1951); it is convenient therefore to reserve the term "cystinuria" for the classical condition leading to

to the extent of 300–400 mg./litre (Dent & Senior, 1954). In patients excreting 0·5–1 g. of cystine/day the concentration of this amino acid will frequently reach saturation level, particularly during the night when the urine passed is most concentrated. Consequently cystine will tend to come out of solution, and this is presumably the prime factor in calculus formation. Lysine, arginine and ornithine, on the other hand, are freely soluble and therefore do not become incorporated in the stones.

Renal and metabolic studies. In the past it had been thought that cystinuria represented a disorder in the intermediary metabolism either of cystine itself or of the other sulphur-containing amino acids, cysteine and methionine (for full reviews see Garrod, 1923, and Bach, 1952). The exact nature of the postulated abnormality had always, however, been obscure, and the discovery that lysine, arginine and ornithine were equally involved introduced further complications, because of the absence of any obvious connection between the intermediary metabolism of these amino acids and the sulphur-containing ones.

An alternative hypothesis now fully proven was put forward by Dent in 1949, who suggested that the abnormality in cystinuria was of renal

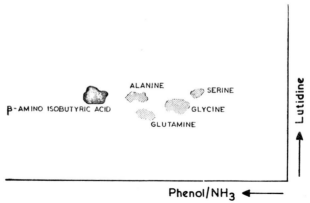

FIG. 16.14. Urine from a healthy individual with an unusual level of β-amino*iso*butyric acid excretion.

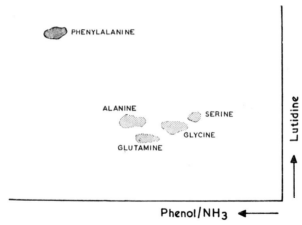

FIG. 16.15. Urine from a patient with phenylketonuria.

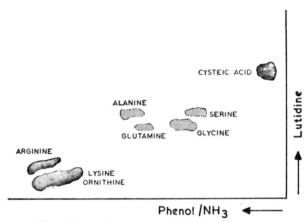

FIG. 16.16. Urine from a patient with cystinuria.

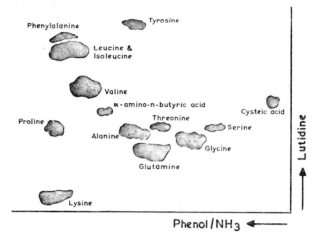

FIG. 16.17. Urine from a patient with the Fanconi syndrome.

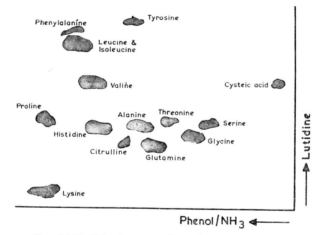

FIG. 16.18. Urine from a patient with Wilson's disease.

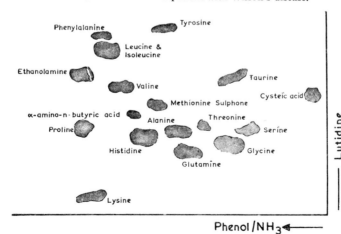

FIG. 16.19. Urine from a patient with acute yellow atrophy.

origin. The renal tubules, he suggested, might be unable to reabsorb the cystine, lysine, arginine and ornithine normally present in the glomerular filtrate, and these substances would therefore appear in large amounts in the urine.

The plasma cystine level has now been measured in a number of cystinuric patients by a variety of different methods (Fowler, Harris & Warren, 1952; Dent, Heathcote & Joron, 1954; Dent, Senior & Walshe, 1954; Stein & Moore, 1954). It is in fact not elevated as would have been expected on the metabolic hypothesis, but is if anything somewhat less than normal as might be anticipated on the renal hypothesis. The same is also true for lysine, arginine and ornithine (Dent & Rose, 1951; Stein & Moore, 1954).

Clearance studies by Dent and his colleagues (1954) have shown that the clearance of cystine is often more than thirty times that found in normal individuals, and indeed is of the same order of magnitude as the expected rate of glomerular filtration. In one subject, where the inulin and cystine clearances were measured simultaneously, almost identical values were obtained.

Many homozygous cystinurics have an even higher cystine clearance, up to twice the glomerular filtration rate (Arrow & Westall, 1958; Frimpter, Horwith, Furth, Fellows & Thomson, 1962). This is not due to artefacts such as solution of cystine from a cystine stone, as diuresis does not appreciably increase urinary cystine output (Dent et al., 1965). The results may represent a true tubular secretion of cystine, conversion of plasma cysteine to cystine within the kidney, or a continuation of cystine efflux from proximal tubular cells with complete absence of influx.

Clearances of dibasic amino acids in cystinuria have been measured by Doolan, Harper, Hutchin & Alpen (1957) using microbiological assay, and by Arrow & Westall (1958) using column chromatography. In homozygotes the cystine clearance approximates to the glomerular filtration rate, only a small fraction of filtered lysine is reabsorbed by the tubules, whilst the clearances of arginine and ornithine are more variable from case to case. Considerable amounts of the latter two amino acids are reabsorbed by the tubules even in the most severe cases of the disease.

The results of experiments involving the feeding of cystine and cysteine to cystinuric subjects have been variously interpreted (Bach, 1952), but can probably be most comprehensively understood on the renal and intestinal theories (Dent et al., 1954; Milne, Asatoor, Edwards & Loughridge, 1961). If cystine itself is fed to cystinuric patients there is little or no rise in the plasma cystine level,

and no increase in the urinary cystine. It appears, however, to be absorbed and metabolized, because an appropriate increase in the urinary sulphate can be demonstrated (Dent et al., 1954; Hele, 1909; Alsberg & Folin, 1906; Lovney, Berglund & Graves, 1923).

Ingestion of cysteine by cystinurics leads to quite different phenomena. There is a rapid rise in the plasma level of cystine (or cysteine) and a very marked increase in excretion of cystine in the urine (Dent et al., 1954; Brand, Cahill & Harris, 1933, 1935; Lewis, Brown & White, 1936). If cysteine is fed to normal subjects there is a similar rise in plasma level, and also an appreciable excretion of cystine in the urine (Dent et al., 1954). In general in these experiments the urinary cystine output varied with the plasma levels. However, for equivalent plasma levels the cystine excretion was much greater in the cystinurics than in the normal subjects. In cystinurics the cystine clearance did not change with increasing plasma levels, but remained virtually constant at a value of the same order of magnitude as the glomerular filtration rate. In normals the clearances were very much lower, but did rise with increasing plasma levels.

These experiments suggest that cystinurics do not differ in any material respect from normal subjects in their intermediary metabolism of cystine, cysteine or methionine. However, for equivalent plasma concentrations of cystine, they excrete it in much greater amounts indicating a defect in renal function.

The renal hypothesis implies that in normal individuals the tubular reabsorption of cystine, lysine, arginine and ornithine has at least one step which is common to and specific for these amino acids, and that in cystinuria this process is in some way defective. An interesting question which arises is what property common to cystine, lysine, arginine and ornithine leads to their being handled by the renal tubules differently from other amino acids. Some evidence for a common reabsorptive mechanism for lysine and arginine in dogs has been obtained (Beyer, Wright, Skeggs, Russo & Shaner, 1947), and these particular substances resemble each other and ornithine sufficiently closely in structure and chemical properties to make this association not very surprising. The specific association of cystine with the basic amino acids is, however, rather unexpected. Dent & Rose (1951) originally suggested, on the basis of the structural formulae (Fig. 16.20), that the important similarity might be the occurrence of two positively charged amino groups separated by a chain of four to six atoms.

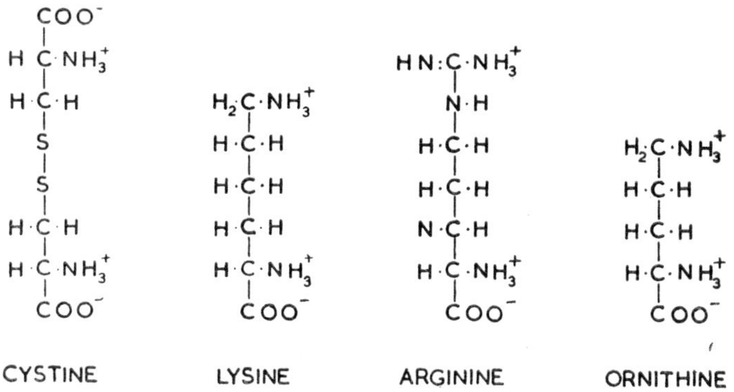

COO⁻ ... (chemical structural formulae)

CYSTINE   LYSINE   ARGININE   ORNITHINE

Fig. 16.20. Formulae of cystine, lysine, arginine and ornithine.

The transport mechanism could perhaps involve the combination of these positively charged amino groups with similarly spaced, negatively charged carboxyl groups projecting from alternate glutamate or aspartate residues on a protein surface.

There are, however, indications that the mechanism of transport of di-sulphur amino acids, although connected with those of lysine, arginine and ornithine, involves a separate mechanism. The dibasic amino acids, but not cystine, are concentrated within renal cortical slices (Rosenberg, Downing, Durant & Segal, 1962). The di-sulphide linkage was found to be essential in the active transport of sulphur-containing amino acids by hamster intestinal sacs (Spencer, Brody & Mautner, 1965).

Frimpter (1961) recognized excess excretion of the mixed disulphide of cysteine and homocystine in cystinuric patients, in amounts of about one-tenth that of cystine. Probably there is a complex equilibrium of the five amino acids cysteine, homocysteine, cystine, homocystine, and the mixed disulphide in plasma. It is known that cystine and cysteine are in highest concentration, the ratio cystine/cysteine averaging 2·5 (Brigham, Stein & Moore, 1960). This equilibrium is controlled by the enzyme cystine reductase, which favours a higher cysteine concentration than would occur by spontaneous chemical equilibrium. If it is assumed that the plasma concentration of cysteine is twenty times that of homocysteine, the relative concentration of cystine : mixed disulphide : homocystine would be expected to be about 400 : 40 : 1. Probably each of the three disulphides is excreted by homozygous cystinurics at a clearance approximating to the glomerular filtration rate. Cystine would, therefore, occur in cystinuric urine at easily detectable concentration, the

mixed disulphide would be detectable with some difficulty, and homocystine would be far below the level of possible recognition. Cystine calculi were found to contain small amounts of the mixed disulphide, which is also an extremely insoluble amino acid.

Many apparently anomalous findings in cystinuria have now been explained by the demonstration that a similar amino acid transport defect is present in the gut as well as in the kidney (Milne et al., 1961; Asatoor et al., 1962). Over 70 years ago Von Udranšky and Baumann (1889) recorded the excretion of the diamines, putrescine and cadaverine, in cases of cystinuria. Later work was reviewed by Garrod (1908). These results until recently were explained as due to degradation of lysine and ornithine in infected and contaminated urine specimens. Investigations in cystinuria have clarified the metabolic pathways of absorbed diamines produced by bacterial action in the colon (Fig. 16.21). They are first oxidized by diamine oxidase to the γ-amino-aldehydes. These are highly reactive compounds and a proportion spontaneously cyclize with formation of Δ_1-pyrroline and Δ_1-piperideine. These compounds are reduced in the body to pyrrolidine and piperidine which are invariably present in normal urine (von Euler, 1945).

After feeding lysine and ornithine to cystinurics abnormal amounts of the unchanged amino acid and of the corresponding diamine are present in the stools. There is also grossly increased urinary output of pyrrolidine or piperidine reaching a maximum about 16 hr. after amino acid ingestion. Similar findings occur after arginine ingestion, and plasma levels of arginine were found to be abnormally low in cystinurics, conclusively proving delayed and incomplete absorption from the gut. Arginine is degraded by colonic bacteria

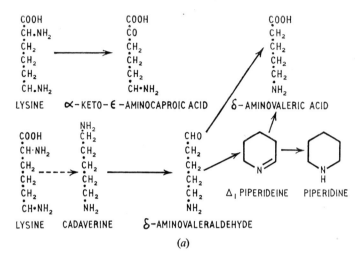

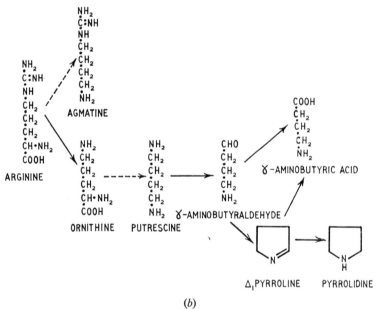

FIG. 16.21. Cystinuria.

(a) Minor pathways of lysine metabolism. Normally this amino acid is degraded *via* α-keto-ε-aminocaproic acid. Lysine reaching the colon is converted to cadaverine. Broken lines indicate pathways confined to bacterial metabolism.

(b) Minor pathways of arginine metabolism. Arginine reaching the colon is converted to ornithine and putrescine.

to ornithine *via* citrulline. In this case, therefore, excess citrulline is also found in faeces, and some may be absorbed and be excreted in the urine as a temporary amino-aciduria of the "overflow" type. Citrullinuria in cystinurics has also been recorded by Visakorpi & Hyrska (1960), and

appears to occur frequently in cystinuric dogs (Treacher, 1962).

Jejunal biopsies from normal controls were found to concentrate the cystine, lysine, arginine and ornithine, but no such active transport occurred in biopsies from many homozygous cystinuric subjects (McCarthy, Borland, Lynch, Owen & Tyor, 1964; Thier, Segal, Fox, Blair, & Rosenberg, 1965). Plasma cystine increases more slowly and to a lower peak after oral cystine in cystinurics as compared to normals (London & Foley, 1965), whereas there was no such difference after cysteine ingestion (Foley & London, 1965).

Genetical studies. It has been known for a long time that cystinuria is genetically determined, and in recent years it has been possible to study more than 30 different families in which this condition

fact, all values may be found between the very low amounts encountered in a random sample of the normal population and the very large amounts in cystinuric patients with stone formation. Determinations on several samples from particular individuals over periods of 2–3 years. showed that each person has a fairly characteristic level of excretion of these amino acids.

Fig. 16.22 shows the relationship between the cystine excretion and the lysine excretion in individual members of these families. There is a

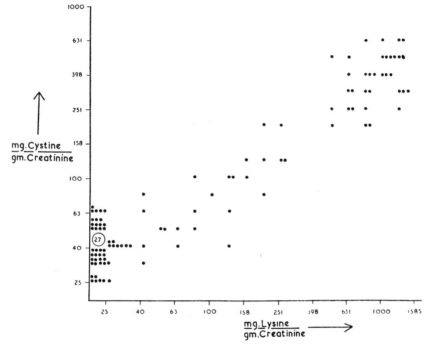

Fig. 16.22. Cystine and lysine contents of urine from a series of cystinuric patients and their relatives. Each point represents a single individual. The concentration of cystine and lysine has been related to the creatinine content in each sample in order to minimize variations due to different rates of urine formation (Harris *et al.*, 1955).

occurred (Harris & Warren, 1953; Harris, Mittwoch, Robson & Warren, 1955). When the urine from healthy relatives of patients with cystine stone formation is examined it is found that a number of them, though clinically quite well, nevertheless excrete cystine and lysine in unusual amounts in their urine, and occasionally arginine and ornithine are found as well. Quantitative estimations of cystine, lysine and arginine have been made on the urines of a large number of such relatives of cystinuric patients, and it is apparent that among them there is a considerable variation in the excretion of these substances. In

very close correlation between the cystine and lysine outputs. Differences between individuals with regard to their cystine excretions are paralleled by equivalent differences in the lysine excretions. On the other hand, abnormal arginine excretion is only consistently found when the cystine and lysine outputs are relatively high (Fig. 16.23). Below these levels, even though the excretion of cystine and lysine may be well above the values found in normal individuals, the arginine output is either within normal limits or is at most only slightly elevated. Apparently the cystine and lysine excretion must be above a certain threshold before

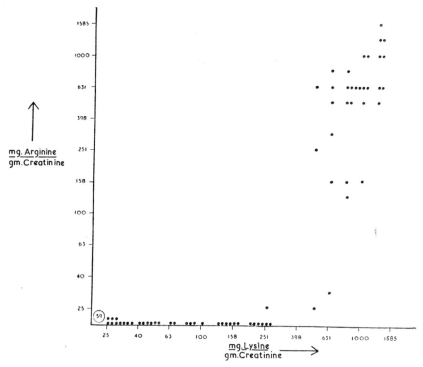

F<small>IG</small>. 16.23. Lysine and arginine contents of urine from a series of cystinuric patients and their relatives. Each point represents a single individual. The concentration of lysine and arginine has been related to the creatinine content in each sample in order to minimize variations due to different rates of urine formation (Harris *et al.*, 1955).

arginine is excreted in excess. The same may be the case for ornithine, but detailed quantitative results are not yet available. Thus, healthy individuals occur in some of these families with a moderately increased but quite definitely abnormal excretion of cystine and lysine, and with normal arginine excretion. Such individuals rarely form stones, presumably because the urinary cystine concentration does not rise to saturation level.

If it is true that in most cystinuric patients with stone formation there is a complete or nearly complete failure to reabsorb in the renal tubules cystine, lysine, arginine and ornithine, then the fact that all degrees of cystine and lysine excretion may be found among their apparently healthy relatives suggests that all degrees of failure of tubular reabsorption may occur. Furthermore, it would appear that when the reabsorptive capacity for these four amino acids is limited, but not completely abolished, then arginine and perhaps ornithine are reabsorbed preferentially to cystine and lysine.

The genetical analysis may be taken much further. It can be shown that the families are heretogeneous with respect to the occurrence of those individuals with moderately increased cystine and lysine excretion, but little or no detectable abnormality in arginine and ornithine excretion. In more than two-thirds of the families such people are not found, and there occurs a sharp segregation between individuals excreting very large amounts of cystine, lysine, arginine and ornithine, and the normals. The familial distribution is typical of a mendelian recessive character (Fig. 16.24). Abnormal individuals are found only in a single sibship in each family; the parents, children and other relatives are normal, and there is an increased incidence of parental consanguinity. Appropriate calculations indicate that the observed segregation ratios are consistent with those theoretically expected. Thus one can conclude that in most cases of cystinuria one is dealing with a rare recessive gene whose effects are only manifested in homozygous individuals. The heterozygotes—that is to say, both parents, all the children and a proportion of the other relatives of the patient—have no detectable abnormality. Thus individuals who carry this

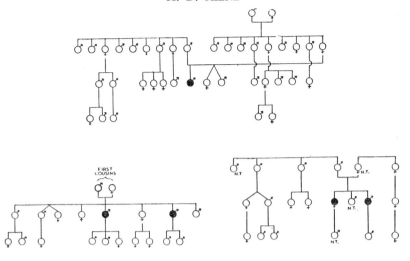

●   GROSSLY ABNORMAL EXCRETION OF CYSTINE,
        LYSINE, ARGININE & ORNITHINE.

○   NORMAL AMINOACID EXCRETION.

N.T.   NOT TESTED.

FIG. 16.24. Typical pedigrees of recessive cystinuria.

abnormal gene in double dose appear to be virtually incapable of tubular reabsorption of these four amino acids, while individuals carrying it only in single dose can do this as efficiently as normal people, at least at normal loads.

In the other families a more complex situation is encountered. Three types of individual may be identified; those with a grossly abnormal excretion of the four amino acids; those with a moderate excretion of cystine and lysine but a normal or only slightly elevated excretion of arginine and ornithine; and those with normal excretion. The intermediate class is somewhat variable and some overlap of the distributions occurs. Nevertheless,

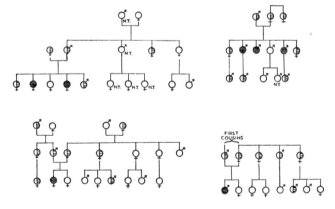

●   GROSSLY ABNORMAL EXCRETION OF CYSTINE,
        LYSINE, ARGININE & ORNITHINE.

◐   ABNORMAL EXCRETION OF CYSTINE & LYSINE.
        ARGININE & ORNITHINE EXCRETION NORMAL OR
        ONLY SLIGHTLY ELEVATED.

N.T.   NOT TESTED.

FIG. 16.25. Typical pedigrees of incompletely recessive cystinuria.

in most instances there is no difficulty in classification.

The familial distribution here (Fig. 16.25) can be readily understood on the hypothesis that the more extreme phenotype, where there is a gross failure to reabsorb the four amino acids, occurs in individuals homozygous for an abnormal gene, whereas the intermediate phenotype with only a moderate failure of lysine and arginine reabsorption occurs in heterozygotes. As in the first group of families, individuals with the abnormal gene in double dose show the complete defect. In contrast to the situation there, however, the gene in single dose also leads to a disturbance of tubular reabsorption.

Whether or not the abnormal genes segregating in the two types of family are at the same chromosomal locus is still unsettled, and no clinical difference has yet been detected between the two groups of homozygotes.

One can perhaps visualize the situation in this second group of families in terms of a fairly simple model. We may suppose that the normal gene at the particular chromosomal locus is in some way concerned with the synthesis of a substance, perhaps an enzyme, which is normally present in the renal tubule cells and is necessary for the active transport of these four amino acids, perhaps because it combines with them specifically; and that the abnormal gene is incapable of carrying out this synthesis. In homozygous individuals carrying no normal gene at this locus the substance will not be formed and so active transport will not take place. Heterozygotes, who have one normal gene and one abnormal one, will perhaps form only limited amounts of the substance, so that the tubular capacity for the reabsorption of these amino acids will be reduced, and only a proportion of these amino acids in the glomerular filtrate will be reabsorbed. Such a substance would presumably have a greater affinity for arginine and perhaps ornithine than for cystine and lysine.

A similar kind of model could also be applied to the first group of families. Here, however, one must assume that if a carrier substance or enzyme is formed in less than normal amounts by the heterozygote, it is nevertheless present in quantities adequate to deal with the normal load of these amino acids.

How far this kind of model will be useful remains to be seen. Nevertheless, it is clear that a particular abnormal gene may lead to a highly specific disturbance in the renal-tubular reabsorptive processes, and that the degree of this disturbance may be related quantitatively to

whether an individual possesses the gene in single or double dose.

Harris & Robson (1955) studied the urinary lysine/arginine ratio in the two types of cystinuria. They found this ratio could vary from $0\cdot8$–$4\cdot2$ in different homozygotes, and observed that the variation was much greater among recessive homozygotes than among incompletely recessive homozygotes, although the mean of the two groups was not significantly different. The ratio in homozygous siblings in recessive cystinuria was very similar, but no such correlation occurred in siblings in the incompletely recessive form of the disease. They concluded that recessive cystinuria is probably not due to a single abnormal gene, and that individuals from different families are, therefore, statistically more dissimilar in the proximal tubular transport of lysine and arginine than are affected siblings with a greater chance of identical hereditary abnormality.

Rosenberg et al. (1966) claim that there are, in fact, three types of human cystinuria. In type I, heterozygotes show no urinary abnormality, and there is complete absence of concentration of cystine and dibasic amino acids by jejunal mucosa. In Types II and III, heterozygotes excrete excess cystine and lysine, but homozygotes differ in jejunal transport. In the former, cystine is concentrated by jejunal mucosa but not the dibasic amino acids, whereas in the latter concentration is normal.

Treatment. Most cases will respond to the high fluid regime of Dent & Senior (1955). Cystine calculi are mainly formed at night when the urine is acidic and there is relative oliguria. It is essential, therefore, that diuresis is maintained during sleep and the patient is awakened once or twice nightly with a full bladder.

In cases in which calculi increase in number and size despite adequate diuresis, penicillamine therapy is indicated (Crawhall, Scowen & Watts, 1963, 1964). Penicillamine, which is dimethylcysteine, reacts with cystine to form the relatively soluble compounds cysteine and the mixed disulphide of penicillamine and cysteine. In normal subjects, urinary cystine output rises considerably on treatment with penicillamine (Hartley & Walshe, 1963), but in cystinuric patients there is a considerable fall in cystine output to values between zero and 200 mg./day. Penicillamine has to be given in doses of over 2 g./day in adults, but this is well tolerated in the majority of patients. Fever, rashes and, occasionally, the production of the nephrotic syndrome are the most important toxic effects. D-penicillamine has proved both more effective and less toxic than the L-isomer.

HARTNUP DISEASE

This condition, named after the first affected family, was first described by Baron, Dent, Harris, Hart & Jepson (1956) in four siblings who were children of first cousins. One other affected family in which the parents were consanguinous has been described (Jonxis, 1957), so that the disease is almost certainly due to a rare recessive gene. Only 36 known cases have been recognized to date.

Clinical aspects. Hartnup disease does not produce very severe disability. The main feature is a pellagrous photosensitive rash, affecting particularly the forearms, legs and face. The rash may be red, dry and scaly, or sometimes raw, blistered and weeping. It responds slowly but satisfactorily to nicotinamide therapy. Attacks of cerebellar ataxia may occur for short periods during the exacerbations of the disease; there is unsteadiness, nystagmus, diplopia and intention tremor. The attacks rarely last longer than a week and do not leave any permanent sequelae. Intelligence is normal, or at most is only slightly impaired. The patients are, on an average, less than average height (Colliss, Levi & Milne, 1963).

Biochemical abnormalities. The essential biochemical abnormality in Hartnup disease is a specific amino-aciduria of the "renal" type. Total amino acid output is over ten times the normal and the ratio of amino N to total urinary N is five to seven times the upper normal figure. Chromatography shows a specific amino acid pattern which varies little from case to case, and chiefly involves alanine, asparagine, citrulline, glutamine, histidine, isoleucine, leucine, phenylalanine, serine, threonine, tryptophan, tyrosine and valine. The defect, therefore, involves monoamino-monocarboxylic amino acids with the exceptions of glycine, proline and hydroxyproline, which are reabsorbed from the glomerular filtrate by a separate transport system. The output of dibasic amino acids involved in the transport defect of cystinuria is normal or at most only very slightly increased. Hydrolysis of urine shows there is no increased peptide excretion, but glutamine and glycine content rise considerably after hydrolysis due to breakdown of organic acid conjugates, e.g. indolylacetylglutamine and hippuric acid.

Plasma amino acids are reduced by about 30% of the average normal (Evered, 1956; Cusworth & Dent, 1960), an abnormality easily explained by the severe amino-aciduria. Clearances of the affected amino acids are, therefore, grossly increased. Histidine clearance is particularly high, corrected figures of 122 ml./min. (Evered, 1956),

and 140 ml./min. (Jonxis, 1957) having been recorded, indicating complete block of the normal reabsorption mechanism of this amino acid. There is no other abnormality of proximal tubular function, i.e. no glycosuria, no phosphate leak or increase of uric acid clearance, and no proteinuria. The increased and rather inconstant excretion of indolic substances in the urine has now been fully explained by the associated jejunal reabsorption defect of the disease.

Reduced transport and absorption of tryptophan in the small intestine has now been conclusively proved (Milne et al., 1960), but probably the other amino acids excreted in excess are also involved. On normal diets, the abnormality of tryptophan absorption in the gut accounts for the increased urinary output of indican, indolyl-3-acetic acid and indolylacetyl-glutamine found in most cases of the disease. Tryptophan is incompletely absorbed in the jejunum, and therefore is in abnormally high concentration in the contents of the colon. Some tryptophan appears unchanged in the faeces, but a greater amount is degraded by colonic bacteria, especially *E. coli*. The principal degradation product is indole, produced by action of the bacterial enzyme, tryptophanase. The faeces in Hartnup disease contain unusually large amounts of indole, but some is absorbed and hydroxylated to indoxyl. This is conjugated with sulphate and excreted as urinary indican. A smaller fraction of indoxyl is excreted as indoxyl-β-glucuronide. Traces of bis-indolyl-indoxyl may also be found in urine specimens from cases of Hartnup disease due to combination of indole and indoxyl during the initial oxidation of indole in the liver. Tryptamine is also found in the faeces of cases of Hartnup disease from bacterial decarboxylation of tryptophan. After absorption this is oxidized by monoamine oxidase and aldehyde oxidase to indolyl-3-acetic acid. If the urine is alkaline this is mainly excreted as the free acid (Milne, Crawford, Girao & Loughridge, 1960). In acid urine the clearance of indolylacetic acid is greatly reduced, and the major fraction is excreted in conjugation with glutamine, as indolylacetylglutamine. There is no excess output of indolyllactic acid as in phenylketonuria and maple syrup urine disease. This proves that urinary indolylacetic acid is derived from tryptamine in Hartnup disease, and from indolylpyruvic acid in the other two conditions (Fig. 16.26). After ingestion of large doses of *l*-tryptophan, cases of Hartnup disease excrete considerable amounts of indolylacrylic acid and its conjugate, indolylacrylylglycine (Milne et al., 1960). This is probably formed by oxidation of indolylpropionic acid

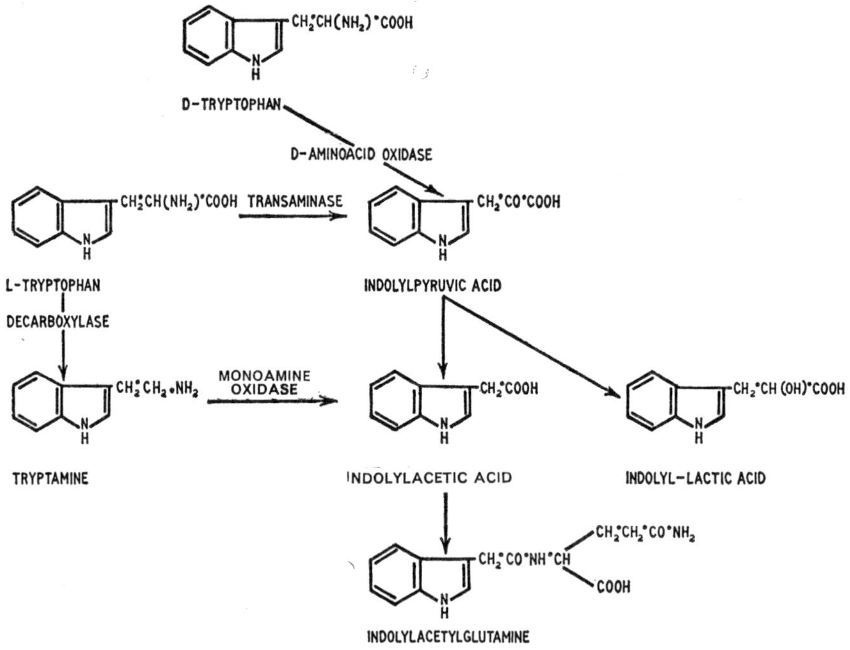

FIG. 16.26. Hartnup Disease. Minor pathways of tryptophan metabolism to indolic acids. If tryptophan is decarboxylated to tryptamine only indolylacetic acid is formed, whereas if first converted to indolylpyruvic acid, both indolylacetic and indolyllactic acids are formed.

formed in small amounts during bacterial degradation of tryptophan.

Some cases of Hartnup disease may excrete indolic metabolites in amounts at the upper limit of the normal range when on a normal diet. After ingestion of excess tryptophan, however, the excretion is always greatly in excess of the normal output. Tryptophan absorption, therefore, may be little impaired at normal dietary levels, but the maximal absorption rate is greatly reduced. After neomycin ingestion the indolic metabolites virtually disappear from the urine (Shaw *et al.*, 1960), proving that their production is dependent on bacterial action within the gut. Unlike the findings in cystinuria, *E. coli* isolated from the stools of cases of Hartnup disease show no evidence of selective enhancement of their capacity to degrade unabsorbed amino acids (Asatoor, Craske, London & Milne, 1963). There is no absolute proof to date of impaired absorption of other amino acids in addition to tryptophan. The stools from cases of Hartnup disease, however, contain excess branched-chain amino acids and phenylalanine (Milne, unpublished observations). Probably, therefore, all the amino acids involved in the renal transport

defect are also less efficiently absorbed from the gut.

At least 36 cases of the disease have now been described (Jepson, 1965). Unlike cystinuria, it is unfortunately unknown to date whether there is concentration of the affected amino acids in jejunal mucosa and renal cortical slices.

Cause of symptoms and treatment. The pellagra of Hartnup disease is easily explained by the abnormalities of tryptophan metabolism. There is wastage of tryptophan by loss in urine and faeces, and by bacterial degradation to indolic metabolites which are useless nutritionally. Less tryptophan is, therefore, available for the main metabolic pathway *via* kynurenine, with consequently impaired formation of nicotinamide. The pellagra usually responds satisfactorily to treatment with nicotinamide. There is less certainty regarding the central nervous manifestations. During exacerbations of Hartnup disease there are short lived attacks of cerebellar ataxia often associated with hallucinations and other psychotic symptoms (Hersov & Rodnight, 1960). The attacks suggest an acute intoxication, and are probably due to excess production by bacteria of toxic substances in the colon which temporarily overwhelm the "detoxication" processes in the liver. Likely metabolites are indole and tryptamine from tryptophan, phenylethylamine from phenylalanine, tyramine from tyrosine, and aliphatic amines from decarboxylation of branched-chain amino acids. There has, however, been no opportunity to re-examine cases of Hartnup disease in relapse, so this remains speculative. Treatment with oral neomycin would obviously be a logical method of therapy in future cases. Cases of Hartnup disease seem to improve with advancing age, possibly due to maturation of enzyme systems. Administration of amine oxidase inhibitors is obviously contra-indicated in Hartnup disease. Further advances in this interesting disease must await recognition of fresh acute cases in young children.

PROLINURIA

Several families have been described in which the homozygotes showed increased urinary output of glycine, proline and hydroxyproline, but the plasma levels of these amino acids were either normal or slightly reduced (Tada, Morikawa, Ando, Yoshida & Minagawa, 1965; Scriver & Wilson, 1967). The heterozygotes had abnormalities of glycine clearance only, proline and hydroxyproline clearances being normal. Some of the patients have been mental defectives whilst others were completely normal. Probably the anomaly is harmless, but has been discovered during screening techniques preferentially used in mentally deficient patients. There appears also to be impaired proline absorption in the gut (Morikawa, Tado, Ando, Yoshida, Yokoyama & Arakawa, 1966; Goodman, Macintyre & O'Brien, 1967) as shown by low plasma proline concentrations after an oral proline load, and the appearance of excess proline in the stools. The condition is, therefore, analogous to cystinuria and Hartnup disease but affects a separate amino acid transport group. Families have been described in which hyperglycinuria has appeared in individuals of several generations (de Vries, Kochwa, Lazebnik, Frank & Djaldetti; 1957). These are probably heterozygotes of prolinuria, falsely simulating the dominant Mendelian heredity of "glycinuria".

GROUP III. RENAL AMINO-ACIDURIA DUE TO NON-SPECIFIC DISORDERS OF AMINO ACID TRANSPORT

The term Fanconi syndrome is difficult to define precisely. It is an eponymous title for a varied pattern of renal tubular malfunction involving tubular transport of amino acids, glucose, phosphate, uric acid and electrolytes, and ability to acidify and concentrate urine. Unnecessary subdivisions based on combinations of functional defects have occurred in the past, e.g. a syndrome of defective reabsorption of glucose and amino acids alone was described as a separate entity (Luder & Sheldon, 1955). The affected individuals later developed increased phosphate clearance with frank rickets (Sheldon, Luder & Webb, 1961), showing that various transport defects may develop at different ages in the same patient.

The various types of the Fanconi syndrome may be classified as follows:

(a) Lignac-Fanconi disease or cystinosis, a recessive hereditary disease of infancy and childhood.

(b) Hereditary types of the adult Fanconi syndrome due to a different recessive gene.

(c) Acquired Fanconi syndrome due to the nephrotic syndrome (Stanbury & Macaulay, 1957), multiple myelomatosis (Engle & Wallis, 1957), or extrinsic poisons, e.g. heavy metals, phenols and maleic acid.

Some authorities (Morgan, Stewart, Lowe, Stowers & Johnstone, 1962) include the renal abnormalities of Wilson's disease and galactosaemia as examples of the Fanconi syndrome. This seems unnecessary as the renal defect is only a small facet of generalized disease, and these conditions therefore will be described separately.

LIGNAC-FANCONI DISEASE

This is a complex syndrome which has been described from different points of view under a variety of different names. These include Lignac-Fanconi disease, the syndrome of de Toni, Fanconi and Debré, cystine rickets, cystinosis, cystine storage disease with amino-aciduria, amino acid diabetes. It is usually encountered in infants and young children. There is a general failure to thrive, and with this is associated a severe form of rickets resistant to ordinary doses of vitamin D, chronic acidosis, polyuria, renal glycosuria, hypophosphataemia, a marked generalized amino-aciduria and often electrolyte disturbances with hypokalaemia. The children usually do quite well for the first few months of life and then may present because of vomiting, failure to grow or polyuria. In other cases the first indication of the disease is a severe resistant rickets with dwarfing and concomitant deformities. A widespread deposition of cystine crystals throughout the tissues (cystinosis) is often found in such children at post-mortem (Abderhalden, 1903; Lignac, 1924, 1926), and it may also be recognized in life by the demonstration of cystine crystals in aspirated bone marrow, in the conjunctiva and cornea, or in lymph nodes removed by biopsy (Esser, 1941; Fanconi, 1946; Burki, 1941; Ullrich, 1948; Douglas & Bickel, 1952; Baar & Bickel, 1952).

Amino-aciduria appears to be a constant feature of the syndrome. A considerable increase in the excretion of glycine, alanine, serine, glutamine, valine, leucine, isoleucine, phenylalanine, lysine, cystine, arginine and proline may be encountered. Histidine, taurine, 1-methylhistidine and β-aminoisobutyric acid are usually not markedly involved (Dent, 1947; Dent & Harris, 1951; Bickel et al., 1952).

Many of the diverse features of this condition can be explained on the hypothesis that there exists a defect in the renal tubular reabsorption of amino acids, glucose, phosphate, water and possibly other substances such as bicarbonate from the glomerular filtrate (Fanconi, 1931, 1936, 1954; McCune et al., 1943; Stowers & Dent, 1947; Dent, 1954a, b; Milne et al., 1952; Anderson et al., 1952). The low renal threshold for phosphate could account for the low plasma phosphate level and this can probably be regarded as determining the rickets or osteomalacia.

That the amino-aciduria is renal has been contested by Bickel et al. (1952) who regard it as of the "overflow" type, and a reflection of some generalized disturbance in protein metabolism. However, Dent and his colleagues (Dent, 1954a, b; Dent & Fowler, 1955) have failed to find any abnormality in the plasma amino acids in a series of children with all the characteristic features of the Fanconi syndrome, including cystinosis. In particular, the level of α-amino nitrogen was found to be within normal limits, and the renal clearance of α-amino nitrogen was much increased. In the adult type of case the same results were obtained (Dent, 1954b). Here it was also shown by elution chromatography that the plasma levels of all the individual amino acids were normal and that the renal clearances of those amino acids occurring in abnormal amounts in the urine were elevated (Evered, 1954). It was also possible to carry out α-amino nitrogen clearances following casein feeding. The patients behaved in the same way as the controls as far as the elevation and subsequent fall of α-amino nitrogen plasma levels following casein feeding were concerned. However, at each level of plasma α-amino nitrogen the clearances of the patients were very much greater than the controls.

Although the amino-aciduria is of the renal or "overflow" type, there are certain slight abnormalities of individual plasma amino acids due to metabolic causes. Plasma cystine is certainly increased, although the cysteine levels are normal (Brigham et al., 1960), and possibly the plasma aspartic acid concentration is above normal (Linneweh, 1961). Plasma cystine was 1·6 and 1·7 mg./100 ml. in two cases, contrasting with an average normal value of 1·0 mg./100 ml. The cystine/cysteine ratio in plasma is about 4·0 (normal value 2·5).

Further support for the renal theory has come from the work of Darmady and his colleagues (Clay, Darmady, & Hawkins, 1953; Darmady, 1954), who have carried out elegant microdissections of the nephrons in the kidneys from such cases. They have found a peculiar and characteristic abnormality of the proximal convoluted tubule (Fig. 16.27). This is shorter than normal and is joined to the glomerulus by a narrow swan-like neck. It is present in all or nearly all the nephrons. This peculiarity was found both in a child of 14 months with cystinosis and in an adult case of the Fanconi syndrome without cystinosis, and this emphasizes the close similarity of two kinds of case.

The renal hypothesis cannot, however, account for all the known features of the disease. It provides, for example, no explanation for the widespread deposition of cystine in the tissues which is found in infants and children with the Fanconi syndrome. So far no satisfactory explanation for this phenomenon is available, but it seems probable that there must be some specific metabolic defect present besides the renal tubular disorder.

Family studies indicate that the syndrome is inherited as a typical mendelian recessive character (Dent & Harris, 1951; Bickel & Harris, 1952). It is probable that the type of case occurring in adult life is genetically distinct from those found in childhood, because they each run true to type within different families. It may be that the abnormal genes concerned in determining the two types are alleles, but no definite evidence is yet available on this point.

Cases vary according to the relative prominence of cystine deposits in the cornea, lymph nodes, bone marrow, liver, spleen and kidneys, and the associated renal tubular defects. Cystinosis is in general more severe in the acute cases with general constitutional upset, and in the more chronic cases associated with renal defects often presenting as resistant rickets and terminating in renal failure with hypertension. Cystine crystals may sometimes be found within leucocytes in the peripheral blood (Korn, 1960).

Several cases of proved cystinosis have been

described in which renal function was apparently normal (Weber, 1953; Bickel, 1962). In addition, the pattern of tubular defect is variable from case to case. This suggests that the renal abnormalities may be secondary to the cystinosis or to an associated metabolic defect. Cystine crystals within the kidney are more profuse in the cortex than in the medulla. Cystine itself has been shown to be nephrotoxic, both glycosuria and amino-aciduria being produced by cystine or methionine feeding in the experimental animal (Stave & Schlaak, 1956; Schwarz-Tiene, Careddu & Cabassa, 1957). The primary abnormality of the disease is, therefore, more likely to be associated with the cystinosis than with abnormalities of renal function.

The intracellular fluid of affected cells must obviously be saturated with cystine, and therefore the concentration must be considerably higher than the raised plasma levels found in cases of the disease. Cystine incorporation into plasma protein is normal, and consequently the defect is more likely to lie in pathways of cystine degradation. The high cystine/cysteine ratio in cystinotic plasma suggested a deficiency in the reduction of cystine to cysteine. Worthen & Good (1961) claimed that cystine reductase was reduced in the plasma of two cases of the disease, and Seegmiller & Howell (1961) reported low activity of an enzymic system catalysing the transfer of H from reduced glutathione to cystine. Patrick (1962) examined samples of liver obtained at necropsy from three cases of the disease. The reduction of cystine to cysteine by cystine reductase and by glutathione-cysteine transhydrogenase was completely normal. Both amino acids were completely oxidized by the cystinotic liver with liberation of normal amounts of H_2S. Transamination of cysteine and cysteic acid with a-keto-glutarate was within normal limits. The in vitro findings agree with the in vivo observations of normal urinary excretion of inorganic sulphate by cystinotic patients. These observations, therefore, do not support an abnormality of cystine reduction or of known pathways of further degradation of cysteine itself. Patrick (1962), however, agrees that cystine deposits are specifically confined to reticulo-endothelial cells, and further work should concentrate on this system rather than on general cellular metabolism.

Increase of plasma pyruvate occurs in the exacerbation of cystinosis, and Clayton & Patrick (1961) found that treatment with dimercaprol (BAL) or penicillamine lowered plasma pyruvate and resulted in some clinical improvement.

Better results might well occur if therapy was started earlier in the disease. Unfortunately, even in a newly-born sib of a known case of cystinosis it is difficult to make a certain early diagnosis. Both criteria of diagnosis, cystine deposits and proximal tubular insufficiency, do not occur in the early weeks of life and it is, therefore, impossible to recognize affected cases in the neonatal period.

A variant of cystinosis with a much more benign course has been described (Cogan, Kuwabara, Kinoshita, Sheehan & Mirola, 1957; Lietman, Frazier, Wong, Shotten & Seegmiller, 1966). The main difference is that the kidneys remain uninvolved, and cystine deposits in other tissues appear to cause only minor disability. This suggests that the fundamental abnormality in cystinosis lies in the affected cells rather than that the disease is due to a circulating toxin. Presumably there is an abnormality in oxidation-reduction potential favouring function of the oxidized disulphide form of sulphydryl compounds. The normal cell chiefly contains cysteine, with very small amounts of the oxidized derivative cystine. This is of practical importance in that it should not prevent late cases of uraemia in cystinosis being treated by renal transplantation. Quite possibly the transplanted kidney would not be susceptible to cystine deposition and subsequent fibrosis, and therefore the prognosis might well be at least as favourable as cases due to chronic nephritis.

Hereditary form of the adult Fanconi syndrome. The adult Fanconi syndrome is characterized by osteomalacia and the typical disorders of proximal and distal tubular function, but there is never associated cystinosis. The condition is much more rare than Lignac-Fanconi syndrome in childhood, and probably a minority of adult cases of the syndrome are due to an inherited defect. Dent & Harris (1956) have described a family in which several siblings were affected, suggesting recessive heredity. The prognosis is much more favourable than in the Lignac-Fanconi syndrome, most cases responding satisfactorily to calciferol therapy, supplemented by potassium and sodium bicarbonate if there is hypokalaemia and acidosis. Occasionally cases may become resistant to calciferol, but still respond favourably to dihydrotachysterol (Cusworth & Dent, 1960).

In a recent analysis of hereditary forms of the adult Fanconi syndrome, Hunt et al. (1966) list six affected families, and claim that the heredity is dominant autosomal in type. Many of the families were also affected by retinitis pigmentosa, but it remains uncertain whether this is due to an associated, but separate, abnormal gene or whether there is a metabolic abnormality resulting in combined retinal and proximal tubular damage.

Acquired forms of the Fanconi syndrome. Proximal tubular defects typical of the Fanconi syndrome can occur due to heavy metal poisoning, e.g. lead and cadmium (Clarkson & Kench, 1956), uranium (Rothstein & Berke, 1949), other known poisons, e.g. lysol (Spencer & Franglen, 1952), oxalic acid (Emslie-Smith, Johnstone, Thomson & Lowe, 1956), phosphorus (Crane, Ebeling & Bentley, 1959), calciferol (von Crefeld & Avons, 1949) and maleic acid (Harrison & Harrison, 1954), the nephrotic syndrome especially in childhood (Stanbury & Macaulay, 1957), multiple myelomatosis (Sirota & Hamerman, 1954; Dragsted & Hjorth, 1956; Engle & Wallis, 1957) and to vitamin C (Jonxis & Huisman, 1954) and vitamin D (Jonxis, Smith & Huisman, 1952) deficiencies. In each case there is presumably some specific damage to proximal tubular cells causing multi-factorial defects of tubular function. Obviously sporadic cases of the hereditary form can also occur with no affected siblings, causing difficulties in differential diagnosis. Cases of the Fanconi syndrome in childhood should not be diagnosed as Lignac-Fanconi disease unless the patient or siblings are proved to have cystinosis. Stanbury (1962) has described two such patients, and in one the aetiology was shown to be an obstructive nephropathy with bilateral ureteric reflux.

LOWE'S SYNDROME
(CEREBRO-OCULO-RENAL DYSTROPHY

Lowe, Terrey & Maclachlan (1952) first described the association of renal tubular defects, mental retardation and severe congenital anomalies of the eyes; and since then about 40 cases have been described (Lowe, 1960). The disease is transmitted by a recessive gene carried on the X-chromosome. The clinical symptoms and signs are more severe than those of the Lignac-Fanconi disease and are often obvious at birth. There may be congenital glaucoma ("buphthalmos"), corneal opacities, and congenital cataracts. The infant is totally blind or suffers from severe visual impairment with coarse nystagmus and photophobia. There is often gross muscular weakness and separation of the recti muscles and an umbilical hernia may occur. Later there is anorexia, failure to thrive, evidence of gross mental retardation, and a vitamin D-resistant rickets.

The proximal tubular defects are similar to those of the Lignac-Fanconi disease but there

is often an especial increase of urinary lysine and tyrosine. Early reports of increased urinary output of other organic acids were not confirmed by Dedmon, Dent, Scriver & Westall (1961). The condition in many clinical respects resembles the multiple defects of infantile galactosaemia, but unfortunately the primary cause is unknown and therefore rational therapy is as yet impossible.

WILSON'S DISEASE
(HEPATOLENTICULAR DEGENERATION)

This is a progressive condition developing in adolescence or early adult life, characterized neurologically by the occurrence of widespread tremor, muscular rigidity and other features indicating dysfunction of the extra-pyramidal motor system. Some degree of dementia and even psychosis may also be found. Pathologically, the lesion consists of a bilaterally symmetrical degeneration of the lenticular and caudate nuclei, with some degenerative changes in the nerve cells of the cerebral cortex. Associated with these changes and often preceding them is a progressive multilobular cirrhosis of the liver.

One curious feature of the condition is the so-called Kayser-Fleischer ring. This is a zone of pigmentation, greenish brown in colour, at the periphery of the cornea.

Biochemical findings in Wilson's disease. Two types of abnormal biochemical findings have been reported in this condition. The first is a gross disorder of Cu metabolism, and the second is a marked generalized aminoaciduria. It now appears certain that the disturbance of Cu metabolism is the primary lesion (see also Chapter 13).

Uzman & Denny Brown (1948) first demonstrated that a gross generalized amino-aciduria may occur in Wilson's disease. This has been widely confirmed (Dent & Harris, 1951; Cooper, Eckhardt, Falcon & Davidson, 1950; Stein, Bearn & Moore, 1954). Though the majority of patients with unequivocal Wilson's disease show such an amino-aciduria, not all do so (Stein, Bearn & Moore, 1954; Cartwright, Hodges, Gubler, Mahoney, Damm, Wintrobe & Bean, 1954). There is also considerable variation in the degree of the amino-aciduria from case to case.

Stein, Bearn & Moore (1954) have carried out a very detailed examination of the urinary amino acids in this condition using ion-exchange chromatography. Typical results are shown in Table 16.5. Most of the amino acids usually found in urine, with the exception of taurine, 1-methylhistidine and 3-methylhistidine, may be encountered in increased amounts. In addition, proline

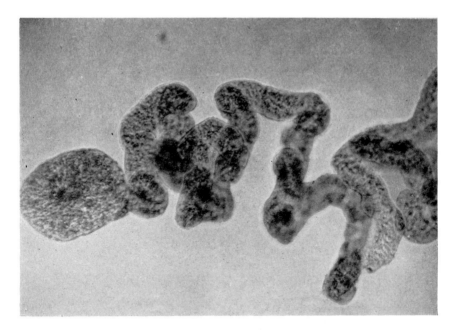

(A)

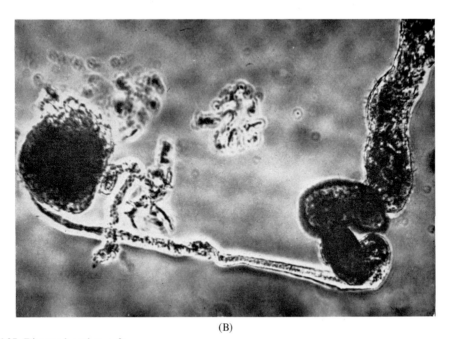

(B)

FIG. 16.27. Dissected nephrons from:
(A) A normal kidney.
(B) A kidney from a patient with the Fanconi syndrome.
In each case a glomerulus and the first part of the proximal convoluted tubule is shown. In the Fanconi syndrome
there is a narrow, elongated neck connecting the glomerulus with a normal-sized proximal convoluted
tubule. (Reproduced by kind permission of Dr. Darmady.)

[To face p. 598.

and citrulline, which are not usually found in appreciable amounts in the normal, may here be excreted in considerable quantities. Besides the amino acids excreted in the free state, there is also an increased excretion of conjugated amino acids. Some of these conjugates may be oligopeptides (Uzman & Hood, 1952).

In contrast to the findings in the urine, the amino acid content of the plasma both qualitatively and quantitatively, and both in the fasting state and after a protein meal, is within normal limits (Cooper et al., 1950; Matthews, Milne & Bell, 1952; Stein, Bearn & Moore, 1954). It appears, therefore, that the amino-aciduria is renal in type and dependent on inefficient reabsorption of amino acids by the renal tubules from the glomerular filtrate.

Multiple defects of tubular function occur in many cases of Wilson's disease in addition to the amino-aciduria (Bearn, Yu & Gutman, 1957; Morgan, Stewart, Lowe, Stowers & Johnstone, 1962). Proximal tubular defects include a high uric acid clearance with an abnormally low plasma uric acid (Bishop, Zimdahl & Talbott, 1954), renal glycosuria with reduction of Tm (Bearn et al., 1957), and an increased phosphate clearance with a reduced plasma phosphate and resultant rickets or osteomalacia (Morgan et al.,

1962). In addition, there may be reduced glomerular filtration rate, renal plasma flow and Tm_{PAH} (Bearn et al., 1957). As in the Fanconi syndrome, there may also be distal tubular defects, e.g. reduction of urinary acidification power with an output of ammonia higher than appropriate for the urinary pH. One characteristic abnormality is hypercalciuria which may lead to renal stone formation and osteoporosis (Litin, Randall, Goldstein, Power & Diesser, 1959; Rosenoer & Michell, 1959). Treatment with penicillamine improves many of the defects of renal function as well as the neurological aspects of the disease. The amino-aciduria usually proves more resistant to treatment than the other renal abnormalities.

These multiple defects of renal function are associated with histopathological abnormalities characteristic of the disease. Unlike the findings in Lignac-Fanconi syndrome, there is no "swan-neck" deformity of the proximal tubule (Morgan et al., 1962), but there may be areas of both proximal and distal tubular disorganization with secondary fibrosis. Histology shows focal areas of tubular epithelial cell degeneration with detachment of epithelial cells from the basement membrane and cellular necrosis (Wolff, 1962). Staining with rubeanic acid shows intracytoplasmic Cu granules within the affected tubular cells.

Probably the multiple defects of renal tubular function are due to toxicity from excess deposition of Cu. This is because Wilson's disease, with characteristic clinical findings and typical disturbance of Cu metabolism, may occur in the absence of any marked amino-aciduria. Furthermore, the amino-aciduria is renal in origin, and other renal amino-acidurias of the same generalized type do not lead either to disturbances of Cu metabolism or to pathological and clinical features of the sort that are found in Wilson's disease. In general, quite severe amino-aciduria may be found without any noticeable effect on the general nutritional state due to chronic loss of amino acids.

Genetics. The disease occurs frequently among brothers and sisters of affected patients; it rarely if ever occurs in more than one generation and there is a very high incidence of parental consanguinity (Matthews, Milne & Bell, 1952; Bearn, 1953). There is little doubt that it is inherited as a typical mendelian recessive character. The affected patients are homozygous for the abnormal gene concerned. The heterozygotes although clinically normal have been shown to have a minor defect in Cu metabolism as indicated by a lower than normal rate of incorporation of ^{64}Cu into caeruloplasmin (Sternlieb et al., 1961). One might

TABLE 16.5

Free amino acids excreted in the urine in three patients with Wilson's disease
(Stein et al., 1954)

	mg./day		
Glutamine and Asparagine	590	710	130
Aspartic acid	< 10	< 10	< 10
Glutamic acid	87	110	21
Glycine	550	900	220
Alanine	230	490	74
Valine	63	110	6
Leucine	25	65	15
Isoleucine	28	66	13
Serine	425	510	95
Threonine	580	860	82
Cystine	120	770	50
Methionine	17	5	5
Taurine	49	130	120
Phenylalanine	120	120	20
Tyrosine	420	270	45
Histidine	580	680	270
1-Methylhistidine	42	77	38
Citrulline	190	440	10
Ornithine	5	130	5
Lysine	79	860	33
Arginine	10	160	10
Total	4195	7480	1225

speculate that the normal gene at this locus is concerned with the synthesis of caeruloplasmin, and that in its absence this synthesis is inefficient so that inadequate amounts of this protein are formed. If the general theory of Cartwright and his colleagues is correct this could set in train all the diverse pathological consequences which may be encountered.

AMINO ACID EXCRETION IN GALACTOSAEMIA

The discovery that amino-aciduria may occur in galactosaemia (Holzel, Komrower & Wilson, 1952) was somewhat unexpected. The amino-aciduria appears to represent only a minor feature of the overall metabolic upset in this condition, and while of considerable theoretical interest is of no great clinical importance.

In galactosaemia there is a marked inability to metabolize galactose completely. After taking galactose by mouth there is a gross elevation of the blood galactose level and a consequent excretion of galactose in the urine. Infants with this condition who are on an ordinary milk diet show a persistent elevation of the blood galactose and a more or less continuous excretion of galac-

tose in the urine. Under these conditions they fail to thrive, their livers become enlarged, they develop cataract and they frequently die in early infancy. If they survive they are liable to show a severe degree of mental retardation. If they are fed a galactose-free diet, the blood galactose falls, galactose disappears from the urine and their physical condition rapidly improves. It has been shown that the primary lesion is an inability to convert galactose-1-phosphate to glucose-1-phosphate (Schwarz et al., 1955) due to a deficiency of the enzyme galactose-1-phosphate uridyl transferase (Kalckar, 1957).

Children with galactosaemia, on a diet containing galactose, excrete abnormal quantities of amino acids in their urine (Holzel et al., 1952; Bickel & Hichmans, 1952). Studies by paper chromatography indicate that there is a relatively large increase in serine, glycine, threonine and alanine, and moderate increases in glutamine, valine, leucine and tyrosine (Holzel et al., 1952; Bickel et al., 1952; Cusworth, Dent & Flynn, 1955).

If galactose is removed from the diet the amino-aciduria eventually disappears, though this may take some days (Cusworth et al., 1955).

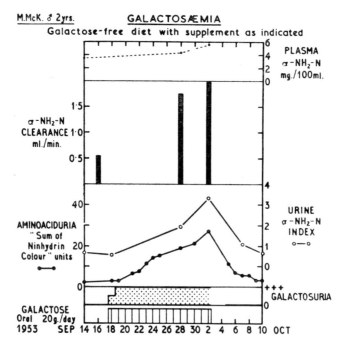

Fig. 16.28. Amino acid clearances and excretions before, during and after addition of galactose to the diet of a patient with galactosaemia. (Cusworth et al., 1955.) (Reproduced by kind permission of the Editors of the Archives of Disease in Childhood.)

If galactose feeding is then reintroduced, the amino-aciduria gradually develops again, but several days elapse before it is clearly apparent. This is in marked contrast to the galactosuria which develops immediately.

When the amino-aciduria is present, the plasma a-amino nitrogen level is in most cases within normal limits (Komrower, 1953; Cusworth et al. 1955; Hsia, Hsia, Green, Kay & Gellis, 1954).

Cusworth et al. (1955) carried out a-amino nitrogen clearance studies in a galactosaemic child on a galactose-free diet, and then during a period when galactose was being fed (Fig. 16.28). On the galactose-free diet the a-amino nitrogen clearance was normal, whereas after 10 days on a diet containing galactose it was distinctly raised. It thus seems likely that defective renal tubular reabsorption is the main cause of the amino-

aciduria, though in view of the known liver damage it is possible that this may contribute in advanced cases. The tubular disorder could perhaps be due to a toxic effect of the raised galactose content of the blood, or to the excessive accumulation of galactose-1-phosphate within the cells.

A similar proximal tubular disorder occurs in hereditary fructose intolerance due to lack of fructose 1-phosphate aldolase. Ingestion of fructose very soon causes proteinuria and a renal type of amino-aciduria (Lelong et al., 1962). The temporary proximal tubular damage is probably due to accumulation of fructose 1-phosphate within the tubule cells. Plasma amino acids may be increased in neglected cases due to liver damage, and this may cause an overflow type amino-aciduria in addition.

References

ABDERHALDEN, E. (1903). *Hoppe-Seyl. Z.*, **38**, 557.

ABRAHAM, D., PISANO, J. J. & UDENFRIEND, S. (1962). *Arch. Biochem. Biophys.* **99**, 210.

ALLAN, J. D., CUSWORTH, D. C., DENT, C. E., & WILSON, V. K. (1958). *Lancet*, **1**, 182.

ALSBERG, C. L. & FOLIN, O. (1906). *Amer. J. Physiol.*, **14**, 54.

AMMON, R. (1961). *Z. physiol. Chem.*, **324**, 129.

ANDERSON, I. A., MILLER, A. & KENNY, A. P. (1952). *Quart, J. Med.*, **21**, n.s., 33.

ARCHIBALD, R. M. (1944). *J. Biol Chem.*, **154**, 643.

ARMSTRONG, M. D. & ROBINSON, K. S. (1954). *Arch. Biochem.*, **52**, 287.

ARMSTRONG, M. D. & TYLER, F. A. (1955). *J. clin. Invest.*, **34**, 565.

ARROW, V. K. & WESTALL, R. G. (1958). *J. Physiol.*, **142**, 141.

ASATOOR, A. M., CRASKE, J., LONDON, D. R. & MILNE, M. D. (1963). *Lancet*, **1**, 126.

ASATOOR, A. M., LACEY, B. W., LONDON, D. R. & MILNE, M. D. (1962). *Clin. Sci.*, **23**, 285.

AUERBACH, V. H., DI GEORGE, A. M., BALDRIDGE, R. C., TOURTELLOTTE, C. D. & BRIGHAM, M. P. (1961). *Clin. Res.*, **9**, 334.

AXELROD, J., UDENFRIEND, S. & BRODIE, B. B. (1954). *J. Pharmacol.*, **111**, 176.

BAAR, H. S. & BICKEL, H. (1952). *Acta paediatr. Stockh.*, **42**, Suppl. 90, 171.

BACH, S. J. (1952). The Metabolism of Protein Constituents in the Mammalian Body. Oxford, Clarendon Press.

BARON, D. N., DENT, C. E., HARRIS, H., HART, E. W. & JEPSON, J. B. (1956). *Lancet*, **2**, 421.

BEARN, A. G. (1953). *Amer. J. Med.*, **15**, 442.

BEARN, A. G. & KUNKEL, H. G. (1954). *J. clin. Invest.*, **33**, 400.

BEARN, A. G., YU, T. F., & GUTMAN, A. B. (1957). *J. clin. Invest.*, **36**, 1107.

BERLOW, S. (1966). *A.M.A. J. Dis. Child.*, **112**, 135.

BERRY, H. K. (1953). *Amer. J. phys. Anthrop.*, **11**, 559.

BERRY, H. K., SUTHERLAND, B. S., UMBARGER, B. & O'GRADY, D. (1967). *A.M.A. J. Dis. Child.*, **113**, 2.

BESSMAN, S. P. & BALDWIN, R. (1962). *Science*, **135**, 789.

BESSMAN, S. P. & TADA, K. (1960). *Metabolism*, **9**, 377.

BEYER, K. H., WRIGHT, L. D., RUSSO, H. F., SKEGGS, H. R. & SHANER, G. A. (1947). *Amer. J. Physiol.*, **151**, 202.

BICKEL, H. (1962). *In* "Renal Disease". Ed. Black, D. A. K. Oxford, p. 247.

BICKEL, H., GERRARD, J. & HICKMANS, E. M. (1954). *Acta paediatr. Stockh.*, **43**, 64.

BICKEL, H. & GRÜTER, W. (1963). "Phenylketonuria." Ed. LYMAN, F. L. Charles C. Thomas, Springfield, Ill.

BICKEL, H. & HARRIS, H. (1952). *Acta paediatr. Stockh.* **42**, Suppl. 90, 22.

BICKEL, H. & HICKMANS, E. M. (1952). *Arch. Dis. Childh.*, **27**, 348.

BICKEL, H., SMALLWOOD, W. C., SMELLIE, J. M., BAAR, H. S. & HICKMANS, E. M. (1952). *Acta paediatr. Stockh.*, **42**, Suppl. 90. 9.

BISHOP, C., ZIMDAHL, W. T. & TALBOTT, J. H. (1954). *Proc. Soc. exp. Biol., N.Y.*, **86**, 440.

BLOCH, K. (1944). *J. Biol. Chem.*, **155**, 255.

BLOCH, R. J., JERVIS, G. A., BOLLING, D. & WEBB, M. (1940). *J. Biol. Chem.*, **134**, 567.

BLUM, L. (1908). *Arch. exp. Path. Pharmak.*, **59**, 268.

BLUMBERG, B. S. & GARTLER, S. M. (1959). *Nature (Lond.)*, **184**, 1990.

BOREK, E., BRECHER, A., JERVIS, G. A. & WAELSCH, H. (1950). *Proc. Soc. exp. Biol., N.Y.*, **75**, 86.

BOSCOTT, J. & BICKEL, H. (1953). *Scand. J. clin. Lab. Invest.*, **5**, 380.

BRAND, E., CAHILL, G. F. & HARRIS, M. M. (1933). *Proc. Soc. exp. Biol., N.Y.*, **31**, 348, 1247.

BRAND, E., CAHILL, G. F. & HARRIS, M. M. (1935). *J. Biol. Chem.*, **109**, 69.

BRIGHAM, M. P., STEIN, W. H. & MOORE, S. (1960). *J. clin. Invest.*, **39**, 1633.

BRIMBLECOMBE, F. S. W., BLAINEY, J. D., STONEMAN, M. E. R. & WOOD, B. S. (1961). *Brit. med. J.*, **2**, 793.

BRIMBLECOMBE, F. S. W., STONEMAN, M. E. R. & MALIPHANT, R. (1959). *Lancet*, **1**, 609.

BRODIE, B. B., AXELROD, J., SHORE, P. A. & UDENFRIEND, S. (1954). *J. biol. Chem.*, **208**, 741.

BUBL, E. C. & BUTTS, J. S. (1949). *J. biol. Chem.*, **180**, 839.

BUDD, M. A., TANAKA, K., HOLMES, L. B., EFRON, M. L., CRAWFORD, J. D. & ISSELBACHER, K. J. (1967). *New England J. Med.*, **277**, 321.

BUERGI, W., RICHTERICH, R. & COLOMBO, J. P. (1966). *Nature (Lond.)*. **211**, 854.

BURKI, E. (1941). *Ann. paediatr.*, **156**, 324.

CANELLAKIS, E. S. & TARVER, H. (1953). *Arch. Biochem. Biophys.*, **42**, 446.

CARSON, N. A. J. (1967). *A.M.A. J. Dis. Child.*, **113**, 95.

CARSON, N. A. J. & NEILL, D. W. (1962). *Arch. Dis. Childhood*, **37**, 505.

CARTWRIGHT, G. E., HODGES, R. E., GUBLER, C. J., MAHONEY, J. P., DAMM, K., WINTROBE, M. M. & BEAN, W. B. (1954). *J. clin. Invest.*, **33**, 1487.

CHANDLER, J. P. & LEWIS, H. B. (1932). *J. biol. Chem.*, **96**, 619.

CHILDS, B. & NYHAN, W. L. (1964). *Pediatrics*, **33**, 403.

CHILDS, B., NYHAN, W. L., BORDEN, M., BARD, L. & COOKE, R. E. (1961). *Pediatrics*, **27**, 522.

CLARKSON, T. W. & KENCH, J. E. (1956). *Biochem. J.*, **62**, 361.

CLAY, R. D., DARMADY, E. M. & HAWKINS, M. (1953). *J. Path. Bact.*, **65**, 551.

CLAYTON, B. E. & PATRICK, A. D. (1961). *Lancet*, **2**, 909.

COCHRANE, W. A., PAYNE, W. W., SIMPKISS, M. J. & WOOLF, L. I. (1956). *J. clin. Invest.*, **35**, 411.

COGAN, D. G., KUWABARA, T., KINOSHITA, J., SHEEHAN, L. & MIROLA, L. (1957). *J. Amer. med. Ass.*, **164**, 394.

COLLISS, J., LEVI, J. & MILNE, M. D. (1963). *Brit. med. J.*, **1**, 590.

COLOMBO, J. P., RICHTERICH, R., DONATH, A., SPAHR, A. & ROSSI, E. (1964). *Lancet*, **1**, 1014.

COON, M. J. & ABRAHAMSEN, N. S. B. (1952). *J. biol. Chem.*, **195**, 805.

COON, M. J., ROBINSON, W. G. & BACKAWAT, B. K. (1955). Symposium on amino acid metabolism. Eds. McElroy, W. D. & Glass, H. B. Johns Hopkins Hospital Press, Baltimore.

COOPER, A. M., ECKHARDT, R. D., FALCON, W. W. & DAVIDSON, C. S. (1950). *J. clin. Invest.*, **29**, 265.

COWIE, V. & PENROSE, L. S. (1951). *Ann. Eugen. Camb.*, **15**, 297.

CRANE, C. W., EBELING, D. & BENTLEY, A. B. (1959). *Aust. Ann. Med.*, **8**, 66.

CRAWHALL, J. C., SCOWEN, E. F. & WATTS, R. W. E. (1963). *Brit. med. J.*, **1**, 588.

CRAWHALL, J. C., SCOWEN, E. F. & WATTS, R. W. E. (1964). *Brit. med. J.* **1**, 1411.

CROME, L. (1962). *J. Neurol. Neurosurg. Psychiat.*, **25**, 149.

CROME, L., DUTTON, G. & ROSS, C. F. (1961). *J. Path. Bact.*, **81**, 379.

CROME, L. & PARE, C. M. B. (1960). *J. ment. Sci.*, **106**, 862.

CROME, L., TYMMS, V. & WOOLF, L. I. (1962). *J. Neurol. Neurosurg. Psychiat.*, **25**, 143.

CRUMPLER, H. R., DENT, C. E., HARRIS, H. & WESTALL, R. G. (1951). *Nature (Lond.)*, **167**, 307.

CUSWORTH, D. C. & DENT, C. E. (1960). *Biochem. J.*, **74**, 550.

CUSWORTH, D. C., DENT, C. E. & FLYNN, F. V. (1955). *Arch. Dis. Childh.*, **30**, 150.

DALGLIESH, C. E. (1954). *Biochem. J.*, **58**, xlv.

DANCIS, J., HUTZLER, J. & LEVITZ, M. (1960). *Biochem. Biophys. Acta*, **43**, 342.

DANCIS, J., LEVITZ, M., MILLER, S. & WESTALL, R. G. (1959). *Brit. med. J.*, **1**, 91.

DANCIS, J., LEVITZ, M. & WESTALL, R. G. (1960). *Pediatrics*, **25**, 72.

DANN, M., MARPLES, E. & LEVINE, S. Z. (1943). *J. clin. Invest.*, **22**, 87.

DARMADY, E. M. (1954). Ciba Foundation Symposium on the Kidney, London, J. &. A. Churchill.

DATTA, S. P. & HARRIS, H. (1951). *Nature (Lond.)*, **168**, 296.

DAVISON, A. N. & SANDLER, M. (1958). *Nature (Lond.)*, **181**, 186.

DEDMON, R. E., DENT, C. E., SCRIVER, C. R. & WESTALL, R. G. (1961). *Clin. Chim. Acta*, **6**, 291.

DENT, C. E. (1946). *Lancet*, **2**, 637.

DENT, C. E. (1947). *Biochem. J.*, **41**, 240.

DENT, C. E. Biochemical Society Symposium No. 3. Cambridge University Press (1949).

DENT, C. E. (1950). *Schweiz. med. Wschr.*, **80**, 752.

DENT, C. E. (1951). In "Recent Advances in Clinical Pathology". 2nd Ed. London, J. & A. Churchill.

DENT, C. E. (1954a). *Exp. Med. Surg.*, **12**, 229.

DENT, C. E. (1954b). In "Lectures on the Scientific Basis of Medicine". London, Athlone Press, **2**, 213.

DENT, C. E. & FOWLER, D. (1955). Personal Communication.

DENT, C. E., FRIEDMAN, M., GREEN, H. & WATSON, L. C. A. (1965). *Brit. med. J.* **1**, 403.

DENT, C. E. HARRIS, H. (1951). *Ann. Eugen., Camb.*, **16**, 60.

DENT, C. E. & HARRIS, H. (1956). *J. Bone Jt. Surg.*, **38B**, 204.

DENT, C. E., HEATHECOTE, J. G. & JORON, G. E. (1954). *J. clin. Invest.*, **33**, 1210.

DENT, C. E. & ROSE, G. A. (1951). *Quart. J. Med.*, **20**, n.s., 205.

DENT, C. E. & SENIOR, B. (1954). Personal Communication.

DENT, C. E. & SENIOR, B. (1955). *Brit. J. Urol.*, **27**, 317.

DENT, C. E., SENIOR, B. & WALSHE, J. M. (1954). *J. clin. Invest.*, **33**, 1216.

DENT, C. E. & WESTALL, R. G. (1961). *Arch. Dis. Childh.*, **36**, 259.

DE VRIES, A., KOCHWA, S., LAZEBNIK, J., FRANK, M. & DJALDETTI, M. (1957). *Amer. J. Med.*, **23**, 408.

DOOLAN, P. D., HARPER, M. A., HUTCHIN, M. E. & ALPEN, E. L. (1957). *Amer. J. Med.*, **23**, 416.

DOUGLAS, A. A. & BICKEL, H. (1952). *Acta paediatr. Stockh.*, **42**, Suppl. 90, 106.

DRAGSTED, P. J. & HJORTH, N. (1956). *Danish med. Bull.*, **3**, 177.

LA DU, B. N. & ZANNONI, V. G. (1955). *J. Biol. Chem.*, **217**, 777.

LA DU, B. N. & ZANNONI, V. G. (1956). *J. Biol. Chem.*, **219**, 273.

DUNN, M. S., AKAWAIE, S., YEH, H. L. & MARTIN, H. J. (1950). *J. clin. Invest.*, **29**, 302.

DUSTIN, J. P., MOORE, S. & BIGWOOD, E. J. (1955). *Metabolism*, **4**, 75.

DU VIGNEAUD, V., KILMIER, G. W., RACHELE, J. R. & COHN, M. (1944). *J. biol. Chem.*, **155**, 645.

ECKHARDT, R. D. & DAVIDSON, C. S. (1949). *J. biol. Chem.*, **177**, 687.

EDWARDS, S. W., HSIA, D. Y-Y. & KNOX, W. E. (1955). *Fed. Proc.*, **14**, 206.

EFRON, M. L. (1965). *New England J. Med.*, **272**, 1243.

EFRON, M. L. (1967). *A.M.A. J. Dis. Child.*, **113**, 166.

EFRON, M. L., BIXBY, E. M., PALLATA, O. L. G. & PRYLES, C. V. (1962). *New England J. Med.*, **267**, 1193.

EFRON, M. L., BIXBY, E. M. & PRYLES, C. V. (1965). *New England J. Med.*, **272**, 1299.

EMBDEN, H. (1893). *Hoppe-Seyl. Z.*, **17**, 182.

EMSLIE-SMITH, D., JOHNSTONE, J. H., THOMSON, M. B. & LOWE, K. G. (1956). *Clin. Sci.*, **15**, 171.

ENGLE, R. L. & WALLIS, L. A. (1957). *Amer. J. Med.*, **22**, 5.

ESSER, M. (1941). *Ann. paediatr.*, **156**, 344.

EVERED, D. F. (1954). "A Study of Amino Acids in Biological Fluids using Ion-exchange Resins." Ph.D. Thesis. London University.

EVERED, D. F. (1956). *Biochem. J.*, **62**, 416.

FALTA, W. (1904). *Dtsch. Arch. klin. Med.*, **81**, 231.

FANCONI, G. (1931). *Jb. Kinderheilk*, **133**, 257.

FANCONI, G. (1936). *Jb. Kinderheilk*, **147**, 299.

FANCONI, G. (1946). *Helv. paediat. Acta*, **1**, 183.

FANCONI, G. (1954). *Arch. Dis. Childh.*, **29**, 1.

FERRARI, V., CAMPAGNARI, F. & GUIDA, A. (1955). *Minerva Med.*, **2**, 119.

FINK, K. (1956). *J. biol. Chem.*, **218**, 9.

FINK, K., CLINE, R. E., HENDERSON, R. B. & FINK, R. M. (1956). *J. biol. Chem.*, **221**, 425.

FINK, R. M., MCCAUGHY, C., CLINE, R. E. & FINK, K. (1956). *J. biol. Chem.*, **218**, 1.

FISHBERG, E. H. (1948). *J. biol. Chem.*, **172**, 155.

FOLEY, T. H. & LONDON, D. R. (1965). *Clin. Sci.*, **29**, 549.

FÖLLING, A. (1934a). *Nord Med. Tidskr.*, **8**, 1054.

FÖLLING, A. (1934b). *Hoppe-Seyl. Z.*, **277**, 169.

FÖLLING, A., CLOSS, K. & GAMMES, T. (1938). *Hoppe-Seyl. Z.*, **256**, 1.

FÖLLING, A., MOHR, O. L. & RUUD, L. (1945). *Norske Videnskaps Akad i Oslo Mat-Naturv. Klasse*, **13**.

FOWLER, D. I., HARRIS, H. & WARREN, F. L. (1952). *Lancet*, **1**, 544.

FREEMAN, J. M., NICHOLSON, J. F., MASLAND, W. S., ROWLAND, L. P. & CARTER, S. (1964). *J. Pediat.*, **65**, 1039.

FRIMPTER, G. W. (1965). *Science*, **149**, 1095.

FRIMPTER, G. W. (1961). *J. biol. Chem.*, **236**, PC52.

FRIMPTER, G. W., HAYMOVITZ, A. & HORWITH, M. (1963). *New England J. Med.*, **268**, 333.

FRIMPTER, G. W., HORWITH, M., FURTH, E., FELLOWS, R. E. & THOMPSON, D. D. (1962). *J. clin. Invest.*, **41**, 281.

FROMHERZ, K. & HERMANNS, L. (1914). *Hoppe-Seyl. Z.*, **91**, 194.

FUHRMANN, W. (1963). *Dtsch. med. Wschr.*, **88**, 525.

GABUZDA, G. J., Jr., ECKHARDT, R. D. & DAVIDSON, C. S. (1952). *J. clin. Invest.*, **31**, 1015.

GARROD, A. E. (1902). *Lancet*, **2**, 1616.

GARROD, A. E. (1908). *Lancet*, **2**, 142 & 214.

GARROD, A. E. (1923). "Inborn Errors of Metabolism." 2nd Ed. London, Oxford University Press.

GARTLER, S. M. (1959). *Arch. Biochem. Biophys.*, **80**, 400.

GENTZ, J., JAGENBURG, R. & ZETTERSTROM, R. (1965). *J. Pediat.*, **66**, 670.

GERRITSEN, T., KAVEGGIA, E. & WAISMAN, H. A. (1965). *Pediatrics*, **36**, 882.

GERRITSEN, T., VAUGHN, J. G. & WAISMAN, H. A. (1962). *Biochem. Biophys. Res. Comm.*, **9**, 493.

GERRITSEN, T. & WAISMAN, H. A. (1966). *New England J. Med.*, **275**, 66.

GHADIMI, H., BINNINGTON, V. I. & PECORA, P. (1965). *New England J. Med.*, **723**, 723.

GHADIMI, H. & PARTINGTON, M. W. (1967). *A.M.A.J. Dis. Child.*, **113**, 93.

GHADIMI, H., PARTINGTON, M. W. & HUNTER, A. (1961). *New England J. Med.*, **265**, 221.

GOODMAN, S. L., MACINTYRE, C. A. & O'BRIEN, D. (1967). *J. Pediat.*, **71**, 246.

GREIBURG, H. (1957). *Klin. Wschr.*, **35**, 889.

GRUNER, H. D. (1961). *Nature (Lond.)*, **189**, 63.

GRUTTERINCK, A. & VAN DEN BERGH, H. (1907). *Ned Tijdschr. Geneesk.*, **2**, 1117.

GRUTTNER, K., MULLER, F. & WALLIS, H. (1958). *Wschr. Kinderh.*, **106**, 41.

HAGER, S. E., GREGERMAN, R. I. & KNOX, W. E. (1957). *J. Biol. Chem.*, **225**, 935.

HAGIHIRA, H., LIN, E. C. C., SAMIY, A. H. & WILSON, T. H. (1961). *Biochem. Biophsy. Res. Comms.*, 478.

HALVORSEN, S. (1967). *A.M.A. J. Dis. Child.*, **113**, 38.

HALVORSEN, S. & GJESSING, L. R. (1964). *Brit. med. J.*, **2**, 1171.

HALVORSEN, S., PANDE, H., LOKEN, A. C. & GJESSING, L. R. (1966). *Arch. Dis. Childh.*, **41**, 238.

HARRIS, H. (1953). *Ann. Eugen. Camb.*, **18**, 43.

HARRIS, H., MITTWOCH, U., ROBSON, E. B. & WARREN, F. L. (1955). *Ann. hum. Genet.*, **19**, 196.

HARRIS, H., PENROSE, L. S. & THOMAS, D. H. H. (1959). *Ann. hum. Genet.*, **23**, 442.

HARRIS, H. & ROBSON, E. B. (1955). *Acta genet.* (*Basel*), **5**, 381.

HARRIS, H. & WARREN, F. L. (1953). *Ann. Eugen. Camb.*, **18**, 125.

HARRISON, H. E. & HARRISON, H. C. (1954). *Science*, **120**, 606.

HARTLEY, B. S. & WALSHE, J. M. (1963). *Lancet*, **2**, 434.

HELE, T. S. (1909). *J. Physiol.*, **39**, 52.

HERSOV, L. A. & RODNIGHT, R. (1960). *J. Neurol. Neurosurg. Psychiat.*, **32**, 40.

HIER, S. W. (1947). *J. biol. Chem.*, **171**, 813.

HOGBEN, L. T., WORRALL, R. L. & ZUEVE, I. (1932). *Proc. roy. Soc. Edinb.*, **52**, 264.

HOLT, L. E., Jr., LUYDERMAN, S. E., DANCIS, J. & NORTON, P. M. (1960). *Fed. Proc.*, **19**, 10.

HOLZEL, A., KOMROWER, G. M. & WILSON, V. K. (1952). *Brit. med. J.*, **1**, 194.

HORNER, F. A. & STREAMER, C. W. (1959). *AMA. J. Dis. Child.*, **97**, 345.

HSIA, D. Y. Y., DRISCOLL, K. W., TROLL, W. & KNOX, W. E. (1956). *Nature*, (*Lond.*), **178**, 1239.

HSIA, D. Y. Y. & GELLIS, S. S. (1954). *J. clin. Invest.*, **33**, 1603.

HSIA, D. Y. Y., HSIA, H. H., GREEN, S., KAY, M. & GELLIS, S. S. (1954). *Amer. J. Dis. Childh.*, **88**, 458.

HSIA, D. Y., KNOX, W. E., QUINN, K. V. & PAINE, R. S. (1958). *Pediatrics*, **21**, 178.

HUISMAN, T. H. J. (1954). *Pediatrics*, **14**, 245.

HUISMAN, T. H. J. & JONXIS, J. H. P. (1957). *Arch. Dis. Childh.*, **32**, 77.

HUNT, D. D., STEARNS, G., McKINLEY, J. B., FRONING, E., HICKS, P. & BONFIGLIO, M. (1966). *Amer. J. Med.*, **40**, 492.

JAGENBURG, O. R. (1959). *Scand. J. clin. Invest.*, **11**, Supp. 43.

JEPSON, J. B. *In* "The Metabolic Basis of Inherited Disease", 2nd Ed. Ed. STANBURY, J. B., WYNGAARDEN, J. B. & FREDERICKSON, D. S. McGraw-Hill Book Co., N.Y. 1966.

JERVIS, G. A. (1937). *Arch. Neurol. Psychiat.*, **38**, 944.

JERVIS, G. A. (1938). *J. biol. Chem.*, **126**, 305.

JERVIS, G. A. (1947). *J. biol. Chem.*, **169**, 651.

JERVIS, G. A. (1950). *Proc. Soc. exp. Biol., N.Y.*, **75**, 83.

JERVIS, G. A. (1952). *Proc. Soc. exp. Biol., N.Y.*, **81**, 715.

JERVIS, G. A. (1953). *Proc. Soc. exp. Biol., N.Y.*, **82**, 514.

JERVIS, G. A. (1954). *Res. Publ. Ass. Nerv. Ment. Dis.*, **33**, 259.

JERVIS, G. A., BLOCK, R. J., BOLLING, D. & KANZE, E. (1940). *J. biol. Chem.*, **134**, 105.

JONXIS, H. P. & HUISMAN, T. H. J. (1953). *Lancet*, **2**, 428.

JONXIS, H. P. & HUISMAN, T. H. J. (1954). *Paediatrics*, **14**, 238.

JONXIS, J. H. P. (1957). *Ned. T. Geneesk*, **101**, 569.

JONXIS, J. H. P., SMITH, P. A. & HUISMAN, T. H. J. (1952). *Lancet*, **2**, 1015.

JOPE, E. M. (1946). *Brit. J. industr. Med.*, **3**, 136.

KALCKAR, H. M. (1957). *Science*, **125**, 105.

KATSCH, G. & METZ, E. (1927). *Dtsch. Arch. klin. Med.*, **157**, 143.

KINNORY, D. S., TAKEDA, Y. & GREENBERG, D. M. (1955). *J. biol. Chem.*, **212**, 385.

KNAPP, A. (1960). *Clin. Chim. Acta*, **5**, 6.

KNOX, W. E. (1961). *In* "Biochemist's Handbook". Ed. Long, C. London.

KOCH, R., ACOSTA, P., FISHLER, K., SCHAEFFLER, G. & WOHLERS, A. (1967). *A.M.A.J. Dis. Child.*, **113**, 6.

KOMROWER, G. M. (1953). *Arch. franç. Pédiat.*, **10**, 185.

KOMROWER, G. M. (1967). *A.M.A.J. Dis. Child.*, **113**, 98.

KOMROWER, G. M. & WESTALL, R. (1967). *A.M.A.J. Dis. Child.*, **113**, 77.

KOMROWER, G. M., WILSON, V., CLAMP, J. R. & WESTALL, R. G. (1964). *Arch. J. Dis. Child.*, **113**, 77.

KOPELMAN, H., ASATOOR, A. M. & MILNE, M. D. (1964). *Lancet*, **2**, 1075.

KORN, D. (1960). *New England. J. Med.*, **262**, 545.

KOTAKE, Y., MASAI, Y. & MORI, Y. (1922). *Hoppe-Seyl. Z.*, **122**, 195.

LA DU, B. N., HOWELL, R. R. & JACOBY, G. A. L. (1962). *Biochem. Biophys. Res. Comms.*, **7**, 398.

LA DU, B. N., O'BRIEN, W. M. & ZANNONI, V. G. (1962). *Arthrit. Rheum.*, **5**, 81

LA DU, B. N. & ZANNONI, V. G. (1955). *J. biol. Chem.*, **217**, 777.

LA DU, B. N., ZANNONI, V. G., LASTER, L. & SEEGMILLER, J. E. (1958). *J. biol. Chem.*, **230**, 251.

LANG, K., KNOPP, K. & WEBER, D. (1957). *Z. Kinderh.*, **80**, 311.

LANGDELL, J. I. (1965). *Arch. Gen. Psychiat.*, **12**, 363.

LANYAR, F. & LIEB, H. (1931). *Hoppe-Seyl. Z.*, **203**, 135.

LEAF, G. & NEUBERGER, A. (1948). *Biochem. J.*, **43**, 606.

LELONG, M., ALAGILLE, D., GENTIL, C., COLIN, J., TUPIN, J. & BOUQUIER, J. (1962). *Bull. et. mém. Soc. méd. hop. Paris*, **113**, 58.

LEVENSON, J., LINDAHL-KIESSLING, K. & RAYNER, S. (1964). *Lancet*, **2**, 756.

LEVIN, B. (1967). *A.M.A. J. Dis. Child.*, **113**, 162.

LEVIN, B., MACKAY, H. M. M. & OBERHOLZER, V. G. (1961). *Arch. Dis. Childh.*, **36**, 622.

LEVINE, S. Z., DANN, M. & MARPLES, E. (1943). *J. clin. Invest.*, **22**, 551.

LEWIS, H. B., BROWN, B. H. & WHITE, F. R. (1936). *J. biol. Chem.*, **114**, 171.

LICHTENSTEIN, L. & KAPLAN, L. (1954). *Amer. J. Path.*, **30**, 99.

LIETMAN, P. S., FRAZIER, P. D., WONG, V. G., SHOTTEN, D. & SEEGMILLER, J. E. (1966). *Amer. J. Med.*, **40**, 511.

LIGNAC, G. O. E. (1924). *Dtsch. Arch. klin. Med.*, **145**, 139.

LIGNAC, G. O. E. (1926). *Krankheitsforschung*, **2**, 43.

LING, N. R. (1955). *Biochem. J.*, **59**, x.

LINNEWEH, F. (1961). Cited by BICKEL, H., in "Renal Disease". Ed. Black, D. A. K. (1962). Oxford, Blackwell.

LITIN, R. B., RANDALL, R. V., GOLDSTEIN, N. P., POWER, M. H. & DIESSNER, G. R. (1959). Amer. J. med. Sci., 238, 614.

LONDON, D. R. & FOLEY, T. H. (1965). Clin. Sci., 29, 133.

LOVNEY, J. M., BERGLUND, H. & GRAVES, R. C. (1923). J. biol. Chem., 57, 515.

LOWE, C. U. (1960). Maandschr. v. Kindergeneesk, 28, 77.

LOWE, C. U., TERREY, M. & MACLACHAN, E. A. (1952). Amer. J. Dis. Child., 83, 164.

LUDER, J. & SHELDON, W. (1955). Arch. Dis. Childh., 30, 160.

MABRY, C. C. & KARAM, E. A. (1963). Southern med. J., 56, 1444.

McCARTHY, C. F., BORLAND, J. L. Jr., LYNCH, H. J. Jr., OWEN, E. E. & TYOR, M. P. (1964). J. clin. Invest., 43, 1516.

McCUNE, D. J., MASON, H. H. & CLARKE, H. T. (1943). Amer. J. Dis. Child., 65, 81.

MACKENSIE, D. Y. & WOOLF, L. I. (1959). Brit. med. J., 1, 90.

McDONALD, L., BRAY, C., FIELD, C., LOVE, G. & DAVIES, B. (1964). Lancet, 1, 745.

McMURRAY, W. C. & MOHYUDDIN, F. (1962). Lancet, 2, 352.

McMURRAY, W. C., MOHYUDDIN, F., ROSSITER, R. J., RATHBUN, J. C., VALENTINE, G. H., KOEGLER, S. J. & ZARFAS, D. E. (1962). Lancet, 1, 138.

MARSDEN, H. B. & WILSON, V. K. (1955). Brit. med. J., 1, 324.

MATTHEWS, W. B., MILNE, M. D. & BELL, M. (1952). Quart. J. Med., 21, n.s., 425.

MEDES, G. (1932). Biochem. J., 26, 917.

MENKES, J. H. (1959). Pediatrics, 23, 348.

MENKES, J. H. (1966). J. Pediat., 69, 413.

MENKES, J. H., HURST P. L. & CRAIG J. M. (1954). Pediatrics, 14, 462.

MILCH R. A. (1961). Arthrit. Rheum., 4, 131.

MILCH, R. A. & MURRAY, R. A. (1961). Arthrit. Rheum., 4, 268.

MILNE, M. D. (1959). Lancet, 2, 467.

MILNE, M. D. (1964). Brit. med. J., 1, 327.

MILNE, M. D., ASATOOR, A. M., EDWARDS, K. D. G. & LOUGHRIDGE, L. W. (1961). Gut, 2, 323.

MILNE, M. D., CRAWFORD, M. A., GIRAO, C. B. & LOUGHRIDGE, L. W. (1960). Quart. J. Med., n.s., 29, 407.

MILNE, M. D., STANBURY, S. W. & THOMPSON, A. E. (1952). Quart. J. Med., 21, n.s., 61.

MITOMA, C., AULD, R. M. & UDENFRIEND, S. (1957). Proc. Soc. exp. Biol., N.Y., 94, 634.

MITOMA, C. & LEEPER, L. C. (1954). Fed Proc., 13, 266.

MIYAMOTO, M. & FITZPATRICK, T. B. (1957). Nature (Lond.), 179, 199

MOHYUDDIN, F. RATHBUN, J. C. & McMURRAY, W. C. (1967). A.M.A. J. Dis. Child., 113, 152.

MONGEAU, J. G., HILGARTNER, M., WORTHEN, H. G. & FRIMPTER, G. W. (1966). J. Pediat., 69, 1113.

MOORE, S. & STEIN, W. H. (1951). J. biol. Chem., 192, 663.

MOORE, S. & STEIN, W. H. (1954). J. biol. Chem., 211, 893.

MORGAN, H. G., STEWART, W. K., LOWE, K. G., STOWERS, J. M. & JOHNSTONE, J. H. (1962). Quart, J. Med., n.s., 31, 361.

MORIKAWA, T., TADA, K., ANDO, T., YOSHIDA, T., YOKOYAMA, Y. & ARAKAWA, T. (1966). Tohoku J. exp. Med., 90, 105.

MORROW, G. (1967). A.M.A. J. Dis. Child., 113, 157.

MOSS, A. R. (1941). J. biol. Chem., 137, 739.

MOSS, A. R. & SCHOENHEIMER, R. (1940). J. biol. Chem., 135, 415.

MUDD, S. H., FINKELSTEIN, J. D., IRREVERRE, F. & LASTER, L. (1964). Science, 143, 1443.

MUDGE, G. H. (1958). Amer. J. Med., 24, 785.

MURPHY, D. (1958). Irish J. med. Sci., 391, 335.

NEUBAUER, O. (1909). Dtsch. Arch. klin. Med., 95, 211.

NEUBAUER, O. (1928). Handb. norm pathol. physiol. Berlin, Julius Springer.

NEUBAUER, O. & FALTA, W. (1904). Hoppe-Seyl. Z., 42, 81.

NEUBERGER, A., RIMINGTON, C. & WILSON, J. M. G. (1947). Biochem. J., 41, 438.

NEWMAN, C. G. H., WILSON, B. D. R., CALLAGHAN, P. & YOUNG, L. (1967). Lancet, 2, 439.

NYHAN, W. L. (1967). A.M.A. J. Dis. Child., 113, 129.

NORTON, P. M., ROITMAN, E., LUYDERMAN, S. E. & HOLT, L. E., Jr. (1962). Lancet, 1, 26.

PARE, C. M. B., SANDLER, M. & STACEY, R. S. (1957). Lancet, 1, 551.

PARE, C. M. B., SANDLER, M. & STACEY, R. S. (1958). Lancet, 2, 1099.

PARKES, W. E. & NEILL, D. W. (1953). Brit. med. J., 1, 653.

PATRICK, A. D. (1962). Biochem. J., 83, 248.

PENROSE, L. S. (1935). Lancet, 1, 23.

PENROSE, L. S. & QUASTEL, J. H. (1937). Biochem. J., 31, 266.

PERRY, T. L., HANSEN, S., TISCHLER, B., BUNTING, R. & BERRY, K. (1967). New England J. Med., 277, 1219.

PERRY, T. L., HARDWICK, D. F., DIXON, G. H., DOLMAN, C. L. & HANSEN, S. (1965). Pediatrics, 36, 236.

PIETER, H. (1925). Pr. méd., 33, 1310.

POMERANZ, M. M., FRIEDMAN, L. J. & TUNICK, I. S. (1941). Radiology, 37, 295.

PRICE, J. M., YESS, M. BROWN, R. R. & JOHNSON, S. A. M. (1967). Arch. Dermatol., 95, 462.

RAVDIN, R. G. & CRANDALL, D. I. (1951). J. biol. Chem., 189, 137.

ROBSON, E. B. & ROSE, G. A. (1957). Clin. Sci., 16, 75.

ROOF, B. S. & TURNER, J. C. (1955). J. clin. Invest., 34, 1647.

ROSE, W. C. (1937). Science, 86, 298.

ROSE, W. C., HAINES, W. J., JOHNSON, J. W. & WARNER, D. T. (1943). J. biol. Chem., 148, 457.

ROSENBERG, L. E., DOWNING, S., DURANT, J. L. & SEGAL, S. (1966). *J. clin. Invest.*, **45**, 365.

ROSENBERG, L. E., DOWNING, S. J. & SEGAL, S. (1962). *J. biol. Chem.*, **237**, 2265.

ROSENOER, V. M. & MICHELL, R. C. (1959). *Brit. J. Radiol.*, **32**, 805.

ROTHSTEIN, A. & BERKE, H. (1949). *J. Pharmacol.*, **96**, 179.

RUSSELL, A., LEVIN, B., OBERHOLZER, V. G. & SINCLAIR, L. (1962). *Lancet*, **2**, 699.

RUSZKOWSKI, M., BAERTL, J. M. & GABUZDA, G. J. (1960). *Pol. Zyg. Lek.*, **15**, 1679.

RUTTINGER, V., MILLER, S., ANDRECOVITZ, M. E. & PERDUE, G. M. (1954). *Proc. Soc. exp. Biol., N.Y.*, **86**, 108.

SANDLER, M. & PARE, C. M. B. (1954). *Lancet*, **1**, 494.

SCHAFER, I. A., SCRIVER, C. R. & EFRON, M. L. (1962). *New England J. Med.*, **267**, 51.

SCHINKE, R. N., MCKUSICK, V. A., HUANG, T. & POLLACK, A. D. (1965). *J. Amer. med. Ass.*, **193**, 711.

SCHREIER, K. & MÜLLER, W. (1964). *Deutsch. Med. Wschr.*, **89**, 1739.

SCHWARZ, V., GOLBERG, L., KOMROWER, G. M. & HOLZEL, A. (1955). *Biochem. J.*, **59**, xxii.

SCHWARZ-TIENE, E., CAREDDU, P. & CABASSA, N. (1957). *Minerv. pediatr.*, **9**, 231.

SCRIVER, C. R., LAROCHELLE, J., & SILVERBERG, M. (1967). *A.M.A. J. Dis. Child.*, **113**, 41.

SCRIVER, C. R., PUESCHEL, S. & DAVIES, E. (1966). *New England J. Med.*, **274**, 636.

SCRIVER, C. R. & WILSON, O. H. (1967). *Science*, **155**, 1426.

SCRIVER, C. R., SCHAFER, I. A. & EFRON, M. L. (1961). *Nature (Lond.)*, **192**, 672.

SEALOCK, R. R. & GOODLAND, R. L. (1951). *Science*, **114**, 645.

SEALOCK, R. R., GOODLAND, R. L., SUMERWELL, W. N. & BRIERLY, J. M. (1952). *J. Biol. Chem.*, **196**, 761.

SEEGMILLER, J. E. & HOWELL, R. R. (1961). *Clin. Res.*, **9**, 189.

SEEGMILLER, J. E., ZANNONI, V. G., LASTER, L. & LA DU, B. N. (1961). *J. biol. Chem.*, **236**, 774.

SHAW, K. N. F., REDLICH, D., WRIGHT, S. W. & JEPSON, J. B. (1960). *Fed. Proc.*, **19**, 194.

SHELDON, W., LUDER, J., WEBB, B. (1961). *Arch. Dis. Childh.*, **36**, 90.

SIDBURY, J. B., SMITH, E. K. & HARLAN, W. (1967). *J. Pediat.*, **70**, 8.

SIROTA, J. H. & HAMERMAN, D. (1954). *Amer. J. Med.*, **16**, 138.

SNYDERMAN, S. E. (1967). *A.M.A. J. Dis. Child.*, **113**, 68.

SPENCER, R. P., BRODY, K. R. & MAUTNER, H. G. (1965). *Nature (Lond.)*, **207**, 418.

SPENCER, A. G. & FRANGLEN, G. T. (1952). *Lancet*, **1**, 190.

STANBURY, S. W. (1962). "Renal Disease." Ed. Black, D. A. K. Oxford, Blackwell, p. 508.

STANBURY, S. W. & MACAULEY, D. (1957). *Quart. J. Med.*, n.s., **26**, 7.

STAVE, U. & SCHLAAK, E. (1956). *Z. Kinderheilk.*, **78**, 261.

STEELE, B., REYNOLDS, M. S. & BAUMANN, C. A. (1950). *J. Nutrit.*, **40**, 145.

STEIN, W. H. (1951). *Proc. Soc. exp. Biol., N.Y.*, **78**, 705.

STEIN, W. H. (1953). *J. biol. Chem.*, **201**, 45.

STEIN, W. H., BEARN, A. G. & MOORE, S. (1954). *J. clin. Invest.*, **33**, 410.

STEIN, W. H. & MOORE, S. (1954). *J. biol. Chem.*, **211**, 915.

STEIN, W. H., PALADINI, A. C., HIRS, C. H. W. & MOORE, S. (1954). *J. Amer. chem. Soc.*, **76**, 2848.

STEIN-PARVÉ, E. P. & BEINERT, H. (1958). *J. biol. Chem.*, **233**, 853.

STERNLIEB, I., MORELL, A. G., BAUER, C. D., COMBES, B., DE BOBES-STEINBERG, S. & SCHEINBERG, I. H. (1961). *J. clin. Invest.*, **40**, 707.

STOWERS, J. M. & DENT, C. E. (1947). *Quart. J. Med.*, **16**, n.s., 275.

TADA, K., ITO, H., WADA, Y., & ARAKAWA, T. (1963). *Tohoku J. exp. Med.*, **80**, 118.

TADA, K., MORIKAWA, T., ANDO, T., YOSHIDA, T. & MINAGAWA, A. (1965). *Tokoku J. exp. Med.*, **87**, 133.

TALLAN, H. H., MOORE, S., STEIN, W. H. (1958). *J. biol. Chem.*, **230**, 707.

TALLAN, H. H., STEIN, W. H. & MOORE, S. (1954). *J. biol. Chem.*, **206**, 825.

TASHIAN, R. E. (1961). *Metabolism*, **10**, 393.

TAWAKA, K., BUDD, M. A., EFRON, M. L. & ISSELBACHER, K. J. (1966). *Proc. Nat. Acad. Sci.*, **56**, 236.

THIER, S. O., SEGAL, S., FOX, M., BLAIR, A. & ROSENBERG, L. E. (1965). *J. clin. Invest.*, **44**, 442.

THIERFELDER, H. & SHERWIN, C. P. (1914). *Ber. Dtsch. chem. Ges.*, **47**, 2630.

THIERFELDER, H. & SHERWIN, C. P. (1915). *Hoppe-Seyl. Z.*, **94**, 1.

TREACHER, R. J. (1962). *Vet. Rec.*, **74**, 503.

UDENFRIEND, S. & BESSMAN, S. P. (1953). *J. biol. Chem.*, **203**, 961.

UDENFRIEND, S. CLARK, C. T., AXELROD, J. & BRODIE, B. B. (1954). *J. biol. Chem.*, **208**, 731.

UDENFRIEND, S. & COOPER, J. R. (1952). *J. biol. Chem.*, **194**, 503.

ULLRICH, O. (1948). *Z. Kinderheilk.*, **66**, 154.

UZMAN, L. L. & DENNY BROWN, D. (1948). *Amer. J. med. Sci.*, **215**, 599.

UZMAN, L. L. & HOOD, B. (1952). *Amer. J. med. Sci.*, **223**, 392.

VAN CREFELD, S. & ARONS, P. (1949). *Ann. paediat.*, **173**, 299.

VISAKORPI, J. K. & HYRSKE, I. (1960). *Ann. Paediat. Fenn.*, **6**, 112.

VON EULER, U. S. (1945). *Acta pharmacol. (Kbh)*, **1**, 29.

VON UDRANSZKY, L. BAUMANN, E. (1889). *Z. physiol. Chem.*, **13**, 562.

WADA, Y., TADA, K., MINAGAWA, A., YOSHIDA, T., MORIKAWA, T. & OKAMURA, T. (1963). *Tohoku J. exp. Med.*, **81**, 46.

WAISMAN, H. A. (1967). *A.M.A.J. Dis. Child.*, **113,** 101.

WAISMAN, H. A., WANG, H. L., PALMER, G. & HARLOW, H. F. (1960). *Nature (Lond.),* **188,** 1124.

WALLACE, H. W., MOLDAVE, K. & MEISTER, A. (1957). *Proc. Soc. exp. Biol., N.Y.,* **94,** 632.

WALLRAFF, E. B. BRODIE, E. C. & BORDEN, A. L. (1950). *J. clin. Invest.,* **29,** 1542.

WALSHE, J. M. (1953). *Quart. J. Med.,* **22,** n.s., 483.

WEBER, H. (1953). *Helv. paediat. Acta,* **8,** 348.

WESTALL, R. G. (1952). *Biochem. J.,* **52,** 638.

WESTALL, R. G. (1955). *Biochem. J.,* **60,** 247.

WESTALL, R. G. (1960). *Biochem. J.,* **77,** 135.

WESTALL, R. G., DANCIS, J. & MILLER, S. (1957). *AMA. J. Dis. Child.,* **94,** 571.

WILSON, V. K., THOMSON, M. L. & DENT, C. E. (1953). *Lancet,* **2,** 66.

WOLFF, S. M. (1962). *Clin. Res.,* **10,** 45.

WOLKOW, M. & BAUMANN, E. (1891). *Hoppe-Seyl. Z.,* **15,** 228.

WOLLASTON, W. H. (1812). *Phil. Trans. Roy. Soc.* p. 223.

WOODY, N. C., HUTZLER, J. & DANCIS, J. (1966). *A.M.A. J. Dis. Child.,* **112,** 577.

WOOD, J. L. & COOLEY, S. L. (1954). *Proc. Soc. exp. Biol., N.Y.,* **85,** 409.

WOOLF, L. I. (1951). *Biochem. J.,* **49,** ix.

WOOLF, L. I. (1962). *Proc. Nitrit. Soc.,* **21,** 21.

WOOLF, L. I. & Edmunds, M. E. (1950). *Biochem. J.,* **47,** 630.

WOOLF, L. I., GRIFFITHS, R. & MONCRIEFF, A. (1955). *Brit. med. J.,* **1,** 57.

WORTHEN, H. G. & GOOD, R. A. (1961). *AMA. J. Dis. Child.,* **102,** 494.

ZANNONI, V. G., SEEGMILLER, J. E. & LA DU, B. N. (1962). *Nature, (Lond.),* **193,** 952.

Chapter 17

LIPIDOSES AND SECONDARY DISORDERS OF LIPID METABOLISM*

by

N. ZÖLLNER and G. WOLFRAM

Medical Polyclinic of the University of Munich

* In this chapter "hyperlipidaemia" is used as a general term, denoting increase in several or all types of plasma lipids. "Hyperlipaemia" is reserved for increases in neutral fat, i.e. the sum of tri-, di-, and monoglycerides, corresponding to "hypercholesterolaemia". Possible "secondary" rises in other lipids, such as phosphatides in hypercholesterolaemia or cholesterol and its esters in hyperlipaemia are not considered in this nomenclature. Hyperlipaemia is preferred to hypertriglyceridaemia since the chemical methods used determine neutral fat glycerol without distinguishing between the tri-, di-, and monoglycerides.

DISEASES associated with the accumulation of lipids in cells of mesenchymal origin or in plasma are called lipidoses. The accumulated lipids may be different in the various disorders, and indeed are specific for the disease in some of them. Lipidoses may be "primary disorders" in which a derangement of lipid metabolism is the cause of the whole pathological picture; however increased concentrations of lipids in serum and/or organs occur also as a consequence of other diseases, and in some of them derangement of lipid metabolism may be a conspicuous finding. As far as these disorders produce abnormal levels of plasma lipids, they will be considered here.

CLASSIFICATION

Lipidoses may be classified according to the type of lipid accumulating, the histological appearance, or by lipid levels in the plasma. A combination of all three principles is most reasonable. Thus we distinguish between sphingolipidoses, in which lipids containing sphingosine accumulate (i.e. Gaucher's disease, Niemann-Pick's disease, Tay-Sachs' disease, metachromatic leucodystrophy and possibly Pfaundler-Hurler's disease), and lipidoses in which cholesterol predominates among the lipids of the affected cells. The latter lipidoses are also called xanthomatoses since their lesions contain typical xanthoma cells whose cytoplasm, after the usual histological procedures, is vacuolar or foamy (in eruptive xanthoma foam cells are rare, but do occur).

The lipidoses may also be differentiated into disorders with increased plasma lipid levels (hyperlipidaemias) and diseases with normal levels. In the diseases with increased lipid levels xanthoma formation is secondary to the increased plasma level which may also exist without recognizable clinical consequences; the increased plasma level and not the intracellular lipid accumulation is the essential feature; xanthoma formation is not a diagnostic *conditio sine qua non*. In the sphingolipidoses increases of total plasma lipids occur only as a consequence of severe malnutrition and bear no relationship to the primary disease mechanism. The various features of eosinophilic granuloma belong to the normocholesterolaemic xanthomatoses.

METABOLISM OF THE PLASMA LIPIDS

Cholesterol

For a survey of steroid chemistry see Fieser & Fieser (1959) or more briefly Klyne (1957).

In the organism, cholesterol is synthesized from acetate (Bloch & Rittenberg, 1945; Cornforth, 1953); most of the details are now known as a result of the work of Bloch, Lynen, Popják and others. In cholesterol biosynthesis (Fig. 17.1) acetoacetate is formed from acetylCoA, and a third acetylCoA is condensed with it to form β-hydroxy-β-methylglutarylCoA. The CoA is split off, and at the same time the carboxyl group is reduced to an alcohol; the product, mevalonic acid, is the key intermediate of steroid synthesis. The next three steps lead to isopentenyl pyrophosphate which is the "active isoprene". Condensations of isopentenylpyrophosphate lead to farnesylpyrophosphate. Two molecules of farnesylpyrophosphate condense "head to head" to form squalene which is cyclized, the first identifiable product being lanosterol. Several oxidations, decarboxylations and reductions then eliminate three methyl groups and a double bond; another double bond must change its position. Figure 17.1 shows the most important reactions. Papers by Cornforth (1959) and Wright (1961) provide important summaries.

Cholesterol synthesis from acetate may be influenced by the quantity of cholesterol already preformed in the liver (Tomkins, Sheppard & Chaikoff, 1953a, b). Fasting reduces cholesterol synthesis. Dietary cholesterol also inhibits cholesterol synthesis (Kritchevsky et al., 1960; Bhattathiry & Siperstein, 1963; Gould & Swyryd, 1966).

[2-^{14}C]-acetate is incorporated in the plasma cholesterol with peak activity after 8 hr. (Hellman et al., 1955), while ester cholesterol shows a peak after 2 days.

Absorption. The absorption of cholesterol is facilitated by the presence in the intestines of neutral fat (Thannhauser, 1923) and of bile (Bollman & Flock, 1951; Siperstein, Chaikoff & Reinhardt, 1952; Kim & Ivy, 1952). Early investigators thought that cholesterol is absorbed as cholesterol ester. Recent experiments show that free cholesterol also may be absorbed (Swell, Boiter, Field & Treadwell, 1955). Indeed about 30% of cholesterol in thoracic duct lymph is free; among the esters those of oleic acid predominate (Blomstrand, 1961). Man absorbs not only cholesterol which is of animal origin, but to a minor degree plant sterols as well (Böhle et al., 1964).

Breakdown. It should be appreciated that cholesterol is the precursor of steroid hormones as well as bile acids, and that the biosynthesis of these substances represents pathways of cholesterol breakdown. For a review the paper by

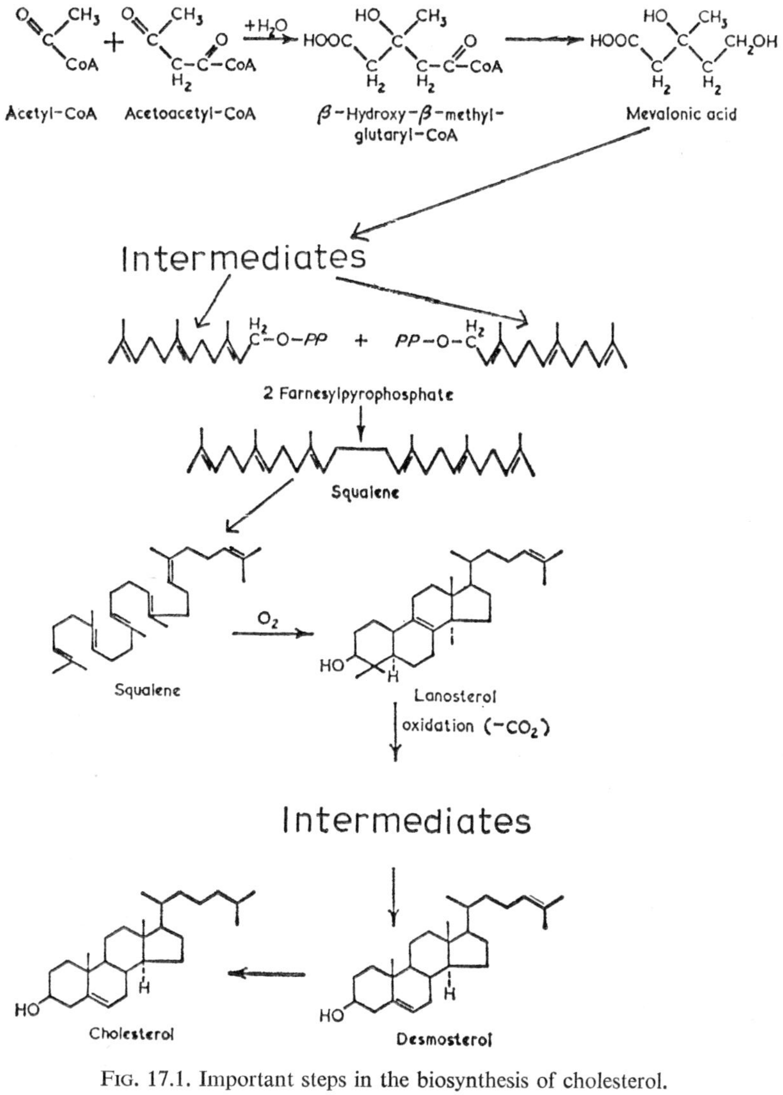

FIG. 17.1. Important steps in the biosynthesis of cholesterol.

Bergström, Daniellsson & Samuelsson (1960) should be consulted.

A disintegration of the ring skeleton of the steroids by enzymic processes in intermediary metabolism is apparently impossible (Chaikoff *et al.*, 1952; Hellman *et al.*, 1955). Bacterial enzymes in the intestine, however, can disintegrate the sterol ring, and convert cholesterol to products not precipitated with the usual reagents for cholesterol determination (Beumer & Fasold, 1933; Nékám & Ottenstein, 1935; Hellman *et al.*, 1955). On the other hand the administration of [4-^{14}C]-cholesterol does not lead to the expiration of radioactive CO_2; this observation indicates that whatever degradation products are formed, they are not metabolized by the body.

Excretion. Several sterols occur in the faeces of man, and the average excretion of total sterols on a mixed diet is estimated to be 1·6–2·2 g./day (Grundy & Ahrens, 1966).

Cholesterol, as well as bile acids, undergoes an enterohepatic circulation. Cholesterol is excreted with the bile and also directly into the intestine. Stanley & Cheng (1956), administering [4-^{14}C]-cholesterol in food to man, estimated this excretion to amount to 1–2 g./day; reabsorption of cholesterol should amount to about 1·5 g. A patient with complete occlusion of the common duct was found to excrete 140 mg. sterol, an amount probably corresponding to that directly excreted into the intestine. Fig. 17.2 gives a schematic representation of the quantitative aspects. In the same figure the enterohepatic circulation of the bile acids is shown. The data for bile acid synthesis and pool size are from Lindstedt (1957); they show that the enterohepatic circulation of bile acid must be very rapid, a conclusion consistent with the finding that 80 to 90% of orally fed

Cholesterol in plasma. In young men the average level of total plasma cholesterol is 170 mg./100 ml.; in financially prosperous populations this average level increases with age to values in the range of 240–260 at the age of 55; in poorer parts of the world the increase is much less pronounced. In women the cholesterol levels are markedly lower only until the menopause. In very old age cholesterol values become lower in both sexes. It should be appreciated that the standard deviation of plasma cholesterol at the age of 50 is rather large, about 30–40 mg./100 ml.; cholesterol

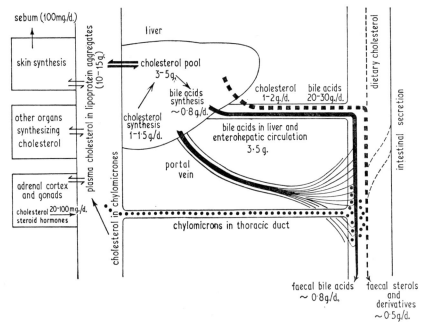

Fig. 17.2. Schematic representation of the pathways and enterohepatic circulation of cholesterol and bile acids in liver and plasma.

labelled bile acid appears within 2 hr. in fistula bile (Sjövall & Åkesson, 1955).

Comparison of the quantitative data for both enterohepatic circulations indicates that about half of the cholesterol synthesized in the liver is metabolized to bile acids, the other half being lost by excretion after bacterial degradation. Since the excretion of bile acids is much larger than that of cholesterol, interruption of the enterohepatic circulation by production of a bile fistula necessarily brings about a larger increase in the conversion of cholesterol to bile acids so that the percentage of cholesterol converted to bile acids increases. Findings in bile fistula patients have to be interpreted in the light of this consideration.

values up to 340 mg./100 ml. may therefore lie within the $m \pm 2\sigma$ limits of the values in an apparently healthy population, i.e. within the "normal range". Obviously the definition of the term "normal value" enters into the discussion, and comparison of central European values with values from Southern Italy would make most of the former appear "elevated".

The factors which increase cholesterol in wealthy populations are only partly understood. It appears that a diet rich in fat containing saturated or mono-unsaturated fatty acids as well as cholesterol is responsible, but the evidence on this point is not complete.

About two-thirds of the plasma cholesterol are

TABLE 17.1

The fatty acids in serum cholesterol esters

	$C_{14:0}$	$C_{15:0}$	$C_{16:0}$	$C_{16:1}$	$C_{17:0}$	$C_{18:0}$	$C_{18:1}$	$C_{18:2}$	$C_{18:3}$	$C_{20:3}$	$C_{20:4}$	$C_{20:5}$	$C_{22:5}$	$C_{22:6}$
Schrade *et al.* (1960)	1·1	—	12·1	6·8	—	2·6	18·9	47·1		0·9	5·0		1·4	—
Hallgren *et al.* (1960)	1·4	0·6	11·0	4·8	1·1	0·8	23·2	46·2	2·1	—	5·9	1·8	0·6	—
Zöllner & Wolfram (Unpublished)	1·3	0·4	12·3	4·1	0·6	0·7	23·8	48·7	0·4	0·6	6·7	0·4	—	—

esterified with fatty acids; Table 17.1 lists the predominating acids as well as their relative amounts. A diet rich in poly-unsaturated acids increases the relative amounts of the respective esters (Ahrens *et al.*, 1959; Cramér & Björntorp, 1962). Strict reduction of dietary linoleate decreases the amount of linoleic acid ester (Zöllner, Wolfram & Londong, 1966). In general, however, it is amazing how close normal values are in a population fed *ad libitum* (Zöllner, Wolfram & Amin, 1962). It is noteworthy that linoleic acid esters do not predominate in the plasma of the new-born (Zöllner & Wolfram, 1962; Zöllner *et al.*, 1966).

Influence of endocrines on the clinical biochemistry of cholesterol. The increase of cholesterol in the serum of hypothyroid patients and its low level in hyperthyroid individuals are well known. It was shown that in myxoedematous patients, the synthesis of cholesterol after ingestion of [1-^{14}C]-acetate is markedly decreased (LeRoy, 1955). In the face of decreased synthesis increased blood levels clearly mean decreased turnover as a result of decreased breakdown. On the other hand the administration of thyroid hormones leads to a decreased half-life of plasma cholesterol in animals (Boyd & Oliver, 1958) and man (Gould, 1959).

After bilateral ovariectomy there is a rise of the plasma cholesterol of about 40 mg./100 ml., to the level observed in post-menopausal women (Oliver & Boyd, 1959). Animal experiments seem to indicate that ovariectomy increases the half-life of plasma cholesterol, while administration of oestrogens in oestrogenic doses seems to decrease it. Less is known about the influence of male sex hormones; Furman *et al.* (1958) have reported that young eunuchs have a significantly lower plasma cholesterol than controls, although late orchidectomy does not appear to lower cholesterol values.

The influence of adrenal hormones is ill-defined. In man, Adlersberg, Schaefer & Drachman (1951) found slight increases in plasma cholesterol after the administration of ACTH or cortisone. On the other hand, Conn *et al.* (1950) and Oliver & Boyd (1956) found that cortisone lowers high cholesterol values. In our experience cortisone effects are quite unpredictable and may be incidental to the influence of cortisone on the disease present.

Plasma Phospholipids

Lipid phosphorus in the plasma is maintained in a rather constant relationship to cholesterol levels. This is true also in the hyperlipidaemias. Indeed, it appears possible that the primary change in these disorders involves phosphatide metabolism or lipoprotein metabolism, thus explaining the correlation. According to Man *et al.* (1945)

[lipid phosphorus] = 0·0294 [total cholesterol] + (3·62 ± 1·04), values being given as mg./100 ml.

Later, Jackson & Wilkinson (1952) found that an even better correlation can be obtained between phospholipids and free cholesterol, i.e.

[phospholipids] = 2·0 [free cholesterol] + 80.

The latter authors claim that this ratio is not influenced by disease.

Turnover. Most phosphatides administered orally are hydrolysed in the gut, so that their influence on total turnover is small. On the other hand, fat absorption leads to an increased synthesis of phosphatides in the intestinal wall (Artom, 1952), presumably because phosphatides are the physiological stabilizer for the chylomicrons in the thoracic duct lymph. In general, phosphatide turnover is rather rapid if measured with ^{32}P. For example, the half-life of phospholipids in the blood of the dog was found by Chaikoff *et al.* (1948) to be only 7·5 hr. For further information a recent monograph (Ansell & Hawthorne, 1964) should be consulted.

Phosphatides in plasma. Until the advent of chromatographic procedures, only lecithin, cephalins and sphingomyelin were known to occur in human plasma. By now it is established that lysolecithins (Phillips, 1958) and lysocephalins are also present. Table 17.2 gives the relative amounts of these substances, obtained from our own studies, the results of which agree with most other investigators. For a compilation of these see Nye et al. (1961).

TABLE 17.2

Composition of serum phosphatides
(from Zöllner & Kirsch, 1960)

	mg./ 100 ml. of plasma	% of total phosphatides
Lecithin[1]	162·2	66·8
Lysolecithin	18·6	7·7
Phosphatidylethanolamine and serine[1]	10·0	4·1
Lysophosphatidylethanolamine	4·7	1·9
Sphingomyelin	40·8	16·8
Unidentified	6·1	2·5
	242·4	99·8

[1] Plasmalogens corresponding to lecithin and cephalins are not enumerated.

Very little is yet known about the behaviour of the different phosphatides under pathological conditions. Phillips (1960) found that in the serum of patients with icteric liver disease the ratio of sphingomyelin to lecithin was decreased, while the relative as well as absolute concentrations of lysolecithin were diminished. His findings have been corroborated in various laboratories (Dienstl et al., 1966; Gjone & Orning, 1966), as well as in our own. So far there appears to be a certain negative correlation with bilirubin levels, while no relationship to the basic disease process is apparent.

Nye & Waterhouse (1961) have shown a relative increase in lysolecithin and sphingomyelin in the nephrotic syndrome. Nothman & Proger (1962) claim that there is an increase of phosphatidyl ethanolamine and phosphatidyl serine in coronary heart disease. On the other hand, Wagener et al (1964) found the relative amounts of all phosphatides to be normal in arteriosclerosis. The fatty acids in total phosphatides behave similarly to those in cholesterol esters; however the extent of changes is usually less pronounced. Phosphatide fractions isolated by thin layer chromatography can be analysed for their fatty acids (Bowyer et al., 1963).

Triglycerides

Chyle and liver are the sources of plasma triglycerides. Thus, next to catabolism, the alimentary supply of fat and hepatic synthesis are the most important factors determining the levels of neutral fat. After a meal containing fat, triglyceride concentration in the plasma rises, reaching its maximum after 2½–4 hr. Return to normal often takes as long as 10 hr. and therefore attention to a sufficient period of fasting is necessary if comparable values for plasma triglycerides are to be obtained. Fasting hypertriglyceridaemia induced by a diet rich in fat undoubtedly occurs; however most authorities agree that carbohydrate-induced hyperlipaemia (Ahrens et al., 1961) is also common (*vide infra*).

Whether hypertriglyceridaemia occurs without a concomitant rise in plasma cholesterol and phosphatides is not certain, since the ranges of "normal" for these various constituents have been determined by different ways. If the usual standards of normal are employed, isolated hypertriglyceridaemia does occur.

The elimination of triglycerides from plasma is enhanced by a lipoprotein lipase which is associated with the clearing factor, inducible by heparin (Review by Robinson, 1963). Upon the injection of heparin, a serum made turbid by the previous alimentary administration of fat becomes translucent. Chemically the level of triglycerides decreases while the levels of monoglycerides, free fatty acids and free glycerol rise. A deficiency of the body to form lipoprotein lipase is presumably the basis of one of the hyperlipidaemias.

Free Fatty Acids

Of the major plasma lipid fractions, free fatty acids are the smallest, but the one turned over most rapidly. In the fasting state, nearly all of this moiety comes from adipose tissue, the liberation from which is influenced by diet, hormones and the sympathetic nerve system. In addition a number of drugs are known to effect lipolysis.

Fatty acids liberated from adipose tissue are either metabolized by the tissues or taken up by the liver, from which they eventually emerge as plasma lipids, mainly triglycerides. Thus increased mobilization of depot fat may lead to hyperlipaemia.

Deviations of the free fatty acid level from normal occurs in diabetes, but markedly so only in frank or latent ketoacidosis. In marked obesity free fatty acids closely correlate with body weight. Other states with increased free fatty acid levels are starvation, pregnancy and acromegaly. All in all, the free fatty acids are of little diagnostic importance, except, in the opinion of some authors, in the evaluation of diabetes. For a review of this subject see Carlson et al. (1965).

Lipoproteins of Plasma

In plasma lipids are associated with proteins. Thus free fatty acids are found in the albumin fraction, while all other major lipids occur together with certain globulins, forming the lipoproteins proper.

Various physical methods have been employed to separate and quantitate the lipoproteins, i.e. low temperature ethanol fractionation, ultracentrifugation and electrophoresis. The results of these methods are not strictly comparable. Usually the results of ultracentrifugation are given in "Svedberg units of flotation" (S_f), since lipoproteins tend to float in solutions of certain density. Very light particles such as chylomicrons have high S_f-values (above 400) while others have values up to this number. Some lipoproteins (high density lipoproteins) sediment.

Electrophoresis separates four types of lipoproteins, namely chylomicrons, β-lipoproteins, pre-β-lipoproteins and α-lipoproteins. None of these classes is homogeneous with respect to the protein moiety, since in immuno-electrophoresis several apoproteins could be demonstrated.

While most authors still classify the hyperlipidaemias according to concentration and behaviour of various lipid fractions, Fredrickson & Lees (1965) have proposed a classification by modified paper electrophoresis of lipoproteins.

Very little is known about the structure of lipoproteins. A recent review is that by Fredrickson et al. (1967). Today it is generally agreed that lipids in lipoproteins are exchanged rapidly with lipids in other lipoproteins or cell membranes, and that covalent bonds do not play a role in lipoprotein structure. It is also accepted that phospholipids provide for the linking of non-polar lipids (e.g. cholesterol, neutral fats) to the protein carrying the lipid, but there is disagreement about the way this link is brought about. For details of this argument a review should be consulted (Zöllner, 1958).

ANALYTICAL METHODS

Minimal lipid analysis of serum consists of judging whether a fasting specimen is clear or turbid and the determination of total cholesterol. Even the slightest turbidity indicates an increased level of neutral fat. For a "complete analysis" triglycerides, total and free cholesterol, lipid phosphorus and free fatty acids might be determined, but such an analysis is rarely necessary. For more specific questions lipoproteins or lipoprotein lipase might be determined and in certain instances further separations by chromatographic procedures are warranted. A compilation of all these methods has recently been published (Zöllner & Eberhagen, 1965).

Neutral fat should be determined as lipid glycerol, either from a lipid extract or as the difference between free glycerol and total glycerol hydrolysable by mild alkali in native serum. In lipid extracts glycerol may be determined either by periodate oxidation (Carlson, 1963) or an enzymic method (Eggstein & Kreutz, 1966), while glycerol in serum can be determined by enzymic means only.

The determination of total lipids by means of the sulphophosphovanillin reaction (Zöllner & Kirsch, 1962) is much easier than weighing a dried lipid extract; it may be performed in very small samples and is sufficient for the detection of more pronounced increases of triglycerides as well as a screening for hyperlipaemia in general.

Various accurate methods for the determination of cholesterol are available; it is very important that they are performed on complete lipid extracts.

The determination of free cholesterol is only necessary if liver diseases are under consideration, where the ratio of free to total cholesterol is increased. Cholesterol esters may easily be separated by thin-layer chromatography. This procedure may be useful in liver disease, nutritional studies and occasionally for the detection of rare lipids. For a review see Zöllner (1964).

The determination of lipid phosphorus should also be done only on lipid extracts. Values should be expressed as lipid phosphorus. It is conventional to use phospholipids after multiplying by a conversion factor of 25, but this introduces some inaccuracy. Phospholipids can also easily be separated and quantitated by thin-layer chromatography, but so far no clinical significance can be attached to this procedure.

Free fatty acids are best titrated according to the method of Trout et al. (1960). It is essential that extraction and separation of the extract are done immediately after obtaining the serum.

Lees & Hatch (1963) have described a method for paper electrophoretic separation of the various lipoproteins. Possibly electrophoresis on agarose gel (Rapp, 1966) is to be preferred. Noble (1968) has recently described an improved technique.

Occasionally the determination of lipoprotein lipase becomes necessary. The method of Fredrickson et al. (1963) is sound and reproducible. We have found that commercial emulsions of fat used for intravenous nutrition may be substituted for the original substrate without appreciably influencing the results.

Gas-liquid chromatography should be employed if the question of abnormal fatty acids arises such as in Refsum's syndrome. For this purpose the fatty acid methyl esters may be prepared from a total lipid extract. Obviously, large enough lipid fractions can also be analysed by this method, but so far no clinical usefulness for this extra work has been demonstrated.

DISEASES INVOLVING ALTERATIONS OF PLASMA LIPID LEVELS

Altered concentrations of lipids in plasma are very common findings in clinical chemistry. However the broad range of the normal is usually not appreciated; thus the standard deviation for serum cholesterol in the same sex and age group is 30–40 mg./100 ml. in all published series. It appears doubtful to us whether values in the statistically normal range are of diagnostic significance, although high normal values may have prognostic significance as far as they seem to be

associated with an increased risk of coronary disease. Table 17.3 shows what we consider to be normal under these considerations.

Abnormal lipid concentrations may be secondary to a number of diseases but may also occur alone. Some of the primary hyperlipidaemias are well established nosological entities, but some are still ill-defined. Therefore in every case diagnosis of primary disease must exclude the secondary involvement of plasma lipids. For this reason the secondary alterations of plasma lipids are discussed first.

Secondary Alterations of Plasma Lipids

The most common cause of secondary hyperlipaemia is diabetes mellitus. In this disease there may be high concentrations of triglycerides, cholesterol, phospholipids and free fatty acids. Xanthoma of the skin can occur. Hypertriglyceridaemia and hypercholesterolaemia usually are found together. If they are marked, they indicate that the primary disease is not well controlled; very high triglyceride levels are only found if the glucose metabolism is severely deranged. On the other hand hypercholesterol-

TABLE 17.3

Normal concentrations of lipids in the plasma

If two figures are given, the method by which the range has been obtained is not stated or there are only a few analyses. If three figures are given, the mean figure gives the mean normal value, the other two figures give the range, determined either by m $\pm$ 2 SD or by the 2·5 and 97·5 percentile.

	mg./100 ml.	mmol./l.	Reference	Comment
Total fatty acids	190–600	6·86–21·63	1	
Neutral fat				Central European type diet
	34– 86–138		2	<30 yr. old
	68–174–280			51–60 yr. old
				Low-fat diet
	44– 68– 92		2	51–60 yr. old
Free fatty acids		0·180–0·560	3	
		–1·060		
Total cholesterol				Central European type diet
	125–213–305		4	men 25–29 yr. old
	148–242–336		4	men 40–59 yr. old
				Low-fat diet
	125–209–293		5	men 40–59 yr. old
Free cholesterol			6	25–30–37% of total cholesterol
Total phosphatides	150–250		6	Parallels cholesterol, cf. Jackson & Wilkinson (1952)
Plasmalogens	2·2–3·0		6	
Cerebrosides	3·5–5·7		7	
Carotenoids	0·025–0·250		8	
Total lipids	400–700		8	

References 1. Thannhauser (1958). 2. Antonis & Bersohn (1960). 3. Stuhlfauth & Zöllner (1959). 4. Lewis *et al.* (1957). 5. Keys *et al.* (1954). 6. Zöllner (1957). 7. Svennerholm & Svennerholm (1956). 8. Zöllner (1959).

aemia and also small increases in neutral fat may be found in aglycosuric patients. Often these patients are overweight. Hyperlipaemia in manifest diabetes should not be confused with primary hyperlipaemias (so called carbohydrate-induced), which often show impaired glucose tolerance tests but no other diabetic manifestations (*vide infra*).

Free fatty acids rise whenever carbohydrate metabolism in diabetes deteriorates and ketoacidosis is imminent. Diabetic subjects tend to have elevated plasma levels of free fatty acids, even if they are in good regulation and examined fasting. Patients in ketosis show marked increases in most cases. A glucose tolerance test or injection of glucagon shows abnormal responses of free fatty acids; the usual sharp fall is delayed and diminished in amplitude (Bierman *et al.*, 1957).

The same findings as in diabetes may be found in von Gierke's disease (glycogenosis type I). Presumably it also is due to the derangement of glucose metabolism.

In hypothyroidism hypercholesterolaemia and hypertriglyceridaemia are common. Hypertriglyceridaemia is rarely pronounced and responds to a low-fat diet, but occasionally it may be the presenting finding. The diagnosis is established by substitution of thyroid hormone. In hypothyroidism secondary to hypopituitarism the same serum lipid alterations are found. It seems possible that hormones other than TSH are involved in their pathogenesis; however in one of our own cases of Sheehan's disease lipids became normal when thyroid hormones were substituted. In the few hypothyroid patients described with skin xanthomata, a creamy serum was observed (Craig *et al.*, 1944; Zöllner, 1955). In hyperthyroidism plasma lipid levels are in the low normal range and this finding is of no diagnostic value.

An increase in all lipids or in cholesterol alone is found in the nephrotic syndrome. Even in this disorder skin xanthomata may occur (Crocker, 1951). Corticosteroid therapy of nephrotic children decreases the neutral fat and cholesterol (Soshea & Farnsworth, 1951; Kramer *et al.*, 1952).

In various pancreatic diseases lipids, particularly triglycerides, may be elevated. This is often true for the pancreatic involvement of the alcoholic. On the other hand abdominal crises of essential hyperlipaemia may closely simulate pancreatitis. Also there are reports in the literature which describe pancreatitis as secondary in familial hyperlipaemia (Klatskin & Gordon, 1952).

Although Keys and his co-workers have shown that there is no correlation between plasma lipids and body weight (Keys, 1954), there remains the fact that obese persons with hyperlipaemia lower their plasma lipid when put on low-calorie diets. Prolonged fasting and starvation are said to lead to high lipid levels. This is certainly so in properly conducted experiments, but in patients deprived of food for a few days hyperlipaemia is not a feature and also in the cachexia of the chronically ill hyperlipaemia is usually not found. A number of other diseases such as haemolytic anaemia and multiple myeloma have been reported to produce increased lipid levels.

In liver disease lipid metabolism is influenced in several ways. Damage of the parenchymal cells usually leads to low lipid concentrations and particularly to low concentrations of cholesterol esters (Thannhauser, 1923), while cholestatic disease produces hypercholesterolaemia and hyperphosphatidaemia. Occasionally lipid levels will be very high, but triglycerides are always normal and the serum is always completely clear unless there is concomitant pancreatic disease such as in the alcoholic.

Xanthomatous biliary cirrhosis (pericholangiolitic biliary cirrhosis with tuberous and plain xanthoma) is a syndrome (Thannhauser, 1950*a*; Thannhauser & Magendantz, 1938; MacMahon & Thannhauser, 1952) characterized by (1) jaundice of several years' duration, (2) hepatosplenomegaly, (3) skin xanthomata over the whole body, (4) a transparent serum, low in neutral fat, (5) extremely high values of total cholesterol with normal percentage of esters, although in the later stages both values decrease, and (6) total phospholipids very high and remaining so throughout the disease. The name "primary biliary cirrhosis" is used to designate the same syndrome (Ahrens *et al.*, 1950). It occurs in females between the ages of 40 and 50. Histologically, changes in the liver consist of a non-specific chronic proliferative inflammatory reaction centred around the terminal bile ducts, i.e. chronic pericholangiolitis without new formation of small bile ducts. Possibly this type of biliary cirrhosis represents the late phase of a hypersensitivity reaction of the cholangioles, since a similar histology is found in cases of jaundice due to hypersensitivity to drugs.

Arsenical hepatitis (Hanger & Gutman, 1940) following arsphenamine intoxication (Stolzer, Miller, White & Zuckerbrod, 1950; Spring, 1950; Roester, 1950) may cause high cholesterol values with skin xanthomata, but the xanthomata disappear if the hepatitis subsides. Males and females may acquire this disease. Presumably other forms of long-continuing, drug-induced cholestatic liver disease may also occasionally lead to xanthoma formation.

Congenital dysplasia of the intralobular bile ducts, resulting in very severe skin xanthomata, was first observed in a 9-year-old boy (MacMahon & Thannhauser, 1952). In contrast to xanthomatous biliary cirrhosis this boy's serum showed high neutral fat as well as high cholesterol and phospholipid levels.

Post-operative biliary obstruction has very occasionally produced skin xanthomata (Eusterman & Montgomery, 1944), which disappear after the reconstruction of the biliary tract. Pigment cirrhosis with haemochromatosis caused skin xanthomata in one case (Cantarow & Bucher, 1938).

In the more common types of liver disease, e.g. viral hepatitis, Laennec's cirrhosis and obstructive jaundice, xanthoma do not occur. In the cellular damage of hepatitis and cirrhosis the levels of all lipids are low, and total cholesterol concentrations below 100 mg./100 ml. are not rare. At the same time the ratio of cholesterol esters to total cholesterol may be reduced. Very often there is a relative reduction of cholesterol linoleate (Zöllner & Wolfram, 1961). In predominantly cholestatic disease, i.e. in obstructive jaundice, but very often also in drug-induced hepatic damage, there is a progressive rise of total cholesterol and phospholipid levels, while neutral fat remains low. If hepatocellular damage supervenes, lipid values may decrease, and the changes described above may become apparent; thus serial determinations of plasma lipids are of prognostic importance. If liver disease is associated with pancreatic disease, the serum may be milky. The combination of this biochemical abnormality with haemolytic anaemia has been described by Zieve (1958).

In Refsum's syndrome a new lipid was found (Zöllner & Wolfram, 1962), which was later shown by Klenk & Kahlke (1963) to be tetramethyl hexadecanoic acid. So far this is the only instance where a plasma lipid that normally occurs only in very minute quantities becomes a major fraction.

Norum & Gjone (1967) described siblings in whom serum cholesterol esters were virtually absent. There was no α-lipoprotein demonstrable. The authors attribute this disorder to a deficiency in lecithin-cholesterol acyl transferase, which they were able to demonstrate.

Primary Hyperlipidaemias

There are at least three, probably five and possibly more diseases in which elevated levels of plasma lipids are the essential feature and the cause of the pathological manifestations. The differentiation of these various disorders at times is difficult. Nevertheless it must always be tried since prognosis and nowadays even the choice of therapy depend on it.

The most important analysis still is total cholesterol. Wherever possible neutral fat should also be determined. If this is not feasible it should be estimated from analyses of total lipids and cholesterol by the formula given by Zöllner & Kirsch (1962), or at least increased concentrations should be checked for by looking for slight turbidity. Electrophoretic separation of lipoproteins seems to be useful. One of the hyperlipaemias certainly is an inborn error of metabolism, since it can be shown to run in families, and such a familial association should indeed be demonstrated as a diagnostic procedure. The classification of the others may depend on the results of therapy.

While we still prefer to classify the hyperlipidaemias by the results of lipid analyses, Fredrickson & Lees (1965) prefer a classification according to the lipoproteins present in increased amounts, and indeed speak of hyperlipoproteinaemias. Doubtless this classification helps to separate idiopathic hyperlipaemia and familial hypercholesterolaemia. However the "mixed forms" are difficult to classify by lipoprotein electrophoresis, and no more reliance should be put on this method than on any selection among the others. As far as has been investigated, subfractionation of the major plasma lipids does not reveal pathological compositions. Therefore such further analyses are of no diagnostic value at the moment.

Idiopathic Familial Hypercholesterolaemia (Hyperlipoproteinaemia Type II)

A fully developed case of idiopathic familial hypercholesterolaemia is characterized by (1) xanthelasma of the eyelids, (2) xanthoma *tuberosum et planum*, (3) tendon xanthoma, (4) xanthoma of blood vessels and endocardium, and (5) familial hypercholesterolaemia. Thannhauser & Magendantz (1938), as well as Müller (1939), demonstrated clinically that these features belong to one clinical syndrome, and may occur singly or in various combinations.

The orange-yellow skin xanthomata are located mainly on the eyelids, the extensor surface of the elbows and knees, and the buttocks. They are often accompanied by fleshy colourless xanthomata in the subcutaneous tissue of the fingers or buttocks. Yellow xanthomatous infiltration of the creases of the palms and fingers occurs only in patients with subcutaneous fleshy xanthomata. The tendon xanthomata are part of the tendons, from which they cannot be mechanically separated. They are localized in the tendons of the fingers, usually above the knuckles, as well as in the Achilles tendon and in other tendons below the knee joint. Brain, meninges, bone, liver, spleen and lymph nodes are never involved, lipoid arcus of the cornea is not an important sign, since in juvenile cases it may be lacking and in adults it occurs at normal plasma cholesterol levels. The inheritance of idiopathic familial hypercholesterolaemia is by an autosomal dominant gene (Hirschhorn & Wilkinson, 1959).

Histological examination of the skin xanthomata reveals foam cells accumulated beneath the layers of the cutis surrounded by fibrous tissue.

The xanthomata of the arterial intima and endocardium are very important because of their frequent occurrence in the coronary vessels, where they may cause angina and coronary occlusion. We have observed a family in which all three children died before the age of 28. The arterial lesions are slightly elevated, and consist of an accumulation of foam cells in the intima beneath the endothelium causing cushion-like elevations. In later phases fibrous tissue and consecutive sclerosis of the vessels develop. Because the arterial xanthoma in idiopathic familial hypercholesterolaemia histologically resembles the arterial lesion produced in herbivorous animals by cholesterol feeding, an identical pathogenesis was assumed for the atheroma formation in idiopathic familial hypercholesterolaemia and the atheromatous lesion in arteriosclerosis (Constantinides et al., 1961). Cholesterol accumulation in the serum would thus be in both instances the primary cause of the changes in the vessel wall. Familial hypercholesterolaemia is a metabolic disorder and cholesterol is indeed the *materia peccans* which infiltrates the intima and incites the tissue to form xanthomata. This disease process occurring in the young should not be confused with the arteriosclerosis (atherosclerosis) of the higher age group, where the primary disorder concerns the elastic structures and ground substance of the vascular wall into which cholesterol infiltrates secondarily and precipitates. It should, however, be emphasized that the two processes (the first due to a disturbance of cholesterol metabolism in idiopathic familial hypercholesterolaemia, and the other arising from primary damage of the arterial wall and secondary cholesterol precipitation) cannot be distinguished histologically in their later stages.

Familial hypercholesterolaemia may occur without skin xanthomata or clinically recognizable cardiac disease, but still may cause atheroma formation in the coronary vessels of young people belonging to families with idiopathic familial hypercholesterolaemia.

Lipid partition (Table 17.4) of the serum in idiopathic familial hypercholesterolaemia shows that the total cholesterol increases 2–4 times over the

TABLE 17.4

Lipid analysis of serum in cases of "idiopathic hyperlipaemia" in an adult, of idiopathic familial hypercholesterolaemia (A) and of idiopathic familial hypercholesterolaemia with secondary hyperlipaemia (B)
(all values as mg./100 ml.)

	12.2.26	After low-fat diet 29.3.46	Idiopathic hyperlipaemia	19.9.46	19.5.47	(A)	(B)
Total fatty acids	5196	480	The eruptive	1171	3100	—	—
Neutral fat	4477	275	xanthomata	—	2525	110	750
Total cholesterol	693	175	gradually	242	375	472	452
Free cholesterol	323	58	disappeared	85	150	133	140
Cholesterol present as esters	396	117	leaving a brownish-red	185	225	339	312
Ditto, % of total	53	67	skin dis-	—	60	72	69
Total phospholipids	810	195	coloration.	—	351	358	341
Lecithin and cephalin	685	175	Then the patient	—	—	—	—
Blood sugar	206	130	gradually	120	—	—	—
Urine sugar	0·2 g.	Negative	stopped keeping to his diet.	Negative	Negative	—	—

Results in the case of idiopathic hyperlipaemia are from Thannhauser (1950*b*), the other results from Zöllner's laboratory.

normal values. The cholesterol esters are in the normal proportion, 70 to 75 % of the total cholesterol (Thannhauser, 1958). The partition of the cholesterol esters is normal (Zöllner, Wolfram & Amin, 1962). Lipid P rises parallel to the cholesterol in the fashion described by Jackson & Wilkinson (1952). From data in Thannhausers's monograph (Thannhauser, 1958) as well as from unpublished experiments of our own it appears that there is predominantly a rise of glycerophosphatides, while sphingomyelin does not increase. An increase of neutral fat is not a feature of the disease and indeed, if present strongly argues against the diagnosis. In paper electrophoresis there is a sharp band of β-lipoprotein (hyperbetalipoproteinaemia).

Therapeutically a diet low in cholesterol is without effect. On the other hand, lowering of fat intake leads to some reduction of plasma cholesterol if the patient adheres to a very strict regimen. If the usual dietary fats are replaced by oils rich in polyunsaturated fatty acids there is also a lowering of cholesterol levels. In patients with high normal cholesterol levels, such a diet leads to low normal or average cholesterol levels (Kinsell et al., 1953; Bronte-Stewart et al., 1956; Ahrens et al., 1959), but in idiopathic hypercholesterolaemia normal cholesterol values cannot be attained. Usually, additional drug therapy is necessary. In our opinion, nicotinic acid (Berge et al., 1961) or its alcohol derivative β-pyridyl carbinol (Zöllner & Gudenzi, 1966) are the drugs of choice. In view of the serious prognosis of idiopathic familial hypercholesterolaemia, the possible, but apparently reversible side-effects of the drugs (cholestatic hepatic disease, diabetes) must be accepted and watched for.

Idiopathic Hyperlipaemia
(Hyperlipoproteinaemia Type I)

Idiopathic hyperlipaemia is a very rare disorder which in childhood is accompanied by hepatosplenomegaly and eruptive xanthomata, while in the adult it may be accompanied by slight glycosuria and hepatosplenomegaly. The accumulation of neutral fat (hyperlipaemia) in the serum (milky serum) is the outstanding change; cholesterol and phospholipids are much less increased (Table 17.4). While the patient is on a normal diet there is massive hyperchylomicronaemia, if a low-fat high-carbohydrate diet is instituted pre-β-lipoproteins may occur. Chylomicrons leave the plasma at a very low speed and there are uniquely low post-heparin lipoprotein lipase activities in the plasma of patients with this disorder (Fredrickson et al., 1963).

This anomaly was first described as "hepatosplenomegalic lipoidosis" by Bürger & Grütz (1932) and by Holt et al. (1936). Familial occurrence has been described by Holt (Holt et al., 1936, 1939), but often no second case can be found in the patient's family.

Freshly erupted transient papulo-nodular yellowish pink xanthomata, unlike the tuberose xanthomata of idiopathic familial hypercholesterolaemia, show on biopsy only a few scattered foam cells. In contrast to the neutral fat accumulation in the serum, the enlarged liver and spleen, in the only autopsied case, contained no neutral fat, but only a few scattered foam cells (Chapman & Kinney, 1941). On the other hand the bone marrow contained foam cells in most cases studied.

This syndrome shows three clinical features (Thannhauser, 1950a): (1) The serum is creamy because of enormously increased fat, which, however, causes no physical discomfort. At high neutral fat levels (higher than 2000 mg./100 ml.) this creaminess may be seen in the ocular fundus; this is called lipaemia retinalis. (2) The eruptive xanthoma appear and disappear with the rise and fall of the level of the neutral fat. (3) The liver and spleen may be enlarged, but they change in size with the fat content of the serum. Jaundice is not present. Attacks of abdominal colic, which may dramatically simulate an acute surgical abdomen, occasionally occur.

In the adult hyperlipaemia may be discovered accidentally by a routine blood examination, since eruptive xanthomata are not always present. Adults, however, suffer less from hepatosplenomegaly and abdominal colic, but tend to show a slight elevation of blood sugar or slight glycosuria. This tendency probably explains why most cases of idiopathic hyperlipaemia have been erroneously classified as "xanthoma diabeticorum" in the older literature. It is now clear (Thannhauser, 1950) that the hyperlipaemia and secondary xanthoma due to diabetes disappear promptly upon insulin treatment, while idiopathic hyperlipaemia does not react to insulin but only to a low-fat diet.

Investigators disagree on whether idiopathic hyperlipaemia causes atheromatous lesions. Thannhauser's (1950) adult cases did not show early angina or myocardial infarction, although other authors differ (Joyner, 1953; Malmros et al., 1954; Schettler et al., 1958). Such discrepancies may arise where cases of mixed type hyperlipidaemias are reported as "idiopathic hyperlipaemia".

A diet containing only 20–30 g. fat/day is effective in returning the neutral fat to near normal values, and all other serum lipids to normal values. These values, however, become high again upon deviation from this low-fat diet. Medium chain-length triglycerides may help the patient to overcome some of the difficulties of a very low fat diet.

Mixed Hyperlipidaemias
(Hyperlipoproteinaemias Types III, IV and V)

These disorders, which account for most of the cases of primary hyperlipidaemias, are characterized by a special lipoprotein (pre-β-lipoprotein) that can be demonstrated by a special technique of paper electrophoresis. On chemical analysis they show increased levels of neutral fat and usually of cholesterol. The elevation of triglycerides can vary considerably but rarely exceeds the concentration of cholesterol by more than a factor of 5 (while in essential hyperlipaemia this factor commonly is around 10). Fredrickson & Lees (1966) state that in all cases hyperlipaemia is carbohydrate-induced, and this correlates somewhat with the well known fact that many cases of hyperlipaemia do not respond to fat restriction (which if done in an isocaloric diet necessarily means an increased administration of carbohydrates). However other authors (Kinsell *et al.*, 1967) state that pure carbohydrate-induced hypertriglyceridaemia is relatively rare. In our opinion it is not certain whether the classification proposed by Fredrickson & Lees is justified. It may be that the mixed hyperlipidaemias are one disease with very different manifestations, or it may be just as well a mixture of even more than three disorders. The biochemical differentiation is mainly based on electrophoretic analysis of the lipoproteins. However, results from this method cannot be used for differential diagnosis because different electrophoretic patterns occur in one family with hyperlipidaemia, selected patients may change from one pattern to another and certain defined diseases such as diabetes, hypothyroidism and nephrosis may each be associated with several lipoprotein patterns, according to data published by Fredrickson & Lees (1966). In our opinion it is therefore much more likely that the primary disorder is one of lipid metabolism inducing changes in the carrier proteins.

Table 17.5 summarizes some of the diagnostic criteria of the mixed hyperlipidaemias. In the last edition of this book we have called these disorders idiopathic familial hypercholesterolemia with secondary hyperlipaemia, and indeed Fredrickson & Lees also found patients without increase in neutral fat in these families.

The clinical consequences of the disorder resemble a combination of the two diseases described above. Xanthoma of all types, hepatosplenomegaly and abdominal crises may occur, but the most common consequences are early manifestations of arteriosclerosis, especially myocardial infarction and peripheral vascular disease. In a high percentage of cases glucose tolerance is impaired but glycosuria is rare. It remains to be seen whether there is a genetic connection with diabetes mellitus or whether these are different diseases.

LIPOPROTEIN DEFICIENCY DISEASES

Lack of certain lipoproteins produces disturbances in lipid transport. Although the diseases are very rare, their study has greatly enhanced our knowledge.

TABLE 17.5

Differential diagnosis of "mixed hyperlipidaemias"

Criterion	Type III	Type IV	Type V
Paper electrophoresis (increased fractions)	Pre β- and β-lipoproteins	Pre-β-lipoproteins only	Pre-β-lipoproteins and chylomicrons
Turbidity	(+)–++	(+)–++	++
Triglycerides (typical ranges)	200–1500	300–8000	normal–3500
Total cholesterol (typical ranges)	350–800	200–1200	generally normal or slightly elevated
Xanthoma	as in familial hypercholesterolaemia		as in essential hyperlipaemia
Seen also in	hypothyroidism nephrosis	nephrosis	nephrosis

Familial High-density Lipoprotein Deficiency
(Tangier Disease)

In Tangier disease (Fredrickson *et al.*, 1961) there is an almost complete absence of plasma high-density lipoprotein. Concomitantly the plasma levels of total cholesterol and of phospholipids are reduced below 100 mg./100 ml. Triglycerides may be normal, but when the patients are given high-carbohydrate diets, intense hypertriglyceridaemia supervenes (Fredrickson, 1966). There is lipid storage, mainly of cholesterol esters, in recitulo-endothelial tissues, leading to enlargement of tonsils and lymph nodes as well as to hepatosplenomegaly. Infiltration of the cornea does occur. In the heterozygote there are low levels of plasma high-density lipoprotein but no lipid depots in the tissues.

Abetalipoproteinaemia
(Bassen-Kornzweig Disease)

In this disease no lipoproteins of a density below 1·063 can be found in plasma; plasma total cholesterol and phospholipid levels are low, and triglycerides are virtually absent (levels below 20 mg. per 100 ml.). If fat is administered orally, the epithelial cells of the villi of the upper intestines become engorged with fat and there will be steatorrhoea, particularly in children (Salt *et al.*, 1960). Malabsorption is the rule. Acanthocytosis may be the first finding noted (Bassen & Kornzweig, 1950). Retinitis pigmentosa and a progressive degeneration of cerebellum and posterolateral columns are further features. Autopsy of a proven case (Sobrevilla *et al.*, 1964) showed extensive demyelination of posterior columns and spinocerebellar tracts, as well as focal demyelination in peripheral nerves. Erythrocyte lipids are low in linoleic and arachidonic acid. For a review see Farquhar & Ways (1966).

LIPIDOSES WITH ABNORMAL FATTY ACID COMPOSITION

Heredopathia Atactica Polyneuritiformis
(Refsum's Disease)

This disease was at first described by Refsum (1946) as a separate entity. The stored lipid, phytanic acid (3,7,11,15-tetramethylhexadecanoic acid), was identified by Klenk & Kahlke (1963). This branched-chain fatty acid was found in different but considerable amounts in total tissue lipids. In serum it may increase up to 20% of the total fatty acids.

The early symptoms are signs of chronic polyneuropathy with distal muscular atrophy and progressive pareses of the distal parts of the extremities (Richterich *et al.* 1965*a*, 1965*b*). Sensory disturbances include paraesthesiae and occasionally severe pain, especially in the knees. Cerebellar involvement causes ataxia and nystagmus. The deep tendon reflexes are weak or absent. Nearly always present are atrophy of muscles, atypical pigmentary retinitis, night blindness and concentric narrowing of the visual fields. There is often impairment of hearing or deafness and anosmia. The cerebrospinal fluid protein is always considerably increased while the cell count is normal. Cardiac involvement may lead to electrocardiographic abnormalities, tachycardias and arrhythmias. Skeletal malformations occasionally occur, which are usually symmetrical, and skin changes resembling ichthyosis. The mental development is normal.

The disease may become manifest at any time from childhood to adult life; a sexual prevalence could not be noted. In some affected families there was consanguinity of the parents. An autosomal recessive mode of transmission is discussed. The demonstration of phytanic acid in plasma or organ lipids is pathognomonic for the disease. For treatment it appears useful to restrict the intake of dietary phytol, the precursor of the phytanic acid (see also Chapter 13).

NORMOCHOLESTEROLAEMIC XANTHOMATOSES

Schüller-Christian's Syndrome. Eosinophilic Xanthomatous Granuloma

In the early literature it had not been established that the histological features in different phases of the disease are very different indeed, and that Schüller-Christian's disease may occur in various forms, namely, as a monosymptomatic form involving a single tissue (skin or bone), in various combinations involving simultaneously several organs, or as a generalized form in infants affecting skin, osseous system, meninges, lungs, pleura, lymph nodes, liver, endocrine organs and in rare cases the brain (Thannhauser, 1940, 1950).

According to Holm *et al.* (1944) one should differentiate histologically four phases: (1) a proliferative phase consisting of an accumulation of reticulum cells and histocytes in the tissue; (2) a granulomatous phase showing numerous eosinophilic cells, leucocytes and giant cells (incipient lipid accumulation in some reticulum cells may already be present); (3) a xanthomatous phase in which intracellular lipid material is definitely evident in the cytoplasm of reticulum cells. The cytoplasm becomes foamy and develops the characteristics of xanthoma cells; (4) a fibrous phase in which the xanthoma cells and endothelial cells are replaced by fibroblasts and connective tissue. These phases are not strictly demarcated, and their histological features may greatly overlap during the disease.

In Schüller-Christian's disease the foam cell develops independently of the normal cholesterol content of the serum. A normal plasma level of cholesterol, phospholipids and neutral fat characterizes this disease. Farber (1941, 1944) assumes that the cholesterol in the foam cells is derived from detritus of focal necrosis in the granulomatous tissue. In eosinophilic xanthomatous granuloma, however, large necrotic areas are rarely, if ever, found, whereas in other granulomas, such as Hodgkin's disease, mycosis fungoides or infectious granulomas, large areas of necrosis are evident, but without foam-cell formation. Chemical analysis of tissue in the xanthomatous phase of Schüller-Christian's disease shows an increase of 10–20 times over that of normal tissue (see Table 17.6). Such an enormous increase cannot be

on the eyelids. The lesions, varying from pinhead to walnut size, are raised, discrete or clustered in ridges or furrows. A rare variety may occur as variola-like papules, also named isolated reticulosis of the skin. The papules may disappear completely or degenerate into permanent xanthomata.

Flat, petechial, reddish-purple disseminated lesions of pinhead size may occur together with fully developed xanthomata (Thannhauser, 1950). Histologically the initial lesion shows some haemorrhagic exudation in a conglomerate of adventitial cells derived from the outer wall of a small artery (Fraser, 1935).

Juvenile xanthoma, a discrete, wart-like papular lesion, is reddish brown or deep orange. This type, belonging clinically to the disseminated group, was erroneously called naevo-xantho-endothelioma.

Osseous lesions appear upon X-ray examination as osteolytic areas. The isolated lesion was described as a separate disease entity, eosinophilic

TABLE 17.6

Lipid partition in specimens of tissue during the xanthomatous phase of eosinophilic xanthomatous granuloma

(values given as percentages of dry weight)

Tissue	Total cholesterol	Free cholesterol	Cholesterol esters	Total phospholipid
Diseased lymph node	17·90	2·20	15·70	6·4
Normal lymph node	0·60–2·30	0·50–1·10	0·20–1·20	5·5–11·0
Dura mater	18·58	3·20	15·30	—
Skin	4·55	3·66	0·89	—
Normal skin	0·15–0·30	—	—	—
Diseased liver	7·25	4·55	2·70	7·4
Normal liver	1·10–2·60	1·50–2·10	0·45–0·55	9·0–11·0

Reprinted from *Xanthomatoses*; Thannhauser (1950*b*).

attributed to cholesterol infiltration from small areas of focal necrosis.

Thannhauser (1950) therefore concluded that the cholesterol originates intrinsically in those cells of the granuloma where it is found. These cells of reticular and histocytic origin maintain the functional possibilities of undifferentiated embryonal reticulum cells (embryonal fat cells of Waldeyer (1871)) to form various kinds of lipids, including cholesterol.

Xanthomata disseminata (Thannhauser, 1950) of the skin are lemon or chamois-coloured, or in later phases maroon. They appear over the whole body, especially around the neck, axillae, trunk and in the antecubital fossae. Xanthelasmas form

granuloma of the bone, but now Lichtenstein (1953) considers it as the monosymptomatic form of Schüller-Christian's disease.

Lesions of lung and pleura show an X-ray pattern similar to that of miliary tuberculosis or diffuse fibrosis.

The granulomatous masses involving the meninges cause raised intracranial pressure and exophthalmos. Diabetes insipidus resulting from pituitary gland involvement is not present in all cases. Involvement of the brain substance is very rare.

Hepatosplenomegaly with lymphadenopathy occurs in children, especially in the generalized form (Letterer-Siwe disease) in infancy. In cases of liver involvement, neither jaundice nor ascites is observed. These cases can be diagnosed only by biopsy. The early histology may show only reticulo-histocytic proliferation. The accumulation of lipids in some cases becomes visible if the child lives long enough. Recently, rare cases of Schüller-Christian's disease have been described complicated by a leukaemic blood picture (Freud et al., 1954; Gray & Taylor, 1953) and bone-marrow reaction.

Differential diagnosis from other fully developed granulomas is not difficult because no other systemic granuloma has a xanthomatous phase. The reticular histocytic proliferative phase, however, is not always easily differentiated from other systemic reticuloses. Repeated biopsies may be needed in all these instances, and the specimens should be analysed chemically.

Xanthoma (Foam) Cells in Inflammatory and in True Tumours

Foam cells may originate in inflammatory, fibromatous, sarcomatous or carcinomatous tissue. Corresponding to the number of reticular cells undergoing xanthomatous transformation, the tumour becomes more yellowish, appearing as a xanthomatous tumour.

Foam cells are observed in the wall of a chronically inflamed gall bladder (so-called strawberry gall bladder), in chronic salpingitis, chronic osteomyelitis or in fibrous dysplasia, in necrotic areas of nodules of rheumatoid arthritis, and in chronic pneumonitis (so-called cholesterol pneumonitis), in inflammatory xanthoma of the breast, and in the intestinal lipodystrophy of Whipple (xanthomatous transformation of the mesentery).

In xantholipoma, xanthomatous polycystic lymphangioma and epithelial tumours with xanthoma cell formation, the level of the serum cholesterol is normal.

THE SPHINGOLIPIDOSES

Classification

The term sphingolipidoses is chosen to indicate that, in all the diseases classified under this heading, there is an accumulation of substances containing sphingosine as a part of their molecule. All known sphingolipids consist of a fatty acid amide of sphingosine, called ceramide, and a more characteristic group, bound to C-1 of the sphingosine, by an ester or glycosidic bond. Each of the known sphingolipids may be accumulated in a single disease (Table 17.7).

TABLE 17.7

The sphingolipidoses and their corresponding lipids

Disease	Lipid accumulated	Group linked to the ceramide
Gaucher's	Cerebroside	Glucose
Niemann-Pick's	Sphingomyelin	Phosphoryl-choline
Tay Sachs'	Ganglioside	
Pfaundler-Hurler's	Ganglioside and Mucopoly-saccharide	Oligosaccharides consisting of hexoses, N-acetyl-hexosamine and neura-minic acid
Metachromatic Leucodystrophy	Sulphatide	Galactose-3-sulphate
Fabry's	Ceramide polyhexosides	digalactoside, galactosyllacto-side

Typical of the sphingolipidoses is the involvement of the brain in cases occurring in infancy. This presumably is due to the fact that at that age the brain is still developing, and therefore the metabolism of its constituents, including sphingolipids, is intensive. A recent text on the special aspects of cerebral lipidoses has been edited by van Bogaert, Cumings & Lowenthal (1957). In many cases the reticulo-endothelial system is also involved. In the old literature some of the sphingolipidoses are considered to be diseases of the central nervous and/or the reticulo-endothelial system, but more recent evidence indicates that like all other inborn disorders of metabolism they are generalized diseases. Such evidence is the finding of abnormal lymphocytes in Tay-Sachs' disease (von Bagh & Hortling, 1948), and the demonstration of increased amounts of sulphatides in the kidney of cases of metachromatic leucodystrophy (Austin, 1959).

Gaucher's Disease (GD) (Cerebrosidosis)

Marchand (1907) attributed the enlarged pale cells to a foreign substance, later identified by Epstein (1924) and Lieb (1924, 1929) as kerasin, a cerebroside. Aghion (1934), as well as Halliday, Douel, Tragerman & Ward (1940), found the cerebrosides in Gaucher cells to be glucocerebrosides, a fact confirmed by others (Carter et al., 1961; Suomi & Agranoff, 1965). Thannhauser (1953) described the accumulation of gangliosides and cerebrosides in GD, and Philippart & Menkes (1964) showed that the splenic glycolipids in GD

TABLE 17.8

Analysis of spleen and serum of an 8-year-old boy with Gaucher's disease

	Spleen	Normal spleen
	(Values given as % of dry weight)	
Total cholesterol	2·7	0·6– 2·3
Free cholesterol	0·5	0·5– 1·1
Ester cholesterol	2·2	0·2– 1·2
Total phospholipids	9·4	5·5–11·0
Sphingomyelin	0·6	0·7– 1·0
Cephalin	1·5	1·6– 4·0
Lecithin	7·3	3·1– 4·0
Lipid fatty acids	6·1	7·0– 9·0
Cerebrosides	6·7	0·1– 0·6

	Serum (mg./100 ml.)	Normal serum (fasting) (mg./100 ml.)
Total cholesterol	145	130–260
Free cholesterol	40	30– 70
Ester cholesterol	105	100–190
Total phospholipids	92	100–250

contain ganglioside (Table 17.8). Recently Svennerholm (1966) reported the occurrence of increased gangliosides in addition to ceramide lactosides and glucocerebrosides in cases of infantile GD.

The large pale Gaucher cell is round, oval or polygonal. Sometimes 10–12 nuclei occur in a very large cell, 70–80 μ in diameter. The Gaucher cell does not stain with Sudan III, scarlet R or Smith-Dietrich. Mallory's stain colours Gaucher cells strongly blue (Morrison & Hack, 1947). Electron microscope studies by Fisher & Reidbord (1962) resulted in the demonstration of mitochondria located within round, oval or irregularly shaped cytoplasmic bodies which probably develop as a result of the metamorphosis to G cells. Histochemical properties suggest that they contain the cerebroside-protein complex. A further significant histochemical finding is the high activity of an acid phosphatase (Crocker & Landing, 1960; Fisher & Reidbord, 1962), which can be demonstrated in 80% of the Gaucher cells (Czitober et al., 1964). Gaucher cells arise from the reticulum and adventitial and periadventitial cells of small arterioles. Gött & Rexa (1964) with the use of a method described by Klima et al. (1956) could demonstrate numerous Gaucher cells in the circulating blood of an affected adult. According to Gerken & Wiedemann (1964) affected siblings, as well as clinically healthy ones and parents, had typical Gaucher cells in the circulating blood.

It is agreed that GD is hereditary, occurring not only in sibs but also in members of different generations of one family.

In the serum of patients with GD, as in normal serum, only small concentrations of cerebrosides are present (Thannhauser, Benotti & Reinstein, 1939). Svennerholm & Svennerholm (1963) found elevated plasma cerebroside levels however. Further data are needed.

Observations of Hillborg & Estborn (1964), who described the development of skeletal changes in relation to splenectomy, support the theory that the absence of the main storage organ may result in compensatory increase of storage by other tissues to effect the removal of excess cerebrosides.

Studies of Brady et al. (1965) with a 1-^{14}C-labelled glucocerebroside support the theory of lack of a glucocerebroside-cleaving enzyme. Purified splenic extracts from Gaucher patients and from subjects with congenital haemolytic anaemia and idiopathic thrombocytopenic purpura were compared as regards the activity of the glucocerebroside-cleaving enzyme. Enzyme activity from Gaucher spleens was only one-fifth to one-tenth that of other splenic extracts. The findings of Patrick are in agreement (1965). Thus the accumulation of a glucocerebroside may be due to an incomplete breakdown of a ganglioside.

An interesting finding was the elevation of serum levels of an acid phosphatase (Tuchman et al., 1956). This enzyme could be differentiated from that increased in other diseases of the bones by the use of differential inhibition and activation (Gründig et al., 1965); for example it is not inhibited by L-tartrate like prostatic phosphatase (Tuchman et al., 1959). Hillborg & Estborn (1964) found decreased activity of the acid phosphatase in red cells of patients with GD. These authors as well as Crocker & Landing (1960) considered the acid phosphatase to originate from the Gaucher cell. Crocker & Landing (1960) observed a decrease of acid phosphatase in serum of patients after splenectomy; the later increase was considered as a sign of the new accumulation of Gaucher cells in other organs. Thus the elevated acid phosphatase in serum may be a secondary effect. In healthy relatives of Gaucher patients no elevation of acid phosphatase was found (Hillborg & Estborn, 1964).

In adults the spleen, lymph nodes, liver and bones are most frequently involved. Other organs, and especially the nervous system, are not implicated. The patients usually do not appear ill.

The spleen may be moderately enlarged or enormous. Splenic puncture reveals the characteristic Gaucher cell. Symptoms of chronic liver disease with decreased liver function are rare. Lymphadenopathy is not outstanding. The osseous system is involved in most cases, due to the infiltration of bone marrow with Gaucher cells.

Thrombocytopenia, and in later stages pancytopenia, may occur if the bone marrow is replaced by numerous Gaucher cells. Myeloid metaplasia has been observed in such cases. Haemorrhages and bruises are later manifestations. The Gaucher cells are recognized in the unstained bone marrow smear by their size and the structure of their protoplasma which is especially well recognized by phase microscopy of supravital preparations. The diagnosis of GD must be made by bone marrow aspiration, or by chemical analysis of a biopsied specimen of an organ (lymph node).

Oberling & Woringer (1927) first distinguished GD in early infancy from GD in children and adults. Severe brain disease is outstanding in infantile GD, despite the fact that Gaucher cells are not found in the brain substance. Muscle rigidity is the main feature, and the infant develops trismus and dysphagia. Later the infant neither sees nor hears. Maloney & Cumings (1960) reported increases in brain kerasin in juvenile patients. The white matter shows a decrease in all lipid classes which is correlated with the severity of the clinical symptoms (Banker et al., 1962).

Niemann-Pick's Disease (NP)
(Sphingomyelinosis)

Klenk (1934) first demonstrated that the increase in the phospholipids in the organs of an infant with this disease was principally due to an accumulation of sphingomyelin.

The NP cell is a large, round cell varying from 20 to 50 μ. After treatment with ordinary fixing reagents, which dissolve fat, the NP cell appears foamy, not unlike the foam cell of a xanthomatous disorder. The characteristic stain for NP cells is the Smith-Dietrich stain showing a deep blue-black colour. NP cell cannot be recovered from circulating blood and the vascular endothelium is not a precursor for these cells (Bloom, 1928).

The sphingomyelin level in the serum is not elevated. NP disease therefore cannot be diagnosed by analysing the serum. Some cases show hyperlipaemia, considered as due to undernutrition. In several patients described by Crocker & Farber (1958) however the degree of hyperlipidaemia paralleled the increase of lipids in tissue. Sweeley (1963) analysed plasma sphingomyelin fatty acids in NP disease and found fatty acids with chain lengths varying from C_{12} to C_{24}; palmitic acid was the main component.

The outstanding accumulation of sphingomyelin in visceral organs must be proved by biopsy of lymph glands or liver. The analyses in Table 17.9 show that in NP disease sphingomyelin accumulates in several organs. Crocker & Farber (1958) found for the grey matter an increased cholesterol content with the sphingomyelin being always at or above the upper limit of normal. According to Cumings (1962) the cortex, if analysed alone, shows a well-marked increase in sphingomyelin and cholesterol. This corroborates the findings of Klenk (1955) that in NP disease the brain contains increased amounts of sphingomyelin and gangliosides. Recent analytical results from Ställberg-Stenhagen & Svennerholm (1965) and Rouser et al. (1965) showed increased proportions of stearic acid, while that of the longer chain fatty acids is decreased. Pilz & Jatzkewitz (1964) found stearyl sphingomyelin increased threefold and lignoceryl and nervonyl sphingomyelin increased 1·5–2 fold.

TABLE 17.9

Sphingomyelin content of organs in Niemann-Pick disease
(all values given as % of dry weight)

The values for brain have been obtained from a sample containing medulla and cortex

	Niemann-Pick spleen	Normal spleen	Niemann-Pick kidney	Normal kidney	Niemann-Pick liver	Normal liver	Niemann-Pick brain	Normal brain
Total cholesterol	6·73	1·8– 2·4	2·82	1·4– 2·8	7·0	2·0– 2·6	6·45	7·3–15·0
Free cholesterol	6·70	1·0– 1·1	2·81	1·0– 1·1	4·5	0·4– 0·5	5·43	1·3– 4·6
Ester cholesterol	0·03	0·7– 1·3	0·01	0·5– 1·7	2·5	1·5– 2·2	1·02	6·1–10·3
Total phospholipids	42·5	5·5–11·0	—	7·0–10·0	37·1	9·0–11·0	61·0	25–35
Sphingomyelin	32·7	0·7– 1·0	—	0·6– 0·8	25·9	0·3– 0·5	4·84	4·5– 7·0

These analyses show that component fatty acids of sphingomyelin in normal viscera and in viscera of NP disease may differ quantitatively.

Every theory of NP disease centres around the accumulation of sphingomyelin. Almost certainly the metabolic error in NP disease consists of an enzymic abnormality. Crocker & Farber (1958) found a normal activity of a phospholipase (in tissues of NP disease), which catalyzes the hydrolytic cleavage of lecithin and sphingomyelin. Brady et al. (1966) found an enzyme in normal human liver which catalyzes the hydrolysis of sphingomyelin. Comparison of enzyme activities in liver and kidney samples of control subjects and of 6 patients with NP disease showed large differences in the hydrolysis of ^{14}C-sphingomyelin (Fredrickson, 1966), while inhibition of the enzyme by the accumulated sphingomyelin of NP tissue could be excluded, lecithin appeared competitively to inhibit the enzyme without being hydrolysed.

Holtz et al. (1964) studied fibroblasts of NP patients in tissue culture and found that their sphingomyelin contained 18% and control cultures 7% of the total lipid phosphorus. In amnion cell cultures of two children whose siblings had NP disease one infant had 7·9% and the other 13% of the lipid phosphorus in sphingomyelin, while in normal cultures 7·4% of the lipid phosphorus was in sphingomyelin. The former child was normal, the latter developed NP disease.

The infants, born with normal weight, develop normally in the first week. However a number of malformations have been reported in affected children (Pick, 1927, 1933; van Bogaert, 1934). Videbaek (1952) found microgyria, polydactyly and cleft formations; bluish-black moles were described by Schiff (1926) in the lumbosacral region and by Thannhauser (1958) in the oral mucosa. The children gradually stop eating. Their abdomens are distended by the enlarged liver and spleen. The lymph nodes enlarge. At the height of the disease the infant is apathetic. In the retina a cherry-red spot with a greyish-green halo, which occupies the place of the macula, is often found. As the eyesight diminishes and inner ear deafness develops, the infant eventually cannot react to voices or sound. Later the motor and psychic functions are lost. The infant becomes completely debilitated, until it dies from cachexia at the age of 20–25 months.

NP disease can be diagnosed early only through bone marrow puncture. Crocker & Farber (1958) found vacuolation of agranulocytes in all their patients. Neither total white cell phospholipids nor the proportion of sphingomyelin was found to be elevated. The search for these cells in parents and siblings of affected children has been unsuccessful.

Several variants of the classical infantile form of the disorder have been described (Crocker & Farber, 1958; Pfändler, 1946) which probably represent genetically distinct subgroups but heterogeny cannot be considered proved to date. Adult cases have been discovered only lately. In a histological and chemical study of two brothers, 29 and 33 years old, Dusendschon & Farverger (1945) and Pfändler (1946) found large accumulations of sphingomyelin in the enlarged liver and spleen. The clinical features differed from those of infantile NP disease. In another adult case the diagnosis was made by biopsy (Sperry, 1953; Terry, Sperry & Brodoff, 1954), and the clinical features included hepatosplenomegaly and fibrosis due to NP cells of the lung. A fourth adult case showed splenomegaly with NP cells and foamy blood (Blum, Thannhauser & Thannhauser, unpublished). Analysis of the extirpated spleen in the last case revealed a sphingomyelin content of 8·6 g./100 g. dry weight, and verified the diagnosis. Unlike the infantile form, brain symptoms were not present in the adult cases. But a female patient exhibited splenomegaly at the age of four and developed progressive neurological defects at the age of 12 (Fredrickson, 1966). Now about 25 years old she is able to live a relatively normal life. A 42 year old male patient was found to have an isolated pulmonary lesion on X-ray examination. Biopsy of lung, bone and liver showed histological and clinical changes compatible with the diagnosis of NP disease.

Amaurotic Familial Idiocy
(Gangliosidosis)

Four different types of this disease occur; in infancy (Tay-Sachs), in late infancy (Bielschowsky), in juveniles (Vogt-Spielmeyer) and in adults (Kufs), respectively. These diseases, which are histologically quite similar, are separate entities with no genetic interrelation (Hanhart, 1954; van Bogaert & Klein, 1955). Available evidence seems to indicate that gangliosides accumulate in all of them (Niemann-Pick's disease also shows some accumulation of gangliosides, but no genetic interrelation with the amaurotic familial idiocies). The finding of an increased ganglioside content of the brain in several diseases has been interpreted as an indication that the accumulation of these substances is brought about by a secondary, nonspecific storage process. However, work initiated by Kuhn et al. (1961) has shown that there are several gangliosides of different chemical constitution. Thus, it is conceivable that the accumulation of each of these substances is based on a different metabolic disorder and leads to a different disease. Since most of the chemical studies have been done in Tay-Sachs' disease, this will be considered in some detail. For a review of the literature, Diezel's paper (1962) may be consulted.

Klenk, who discovered gangliosides in the brain, was also the first to demonstrate their increase in Tay-Sachs' disease (TS disease). Considerably increased amounts of gangliosides can be demonstrated in the cerebral cortex in cases of Tay-Sachs' disease. By means of thin-layer chromatography Müldner et al. (1962) have shown that this increase is due to a specific ganglioside. Recently Booth et al. (1966) reported the analysis of this substance as well as of the gangliosides increased in Niemann-Pick's and in Pfaundler-Hurler's disease.

The findings of abnormal lymphocytes in amaurotic familial idiocy, which originally had been described by von Bagh & Hortling (1948) in the juvenile disease (Spielmeyer-Vogt), have also been observed in Tay-Sachs' disease (Spiegel-Adolf et al., 1959). In the juvenile form these vacuolated lymphocytes have also been found in the mother of the patient (Derwort & Noetzel, 1959; Derwort & Deterling, 1959). They may possibly become useful as a means of identifying the heterozygous carrier of the disease.

There are no significant abnormalities of the main serum lipid classes in TS disease. An increased N-acetylneuraminic acid content is found in a variety of diseases, but an elevated globulin neuraminic acid:globulin protein ratio was found to be a good statistical indicator for biochemical differentiation of amaurotic family idiocy from other disease groups (Saifer & Gerstenfield, 1962).

Recently an increase of a number of enzymes in the plasma and cerebrospinal fluid has been found and claimed to be important in the differential diagnosis of TS disease from Niemann-Pick's disease (Aronson et al., 1961).

Of great interest is the discovery of a deficiency or absence of fructose-1-phosphate aldolase in TS disease serum (Volk, 1964). It is also absent in mothers and fathers of the patients, and approximately 50% of paternal and maternal grand parents had no serum fructose-1-phosphate aldolase activities, while the same was found in about 25% of unaffected siblings.

At autopsy ganglion cells are swollen and rounded, with ballooning of the dendritic process. Nuclei are displaced to the periphery, though deposition of abnormal material within the nucleus has not been observed, and the nucleoli are normal (Terry & Weiss, 1963). The typical ultrastructural ganglion cell abnormalities consist of membranous cytoplasmic bodies (Terry & Weiss, 1963; Samuels et al., 1965). They are round or oval, 0·5 to 2·0 μ in diameter, and can occupy a considerable portion of the cytoplasm.

Metachromatic Leucodystrophy (ML)
(Sulphatidosis)

This disease, which is a degenerative diffuse demyelinating disorder, is characterized by an increase of sulphatides (Jatzkewitz, 1958, 1960). In this group of substances the galactose of cerebroside is esterified with sulphuric acid; hence, they are also called cerebron sulphates. (The term 'sulphatide' however is preferable because it does not involve an assumption about the type of fatty acid contained in the molecule.) The material stored in metachromatic leucodystrophy contains galactose (Jatzkewitz, 1960), and therefore the basic metabolic defect bears no relation to the defect of Gaucher's disease.

The clinical picture shows a great variability, nevertheless certain signs can be consistently observed. Hagberg (1963) proposed a division of the clinical course into four stages. One of the first signs in children is impairment of motor function with arrest of physiological development followed by loss of acquired skills, difficulties with speech and arrest of mental development. Often diplegic or tetraplegic paralysis develops, together with ataxia, paralysis of ocular muscles, nystagmus and progressive impairment of speech. Muscular hypotonicity, spasticity, diminution or absence of tendon reflexes and myoclonic movements can complete the neurological picture. Optic atrophy results in impairment of vision. The final stage is characterized by decerebrate rigidity, blindness and deafness; ultimately intercurrent infections or cerebral hyperpyrexia terminate the disease. In juvenile cases visual and auditory disturbances may occur early but the progression of the disease may be slower. At the end there is ataxia and spasticity. In the adult form, the onset of which is after puberty, there is a slowly progressing symptomatology, and clinical pictures like schizophrenia, paralysis and dementia have been described.

In blood there are no characteristic abnormalities (Hagberg, 1963); in urine a typical urinary sulphatide pattern with a second spot with lower R_f-value in addition to the larger sulphatide spot in the normal urine is found. According to Svennerholm & Svennerholm (1963) it is N-acylsphingosine-glucose-galactose-sulfate; it has also been isolated from normal and pathological kidneys (Mårtensson et al., 1966). Austin et al.

(1964) found in the urine of patients with ML a diminution of sulphatase A activity to about 2% of normal, so that the determination of urinary sulphatase A may be a screening test for ML.

It appears certain that the stored sulphatide in ML is identical with the normal sulphatide. Mårtensson *et al.* (1966) showed in kidney sulphatides some differences of the fatty acid content between normals and patients with ML. These findings indicate that metachromatic leucodystrophy is also a generalized lipidosis, and probably an inborn disorder of metabolism.

Several studies examined enzymes of sulphatide catabolism. Mehl & Jatzkewitz (1963) isolated fractions with cerebroside-sulphatase activity from pig kidneys. In 1965 the same authors succeeded in finding a difference in the arylsulphatase activities in normal kidneys and in kidneys of ML patients.

Angiokeratoma Corporis Diffusum (*Fabry's Disease*)

This disease was first described in 1898 by Fabry. It is a familial sphingolipidosis with the storage of ceramide-dihexoside and ceramide-trihexoside (Sweeley & Klionsky, 1963, 1964). The histological changes are thickening of the walls of blood vessels of skin and other organs, occurrence of storage cells in reticulo-endothelial tissues, and ganglion cell storage.

The first typical signs are the angiokeratomas, which occur in all male patients. These skin lesions consist of numerous small spots or papules with a colour ranging from purple to black. They are diffusely distributed over the lower parts of the body, particularly the lumbosacral, umbilical and genital areas and the buttocks. Angiokeratomas are rarely seen on the face or on hands or feet. The clinical picture is characterized by pain in the extremities and signs resulting from involvement of the vasculature, the heart and the kidneys which determine the course and prognosis. The symptomatology includes impairment of sweat secretion, fever, anaemia, vasomotor, gastro-intestinal and cerebrovascular disturbances, with headache, acute hemiparaesthesiae, hemiparesis and hemiplegia. Slight corneal opacity is uniformly present, but visual acuity is not impaired.

Angiokeratomas appear with the onset of puberty, and most patients die between the 30th and 60th year of life. While the occurrence of the full syndrome is restricted to men, an incomplete form of the disorder often without the typical skin lesions may be found in women. There is no specific treatment. For a review see De Groot (1964) and Sweeley & Klionsky (1966).

Pfaundler-Hurler's Disease

The characteristic features of this disease are dwarfism, skeletal deformities (among which a flat bridge of the nose, widely spaced eyes, a short neck, short long-bones, wide hands with short fingers and typical X-ray changes are most prominent), limited range of joint motion (often combined with flexion contractures of hips and knees), hepatosplenomegaly, cardiac enlargement and (later) failure, clouding of the cornea and mental retardation. Not all of these need be present and especially the last two may be lacking. The typical appearance of the unfortunate children led Ellis *et al.* (1936) to coin the term "gargoylism" for the disease, but we agree with McKusick (1959, 1960), that the use of this gruesome term should be discontinued. The disease is a familial disorder. McKusick (1959, 1960) differentiates an autosomal, recessive disorder in which corneal clouding and mental retardation are common and which usually occurs before the age of 20, from a less common sex-linked-recessive disorder with less of the named changes and a relatively good prognosis, patients surviving beyond adulthood (Gills *et al.*, 1965). The patients described by Hurler (1919) belong to the first type; possibly Hunter's (1917) cases are instances of the second (Goldberg *et al.*, 1965). This second type represents about one third of cases of Hurlers disease (Maroteaux & Lamy, 1965).

Histologically, cytoplasmic swelling of the cells is characteristic, especially of the epithelial cells of the liver, pituitary gland, reticulo-endothelial cells as well as of the mesodermal connective tissue cells. The cytoplasm of these large cells may be vacuolated, and thus give the impression of a foamy or granular structure. It was therefore suggested that Pfaundler-Hurler's disease might belong to the lipid diseases (Ellis *et al.*, 1936). Washington (1942) even coined the name "lipochrondrodystrophy". Electron microscope studies show similarities with Tay-Sachs' disease, particularly as regards the appearance of typical membranous cytoplasmic bodies (Gonatas & Gonatas, 1965; Aleu *et al.*, 1965). Earlier tissue analyses (Henderson *et al.*, 1952; Straus *et al.*, 1947) showed no lipid increase in the involved organs; however, several authors demonstrated increased amounts of gangliosides, which had not been considered in the earlier papers, in brain (Kutzim, 1946; Brante, 1951, 1952, 1957; Klenk & Löhr, 1955; Klenk, 1957) as well as in liver and spleen (Uzman, 1955). The alteration of ganglioside concentration is not caused by one ganglioside, but involves several (Booth *et al.*, 1966; Suzuki, 1966). A structural abnormality of gangliosides is unlikely (Ledeen *et al.*, 1965).

Brante (1952) isolated very large amounts (10% of dry weight) of mucopolysaccharides from the liver, and since then the disease has been considered to be an inherited disorder of mucopolysaccharide metabolism, a mucopolysaccharidosis. Stacey & Barker (1956), as well as Brown (1957) have published further analyses of these substances, which are considered to consist of several fractions containing various amounts of sulphate. From the urine, considerable amounts of mucopolysaccharides could be isolated (200–300 mg./day), consisting of chondroitin sulphate and heparitin sulphate (Dorfman & Lorincz, 1957; Meyer *et al.*, 1958). The occurrence of both

mucopolysaccharides is used for distinction of Hurler's disease from other mucopolysaccharidoses or other disorders associated with increased mucopolysaccharide excretion, such as Marfan's syndrome (Berenson & Dalferes, 1965). Austin *et al.* (1964) found an increased arylsulphatase B activity in the urine of patients with Hurler's disease. The relationship between the acid mucopolysaccharides and gangliosides is not known. Doss & Matiar-Vahar (1965) speculate that gangliosides accumulate in the brain, because the ganglion cell has no other way to metabolize polysaccharide fragments except by using them for ganglioside synthesis. Dorfman (1966) suspects a deficiency of protein-binding for chondroitinsulphate with the result that it is not retained properly in connective tissues, leading to increased concentrations in serum, organs, and urine.

References

ADLERSBERG, D., SCHAEFER, L. E. & DRACHMAN, S. R. (1951). *J. clin. Endocrinol.*, **11**, 67.

AGHION, H. (1934). "La Maladie de Gaucher dans l'enfance." Thèse de Paris.

AHRENS, E. H., Jr., INSULL, W., Jr., HIRSCH, J., STOFFEL, W., PETERSON, M. L., FARQUHAR, J. W., MILLER, T. & THOMASSON, H. J. (1959). *Lancet*, **1**, 115.

AHRENS, E. H., Jr., PAYNE, M. A., KUNKEL, H. G., EISENMENGER, W. J. & BLONDHEIM, S. H. (1950). *Medicine*, **29**, 299.

AHRENS, E. H., Jr., HIRSCH, J., OETTE, K., FARQUHAR, J. W. & STEIN, Y. (1961). *Trans. Ass. Amer. Phycns*, **74**, 134.

ALEU, F. P., TERRY, R. D. & ZELLWEGER, H. (1965). *J. Neuropath. exp. Neurol.*, **24**, 304.

ANSELL, G. B. & HAWTHORNE, J. N. (1964). "Phospholipids." B. B. A. Library Vol. 3, 19, Amsterdam-London-New York Elsevier.

ANTONIS, A. & BERSOHN, I. (1960). *Lancet*, **1**, 998.

ARONSON, S. M., SAIFER, A., PERLE, G. & VOLK, B. W. (1961). *Amer. J. clin. Nutr.*, **9**, 103.

ARTOM, C. (1952). "Formation of Phospholipids in Animal Tissue", in "Phosphorus Metabolism", Vol. I., Ed. McElroy, W. D. & Glass, B., Baltimore, Johns Hopkins Press.

AUSTIN, J. H. (1959). *Proc. Soc. exp. Biol.*, (*N.Y.*), **100**, 361.

AUSTIN, J., MCAFEE, D., ARMSTRONG, D., O'ROURKE, M., SHEARER, L. & BACHHAWAT, B. (1964). *Biochem. J.*, **93**, 15c.

VON BAGH, K. & HORTLING, H. (1948). *Nord. Med.*, **38**, 1072.

BANKER, B. Q., MILLER, J. Q. & CROCKER, A. C. (1962). In "Cerebral Sphingolipid." Ed. Aronson, S. M. & Volk, B. W. New York, Academic Press.

BASSEN, F. A. & KORNZWEIG, A. L. (1950). *Blood*, **5**, 381.

BERGE, K. G., ACHOR, R. W. P., CHRISTENSEN, N. A., MASON, H. L. & BARKER, N. W. (1961). *Am. J. Med.*, **31**, 24.

BERGSTRÖM, S., DANIELSSON, H. & SAMUELSSON, B. (1960). In "Lipid Metabolism", Ed. Bloch. K., New York, K. Wiley & Sons.

BERENSON, G. S. & DALFERES, E. R. (1965). *Biochem. biophys. ACTA.*, (Arnst), **101**, 183.

BEUMER, H. & FASOLD, H. (1933). *Biochem. Z.*, **259**, 471.

BHATTATHIRY, E. P. M. & SIPERSTEIN, M. D. (1963). *J. clin. Invest.*, **42**, 1613.

BIERMAN, E. L., DOLE, V. P. & ROBERTS, T. N. (1957). *Diabetes*, **6**, 475.

BLOCH, K. & RITTENBERG, D. (1945). *J. biol. Chem.*, **159**, 45.

BLOMSTRAND, R. (1961). "Klinische Studien über Fettsäuremetabolismus mit Hilfe von Gaschromatographie, in "Die Bedeutung der Nahrungsfette in der Pädiatrie." Ed. Jochims, J. Stuttgart, Enke.

BLOOM, W. (1928). *Arch. Path.*, **6**, 827.

BÖHLE, E., HARMUTH, E. & RAJEWSKY, (1964). *Z. Klin. Chem.*, **2**, 105.

VAN BOGAERT, L. (1934). *Bull. Acad. roy. Med. Belg.*, **14**, 323.

VAN BOGAERT, L., CUMINGS, J. N. & LOWENTHAL, A. Eds. (1957). "Cerebral lipidoses." Oxford, Blackwell.

VAN BOGAERT, L. & KLEIN, D. (1955). *J. génét. human.*, **4**, 23.

BOLLMAN, J. L. & FLOCK, E. V. (1951). *Amer. J. Physiol.*, **164**, 480.

BOOTH, D. A., GOODWIN, H. & CUMINGS, J. N. (1966). *J. Lipid. Res.*, **7**, 337.

BOWYER, D. E., LEAT, W. N. F., HOWARD, A. N. & GRESHAM, G. A. (1963). *Biochim. Biophys. Acta.*, **70**, 423.

BOYD, G. S. & OLIVER, M. F. (1958). *Brit. med. Bull.*, **14**, 239.

BRADY, R. O., KANFER, J. N. & SHAPIRO, D. (1965). *J. biol. Chem.*, **240**, 39.

BRADY, R. O. MOCK M. B. & FREDRICKSON, D. S. (1966). *Proc. nat. Acad. Sci.*, (Wash.), **55**, 366.

BRANTE, G. (1951). *Fette u. Seif.*, **53**, 457.

BRANTE, G. (1952). *Scand. J. clin. lab. Invest.*, **4**, 43.

BRANTE, G. (1957). Chemical pathology in gargoylism. In "Cerebral lipidoses", p. 164. Ed. Cumings, J. M. & Lowenthal, M. Oxford, Blackwell.

BRONTE-STEWART, B., ANTONIS, A., EALES, L. & BROCK, J. F. (1956). *Lancet*, **1**, 521.

BROWN, D. H. (1957). *Proc. nat. Acad. Sci.*, **43**, 783.

VAN BRUGGEN, J. T., HUTCHENS, T. T., CLAYCOMB, C. K., CATHEY, W. J. & WEST, E. S. (1952). *J. biol. Chem.*, **196**, 389.

BÜRGER, M. & GRÜTZ, O. (1932). *Arch. Derm. Syph.*, (Wien), **166**, 542.

CANTAROW, A. & BUCHER, C. J. (1938). *Arch. intern. Med.*, **67**, 333.

CARLSON, L. A. (1963). *J. Atheroscler. Res.*, **3**, 334.

CARLSON, L. A., BOBERG, J. & HÖGSTEDT, H. (1965). In "Handbook of physiology." Ed. Renold, A. E. & Cahill, G. F. sect. 5, p. 625. Baltimore, Waverly Press Inc.

CARTER, H. E., ROTHFUS, J. A. & GIGG, R. (1961). *J. Lipid Res.*, **2**, 228.

CHAIKOFF, I. L., SIPERSTEIN, M. D., DAUBEN, W. G., BRADLOW, H. L., EASTHAM, J. F., TOMKINS, G. M., MEIER, J. R., CHEN, R. W., HOTTA, S. & SRERE, P. A. (1952). *J. biol. Chem.*, **194**, 413.

CHAIKOFF, J. L., ZILVERSMIT, D. B. & ENTENMAN, C. (1948). *Proc. Soc. exp. Biol.*, *N.Y.*, **68**, 6.

CHAPMAN, F. D. & KINNEY, T. D. (1941). *Amer. J. Dis. Child.*, **62**, 1014.

CONN, J. W., VOGEL, W. C., LOUIS, L. H. & FAJANS, S. S. (1950). *J. Lab. clin. Med.*, **35**, 504.

CONSTANTINIDES, P., BOOTH, J. & CARLSON, G. (1961). "Advanced atherosclerosis of the human type in the rabbit", in "Drugs affecting lipid metabolism." Amsterdam, London, New York, Princeton, Elsevier Pub. Co.

CORNFORTH, J. W. (1959). *J. lipid. Res.*, **1**, 3.

CORNFORTH, J. W., HUNTER, G. D. & POPJÁK, G. (1953). *Arch. Biochem.*, **42**, 481.

CRAIG, L. S., LISSER, H. & SOLEY, M. H. (1944). *J. Clin. Endocrin.*, **4**, 12.

CRAMÉR, K. & BJÖRNTORP, P. (1962). *Acta med. scand.*, **171**, 441.

CROCKER, A. C. (1951). *Pediatrics*, **8**, 573.

CROCKER, A. C. & FARBER, S. (1958). *Medicine*, (Baltimore), **37**, 1.

CROCKER, A. C. & LANDING, B. H. (1960). *Metabolism*, **9**, 341.

CUMINGS, J. N. (1962). In "Erbliche Stoffwechselkrankheiten." München, Urban & Schwarzenberg.

CZITOBER, H., GRÜNDIG, E. & SCHOBEL, B. (1964). *Klin. Wschr.*, **42**, 1179.

DE GROOT, W. P. (1964). *Dermatologica* (Basel), **128**, 321.

DERWORT, A. & DETERLING, K. (1959). *Nervenarzt*, **30**, 442.

DERWORT, A. & NOETZEL, H. (1959). *Dtsch. Z. Nervenhk.*, **179**, 232.

DIENSTL, F., KUNZ, F. & MAIZER, H. A. (1966). *Klin. Wschr.*, **44**, 967.

DIEZEL, P. (1962). In "Grundlagenforschung IV." Georg Thieme. Verlag, Stuttgart,

DORFMAN, A. & LORINCZ, A. E. (1957). *Proc. nat. Acad. Sci.*, **43**, 443.

DORFMAN, A. (1966). In "The Metabolic basis of inherited disease." p. 963. Ed.: Stanbury, J. B. Wyngaarden, J. B. & Fredrickson, D. S. New York, McGraw-Hill Book Company.

DOSS, M. & MATIAR-VAHAR, H. (1965). *Fortschr. Neurol. Psychiat.*, **33**, 671.

DUSENDSCHON, A. & FARVERGER (1945). "Deux cas familiaux de maladie de Niemann-Pick chez adulte." Thèse, Faculté de Médecine, Génève.

EGGSTEIN, M. & KREUTZ, F. H. (1966). *Klin. Wschr.*, **44**, 262.

ELLIS, R. W. B., SHELDON, W. & CAPON, N. B. (1936). *Quart. J. Med.*, **5**, n.s., 119.

EPSTEIN, E. (1924). *Biochem. Z.*, **145**, 398.

EUSTERMAN, G. B. & MONTGOMERY, H. (1944). *Gastroenterology*, **3**, 275.

FABRY, J. (1898). *Arch. Derm. Suppl.* **43**, 187.

FARBER, S. (1941). *Amer. J. Path.*, **17**, 625.

FARBER, S. (1944). *Amer. J. Dis. Child.*, **68**, 350.

FARQUHAR, J. W. & WAYS, P. (1966). Abetalipoproteinemia. In Stanbury-Wyngaarden-Fredrickson. "The Metabolic Basis of Inherited Disease." 2nd ed. McGraw-Hill, New York-London.

FIESER, L. F. & FIESER, M. (1959). "Steroids." New York, Reinhold.

FISHER, E. R. & REIDBORD, H. (1962). *Am. J. Path.*, **41**, 679.

FRASER, J. (1935). *Brit. J. Surg.*, **22**, 800.

FREDRICKSON, D. S., ALTROCCHI, P. H., AVIOLI, L.-V., GOODMAN, DeW. S. & GOODMAN, H. C. (1961). *Ann. Int. Med.*, **55**, 1016.

FREDRICKSON, D. S., ONO, K. & DAVIS, L. L. (1963). *J. Lipid. Res.*, **4**, 24.

FREDRICKSON, D. S. & LEES, R. S. (1965). *Circulation*, **31**, 326.

FREDRICKSON, D. S. (1966). Familial High-Density Lipoprotein Deficiency: Tangier Disease. In: Stanbury-Wyngaarden-Fredrickson. "The Metabolic Basis of Inherited Disease." 2nd ed. McGraw-Hill, New York-London.

FREDRICKSON, D. S. (1966). In "The Metabolic Basis of Inherited Disease." p. 580. Eds.: Stanbury, J. B. Wyngaarden J. B. & Fredrickson, D. S. New York, McGraw-Hill, 2nd Edition.

FREDRICKSON, D. S. & LEES, R. S. (1966). Familial Hyperlipoproteinaemia. In Stanbury-Wyngaarden-Fredrickson. "The Metabolic Basis of Inherited Disease." 2nd ed. McGraw-Hill, New York-London.

FREDRICKSON, D. S., LEVY, R. I. & LEES, R. S. (1967). *New Engl. J. Med.*, **276**, 32.

FREUD, P., PLACHTA, A., SPEER, F. D. & LUHBY, A. L. (1954). *Amer. J. Dis. Child.*, **88**, 43.

FURMAN, R. H., HOWARD, R. P., SHETLAR, M. R., KEATY, E. C. & IMAGAWA, R. (1958). *Circulation*, **17**, 1076.

GERKEN, H. & WIEDEMANN, H. R. (1964). *Ann. paediat.* (Basel), **203**, 328.

GILLS, J. P., HOBSON, R., HANLEY, W. B. & McKUSICK, V. A. (1965). *Arch. Ophthal.*, **74**, 596.

GJONE, E. O. & ORNING, M. (1966). *Scand. J. clin. Lab. Invest.*, **18**, 209.

GÖTT, E. & REXA, H. (1964). *Acta haemat.*, **31**, 113.

GOLDBERG, M. F., MAUMENEE, A. E. & McKUSICK, V. A. (1965). *Arch. Ophthal.*, **74**, 516.

GONATAS, N. K. & GONATAS, J. (1965). *J. Neuropath. exp. Neurol.*, **24**, 341.

GOULD, R. G. (1959). In "Hormones and Atherosclerosis." Ed. Pincus, G., New York, Academic Press.

GOULD, R. G. & SWYRYD, E. A. (1966). *J. Lipid. Res.*, **7**, 698.

GRAY, J. D. & TAYLOR, S. (1953). *Cancer*, **6**, 333.

GRÜNDIG, E., CZITOBER, H. & SCHOBEL, B. (1965). *Clin. Chim. Acta*, **12**, 157.

GRUNDY, S. M. & AHRENS, E. H., Jr. (1966). *J. Clin. Invest.*, **45**, 1503.

HAGBERG, B. (1963). In "Brain lipids and lipoproteins, and the leucodystrophies." p. 134. Eds: Folch-Pi, J. & Bauer, H. J. Amsterdam, Elsevier Publishing Co.

HALLGREN, B., STENHAGEN, S., SWANBORG, A. & SVENNERHOLM, L. (1960). *J. clin. Invest.*, **39**, 1424.

HALLIDAY, N., DEUEL, H. J., Jr., TRAGERMAN, L. J. & WARD, W. E. (1940). *J. biol. Chem.*, **132**, 171.

HANGER, F. M., Jr. & GUTMAN, A. B. (1940). *J. Amer. med. Ass.*, **115**, 263.

HANHART, E. (1954). *Acta genet.*, **3**, 331.

HELLMAN, L., ROSENFELD, R. S., EIDINOFF, M., FUKUSHIMA, N. & GALLAGHER, T. (1955). *J. clin. Invest.*, **34**, 48.

HENDERSON, J. L., MACGREGOR, A. R., THANNHAUSER, S. J. & HOLDEN, R. (1952). *Arch. Dis. Childh.*, **27**, 230.

HILLBORG, P. O. & ESTBORN, B. (1964). *Acta paediat.* (Uppsala), **53**, 558.

HIRSCHHORN, K. & WILKINSON, F. C. (1959). *Amer. J. Med.*, **26**, 60.

HOLM, J. E., TEILUM, G. & CHRISTENSEN, E. (1944). *Acta med. scand.*, **118**, 292.

HOLT, L. E., Jr., AYLWARD, F. X. & TIMBRES, H. G. (1936). *J. clin. Invest.*, **15**, 451.

HOLT, L. E., Jr., AYLWARD, F. X. & TIMBRES, H. G. (1939). *Bull. Johns Hopk. Hosp.*, **64**, 279.

HOLTZ, A. J., UHLENDORF, W. & FREDRICKSON, D. S. (1964). *Fed. Proc.*, **23**, 128.

HUNTER, C. (1917). *Proc. R. Soc. Med.*, **10**, I, 104.

HURLER, G. (1919). *Z. Kinderheilk.*, **24**, 220.

JACKSON, R. S. & WILKINSON, C. F. (1952). *Ann. intern. Med.*, **37**, 1162.

JATZKEWITZ, H. (1958). *Z. physiol. Chem.*, **311**, 279.

JATZKEWITZ, H. (1960). *Z. physiol. Chem.*, **320**, 134.

JOYNER, C. R. (1953). *Ann. intern. Med.*, **38**, 759.

KEYS, A. (1954). *Am. J. Publ. Health.*, **44**, 864.

KEYS, A., VIVANCO, F., RODRIGUEZ MIÑON, J. L., KEYS, M. H. & CASTRO MENDOZA, H. (1954). *Metabolism*, **3**, 195.

KIM, K. S. & IVY, A. C. (1952). *Amer. J. Physiol.*, **171**, 302.

KINSELL, L. W., MICHAELIS, G. D., PATRIDGE, J. W., BOLING, L. A., BALCH, H. E. & COCHRANE, G. C. (1953). *J. clin. Nutr.*, **1**, 224.

KINSELL, L. W., SCHLIERF, G., KAHLKE, W. & SCHETTLER, G. (1967). Essential Hyperlipaemia. In "Lipids and Lipidoses." Schettler. Springer-Verlag, Berlin-Heidelberg, New York.

KLATSKIN, G. & GORDON, M. (1952). *Amer. J. Med.*, **12**, 3.

KLENK, E. (1934). *Hoppe Seyl. Z.*, **229**, 151.

KLENK, E. (1955). "The pathological chemistry of the developing brain", in "Biochemistry of the developing nervous system." New York, Academic Press.

KLENK, E. & LÖHR, H. (1955). Unpublished results; cit. by KLENK 1955.

KLENK, E. (1957). *Wien. Z. Nervenhk.*, **13**, 309.

KLENK, E. & KAHLKE, W. (1963). *Z. physiol. Chem.*, **333**, 133.

KLIMA, R., BEYREDER, J. & HERZOG, E. (1956). *Wien. med. Wschr.*, **106**, 809.

KLYNE, W. (1957). "The Chemistry of the Steroids." London, Methuen.

KRAMER, B., CASDEN, D. D., GOLDMAN, H. & SILVERMAN, S. H. (1952). *Postgrad. med.*, **11**, 439.

KRITCHEVSKY, D., STAPLE, E. & WHITEHOUSE, M. W. (1960). *Amer. J. clin. Nutr.*, **8**, 411.

KUHN, R., WIEGANDT, H. & EGGE, H. (1961). *Angew. Chem.*, **73**, 580.

KUTZIM, H. (1946). M.D.-thesis, Köln.

LEDEEN, R., SALZMAN, K., GONATAS, J. & TAGHAVY, A. (1965). Part 1. *J. Neuropath. exp. Neurol.*, **24**, 341.

LEES, R. S. & HATCH, F. T. (1963). *J. Lab. clin. Med.*, **61**, 518.

LEROY, G. V. (1955). *Ann. intern. Med.*, **42**, 239.

LETTERER, E. (1934). Veröffentlichungen aus der Gewebe- und Konstitutions Pathologie, Heft 36 (Band 8, Heft 4).

LEWIS, L. A., OLMSTED, F., PAGE, I. H., LAWRY, E. Y., MANN, G. V., STARE, F. J., HANIG, M., LAUFFER, M. A., GORDON, T. & MOORE, F. E. (1957). *Circulation*, **16**, 227.

LICHTENSTEIN, L. (1953). *Arch. Path.*, **56**, 84.

LIEB, H. (1924). *Hoppe Seyl. Z.*, **140**, 305.

LIEB, H. (1929). *Hoppe Seyl. Z.*, **181**, 280.

LINDSTEDT, S. (1957). *Acta physiol. scand.*, **40**, 1.

McKUSICK, V. A. (1959). "Vererbbare Störungen des Bindegewebes." Verlag, Stuttgart, Georg Thieme.

McKUSICK, V. A. (1960). "Heritable Disorders of Connective Tissue." 2nd ed. St. Louis, Mosby.

MacMAHON, H. E. & THANNHAUSER, S. J. (1952). *Gastroenterology*, **21**, 488.

MALMROS, H., SWAIIN, B. & TRUEDSSON, E. (1954). *Acta med. scand.*, **149**, 91.

MALONEY, A. F. J. & CUMINGS, J. N. (1960). *J. Neurol. Neurosurg. Psychiat.*, **23**, 207.

MAN, E. B., KARTIN, B. L., DURLACHER, S. H. & PETERS, J. P. (1945). *J. clin. Invest.*, **24**, 623.

MARCHAND, F. (1907). *Münch. med. Wschr.*, **54**, 1102.

MAROTEAUX, P. & LAMY, M. (1965). *J. Pediat.*, **67**, 312.

MÅRTENSSON, E., PERCY, A. & SVENNERHOLM, L. (1966). *Acta paediat.* (Uppsala), **55**, 1.

MEHL, E. & JATZKEWITZ, H. (1963). *Hoppe Seyl. Z. physiol. Chem.*, **331**, 292.

MEHL, E. & JATZKEWITZ, H. (1965). *Biochem. biophys. Res. Commun.*, **19**, 407.

MEYER, K., GRUMBACH, M. M., LINKER, A. & HOFFMANN, P. (1958). *Proc. Soc. exp. Biol., N.Y.*, **97**, 273.

MORRISON, R. W. & HACK, M. H. (1947). *Amer. J. Path.*, **25**, 597.

MÜLDNER, H. G., WHERRETT, J. R. & CUMINGS, J. N. (1962). *J. Neurochem.*, **9**, 607.

MÜLLER, C. (1939). *Nord. med.* (*Norsk mag. f. laegevidensk.*), **2**, 1183.

NÉKÁM, L., Jr. & OTTENSTEIN, B. (1935). *Klin. Wschr.*, **14**, 641.

NOBLE, R. P. (1968). *J. Lipid Res.* **9**, 693.

NORUM, K. R. & GJONE, E. (1967). *Scand. J. clin. Lab. Invest.*, **20**, 231.

NOTHMAN, M. M. & PROGER, S. (1962). *J. Amer. med. Ass.*, **179**, 40.

NYE, W. H. R. & WATERHOUSE, C. (1961). *J. clin. Invest.*, **40**, 1202.

NYE, W. H. R., WATERHOUSE, C. & MARINETTI, G. V. (1961). *J. clin. Invest.*, **40**, 1194.

OBERLING, C. & WORINGER, P. (1927). *Rev. franç. Pédiat.*, **3**, 475.

OLIVER, M. F. & BOYD, G. S. (1956). *Lancet*, **2**, 1273.

OLIVER, M. F. & BOYD, G. S. (1959). *Lancet*, **2**, 690.

PATRICK, A. D. (1965). *Biochem. J.*, **97**, 17c.

PFÄNDLER, U. (1946). *Schweiz. med. Wschr.*, **76**, 1128.

PHILLIPPART, M. & MENKES, J. H. (1964). *Biochem. biophys. Res. Commun.*, **15**, 551.

PHILLIPS, G. B. (1958). *Biochim. Biophys. Acta*, **29**, 594.

PHILLIPS, G. B. (1960). *J. clin. Invest.*, **39**, 1639.

PICK, L. (1927). *Med. Klinik*, **23**, 1483.

PICK, L. (1933). *Amer. J. med. Sci.*, **185**, 453, 601.

PILZ, H. & JATZKEWITZ, H. (1964). *J. Neurochem.*, **11**, 603.

RAPP, W. (1966). *Clin. chim. Acta*, **15**, 177.

REFSUM, S. (1946). *Acta psychiat. scand. Suppl.* 38.

RICHTERICH, R., VAN MECHELEN, P. & ROSSI, E., (1965a)., *Amer. J. Med.* **39**, 230.

RICHTERICH, R., MOSER, H. & ROSSI, E. (1965b)., *Humangenetik*, **1**, 322.

ROBINSON, D. S. (1963). *Advances Lipid Res.*, **1**, 133.

ROESTER, L. (1950). *Dtsch. Ges. Verdau.-u. Stoffwechselkr.*, **10**, 193.

ROUSER, G., GALLI, C. & KRITCHEVSKY, G. (1965). *J. Am. Oil Chemists' Soc.*, **42**, 404.

SAIFER, A. & GERSTENFIELD, S. (1962). *Clin. chim. Acta*, **7**, 467.

SALT, H. B., WOLFF, O. H., LLOYD, J. K., FOSBROOKE, A. S., CAMERON, A. H. & HUBBLE, D. V. (1960). *Lancet*, **2**, 325.

SAMUELS, S., GONATAS, N. K. & WEISS, M. (1965). *J. Neuropath. exp. Neurol.*, **24**, 256.

SCHETTLER, G., EGGSTEIN, M. & JOBST, H. (1958). *Dtsch. med. Wschr.*, **83**, 1.

SCHIFF, F. (1926). *Jb. Kinderheilk*, **112**, 1.

SCHRADE, W., BÖHLE, E., BIEGLER, R., TEICKE, R. & ULLRICH, B. (1960). *Klin. Wschr.*, **38**, 739.

SIPERSTEIN, M. D., CHAIKOFF, I. L. & REINHARDT, W. O. (1952). *J. biol. Chem.*, **198**, 111.

SJÖVALL, J. & ÅKESSON, I. (1955). *Acta physiol. scand.*, **34**, 273, 279.

SOBREVILLA, L. A., GOODMAN, M. L. & KANE, C. A. (1964). *Amer. J. Med.*, **37**, 821.

SOSHEA, J. W. & FARNSWORTH, E. B. (1951). *J. Lab. clin. Med.*, **38**, 414.

SPERRY, W. M. (1953). *Proc. Ass. Res. Nerv. Ment. Dis.*, **32**, 262.

SPIEGEL-ADOLF, M., BAIRD, H. W., KOLLIAS, D. & SZEKELY, E. G. (1959). *Amer. J. Dis. Child.*, **97**, 676.

SPRING, H. (1950). *Med. Mschr., Stuttgart*, **4**, 454.

SUOMI, W. D. & AGRANOFF, B. W. (1965). *J. Lipid Res.*, **6**, 211.

SUZUKI, K. (1966). In "Sphingolipidoses," 1965. Ed.: Aronson, S. M. & Volk, B. W. New York, Pergamon Press.

STACEY, M. & BARKER, S. A. (1956). *J. clin. Path.*, **9**, 314.

STÄLLBERG-STENHAGEN, S. & SVENNERHOLM, L. (1965). *J. Lipid. Res.*, **6**, 140.

STANLEY, M. M. & CHENG, S. (1956). *Gastroenterology*, **30**, 62.

STOLZER, B. L., MILLER, G., WHITE, W. A. & ZUCKERBROD, M. (1950). *Amer. J. Med.*, **9**, 124.

STRAUS, R., MERLISS, R. & REISER, R. (1947). *Amer. J. clin. Path.*, **17**, 671.

STUHLFAUTH, K. & ZÖLLNER, N. (1959). *Klin. Wschr.*, **37**, 1162.

SVENNERHOLM, E. & SVENNERHOLM, L. (1956). *Acta chim. scand.*, **10**, 1048.

SVENNERHOLM, E. & SVENNERHOLM, L. (1963). *Nature* (Lond.), **198**, 688.

SVENNERHOLM, L. (1966). *Biochem. J.*, **98**, 20.

SWEELEY, C. C. (1963). *J. Lipid. Res.*, **4**, 402.

SWEELEY, C. C. & KLIONSKY, B. (1963). *J. biol. Chem.* **238**, 3148.

SWEELEY, C. C. & KLIONSKY, B. (1964). Abstracts 6th Internat. Congr. Biochem. New York.

SWEELEY, C. C. & KLIONSKY, B. (1966). In "The Metabolic Basis of Inherited Disease, p. 618. Eds.: Stanbury, J. B., Wyngaarden, J. B., Fredrickson, D. S. New York. McGraw-Hill Book Co.

SWELL, L., BOITER, R. A., FIELD, H., Jr. & TREADWELL, C. R. (1955). *Amer. J. Physiol.*, **180**, 129.

TERRY, R. D., SPERRY, W. M. & BRODOFF, B. (1954). *Amer. J. Path.*, **30**, 263.

TERRY, R. D. & WEISS, M. (1963). *J. Neuro-path. exp. Neurol.*, **22**, 18.

THANNHAUSER, S. J. (1923). *Dtsch. Arch. klin. Med.*, **141**, 290.

THANNHAUSER, S. J. (1940). "Lipidoses." New York, Oxford University Press, pp. 257–84.

THANNHAUSER, S. J. (1950a), "Lipidoses." New York, Oxford University Press.

THANNHAUSER, S. J. (1950b). *J. Mt. Sinai Hosp., N.Y.*, **17**, 90.

THANNHAUSER, S. J. (1953). *Proc. Ass. Res. Nerv. Ment. Dis.*, **32**, 238.

THANNHAUSER, S. J. (1958). "Lipidoses," 3rd ed. New York & London, Grune & Stratton.

THANNHAUSER, S. J., BENOTTI, J. & REINSTEIN, H. (1939). *J. biol. Chem.*, **129**, 709.

THANNHAUSER, S. J. & MAGENDANTZ, H. (1938). *Ann. intern. Med.*, **11**, 1662.

TOMKINS, G. M., SHEPPARD, H. & CHAIKOFF, I. L. (1953a). *J. biol. Chem.*, **201**, 137.

TOMKINS, G. M., SHEPPARD, H. & CHAIKOFF, I. L. (1953b). *J. biol. Chem.*, **203**, 781.

TROUT, D. L., ESTES, E. H. & FRIEDBERG, S. J. (1960). *J. Lipid Res.* **1**, 199.

TUCHMAN, L. R., SUNA, H. & CARR, J. J. (1956). *J. Mt. Sinai Hosp., N.Y.*, **23**, 227.

TUCHMAN, L. R., GOLDSTEIN, G. & CLYMAN, M. (1959). *Amer. J. Med.*, **27**, 959.

UZMAN, L. L. (1955). *Arch. Path.*, **60**, 308.

VIDEBAEK, A. (1952). *Acta paediat.* (Uppsala), **41**, 355.

VOLK, B. W. (1964). Path. anatomy. In "Tay-Sachs Disease." Ed. Volk, B. W. New York, Grune & Stratton.

WAGENER, H., LANG, D. & FROSCH, B. (1964). *Z. ges. exp. Med.*, **138**, 425.

WALDEYER, N. (1871). *Virchows Arch.*, **52**, 318.

WASHINGTON, J. (1942). In "Brenneman's Practice of Pediatrics," Vol. 4, Chapter 30. Hagerstown, Md., Prior.

WRIGHT, L. D. (1961). *Annu. Rev. Biochem.*, **30**, 525.

ZIEVE, L. (1958). *Ann. intern. Med.*, **48**, 471.

ZÖLLNER, N. (1955). *Dtsch. med. Wschr.*, **80**, 128.

ZÖLLNER, N. (1957). In "Thannhauser's Lehrbuch des Stoffwechsels und der Stoffwechselkrankheiten". Stuttgart, Georg Thieme.

ZÖLLNER, N. (1958). *Dtsch. med. Wschr.*, **83**, 448.

ZÖLLNER, N. (1959). *Dtsch. med. Wschr.*, **84**, 386.

ZÖLLNER, N. & KIRSCH, K. (1960). *Zschr. exp. Med.*, **134**, 10.

ZÖLLNER, N. & WOLFRAM, G. (1961). *Klin. Wschr.*, **39**, 817.

ZÖLLNER, N. & KIRSCH, K. (1962). *Z. ges. exp. Med.* **135**, 545.

ZÖLLNER, N. & WOLFRAM, G. (1962). *Klin. Wschr.*, **40**, 267 and 1101.

ZÖLLNER, N. (1964). *Dtsch. Med. Wschr.*, **89**, 731.

ZÖLLNER, N. & EBERHAGEN, D. (1965). "Untersuchung und Bestimmung der Lipoide im Blut." Springer-Verlag, Berlin-Heidelberg-New York.

ZÖLLNER, N., WOLFRAM, G. & AMIN, G. (1962). *Klin. Wschr.*, **40**, 273.

ZÖLLNER, N., WOLFRAM, G., LONDONG, W. & KIRSCH, K. (1966). *Klin. Wschr.*, **44**, 380.

ZÖLLNER, N., WOLFRAM, G. & LONDONG, W. (1966). *Z. ges. exp. Med.*, **140**, 24.

ZÖLLNER, N. & GUDENZI, M. (1966). *Med. Klin.*, **61**, 1996.

Chapter 18

ATHEROSCLEROSIS

by

GEORGE S. BOYD

Department of Biochemistry, Edinburgh University

THE elimination of many infectious diseases has accentuated the importance of certain changes associated with advancing years, often termed the diseases of ageing. The future control of these processes presents a challenge to all who are interested in metabolism.

The most prevalent degenerative change observed in the cardiovascular system is atherosclerosis, which affects the main arteries, and leads to ischaemic changes in the myocardium, brain or limbs. A study group of WHO defined atherosclerosis as "A variable combination of changes of the intima of arteries (as distinct from arterioles) consisting of the focal accumulation of lipids, complex carbohydrates, blood and blood products, fibrous tissue and calcium deposits, and associated with medial changes" (WHO Technical Report, 1958). This definition emphasizes the pleomorphic character of the arterial lesion, which is often overlooked in studies on atherosclerosis. It is now generally accepted that there are both vascular and blood factors involved in the process of atheromatosis.

The fundamental problem in elucidating the pathogenesis of atherosclerosis is to identify dependent and independent variables operative within the complex physio-pathological situation which prevails in atherosclerosis. As a result of extensive scientific studies on atherosclerosis, evidence has accrued that a large variety of factors are operative in this situation. These factors include plasma hyperlipaemia, hypertension and accelerated blood clotting tendencies. It is for this reason that there have been a great many studies on the relationship between dietary fats and plasma lipids; dietary lipids and thrombosis, and similarly studies on the inter-relationships of hypertension, plasma lipids and atherosclerosis. The complex interplay of these parameters constitutes the complicated problem of atherosclerosis.

Morphology

Before attempting to discuss the possible biochemical abnormalities found in association with atherosclerosis it is essential to give some consideration to the main morphological features of this situation. Atherosclerosis affects the intima of the larger arteries, and may be observed by the naked eye as raised plaques of lipid or other material encroaching on the lumen of the vessel. Pathologists frequently classify these intimal lesions into several discrete categories.

The earliest observable lesions (found in children) are those classified as fatty streaks. These superficial pale yellow intimal lesions are easily identified by the topical application of fat stains applied to the intimal surface of arteries. When the fatty streak is examined microscopically it is often found to consist of macrophages which are apparently laden with lipid droplets.

The second type of intimal lesion frequently observed by pathologists is the fibrous plaque. These intimal vascular lesions are firm and appear as grey elevated areas of thickening, and upon examination by the light microscope or by the electron microscope they can be shown to consist of collagen and elastic fibres; they also contain smooth muscle cells. As a rule these fibrous plaques contain a variable amount of fat, but proportionately they contain less lipid than the fatty streaks.

The third type of vascular lesion frequently found is that which is often referred to as atheroma. In this case the lesions consist of soft fatty raised areas, and are frequently found in association with other somewhat complex lesions in which there may be evidence of intimal haemorrhage with superimposed thrombosis. The atheroma and complex lesions sometimes have evidence of calcification and/or ulceration.

In certain experimental atheroma studies in animals it can be shown that the fatty streaks may be the precursors of the fibrous plaques, and that the fibrous plaques perhaps are the precursors of the other more complex ulcerative type of lesions. It will be appreciated that it is difficult, in fact almost impossible, to establish whether the fatty streaks are the precursors of the fibrous plaques in man. Evidence has been presented that the fatty streaks and the fibrous plaques appear to occur at different sites in the arterial tree in man (Schwartz & Mitchell, 1962). A similar conclusion has been obtained from studies on the chemical composition of the different lesions (Smith, 1965; Smith, Slater & Chu, 1968).

Since the atherosclerotic lesion contains appreciable amounts of lipid, various theories have evolved around the general lipid infiltration concept. It is usually implied in this theory that the primary cause of atherosclerosis is an infiltration of lipids (from the blood plasma) into the intimal tissues, and as a result intimal lipid

deposition occurs giving rise to fatty flecks or fatty streaks. Attempts are then made to produce arguments connecting the lipid deposition with the subsequent appearance of fibrous plaques. In the fibrous plaque the lipid component is less and there is degeneration of intimal connective tissue with the appearance of smooth muscle cells. It is not clear at the present time which cells in the arterial intima are the site of production of collagen, but it has been suggested that the smooth muscle cells seen in these lesions may be responsible.

As a result of studies performed over the last few decades it now seems clear that mural thrombi appear at the site of atheromatous plaques and subsequently these thrombi are incorporated into the intima of the vessel. Pathologists are familiar with the laminated appearance of many of the older atheromatous lesions observed in the intima of arteries. This has been explained as being due to recurring thrombotic events where in each instance the resultant mural thrombi become incorporated into the vessel wall. The endothelium grows over the thrombi and this alteration to the vasculature may be the site of subsequent thrombotic events and hence additional thrombi become incorporated into the wall in a serial fashion. This process is thought to be the mechanism which gives rise to the laminated appearance of the "older" complex lesions (Duguid, 1948).

As a result of pathological, histochemical and microanalytical studies it has been possible to subject the vascular lesions occurring in the arterial system to a fairly detailed chemical analysis. The early fatty flecks or fatty streaks contain mainly lipids, and the lipids which are found in these fatty streaks have a composition somewhat similar to the lipid composition of blood plasma (Böttcher & Van Gent, 1961; Smith, 1965). These findings gave support to the concept that the fatty streaks were generated by the passive deposition of plasma lipids in the vessel wall. It has been possible to show that the fibrous plaques contain connective tissue, collagen, and fibrin. The fibrin could arise by the incorporation of mural thrombi into the intima of the vessels, or it may have arisen as a result of the conversion of fibrinogen from blood plasma being converted into fibrin by reactions within the intima. The complex lesions contain connective tissue, muscle cells and lipids. Under certain circumstances there is a marked increase in the calcium content of these lesions.

In order to produce a biochemical basis for the complicated pathological situation embracing atherosclerosis it is necessary to explain the increase in the appearance of fatty flecks or fatty streaks with advancing years, the appearance in the intima of the fibrous plaques and also the complex ulcerative type of atheromatous plaques. Since the accumulation of lipids in the intimal layer of the vessels has been regarded by many as an early event in the process of atherosclerosis, it is important that this event should be considered at the outset. Futhermore it is possible to induce in experimental animals aortic fatty streaks using various dietetic manipulations. Some arterial intimal lesions in experimental animals have a similarity to human atherosclerosis in that chemically and histologically these early lesions resemble the situation in man. This subject has been reviewed by Adams (1964).

Aetiology

The aetiology of atherosclerosis has been the subject of controversy for over a century. The mechanism of the arterial changes has been "explained" by a variety of theories.

One of the earliest studies on atherosclerosis is that of Rokitansky (1852), who considered that the thickening of the intima was due to the deposition of material derived from blood. This view was contested by Virchow (1856), who attributed the vascular lesions to a manifestation of inflammatory processes which were followed by fatty degeneration.

Leary (1941) put forward the view that the process of atheromatosis was due to a type of fatty infiltration of the vessels, while Duguid (1946, 1948) advanced an alternative explanation for the process of atherosclerosis. He revived interest in the theory of Rokitansky, and presented evidence for the presence of fibrin in arterial lesions. This theory stresses the importance of thrombosis in the aetiology, and has come to be known as the "thrombogenic" theory of atherosclerosis.

Wilens (1951) drew attention to the slowly developing increase in the thickness of the arterial intima, which proceeds throughout life. Since the arterial intima of males appears to thicken faster than the arterial intima of females, Wilens suggested that this may explain the difference between the sexes in their presentation with the clinical manifestations of atherosclerosis. Wilens considered that the appearance of arterial lipid-laden plaques was a natural consequence of the age-dependent intimal thickening, and his views have come to be regarded as a "senescence" theory of atherosclerosis. Some of the evidence for and against these different theories has been

reviewed at length by Crawford (1961), Constantinides (1965) and Mitchell & Schwartz (1965).

The cholesterol ester content of normal intima increases with age and the fatty acid moiety of the esters also changes with age. In middle age the cholesterol ester pattern of the intima resembles the cholesterol ester pattern in certain low-density plasma lipoproteins (see later section on plasma lipids).

The earliest microscopic lesion observable in human arteries is possibly the appearance of minute lipid droplets within the intima. Whether the presence of this lipid can be considered a pathological change is in doubt, but, by analogy with other tissues, in all probability these fatty droplets can be metabolized and hence they may appear and disappear from the tissue fairly freely. Most arterial tissues exhibit another type of lipid infiltration, demonstrable as the appearance of small fatty streaks of variable length and width. These lipid lesions are found in arteries of children (Schwartz, 1967), and the problem is to establish whether these fatty streaks are generated from the minute fatty droplets, and, if so, are they the precursors of atheromatous lesions?

Holman, McGill, Strong & Geer (1958) subscribe to the view that the vascular changes can be explained on the basis of lipid infiltration producing fatty streaks, and these in turn develop into atheromatous plaques. It is known that the lipid composition of the plasma in contact with the plaque resembles the lipid composition of the intima (Weinhouse & Hirsch, 1940; Buck & Rossiter, 1951; Smith, 1965), and isotopic evidence has been cited in support of the concept that the circulating plasma lipids can be deposited within the atheromatous material (Biggs, Kritchevsky, Colman, Gofman, Jones, Lindgren, Hyde & Lyon, 1952).

The theory of lipid infiltration, in which the severity of a type of vascular lesion is related to the concentration of certain lipids in plasma, would be consistent with the hypothesis that by lowering the plasma lipid level the lipid contained in the lesion might be made to regress. There is evidence that in certain experimental animals rendered atherosclerotic by dietary means, the degree of atheromatosis can be reduced by reversion to normal plasma lipid levels. Furthermore, in man it is often observed that the macroscopic appearance of the arteries of individuals dying of "wasting diseases" is relatively free from superficial lipid-laden streaks (Wilens, 1947). Additional evidence on this point also came from studies on German prisoners of war dying during internment under conditions described as nutritionally inadequate. In this case, the degree of atheromatosis observed in these men was less than would be encountered under more normal conditions (Schettler, 1961).

There are many points of weakness in the lipid infiltration theory of atherosclerosis, and these have been exposed by the thrombotic theory proposed by Duguid (1946, 1948) and Duguid & Robertson (1957). These authors point out that in many atheromatous vessels it is possible to identify material having histological and chemical properties comparable to those of fibrin, and in many lesions the bulk of the atheromatous mass is proteinaceous. Duguid has shown in human and in experimental material many instances of mural thrombi in various stages of organization, and which are covered by a layer of endothelium. In the "thrombogenic theory" the emphasis is on blood factors which predispose to thrombosis on the one hand and fibrinolysis on the other; the thrombotic theory of atherosclerosis has evolved into a concept of an imbalance between the rate of deposition and the rate of dissolution of fibrin. Duguid points out that the clinical sequelae to atheroma are frequently thrombotic in origin, and emphasizes that in almost all instances of myocardial infarction he can establish the presence of a thrombus. This high incidence of thrombosis in fatal myocardial infarcts has not been recorded by all observers; for example, Master, Gulner, Dack & Jaffe (1941), Branwood & Mongomery (1956) and Crawford, Dexter & Teare (1961) were only able to establish the presence of an occlusive thrombus in about 40% of their cases.

Within the last decade considerable support has accrued in favour of the importance of thrombosis in the development of atherosclerotic lesions (see reviews by Mustard, 1961, and Mustard, Rowsell & Murphy, 1964). This is due to electron microscopic studies on platelet plugs *in vivo* and platelet behaviour *in vitro*. The interaction between platelets and the blood clotting mechanism leading to fibrin formation has been extensively studied, and conversely the effect of fibrin on the behaviour of platelets has been investigated (French & Poole, 1963; French, MacFarlane & Sanders, 1964).

There is evidence that in subjects with atherosclerosis (clinical evidence of ischaemic heart disease) the blood clotting mechanism deviates from normality in that heparin is not so effective in these subjects. Similarly the blood platelets in these subjects exhibit an increased stickiness to glass (McDonald, 1957). Laboratory studies

along these lines taken in conjunction with the pathological data have directed attention to the thrombotic component in the aetiology of atherosclerosis.

The abundant evidence suggesting that atheromatous lesions are rich in both protein and lipid presents a major problem in attempts to reconcile all the variants of the lipid infiltration theory on the one hand, with the thrombogenic theory on the other. The usual histological interpretation that the thrombus undergoes "fatty degeneration" is difficult to explain on a metabolic basis; while, conversely, the deposition of lipids in vessels, which apparently predisposes to thrombus formation, is also difficult to explain. This has led many to the acceptance of a compromise explanation, in which the appearance of fatty flecks and lipid-laden streaks is ascribed to the passive lipid deposition or lipid infiltration, while the thrombus formation is considered as a different process but causally related to the vascular lipid changes. The lipid lesions may then be considered as a site for the "trigger reaction" involved in the blood clotting process by some mechanism as yet unexplained.

The pleomorphism of the lesion is unlikely to arise from a single factor, but rather from multicausal origins. The atheromatous process is a complex sequence involving various factors which may operate at widely different periods throughout the life-span of the individual.

Many studies have been conducted relating deaths due to ischaemic heart disease to various environmental, dietary, and other factors in different communities. If the percentage of calories ingested as fats in different communities is contrasted with the incidence of clinical manifestations of atherosclerosis, there is a positive correlation between these parameters. Thus the percentage caloric fat intake is low in Japan and in the Bantu community in South Africa, while the intake of fat is high in the United States, Canada and Britain. The mortality from ischaemic heart disease is much higher in these latter countries than it is in Japan or in the Bantu community in South Africa. A great deal of attention has been focused on figures of this sort, and many observers have stressed the role of fat intake in the diet to a point which suggests that the only important causative agent is the lipid content of the diet.

Various attempts have been made to check the reliability of this hypothesis, and to annul differences in hereditary factors prevailing in different communities by a variety of crossover or translocation studies. Observations have been made upon the incidence of atherosclerotic diseases and lipid intake in Japanese subjects resident in their homeland, and Japanese who emigrated to the United States (Keys, Kimura, Kusukawa, Bronte-Stewart, Larsen & Keys, 1958). Similarly, Puerto Ricans resident in Puerto Rico have been contrasted with Puerto Ricans who have emigrated to the United States, while recent central European emigrants to Israel have been contrasted with more long-standing immigrants to that country (Toor, Katchalsky, Agmon & Allalouf, 1957).

All these studies have tended to support the thesis that racial or hereditary factors can be cancelled by environmental and/or dietetic factors, because an individual belonging to a community in which the prevalence of this disease is low very rapidly acquires the almost identical disease rate of the group in which he elects to live.

The major effort in much cardiovascular research is to establish the relative significance of the environmental or socio-economic factors, including physical exercise, smoking and the consumption of diets higher in calories than the energy expenditure requires. The diets often contain a high percentage of calories from lipids, and the latter usually are dairy products of animal fats which have a high percentage of saturated fatty acids in the dietary triglycerides. This subject has been studied in depth in a great many centres and it has been suggested that the consumption of frugal vegetarian diets in the "underdeveloped countries" contributes to their relative immunity from atherosclerosis.

If the concept is correct that some dietary factor or factors are causally related to the production of arterial lesions, then it should be possible to influence the production of these lesions by manipulation of the amount of the dietary factors ingested by a population. On the basis of the epidemiological studies cited previously, the causative agent might be assumed to be some constituent of the lipid portion of the diet, or a critical concentration of the dietary calories ingested as lipid. This will be discussed in a later section.

During the second world war, certain European communities were subjected to dietary restriction in which the amount of lipid available to the community was drastically reduced. The very dramatic decrease in death rate from vascular diseases in Norway and Finland during this period has been attributed to the fall in consumption of dairy produce (Malmros, 1950; Strøm & Jensen, 1951). Unfortunately, while these figures are very impressive, the observations suffer from the major

defect that the community was not merely subjected to a change in diet during this period, as many other alterations to environmental factors were also operative. Obviously it is exceedingly difficult to achieve a major change in the dietary intake of a community under conditions in which the individuals in that community are free to choose their way of life and diet for themselves. The ideal situation would be one in which it was possible to manipulate the content of the diet of one group of *normal* individuals, and observe the prognosis of this group when contrasted with a similar matched group drawn from the same community balanced with respect to age, sex, etc. Various studies along these general lines are at present being made throughout the world, and when the results of studies such as these emerge (in general a study of this sort may take from five to ten years) we should be in a much stronger position in our assessment of the role of certain dietary factors in the aetiology of atherosclerosis. This will be discussed in a subsequent section dealing with preventative measures.

It has been known for centuries that certain degenerative changes in arteries are associated with the appearance of lipids in the lesions, and Vogel (1847) discovered that cholesterol was a constituent of atheromatous plaques. Anitschkow (1913) performed the experiment which has been repeated countless times since, namely the feeding of cholesterol to rabbits, which produces arterial lesions bearing a close similarity to certain lesions occurring spontaneously in man. Much of the older literature on this aspect of the subject has been reviewed in monographs (Cowdry, 1933, Mitchell & Schwartz, 1965, Constantinides, 1965).

The administration of cholesterol to the rabbit results in a marked plasma hypercholesterolaemia, and the severity of the arterial lesion produced in this species correlates fairly well with both the plasma cholesterol level and with the length of the period of sustained hypercholesterolaemia. Using modified dietary techniques, this generalization is true for various other species such as the rat (Wissler, Eilert, Schroeder & Cohen, 1954), dog (Steiner & Kendall, 1946), chick (Kesten, Meeker & Jobling, 1936), monkey (Mann, Andrus, McNally & Stare, 1953) and many other birds and mammals. Experimental atherosclerosis has been reviewed by Katz & Stamler (1953), Constantinides (1965), and Sandler & Bourne (1963).

There is considerable evidence that in certain humans, in whom there is present marked plasma hypercholesterolaemia, such as in "familial

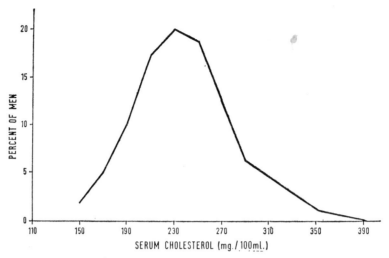

FIG. 18.1. Distribution of serum cholesterol levels in 1875 men, by age. Framingham study (redrawn).

hypercholesterolaemia'', xanthomatosis, etc., these individuals exhibit an arterial lesion comparable to the cholesterol-fed rabbit. Also these subjects present with clinical evidence of atheroma, such as coronary artery disease, at an earlier age than comparable individuals who are not hyperlipaemic.

Furthermore, in a fairly large section of the population, who present with clinical evidence of coronary artery disease and in whom it is assumed there is greater than average coronary atheroma present, there is evidence of elevation of the plasma cholesterol level above that

prevailing in "normal" individuals derived from the same population.

The National Heart Institute of the Public Health Service (United States) acting through the Massachusetts Department of Public Health and the Framingham Health Department conducted a long term study of coronary heart disease over a period of at least twelve years in the town of Framingham. This longitudinal community study has provided unique data on the natural history of this disease. Through a prospective study of the general adult population of this town it has been possible to assess the significance of factors

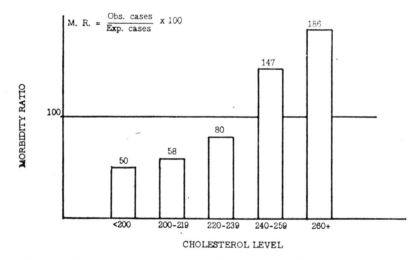

FIG. 18.2. Relation between plasma cholesterol levels and morbidity. Framingham study

in the host and in the environment which influence the incidence of coronary artery disease. By the judicious selection of a limited series of tests it has been shown that certain parameters are positively correlated with the incidence of this disease. Two important factors in this connection, which can be deemed to fall within the category of the biochemical basis of metabolic disease, are hypertension and hypercholesterolaemia. The former will be considered in another chapter of this book; the latter will be dealt with in this section.

The Framingham study indicated that healthy males showed an increased susceptibility to ischaemic heart disease with increasing plasma cholesterol concentration (Dawber, Kannell & Lyell, 1963). It was shown in this study that males having plasma cholesterol concentrations less than 200 mg./100 ml. had about one half of the average morbidity of the group. By contrast those men with plasma cholesterol concentrations exceeding 260 mg./100 ml. had nearly double the average morbidity of the group. (See Figs. 18.1 and 18.2.) This study has extremely important implications because it demonstrates that the subjects who presented prematurely with clinical evidence of atherosclerosis had elevated plasma lipid levels prior to the clinical presentation with the disease.

Plasma Lipids

The relationship between the plasma lipids and atherosclerosis has been extensively investigated for many years. If the blood plasma from a normal fasting subject is examined microscopically under dark ground illumination, small refractile particles can be seen. These spherical lipid particles are termed chylomicrons and consist mainly of triglyceride. These lipid particles only represent a small fraction of the total lipid present in normal fasting plasma, as most of the lipids in plasma are found in association with certain proteins. The lipid-protein molecules present in plasma are termed lipoproteins. Thus most of the plasma lipids are associated with the α and β globulins and this association of lipids with these specific proteins gives rise to a classification of the lipoproteins into α and β-lipoproteins. These macromolecular complexes consist of cholesterol, cholesterol esters, phospholipids, triglycerides and other lipids bound to the protein by secondary valence type bonds. A large number of reviews on lipoprotein structure have been published (Cornwell, 1967; Fredrickson *et al.*, 1967; Van den Heuvel, 1962; Lindgren & Nichols, 1960; Oncley, 1956).

In general, the ratio cholesterol:phospholipid (both expressed in mg.) present in the plasma β-lipoprotein is greater than 1:1 while the cholesterol:phospholipid ratio present in the plasma α-lipoprotein is about 1:2.

In most mammalian species both α- and β-lipoproteins are present in plasma, but the ratio of $\alpha:\beta$ varies considerably. For example, the average $\alpha:\beta$ lipoprotein ratio in man is about 30:70, in the rabbit it is about 50:50, while in the rat it is in the region of 90:10.

The plasma lipoproteins have been shown to be exceedingly heterogeneous, and the techniques of lipoprotein separation utilizing the ultra-centrifuge have given rise to a classification of the lipoproteins according to their sedimentation characteristics in media of different densities (Gofman, Lindgren, Elliott, Mantz, Hewitt, Strisower, Herring & Lyon, 1950; Lindgren, Elliott & Gofman, 1951).

The lipids in blood plasma can be classified into four main groups. These comprise the chylomicrons, the β-lipoproteins or low density lipoproteins, the pre-β-lipoproteins or very low density lipoproteins and the high density lipoproteins or α-lipoproteins. The plasma from a normal fasting subject may contain only β-lipoproteins and α-lipoproteins. After a fatty meal, a normal subject responds with an increase in the plasma chylomicron concentration which disappears a few hours after the fatty meal. The chemical composition of the plasma lipoproteins is shown in Table 18.1. In normal subjects the plasma β- and α-lipoproteins remain surprisingly constant throughout adulthood. Since it is known that certain hyperlipaemic states appear to be correlated with premature atherosclerosis or premature onset of the consequences of atherosclerosis, a great deal of attention has been given to the possibility of devising adequate biochemical screening techniques which could be applied to human plasma as possible diagnostic tests of the atherosclerotic state or pre-atherosclerotic states. In the opinion of many investigators the plasma cholesterol concentration remains the best single measurement for the detection of hyperlipaemic states. The frequency distribution pattern of plasma cholesterol in healthy American adult males is shown in Fig. 18.1, and the risk of developing "heart attack" compared with plasma cholesterol concentration in Fig. 18.2.

A number of investigators have preferred to use somewhat more sophisticated and certainly more complex techniques involving the use of the analytical ultra-centrifuge or zonal electrophoresis using different types of support and electro-

TABLE 18.1

Lipoprotein class	Chylomicrons	Very low-density lipo-proteins	Low-density lipoproteins	High-density lipoproteins
Specific gravity	0·94–0·98	0·98–1·006	1·006–1·063	1·063–1·21
Sf	400–40,000	20–400	0–20	—
Electrophoretic mobility	origin or a_2	pre-β or a_2	β_1	a_1
Approx. diameter (Å)	500–5000	ca. 400	ca. 200	ca. 100
Mol. wt.	ca. $4 \cdot 10^{10}$	$6 \cdot 10^{6}$	$2 \cdot 10^{6}$	$2 \cdot 10^{5}$
Percentage Chemical Composition				
Triglyceride	85	50	11	8
Cholesterol	2	7	8	3
Ester cholesterol	5	12	37	14
Phospholipid	6	18	22	22
NEFA	—	2	1	3
Protein	2	10	21	50
Apo-protein classification	A + B	A, B + C	B	A
N-Terminal amino acid	Asp + Glu	Asp + Glu + Ser + Thr	Glu	Asp
C-Terminal amino acid			Ser	Thr

phoretic conditions. The method which has become popular within recent years for screening plasma lipoprotein patterns in man (Lees & Hatch, 1963) is a modification of the paper electrophoretic method devised many years ago (see review by Pezold, 1961). By paper electrophoresis it is possible using a small amount of plasma to rapidly screen the sample to establish whether the lipoprotein pattern is that seen in normal young healthy subjects or whether the pattern is abnormal. Thus this semi-quantitative technique can rapidly demonstrate the presence of chylomicrons in a fasting plasma sample, the amount of β-lipoprotein present, the appearance of pre-β or very low density lipoprotein or the presence or absence of normal amounts of α-lipoprotein. This method has been simplified and

widely used by Fredrickson and colleagues and in their hands it has proved to be a useful screening method in order to obtain information for the possible phenotyping of plasma samples (Fredrickson, Levy & Lees, 1967). Fig. 18.3 shows a series of electrophoretograms obtained from normal subjects and from subjects with certain well characterized lipoprotein abnormalities. From a biochemical standpoint, when an investigator is confronted with a human plasma sample for evaluation of plasma lipids it is usually easier first to determine the plasma cholesterol concentration. If the plasma cholesterol concentration falls within the limits of normal values for the laboratory and in Britain this will usually be about 190 mg. ±35 mg. %, then there is usually little further requirement to pursue the

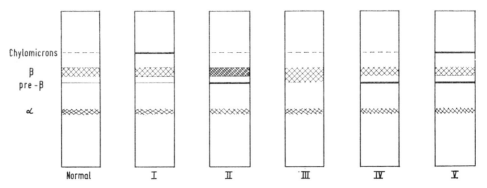

FIG. 18.3. Phenotyping of plasma lipoproteins—after Fredrickson & Lees (1965).

investigations. On the other hand, if the plasma cholesterol concentration is elevated it will be desirable to investigate the plasma hyperlipaemic situation. If the laboratory has facilities for the investigation of triglycerides then the plasma triglyceride concentration should be determined. If the plasma triglyceride concentration in a fasting subject exceeds 130 mg./100 ml. then this would be considered by many to be an abnormal state.

On the assumption that the plasma cholesterol concentration is raised and the plasma triglyceride concentration is normal or raised, it is then essential to investigate the situation to establish whether the hyperlipaemia is primary or secondary. Thus in the hypothyroid state, in biliary obstruction, in diabetes and many other pathological cirumstances there is a tendency towards elevated plasma lipid levels. In these conditions the plasma hyperlipaemia would be considered to be "secondary" because when the metabolic abnormality in the individual is corrected, either by the administration of thyroid hormone, by surgical intervention in biliary obstruction or by the treatment of the diabetic state then the plasma lipid levels will usually return to normal. If there is no known metabolic cause for the hyperlipaemic state then the hyperlipaemia is classified as primary and the investigator is then required to establish whether the abnormality is due to a familial factor or due to some other environmental factor such as a dietetic factor.

In the terminology of Fredrickson et al. (1967) Type 1 hyperlipaemia is due to an impairment in the ability to remove exogenous or dietary fat from plasma. In this situation the plasma chylomicron concentration is elevated and the serum cholesterol concentration is usually increased. In the Type 1 lipoprotein disorder the plasma triglycerides may be elevated about 18 hours after the last meal and this is thought to be due to the inability of the individual to clear the chylomicrons from the plasma. Under these circumstances the paper electrophoretogram shows a clear "chylomicron band" located at the origin. It is thought that the physiological removal of chylomicrons from blood plasma is due to a lipoprotein lipase which effects a "clearing reaction". In normals this enzyme can be induced by the administration of a small dose of heparin. The post-heparin lipoprotein lipase activity of the plasma sample is low in the Type 1 disorder.

In Type 2 lipoprotein disorder, the plasma cholesterol concentration is elevated. The fasting plasma triglyceride concentration is normal or only slightly elevated. The plasma electrophoretogram demonstrates a markedly elevated β-lipoprotein band and there may be evidence of a pre-β or very low density lipoprotein band on the paper electrophoretogram. The α-lipoprotein is normal. The post-heparin lipoprotein lipase activity of the plasma sample is normal.

In the Type 3 lipoprotein disorder the plasma cholesterol concentration and the plasma triglyceride concentration are both elevated. The appearance of the plasma may be either milky or clear. The electrophoretogram shows an elevated β-lipoprotein which extends into the pre-β or very low density lipoprotein zone on the paper strip. There is collateral evidence that the β-lipoprotein in this situation is abnormal in that it has a triglyceride content many times that observed in the normal β-lipoprotein. The post-heparin lipoprotein lipase activity in this situation is low.

The Type 4 plasma lipoprotein abnormality is again associated with an elevated plasma cholesterol concentration. In this instance the plasma triglyceride elevation is proportionately much greater than the elevation seen in the plasma cholesterol concentration and hence the plasma may be turbid. The paper electrophoresis findings on the plasma lipoproteins demonstrate a marked elevation of the pre-β or very low density lipoprotein concentration. The post-heparin lipoprotein lipase activity is usually normal in this situation.

The Type 5 lipoprotein abnormality is sometimes classified as a mixed hyperlipaemia. In this situation the plasma cholesterol concentration and the plasma triglyceride concentration are both elevated. As in the Type 4 situation the elevation of the plasma triglycerides greatly exceeds the elevation observed in the plasma cholesterol concentration. The plasma is invariably turbid and the electrophoretogram demonstrates a prominent chylomicron band and also a marked elevation in the pre-β or very low density lipoprotein band. As a rule the post-heparin lipoprotein lipase activity is low.

As far as can be established the Type 1 and Type 5 lipoprotein abnormalities are very rare. By contrast Types 2 and 4 are the principal abnormalities encountered in the hyperlipaemic states. Thus, when an investigator is confronted with a particular hyperlipaemic situation the problem is to devise a therapeutic procedure which will result in normalizing the plasma lipid pattern. Fortunately some of the plasma lipid abnormalities encountered in man can be corrected

TABLE 18.2

Types of hyperlipoproteinaemia as defined by various indexes to plasma lipoprotein concentrations[1]

Type	Appearance	Plasma lipids		Paper electrophoretic bands	Analytical ultracentrifuge Sf	Precipitation with high-molecular weight polymers	Immuno-precipitation (antiserum to β-lipoproteins)
		Cholesterol	Triglyceride				
I	Milky	↓	↑	Chylomicrons present; all other lipoproteins	100–400 ↑	Massive	Variable
II	Clear	↑	Normal or ↑	β↑ Pre-β↑	0–12 ↑ 100 ↑	Heavy	Heavy
III	Turbid	↑	↑	"Broad β" pre-β↑	0–12 ↓ 12–100 ↑	Heavy	Heavy
IV	Turbid	↑	↑	Pre-β↑	0–20 normal 20–400 ↑	Heavy	Variable
V	Turbid or milky	↑	↑	Chylomicron band present; pre-β↑	20–400 ↑	Heavy	Variable

[1] ↑ increased: ↓ decreased. (From Fredrickson *et al.* 1967.)

by various manipulations, however there are certain situations in which it seems impossible at the present time to correct the lipoprotein abnormality.

The various types of hyperlipoproteinaemia as defined by Fredrickson *et al.* (1967) are tabulated in Table 18.2.

Diagnostic Tests for Atherosclerosis

Many studies have been made within recent years to attempt to establish quantitative relevance to various physiological factors, in groups of individuals, to assess which factor or factors correlate best with the clinical or pathological evaluation of the degree of atherosclerosis present in different groups. Most of the comparative metabolic studies are designed either to elucidate the significance of a parameter in the pathogenesis of the process, or to establish the magnitude of the parameter's deviation from "normality" prevailing in an affected group. The aim of many investigations has been to find some simple "test", which would be indicative of atheromatous arterial involvement, and then to apply this to clinically normal subjects to predict future clinical events.

As discussed previously there is a great deal of support for the general thesis that the plasma cholesterol concentration tends to be higher in individuals presenting with coronary artery disease than in "normals" matched for age, sex, weight, etc. (Morrison, Hall & Chaney, 1948; Steiner, Kendall & Mathers, 1952). The difference between the average plasma cholesterol concentrations of the two groups is highly significant, but the overlap is great, and hence the plasma cholesterol concentration has a limited value as a prognostic test when applied to a given individual. Variants on this simple test have been proposed, such as the cholesterol/phospholipid (C/P) ratio, but once again there is little gain if any in discrimination between the total cholesterol and the C/P ratio (Ahrens & Kunkel, 1949).

As discussed previously, almost all the plasma cholesterol is carried as lipoprotein complexes with the α- and β-globulins. This has led to attempts to describe the plasma cholesterol in terms of cholesterol bound to the α-lipoprotein, compared to cholesterol bound to the β-lipoprotein, i.e. α/β ratio. Once again the α/β lipoprotein ratio is of interest in so far as it is reduced in subjects with clinical coronary artery disease (Barr, Russ, & Eder, 1951; Oliver & Boyd, 1953), but the α/β lipoprotein ratio is no better as a predictor of atherosclerosis than the plasma cholesterol level.

The heterogeneity of the β-lipoproteins suggested that perhaps there may be certain lipoproteins circulating which predispose the subjects to atherosclerosis. This led to descriptions of the β-lipoproteins in terms of their flotation characteristics in the ultracentrifuge (cf. Gofman *et al.*, 1954).

These studies by Gofman and collaborators resulted in the critical examination of different analytical techniques to establish whether any given plasma lipid determination was superior to another. A comprehensive study showed that the simple determination of the serum cholesterol level had as useful a "predictive" value, in terms of assessing the degree of atherosclerosis in an individual, as had the much more complex analysis involving for instance the ultracentrifugal separation of certain selected lipoproteins within the β-lipoprotein complex (Technical Group of the Committee on Lipoproteins and Athero-sclerosis, 1956).

The development of rapid and precise methods for the determination of plasma triglycerides has also led to the use of this parameter in the screening of the population. The re-introduction of paper electrophoresis has resulted in the differentiation of the plasma hyperlipaemia becoming greatly simplified. This subject was discussed previously and has been reviewed by Fredrickson *et al.* (1967).

Hereditary Aspects of Atherosclerosis

There is a great deal of evidence to support the hypothesis that in certain instances metabolic abnormalities, which lead to the production of plasma hyperlipaemias are under genetic in-fluences. The plasma cholesterol levels are known to be elevated in xanthoma tuberosum and in xanthoma tendinosum. In both these conditions there is usually present premature athero-sclerosis, as well as the deposition of lipids in-cluding cholesterol in certain other non-vascular sites (Fagge, 1873; Montgomery, 1940).

There are instances in which plasma hyper-cholesterolaemia occurs as a genetic expression, without evidence of xanthomatosis, as a com-plicating factor. Nevertheless, in those families in which familial hypercholesterolaemia is pre-sent, there is a predisposition to premature atheromatous complications.

The mode of inheritance of familial hyper-cholesterolaemia has been the subject of a large number of studies. The precise genetic mechanism, especially with regard to the problem of hyper-cholesterolaemia occurring with and without xanthomatosis, has not yet been settled. In view of the complications arising out of the degrees of severity of hypercholesterolaemia observed in certain families, theories have been advanced that the xanthomatosis could be explained on

the basis of a single dominant gene (Stecher & Hersh, 1949), or due to a single gene, or the concurrence of two abnormal alleles (Epstein, Block, Hand & Francis, 1959), or that the gene is incompletely dominant (Adlersberg, Parets & Boas, 1949; Wilkinson, 1950).

In a number of instances of essential hyper-cholesterolaemia, a continuous transition can be observed relating the degree of hypercholesterol-aemia, or the period of hypercholesterolaemia, to the severity of the xanthomatosis, and for the production of xanthoma tendinosum the time factor has been stressed by Hood & Angerval, (1959).

The genetic factors which influence the plasma lipids can be considered apart from the environ-mental or dietetic factors. Nevertheless, there is a marked interrelationship between genetic and environmental factors, because the hereditary factors influence markedly the susceptibility of an individual in an unfavourable environment. It is unfortunate that the precise biochemical defect underlying the genetic differences which exist in the handling of the plasma lipids has not been more clearly defined.

Platelets

It was shown by Born (1956) that blood pla-telets have a high ATP concentration. It was later shown by the same worker (Born, 1958), that the concentration of ADP in platelets de-creased during the clotting of platelet-rich plasma. In 1961, Gaarder, Jonsen, Laland, Hellem & Owren discovered that very low con-centrations of ADP affect blood platelets and bring about an adhesion and aggregation of the platelets. These authors concluded that the release of ADP may play an important role in the trigger mechanism of the initial phases of the thrombotic reaction. Later, Born (1962) investi-gated the mechanism of platelet adhesion and aggregation. By the use of a spectrophotometric method this worker was able to show that concentrations of about 2.5×10^{-7}M ADP were sufficient to influence platelet behaviour *in vitro*. Under the conditions of this platelet assay it was shown that at 2.5×10^{-6}M ADP the maximum effect of this nucleotide on blood platelets was achieved. These *in vitro* studies suggested that the stickiness or adhesiveness of blood platelets was markedly affected by nucleo-tides such as ADP. When the concentration of ADP was low, the platelets could be shown to aggregate, and after an interval of several minutes the platelets tended to dis-aggregate and return to their initial physiological state. If the con-

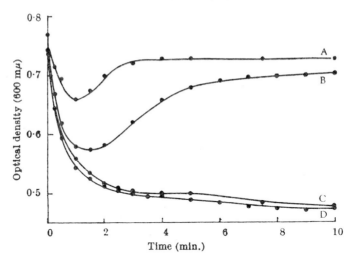

FIG. 18.4. The effect of varying concentration of ADP on platelet aggregations *in vitro*. (Born)

centration of ADP was higher then the platelets aggregated and there was no subsequent dis-aggregation (see Fig. 18.4). Born & Cross (1963) showed that ADP affected platelets similarly *in vivo*.

It has been known for a long time that when platelets adhere to charged surfaces, such as discontinuities in the intimal surface of the arterial system, or collagen (Zucker & Borelli, 1962), then the platelets form into a platelet mass. After a period of adhesion the platelets may undergo a morphological change which is sometimes termed platelet viscous metamor-phosis (Eberth & Schimmelbusch, 1889). As a result of electron microscope studies coupled to biochemical and physiological investigations on the role of nucleotides, such as ADP, in platelet behaviour, it has been possible to arrive at a working hypothesis which serves as a basis for atherosclerosis research (Hellem & Owren, 1964).

As a result of epidemiological investigations which have been conducted in the United States, there is now little doubt that hyperlipaemic and hypertensive phases precede the clinical presen-tation or thrombotic tendency in most indivi-duals presenting with a myocardial infarction. Thus, from the Framingham studies (Dawber, Kannel & Lyell, 1963) it has become clear that if an individual has an elevated plasma lipid concentration and is also hypertensive, then the probability of this individual presenting pre-maturely with coronary artery disease, or some other manifestation of atherosclerosis, is much greater than in an individual whose plasma lipid concentration is normal and who is normo-tensive. Furthermore, there seems little doubt that the combination of hyperlipaemia and hypertension predisposes experimental animals to the deposition of lipids in the arterial intima giving rise to fatty flecks and fatty streaks. The question then arises regarding the possibility that the impairment of the endothelial lining by the deposition of the fatty material is a sufficient alteration to the intimal surface to pro-duce a situation which predisposes to the aggregation and perhaps increased adhesiveness of the passing blood platelets (see Mustard, 1961; Haslam, 1964). If the alteration to the vascular wall is sufficient to change the blood platelets then the platelets may stick to the arterial intima and in sticking they may release ADP and other nucleotides. Consequently the elevated local concentration of ADP will bring about an in-creased stickiness of platelets in the immediate vicinity. This explanation hints at a type of chain reaction in which a platelet, on sticking to a rough or charged surface, releases ADP which influences the stickiness of nearby platelets. This explanation is in fact the basis of some of the modern views on the role of platelets in the aetiology of atherosclerosis. Therefore, a great deal of effort has been expended on the investi-gation of compounds which may antagonize ADP-mediated platelet adhesiveness. Adenosine and derivatives of adenosine have been studied with a view to the development of substances of potential therapeutic usefulness in the control of platelet adhesion and cohesion (Clayton, Born & Cross, 1963; Born, Honour & Mitchell, 1964).

While platelet aggregation as such does not necessarily promote fibrin formation, nevertheless platelets and platelet factors play an important role in blood coagulation and thrombus formation. For instance, the blood clotting system is activated by enzymes and phospholipids released by damaged tissues and by blood platelets.

One question which has occupied the attention of investigators is the possibility that the blood platelets in patients presenting with ischaemic heart disease may have characteristics different from those found in normal individuals. In much the same way the blood clotting mechanism has also been extensively investigated to contrast patients with "normals". It is well known that heparin is less effective as an anti-coagulant in patients with ischaemic heart disease than in normal subjects, and this expression of heparin resistance is apparent when studied by *in vivo* and by *in vitro* methods. In much the same way the blood platelets from subjects with ischaemic heart disease appear to be much more adhesive to foreign surfaces such as glass than the blood platelets from normal subjects (MacDonald, 1957). However the blood platelets from individuals with ischaemic heart disease show a normal reaction towards exogenous ADP. Minor lesions within the intimal surface of the arterial system will result in a change in the characteristics of the endothelial lining which may activate the clotting mechanism and influence platelet adhesion. This combination of a change in the blood clotting mechanism and increased platelet adhesiveness may well be an important factor in the production of thrombosis at certain specific arterial sites. At the present time there is considerable interest in the control of platelet stickiness and aggregation under the influence of hormones such as adrenaline and the prostaglandins (Kloeze, 1966; Emmons, Hampton, Harrison, Honour & Mitchell, 1967; Clayton & Cross, 1963).

Thrombosis

The morphological evidence cited previously emphasized that thrombosis may be an important factor in the development of advanced vascular lesions. It is well known that there are a number of factors involved in the production of thrombosis. These include the protein factors present in blood plasma some of which lead to the ultimate conversion of soluble plasma fibrinogen into plasma fibrin, which is insoluble and fibrous in nature. Apart from factors in blood plasma involved in the thrombotic process it is also well known that the thrombocytes or platelets are also implicated in the thrombotic process, as cited previously. When a vessel wall is damaged, the platelets adhere to the area of endothelial injury and also adhere to one another and build up a microscopic entity sometimes termed a white body. These white bodies are composed almost entirely of platelets without any adhering fibrin. The aggregation of platelets which may be observed *in vitro* has much in common with the platelet thrombi observed *in vivo*. The *in vitro* aggregation can be accelerated by adenosine diphosphate in low concentrations. During thrombus formation some of the formed elements present in normal blood such as the red blood cells, the white blood cells or the platelets may disrupt and release adenosine diphosphate into the blood plasma. Thus any situation which results in the release of ADP into plasma could trigger off platelet aggregation. It is therefore inferred that adhesion and aggregation of platelets may be initial stages in the production of haemostatic plugs and thrombi. Various *in vitro* studies have emphasized however that certain stages of platelet aggregation may in fact be reversible. The end-product of the activity of a cascade of enzymes involved in blood coagulation is of course the conversion of fibrinogen to fibrin. The platelet aggregation appears to be independent of the clotting mechanism, but the formation of effective haemostatic plugs and thrombi requires clotting for its completion. There is evidence that when platelets undergo aggregation under the influence of ADP a specific phospholipid may be released during this process. It seems possible that the platelets participate in the clotting mechanism by the provision of such a specific phospholipid essential for the normal clotting process.

The blood clotting mechanism can also be activated by certain saturated fatty acids and these fatty acids can also bring about aggregation of platelets. It has been shown that the rapid infusion of saturated fatty acids into the blood of animals can produce thrombosis.

It has been suggested that atheromatous lesions may present to the elements in the blood an abnormal surface which results in activation of the clotting mechanism as well as promoting platelet adhesion. These circumstances could result in an increased coagulability of the blood in the presence of the increased platelet stickiness.

Dietary Aspects of Atherosclerosis

Various studies have been performed on the relationship of certain dietary factors to the plasma lipids in man and experimental animals. Since much of the early interest in atherosclerosis and the plasma lipids centred on the plasma cholesterol concentration, it was reasonable that the cholesterol content of the diet should be suspected as a factor influencing the plasma cholesterol concentration.

It is known that possibly all mammalian nucleated cells have the ability to synthesize cholesterol from non-sterol precursors, and from a quantitative standpoint the plasma lipoproteins and hence the plasma cholesterol largely originate by hepatic synthesis. There is, however, growing evidence for the contribution to the plasma cholesterol compartment by cholesterol synthesis in the gut.

It is also known that, from a quantitative aspect, the bile acids are the principal degradation products of cholesterol metabolism (see review by Danielsson, 1968). Since the plasma and liver cholesterol contents can be treated as a single metabolic pool, the concentration of the circulating cholesterol is therefore dependent upon two opposing processes, namely the rate of cholesterol synthesis and the rate of cholesterol removal or degradation. Much of the newly synthesized cholesterol from the liver is discharged into the bile, together with bile salts formed by hepatic degradation of cholesterol. The biliary cholesterol and bile salts mix with the dietary cholesterol and other lipids and the bile salts discharge their function as surface active agents in facilitating the absorption of triglycerides, cholesterol and other lipids from the small intestine. Thus, the endogenous and exogenous cholesterol become equilibrated and, as the amount of cholesterol synthesized by an adult man is of the order of 1–3 g./day, the contribution of cholesterol derived from the diet to this pool rarely exceeds half the endogenous contribution. Furthermore, experiments have shown that the rate of cholesterol synthesis can be influenced by dietary cholesterol, which acts as a feed-back mechanism on the synthetic process (Gould & Taylor, 1950; Gould & Swyrd, 1967; Wilson, 1964).

The results of a large number of experiments, in which the dietary intake of cholesterol has been varied within the usual limits of the normal diet, suggest that the amount of cholesterol present in the diet exerts little influence on the plasma cholesterol concentration (Keys, Anderson, Mickelsen, Adelson & Fidanza, 1956).

From a quantitative standpoint the principal lipid in the normal diet is of course triglyceride. The concentration of triglyceride in the diet has been implicated in the aetiology of atherosclerosis for many years. In general, support for this thesis has been derived from the epidemiological studies which have been cited previously. It has been shown that if other factors are held constant, then, as the percentage of calories in the diet derived from triglyceride increases, the serum cholesterol concentration also increases. It is well known that the saturated fatty acids and the mono-unsaturated acids tend to elevate the plasma cholesterol concentration, whereas the poly-unsaturated fatty acids of the linoleic acid, linolenic or arachidonic acid type tend to decrease the plasma cholesterol concentration (Kinsell et al., 1953; Kingsbury, 1961). Since the latter acids are essential for the growth and well-being of certain species (Burr & Burr, 1929) they have been termed the essential fatty acids. These acids have not yet been definitely demonstrated to be essential in adult man, but as they exert an effect as plasma cholesterol concentration depressants, this action has been cited by certain authors as support of the thesis that poly-unsaturated fatty acids are essential dietary factors. The difficulty in assessing the "essential" nature of these acids in human nutrition arises out of the difficulty of obtaining an edible diet utilizing purified ingredients, which can be shown to be devoid of extraneous trace amounts of poly-enoic acids. Until a diet of this type is available in quantity and fed to humans for fairly long periods it will be impossible to assess accurately the claim that essential fatty acids have a vitamin-like role in adult human nutrition. While certain poly-unsaturated fatty acids achieve a depression in the concentration of the circulating cholesterol, they also bring about an alteration to the types of fatty acid esterified as cholesterol esters. When the dietary intake of linoleic acid is raised above the normal level for a given individual, the plasma cholesterol concentration decreases and the proportion of cholesterol linoleate in the cholesterol ester fraction increases (Schrade, Böhle & Biegler, 1961). It has therefore been concluded that in a normal diet one of the factors which dictates the plasma cholesterol concentration is the ratio of the long-chain saturated acids plus the mono-enoic acids contrasted with the dietary poly-unsaturated fatty acids (Ahrens, Hirsch, Insull & Peterson, 1958). The compositions of animal and vegetable triglycerides are very different; also the fatty acid composition within these two classes varies with the source of the triglycerides. As a general rule the vegetable triglycerides tend to contain higher proportions of unsaturated fatty acids. However the range of fatty acids found in different plant sources can vary a great deal. For example olive oil contains about 80% oleic acid (mono-unsaturated) while safflower seed oil contains about 80% linoleic acid (di-unsaturated).

It has been shown that mammals can synthesize long-chain saturated and mono-unsaturated fatty acids of the oleic acid type (Mead, 1960). The available evidence suggests that the endogenous synthesis of poly-unsaturated fatty acids (of the methylene-interrupted type) such as linoleic acid does not occur in mammalian tissues to an appreciable extent (Mead, 1960). Using the formula-type diets and specially purified single fatty acids or triglycerides synthesized with specific fatty acid compositions, an attempt has been made to establish whether a given dietary regimen or purified fatty acid influences the plasma cholesterol level in man (Ahrens, Hirsch, Insull & Peterson, 1958). The long-chain saturated fatty acids and the mono-enoic fatty acids tend to elevate the plasma cholesterol concentration in man while the polyenoic fatty acids tend to lower the plasma cholesterol concentration.

The precise mechanism by which the polyunsaturated fatty acids influence the cholesterol concentration has not yet been elucidated. While there is evidence from various sources that by increasing the linoleate content of the diet in certain animals, the rate of cholesterol synthesis can be increased, the rate of cholesterol removal and/or catabolism is accelerated to an even greater

degree. Thus the turnover rate of the plasma cholesterol is increased when the linoleate content of the diet is increased. At the present time it is not yet known whether linoleate influences the excretion of cholesterol as neutral sterols (Spritz, Ahrens & Grundy, 1965) or alternatively increases the breakdown of cholesterol to bile acids (Lewis, 1959; Wood, Shioda & Kinsell, 1966). Evidence has been presented in support of both mechanisms.

It has been known since the early 1930's that human seminal plasma contained a vasodepressor and smooth-muscle stimulating substance. It was discovered in the 1940's that the substance was lipid-soluble and acidic. Two biologically active acids were isolated in crystalline form by Bergström & Sjövall (1957). The acids were shown to be C_{20}, contained a five membered ring and were named prostaglandin E_1 (PGE$_1$) and prostaglandin $F_{1\alpha}$ (PGF$_{1\alpha}$). This subject has been reviewed by Bergström & Samuelsson (1967).

Due to the studies of Bergström and colleagues (Bergström, Danielsson & Samuelsson, 1964) and van Dorp and colleagues (Dorp, Beerthuis, Nugteren & Vonkeman, 1964) it has been established that certain of the essential fatty acids are precursors of the prostaglandins. This group of novel compounds exerts a marked effect on smooth muscle and this is shown by their influence on blood pressure and certain other parameters. The structure of prostaglandin E_2 (PGE$_2$) is shown in Fig. 18.5. The relationship between arachidonic acid and PGE$_2$ is also shown in the figure. The

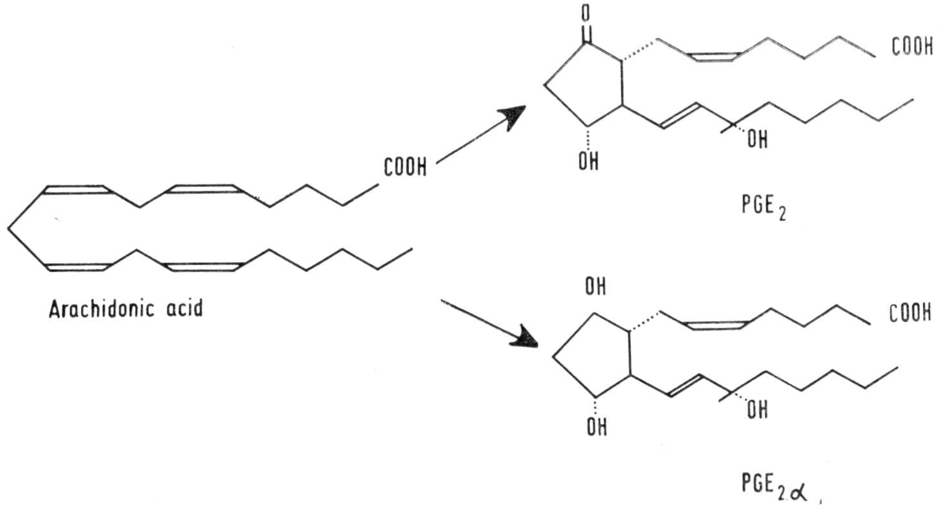

FIG. 18.5. Structure of Prostaglandin E_2.

prostaglandins are rapidly metabolized in tissues such as the lungs to products of the type shown in Fig. 18.5.

The prostaglandins decrease the blood pressure and also decrease platelet stickiness. Thus from the standpoint of experimental atherosclerosis the essential fatty acids as precursors of these hormones would at least (in theory) have an extremely beneficial effect because, if the release of prostaglandins could be a factor of physiological significance in lowering blood pressure and decreasing platelet stickiness *in vivo*, and as both these effects are in a direction deemed to be "anti-atherogenic", then the essential fatty acids would appear to be very desirable. This does not of course explain the mechanism of the lowering of the plasma cholesterol concentration in individuals where essential fatty acids have been administered as a substitute for saturated fatty acids or mono-unsaturated fatty acids in the diet. It is possible that the lowering of the plasma cholesterol concentration is a secondary effect or unrelated to the prostaglandin effects. It is obvious that this will be an extremely fruitful field for further investigation during the next few years.

Plasma Enzyme Studies

The most serious complication of atheromatous involvement of the coronary vessels is the tendency to occlusive thrombosis in these vessels. The resultant ischaemia frequently produces pain, ECG changes and other effects secondary to the anoxia of the myocardium. The myocardium is known to be rich in the enzymes of the transaminase group (Cohen & Hekhuis, 1941). It was shown by LaDue, Wroblewski & Karmen (1954) that plasma transaminase levels were elevated in subjects experiencing a myocardial infarction. The plasma enzymic activity reached a peak about 24–28 hr. after the predicted coronary occlusive incident, and then declined to the pre-ischaemic level within 4 to 6 days (Steinberg & Ostrow, 1955). (See Fig. 18.6). These results were interpreted as due to the release of the enzyme from the cells of the myocardium which were undergoing necrotic change. It was subsequently shown that this change in plasma transaminase could be a useful adjunct to other tests for diagnosis of coronary occlusion in instances where the ECG evidence or other clinical findings required substantiation. This test is complicated if there is evidence of liver dysfunction, or in instances in which there may be other ischaemic areas apart from the myocardium (Wroblewski, 1959). Acute tissue breakdown in heart, liver,

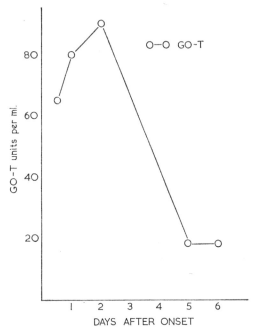

FIG. 18.6. The changes in glutamic-oxaloacetic transaminase in the serum of patients who have suffered a myocardial infarction.
Redrawn with permission of the author—Alldis, D. (1962). *Proc. Assoc. Clin. Bioch.* **II**, 21–26.

skeletal muscle, kidney or brain, may cause elevated serum levels by release of enzymes from the damaged tissue.

Animal studies have indicated that as little as 1 g. of infarcted heart muscle may be detected by this method. The degree and duration of serum enzyme elevations are roughly proportional to the mass of infarcted muscle.

There have been many refinements to the original enzymic assay, and most of these have been aimed at creating a simplified version of the test suitable for routine use. Most of the assays in use employ the technique whereby the activity of the transaminase enzyme can be measured in terms of a change in the NAD:NADH coenzyme system, and hence the assay can be conducted in a spectrophotometer cell (Karmen *et al.*, 1955). The transaminase enzyme of heart muscle catalyses the transference of an amino group from an L-α-amino acid to a suitable keto-acid acceptor, e.g.

l-aspartate + α-ketoglutarate $\rightleftharpoons$ oxaloacetate + l-glutamate
oxaloacetate + NADH + H^+ $\rightleftharpoons$ malate + NAD^+

In the presence of an excess of malate dehydrogenase, and if adequate controls are inserted in the assay procedure, it is possible to measure the activity of the transaminase enzyme in terms of the change in the absorption band of NADH at 340 mμ. This subject has been reviewed by Aspen & Meister (1958) and by Halmolsky (1967, 1968).

Since the original introduction of the serum transaminase enzyme assay into cardiological practice the search has continued for other enzymes in plasma which may be easier to determine or more specific for myocardium undergoing necrotic changes (see Halmolsky, 1967, 1968).

Many enzymes have been investigated in this connection.

Lactic dehydrogenase values are generally increased within the first 18 hours after myocardial infarction. The peak is reached in 2 to 4 days, and returns to normal by 14 days.

The concept of isoenzymes has stimulated research for methods to detect in serum a component specific for the myocardium.

Creatine phosphokinase (CPK) catalyses the phosphorylation of creatine with ATP. This enzyme is present in high concentration in the myocardium. Serum CPK increases about 6 hours after infarction and reaches a maximum after 18 hours. It is claimed by some authors, (Konttinen & Halonen, 1962; Sorensen, 1963) that this enzyme is more sensitive and selective for myocardial infarction than most of the others studied.

At the present time SGOT and SCPK appear to be the tests of choice within the first two days of suspected infarction.

Preventive Measures for Atherosclerosis

There is considerable interest in possible preventive measures, which may be instituted either to arrest the process of atheromatosis, or to achieve regression of the lesions.

Unfortunately it is not possible as yet to obtain direct objective evidence of the degree of vascular involvement in an individual during life. Consequently, the reasoning behind most of the studies is dependent upon the acceptance of the hypothesis that presentation with the clinical manifestations of atherosclerosis can be used as a measure of the degree of atheromatosis in the individual. Secondly, the hypothesis depends upon the theory that the degree of atheromatosis is a function of some factor in the blood plasma such as the plasma lipids. Thirdly, the

hypothesis requires that atheromatous lesions be amenable to arrest or regression.

There is little doubt that the early uncomplicated fatty streaks, which are produced in hyperlipaemic animals and individuals, can be made to regress. However, the more complex pleomorphic lesions which comprise the atheroma present in, for example, the coronary arteries of adults, present a different problem, and whether these lesions will diminish or their development can be arrested, by, for example, plasma lipid changes, is a question which cannot be definitely answered at the moment. Nevertheless, a great deal of effort has been put into the design and execution of experiments in attempts to tackle some of these questions, and to this end a number of dietary and drug trials have been conducted to depress the plasma cholesterol of humans on a long-term basis in order to investigate the influence of these measures on the morbidity and mortality of the subjects. Only a few of these regimens and drugs will be considered in this chapter.

Diet

The problem which confronts the clinical investigator involved in plasma cholesterol-lowering studies is to decide on which section of the community the regimen will be applied. In most of the larger centres it is possible to obtain fairly substantial numbers of patients who have experienced a myocardial infarction and who are amenable to suggestions regarding manipulation of their diets. The subjects are well motivated, because it can be explained to them that a change in their dietary habits might be to their advantage. From a large number of studies conducted in many centres throughout the world it is now well documented that by lowering the total fat intake of the diet and substituting triglycerides containing polyunsaturated fatty acids for triglycerides containing monoenoic fatty acids or saturated fatty acids then the plasma cholesterol concentration can be lowered. Furthermore it is possible to keep the plasma cholesterol concentration fairly steady at this lower level for periods of many years. In most studies conducted along these lines where the individuals have received instruction on the selection of their diet and have received a suitable polyunsaturated fatty acid supplement to their diet the results in terms of alteration to the morbidity and mortality of the "test" group have been equivocal.

Hood (1965) presented evidence on a follow-up on over one hundred individuals who had suffered a myocardial infarction and who had been given advice on alteration to the diet. Although the numbers in this study were small the outcome was in favour of the subjects who had achieved a lowering of the plasma cholesterol concentration in that there were fewer myocardial infarctions in the dietary controlled group than in the control group. Also from Scandinavia, Leren (1966) presented evidence on the effect of a plasma cholesterol-lowering diet in one half of a group of 412 male survivors of myocardial infarction. This investigator found that the cholesterol-lowering diet marginally reduced the incidence of total coronary heart disease relapses when studied over a period of five years. Similarly Christakis *et al.* (1966) have shown that in their study in the New York Anti-coronary Club beneficial effects have been found using a dietary approach to the prevention of coronary heart disease when studied over a seven-year period.

A report of a research committee to the Medical Research Council, London (1968) used an experimental design similar to that employed by Leren (1966). Again, this trial was designed to test the value of a serum cholesterol-lowering diet in the prevention of relapse in men aged under 60 who were recently recovered from a first myocardial infarction. There were 199 men in the experimental group who were given a diet low in saturated fats and containing 85 g. of soya bean oil daily. The control group contained 194 men who consumed their ordinary diet. Both groups were studied regularly and clinical examinations as well as plasma lipid studies investigated. These investigators concluded that this trial gave little support to the suggestion that a diet of the kind used in trial could be recommended in the treatment of patients who had suffered a myocardial infarction. They conclude that, taken in conjunction with the study of Leren, there is no indication that a diet of this sort affects the mortality of the subjects. The authors conclude that this diet may affect a proportion of non-fatal re-infarctions but the numbers were too small to merit high statistical significance to this point. The authors of this report are cautious because they conclude "it must be emphasized finally that these results apply to secondary prevention, that is to the treatment of men who have had an attack of coronary heart disease". The importance of such diets in primary prevention remains to be assessed. The results of these studies are summarized in Table 18.3. Therefore in some studies there has been a marginal benefit on the side of the subjects who have altered their diet (Leren 1966) and in other studies the outcome has been less

TABLE 18.3

	London study	Oslo study
Number of men in trial	393	412
Number aged less than 60 at entry to trial	390	257
Initial plasma cholesterol concentration		
(a) test group	272	296
(b) control group	273	296
Soya bean oil in test diet (g./day)	85	75
Ratio of saturated fatty acids/ poly-unsaturated fatty acids in the test diet	1:1·8	1:2·4
Period of observation (years)	2 to 6	5

(Extract from a table in the *Lancet* September 28th, 1968, page 693).

clear (Research Comm. M.R.C., 1968). The essential problem is that after a myocardial infarction the survival of a subject may not be dictated by the same set of parameters which lead to the initial clinical incident or myocardial infarction. Thus, if coronary thrombosis is related to coronary atherosclerosis and if the degree of coronary atherosclerosis is in some way either directly or indirectly related to the plasma lipid concentrations, then it would seem possible that by lowering the plasma lipid concentration it might be possible to influence the rate of progress of the coronary atherosclerotic process. However, the clinical progress of the disease is discontinuous in that after the acute episode, such as a myocardial infarction, in which a portion of the myocardium is irreversibly damaged, then the prognosis of the individual may no longer be a function of the factors which are involved in the progress of coronary atherosclerosis. It is for this reason that investigators wish to study a population in the pre-ischaemic state. Ideally, the best population would be one in which the subjects were "at risk". This would be a population where the plasma lipid concentrations were perhaps higher than usual and a population where the subjects were "healthy". If the original premise is correct that the rate of increase of coronary atherosclerosis is a function of the plasma lipid concentration, then by lowering the plasma lipids it should be possible to arrest or even cause regression of the coronary atheroma. If the stage of development of the coronary atheroma is related to the clinical incidence of myocardial infarction, then in such a group of "at risk" subjects, manipulation of the plasma lipids should alter the morbidity and mortality of the group. An ambitious scheme along these lines has been projected in the United States called the National Diet-Heart Study and a feasibility trial has been completed (Circulation, Supplement 1, 1968). In this feasibility trial a large number of subjects were studied in different centres and their diet was manipulated using a method whereby the foodstuffs purchased by given families had been prepared from materials of vegetable origin and of known polyunsaturated fatty acid composition. Thus the community was divided into a "test" section whose percentage intake of polyunsaturated fatty acids was higher than the other "control" section of the community, and furthermore the total fat content of the "test" diet was lower than that prevailing in the "control" section. This type of experiment is expensive to design and execute; it requires the collaboration of a large number of investigators and subjects.

It has been suggested from the data obtained in the feasibility study that if about 50,000 volunteers could be obtained for such an experiment and if the volunteers could adhere to the diet for periods of perhaps five years, then it would be possible to obtain definitive evidence on the effect of lowering and altering (qualitatively) the fat intake in the diet. This raises an important issue because many organizations and governments are pondering on the issue regarding the advisability of waiting for the outcome of an experiment of this sort when it is known that the result cannot be obtained for five years after the start of the study, and this investigation has not yet started. Many feel that the situation is sufficiently clear to allow advice to be given that the fat intake in the diet should be decreased and the intake from polyunsaturated fatty acids be elevated. This attitude is not universally accepted in that many wish to adopt an extremely cautious attitude on the basis that the polyunsaturated fatty acids are substances present in a normal diet, and we have no evidence of a sub-clinical deficiency state in man. These fatty acids are non-toxic components of the diet and are known to be essential precursors of a group of hormones termed prostaglandins. It seems reasonable that the suggestion that the polyunsaturated fatty acid intake might be elevated should be actively considered as the most rational way to the manipulation of plasma lipid concentrations at the present time. By contrast with all the known drugs, the polyunsaturated fatty acids are completely devoid of side effects. This cannot be said of any of the drugs in use at the present time.

We are therefore left with an important problem: by lowering the caloric intake from lipids in the diet and by the substitution of polyunsaturated fatty acids for monoenoic fatty acids or saturated fatty acids in the diet it is possible to reduce the plasma lipid concentration. Until the National Diet-Heart Study is complete we will not be in a position to assess the significance of dietary manipulations of this sort to individuals in the pre-ischaemic state.

Many will wish to accept the interim recommendations of bodies such as the American Heart Association that, although absolute evidence on these points has not yet been obtained, in the meantime many individuals might benefit by altering their dietary habits now. It is for this reason that a considerable burden falls upon governments, and indeed on the food industry, to examine the possible ways in which a cooperative effort might achieve the end which is desired by many.

Drugs

The possible application of drugs to the problem of atherosclerosis has occupied the attention of the pharmaceutical industry for some time. On the thrombotic aspect of this disease many substances have been produced which affect the blood clotting mechanism but this aspect will not be dealt with in this chapter. The implication of platelet adhesiveness in the problem of atherosclerosis has only recently been developed as a possible area in which the drug industry might attempt to produce substances capable of modifying platelet behaviour.

The aspect of atherosclerosis research in which the pharmaceutical industry has been most active is in the exploration of drugs capable of lowering the plasma lipid concentration. This has proved such an important aspect of research that international meetings have been held in 1961, 1965 and 1968 dealing specifically with drugs affecting lipid metabolism (see Garattini & Paoletti, 1961; Kritchevsky, Paoletti & Steinberg, 1967; Holmes & Paoletti, 1969).

Only a few of the many drugs which have been examined as potentially useful hypolipidaemic agents will be considered in this section.

Triparanol

Triparanol is the name given to a substituted amino-alkoxy-triaryl-ethanol, which was shown by Blohm & McKenzie (1959) to be capable of reducing the serum cholesterol concentration in experimental animals. It was subsequently shown that this substance also lowered the serum cholesterol in man. The mechanism by which this effect is achieved was investigated by Frantz, Mobberley & Schroepfer (1960) and Avigan, Steinberg, Thompson & Mosettig (1960). These workers demonstrated that triparanol produced a block in cholesterol biosynthesis, after the cyclization of squalene, and the sterol desmosterol (24-dehydrocholesterol) accumulated in the plasma and tissues. Triparanol seemed therefore to inhibit the conversion of desmosterol to cholesterol (see review in "Progress in Cardiovascular Disease", 1960).

Unfortunately, the administration of this substance to humans for long periods produced a series of side-effects which were deemed highly undesirable, and consequently the substance was withdrawn.

Atromid

Atromid is the name given to p-chlorophenoxy-isobutyric acid, one of a series of aryl-isobutyric acids which were shown by Thorp & Waring (1962) to reduce the plasma lipids of rats maintained on a normal diet. The effects of this substance on the plasma lipids fluctuated seasonally, and it appeared to potentiate the metabolic effects of exogenous steroids. The work of Hellman, Bradlow, Zumoff, Fukushima & Gallagher (1959) had shown that androsterone would depress the plasma lipids in man, and this prompted the administration of atromid together with androsterone to humans. In a preliminary study using this combination, Oliver (1962) has shown that it is possible to depress the plasma cholesterol in man and maintain the lowered level for periods of many months. Subsequently it was found that the androsterone was unnecessary.

A symposium on this drug was produced as an unedited supplement to the Journal of Atherosclerosis Research, 1963. This compound is now widely used as a plasma cholesterol-lowering agent. The mode of action is not known; it is claimed to be free from side-effects (Oliver 1967). Recently this has been challenged (3rd International Symposium on drugs affecting lipid metabolism, Milan, 1968), as investigators have reported increases in plasma creatine phosphokinase during atromid treatment. This drug produces fatty livers in experimental animals. Regrettably no serious studies have been reported on the mode of action of this compound before its vigorous promotion as "the drug of choice for lowering plasma cholesterol".

Cholestyramine

Cholestyramine is a quaternary amino resin with characteristics which enable it to bind bile salts at the pH prevailing in the small intestine. The administration of this resin to man and other animals at a suitable dosage level results in an effective break in the entero-hepatic circulation of bile salts. Hashim, Bergen & Van Itallie (1961) have demonstrated that when this substance is administered to humans at a dose level of 10–15 g./day there is a marked drop in the serum cholesterol level. This is presumably due to the sequestration of the bile salts in the gut, with a resultant failure in the reabsorption of dietary and biliary cholesterol. The subjects exhibit steatorrhoea of varying degrees, because the absorption of triglyceride is also impaired by this regimen. The possible usefulness of substances of this general type in the treatment of hypercholesterolaemia is still under study.

Oestrogens

Many studies have emphasized that the clinical manifestations of atherosclerosis are rare in women before the menopause, and these observations, together with various experimental findings, prompted a number of investigators in different centres to study the effects of oestrogens on the plasma lipids of men. When oestrogens are administered to human males at a dose level in excess of the oestrogenic threshold dose, the plasma cholesterol concentration is dramatically reduced (Eilert, 1949). The mechanism by which oestrogens lower the plasma lipids has not been discovered, but a great deal of effort has been applied to the problem of attempting to obtain a substance, structurally related to the oestrogens, which might exert this hypolipaemic action without oestrogenic side effects. These studies have been summarized by Drill & Riegel (1958) and Cook (1961).

A number of long-term studies on the usefulness of oestrogens in the treatment of atheromatous disease processes have been conducted in various parts of the world. For obvious reasons the oestrogens were administered to individuals who already had clinical evidence of the disease, and in most studies, despite sustained plasma lipid depressions for periods up to 5 years, little evidence emerged which would suggest that the administration of oestrogens to human males exerted any beneficial effect on the prognosis after myocardial infarction (Oliver & Boyd, 1961; Stamler, Katz, Pick, Lewis, Page, Pick, Kaplan, Berkson & Century, 1961). It may be that, if this type of therapy had been instituted in hypercholesterolaemic "high risk" human males in the pre-ischaemic state, the outcome would have been different. These studies therefore suffer from the same defect as many other dietary and drug trials in that they are "secondary prevention" studies. This has been discussed previously.

Thyroid

The very dramatic effect of the thyroid hormone on the plasma lipids has been known for many years (Levy & Levy, 1931; Turner & Steiner, 1939), but this hormone is of limited value as a plasma cholesterol depressant because it also produces a profound increase in the basal metabolism of the individual, and unfortunately there is a disproportionate increase in the oxygen consumption rate of the myocardium when contrasted with other tissues. These facts make the use of thyroxine, for instance, of very limited value in the treatment of hypercholesterolaemia in most cases. However, within recent years a number of compounds have been developed which bear a structural resemblance to the thyroid hormone, and these thyroxine analogues appear to influence metabolic processes in a quantitatively different fashion from the parent hormone (Duncan & Best, 1958; Rawson, Money, Kroc, Kumaoka, Benua & Leeper, 1959; Ruegamer, Alpert & Silverman, 1959; Boyd & Oliver, 1960a, b; Cuthbertson, Elcoate, Ireland, Mills & Shearley, 1960a, b). A number of these substances, such as *dextro*-thyroxine, influence the plasma lipid levels to a proportionately higher degree than they elevate the metabolic rate (Starr, Roen, Freibrun & Schleissner, 1960). This fact raised hopes that it would be possible to devise a thyroxine analogue capable of depressing the plasma cholesterol concentration without markedly influencing the oxygen demands of the myocardium. Unfortunately, while the biological effects of these analogues can be quantitatively separated in animals and man, the level of discrimination is still not good enough (Boyd & Oliver, 1960a, b). In the case of *dextro*-thyroxine it is possible to achieve effective lowering of the plasma cholesterol concentration without an observable elevation of the basal metabolic rate, but as many of the subjects treated with this compound exhibit an increase in the frequency and severity of anginal attacks this may indicate that the metabolic requirements of the myocardium have been elevated by the thyroxine analogue (Oliver & Boyd, 1961).

Nicotinic Acid

The substance nicotinic acid was shown by Altschul, Hoffer & Stephen (1955) to depress the plasma cholesterol level in the rabbit and subsequently this compound was shown to be effective in controlling the hypercholesterolaemia occurring in certain humans. The dose of nicotinic acid required to influence the serum cholesterol concentration is of the order of 1–9 g./day. This quantity is vastly in excess of the amount of the substance required in its role as a vitamin. The administration of nicotinic acid at this dose level results in marked peripheral vasodilatation due to a direct effect on the smooth muscle of the vessel wall. Consequently nicotinic acid can be considered to be a drug affecting the peripheral autonomic nervous system. The mechanism of action of this compound on lipid metabolism is not yet established but a variety of theories have been advanced. Kritchevsky *et al.* (1962), showed that nicotinic acid appeared to accelerate cholesterol oxidation in rats. The observations of Carlson & Oro (1962); Carlson (1963) showed that the mobilization of plasma free fatty acids could be blocked by nicotinic acid.

Long-term studies have been instituted in the assessment of nicotinic acid as an anti-atherogenic agent (Berge, Achor, Christensen, Mason & Barker, 1961), but once again the morbidity and mortality of the group tested were not materially influenced by this treatment.

It has been repeatedly shown that nicotinic acid treatment at a dosage adequate to influence plasma lipids results in alterations to carbohydrate. In a recent study in man Zöllner & Wernekke (1963) noted a diminished glucose tolerance in certain subjects. This drug is quite widely used in the "treatment" of hyperlipaemic states.

Sitosterol

Sitosterol is a 24-ethyl-analogue of cholesterol, which is found in grain. This sterol is absorbed to a very limited degree by mammals and birds. The presence of sitosterol in the diet interferes with the absorption of the dietary and biliary cholesterol, which is participating in the enterohepatic circulation of cholesterol (Peterson, 1951). It has been established that the administration of about 10 g./day of sitosterol can increase the faecal excretion of cholesterol, and at the same time the plasma cholesterol concentration is reduced, provided that other factors in the diet (such as the quantity and type of triglyceride) remain unchanged (Pollak, 1953; Best & Duncan, 1956).

Unfortunately, the quantitative effect produced by sitosterol is not very large, and the considerable amount of sitosterol which must be ingested to produce this decrease is unpalatable to many.

Summary

There is evidence in man that arterial changes classified as atherosclerosis are more prevalent in some parts of the world than in others. The reason for this geographical distribution of the disease is unknown. The disease is more prevalent in the "privileged" communities in which starvation is practically non-existent, and, conversely, it is rare in countries afflicted by undernutrition. It is well documented that the plasma lipids correlate with the nutritional status.

It is now well established that the plasma lipid increment observed in populations exhibiting atheroma is causally related to the disease. The elevation of the plasma lipids is one of the few metabolic abnormalities detected in this condition. Agents have been studied which achieve a reduction in the concentration of the plasma lipids of humans. Some plasma lipid depressants also influence certain *in vitro* blood clotting tests in a direction thought to diminish thrombotic tendencies *in vivo*. One important factor is the consumption of diets isocaloric to energy requirements, while other dietary factors which have achieved prominence are the lipid content and the degree of unsaturation in the dietary fatty acids.

Many studies have accentuated the importance of endocrine factors in the aetiology of atherosclerosis, because this disease is a major complicating factor in the most widespread endocrine disorder—diabetes. There is also evidence implicating oestrogens in the clinical presentation of atherosclerosis, because these hormones appear to have a "protective" effect in so far as it is not until some time after their withdrawal at the menopause that women present with the clinical features of the disease. Other endocrine factors have been suggested as influencing atheromatosis, in particular, the role of the thyroid has been emphasized by many, but it is not yet established whether the degree of arterial involvement present in hypothyroid individuals is greater than that which one would expect to find in subjects of the same age, sex, etc.

Many individuals presenting with clinical evidence of atherosclerosis are hypertensive, and since a high percentage of these subjects may also be hyperlipaemic to varying degrees, it is interesting to speculate whether the hypertension and hyperlipaemia are causally related or whether both may be under the control of a common aetiological factor.

The difficulties experienced in establishing with certainty any single causative factor in atherosclerosis have led to a theory that the apparent increase in this disease within recent years is due to the increase in "stress" experienced by the population in the civilization which has evolved. The problem of obtaining an objective measure of "stress" presents difficulties in evaluating the significance of this quantity.

If the percentage of calories consumed as lipids by individuals could be fairly drastically reduced, and also if the percentage of polyunsaturated fatty acids in the lipids of the diet could be increased, this would achieve a diminution in the circulating lipids of most subjects. These measures would have to be undertaken in young, healthy adult subjects who were prepared to consume this diet for many years in order to establish the efficacy of the regimen as a possible method of arresting the atheromatous process. It is hoped that the National Diet-Heart Study may produce definitive results in this area.

References

ADAMS, C. W. M. (1964). *Biol. Rev.*, **39**, 372.

ADLERSBERG, D., PARETS, A. D. & BOAS, E. P. (1949). *J. Amer. med. Ass.*, **141**, 246.

AHRENS, E. H., HIRSCH, J., INSULL, W. & PETERSON, M. L. (1958). In "Chemistry of Lipids as related to Atherosclersis", ed. I. H. Page, p. 222. Springfield, Illinois, C. C. Thomas.

AHRENS, E. H. & KUNKEL, H. G. (1949). *J. exp. Med.*, **90**, 409.

ALTSCHUL, R., HOFFER, A. & STEPHEN, J. D. (1955). *Arch. Biochem.*, **54**, 558.

ANITSCHKOW, N. (1913). *Beitr. Path. Anat.*, **56**, 379.

ASPEN, A. J. & MEISTER, A. (1958). *Methods in Biochem. Analysis*, **6**, 131.

AVIGAN, J., STEINBERG, D., THOMPSON, M. J. & MOSETTIG, E. (1960). *Prog. Card. Disease*, **2**, 525.

BARR, D. P., RUSS, E. M. & EDER, H. A. (1951). *Amer. J. Med.*, **11**, 480.

BERGE, K. G., ACHOR, R. W., CHRISTENSEN, N. A., MASON, H. L. & BARKER, N. W. (1961). *Amer. J. Med.*, **31**, 24.

BERGSTRÖM, S., DANIELSSON, H. & SAMUELSSON, B. (1964). *Biochim. Biophys. Acta*, **90**, 207.

BERGSTRÖM, S. & SAMUELSSON, B. (1967). "The Prostaglandins", Nobel Symposium II. New York, Wiley.

BERGSTRÖM, S. & SJÖVALL, J. (1957). *Acta Chem. Scand. II*, 1086.

BEST, M. M. & DUNCAN, C. H. (1956). *Circulation*, **14**, 911.

BIGGS, M. W., KRITCHEVSKY, D., COLMAN, D., GOFMAN, J. W., JONES, H. B. LINDGREN, F. T., HYDE, G. & LYON, T. P. (1952). *Circulation*, **6**, 359.

BLOHM, T. R., MACKENZIE, R. D., (1959). *Arch. Biochem. Biophys.*, **85**, 245.

BORN, G. V. R. (1956). *Biochem. J.*, **62**, 33P.

BORN, G. V. R. (1958). *Biochem. J.*, **68**, 695.

BORN, G. V. R. (1962). *Nature*, **194**, 927.

BORN, G. V. R. & CROSS, M. J. (1963). *Nature*, **197**, 974.

BORN, G. V. R., HONOUR, A. J. & MITCHELL, J. R. A. (1964). *Nature*, **202**, 761.

BÖTTCHER, C. F. J. & VAN GENT, C. M. (1961). *J. Atherosclerosis Res.*, **1**, 36.

BOYD, G. S. & OLIVER, M. F. (1960a) *J. Endocrin.*, **21**, 25.

BOYD, G. S. & OLIVER, M. F. (1960b) *J. Endocrin.*, **21**, 33.

BRANWOOD, A. W. & MONTGOMERY, G. L. (1956). *Scot. med. J.*, **1**, 367.

BUCK, R. C. & ROSSITER, R. J. (1951). *Arch. Path.*, **51**, 224.

BURR, G. O. & BURR, M. M. (1929). *J. biol. Chem.*, **82**, 345.

CARLSON, L. A. (1963). *Acta Med. Scand.*, **173**, 719.

CARLSON, L. A. & ORÖ, L. (1962). *Acta Med. Scand.*, **172**, 641.

CHRISTAKIS, G., RINZLER, S. H., ARCHER, M., WINSLOW, B., JAMPER, S., STEPHENSON, J., FRIEDMAN, G., FEIN, H., KRAUS, A. & JAMES, G. (1966). *Amer. J. Pub. Hlth.*, **56**, 299.

CIRCULATION (1968). Supplement 1.

CLAYTON, S. & CROSS, M. J. (1963). *J. Physiol.*, **169**, 82.

COHEN, P. P. & HEKHIUS, G. L. (1941). *J. biol. Chem.*, **140**, 711.

CONSTANTINIDES, P. (1965). "Experimental atherosclerosis", Amsterdam, Elsevier.

COOK, D. L. (1961). In "Drugs Affecting Lipid Metabolism", p. 204, ed. Garattini and Paoletti. Amsterdam, Elsevier.

CORNWELL, D. G. (1967). In "Lipids and Lipidoses", p. 168, ed. G. Schettler. Berlin, Springer Verlag.

COWDRY, E. V. (1933). "Arteriosclerosis". New York, Macmillan Co.

CRAWFORD, T. (1961). *J. Atheroscler. Res.*, **1**, 3.

CRAWFORD, T., DEXTER, D. & TEARE, R. D. (1961). *Lancet*, **i**, 181.

CUTHBERTSON, W. F. J., ELCOATE, P. V., IRELAND, D. M., MILLS, D. C. B. & SHEARLEY, P. (1960a). *J. Endocrin.*, **21**, 45.

CUTHBERTSON, W. F. J., ELCOATE, P. V., IRELAND, D. M., MILLS, D. C. B. & SHEARLEY, P. (1960b). *J. Endocrin.*, **21**, 69.

DANIELSSON, H. (1968). In "Metabolic Pathways", 2nd Edition, Greenberg, D. M. London, Academic Press.

DAWBER, T. R., KANNEL, W. B. & LYELL, L. P. (1963). *Ann. N.Y. Acad. Sci.*, **107**, 539.

DORP, D. A., VAN, BEERTHUIS, R. K., NUGTEREN, D. H. & VONKEMAN, H. (1964). *Biochim. Biophys. Acta*, **90**, 204.

DRILL, V. A. & RIEGEL, B. (1958). *Rec. Progr. Hormone Res.*, **14**, 29.

DUGUID, J. B. (1946). *J. Path. Bact.*, **58**, 207.

DUGUID, J. B. (1948). *J. Path. Bact.*, **60**, 57.

DUGUID, J. B. & ROBERTSON, W. B. (1957). *Lancet*, **i**, 1205.

DUNCAN, C. H. & BEST, M. M. (1958). *Endocrinology*, **63**, 169.

DUNCAN, C. H. & BEST, M. M. (1962). *Amer. J. Clin. Nutr.*, **10**, 297.

EBERTH, J. C. & SCHIMMELBUSCH, C. (1889). *Virchow's Arch. Path. Anat.*, **116**, 327.

EILERT, M. L. (1949). *Amer. Heart J.*, **38**, 472.

EMMONS, P. R., HAMPTON, J. R., HARRISON, M. J. G., HONOUR, A. J. & MITCHELL, J. R. A. (1967). *Brit. med. J.*, **ii**, 468.

EPSTEIN, F. H., BLOCK, W. D., HAND, E. A. & FRANCIS, T., Jr. (1959). *Amer. J. Med.*, **26**, 39.

FAGGE, C. H. (1873). *Trans. Path. Soc., London*, **24**, 242.

FRANTZ, I. D., MOBBERLY, M. L. & SCHROEPFER, G. J. (1960). *Prog. Cardiovasc. Dis.*, **2**, 511.

FREDRICKSON, D. S. & LEES, R. S. (1965). *Circulation*, **31**, 321.

FREDRICKSON, D. S., LEVY, R. I. & LEES, R. S. (1967). *New Engl. J. Med.*, **276**, 32.

FRENCH, J. E., MACFARLANE, R. G. & SANDERS, A. G. (1964). *Brit. J. exp. Path.*, **45**, 467.

FRENCH, J. E. & POOLE, J. C. F. (1963). *Proc. Roy. Soc. B.*, **157**, 170.

GAARDER, A., JONSEN, J., LALAND, S., HELLEM, A. & OWREN, P. A. (1961). *Nature*, **192**, 531.

GARATTINI, S. & PAOLETTI, R. (1961). "Drugs affecting Lipid Metabolism". Amsterdam, Elsevier.

GOFMAN, J. W., GLAZIER, F., TAMPLIN, A. R., STRISOWER, B. & DE LALLA, O. (1954). *Physiol. Rev.*, **34**, 589.

GOFMAN, J. W., LINDGREN, F. T., ELLIOTT, H. A., MANTZ, W., HEWITT, J., STRISOWER, B., HERRING, V. & LYON, T. (1950). *Science*, **111**, 166.

GOULD, R. G. & SWYRD, E. A. (1967). *J. Lipid Res.*, **7**, 698.

GOULD, R. G. & TAYLOR, C. B. (1950). *Fed. Proc.*, **9**, 179.

HALMOLSKY, M. W. (1967). *Circulation*, **35**, 427.

HALMOLSKY, M. W. (1968). Symposium on coronary heart disease, A. H. A. New York.

HASHIM, S. A., BERGEN, S. S., VAN ITALLIE, T. B. (1961). *Proc. Soc. Exp. Biol., N.Y.*, **106**, 173.

HASLAM, R. J. (1964), *Nature*, **202**, 765.

HELLEM, A. & OWREN, P. A. (1964). *Acta Haematol.*, **31**, 230.

HELLMAN, L., BRADLOW, H. L., ZUMOFF, B., FUKU-SHIMA, D. K., & GALLAGHER, T. F. (1959). *J. clin. Endocrin.* **19**, 936.

HOLMAN, R. L., McGILL, H. C., STRONG, J. P. & GEER, J. C. (1958). *Amer. J. Path.*, **34**, 209.

HOLMES, W. L., and PAOLETTI, R. (1969). Proceedings of 3rd Conference on Drugs affecting lipid metabolism. In press.

HOOD, B. (1965). *Acta med. Scand.* **178**, 161.

HOOD, B. & ANGERVALL, G. (1959). *Amer. J. Med.*, **26**, 30.

JOURNAL OF ATHEROSCLEROSIS RESEARCH (1963). Supplement.

KARMEN, A. (1955). *J. clin. Invest.*, **34**, 131.

KARMEN, A., WROBLEWSKI, F. & LADUE, J. S. (1955). *J. clin. Invest.*, **34**, 126.

KATZ, L. N. & STAMLER, J. (1953). "Experimental Atherosclerosis", Springfield, Illinois, C. C. Thomas.

KESTEN, H. D., MEEKER, D. R. & JOBLING, J. W. (1936). *Proc. Soc. exp. Biol., N.Y.*, **34**, 818.

KEYS, A., ANDERSON, J. T., MICKELSEN, O., ADELSON, S. F. & FIDANZA, F. (1956). *J. Nutr.*, **59**, 39.

KEYS, A., KIMURA, N., KUSUKAWA, A., BRONTE-STEWART, B., LARSEN, N. & KEYS, M. H. (1958). *Ann. intern. Med.*, **48**, 83.

KINGSBURY, K. J. (1961). In "Drugs Affecting Lipid Metabolism", p. 502, ed. Garattini & Paoletti. Amsterdam, Elsevier.

KINSELL, L. W., MICHAELS, G. D., PARTRIDGE, J. W., BOLING, L. A., BALCH, H. E. & COCHRANE, G. C. (1953). *J. clin. Nutr.*, **1**, 224.

KLOEZE, J., (1966). In "The Prostaglandins", Nobel Symposium II, ed. Bergström & Samuelsson. New York, Wiley.

KONTTINEN, A. AND HALONEN, P. I. (1962), *Amer. J. Cardiol.* **10**, 525.

KRITCHEVSKY, D., COTTRELL, M. C., TEPPER, S. A. (1962). *J. Cell Comp. Physiol.* **60**, 105.

KRITCHEVSKY, D., PAOLETTI, R. & STEINBERG, D. (1967). "Progress in Biochemical Pharmacology". Basel, S. Karger.

LADUE, J. S. WROBLEWSKI, F. & KARMEN, A. (1954). *Science*, **120**, 497.

LEARY, T. (1941). *Arch. Path.*, **32**, 507.

LEES, R. S. & HATCH, F. I. (1963). *J. Lab. clin. med.* **61**, 518.

LEREN, P. (1966). *Acta Medica Scand. Supplement* 466.

LEVY, M. & LEVY, M. (1931). *Bull. Acad. Med. Paris*, **105**, 666.

LEWIS, B. (1959). *Postgrad. med. J.*, **35**, 208.

LINDGREN, F. T., ELLIOTT, H. A. & GOFMAN, J. W. (1951). *J. phys. Chem.* **55**, 80.

LINDGREN, F. T., & NICHOLS, A. V., (1960). The plasma proteins **2**, edited F. W. Putnam. New York, Academic Press.

MACDONALD, L. (1957). Lancet ii, 457.

MALMROS, H. (1950). *Acta med. Scand., suppl.*, **246**, 137.

MANN, G. V., ANDRUS, S. B., McNALLY, A. & STARE, F. J. (1953). *J. exp. Med.*, **98**, 195.

MASTER, A. M., GUBNER, R., DACK, S. & JAFFE, H. L. (1941). *Arch. intern. Med.*, **67**, 647.

MEAD, J. F. (1960). In "Lipide Metabolism", p. 41, ed. K. Bloch. New York, Wiley.

MITCHELL, J. R. A. & SCHWARTZ, C. J. (1965). "Arterial Disease". Oxford, Blackwell.

MONTOGOMERY, H. (1940). *Med. Clin. N. Amer.*, **24**, 1249.

MORRISON, L. M., HALL, L. & CHANEY, A. L. (1948). *Amer. J. Med. Sci.*, **216**, 32.

MUSTARD, J. F. (1961). *Canad. med. Ass. J.*, **85**, 621.

MUSTARD, J. F., ROWSELL, H. C. & MURPHY, E. A. (1964). *Amer. J. med. Sci.*, **248**, 469.

OLIVER, M. F. (1962). *Lancet*, **i**, 1321.

OLIVER, M. F. (1967). *Circulation*.

OLIVER, M. F. & BOYD, G. S. (1953). *Brit. Heart J.*, **15**, 387.

OLIVER, M. F. & BOYD, G. S. (1961). *Lancet*, **i**, 783.

ONCLEY, J. L. (1956). Harvey Lectures **50**, 71.

PETERSON, D. W. (1951). *Proc. Soc. exp. Biol., N.Y.*, **78**, 143.

PEZOLD, F. A. (1961). "Lipids and Lipoproteins in blood plasma." Heidelberg, Springer Verlag.

POLLAK, O. J. (1953). *Circulation*, **7**, 696.

Progress in Cardiovascular Disease, (1960), Vol. 2.

RAWSON, R. W., MONEY, W. L., KROC, R. L., KUMAOKA, S., BENUA, R. S. & LEEPER, R. D. (1959). *Amer. J. med. Sci.*, **238**, 261.

Research Committee of the Medical Research Council (1968). *Lancet*, **ii**, 693.

ROKITANSKY, C. VON (1852). "Über einige der wichtigsten Krankheiten der Arterien". Vienna, Meidinger.

RUEGAMER, W. R., ALPERT, M. & SILVERMAN, F. R. (1959). *Fed. Proc.*, **18**, 313.

SANDLER, M. & BOURNE, G. H. (1963). "Atherosclerosis and its Origin". New York, Academic Press.

SCHETTLER, G. (1961). "Arteriosclerosis". Stuttgart, Thieme.

SCHRADE, W., BÖHLE, E. & BIEGLER, R. (1961). In "Drugs Affecting Lipid Metabolism, p. 454, ed. Garattini and Paoletti. Amsterdam, Elsevier.

SCHWARTZ, C. J. (1967). *Arch. Path.*, **83**, 325.

SCHWARTZ, C. J. & MITCHELL, J. R. A. (1962). *Circulation Res.*, **11**, 63.

SMITH, E. B. (1965). *J. Atherosclerosis Res.*, **5**, 224.

SMITH, E. B., SLATER, R. S. & CHU, P. K. (1968). *J. Atherosclerosis Res.*, **8**, 399.

SORENSEN, N. S. (1963). *Acta Med. Scand.*, **174**, 725.

SPRITZ, N., AHRENS, E. H. & GRUNDY, S. (1965). *J. clin. Invest.*, **44**, 1482.

STAMLER, J., KATZ, L. N., PICK, R., LEWIS, L. A., PAGE, I. H., PICK, A., KAPLAN, B. M., BERKSON, D. M. & CENTURY, D. (1961). In "Drugs Affecting Lipid Metabolism", p. 432, ed. Garattini and Paoletti. Amsterdam, Elsevier.

STARR, P., ROEN, P., FREIBRUN, J. L. & SCHLEISSNER, L. A. (1960). *Arch. intern. Med.*, **105**, 830.

STECHER, R. M. & HERSH, A. H. (1949). *Science*, **109**, 61.

STEINBERG, D. & OSTROW, B. H. (1955). *Proc. Soc. exp. Biol., N.Y.*, **89**, 31.

STEINER, A. & KENDALL, F. E. (1946). *Arch. Path.*, **42**, 433.

STEINER, A., KENDALL, F. E. & MATHERS, J. A. L. (1952). *Circulation*, **5**, 605.

STRØM, A. & JENSEN, A. R. (1951). *Lancet*, **i**, 126.

Technical Group of the Committee on Lipoproteins and Atherosclerosis (1956). *Circulation*, **14**, 691.

THORP, J. M. & WARING, W. S. (1962). *Nature (Lond.)*, **194**, 948.

TOOR, M., KATCHALSKY, A., AGMON, J. & ALLALOUF, D. (1957). *Lancet*, **i**, 1270

TURNER, K. B. & STEINER, A. (1939). *J. clin. Invest.*, **18**, 45.

VAN DEN HEUVEL, F. A., (1962). *Canad. J. biochem.* **40**, 1299.

VIRCHOW, R. (1856). "Gesammelte Abhandlungen zur wissenschaftlichen Medizin". Frankfurt, Straatsdruckerei.

VOGEL, J. (1847). "The Pathological Anatomy of the Human Body". Philadelphia, Lea and Blanchard.

WEINHOUSE, S. & HIRSCH, E. F. (1940). *Arch. Path.*, **29**, 31.

WILENS, S. L. (1947). *Arch. intern. Med.*, **79**, 129.

WILENS, S. L. (1951). *Science*, **114**, 389.

WILKINSON, C. F. (1950). *Bull. N.Y. Acad. Med.*, **26**, 670.

WILSON, J. (1964). *J. Lipid Res.*, **5**, 409.

WISSLER, R. W., EILERT, M. L., SCHROEDER, M. A. & COHEN, L. (1954). *Arch. Path.*, **57**, 333.

WOOD, P. D. S., SHIODA, R. & KINSELL, L. W. (1966). *Lancet*, **ii**, 604.

World Health Organization Tech. Rep. Series (1958), 143. Geneva.

WROBLEWSKI, F. (1959). *Amer. J. Med.*, **27**, 911.

ZUCKER, M. B. & BORELLI, J. (1962). *Proc. Soc. exp. Biol., N.Y.*, **109**, 779.

ZÖLLNER, N., & WERNEKKE, G (1963). 6th Internat. Congr, Gerontol., Copenhagen.

Chapter 19

DISORDERS OF THE GASTRO-INTESTINAL TRACT

by

O. M. Wrong, H. S. Wiggins and I. D. P. Wootton

Royal Postgraduate Medical School, London, and the M.R.C. Gastro-enterology Research Unit,
Central Middlesex Hospital, London

I. WATER AND ELECTROLYTE METABOLISM

PRIMARY disease of the alimentary tract is one of the main clinical causes of water and electrolyte disturbance, and this fact justifies the otherwise rather artificial division of this chapter into "water and electrolytes" and "non-electrolytes". To the clinician with an interest in salt and water metabolism the alimentary tract appears as an enormous exchange surface, through which vast losses of isotonic fluid can arise with alarming rapidity. Much of this section is concerned with the effects of these losses on the body as a whole, rather than the detailed pathophysiology of ion and water transport through the mucous membranes and secretory cells of the alimentary tract.

Most foods are consumed as solids or semi-solids, but digestion can only occur in a fluid medium, and large volumes of fluid are secreted into the alimentary tract to render the contents fluid. In Table 19.1 are listed the volumes and composition of the main alimentary secretions in man. It can be seen that 6 or more litres of fluid are secreted into the alimentary tract each day, whereas an average of only 1·5 litres are ingested by mouth, and 150 ml. are lost in the faeces. Thus a volume approximately double the plasma volume is normally secreted each day into the gastro-intestinal tract and reabsorbed.

Most alimentary secretions are isotonic with plasma, and when fluids which are not isotonic are introduced into the lumen a rapid passive movement of water through the membrane occurs, and the fluid remaining in the lumen

becomes isotonic. The only real exception to this general rule is saliva, which in man is invariably hypotonic; the relative impermeability of the squamous oral mucosa appears to prevent rapid osmotic equilibration of saliva with plasma. The contents of all other parts of the alimentary tract are close to isotonicity, and such slight differences as do occur arise because passive water movements are not always rapid enough to maintain osmotic equilibrium. Because these alimentary juices are essentially isotonic, a loss of known volume from the body causes a loss of a predictable amount of electrolyte. The main cations are sodium and potassium, and in the stomach hydrogen ion; and the main anions are chloride and bicarbonate, and various organic anions in biliary tract and colon. At most levels of the alimentary tract sodium is more prominent than potassium; the one conspicuous exception is faeces. This replacement of sodium by potassium in the faeces may have had survival value in the past, for until recent times many communities have had a very low sodium intake but no shortage of potassium, and this is the one alimentary secretion which is inevitably lost from the body.

WATER AND ELECTROLYTE INTAKE

Intake of fluid and electrolytes is largely governed by habit. Man has a well developed thirst mechanism which rapidly informs him when he needs water, but many normal people

TABLE 19.1

Average daily volume and composition of main alimentary secretions. Data are from various sources, including Shohl (1939); Sunderman & Boerner (1949); Gamble (1951); Lans, Stein & Meyer (1952a) and Davenport (1966). Figures for succus entericus are not included, as the composition varies at different levels of the small intestine, and the volume of the normal secretion is not known

| | | Gastric Juice | | | Bile | |
	Mixed saliva	Parietal	Non-parietal	Pancreatic juice	Hepatic	Gall Bladder
Volume, ml.	1500	2500		700	1000	400
pH	6·5	0·9	7·6	7·5–8·8	7·7	7·4
Osmolality, mOsm/kg.	90–180	285	285	285	285	285
Na^+ mEq./l.	30	6	155	130	150	150
K^+ ,,	20	10	15	10	10	12
Cl^- ,,	30	165	125	70	95	17
HCO_3^- ,,	20	0	45	85	22	10
Remarks	Na^+ and Cl^- concentrations rise steeply with increasing flow	H^+ is main cation (155 mEq./l.) in parietal secretion		Composition depends largely on whether, and how, stimulated	Bile anions 20–30 m-mole/l.	Bile anions 150–210 m-mole/l.

drink sufficiently with meals and refreshments to satisfy their water needs, and are seldom conscious of the sensation of thirst. Water intake is normally 1–2 litres, but may be as much as 8–15 litres/day in the subject with obsessional polydipsia or the man who drinks 16 pints of beer every evening. The ability of the kidney to achieve a maximum water diuresis of about 20 litres a day protects against the water intoxication which would otherwise be a danger of these high fluid intakes, and it may be an indication of our primitive ancestors' drinking habits that this ability persists in all of us.

Electrolyte intake is also largely determined by habit. Potassium intake is normally 70–100 mEq./day, and exists mainly in the form of animal protoplasm. Intake of sodium and chloride varies over a wide range (50–400 mEq./day) as it is largely in the form of sodium chloride added to foods during processing, cooking, or at the table. Most diets are acid-producing, giving rise on metabolism to 50–80 mEq./day of hydrogen ion, which is derived from the oxidation of sulphur, and to a lesser extent phosphorus, in animal protein to sulphuric and phosphoric acids; however some mainly vegetable diets may give rise to net alkali production, their content of inorganic cation (mainly potassium) being balanced largely by organic anion, which in the body is oxidized to bicarbonate.

Thirst. The desire to drink water may arise from local causes, in particular dryness of the mouth or pharynx, or a sensation of food sticking in the oesophagus. However in health hypertonicity of body fluids is a more important and effective cause, and produces the sensation of thirst by acting on the central nervous system directly, most probably through a centre in the anterior hypothalamus which is close to the supra-optic nucleus. Andersson, Larsson & Persson, (1960) found that electrical stimulation of this area in goats led to the drinking of enormous volumes of water, whereas destruction prevented the animals from drinking even when dying of water depletion.

It has long been suspected that the hypothalamic thirst "centre" and the "osmoreceptor" which stimulates release of antidiuretic hormone (Jewell & Verney, 1957) are closely related anatomically. Both in health and disease thirst and antidiuresis go hand-in-hand; both are normally stimulated by an increase in plasma osmolality which is so slight that it can be measured only with difficulty, both can also be stimulated by hypovolaemia even when no increase in plasma osmolality occurs (for example

the thirst and antidiuresis which accompany sudden haemorrhage) and both are suppressed by a fall in plasma osmolality. Certainly the two functions are extremely closely related anatomically, so much so that diseases of the hypothalamus causing loss of thirst are nearly always accompanied by diabetes insipidus, and it seems inherently unlikely that two separate structures, both exquisitely sensitive to changes in plasma osmolality, are situated in such close proximity where one structure could perform both functions.

Abnormal lack of thirst. In temperate climates the commonest cause of lack of thirst is impaired consciousness from any cause. It may be argued, depending on how thirst is defined, whether such patients do not experience thirst, or are unable to respond adequately to the sensation. Absence of thirst may arise also in fully conscious patients with lesions of the hypothalamus, usually eosinophil granuloma or craniopharyngioma. The fact that such patients usually have diabetes insipidus as well makes their condition precarious for they may rapidly become severely depleted of water without experiencing any sensation of thirst (Engstrom & Liebman, 1953), and the first sign of their water deficit may be clouding of consciousness or epilepsy, which may mistakenly be attributed to a direct effect of their brain disease, or the chance finding of hypernatraemia. The classical signs of "dehydration", such as hypotension or reduced tissue turgor, are not usually present in these patients, for these are signs of a reduced extracellular fluid volume (i.e. saline depletion). These patients suffer from a pure water deficit, which is sustained mainly by the intracellular space, and hypernatraemia develops long before the signs of an extracellular fluid deficit.

Abnormal thirst, usually accompanied by antidiuresis, can occur in acute hypovolaemia, such as haemorrhage, in various states of chronic hypovolaemia such as nephrotic syndrome and hepatic cirrhosis, and in congestive cardiac failure, where blood volume is usually increased. The one common factor to these different states is failure of some critical part of the circulation. The usual evidence that such patients have an abnormal thirst is not the complaint of thirst, but the fact that they continue to drink normal volumes of fluid despite hyponatraemia, which in normal circumstances inhibits thirst, and become intensely thirsty if an attempt is made to raise their serum sodium to normal by water restriction or infusion of hypertonic saline. Increased plasma renin, caused by inadequate renal perfusion, may be the stimulus to thirst in these situations, for it is now known that renin release is increased by these conditions, and there is evidence from animal experiments (Fitzsimons, 1969) that renin and angiotensin stimulate thirst, perhaps through the action of aldosterone.

Salt appetite. Most people like their food to contain some sodium chloride, but the amount taken spontaneously varies over a very wide range, from about 50 to 400 mEq./day, and this variation is mainly caused by habit, rather than varying physiological need. The minimal daily loss of sodium from the body, by all routes (urine, faeces and sweat) is of the order of 4 mEq./day, and healthy subjects achieve this level of conservation when they are depleted of only 200 mEq. of sodium, a loss which produces no evidence of ill effect. Thus dietary intake of sodium, at least in most civilized communities, is greatly in excess of body needs, and the possession of a specific sodium appetite, responding to the needs of the body, would seem to confer little benefit in terms of survival. Despite these considerations, man does have a sodium appetite which can, in some circumstances, be stimulated by sodium deficiency. But because of the strong influence of suggestion on matters of taste, and the difficulty in maintaining human subjects in a prolonged state of sodium deficiency, most of the work on sodium appetite has been done on animals (Denton, 1967).

Although sodium chloride is the form in which most sodium is consumed by animals and man, there is no evidence as yet for the existence of a specific chloride appetite. Many years ago Richter & Eckert (1938) showed that adrenalectomized rats (which were presumably deficient of both sodium and chloride) had an increased preference for solutions of sodium chloride, sodium lactate, and sodium phosphate, but not for solutions of other chlorides. More recently sodium-deficient rabbits have been shown to have an increased appetite for both sodium chloride and sodium bicarbonate, but to ignore the chlorides of potassium and magnesium (Blair-West *et al.*, 1968). Hence, in experiments of this sort, although sodium chloride has been the usual sodium salt studied, it has been assumed that the appetite observed has been for the sodium rather than for the chloride ion. Even though human consumption of sodium salts is not strictly comparable, for it is not usually in response to a physiological need, it is nevertheless of interest that a normal diet contains appreciable amounts of sodium bicarbonate and sodium glutamate, in addition to sodium chloride, which suggests that in man too the appetite is for the sodium ion rather than for chloride.

There are two quite distinct changes in salt appetite caused by sodium deficiency—an enhanced ability to taste low concentrations of sodium ion, and an increased desire to ingest sodium (Denton, 1967). Although in man the taste buds responsible for detection of salt travel mainly in the chorda tympani, very little is known about the neural pathways responsible for the two responses. Whether humoral factors are involved is also uncertain. Sodium deficiency causes increased secretion of renin and aldosterone, and in the rat aldosterone has been shown to stimulate sodium appetite (Wolf & Handal, 1966). Evidence from the sheep suggests that neither of these hormones, nor angiotensin, is involved in the increased sodium appetite caused by sodium deficiency in this animal (Bott, Denton & Weller, 1967). In man, an increased desire for salt has occasionally been seen in patients with hyperaldosteronism secondary to renal artery stenosis and accelerated hypertension, which suggests that in this species renin or aldosterone might stimulate salt appetite.

In some primitive human communities—such as the Chimbu of New Guinea, the tribes of mountainous parts of China, and the Australian aboriginals—the basic dietary intake of sodium is so low that the possession of an efficient salt appetite is necessary for survival. The same was true until quite recent times of parts of central Africa, India and the Americas. Lack of dietary sodium has been particularly a problem in people subsisting entirely on foods of plant origin, for unlike animal carcasses some plants contain virtually no sodium. Many of these communities have placed great value on salt, and have exchanged wives or fought wars on account of it (Dahl, 1958). In such people, attacks of gastro-enteritis, by increasing faecal loss of sodium, must have been a particularly dangerous threat to life; pregnancy and loss of blood from wounds must have also caused a drain of precious sodium from the body.

In adult humans who are used to a high salt intake the sodium appetite may be so suppressed that they do not experience a yearning for salt even when seriously sodium-depleted. Thus patients with adrenal insufficiency, or sodium-losing renal disease, seldom admit to an increased desire for salt, although they may tolerate very large oral salt supplements without complaint. Only one of the three normal subjects studied by McCance (1936) developed an increased desire for salt when subjected to experimental sodium depletion, and Yensen (1959) remarked on the absence of a craving for salt in his similar experiments. It is possible that the salt appetite is more easily developed (or preserved) in the very young, for spontaneous salt-craving has been a feature of some children with adrenal insufficiency, either congenital or acquired early in life (Richter, 1943).

Potassium, the main intracellular electrolyte, is present in large amounts in all natural foods, for unlike sodium it is an essential constituent of both plant and animal protoplasm. It is therefore not surprising that man does not possess a specific potassium appetite, which would have no obvious biological advantage, and does not deliberately add potassium to his food.

SECRETION AND ABSORPTION OF ELECTROLYTES AND WATER

Saliva

In man saliva is unique among alimentary secretions in being markedly hypotonic (average about 150 mOsm./kg.). This characteristic is not shared with all other mammals; the saliva of sheep, for example, is isotonic with plasma. Human saliva varies in ionic composition between the different salivary glands, and is also greatly influenced by the rate of salivary flow. In resting conditions about 25% of the salivary volume comes from the parotid glands, and most of the remainder from the submandibular glands, but the parotid glands contribute a larger proportion at higher rates of flow. The average composition of resting human parotid saliva is approximately Na^+ 30, K^+ 20, HCO_3^- 40 and Cl^- 10 mEq./l. (Thaysen, Thorn & Schwartz, 1954). With increasing flow salivary osmolality rises to approach isotonicity, mainly because of a steady increase in the concentrations of sodium and chloride (Thaysen et al., 1954; Schneyer & Schneyer, 1967). The pH of saliva varies between 6 and 8, the optimum range for the activity of salivary amylase. However, in man this enzyme plays only a minor part in the digestion of starch, and the main function of saliva is to provide lubrication by means of mucin. The concentration of calcium in saliva is about 3 mEq./l.; this prevents the slow erosion of dental enamel which would occur in a calcium-free medium, but leads to the precipitation of "tartar" (calcium carbonate) around the teeth.

The exact details of formation of saliva are still not fully understood. Most experimental studies have been made in the rat (Burgen, 1967). It appears that an active process of ion secretion occurs in the acini of the glands, with a resultant passive influx of water. The sodium and potassium concentrations of the acinar fluid are similar to those of plasma, but there is relatively more bicarbonate and less chloride. The lining cells of the intercalating and main salivary ducts actively absorb sodium and to a lesser extent secrete potassium, and a hypotonic fluid is thus formed. One curious property of the salivary glands is their ability to concentrate iodide in the saliva, and this process can be depressed by drugs which inhibit uptake of iodide by the thyroid (Rowlands, Edwards & Honour, 1953).

Stomach

Anatomically the stomach appears to be a simple organ, but its secretions, and their formation, are astonishingly complex. There are three main types of cell—the parietal (oxyntic) cells which secrete hydrochloric acid, the chief cells which secrete pepsinogen, and the mucus-secreting cells situated both in the necks of the gastric glands and on the epithelial surface. It is now well established that the parietal cells secrete what is virtually isotonic hydrochloric acid (pH 0·9, containing 155 mEq./l. of both hydrogen ion and chloride) and that the maximum output of acid is proportional to the total mass of such cells (Card & Marks, 1960). The chief cells secrete pepsinogen with very little accompanying water and electrolyte (Hunt, 1959). The mucus-producing cells, which are responsible for most of the surface secretion under resting conditions, produce an alkaline fluid (pH approximately 8·0) with an electrolyte composition very like plasma—Na^+ 130, K^+ 5, Cl^- 120, HCO_3^- 15 mEq./l. (Hunt, 1959; Hollander, 1963). The electrolyte composition of whole gastric juice varies widely, partly because of variations in the volumes contributed by the different cell types but also from the effects of swallowed food and saliva, and regurgitated duodenal juice. The osmolality is usually very slightly below that of plasma (Hollander, 1963) even when dilution with swallowed saliva or water can be excluded, probably because of neutralization of solute during the mixing of alkaline and acid fluids from the two main cell types, i.e. $HCO_3^- + H^+ \rightarrow H_2CO_3 \rightarrow CO_2 + H_2O$ (Davenport, 1966). Occasionally the osmolality is slightly greater than plasma, a finding which suggests that passive movement of water into the gastric lumen is not always able to keep pace with active electrolyte secretion (Hunt & Wan, 1967).

The exact mechanism by which the parietal

cells secrete hydrochloric acid is not finally settled, although the problem has attracted more attention than almost any other in alimentary physiology. The interested reader is referred to reviews by James (1957), Hogben (1960) and Hunt & Wan (1967). Secretion of both chloride and hydrogen ion appears to be active.

Absorption from the stomach is very limited. Water moves passively in both directions across the mucosa but net absorption is slow and for most clinical purposes can be disregarded. Fat-soluble substances, such as ethanol, are more readily absorbed. Most electrolytes are only very slowly absorbed by diffusion, but some organic electrolytes may pass through the mucosa by non-ionic diffusion (Milne, Scribner & Crawford, 1958) which is greatly enhanced by the enormous pH difference between gastric contents and plasma; weak acids which are lipid-soluble in the undissociated state (such as acetylsalicylic acid and antipyrine) are readily absorbed from the stomach, whereas weak bases, such as ammonia and dimethylamine, pass readily into the stomach from the blood stream and may attain higher concentrations in gastric juice than in plasma.

Assessment of acid secretion. The assessment of gastric capacity to secrete acid is still a useful clinical investigation, although it has yielded much less information than originally hoped. Duodenal ulcer, particularly when associated with Zollinger-Ellison syndrome, is accompanied by a secretion of greater than normal amounts of hydrochloric acid (*not* a more acid secretion, as this could not be achieved unless the stomach could secrete a hypertonic fluid), whereas in pernicious anaemia secretion of acid is usually impaired. It is important to note that absence of gastric intrinsic factor is now considered to be the underlying defect in pernicious anaemia, and that this is usually, *but not invariably* accompanied by defective acid secretion; some young patients with pernicious anaemia have been reported to have well preserved acid secretion (Mollin, Baker & Doniach, 1955; Lambert, Prankerd & Smellie, 1961).

Measurement of gastric secretion by aspiration after a gruel meal, with or without stimulation by histamine, has now been largely abandoned in place of the augmented histamine test, in which the patient is given a very large amount of histamine (0·04 mg./kg.) and protected against the systemic effects by an antihistamine drug (Conard, Kawalewski & Van Geertruyden, 1949; Kay, 1953). Alternatively gastric secretion of acid may be stimulated by gastrin (Makhlouf, McManus & Card, 1967) or the synthetic analogue pentagastrin (Mason, Giles & Clark 1969) which cause even less systemic disturbance. Measurement of "true" acid by titration with Töpfer's indicator, which changes colour at pH 3, and of "total" acid by phenolphthalein (pH 8) has also been abandoned, and replaced by measurements of the pH value of gastric contents, and the rate of acid secretion, which is obtained by measuring the volume of the secretion and determining its total acid content by titration to pH 7·4, just as urinary titratable acid is determined. By convention gastric acid content has been expressed as the number of millilitres of 0·1 N NaOH required to neutralize 100 ml. of gastric juice, but fortunately this figure is the same as the gastric acid expressed in mEq./l. One suspects that Davenport (1966) is right in claiming that "if the person who coined the definition had realized it would give such a sensible result, he would have changed his definition". Certainly the rate of acid secretion should be expressed in mEq. or μEq. of acid per unit time, a usage which is immediately comprehensible to those familiar with general acid-base terminology.

Bile

About 500 ml. of bile pass into the duodenum each day. This fluid has a cation composition which is very close to that of plasma, but a markedly different anion composition (Table 19.1). Calculation of osmolality suggests that the fluid is hypertonic to plasma, but it is, in fact, isotonic; the discrepancy arises because the formation of micelles by the bile anions reduces their osmotic contribution, and in addition the bile anions reduce the activity coefficients of the other ions present (Wheeler, 1968). In passing it should be noted that neither in bile nor in plasma are bile "acids" present as *acids*. The pK_a of the glycine conjugates is about 3·6, and that of the taurine conjugates about 1·5, so at the pH of all body fluids except gastric juice, bile "acids" must be present largely as charged *anions*.

Hepatic bile is similar to gall bladder bile in cation concentration, but contains lower concentrations of bile anions (Table 19.1). While in the gall bladder bile is concentrated between three and six times by active absorption of sodium, chloride and bicarbonate (Diamond, 1968), all of which are absorbed against their electrochemical gradient; water absorption appears to be a passive consequence of active ion transport. In addition a small amount of fluid and mucin is secreted by the gall bladder mucosa.

Pancreatic Juice

About 700 ml. of pancreatic juice pass into the duodenum each day. The fluid is the most alkaline of all the intestinal juices, and contains high concentrations of bicarbonate (Janowitz & Dreiling, 1962) with correspondingly low concentrations of chloride (Table 19.1). Sodium and potassium concentrations are close to plasma values, and the fluid is isotonic. For details of secretion, and the factors that influence composition, the reader is referred to Chapter 20.

Small Intestine

The small intestine is a difficult part of the body to study, partly by reason of its inaccessibility, but also because the secretions of the mucosa, unlike pancreatic juice and bile, cannot be easily separated from the fluid which constantly passes through the intestine. Fortunately in most respects the small intestine of man appears to be similar to that of other mammals, and much of our knowledge comes from *in vitro* work on the intestine of small animals (particularly rat and hamster) and study of artificial fistulae or isolated loops (e.g. Thiry-Vella loops) in otherwise intact dogs (Wilson, 1962). When man has been studied, either by use of the Miller-Abbott tube (Miller, 1937) or during the course of some surgical procedure, he has shown results similar to those yielded by animal experiments.

The contents of the small intestine are isotonic with plasma, except in the duodenum where they are frequently hypotonic, as low as 140 mOsm./kg. (Karr & Abbott, 1935). The cause of this hypotonicity may partly be swallowed hypotonic fluids, including saliva, but probably a more important cause is neutralization of osmoles by the interaction of gastric hydrochloric acid with pancreatic bicarbonate: $H^+ + HCO_3^-$ $\rightarrow H_2CO_3 \rightarrow CO_2 + H_2O$.

The reaction of the contents of the small intestine is about pH 6·0 in the duodenum, but may be as low as pH 3·2 (Breuhaus & Eyerly, 1943) depending on the flows of gastric and pancreatic juice. At lower levels in the intestine pH gradually increases to the region of pH 6·5–8·0 by the level of the ileocaecal valve (Mann & Bollman, 1930; Robinson, 1935). There is a corresponding increase in bicarbonate concentration from duodenum to terminal ileum and a reciprocal fall in chloride. These changes are largely dependent on secretion, rather than absorption, for they occur in isolated intestinal loops of dogs even months after continuity of the bowel has been interrupted (de Beer, Johnston & Wilson, 1935; Schiffrin & Nasset, 1939; Swallow & Code, 1967).

Electrolyte movements across the intestinal mucous membrane are exceedingly complex. The physicochemical laws which govern movements of water and ions across membranes, and the characteristics of the several different types of movement, have recently been reviewed by Curran & Schultz (1968) and it is impossible to do justice to this complex subject here. In this section the term "active transport" is used, as suggested by Rosenberg (1948), for a process which brings about net transfer of a substance against its electrochemical potential difference, though even this definition has drawbacks (Curran & Schultz, 1968)—for example, movement of an ion against its electrochemical potential may occur as a result of bulk flow of solvent through a membrane, even in artificial membranes, a phenomenon known as "solvent drag". It should be noted that in life the mucosa of the alimentary tract carries a negative charge with respect to the serosal surface. This charge varies between 5 and 40 mV, being greater in colon than in small intestine (Schultz & Curran 1968); it is an important factor in electrolyte movement, for it is produced by active ion transport, and is itself an important determinant of passive electrolyte movement.

Water. Isotope studies have shown that water flux occurs in both directions across all parts of the small intestine. Net absorption has been the subject of many irreconcilable observations (Schultz & Curran, 1968), but in most circumstances appears to be the result of osmotic gradients caused by solute movement, especially that of sodium (Fordtran & Ingelfinger, 1968). From a comparison of the net water movements created by hypertonic solutions of mannitol, erythritol and urea, Fordtran & Dietschy (1966) have calculated that the effective radius of pores in the jejunum is about 7·5Å, whereas in the ileum it is approximately 3·4 Å. The difference in net water flow in response to osmotic gradients in these two regions is less than these figures would suggest, a finding which implies that jejunal cell pores are either fewer in number or longer than ileal pores.

Ions. Isotopic studies show large sodium fluxes across the mucosa in both directions, greater in jejunum than ileum. Net absorption of sodium, which is active, and inhibited by metabolic poisons, is about half the flux rate from lumen to blood stream, and is also greater in jejunum than ileum. These findings are in keeping with the observation that in man the upper half of the small intestine is the major site of fluid absorption (Borgström *et al.*, 1957). Potassium movements also occur in both directions, but the fluxes are much less than those of sodium, and the movements appear to be passive. Bicarbonate also moves across the intestinal mucosa in both directions; in isolated sections of the small bowel it accumulates in the lumen (de Beer *et al.*, 1935; Schiffrin & Nasset, 1939), and it is accompanied by a carbon dioxide tension considerably higher than that of blood (McGee & Hastings, 1942). The exact mechanism of bicarbonate secretion has not been elicited, but it is likely that the large amounts of carbonic anhydrase in the intestinal mucosa play some part. Chloride also moves across the mucosa in both directions; *in vitro* work (Curran & Solomon, 1957; Kinney & Cole, 1964) indicates that absorption of chloride can take place against the electro-chemical potential difference, but in most circumstances the movement may be passive, and active *secretion* has even been reported (Tidball, 1961). It is possible that chloride and bicarbonate move in opposite directions by an anion-exchange mechanism.

Fordtran & Locklear (1966) have studied the osmolality and electrolyte composition of intestinal chyme from various levels in human subjects fed hypotonic (steak, bread and tea) and hypertonic (milk and doughnuts) meals. With both meals isotonicity was established, not in the stomach (in contrast with the findings of some earlier experiments), but high in the small intestine. A significant component of the total osmotic activity proximal to the jejunum was non-electrolyte, presumably carbohydrates, fats, proteins, and their hydrolytic products. Sodium and chloride concentrations rose rapidly as the meal traversed the duodenum and upper jejunum, to equal (or, in the case of chloride, exceed) the plasma levels by mid-jejunum; lower in the ileum chloride levels fell to 40–90 mEq./l. Potassium concentrations were high (mean 26 mEq./l.) in the stomach, presumably derived from the meal itself, but fell in the upper intestine to 5–10 mEq./l. and remained at that level throughout the ileum. By use of a non-absorbable marker Fordtran & Locklear were able to calculate that the hypotonic meal, which had an initial volume of 645 ml. was represented by 2000 ml. of fluid in the proximal duodenum and about 200 ml. in the terminal ileum (Fordtran & Ingelfinger, (1968).

Colon

The adult human colon normally receives each day from the ileum about 600 ml. of fluid, containing approximately 60 mEq. of sodium, 4 mEq. of potassium, and 30–35 mEq. of both chloride and bicarbonate (Fordtran & Ingelfinger, 1968). The discharge from long-standing ileostomies often is less in volume with less sodium and more potassium, probably because of the effects of chronic mild sodium depletion which is a common consequence of an ileostomy (see below). From a comparison of these figures with the composition of stool it can be calculated that the normal colon absorbs each day about 500 ml. of water, 50 mEq. of sodium, and 30 mEq. of chloride. A further 30 mEq. of bicarbonate also disappear from colonic contents, but this is probably lost by combination with organic acids derived from bacterial action on carbohydrate residues, rather than by absorption. In addition about 6 mEq. of potassium is added to colonic contents by secretion. These activities are the most important and perhaps the only real function of the human colon.

In vitro work on the colon of several small animal species has shown that sodium absorption is active but that potassium secretion can be accounted for by the negative intraluminal potential (about 40 mV) created by active sodium absorption (Ussing & Andersen, 1955; Cooperstein & Hogben, 1959). However in the rat Edmonds (1967) found that potassium secretion is too great to be accounted for by passive movement, and it may well be that potassium secretion is normally dependent on the provision of metabolic energy, but is not usually of sufficient magnitude to demonstrate net movement of potassium against its electrochemical potential. Water absorption appears to be passive and determined by osmotic gradients.

In order to study colonic movements of ions and water *in vivo*, without the complications caused by the presence of food residues, much work has been done on colons "defunctioned" by an ileostomy, or on isolated sections of the colon. In the dog de Beer, Johnston & Wilson showed in 1935 that an isolated segment of the colon secreted a fluid with a pH of 8·0, containing 90 mEq./l. of bicarbonate. More recently d'Agostino, Leadbetter & Schwartz (1953) infused physiological saline into the isolated entire colon of this species, and demonstrated that the chloride in the solution was rapidly replaced by bicarbonate and the sodium was replaced, slightly less rapidly and less completely, by potassium. Studies in the intact dog have since

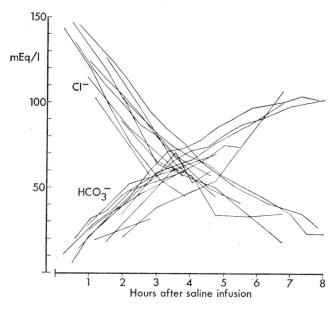

FIG. 19.1. Changes in Cl$^-$ and HCO$_3$$^-$ concentrations in physiological saline infused into the human colon. The subjects were 10 patients with mid-transverse colostomies performed some weeks earlier for localized diverticulitis. At zero time the distal loop of defunctioned colon was filled with as much saline as it could hold (400–800 ml.) and this fluid was then repeatedly sampled through a catheter until no more could be obtained. Note the reciprocal increase in bicarbonate concentration as chloride concentration falls; chloride reabsorption must be greater in amount than bicarbonate secretion because the volume of fluid in the colon is shrinking throughout the experiment (from Wrong, unpublished studies).

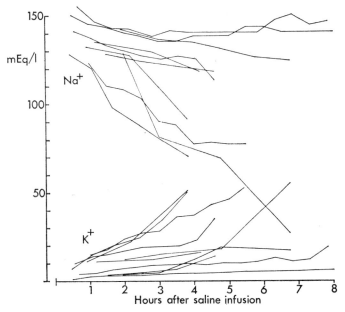

FIG. 19.2. Changes in Na$^+$ and K$^+$ concentrations in physiological saline infused into the human colon. Same experiments as in FIG. 19.1. The changes in concentration are more variable and less marked than those in Cl$^-$ and HCO$_3$$^-$.

shown that secretion of bicarbonate, in addition to sodium absorption, is active (Cooperstein & Brockman, 1959). The accompanying Figures 19.1 and 19.2 show the fate of physiological saline in the defunctioned colon of man; the results are very similar to those of d'Agostino *et al.* in the dog, and suggest that the conclusions from the experiments in that species are applicable to man. It should be noted that the sodium and potassium *concentrations* in the fluid infused into the colon show reciprocal changes, just as do those of chloride and bicarbonate, and thus the fluid in the colon remains isotonic. However, the *total amount* of potassium secreted into the colon is less than the amount of sodium reabsorbed, for the volume in the colon is contracting throughout the experiment; likewise bicarbonate secretion is less in amount than chloride absorption.

Absorption and secretion in the intact human colon has been studied by Levitan, Fordtran Burrows & Ingelfinger (1962), using a technique in which the caecum is first intubated from above, and the colon is next thoroughly washed out. Solutions are then introduced into the lumen and subsequently collected by rectal tube; by use of radioactive isotopes it has been possible to calculate water and ion fluxes as well as net absorption and secretion. The use of this technique has shown that the entire colon can absorb about 3 litres of water a day, but that bidirectional fluxes of water through the mucosa are about three times this figure. Net sodium absorption is about 450 mEq. and net potassium secretion 30 mEq./day; the bidirectional fluxes of these ions are approximately twice as great (Levitan *et al.*, 1962; Shields & Miles, 1965; Levitan, 1967). It should be noted that colonic capacity to absorb sodium and water is not infinite, but is 5–10 times the load which normally reaches it from the ileum. Maximum colonic ability to secrete potassium is never realised, except perhaps in diarrhoea or after administration of ion-exchange resins; when the colon is completely defunctioned it produces small quantities of mucinous fluid containing about 1 mEq./day of potassium (Welch, Wakefield & Adams, 1936).

THE COMPOSITION OF FAECES

Whole faeces. Normal stool has a water content of 70 to 85% and a pH of 5·8–7·9 (Robinson, 1922; Shoshkes, 1947). The daily volume of faeces is normally so small (100–150 ml.) in comparison with the volumes of fluid that are secreted and absorbed into the alimentary tract, that it is tempting to disregard faecal losses

altogether when studying water and electrolyte balance. This oversimplification may be justifiable when considering sodium and chloride, for the normal daily loss of these ions is less than 5 mEq. But the average daily faecal loss of potassium is several times larger, and the faecal content of magnesium, calcium and phosphorus is so great that it represents 50% or more of dietary intake, and is therefore a major factor in the calculation of metabolic balance data.

TABLE 19.2

Partition of electrolyte excretion between urine and faeces. It has been assumed that excretion by other routes is negligible. (From Shohl, 1939.)

| | % of total excretion in | |
	Urine	Faeces
Na$^+$	95	5
K$^+$	79	21
Ca^{++}	12	88
Mg^{++}	31	69
Cl$^-$	98	2
Total P	57	43
Total S	83	17

Berger (1960) collected together all the values from the world literature and found that the normal range of faecal losses was sodium 0·5–5·0 mEq., potassium 5–15 mEq., chloride 0·5–3·0 mEq., magnesium 10–30 mEq., calcium 15–65 mEq., and phosphorus 10–25 m-mole/day. These figures suggest that the bowel is the main route by which calcium, magnesium and phosphorus are lost from the body, whereas the other electrolytes are mainly eliminated through the kidneys; Table 19.2, from Shohl (1939), gives the relative contributions of the two routes to the total excretion of these substances, calculated from data collected by Clark (1926) from inmates of San Quentin prison. Studies such as these involve prolonged periods of collection, usually with faecal markers, to make sure that the calculated daily faecal loss is truly representative. After collection, pooling, and homogenization of faeces an aliquot is either dried and incinerated or digested with concentrated nitric acid; both procedures destroy all organic material and therefore cannot be used to determine stool losses of some substances of great physiological interest—such as bicarbonate, urea, ammonium and organic anion. Thus very little is known about the composition of faeces, in comparison with other body fluids, and this lack of information arises from the technical difficulties of analysing an aesthetically offensive substance which has the texture of a solid (whereas most analytical methods are designed for fluids), with a strong and variable colour which prevents application of most colorimetric methods, and which in addition is the seat of intense continuing bacterial activity. Even what information exists on faecal electrolytes states only the daily excretion, and does not reveal the physical state of each substance, i.e. what proportion is in true solution in faecal water and what proportion is in precipitated form.

Faecal water. Because of the above problems various well-known physical methods of separation have been applied to whole stool in attempts to obtain faecal water free of solid material. Centrifugation, ultrafiltration and dialysis have all been used. Separation of faecal water by centrifugation is only possible in stools containing more than the normal proportion of water, but has proved very useful in the analysis of diarrhoeal stools. Some years ago the author and his colleagues attempted ultrafiltration of normal faeces through a cellophane membrane, using a pressure of one atmosphere and an area of about 100 cm². The procedure was found to be offensive and time-consuming, yielding only 1–2 ml. of ultrafiltrate after 14–16 hours, and it was unsuccessful with stools of more solid than average consistency. Unless ultrafiltration was carried out in the cold, the length of time required was accompanied by steadily increasing concentrations of ammonia and total nitrogen in the filtrate, probably because of continuing bacterial autolysis. The concentrations of other electrolytes were of the same order as those found in faecal dialysate (see below) and the latter method was therefore preferred as it was more generally applicable and yielded larger amounts of fluid.

In-vivo dialysis of faeces. Dialysis of faeces can be performed *in vitro* if the faeces are semi-fluid, but it is more easily carried out *in vivo*. The subject swallows small dialysing capsules, each 6 cm. in length, consisting of cellophane tubing containing a colloidal substance, either dextran or polyvinyl pyrrolidone (Wrong, Metcalfe-Gibson, Morrison, Ng & Howard, 1965). The contents of these capsules rapidly reach diffusion equilibrium with their environment and are in equilibrium with faeces when these are passed per rectum. Table 19.3 gives the values of the most important electrolytes, and related variables, in faecal dialysate collected in this way from a large number of normal subjects. It also gives values for the diffusibility of several different faecal substances; this figure represents the concentration of a substance in faecal dialysate as a percentage of the concentration in the

TABLE 19.3

Average composition of faecal dialysate from normal subjects taking diets of their own choosing. (From Wrong et al., 1965; Wilson et al., 1968a; Charron et al., 1969; and Rubinstein et al., 1969.)

		Concentration	Diffusibility $\left[\dfrac{\text{concentration in faecal dialysate per kg. of water}}{\text{concentration in surrounding faeces per kg. of water}} \times 100 \right]$
Cations	Na^+	18·5 mEq./l.	107%
	K^+	79 mEq./l.	74%
	Na^+/K^+	0·24	—
	NH_4^+	11·2 mEq./l.	—
	Mg^{++}	38 mEq./l.	38%
	Ca^{++}	49 mEq./l.	14%
Anions	Cl^-	14·4 mEq./l.	—
	Total CO_2	39 m-mole/l.	—
	$PO_4^{\equiv}$	2·3 mEq./l.	—
	$SO_4^{=}$	2·8 mEq./l.	—
	Organic anion	172 mEq./l.	—
Etcetera	pH	7·18	—
	Osmolality	357 mOsm./kg.	—
	Urea	nil	—
	Total N	95 m-mole/l.	7·9%
	Total P	3·6 m-mole/l.	5·3%
	Total S	26 m-mole/l.	—

immediately adjacent whole stool, and can only be determined for substances which can be measured with accuracy in both materials.

Calcium, magnesium and phosphate (and probably also carbonate, which in Table 19.3 accounts for part of the total CO_2) tend to precipitate as insoluble salts inside the dialysis capsules, and consequently the figures given for these ions are greater than the diffusible concentrations in faecal water. This problem does not arise with other faecal ions, for the concentrations present of the various ion pairs are well below their solubilities.

Faecal dialysate is unusual among intestinal juices in being hypertonic; this slight hypertonicity can be abolished by intestinal antibiotics, and is therefore probably the result of bacterial activity in the colon, which increases osmolality by breaking down large molecules into a larger number of smaller ones (Wilson, Ing, Metcalfe-Gibson & Wrong, 1968a). An example of this activity is the destruction of urea, a substance which cannot be demonstrated in faecal dialysate from normal subjects. During antibiotic administration urea appears at close to plasma values, and simultaneously the concentration of ammonium falls, but not to zero. It seems likely that urea is normally destroyed by bacterial urease in the colon, being converted to ammonium carbonate; some ammonium may also arise, independently of bacterial action, from peptic digestion of glutamine residues (Melville, 1935).

Table 19.3 shows that most of the anion in faeces is organic. Much of this has not yet been identified, but about one third is acetate, and also present are smaller amounts of many other lower fatty acid anions, and lactate, succinate and fumarate. (The higher fatty acid anions, such as stearate and palmitate, are present in whole stool, but mainly as insoluble calcium soaps, and therefore do not diffuse into faecal dialysate). The main source of these organic anions appears to be food residues, especially carbohydrates, though a small component is produced by the intestinal mucosa (Rubinstein, Howard & Wrong, 1969). Lennon, Lemann & Litzow (1966) have pointed out that the loss of organic anion in faeces represents a gain of hydrogen-ion to the body, which must be taken in account in acid-base balance studies—for each mEq. or organic anion is derived from a m-mole of organic acid which has donated a mEq. of hydrogen ion to the body.

Attempts have been made, by feeding different electrolytes or omitting them from the diet, to discover the origin of the electrolytes in faecal

dialysate (Metcalfe-Gibson et al., 1967). As might be expected, the concentrations of ions which are normally secreted into the alimentary tract (sodium, potassium, chloride, bicarbonate) were little influenced by such manoeuvres, but the concentrations of most other ions was clearly largely determined by oral intake. Adrenal steroids and renal failure cause interesting changes in the composition of both whole faeces and faecal dialysate, and these are considered below.

ABNORMAL LOSSES OF ALIMENTARY SECRETIONS

The effects of loss of alimentary secretions depend on the ionic composition of the fluid lost. Sodium is abundant in most alimentary juices, and deficiency of this ion develops early; the chief consequence is an isotonic contraction of the extracellular fluid (McCance, 1938) accompanied by the symptoms and signs of what is usually known as "dehydration". This term is etymologically incorrect, in that the deficiency is not simply or primarily one of water, and "saline depletion" is a more accurate descriptive term. The clinical features of this state—chiefly fatigue, hypotension, reduced tissue turgor, and azotaemia caused by reduced renal perfusion —are notoriously difficult to evaluate, and unless gross, can easily be overlooked.

Most alimentary secretions contain potassium, although usually the concentration is less than that of sodium, and sustained loss of secretions can lead eventually to a severe potassium deficit. Although most of these patients have an accompanying sodium deficit, this may not develop, or may be very slight, either because the oral intake of sodium is normally greater than that of potassium or because the kidneys conserve sodium much more efficiently than potassium. Alternatively a patient may first develop overt saline depletion, which is corrected by administration of oral or intravenous sodium; only later does the continuing loss of potassium cause trouble. Most cases of potassium deficiency of alimentary origin are complicated by acidosis or alkalosis, and it should be remembered that acidosis increases the plasma potassium level, and may thereby mask a potassium deficit, whereas alkalosis has the opposite effect (Burnell, Villamill, Uyeno & Scribner, 1956).

Acid-base disturbances are a common result of loss of alimentary secretions. Alkalosis may arise from loss of hydrogen ion (usually gastric hydrochloric acid), or as a direct result of potassium deficiency itself (the so-called "hypokalaemic alkalosis"). In the latter condition the prime cause of the alkalosis appears to be a deficiency of intracellular potassium, which is partly replaced by hydrogen ion from the extracellular fluid (Cooke, Segar, Cheek, Coville & Darrow, 1952; Gardner, MacLachlan & Berman, 1952; Irvine, Saunders, Milne & Crawford, 1961); the resulting intracellular acidosis stimulates renal tubular secretion of hydrogen ion, with the consequent development of metabolic alkalosis. Alternatively the loss of large volumes of alkaline intestinal secretion may lead to a metabolic acidosis, or acidosis may develop as a result of the renal failure caused by severe saline depletion of alimentary origin.

Saliva. Saliva is seldom lost from the body in sufficient amount to cause electrolyte deficits. However patients with a complete oesophageal stricture, who are totally unable to swallow their saliva, may lose 20–40 mEq./day of both sodium and potassium in the saliva they expectorate, and these losses may occasionally be important in contributing to electrolyte depletion.

Gastric juice. Repeated or chronic loss of gastric juice by vomiting, leading to severe deficiencies of electrolytes and water, most often results from pyloric stenosis, but may occur in other conditions, such as adrenal insufficiency and anorexia nervosa (Wolff *et al.*, 1968). In the latter condition vomiting is sometimes deliberately concealed by the patient, and without an accurate history it may be very difficult for the physician to diagnose the cause of the metabolic disturbance (Wallace, Richards, Chesser & Wrong, 1968; Hannigan, Frost & Perkins, 1963).

The classical picture of the patient with untreated pyloric stenosis is one of severe saline depletion, with hypochloraemia, marked alkalosis, hypokalaemia and pre-renal uraemia (Burnett, Burrows, Commons & Towery, 1950). Such patients have not only the alkalosis which is to be expected from loss of gastric hydrochloric acid, but are also depleted of both sodium and potassium. Until recently it has been difficult to establish the exact mechanisms leading to deficiencies of these two cations, but the factors considered important have included reduced electrolyte intake (Tarail & Elkinton, 1949; Black, 1964), excessive loss of cation in vomitus (Lans, Stein & Meyer, 1952*b*; Black & Jepson, 1954) and the renal effects of both alkalosis and aldosterone. The rather surprising fact that some of these severely alkalotic and potassium-depleted patients pass a relatively acid and potassium-rich urine was noted 20 years ago by

Burnett *et al.* (1950), but the significance of this finding has been only recently appreciated, largely owing to the studies of Kassirer and Schwartz and their colleagues. These workers showed, both in dog and man, that selective depletion of gastric hydrochloric acid was accompanied by continued losses of sodium and potassium in the urine (Needle, Kaloyanides & Schwartz, 1964; Kassirer & Schwartz 1966*a*), which could be entirely reversed by replacement of chloride (Kassirer & Schwartz, 1966*b*). The main culprit appears to be the hypochloraemic alkalosis, which the kidneys partially correct by the usual renal defence of excreting bicarbonate, a process which inevitably leads to urinary loss of sodium or potassium, for the bicarbonate must be accompanied by a cation. Kassirer & Schwartz suggest that the exact intrarenal mechanism causing increased potassium excretion is a reduced renal tubular reabsorption of sodium with chloride (because less chloride is available for absorption) and an increased reabsorption of sodium at a more distal tubular site where it is exchanged for potassium and hydrogen ion —changes in tubular function which together lead to an increased renal bicarbonate threshold and a negative potassium balance. These observations emphasizing the importance of chloride deficiency in the alkalosis resulting from loss of gastric juice have been amply confirmed by other workers (Aber, Sampson, Whitehead & Brooks, 1962; Howe & Le Quesne, 1964; Grantham & Schloerb, 1964; Lemieux & Gervais, 1964), although there appear to be a few patients in whom potassium deficiency plays a major part in maintaining alkalosis and chloride repletion alone will not correct the disturbance (Davies, Jepson & Black, 1956).

It is likely that excess secretion of aldosterone plays some role in the high urinary losses of potassium which occur in subjects losing gastric hydrochloric acid. Patients vomiting from pyloric stenosis develop clinical evidence of sodium depletion, but nevertheless continue to lose large amounts of sodium in their urine (Burnett *et al.*, 1950; Howe & Le Quesne, 1964; Wallace *et al.*, 1968). Even the subjects of Kassirer & Schwartz, who were on a diet containing only 10 mEq. of sodium a day, increased their urinary sodium losses, and went into negative sodium balance, during removal of gastric hydrochloric acid. This sodium diuresis is a normal renal response to a metabolic alkalosis, but tends to cause saline depletion, and hence stimulate renin and aldosterone secretion (Wallace *et al.*, 1968). The action of aldosterone on the renal tubule is to increase sodium-potassium exchange, and hence it decreases urinary losses of sodium at the expense of potassium. Kassirer, Appleton, Chazan & Schwartz (1967) studied aldosterone in their subjects during hydrochloric acid depletion, and found that the aldosterone secretion rate was initially high, in keeping with the low sodium intake, but fell as alkalosis and potassium depletion developed. They concluded from this and other evidence that increased secretion of aldosterone is not responsible for the alkalosis caused by loss of gastric acid; on the other hand they were able to prevent potassium repletion by giving aldosterone or DOCA during recovery from gastric alkalosis, and this finding is further evidence that increased secretion of aldosterone plays a role in the potassium depletion of pyloric stenosis.

Treatment of the electrolyte deficiences of pyloric stenosis consists of administering chloride parenterally, particularly as the sodium salt, although parenteral potassium may be required if potassium depletion is severe. When adequate chloride is available the kidney rapidly corrects the alkalosis by excreting a bicarbonate-rich urine, and it is not necessary to administer hydrogen ion in the form of hydrochloric acid or ammonium chloride.

Small intestine. Persistent vomiting is now seldom a feature of intestinal obstruction owing to widespread therapeutic use of intestinal or gastric suction. Reduction of distension by aspiration does more than relieve the patient of the discomfort of distension and vomiting, for it has been shown experimentally that the small intestine immediately above an obstruction absorbs less sodium and water and secretes more sodium, potassium and water than it does normally (Shields, 1965) perhaps as a result of venous distension of the bowel. In practice it is not usually possible to deflate the bowel immediately above an intestinal obstruction by aspiration, unless the obstruction is high in the small intestine, and even if this were always possible the changes of electrolyte depletion would not be averted, for large amounts of water and electrolyte are secreted by the normal ileum. Loss of these secretions leads to a clinical picture which is dominated by depletion of sodium, the principal ion in normal ileal contents. In addition acidosis is usual, because of losses of bicarbonate and bile anions. Potassium depletion may become a problem after several days, partly because of reduced intake and a high renal excretion of potassium as part of the metabolic response to surgery. An indication of the severity of the

electrolyte losses is given by Le Quesne (1967) who found that one patient with intestinal obstruction lost 6810 ml. of fluid into the intestine above the obstruction, containing 865 mEq. of Na, 116 of K, and 612 of chloride.

Loss of ileal contents through an external ileal fistula has the same metabolic effects as loss of intestinal contents by gastric suction, except that the amounts lost are often less though they may continue over a longer time.

Ileostomy. Ileostomized subjects taking a diet of their own choosing pass an average of about 500 ml. of liquid stool a day, containing about 55 mEq. of Na, and 5 mEq. of potassium (Nuguid, Bacon & Boutwell, 1961; Kramer, Kearney & Ingelfinger, 1962; Kanaghinis, Lubran & Coghill, 1963). The old surgical folklore that the terminal ileum assumes the function of the colon soon after ileostomy, and the faeces then become more solid, seems to be largely a fiction; in most patients this does not happen, and in those in whom it does it is probable that the continued loss of sodium in the ileostomy fluid has led to sodium depletion with secondary hyperaldosteronism, and that this increases ileal sodium reabsorption and so reduces faecal volume. Certainly features of sodium depletion, such as postural hypotension, weight loss, cramps, and a low urinary sodium, are present in many patients with ileostomies (Gallagher, Harrison & Skyring, 1962; Clarke, Chirnside, Hill, Pope & Stewart, 1967), or can be precipitated by dietary sodium restriction (Kramer, 1966).

Diarrhoea. When stool volume increases during diarrhoea from any cause, the resultant stool usually contains a higher sodium and chloride concentration and lower potassium concentration than normal stool (Fordtran & Dietschy, 1966). Consequently there is a greatly increased loss of sodium and chloride, which is in proportion to the water content of the stool, and a moderate increase in total potassium loss. Usually the sum of sodium and potassium greatly exceeds the faecal chloride; the anions are made up by increased loss of bicarbonate or organic anion (Fordtran, 1967), loss of either of which predisposes to acidosis. An exception to this rule is the rare chloride diarrhoea, discussed below, in which faecal chloride exceeds the sum of sodium and potassium, and alkalosis results, either from faecal loss of hydrogen ion as ammonium, or a result of potassium depletion itself.

Cholera. This form of diarrhoea has recently been intensely studied, particularly by Watten & Phillips and their colleagues (Phillips, 1966).

Although it clearly results from a disease of the small intestine, it can be regarded, at least in terms of electrolyte loss, as an extreme example of a diarrhoea originating from disease of either small or large intestine.

O'Shaughnessy (1832) first recognized that choleraic diarrhoea contains large amounts of sodium and bicarbonate, and remarked on the deficiency of these substances in the blood. Recent studies in a Bangkok epidemic (Watten, Morgan, Songkhla, Vanikiati & Phillips, 1959) have shown mean faecal concentrations of sodium 114; potassium 26; chloride 89 and bicarbonate 44 mEq./1.; stool volumes were as great as 21 litres a day, and stool osmolality varied from 232 to 288 mosm./kg. Patients invariably appeared exceedingly saline-depleted, and showed extreme haemoconcentration (serum proteins as high as 14 or 16 g./100 ml.), with raised plasma sodium and chloride and reduced plasma bicarbonate. Stools appeared to be slightly hypotonic to plasma, even when nothing was taken by mouth, but unfortunately it is not possible to work out the exact difference from the data given by these workers.

The exact pathogenesis of cholera is still in doubt. The vibrio does not invade the intestinal lumen, nor is the intestine ulcerated, and the diarrhoea is therefore believed to be the result of bacterial toxins. It is still not clear (Phillips, 1966; Gordon et al., 1966; Love, 1969) whether the diarrhoea is a result of reduced intestinal absorption of sodium, increased intestinal secretion, or increased mucosal permeability to sodium ("transudation").

Untreated cholera has a very high mortality because of the profound salt and water deficiency it produces. Oral administration of sodium and water is ineffectual in replacing losses, as the administered solutions are not absorbed. Treatment must therefore be intravenous, a fact which was realized over a hundred years ago by O'Shaughnessy (1832) and put into practice by Latta (1832). The early history of treatment has been well described by Gamble (1953). Recently, Gordon et al. (1966) have stated that the ideal fluid for intravenous replacement contains sodium 133, potassium 7, chloride 90 and lactate (or bicarbonate) 50 mEq./1. The amount of fluid required can be determined by measuring either faecal losses or plasma specific gravity (Phillips 1966).

Purgative addiction. Self-administration of purgatives, continued over many years, is a common cause of chronic potassium depletion (Schwartz & Relman, 1953; Relman & Schwartz, 1956).

These patients are usually women, and have often been brought up as children to believe that it is unhealthy not to open the bowels several times a day. The purgatives they take may appear to be harmless or even health-giving; for example two patients known to the author took proprietary preparations with the innocuous labels "vegetable laxative", and "bile-beans", both of which contain the drastic purgatives colocynth and jalap, and the cytotoxic drug podophyllum. Diagnosis is made more difficult by the refusal of many patients to admit that they take purgatives, and the correct diagnosis may only be made by chance discovery (Cope, 1966) or subterfuge. The clinical situation is made even more confusing by the fact that a few of these patients also have anorexia nervosa, or vomit deliberately, or administer diuretic drugs to themselves (Wolff et al., 1968).

The clinical picture of purgative addiction is usually that of a wasted woman, with symptoms and signs of potassium depletion, often a mild extracellular alkalosis, but little evidence of saline depletion. Urinary potassium is usually below 10 mEq./day, but renal damage may eventually lead to impairment of renal potassium conservation, with higher urinary figures (de Graeff & Schuurs 1960). In hospital the metabolic disturbance may correct itself if the patient stops taking purges, but frequently surreptitious self-administration continues, and it has sometimes been impossible to persuade patients to abandon the habit. Patients run a high risk of developing chronic pyelonephritis, a recognized complication of chronic potassium deficiency (Muehrcke & McMillan, 1963), and may die of eventual renal failure from this cause (Cope, 1966).

Papillary adenoma and carcinoma of the colon. These well differentiated neoplasms may secrete so much potassium into the lumen of the colon that the patient develops potassium depletion. Diarrhoea is invariably present, but the lesion may be low in the large intestine, or even in the rectum, and the mucous fluid secreted by the tumour may be passed in large volumes per rectum (up to 3 litres/day) almost without accompanying faecal matter (Shnitka, Friedman, Kidd & MacKenzie, 1961). Unlike the fluid secreted by the normal colon, the fluid formed by these tumours contains large amounts of sodium (Duthie & Atwell, 1963) and saline depletion may result from its loss. Roy & Ellis (1959) found that fluid collected from the surface of two such tumours contained 96 and 122 mEq./1. of sodium, 54 and 25 of potassium, and 114 and 92 of chloride respectively.

Chloride diarrhoea. The composition of most diarrhoeal stools resembles that in cholera (see above), in which the sum of the concentrations of sodium and potassium is considerably greater than the chloride concentration (Evanson & Stanbury, 1965) and the stool is alkaline. Rarely a different picture is seen, the chloride concentration is greater than the sum of sodium and potassium, and the stool is relatively acid. These findings inevitably must mean that there is an increase in faecal unmeasured cation (partly ammonium), whereas normally the unmeasured faecal anion (bicarbonate and organic anion) is more conspicuous. Patients with chloride diarrhoea usually become very alkalotic, whereas most forms of diarrhoea lead to acidosis, or at most the mild alkalosis caused by potassium deficiency.

Chloride diarrhoea may be acquired or congenital. Acquired chloridorrhoea is very uncommon, but has been described in patients with primary colonic disease who have become potassium-depleted from long continued diarrhoea (Lancet, 1966). There is some evidence that the increased faecal chloride is a direct effect of potassium depletion, but it is not known how potassium depletion exerts this effect.

Congenital chloridorrhoea is a rare familial disease, in which chloride diarrhoea is apparent from birth or very shortly afterwards. Affected children are liable to attacks of vomiting, pyrexia, diarrhoea and saline depletion, during which they show hypokalaemia and a disproportionately severe alkalosis. The chloride concentration of the diarrhoeal stool is 100–190 mEq./1., and faecal ammonium may be as high (Evanson & Stanbury, 1965). However faecal ammonium is not always markedly increased— in a typical patient studied by Dr. J. T. Harries and the author, the concentration was 14–22, while faecal chloride was 96–139 mEq./1.

The pathogenesis of congenital chloridorrhoea is not fully understood, though several theories have been proposed (Lancet, 1966). With increasing age the severity and frequency of attacks of diarrhoea subside, and those patients who survive appear to become normal adults.

THE EFFECTS OF ALDOSTERONE AND RELATED STEROIDS

The renal tubule is rightly regarded as the most important site of action of salt-active steroids such as aldosterone, but these substances also influence electrolyte movements in other epithelia, including those of sweat glands, ciliary body, avian salt-gland, fish gills, toad bladder and frog skin. The composition of many alimentary secretions is influenced by these steroids; the change in composition is similar to that of urine, in that sodium concentrations are reduced and potassium concentrations increased, and the action on the gut therefore reinforces the renal effect in increasing total body sodium, and hence extracellular fluid volume, at the expense of potassium.

Not all alimentary secretions have been adequately studied for a mineralocorticoid effect, but it appears that the organs most influenced are the salivary glands and the colon. Thus the hormones have their main effect where secretions which may be lost from the body are elaborated, the only sites where sodium conservation plays a homeostatic role.

Saliva. Adrenal steroids lower the sodium and increase the potassium concentration of mixed saliva (White, Entmacher, Rubin & Leiter, 1955) and the salivary Na/K ratio has therefore been advocated as a means of diagnosing increased mineralocorticoid activity (Frawley & Thorn, 1951; Lauler, Hickler & Thorn, 1962). Conditions known to be accompanied by secondary hyperaldosteronism, such as experimental salt depletion and congestive heart failure, have also been shown to be accompanied by a low Na/K (White, Gordon & Leiter, 1950). Unfortunately in man the salivary sodium concentration, and hence Na/K ratio, is profoundly influenced by slight changes in rate of flow (Thaysen et al., 1954) except at high flow rates which are difficult to achieve in clinical practice. Hence saliva has not been of much help in detecting increased mineralocorticoid activity in man (Prader et al., 1955), although it has been a very useful guide to this state in physiological studies on the sheep (Blair-West, Coghlan, Denton & Wright, 1967). Despite the limitations of human studies it can be safely asserted that an Na/K value of 0·25 or less is evidence of increased mineralocorticoid activity, whereas a value of 1·0 or more excludes it (Lauler et al., 1962); unfortunately in practice many values are found to lie between these figures.

Stomach. There are many studies showing that all the secretory functions of the stomach are depressed in the absence of cortisol, but it is not clear whether mineralocorticoids have an influence on the electrolyte composition of gastric juice. McCance (1938), in his classic studies of human salt depletion, found a slight reduction in the acid, chloride and sodium concentrations of histamine-stimulated gastric juice, with an increase in potassium concentration, but pointed out that these changes could be the result of admixture with swallowed saliva. Lipsett, Schwartz & Thorn (1961) summarized the scanty evidence then available, from which it was not possible to state whether aldosterone definitely has an effect, and Gilder & Moody (1966) have since been unable to demonstrate an effect of aldosterone on the gastric juice of the dog.

Pancreatic juice and bile. No convincing evidence has yet been produced showing whether mineralocorticoids influence the electrolyte composition of these secretions.

Ileum. Study of the effect of mineralocorticoids on sodium and potassium movements in the ileum has not been rewarding, perhaps because variations in ionic flux are so great that small changes are easily obscured. In the dog Berger, Kanzakie & Steele (1952) found no change in sodium or potassium fluxes after DOCA, but Shields, Mulholland & Elmslie (1966) found that administration of aldosterone increased ileal secretion of potassium, without a change in sodium movement.

Studies of ileostomy fluid have been more consistent, though even here the effects o mineralocorticoids are less impressive than further down the bowel. Sodium depletion has been shown to reduce ileostomy losses of sodium and water, and to increase losses of potassium, in both animals and man (Field *et al.*, 1955; Gallagher *et al.*, 1962; Goodall & Kay, 1965; Clarke, Hill & Macbeth, 1967), changes which can be reversed by intravenous salt loading (Clarke & Hill, 1966). Similar changes have followed administration of cortisone (Smiddy, Gregory, Smith & Goligher, 1960) and fludrocortisone (Goulston, Harrison & Skyring, 1963). Levitan & Goulston (1967) failed to demonstrate an effect with aldosterone, but they gave the hormone in a single daily intravenous injection, and it is likely that the short-lived effect of this hormone (usually about 8 hr.) would not be observed in these circumstances.

Colon. Aldosterone and related steroids have profound effects on the colon, although there is some uncertainty as to whether the effect on sodium or potassium movement is the more marked. Increased net absorption of sodium and water has been demonstrated (Levitan & Ingelfinger, 1965; Wrong, 1968) and appears to be the result of increased unidirectional movement of sodium from the lumen (Levitan, 1967). Levitan was unable to demonstrate an effect on potassium movement; however, in the rat Edmonds & Marriott (1967) found an increase in both the net absorption of sodium and the net secretion of

potassium, but no effect on bicarbonate. Shields and his colleagues have found increased potassium secretion, but no effect on sodium, in normal subjects given aldosterone (Shields, Mulholland & Elmslie, 1966) and in a patient with primary aldosteronism (Shields, Miles & Gilberton, 1968). It is likely that these differences between the results of these groups of workers are partly caused by slight differences in experimental technique.

Faeces. The effect of adrenal steroids on faecal composition must be largely a result of the colonic effect, as the influence of these hormones on ileal contents is so slight.

Administration of aldosterone, and conditions associated with increased aldosterone secretion, are accompanied by a low faecal sodium, a high faecal potassium, and a low Na/K ratio. This effect was first observed when ion-exchange resins were used to remove sodium from the body, when it was noted that the sodium yield was disappointingly low in cardiac failure and hepatic cirrhosis (Berger & Steele, 1952; Duncan, 1953) but was high in adrenal insufficiency (Emerson, Kahn & Jenkins, 1953). It has since been realized that patients with primary aldosteronism sometimes have a high daily faecal potassium excretion (Mader & Iseri, 1955; Milne, Muehrcke & Aird, 1957; Brooks, McSwiney, Prunty & Wood, 1957), and that experimental circumstances associated with secondary hyperaldosteronism are associated with a low faecal sodium or Na/K ratio (Duncan, Liddle & Bartter, 1956; Davis, Ball, Bahn & Goodkind, 1959).

The effects of mineralocorticoids on faecal composition have been particularly apparent in specimens obtained by *in vivo* faecal dialysis (Wrong, Morrison & Hurst, 1961; Wrong & Metcalfe-Gibson, 1965; Richards, 1969; Charron *et al.*, 1969). This technique has shown a marked fall in sodium concentration, a smaller percentage increase in potassium concentration, and little or no effect on the concentrations of other ions. In untreated patients with primary aldosteronism the changes were similar to those seen in normal subjects given aldosterone or fludrocortisone, a finding which suggests that escape from the action of aldosterone (which is characteristic of the renal effect of the hormone) is not a feature of the bowel. All the effects of aldosterone on faecal dialysate could be prevented by the aldosterone-antagonist spironolactone, but this substance had little effect on the faecal dialysate of normal subjects who were not receiving aldosterone.

The technique of *in vivo* dialysis of faeces promises to be of value in the diagnosis of primary aldosteronism (Charron *et al.*, 1969; Richards, 1969) but it is possible that a simple determination of Na/K ratio on a sample of whole stool, which is even easier to perform, will be as helpful (Charron *et al.*, 1969).

ALIMENTARY AMMONIA AND UREA; THE EFFECTS OF RENAL FAILURE

Ammonia production. Ammonia in the alimentary tract is derived from at least four sources:

(1) Ingested ammonia. Normal food contains very little free ammonia, but it may be derived from ammonium chloride, administered as a diuretic, or cation-exchange resins in the ammonium form.

(2) Bacterial breakdown of urea. This is the major source of ammonia in the alimentary tract. Many commensal bacteria normally present in the alimentary tract, particularly in the colon and mouth, produce ureases which convert urea to ammonium carbonate. Walser & Bodenlos (1959) showed that at least 20% of the daily production of urea (equivalent to over 40% of the urea pool) is normally destroyed each day in the body. This urea breakdown can be prevented by intestinal antibiotics (Walser & Bodenlos, 1959) or in animals by evisceration or rearing in a germ-free environment (Chao & Tarver, 1953; Levenson, Crowley, Horowitz & Malm, 1959), findings which show that urea destruction depends on the presence of bacteria in the gut. Although urea may be broken down at all levels in the gut, in man the colon appears to be the main site of ammonia production from urea (Folin & Denis, 1912; Silen, Harper, Mawdsley & Weirich, 1955). This organ is particularly abundant in urease-producing bacteria, and urea breakdown is sufficiently rapid and complete to prevent urea normally appearing in detectable quantities in faecal dialysate, although it appears in concentrations close to plasma levels during administration of intestinal antibiotics (Wilson, Ing, Metcalfe-Gibson & Wrong, 1968a).

(3) Ammonia is also produced by peptic digestion of proteins, and is probably derived from the amide group of glutamine radicals (Melville, 1935; Webster, Davidson & Gabuzda, 1958).

(4) Ingraham & Visscher (1938) found that ammonia was directly produced by the mucosa of the ileum, and that this process could be prevented by metabolic inhibitors, suggesting that the ammonia was produced by active metabolism of the mucosa. However *in vitro* work, in a solution containing no urea, would be necessary to prove that this ammonia is not the result of bacterial action.

Ammonia absorption. The major site of ammonia absorption in man is the colon (Folin & Denis, 1912; Silen *et al.*, 1955). However it is probable that ammonia is absorbed from most other parts of the alimentary canal. Drs. J. Kopstein and J. D. Swales (unpublished) have shown in the author's laboratory that ammonia is absorbed from saliva, where it is derived from bacterial breakdown of urea (Schmitz, 1922; Updegraff & Lewis, 1924), through the oral mucosa by a process of non-ionic diffusion.

Ammonia is also absorbed from jejunum and ileum. Kettering & Summerskill (1967) found no evidence in man that absorption at the former site was pH-dependent, and therefore considered that non-ionic diffusion was not important. Mossberg (1967), using metabolic inhibitors in everted sacs of hamster ileum, concluded that ammonia absorption was active and uninfluenced by non-ionic diffusion, although he did note that absorption required the presence of bicarbonate. On the other hand Price *et al.* (1967) found evidence of pH-dependence of ammonia absorption in hamster ileum and dog jejunum, and concluded that the mechanism of absorption was by non-ionic diffusion.

Active secretion of bicarbonate, which occurs in all parts of the intestine, probably plays a major part in facilitating non-ionic diffusion of ammonia, and may reconcile the discrepancies reported above. Rosenfeld, Aboulafia & Schwartz (1963) have pointed out that even such an impermeable membrane as dog bladder may permit rapid passive diffusion of ammonia, provided that bicarbonate is also present. Ammonia and carbon dioxide will diffuse together from such a solution according to the reaction

$$NH_4^+ + HCO_3^- \xrightarrow{\text{non-ionic diffusion}} NH_3 \nearrow + CO_2 \nearrow + H_2O$$

The simultaneous loss of carbon dioxide and ammonia causes no pH change in the solution, and so these two non-ionic species will continue to be generated as long as ammonium and bicarbonate ions are both present. This reaction ("paired non-ionic diffusion") might occur in the interstices of the mucosal surface, where secreted bicarbonate first meets ammonium ion, and the bicarbonate secreted by the mucosa would in this case not gain access to the main lumen of the intestine, and ammonia absorption might appear to be uninfluenced by pH. The finding of Mossberg (1967) that metabolic inhibitors reduced

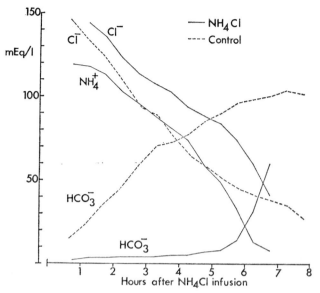

FIG. 19.3. Comparison of the effects of colonic infusion of isotonic ammonium chloride (continuous lines) with sodium chloride (interrupted lines). Note that in the NH₄Cl experiment HCO₃⁻ did not accumulate in the colon until NH₄⁺ had largely disappeared. Osmolalities (260–290 mOsm./kg.) were not significantly different in the two studies, but pH was 7·3–8·2 in the control and 5·8–6·7 in the NH₄Cl experiment.

ammonia absorption can be attributed to their effect in inhibiting active bicarbonate secretion. Unpublished work by Drs. M. Papadimitriou and J. D. Swales, in the author's department, on *in vivo* preparations of human and rat ileum, support the above hypothesis.

In the colon ammonia absorption appears to be by passive non-ionic diffusion (Price *et al.*, 1967). Wherever ammonia is derived by bacterial breakdown from urea the medium is alkaline, and this itself favours non-ionic diffusion. The additional facilitation provided by active bicarbonate secretion is well shown in Figure 19.3, which shows the contrasting fate of isotonic sodium chloride and ammonium chloride solutions in the defunctioned human colon. Note that the bicarbonate which accumulates rapidly after infusion of sodium chloride (and see Fig. 19.1) fails to accumulate in the colon after infusion of ammonium chloride, until almost all the infused ammonium has been absorbed. The likely explanation is that bicarbonate secretion is equal in both studies, but that in the presence of ammonium ion bicarbonate disappears, as a result of paired non-ionic diffusion, as rapidly as it is secreted.

The fate of absorbed ammonia. Except in the mouth and terminal part of the rectum all absorbed ammonia enters the portal circulation

and reaches the liver, where it normally is largely reconverted to urea. However this ammonia can be utilized in protein synthesis, and ingested ammonia or urea is known to make a major contribution to the protein economy of many animals (Liu *et al.*, 1955; Rose & Dekker, 1956; Houpt, 1963). Recently Richards *et al* (1967) studied this phenomenon in man and found that normal subjects could incorporate 4% of an oral load of ammonia nitrogen into serum albumin; this figure was increased to 12% by three weeks of a very low protein diet. These workers suggested that ammonia utilization could be further stimulated by removing all protein from the diet and supplying essential amino acids as keto acids, for with the exceptions of lysine and threonine all essential amino acids can be transaminated in the liver (Meister, 1965).

The above comments suggest that one biological advantage of active bicarbonate secretion throughout the intestine is that it facilitates ammonia reabsorption, and hence assists animals to re-utilize their own urea nitrogen in protein synthesis. This mechanism has obvious biological benefits for the many animals which subsist on very low protein diets, even though it may confer little advantage on Western man.

The gut in uraemia. In renal failure the increased plasma concentration of urea is accompanied by a parallel increase in the urea concentration of most intestinal fluids. In parotid saliva Forland, Shannon & Katz (1964) found urea concentrations close to those in plasma, but in mixed saliva, collected from the mouth, urea concentrations are lower, and ammonia concentrations higher, as a result of bacterial breakdown (Schmitz, 1922; Updegraff & Lewis, 1924). Urea and ammonia concentrations are known to be increased in gastric juice (Lieber & Lefèvre, 1959; Fillastre, Blaise, Ardaillou & Richet, 1965), but it is not known whether the urea is destroyed by ureases of bacterial origin or those normally present in the cells of the gastric mucosa. Lieber & Lefèvre (1959) have suggested that the diminished gastric acidity of uraemia is the result of neutralization of gastric hydrochloric acid by products of urea breakdown.

A few years ago the author was fortunate in having the opportunity to study hepatic bile in a patient recovering from acute renal failure after cholecystectomy, and the urea concentration in the bile was noted to be close to plasma values (Fig. 19.4). Information on urea and ammonia concentrations from small bowel contents and pancreatic juice in renal failure is apparently not available.

Despite the enormous amounts of urea which must enter the gut in renal failure, there is usually no increase in faecal nitrogen (Stanbury & Lumb, 1962) and faecal dialysate urea, pH and ammonia concentrations are only slightly higher than normal (Wilson, Ing, Metcalfe-Gibson &

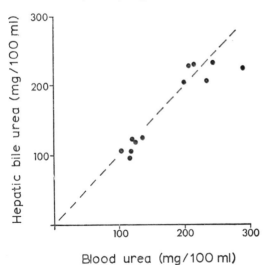

FIG. 19.4. Concentrations of urea in hepatic bile from a patient recovering from acute renal failure.

Wrong, 1968b). However in renal failure faecal dialysate urea concentrations have been shown to increase to close to plasma levels during administration of intestinal antibiotics (Wilson et al., 1968b), a finding which shows that bacterial breakdown of urea in the intestine must be enormously increased. Turnover measurements of labelled urea in uraemia have shown that this is indeed the case, the endogenous destruction of urea being increased in proportion to the increase in plasma urea concentration (Scholtz, 1968; Deane, Desir & Umeda, 1968; Robson, Kerr & Ashcroft, 1968). As might be expected, incorporation of urea nitrogen into plasma albumin is also increased in these circumstances (Richards et al., 1967).

The part played by increased intestinal pH and ammonia concentrations in producing the clinical picture of uraemia is uncertain, but stomatitis, gastritis and colitis have all been attributed to these biochemical changes (Schreiner & Maher, 1961).

Faecal potassium is increased in renal failure (Hayes, McLeod & Robinson, 1967) and sodium is reduced (Wilson et al., 1968b). These changes are similar to those induced by aldosterone, and have been attributed by Wilson et al (1968b) to a chronic state of hyperaldosteronism caused by mild potassium retention.

EFFECTS OF DIVERSION OF URINE INTO THE ALIMENTARY TRACT

In disease of the ureters, bladder, or urethra it may become necessary to divert urine into the bowel by ureteral transplantation. The underlying conditions for which this surgical procedure is most often undertaken are carcinoma of the bladder, tuberculous contracture of the bladder, congenital ectopia vesicae, and intractable fistula of the lower urinary tract. Patients with transplanted ureters are liable to mechanical problems at the site of the anastomosis, and these include stenosis and ureteric reflux, either of which may lead to severe and recurrent renal infection and eventual renal failure; there is also a long-term risk of malignancy developing at the site of the anastomosis (Kille & Glick, 1967). In addition the special absorptive and secretory properties of the gut lead to the development of various predictable electrolyte disturbances, the exact nature of which depends on the segment of bowel used, and the length of time that urine remains within the bowel. The subject has been well reviewed by Schwartz & Kassirer (1963).

Uretero-colic anastomosis. Until the last 15

years the ureters were usually implanted into the sigmoid colon. This operation enables patients to remain continent, for they use the lower bowel as a reservoir which is under voluntary control, but the operation is attended by a high rate of attacks of ascending renal infection, perhaps because colonic contents are normally heavily infested with urinary pathogens, and during straining a positive pressure of up to 120 mm. of water (Keith, 1907) may develop in the colon. In addition such patients, particularly those who do not make a deliberate effort to empty their rectum frequently, are liable to attacks of proctitis, often haemorrhagic, a direct result of the irritant effect of urine on the rectal mucosa.

The metabolic effects of uretero-sigmoid anastomosis include moderate azotaemia (blood urea 50–150 mg./100 ml.), hyperchloraemic acidosis, and less frequently hypokalaemia (about one third of patients) and rarely osteomalacia or rickets, with a low serum inorganic phosphate and a high alkaline phosphatase (Harrison, 1958; Green & Boyd, 1959). These same changes all occur in renal tubular acidosis (see Chapter 10), and hence there was for many years a belief that their development after ureterosigmoid anastomosis was a result of renal damage from ascending infection. It is impossible to deny that this process may play a role in some patients, but it is now clear that the biochemical changes can all be explained as the result of the changes undergone by urine in the colon (Parsons, Powell & Pyrah, 1952; Annis & Alexander, 1952; d'Agostino, Leadbetter & Schwartz, 1953) and it is not necessary to invoke a renal mechanism. The raised blood urea results from colonic reabsorption of urea, both as such (Annis & Alexander, 1952; Bohne & Rupe, 1953), and as ammonia after bacterial degradation (Rosenberg, 1953; Mathisen et al., 1957). Creatinine is not appreciably absorbed from the colon (Bollman & Mann, 1926; Parsons et al., 1952), and if the plasma creatinine is raised above normal this finding suggests true renal impairment. Hyperchloraemic acidosis, almost a constant finding except in patients given prophylactic alkali, is the result of colonic secretion of bicarbonate and reabsorption of urinary chloride. Hypokalaemia is due to potassium depletion caused by colonic secretion of potassium into the urine; the depletion of potassium is more frequent and severe than the plasma potassium concentrations would suggest, for the accompanying acidosis increases the plasma concentration, and a low plasma level may be observed for the first time only when acidosis is corrected. Osteomalacia is probably caused by the chronic acidosis; like the osteomalacia of renal tubular acidosis (Wrong, 1967) it does not develop in patients in whom acidosis is prevented by alkali treatment.

The above sequelae are so common after uretero-sigmoidostomy that the operation has largely been replaced by one in which the ureters are placed into a loop of ileum, rather than colon. However there are a large number of patients with uretero-colic anastomoses functioning at the present time, and the care of their metabolic problems is still important. The majority can be kept free of acidosis on 6–12 grams of sodium bicarbonate (72–145 mEq.) daily, and a potassium supplement is not usually needed. The metabolic effects of the operation can be reduced by frequent emptying of the bowel, which also reduces the risk of colitis and renal infection.

Uretero-ileal anastomosis. Animal experiments, performed many years ago, showed that urine diverted into the intact ileum is almost completely absorbed, and the effect of this operation is therefore tantamount to nephrectomy. In fact this operation, or anastomosis of the ureters with a vein, has been used experimentally when it has been desired to obliterate the effects of urine secretion without damaging renal integrity.

However, an isolated loop of ileum may be used as a conduit for the urine (Brickler, Butcher & McAfee, 1954), and this operation has been much employed in recent years and appears to have fewer serious complications than ureterosigmoidostomy. The principle is different in that the ileum does not act as a reservoir, and merely leads urine into a bag attached to the abdominal wall. Consequently urine does not stagnate in the bowel, and the effects of mucosal absorption and secretion are lessened. In addition there is a lower incidence of renal infection, perhaps because the ileum is not normally the seat of intense bacterial activity, and reflux of infected material into the ureters is less common.

Secretions obtained from isolated ileal loops have bicarbonate concentrations of up to 90 mEq./l. (de Beer, Johnston & Wilson, 1935; Schiffrin & Nasset, 1939), and it might therefore be expected that after this operative procedure patients might still develop hyperchloraemic acidosis because of secretion of bicarbonate into the urine passing through the ileal loop. This complication has been reported (Bricker et al., 1954; Smith & Galante, 1958; Creevy, 1960), but much less frequently than after uretero-sigmoidostomy. Normal ileal contents contain much less potassium than colonic contents, and potassium deficiency does not usually occur after this operation (Geist & Ansell, 1961). The flow of urine through an ileal conduit is sufficiently rapid to prevent significant reabsorption of urea, and an increase in the blood urea concentration of such a patient is good evidence of renal insufficiency.

Further observations are obviously needed, but ileal diversion (uretero-ileostomy) appears to be a considerable improvement on uretero-sigmoidostomy. However the older operation will continue to be preferred by some patients who are not prepared to tolerate an abdominal stoma at any price.

USE OF ION-EXCHANGE RESINS

In clinical medicine ion-exchange resins are employed only in the alimentary tract and it is therefore appropriate to consider their use here.

All the synthetic resins used clinically, with the exception of the weakly acidic polymethacrylate resins (see below) have an insoluble polystyrene matrix having the general formula shown in Figure 19.5. Various ionizable groups, such as

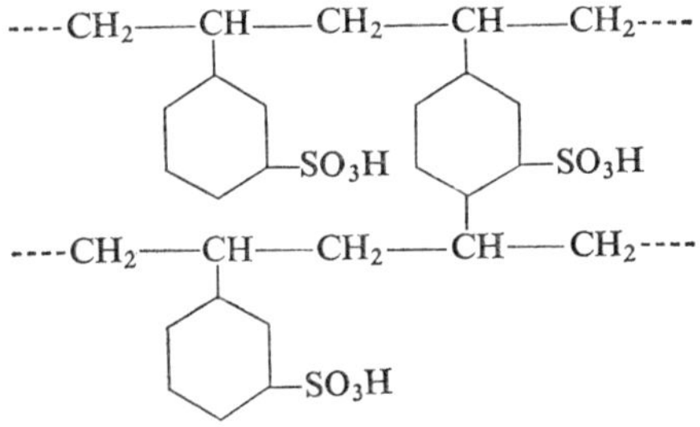

FIG. 19.5. Polystyrene skeleton of a typical ion-exchange resin. In this case the exchange groups are shown as sulphonic acid (RSO_3H) as the resin depicted is a strongly acidic cation-exchanger.

the sulphonic acid group ($-SO_3H$) shown, can be attached to the benzene rings during the process of manufacture, and the properties of these groups determine the exchange properties of the final resin. Thus, if the active group is an acid the resin can exchange its hydrogen ion for other cations, and is known as a cation-exchange resin, whereas if the active group is a base it can reversibly combine with different anions, and is known as an anion-exchange resin. At the present time all resins in clinical use are monofunctional; i.e. they contain only one type of functional group. Most ion-exchange resins have an ion-binding capacity of about

4 mEq. per gram of dried resin; the binding capacity of the weakly acidic polymethacrylate resins is greater, about 12 mEq./g.

The open structure of a resin permits the entrance of a large amount of water, and some resins are more stable in this form. The closeness of the resin structure, and hence the ease with which water and ions can penetrate the matrix, depends on the number of cross-links between the benzene rings, and this is determined during manufacture. Most resins are marketed containing a variable amount of water, up to 50% of their weight, and unless this factor is taken into account a comparison of the capacities of different resins may be misleading.

Binding of ions by ion-exchange resins depends mainly on two factors—(1) the affinity of the resin for different ions, and (2) the ionic composition of the ambient solution. In general the higher the valency of an ion the more tightly it will be bound to a resin. For ions of the same valency the affinity of the resin decreases as the size of the hydrated ion increases, i.e. within the same group of the periodic table the heavier members are usually bound more firmly. However, the affinity for very large ions may be low because the ion may be too large to enter the resin matrix freely. With ions of physiological interest the affinity of most strongly acid cation-exchange resins is in the approximate descending order $Al^{+++} > Sr^{++} > Ca^{++} > Mg^{++} > Cs^+ > Rb^+ > NH_4^+ = K^+ > Na^+ > H^+ > Li^+$, and for strongly basic anion-exchange resins is $PO_4^{\equiv} > SO_4^= > $ citrate$^{\equiv} > CO_3^= > Cl^- > HCO_3^- > $ acetate$^- > OH^-$.

In clinical practice the affinity of a resin for different ions is rather less important in determining what ions become attached to the resin than is the composition of the fluid surrounding the resin. Even ions with a high affinity for a resin can be replaced by other ions if their concentration in the surrounding solution is negligible. Most resins are taken by mouth, and reach ionic equilibrium with the fluid at various levels of the alimentary tract, but the form in which they are excreted in the faeces depends mainly on the ionic composition of colonic contents, for even in this distal part of the alimentary tract the contents are still sufficiently fluid for ionic exchange to occur. Resins are rather unpalatable to take by mouth, having a sandy consistency which the pharmaceutical companies have only partly managed to disguise by grinding and flavouring.

In the following sections the main clinical uses of resins are considered. The principles of all the main types of resin are discussed, even those which are little used, for the clinical uses of resins are likely to increase and their potentialities have not yet been fully explored. For further details of structure and chemical properties the reader is referred to Kitchener (1957), and for clinical applications to Miner (1953).

Cation-exchange Resins

Weakly acidic resins. These are either polymethacrylate resins containing carboxyl groups (RCOOH) or polystyrene resins with phenolic groups attached to the benzene ring (ROH). These resins dissociate and contribute hydrogen to an alkaline medium (over pH 7·0) but return to their original form at lower pH. The polymethacrylate carboxylic resins have a high *in vitro* cation-exchange capacity, about 12 mEq./g. dried resin, and for this reason were one of the first resins used to remove sodium from the body (Feinberg & Rosenberg, 1951; Klingensmith & Elkinton, 1952); they have also been used, in the sodium form, to remove potassium (Elkinton, Clark, Squires, Bluemle & Crosley, 1950). However the full exchange capacity of these resins is not realized at the pH of intestinal fluids (McChesney, Nachod & Tainter, 1953), and they have therefore been largely replaced by the sulphonic acid resins (see below) which are just as efficient as ion-exchangers *in vivo*, and are less bulky and cause fewer gastro-intestinal symptoms.

The tendency of carboxylic resins to revert to the RCOOH form at low pH has been exploited in various "tubeless" tests of gastric analysis, in which a carboxylic resin combined with a non-toxic and easily detected cationic dye is taken by mouth. The amount of dye released by the resin in the stomach, and hence the amount which appears in the urine, is determined by the hydrogen ion concentration of the gastric contents, and a variety of different dyes and carboxylic resins have been used for this purpose (Segal, Miller & Morton, 1950). Unpredictable variations in gastric emptying time and small intestine mobility make it impossible to estimate the excretion of gastric hydrochloric acid in quantitative terms, but do permit a rough estimation of gastric pH which is sufficiently reliable for some clinical purposes.

Strongly acidic resins. In these resins the active radicals are sulphonic acid groups (Fig. 19.5) which are ionized in all but the most acid media; in the hydrogen ion form they will donate hydrogen ion according to the order of affinities shown above, and therefore behave as strong acids. They have been widely used to

remove sodium from the body in oedematous states (Dock & Frank, 1950; Irwin, Berger, Roseberg & Jackenthal, 1949) and have largely replaced carboxylic acid resins for this purpose. Originally they were used in the hydrogen ion or ammonium forms, in amounts up to 75 g./day by mouth, but it was found that many patients became potassium-depleted because of the potassium removed by the resin. The practice was therefore adopted of giving a proportion of the resin in the potassium form; "Katonium" (Bayer Winthrop) is such a resin, and is 25% in the potassium form and 75% in the ammonium form. Such resins are liable to cause acidosis in patients with renal disease, or intensify acidosis already present, because the ammonium contributed to body fluids is converted to hydrogen ion which cannot be excreted by the kidneys. Although these resins are effective in correcting the sodium retention of most oedematous states they are now little used because of the advent of powerful new oral diuretics such as the thiazides and frusemide.

Strongly acidic cation-exchange resins are now chiefly used to prevent dangerous hyperkalaemia in those with potassium retention caused by renal failure (Evans, Hughes-Jones, Milne & Yellowlees, 1953). This problem has been particularly common in patients maintained on very low protein diets (20 g./day or less) which permit survival when it would otherwise be impossible without some form of renal replacement. The resin has usually been given in the sodium form (e.g. "Resonium A", "Kayexelate"), and is effective whether given by mouth or enema; oral administration is slightly more effective, probably because the resin remains longer in the proximal part of the colon, where potassium secretion is active, whereas resin given by enema is apt to be expelled before it exerts its full exchange potential. The yield of potassium when the resin is given by mouth is about 1 mEq./g. of dried resin.

Although sodium cycle resins have undoubtedly prevented many deaths from hyperkalaemia, it has recently been pointed out (Berlyne, Janabi & Shaw, 1966) that the sodium which is released by the resin in the gut may lead to dangerous sodium retention in patients with impaired ability to excrete sodium, and hence contribute to oedema and hypertension. Berlyne *et al.* (1966) suggested that calcium might be a more suitable form of resin for such patients, for calcium is known to be absorbed poorly from the intestine in renal failure. (Magnesium is contraindicated because magnesium retention is a feature of renal failure, and hydrogen ion and ammonium because of the acidosis they cause). Calcium resin has now been used in many centres, but unfortunately has precipitated hypercalcaemia in some patients (Papadimitriou, Gingell & Chisholm, 1968; Sevitt & Wrong, 1968), and so it is clear that the calcium released by the resin in the gut cannot be entirely disregarded. Chugh, Swales, Brown & Wrong (1968) have suggested that the ideal form of cation-exchange resin might be the aluminium phase, which would replace potassium in the gut by a cation which has advantages of its own, for aluminium is not absorbed and precipitates in the gut as insoluble aluminium phosphate, which is advantageous in the treatment of the phosphate retention of renal failure. However the ideal form of cation-exchange resin for potassium removal may not yet have been found, and patients might do best with tailor-made resins to suit individual requirements, containing various proportions of calcium, magnesium, sodium and aluminium.

Anion-exchange Resins

Weakly basic resins. In these the active groups are secondary or tertiary amines, which can take up hydrogen ion, and so associate with an anion, in a medium more acid than pH 7 (e.g. $RN(CH_3)_2 \rightarrow RN(CH_3)_2H^+Cl^-$) but revert to the undissociated amine at higher pH values. Such resins should theoretically be useful in neutralizing gastric hydrochloric acid in patients with peptic ulcer, for they would neutralize gastric acid but have no effect on systemic acid-base metabolism (Martin & Wilkinson, 1946). However, in practice these resins have not been very useful, mainly because of the large doses of resin required and the many cheaper preparations which are as effective in neutralizing gastric acid.

Strongly basic resins. The active group in these resins is the quaternary ammonium radical $(RN(CH_3)_3^+)$ which remains ionized over the entire pH range. They have the disadvantage, for clinical use, that they slowly decompose, yielding trimethylamine which has an unpleasant fishy odour and taste. These resins have been used clinically to reduce the acidosis caused by sulphonic and carboxylic resins in the hydrogen ion cycle (Greenman, Frey, Lewis, Sakol & Danowski, 1953), in the proportions 88% cation-exchanger, 12% anion-exchanger, the anion-exchange resin being in forms such as acetate, lactate, or carbonate which would correct acidosis when exchanged for chloride or phos-

phate from body fluids. Unfortunately the capacity of these resins to correct acidosis is severely limited, being of the order of 1 mEq./g. or less, because during transit through the bowel most of their exchange capacity is taken up by organic anions and bicarbonate (Hurst, Morrison, Timoner, Metcalfe-Gibson & Wrong, 1953) which as we have seen, are the predominant anions in the colon. The relative failure of this form of resin emphasizes an important principle of treatment by oral resins: a resin can only remove from the body ions which are normally present in the bowel lumen at the most distal site where free ionic change is possible. Thus anion-exchange resins remove little chloride from the body, even though they must be converted almost fully to the chloride form in the stomach, because they yield up their chloride content lower down in the intestine where the concentrations of this ion are extremely low.

Strongly basic anion-exchange resins are also used to lower the bile anion concentration of patients with biliary obstruction and intolerable itching, or the serum cholesterol in patients with hypercholesterolaemia. The principle in treatment of the latter condition is that the resin prevents reabsorption of bile anions which are normally reabsorbed in the distal ileum, and thus reduces the cholesterol pool. The resin mainly used for these purposes has been "cholestyramine" (Merck) but other strongly basic anion-exchange resins would probably be as effective. "Cholestyramine" is in the chloride form, and is taken in a dose of about 12 g./day. This treatment has the theoretical hazard of producing a hyperchloraemic acidosis in patients with renal impairment, a danger which could be circumvented by using the resin combined with a metabolizable anion, such as carbonate or acetate.

Ion-exchange resins have numerous other theoretical uses in clinical medicine. An interesting possibility is that they might play a useful role in the treatment of drug overdose (Edwards & McCredie, 1967), for most drugs are either anions or cations and can be bound by the appropriate resin. A cation-exchange resin will bind cations such as quinine, mecamylamine, strychnine and morphine; whereas an anion-exchange resin could be used to bind barbiturates, salicylates, or iodide. Resins could be used either to prevent absorption of a drug from the alimentary tract or, in the case of drugs which are present in intestinal secretions, to increase elimination even after absorption. The use of ion-exchange materials as antidotes to poisoning goes back to medieval times, when the natural earth *terra sigillata* was popular for this purpose (Berger, 1953).

Ion-exchange resins can be manufactured containing radicals which bind ions with a high degree of specificity (Kitchener, 1957) but the clinical uses of such resins have not been explored.

Soluble aluminium and calcium salts, when taken by mouth, behave like highly selective resins, binding phosphate and carbonate respectively. Aluminium phosphate is almost totally insoluble and thus any free aluminium ion in the intestine will bind phosphate and prevent its absorption (Kirsner, 1941); aluminium hydroxide gel is the usual preparation used, and it is employed to reduce the phosphate retention of renal failure (Mallick & Berlyne, 1968). Calcium salts, such as calcium chloride, combine with bicarbonate in the intestine to form insoluble calcium carbonate (Haldane, Hill & Luck, 1923) a reaction which can readily be observed *in vitro* ($Ca^{++} + 2HCO_3^- \rightarrow CaCO_3 + CO_2 + H_2O$). Oral calcium chloride is therefore a very effective acidifying stimulus, for it replaces bicarbonate derived from body fluids by chloride, and it is as effective in producing acidosis as an equivalent amount of oral ammonium chloride (Gamble, Blackfan & Hamilton, 1925). Christensen (1959) has suggested that calcium chloride has an acidifying effect because it is precipitated as tribasic calcium phosphate ($3\,Ca^{++} + 2\,HPO_4^- \rightarrow Ca_3(PO_4)_2 + 2H^+$); but although this reaction, probably occurs to a small extent (Hurst *et al.*, 1963) it does not contribute enough hydrogen ion to the body to explain the full acidifying effect of calcium chloride.

References

ABER, G. M., SAMPSON, P. A., WHITEHEAD, T. P. & BROOKE, B. N. (1962). *Lancet*, **2**, 1028.

ANDERSSON, B., LARSSON, S. & PERSSON, N. (1960). *Acta Physiol. Scand.*, **50**, 140.

ANNIS, D. & ALEXANDER, M. K. (1952). *Lancet*, **2**, 603.

BERGER, E. Y. (1953). *Ann. New York Acad. Sci.*, **57**, 305.

BERGER, E. Y. (1960). In "Mineral Metabolism." Ed. Comar, C. L. & Bronner, F. Academic Press, New York, Vol. 1A, p. 249.

BERGER, E. Y., KANZAKI, G. & STEELE, J. M. (1952). *J. Physiol.* (Lond.), **151**, 352.

BERGER, E. Y. & STEELE, J. M. (1952). *J. Clin. Invest.*, **31**, 451.

BERLYNE, G. M., JANABI, K. & SHAW, A. B. (1966). *Lancet*, **1**, 167.

BLACK, D. A. K. (1964). In "The Scientific Basis of Medicine Annual Reviews," Athlone Press, London, p. 291.

BLACK, D. A. K. & JEPSON, R. P. (1954). *Quart. J. Med.*, **23**, 367.

BLAIR-WEST, J. R., COGHLAN, J. P., DENTON, D. A., NELSON, J. F., ORCHARD, E., SCOGGINS, B. A., WRIGHT, R. D., MYERS, K. & JUNQUEIRA, C. L. (1968). *Nature*, **217**, 922.

BLAIR-WEST, J. R., COGHLAN, J. P., DENTON, D. A. & WRIGHT, R. D. (1967). From "Handbook of Physiology," Sect. 6, Vol. 2, 633. Amer. Physiol. Soc., Washington, D.C.

BOHNE, A. W. & RUPE, C. E. (1953). *Surg. Gynec. Obst.*, **96**, 541.

BOLLMAN, J. L. & MANN, F. C. (1926). *Proc. Soc. Exper. Biol. Med.* (N.Y.), **24**, 923.

BORGSTRÖM, B., DAHLQVIST, A., LUNDH, G. & SJÖVALL, J. (1957). *J. Clin. Invest.*, **36**, 1521.

BOTT, E., DENTON, D. A. & WELLER, S. (1967). *Aust. J. exper. Biol. med. Sci.*, **45**, 595.

BREUHAUS, H. C. & EYERLY, J. B. (1943). *Gastroenterology*, **1**, 583.

BRICKER, E. M., BUTCHER, H. & McAFEE, C. A. (1954). *Surg. Gynec. Obst.*, **99**, 469.

BROOKS, R. V., McSWINEY, R. R., PRUNTY, F. T. G. & WOOD, F. J. Y. (1957). *Amer. J. Med.*, **23**, 391.

BURGEN, A. S. V. (1967). From "Handbook of Physiology," Sec. 6, Vol. 2, p. 561, Amer. Physiol. Soc., Washington, D.C.

BURNELL, J. M., VILLAMILL, M. F., UYENO, B. T. & SCRIBNER, B. H. (1956). *J. Clin. Invest.*, **35**, 935.

BURNETT, C. H., BURROWS, B. A., COMMONS, R. S. & TOWERY, B. J. (1950). *J. Clin. Invest.*, **29**, 175.

CARD, W. I. & MARKS, I. N. (1960). *Clin. Sci.*, **19**, 147.

CHAO, F. C. & TARVER, H. (1953). *Proc. Soc. Exp. Biol. Med.* (N.Y.), **84**, 406.

CHARRON, R. C., LEME, C. E., WILSON, D. R., ING, T. S. & WRONG, O. M. (1969). *Clin. Sci.*, **37**, 151.

CHRISTENSEN, H. N. (1959). "Diagnostic Biochemistry." Oxford University Press, p. 126.

CHUGH, K. S., SWALES, J. D., BROWN, C. L. & WRONG, O. M. (1968). *Lancet*, **2**, 952.

CLARK, G. W. (1926). *Univ. Calif. Publ. Physiol.*, **5**, 195.

CLARKE, A. M., CHIRNSIDE, A., HILL, G. L., POPE, G. & STEWART, M. K. (1967). *Lancet*, **2**, 740.

CLARKE, A. M. & HILL, G. L. (1966). *Proc. Univ. Otago med. Sch.*, **44**, 51.

CLARKE, A. M., HILL, G. L. & MACBETH, W. A. A. G. (1967). *Gastroenterology*, **53**, 444.

CONARD, V., KAWALEWSKI, K. & VAN GEERTRUYDEN, J. (1949). *Acta gastro-ent.belg.*, **12**, 97.

COOKE, R. E., SEGAR, W. E., CHEEK, D. B., COVILLE, F. E. & DARROW, D. C. (1952). *J. Clin. Invest.*, **31**, 798.

COOPERSTEIN, I. L. & BROCKMAN, S. K. (1959). *J. Clin. Invest.*, **38**, 435.

COOPERSTEIN, I. L. & HOGBEN, C. A. M. (1959). *J. gen. Physiol.* **42**, 461.

COPE, C. L. (1966). *Brit. med. J.*, **1**, 1344.

CREEVY, C. D. (1960). *J. Urol.* **83**, 394.

CURRAN, P. F. & SCHULTZ, S. G. (1968). In "Handbook of Physiology," Sect. 6, Vol. III, p. 1217, Amer. Physiol. Soc., Washington, D.C.

CURRAN, P. F. & SOLOMON, A. K. (1957). J. gen. Physiol., **41**, 143.

D'AGOSTINO, A., LEADBETTER, W. F. & SCHWARTZ, W. B. (1953). J. Clin. Invest., **32**, 444.

DAHL, L. K. (1958). New Engl. J. Med., **258**, 1152.

DAVENPORT, H. W. (1966). "Physiology of the Digestive Tract," Year Book Medical Publishers, Chicago, 2nd Edition.

DAVIES, H. E. F., JEPSON, R. P. & BLACK, D. A. K. (1956). Clin. Sci., **15**, 61.

DAVIS, J. O., BALL, W. C., BAHN, R. C. & GOODKIND, M. J. (1959). Amer. J. Physiol., **196**, 149.

DEANE, N., DESIR, W. & UMEDA, T. (1968). Proc. Eur. Dial. Transpl. Assoc., **4**, 245.

DE BEER, E. J., JOHNSTON, C. G. & WILSON, D. W. (1935). J. biol. Chem., **108**, 113.

DE GRAEFF, J. & SCHUURS, M. A. M. (1960). Acta Med. Scand., **166**, 407.

DENTON, D. A. (1967). "Handbook of Physiology," Sect. 6, Vol. 1, p. 433, Amer. Physiol. Soc., Washington, D.C.

DIAMOND, J. M. (1968). From "Handbook of Physiology," Sect. 6, Vol. 5, p. 2451, Amer. Physiol. Soc., Washington, D.C.

DOCK, W. & FRANK, N. R. (1950). Amer. Heart J., **40**, 638.

DUNCAN, L. E. (1953). Amer. Heart J., **45**, 802.

DUNCAN, L. E., LIDDLE, G. W. & BARTTER, F. C. (1956). J. Clin. Invest., **35**, 1299.

DUTHIE, H. L. & ATWELL, J. D. (1963). Gut, **4**, 373.

EDMONDS, C. J. (1967). J. Physiol. (Lond.), **193**, 571.

EDMONDS, C. J. & MARRIOTT, J. C. (1967). J. Endocr., **39**, 517.

EDWARDS, K. D. G. & McCREDIE, M. (1967). Med. J. Aust., **i**, 534.

ELKINTON, J. R., CLARK, J. K., SQUIRES, R. D., BLUEMLE, L. W. & CROSLEY, A. P. (1950). Amer. J. med. Sci., **220**, 547.

EMERSON, K., KAHN, S. S. & JENKINS, D. (1953). Ann. N.Y. Acad. Sci., **57**, 280.

ENGSTROM, W. W. & LIEBMAN, A. (1953). Amer. J. Med., **15**, 180.

EVANS, B. M., HUGHES-JONES, N. C., MILNE, M. D. & YELLOWLEES, H. (1953). Lancet, **2**, 791.

EVANSON, J. M. & STANBURY, S. W. (1965). Gut, **6**, 29.

FEINBERG, A. W. & ROSENBERG, B. (1951). Amer. Heart J., **42**, 698.

FIELD, H., SWELL, L., DAILEY, R. E., TROUT, E. C. & BOYD, R. S. (1955). Circulation, **12**, 625.

FILLASTRE, J. P., BLAISE, P., ARDAILLOU, R. & RICHET, G. (1965). Rev. franc. Étud. clin. biol., **10**, 180.

FITZSIMONS, J. T. (1969). J. Physiol. (Lond.), **201**, 349.

FOLIN, O. & DENIS, W. (1912). J. biol. Chem., **11**, 527.

FORDTRAN, J. S. (1967). Fed. Proc., **26**, 1405.

FORDTRAN, J. S. & DIETSCHY, J. M. (1966). Gastroenterology, **50**, 263.

FORDTRAN, J. S. & INGELFINGER, F. J. (1968). From "Handbook of Physiology," Sect. 6, Vol. III, p. 1457, Amer. Physiol. Soc., Washington, D.C.

FORDTRAN, J. S. & LOCKLEAR, T. W. (1966). Amer. J. digest. Dis., **11**, 503.

FORLAND, M., SHANNON, I. L. & KATZ, F. H. (1964). New Engl. J. Med., **271**, 37.

FRAWLEY, T. F. & THORN, G. W. (1951). In "Proceedings of the 2nd Clinical ACTH Conference," Ed. Mote, J. R., London, Churchill, p. 115.

GALLAGHER, N. D., HARRISON, D. D. & SKYRING, A. P. (1962). Gut, **3**, 219.

GAMBLE, J. L. (1951). "Chemical Anatomy, Physiology and Pathology of Extracellular Fluid," 5th Edit., Harvard University Press.

GAMBLE, J. L. (1953). Pediatrics, **11**, 554.

GAMBLE, J. L., BLACKFAN, K. D. & HAMILTON, B. (1925). J. Clin. Invest., **1**, 359.

GARDNER, L. I., MacLACHLAN, E. A. & BERMAN, H. (1952). J. gen. Physiol., **36**, 153.

GEIST, R. W. & ANSELL, J. S. (1961). Surg. Gynec. Obst., **113**, 585.

GILDER, H. & MOODY, F. G. (1966). Proc. Soc. Exp. Biol. Med. (N.Y.), **121**, 913.

GOODALL, E. D. & KAY, R. N. (1965). J. Physiol. (Lond.), **176**, 12.

GOULSTON, K., HARRISON, D. D. & SKYRING, A. P. (1963). Lancet, **2**, 541.

GORDON, R. S., FEELEY, J. C., GREENOUGH, W. B., SPRINZ, H. & OSEASOHN, R. (1966). Ann. Intern. Med., **64**, 1328.

GRANTHAM, J. J. & SCHLOERB, P. R. (1964). Amer. J. Physiol., **207**, 619.

GREEN, R. C. & BOYD, J. A. (1959). Arch. intern. Med., **103**, 807.

GREENMAN, L., FREY, W. A., LEWIS, R. E., SAKOL, M. J. & DANOWSKI, T. S. (1953). J. Lab. Clin. Med., **41**, 236.

HALDANE, J. B. S., HILL, R. & LUCK, J. M. (1923). J. Physiol. (Lond.), **57**, 301.

HANNIGAN, C. A., FROST, R. A. & PERKINS, W. B. (1963). J. Maine med. Ass., **54**, 76.

HARRISON, A. R. (1958). Brit. J. Urol., **30**, 455.

HAYES, C. P., McLEOD, M. E. & ROBINSON, R. R. (1967). Clin. Res., **15**, 50.

HOGBEN, C. A. M. (1960). Amer. J. Med., **29**, 726.

HOLLANDER, F. (1963). Ann. N.Y. Acad. Sci., **106**, 757.

HOUPT, T. R. (1963). Amer. J. Physiol., **205**, 1144.

HOWE, C. T. & LE QUESNE, L. P. (1964). Brit. J. Surg., **51**, 923.

HUNT, J. N. (1959). Physiol. Reviews, **39**, 491.

HUNT, J. N. & WAN, B. (1967). From "Handbook of Physiology," Sect. 6, Vol. II, p. 781, Amer. Physiol. Soc., Washington, D.C.

HURST, P. E., MORRISON, R. B. I., TIMONER, J., METCALFE-GIBSON, A. & WRONG, O. (1963). Clin. Sci., **24**, 187.

INGRAHAM, R. C. & VISSCHER, M. B. (1938). Amer. J. Physiol., **121**, 771.

IRVINE, R. O. H., SAUNDERS, S. J., MILNE, M. D. & CRAWFORD, M. A. (1961). Clin. Sci., **20**, 1.

IRWIN, L., BERGER, E. Y., ROSEBERG, B. & JACKENTHAL, R. (1949). J. Clin. Invest., **28**, 1403.

JAMES, A. H. (1957). "The Physiology of Gastric Secretion," Arnold, London.

JANOWITZ, H. D. & DREILING, D. A. (1962). In "The Exocrine Pancreas." Ed. de Reuck, A. V. S. & Cameron, M. P. Churchill, London.

JEWELL, P. A. & VERNEY, E. B. (1957). *Phil. Trans. roy. Soc. B*, **240**, 197.

KANAGHINIS, T., LUBRAN, M. & COGHILL, N. F. (1963). *Gut*, **4**, 322.

KARR, W. G. & ABBOTT, W. O. (1935). *J. Clin. Invest.*, **14**, 893.

KASSIRER, J. P., APPLETON, F. M., CHAZAN, J. A. & SCHWARTZ, W. B. (1967). *J. Clin. Invest.*, **46**, 1558.

KASSIRER, J. P. & SCHWARTZ, W. B. (1966a). *Amer. J. Med.*, **40**, 10.

KASSIRER, J. P. & SCHWARTZ, W. B. (1966b). *Amer. J. Med.*, **40**, 19.

KAY, A. W. (1953). *Brit. med. J.*, **2**, 77.

KEITH, A. (1907). In "System of Medicine." Ed. Albutt, T. C. & Rolleston, H. D. 2nd Edit. Macmillan, London. Vol. III, p. 867.

KETTERING, R. F. & SUMMERSKILL, W. H. J. (1967). *Medicine* (Baltimore), **46**, 91.

KILLE, J. N. & GLICK, S. (1967). *Brit. med. J.*, **4**, 783.

KINNEY, V. R. & CODE, C. F. (1964). *Amer. J. Physiol.*, **207**, 998.

KIRSNER, J. B. (1941), *J. Clin. Invest.*, **22**, 47.

KITCHENER, J. A. (1957). "Ion Exchange Resins," Methuen, London.

KLINGENSMITH, W. C. & ELKINTON, J. R. (1952). *Circulation*, **5**, 842.

KRAMER, P. (1966). *J. Clin. Invest.*, **45**, 1710.

KRAMER, P., KEARNEY, M. M. & INGELFINGER, F. J. (1962). *Gastroenterology*, **42**, 535.

LAMBERT, H. P., PRANKERD, A. J. & SMELLIE, J. M. (1961). *Quart. J. Med.*, **30**, 71.

LANCET (1966). Leading article. *Lancet*, **1**, 1305.

LANS, H. S., STEIN, I. F. & MEYER, K. A. (1952a). *Surg. Gynec. Obst.*, **95**, 321.

LANS, H. S., STEIN, I. F. & MEYER, K. A. (1952b). *Ann. Surg.*, **135**, 441.

LATTA, T. (1831–32). *Lancet*, **2**, 274.

LAULER, D. P., HICKLER, R. B. & THORN, G. W. (1962). *New Engl. J. Med.*, **267**, 1136.

LEMIEUX, G. & GERVAIS, M. (1964). *Amer. J. Physiol.*, **207**, 1279.

LENNON, E. J., LEMANN, J. & LITZOW, J. R. (1966). *J. Clin. Invest.*, **45**, 1601.

LE QUESNE, L. P. (1967). *Brit. J. Surg.*, **54**, 449.

LEVENSON, S. M., CROWLEY, L. V., HOROWITZ, R. E. & MALM, O. J. (1959). *J. biol. Chem.*, **234**, 2061.

LEVITAN, R. (1967). *J. Lab. Clin. Med.*, **69**, 558.

LEVITAN, R., FORDTRAN, J. S., BURROWS, B. A. & INGELFINGER, F. J. (1962). *J. Clin. Invest.*, **41**, 1754.

LEVITAN, R. & GOULSTON, K. (1967). *Gastroenterology*, **52**, 510.

LEVITAN, R. & INGELFINGER, F. J. (1965). *J. Clin. Invest.*, **44**, 801.

LIEBER, C. S. & LEFÈVRE, A. (1959). *J. Clin. Invest.*, **38**, 1271.

LIPSETT, M. B., SCHWARTZ, I. L. & THORN, N. A. (1961). In "Mineral Metabolism." Ed. Comar, C. L. & Bronner, F. Academic Press, New York, p. 473.

LIU, C. H., HAYS, V. W., SVEC, H. J., CATRON, D. V., ASHTON, G. C. & SPEER, V. C. (1955). *J. Nutr.*, **57**, 241.

LOVE, A. H. G. (1969). *Gut*, **10**, 63.

McCANCE, R. A. (1936). *Proc. roy. Soc. Lond. B*, **119**, 245.

McCANCE, R. A. (1938). *J. Physiol. (Lond.)*, **92**, 208.

McCHESNEY, E. W., NACHOD, F. C. & TAINTER, M. L. (1953). *Ann. N.Y. Acad. Med.*, **57**, 252.

McGEE, L. C. & HASTINGS, A. B. (1942). *J. Biol. Chem.*, **142**, 893.

MADER, I. J. & ISERI, L. T. (1955). *Amer. J. Med.*, **19**, 976.

MAKHLOUF, G. M., McMANUS, J. P. A. & CARD, W. I. (1967). From "Gastric Secretion." Ed. Schitka, T. K. Gilbert, J. A. L. & Harrison, R. C. Pergamon, London.

MALLICK, N. P. & BERLYNE, G. M. (1968). *Lancet*, **2**, 1316.

MANN, F. C. & BOLLMAN, J. L. (1930). *J. Amer. med. Assoc.*, **95**, 1722.

MARTIN, G. J. & WILKINSON, J. (1946). *Gastroenterology*, **6**, 315.

MASON, M. C., GILES, G. R. & CLARK, G. G. (1969). *Gut*, **10**, 34.

MATHISEN, W., WHITMORE, W. F., RANDALL, H. T. & ROBERTS, K. E. (1957). *J. Urol.*, **77**, 27.

MEISTER, A. (1965). "Biochemistry of the Amino-acids," Academic Press, New York, p. 223.

MELVILLE, J. (1935). *Biochem. J.*, **29**, 179.

METCALFE-GIBSON, A., ING, T. S., KUIPER, J. J., RICHARDS, P., WARD, E. E. & WRONG, O. M. (1967). *Clin. Sci.*, **33**, 89.

MILLER, T. G. (1937). *Rev. gastroenterol.*, **4**, 115.

MILNE, M. D., MUEHRCKE, R. C. & AIRD, I. (1957). *Quart. J. Med.*, **26**, 317.

MILNE, M. D., SCRIBNER, B. H. & CRAWFORD, M. A. (1958). *Amer. J. Med.*, **24**, 709.

MINER, R. W. (1953). *Ann. New York Acad. Sci.*, **57**, 61.

MOLLIN, D. L., BAKER, S. J. & DONIACH, I. (1955). *Brit. J. Haematol.*, **1**, 278.

MOSSBERG, S. M. (1967). *Amer. J. Physiol.*, **213**, 1327.

MUEHRCKE, R. C. & McMILLAN, J. C. (1963). *Ann. Intern. Med.*, **59**, 427.

NEEDLE, M. A., KALOYANIDES, G. J. & SCHWARTZ, W. B. (1964). *J. Clin. Invest.*, **43**, 1836.

NUGUID, T. P., BACON, H. E. & BOUTWELL, J. (1961). *Surg. Obst. Gynec.*, **113**, 733.

O'SHAUGHNESSY, W. B. (1831–32). *Lancet*, **1**, 490.

PAPADIMITRIOU, M., GINGELL, C. & CHISHOLM, G. (1968). *Lancet*, **2**, 948.

PARSONS, F. M., POWELL, F. J. N. & PYRAH, L. N. (1952). *Lancet*, **2**, 599.

PHILLIPS, R. A. (1966). *Ann. Intern. Med.*, **65**, 922.

PRADER, A., GAUTIER, E., GAUTIER, R., NÄF, D., SEMER, J. M. & ROTHSCHILD, E. J. (1955). In Ciba Foundation Colloquia on Endocrinology. Ed. Wolstenholme, G. E. W. & Cameron, M. P. Vol. 8, p. 382, Churchill, London.

PRICE, J. B., SCHWARTZ, G. F., MOLAVI, A., BRITTON, R. C. & VOORHEES, A. B. (1967). *Surg. Forum*, **18**, 331.

RELMAN, A. S. & SCHWARTZ, W. B. (1956). *New Engl. J. Med.*, **255**, 195.

RICHARDS, P. (1969). *Lancet*, **1**, 437.

RICHARDS, P., METCALFE-GIBSON, A., WARD, E. E., WRONG, O. & HOUGHTON, B. J. (1967). *Lancet*, **2**, 845.

RICHTER, C. P. (1942–43). *Harvey Lect.*, **38**, 63.

RICHTER, C. P. & ECKERT, J. F. (1938). *Endocrinology*, **22**, 214.

ROBINSON, C. S. (1922). *J. biol. Chem.*, **52**, 445.

ROBINSON, C. S. (1935). *J. biol. Chem.*, **108**, 403.

ROBSON, A. M., KERR, D. N. S. & ASHCROFT, R. (1968). In "Nutrition in Renal Disease." Ed. Berlyne, G. M. Livingstone, Edinburgh.

ROSE, W. C. & DEKKER, E. E. (1956). *J. biol. Chem.*, **223**, 107.

ROSENBERG, M. L. (1953). *J. Urol.*, **70**, 569.

ROSENBERG, T. (1948). *Acta Chem. Scand.*, **2**, 14.

ROSENFELD, J. B., ABOULAFIA, E. D. & SCHWARTZ, W. B. (1963). *Amer. J. Physiol.*, **204**, 568.

ROWLANDS, E. N., EDWARDS, D. A. W. & HONOUR, A. J. (1953). *Clin. Sci.*, **12**, 399.

ROY, A. D. & ELLIS, H. (1959). *Lancet*, **1**, 759 and 1056.

RUBINSTEIN, R., HOWARD, A. V. & WRONG, O. M. (1969). *Clin. Sci.*, **37**, 549.

SCHIFFRIN, M. J. & NASSET, E. S. (1939). *Amer. J. Physiol.*, **128**, 70.

SCHMITZ, H. W. (1922). *J. Lab. Clin. Med.*, **8**, 78.

SCHNEYER, L. H. & SCHNEYER, C. A. (1967). From "Handbook of Physiology," Sect. 6, Vol. 2, p. 497, Amer. Physiol. Soc., Washington, D.C.

SCHOLTZ, A. (1968). *Proc. Eur. Dial. Transpl. Assoc.*, **4**, 204.

SCHREINER, G. E. & MAHER, J. F. (1961). "Uremia," Thomas, Springfield.

SCHULTZ, S. G. & CURRAN, P. F. (1968). From "Handbook of Physiology," Sect. 6, Vol. III, p. 1245, Amer. Physiol. Soc., Washington, D.C.

SCHWARTZ, W. B. & KASSIRER, J. P. (1963). In "Diseases of the Kidney." Ed. Strauss, M. B. & Welt, L. G. Little, Brown, Boston.

SCHWARTZ, W. B. & RELMAN, A. S. (1953). *J. Clin. Invest*, **32**, 258.

SEGAL, H. L., MILLER, L. L. & MORTON, J. I. (1950). *Proc. Soc. Exp. Biol. Med.* (N.Y.), **74**, 218.

SEVITT, L. H. & WRONG, O. M. (1968). *Lancet*, **2**, 950.

SHIELDS, R. (1965). *Brit. J. Surg.*, **52**, 774.

SHIELDS, R. & MILES, J. B. (1965). *Postgrad. med. J.*, **41**, 435.

SHIELDS, R., MILES, J. B. & GILBERTSON, G. (1968). *Brit. med. J.*, **1**, 93.

SHIELDS, R., MULHOLLAND, A. T. & ELMSLIE, R. G. (1966). *Gut*, **7**, 686.

SHNITKA, T. K., FRIEDMAN, M. H. W., KIDD, E. G. & MACKENZIE, W. C. (1961). *Surg. Gynec. Obst.*, **112**, 608.

SHOHL, A. T. (1939). "Mineral Metabolism," Reinhold, New York.

SHOSHKES, M. (1947). *Gastroenterology*, **9**, 765.

SILEN, W., HARPER, H. A., MAWDSLEY, D. L. & WEIRICH, W. L. (1955). *Proc. Soc. Exper. Biol. Med.* (N.Y.), **88**, 138.

SMIDDY, F. G., GREGORY, S. D., SMITH, I. B. & GOLIGHER, J. C. (1960). *Lancet*, **1**, 14.

SMITH, D. R. & GALANTE, M. (1958). *Amer. J. Surg.*, **96**, 254.

STANBURY, S. W. & LUMB, G. A. (1962). *Medicine* (Baltimore), **41**, 1.

SUNDERMAN, F. W. & BOERNER, F. (1949). "Normal Values in Clinical Medicine," Saunders, Philadelphia.

SWALLOW, J. H. & CODE, C. F. (1967). *Amer. J. Physiol.*, **212**, 717.

TARAIL, R. & ELKINTON, J. R. (1949). *J. Clin. Invest.*, **28**, 99.

THAYSEN, J. H., THORN, N. A. & SCHWARTZ, I. L. (1954). *Amer. J. Physiol.*, **178**, 155.

TIDBALL, C. S. (1961). *Amer. J. Physiol.*, **200**, 309.

UPDEGRAFF, H. & LEWIS, H. B. (1924). *J. biol. Chem.*, **61**, 633.

USSING, H. H. & ANDERSEN, B. (1955). Proceedings 3rd Internat. Cong. Biochem., Brussels, Academic Press, New York.

WALLACE, M., RICHARDS, P., CHESSER, E. & WRONG, O. (1968). *Quart. J. Med.*, **37**, 577.

WALSER, M. & BODENLOS, L. J. (1959). *J. Clin. Invest.*, **38**, 1617.

WATTEN, R. H., MORGAN, F. M., SONGKHLA, Y. N., VANIKIATI, B. & PHILLIPS, R. A. (1959). *J. Clin. Invest.*, **38**, 1879.

WEBSTER, L. T., DAVIDSON, C. S. & GABUZDA, G. J. (1958), *J. Lab. Clin. Med.*, **52**, 501.

WELCH, C. S., WAKEFIELD, E. G. & ADAMS, M. (1936). *Arch. Intern. Med.*, **58**, 1095.

WHEELER, H. O. (1968). From "Handbook of Physiology," Sect. 6, Vol. 5, p. 2409, Amer. Physiol. Soc., Washington, D.C.

WHITE, A. G., ENTMACHER, P. S., RUBIN, G. & LEITER, L. (1955). *J. Clin. Invest.*, **34**, 246.

WHITE, A. G., GORDON, H. & LEITER, L. (1950). *J. Clin. Invest.*, **29**, 1445.

WILSON, D. R., ING, T. S., METCALFE-GIBSON, A. & WRONG, O. M. (1968a). *Clin. Sci.*, **34**, 211.

WILSON, D. R., ING, T. S., METCALFE-GIBSON, A. & WRONG, O. M. (1968b). *Clin. Sci.*, **35**, 197.

WILSON, T. H. (1962). "Intestinal Absorption," Saunders, Philadelphia.

WOLF, G. & HANDAL, P. J. (1966). *Endocrinology*, **78**, 1120.

WOLFF, H. P., VESCEI, P., KRÜCK, F., ROSCHER, S., BROWN, J. J., DÜSTERDIECK, G. O., LEVER, A. F. & ROBERTSON, J. I. S. (1968), *Lancet*, **1**, 257.

WRONG, O. M. (1967). *Bull. post-grad. Comm. Med.*, Sydney, **23**, 233.

WRONG, O. M. (1968). *Brit. med. J.*, **1**, 379.

WRONG, O. M. & METCALFE-GIBSON, A. (1965). *Proc. roy. Soc. Med.*, **58**, 1007.

WRONG, O. M., METCALFE-GIBSON, A., MORRISON, R. B. I., NG, S. T. & HOWARD, A. V. (1965). *Clin. Sci.*, **28**, 357.

WRONG, O. M., MORRISON, R. B. I. & HURST, P. E. (1961). *Lancet*, **1**, 1208.

YENSEN, R. (1959). *Quart. J. exper. Psychol.*, **11**, 230.

II. ABSORPTION AND MALABSORPTION OF FAT, CARBOHYDRATE AND PROTEIN

Fat Digestion

Fat provides calories and essential fatty acids, and acts as a vehicle for the absorption of fat-soluble vitamins. The greater part of our dietary fat intake is, however, not essential, since Winitz, Graff, Gallagher, Norkin & Seedman (1965) showed that no detrimental effects resulted when human volunteers were maintained for a period of 19 weeks on a diet in which the only lipid was 2 g. per day of ethyl linoleate containing the fat-soluble vitamins. From the diagnostic point of view the failure of efficient fat absorption is of prime importance. The currently accepted theory of the mechanism of fat absorption has been well reviewed by Senior (1964) and by Johnston (1968). Most of the experimental data has been obtained from animals, but when it has been possible to check these in man (Blomstrand, Gurtler & Werner, 1965; Kayden, Senior & Mattson, 1967) the results support the general conclusions.

Dietary fat consists essentially of the triglyceride esters of long chain fatty acids; in triglycerides 95% of the calories are in the fatty acid portion of the molecules, and it is the absorption of these fatty acids which is important. That pancreatic lipase is of major importance in the absorption of fat is clear from the very gross steatorrhoea which results in patients with pancreatic atrophy. Pancreatic lipase is a hydrolytic enzyme that attacks primary ester bonds of fatty acid esters at the oil-water interface. It shows little specificity in regard to the nature of the fatty acid for fatty acids with chain lengths greater than 12. However, it exhibits a very pronounced specificity for the fatty acids located in the 1 and 3 positions of the triglyceride. Thus, the immediate result of the action of pancreatic lipase on triglyceride emulsions is to produce a mixture of 1-2-diglyceride, 2-monoglyceride and free fatty acid as well as some unchanged triglyceride. Since the fatty acids in the 2 position of glycerides show a tendency to isomerize spontaneously to the 1 or 3 position, should these be vacant, the ultimate mixture in the small intestinal contents may also contain 1-3-diglyceride and 1-monoglyceride. These latter compounds are capable of being completely hydrolysed by pancreatic lipase. These isomerization reactions are relatively slow compared with the action of pancreatic lipase, and their significance in fat absorption is still not clear. If adequate precautions are taken to prevent isomerization during the isolation procedure, the majority of the monoglyceride isolated from intestinal contents is found to be the 2 isomer (Hofmann & Borgstrom, 1964). These reactions have been shown to take place extremely rapidly, and in samples isolated from the duodenum after administering a fat-containing meal a very considerable proportion of the fatty acids is already present as free fatty acids, although the amount of hydrolysis which takes place in the stomach is usually very small. The rate at which pancreatic lipase attacks triglyceride is very dependent upon the degree of emulsification of the triglyceride substrate which determines the area of the oil-water interface. It is probable that the presence of bile salts in the duodenum, by aiding the emulsification of the triglyceride, accounts for the very rapid hydrolysis which occurs, although it is difficult to demonstrate an effect of bile salts in vitro when finely emulsified triglyceride substrates are used.

The composition and metabolism of human bile salts is discussed on pp. 695-700, and their relationship to fat absorption has been reviewed by Hofmann & Small (1967). Bile salts are planar molecules with the polar groups located on one side of the plane and the non-polar groups on the other. The amphipathic nature of the bile salts is expressed by the formation of micelles in solution by the association of two or more molecules depending on the particular bile salt. The concentration at which micelle formation occurs is between 2–8 millimolar depending on the bile salts. Since this critical micellar concentration is exceeded in the normal small intestinal contents after a meal, bile salts in intestinal contents exist in the micellar form. It is assumed that micelles form by association of the non-polar surfaces of the bile salt molecules and a micelle consisting of several molecules of bile salts has at its centre a micro non-polar region surrounded by the multiple polar groups of the bile salt molecules which maintain the complex in aqueous solution. Other lipid-soluble molecules can enter this non-polar central portion of the micelle and thus form mixed micelles with diameters up to 100 Å in which water-insoluble lipids are essentially in aqueous solution. Triglyceride and its digestion products can all be held in a mixed micellar solution by bile salts, but much greater quantities of monoglyceride and free fatty acids are solubilized than di- and triglyceride. The amount of mixed glyceride and fatty acid that can be solubilized into micellar solution by bile salts is slightly greater than the weight of bile salt present. If all the 120–140 g. of fat in the Western diet is to pass through a micellar phase before absorption, each molecule in the 2–4 g. pool will be used 30–50 times a day. Except in samples obtained in the early stages of digestion during emptying of the gall bladder the concentration of bile salts in post-prandial small intestinal contents is from 2–5 mg./ml. (5–12 m.mol.). When the fat concentration, as frequently occurs, exceeds this figure only a portion of the fat is held in micellar solution, the remainder being present as an emulsion. As a result of the combined action of pancreatic lipase and bile salts the fatty acids of dietary triglyceride are rapidly distributed into a complex mixture of digestion products which are found in both emulsion and mixed micellar phases. Free fatty acids and monoglyceride predominate in the micellar phase and the majority of the di- and triglycerides are found in the emulsion phase (Hofmann & Borgstrom, 1964). It is from this mixture that absorption occurs.

Fat Absorption

It has proved difficult to elucidate the chemical form in which the fatty acids pass through the luminal membrane of the mucosal cell, since the reactions catalysed by pancreatic lipase in the lumen of the small intestine are reversible and the fatty acids of dietary triglyceride leave the intestinal mucosa via the lymphatics as triglyceride or as free fatty acids in the portal blood. The mucosal epithelial cells contain all the necessary enzyme systems to synthesize this triglyceride from fatty acids and glycerol or monoglyceride or diglyceride, as well as a lipase that will hydrolyse monoglyceride or di- or triglyceride to free fatty acids and glycerol. Thus metabolic pathways exist in the mucosal cell which can convert any or all the intraluminal lipids to triglycerides from any mixture that may be absorbed. The currently accepted theory is based on studies of the appearance of glycerol and fatty acids in lymph triglyceride after feeding triglyceride labelled in both the glycerol and fatty acid moiety. This experiment shows that the ratio of labelled glycerol to labelled fatty acid in the lymph is about half that of the fed triglyceride, indicating that half the triglyceride is completely hydrolysed during the absorptive process. Taken in conjunction with the predominance of monoglycerides and free fatty acids in the lumen, this has led to the view that the majority of the fatty acids are absorbed either as free fatty acids or 2-monoglyceride. No active process for the transport of fatty acids or mono-glyceride across the small intestinal mucosa cell has been demonstrated. Being lipid-soluble these compounds should be readily transported across the membrane by passive diffusion. The rate of this process will depend upon the concentration of the molecules in the intraluminal solution. As the solubility of monoglyceride and of free fatty acids in water at the pH of the small intestine is extremely small, the micelles, which are not themselves absorbed intact, probably function by maintaining the concentration of monoglyceride and free fatty acid at the limiting membrane of the mucosal cell, since their small size enables them to penetrate much more closely than the particles of an emulsion could do, even into the spaces between the microvilli.

Once within the intestinal cell triglyceride is synthesized from the absorbed compounds. This triglyceride leaves the mucosal cell incorporated into chylomicrons, and it has been shown that the synthesis of β-lipoprotein is essential for the formation of chylomicrons. The chylomicrons are released into the extracellular spaces of the mucosa, find their way into the lymphatics and are carried via the lymphatic trunk into the thoracic duct and eventually into the circulation. Some of the fatty acids however leave the small intestine via the portal vein and the partition between the portal and lymphatic routes is determined by the chain length of the fatty acid; fatty acids with 14 carbon atoms or more are thought to enter the circulation predominantly via the lymphatics although this route may be less important in some individuals, whereas fatty acids with 10 carbon atoms or less would be absorbed by the portal route. Since the majority of dietary fatty acids have a chain length greater than 14 carbon atoms these medium-chain fatty acids are under normal circumstances of negligible importance. However, the recent introduction of medium-chain triglycerides for the treatment of malabsorption syndromes (Iber, Hardoon & Sangree, 1963; Holt, Hashim & Van Itallie, 1965) in which 90% of the fatty acids are 10 or 8 carbon compounds has given the absorption of these fatty acids more than theoretical interest. Medium-chain triglycerides are well hydrolysed by pancreatic lipase, and since the hydrolysis products are much more water-soluble than their long-chain counterparts, they are less dependent on bile salts for their rapid absorption and are removed from the intestinal mucosa via the portal vein. Their greater water-solubility ensures a higher concentration at the limiting membrane of the mucosal cell and thus presumably accounts for their rapid absorption.

Detection of Steatorrhoea

The only way in which steatorrhoea can be detected with complete confidence is by analysis of the stool samples for fat content, and the only reliable index is the amount of fat excreted per day. Because of irregularities in the daily output of faeces a minimum collection period of three days is required for diagnostic purposes and for following progress of treatment five-day periods are required. The diet should contain 100 g. of fat per day during the collection period. The need for timed collections can be overcome if a non-absorbable marker is incorporated in the diet. If a known amount of marker is ingested each day then the total amount of marker in a stool specimen would indicate the number of days of diet from which this specimen had been derived. Chromium sesquioxide has been used as a non-absorbable marker (Whitby & Lang, 1960). Since the colon acts as a mixing chamber, i.e. the contents already present are mixed with those that enter, a regime of constant fat, constant marker diet must be maintained for two days before the sample is obtained on the third day to allow equilibration of colonic contents.

The method most widely used for determination of faecal fat is that of van de Kamer, Huinick & Weyers (1949). The fatty acid content of a light petroleum extract of a saponified aliquot of the stool sample is determined by titration. What is determined is the number of milli-equivalents of titratable acid that can be extracted into light petroleum. This is usually converted to grams of fatty acid by assuming an arbitrary equivalent weight of 284. This method is of little use for determining steatorrhoea following medium-chain triglyceride feeding, since the fatty acids from the medium-chain triglycerides extract less readily into light petroleum and their equivalent weight is much less than that which is assumed in the calculation. Normal subjects on a diet containing 100 g. fat excrete up to 6 g. of fat a day and values above this level, when the collection periods are known to be accurate, indicate malabsorption.

The difficulties and economics of obtaining a complete and accurately timed faecal collection, although to some extent relieved by the use of non-absorbable markers, has led to many attempts at shortened procedures to demonstrate malabsorption of fat. In the vitamin A tolerance test a large known dose of vitamin A ester in oil is administered in a test meal, and the increase over the fasting level of vitamin A in the plasma at four or five hours after the test meal is determined (Wormsley, 1963). Provided that an adequate amount of fat is included in the test meal an increase of more than 600 I.U. following a dose of 5,000 I.U./kg. indicates the absence of steatorrhoea. Values below 600 I.U. may be found in

some cases without steatorrhoea, and the test is quite valueless following surgical procedures in the alimentary tract. Radioiodine-labelled triolein has also been used (Wormsley, 1963), and the blood levels when expressed as the percentage of the administered dose compare closely to the dose of vitamin A expressed in the same way in the same subject, and similar limitations apply to the two procedures (French, 1960). Blood levels do not appear to be related to the severity of the steatorrhoea, and although the measurement of faecal radioactivity, or the appearance of radioactive iodide resulting from the metabolism of the labelled fatty acid over a 72-hour period in the urine, corresponds more closely with the percentage of fat absorbed, the correspondence is not sufficiently close to define the severity of steatorrhoea with any precision, and the difficulty of collecting stool samples uncontaminated by urine in ill patients limits their usefulness.

Causes of Steatorrhoea

There are many points at which pathological changes can disorganize the complex series of reactions involved in fat absorption, and the diverse diseases in which steatorrhoea is a symptom will be considered in groupings determined by the probable site of the defect. It must be borne in mind that in a complex series of reactions disorganisation at any point may distort preceding as well as subsequent reactions, and steatorrhoea will seldom be due to a single malfunction.

Any interference with the lymphatic drainage of the small intestine as sometimes occurs in tuberculosis or Hodgkin's disease will cause steatorrhoea. The gross steatorrhoea of Whipple's disease, the invasion of the intestinal mucosa by an as yet unidentified organism causing changes in the lymphatic tissue, is also probably due to obstruction of the lymph flow, although the mucosal cells may also be affected. Intestinal lymphangiectasia is associated with excessive protein loss into the gut with rapid albumin turnover and steatorrhoea. It has been shown that the elimination of fat from the diet (Jeffries, Chapman & Sleisenger, 1964), or its replacement by medium-chain triglycerides (Jarnum & Jensen, 1966) the fatty acids of which leave by the portal route, causes a marked decrease in albumin loss into the small intestine.

In the rare condition acanthocytosis or congenital β-lipoprotein deficiency associated with mild steatorrhoea Dobbins (1966) has shown by electron micrographic studies that the defect in fat absorption is in the exit of triglyceride from the mucosal cells presumably related to the failure of β-lipoprotein synthesis for the formation of chylomicrons. The very mild degree of steatorrhoea that is found in this condition raises some doubts as to the importance of the lymphatic pathway of fat absorption. Whilst in non-tropical sprue or adult coeliac disease the steatorrhoea is undoubtedly due to a mucosal defect, the precise nature of the biochemical lesion is still in doubt. Indeed steatorrhoea is not always present in this disease and frequently is mild (Stewart, Pollock, Hoffbrand, Mollin & Booth, 1967).

Fibrocystic disease, severe chronic pancreatitis or destruction of the pancreatic duct may result in such low levels of pancreatic lipase that steatorrhoea occurs due to the failure of hydrolysis of the dietary triglyceride. The deficiency of pancreatic enzymes must be severe before malabsorption occurs. Cook, Lennard-Jones, Sherif & Wiggins (1967) showed that steatorrhoea did not occur in chronic pancreatitis until the response of pancreatic enzymes induced by a test meal was reduced to 25% of the lower limit of the normal range.

Obstructive jaundice and consequent absence of bile salts from the small intestine in the absence of pancreatic disease produces a less severe steatorrhoea than pancreatic deficiency. Interruption of enterohepatic circulation of bile salts by ileal disease or resection has been shown to lower the intraluminal concentration to below the critical micellar concentration (Van Dest, Fordtran, Morowski & Wilson, 1968), and the micellar phase is absent in these patients (Hardison & Rosenberg, 1967). Steatorrhoea was, however, mild in those cases where the resection or disease was limited in extent.

Carbohydrate Digestion

Carbohydrate in the western diet is principally starch, sucrose and lactose. The polysaccharide starch is a mixture of amylose, a straight chain polymer of glucose with 1–4 glucosidic linkages and amylopectin with similar chains crosslinked with 1–6 glucosidic bonds producing a branch chain structure. These polysaccharides are attacked by amylase present in the saliva, but the duration of this action is short since gastric acidity inactivates the enzyme. Pancreatic amylase continues the hydrolysis in the small intestine. Pancreatic and salivary amylases have the same specificity (Fischer & Stein, 1960), i.e. they hydrolyse the 1:4 glucosidic bonds randomly in the polysaccharide chains and have low activity towards the trisaccharide and low activity towards

maltose. They do not hydrolyse the 1–6 links. The final result of the action of amylase is to produce a mixture of maltose and glucose and some isomaltose and limit dextrins from amylopectin, with maltose predominating. The glucose so produced, the small quantity of monosaccharide existing in the diet and a minor amount produced by the low levels of disaccharidases found in intestinal contents (Borgstrom, Dahlquist, Lundh & Sjovall, 1957) are the only monosaccharides presented to the intestinal mucosa for absorption, and under normal conditions disaccharide is the predominant carbohydrate available for absorption. Only very small quantities of disaccharide, however, enter the blood and it has been shown by Weser & Sleisenger (1967) that 90% of lactose or sucrose given intravenously can be recovered in the urine over 24 hours although maltose was metabolized. Since these sugars, although present in the diet, are found in only trace amounts in normal urine a system must exist for the hydrolysis of disaccharide between the lumen of the small intestine and the blood. The present knowledge of the location and activity of disaccharidases has been recently reviewed by Semenza (1968).

The disaccharidases are located at the external membrane of the brush border of the mucosal cell and the activities are recovered in particulate fractions of homogenates. Various methods of solubilization have been used to isolate the activities, and thermal stability and inhibitor studies have been used to characterize the different activities in various species. The results of the different methods show few discrepancies. The following activities have been located in human intestinal mucosal brush borders (Auricchio, Semenza & Rubino, 1965; Dahlquist, 1962):

(1) Sucrase, which also hydrolyses maltose and maltotriose.

(2) Isomaltase, which also hydrolyses maltose, maltotriose and palatanose.

(3) Trehalase.

(4) Lactase.

(5) Maltases, two other maltases in addition to the activity shown by sucrase and isomaltase have been detected.

Although these enzymes are usually referred to as disaccharidases they possess activity towards larger oligosaccharides, and maltases probably have some amylase activity. Isomaltase can hydrolyse the limit dextrans from the 1–6 branched amylopectin. The combination of amylase in the intestinal lumen and the disaccharidases at the absorptive membrane reduce the carbohydrate of the diet to the monosaccharides glucose, fructose, and galactose, that enter the mucosal cell.

Monosaccharide Absorption

Crane (1968) has reviewed the extensive literature in this field. Glucose and galactose are actively absorbed, i.e. they can be transferred from the mucosal to the serosal side of the small intestinal mucosa when the concentration in the serosal solution exceeds that of the mucosal solution, and the mechanism is saturatable, i.e. the rate of absorption increases with increase in the concentration up to a level where further increases in concentration produce no increase in absorption. The situation where the intraluminal concentration of glucose is less than the plasma concentration seldom occurs in physiological circumstances (Dahlquist & Borgstrom, 1961), except perhaps towards the end of the absorption of a meal, and the significance of the transport mechanism is rather that it enables these monosaccharides to cross the external membrane of the mucosal cell at a much greater rate than simple diffusion would allow. The same transport mechanism is shared by glucose and galactose and is sodium-dependent. Fructose is absorbed by a different mechanism for which the characteristics of active absorption have not been demonstrated. The rate is slower than for glucose and galactose but still more rapid than simple diffusion could achieve. These characteristics of monosaccharide absorption in man as determined by intestinal perfusion techniques have been described by Holdsworth & Dawson (1964). Disaccharide absorption in man has also been studied by intestinal perfusion techniques by Gray & Ingelfinger (1965), and the results show that under these conditions some monosaccharides diffuse back into the luminal fluid. The proportion of fructose to glucose found in the recovered perfusion fluid agreed well with the results of Holdsworth & Dawson on the relative rates of absorption of these two monosaccharides.

Tests of Carbohydrate Absorption

Because all carbohydrates are extensively metabolized by the bacterial population of the small intestine measurements of faecal output are impossible. The glucose tolerance test gives poor discrimination for carbohydrate malabsorption. The starch tolerance test, in which the blood glucose levels after ingestion of a standard load of starch are compared with those following an equivalent quantity of glucose, has also been found to be unreliable as an index of amylase activity in the small intestine (Drieling, Janowitz & Pernier, 1964). The D-xylose test was originally

used on the assumptions that this pentose is absorbed by passive diffusion, is not metabolized, and is excreted in the urine. The first two of these assumptions are now known to be untrue (Csaky & Lassen, 1964; Pitkanen & Svinhufvud, 1965), and the excretion in the urine is dependent on good kidney function. However, this test is still of great value in determining upper small intestinal mucosal function. About 60% of an oral dose is absorbed in the normal subject (Fordtran, Soegal & Ingelfinger, 1962) and about 50% of this is metabolized (Wyngaarden, Segal & Foley, 1957). The majority of the absorbed and non-metabolized xylose is excreted in the 5-hr. period following ingestion of the test dose. The mean 5-hr. urinary excretion of D-xylose after a 25 g. oral dose have been reported as being between 5·6 and 7·5 g. (Christiansen, Kirsner & Ablaza, 1959) in normal subjects and in practice the lower limit of normal is taken as 5 g. The lactose tolerance test as a measure of lactase deficiency has been well investigated by McGill & Newcomer (1967). The result of this test is interpreted as normal if a rise in blood glucose is more than 20 mg./100 ml. over the fasting level after a 50 g. oral dose of lactose. It was found that using venous blood 20% of subjects known to have normal jejunal lactase activity showed an abnormal result, while one out of 18 patients with low jejunal enzyme levels gave a false positive. Using capillary bloods there were no false positives but the false negatives increased to 40%. Assay of disaccharidase activity in peroral biopsy specimens of the jejunal mucosa (Dahlquist, 1966) is the most reliable method of studying disaccharidase deficiency, since activity of this enzyne is normally low in the duodenum and ileum (Newcomer & McGill, 1966) and the tissue should be assayed or deep frozen at once. Disaccharidase activities are expressed on a nitrogen or wet weight basis, although relating them to the alkaline phosphatase activity would seem to have some theoretical advantages (Plotkin & Isselbacher, 1964). Each laboratory prepares its own normal series.

Malabsorption of Carbohydrates

A deficiency of pancreatic amylase should result in starch malabsorption but very little information is available on this subject. Most mammals lose their intestinal lactase early in life and this seems also to be true in the majority of the human population of the world. In the Western societies however, lactase is usually retained throughout life and those few individuals who lose their lactase may present as cases of primary acquired lactose intolerance. A secondary lactase deficiency is a feature of a number of diseases of the intestinal mucosa. In non-tropical sprue levels of all disaccharidases may be depressed, but lactase is usually the most severely affected (Plotkin & Isselbacher, 1964). Deficiency of sucrase, usually accompanied by isomaltase deficiency, is a rare genetically determined disease (Dahlquist, Auricchio, Semenza & Prader, 1963). The rare condition of glucose–galactose malabsorption has been reported (Schneider, Kintner & Stirling, 1966). Fructose absorption is normal in these patients. All these isolated carbohydrate absorption defects are usually manifested in early life at the first exposure to the substrate for the absent system. The unabsorbed carbohydrates are subjected to bacterial metabolism and these metabolites may produce osmotic or pharmacological diarrhoea (Weijers, Van de Kamer, Dicke & Ijsseling, 1961). In children an excess of lactic acid in the stools is a frequent finding.

Protein Absorption and Malabsorption

The amino acids in the diet are predominantly in the form of protein and it is necessary that the peptide bonds should be split before absorption can take place, although there is some doubt as to whether it is necessary for the protein to be reduced to its constituent amino acids before these can be absorbed (Fisher, 1967). In contrast to the situation with dietary polysaccharides which are polymers of a single molecule, glucose, the proteins are polymers of at least 20 different amino acids and individual proteolytic enzymes split the peptide bonds between certain amino acids only and also show specificity for certain situations in the peptide molecules. The intestinal secretions contain an array of proteolytic enzymes which may be broadly classified as exopeptidases which can split peptide bonds located at the end

of the polypeptide chains and endopeptidases that can act at positions along the chain. The pepsins of gastric juice are endopeptidases with specificity towards peptide bonds involving aromatic amino acids and are active from pH 2 to pH 4 (Taylor, 1968); thus in a normal stomach a limited amount of proteolysis can occur. The pancreatic juice contains three other endopeptidases, trypsin, chymotrypsin and elastase and two exopeptidases, carboxypeptidase A and B (Keller, 1968). Trypsin splits peptide bonds of basic amino acids, chymotrypsin of aromatic amino acids and elastase of non-polar amino acids. Carboxypeptidase A removes aromatic or non-polar amino acids from the carboxyl ends of peptides, and carboxypeptidase B removes basic amino acids from the carboxyl end. The combined action of all these enzymes should be capable of hydrolysing most proteins to their constituent amino acids, but this has never been satisfactorily demonstrated (Crane & Neuberger, 1960).

The absorption of amino acids has been extensively studied in animals and to a lesser extent in man and has been recently reviewed (Wiseman, 1968). There appears to be a special active transport mechanism for neutral amino acids and another for basic amino acids. The dicarboxylic amino acids probably have a special transport mechanism also. There is some evidence for the absorption of small peptides (Craft, Geddes & Matthews, 1968) but little doubt that free amino acids enter the circulation.

Deficiency of pepsin has no effect on protein absorption, but pancreatic deficiency results in excessive losses of nitrogen in the stool. Apart from general malfunctioning of intestinal mucosa as in non-tropical sprue, specific deficiencies in amino acid transport systems are rare, are associated with renal disease rather than malabsorption and are dealt with in Chapter 16.

References

AURICCHIO, S., SEMENZA, G. & RUBINO, A. (1965). *Biochim. Biophys. Acta*, **96**, 498.

BLOMSTRAND, R., GURTLER, J. & WERNER, B. (1965). *J. Clin. Invest.*, **43**, 247.

BORGSTROM, B., DAHLQUIST, A., LUNDH, G. & SJOVALL, J. (1957). *J. Clin. Invest.*, **36**, 1521.

CHRISTIANSEN, P. A., KIRSNER, J. B. & ABLAZA, J. (1959). *Amer. J. Med.*, **27**, 443.

COOK, H. B., LENNARD-JONES, J. E., SHERIF, S. M. & WIGGINS, H. S. (1967). *Gut*, **8**, 408.

CRAFT, I. L., GEDDES, D. & MATTHEWS, D. M. (1968). *Gut*. **9**, 425.

CRANE, C. W. & NEUBERGER, A. (1960). *Biochem. J.*, **74**, 313.

CRANE, R. K. (1968). "Handbook of Physiology," Sect. 6, 1323, Amer. Physiol. Soc., Washington, D.C.

CSAKY, T. Z. & LASSEN, U. V. (1964). *Biochim. Biophys. Acta*, **82**, 215.

DAHLQUIST, A. (1962). *J. Clin. Invest.*, **41**, 463.

DAHLQUIST, A. (1966). *Anal. Biochem.*, **14**, 376.

DAHLQUIST, A., AURICCHIO, S., SEMENZA, G. & PRADER, A. (1963). *J. Clin. Invest.*, **42**, 566.

DAHLQUIST, A. & BORGSTROM, B. (1961). *Biochem. J.*, **81**, 411.

DOBBINS, W. O. (1966). *Gastroenterology*, **50**, 195.

DRIELING, D. A., JANOWITZ, H. D. & PERNIER, C. V. (1964). "Pancreatic Inflammatory Disease," Harper, New York.

FISCHER, E. H. & STEIN, E. A. (1960). "The Enzymes," Vol. 4, 313, Academic Press, New York.

FISHER, R. B. (1967). *Brit. Med. Bull.*, **23**, 241.

FORDTRAN, J. S., SOEGAL, K. H. & INGELFINGER, F. J. (1962). *New Eng. J. Med.*, **267**, 274.

FRENCH, A. B. (1960). Personal communication.

GRAY, G. M. & INGELFINGER, F. J. (1965). *J. Clin. Invest.*, **44**, 390.

HARDISON, W. G. M. & ROSENBERG, I. H. (1967). *New Engl. J. Med.*, **277**, 337.

HOFMANN, A. F. & BORGSTROM, B. (1964). *J. Clin. Invest.*, **43**, 247.

HOFMANN, A. F. & SMALL, D. M. (1967). *Ann. Rev. Med.*, **18**, 333.

HOLDSWORTH, C. D. & DAWSON, A. M. (1964). *Clin. Sci.*, **27**, 371.

HOLT, P. R., HASHIM, S. A. & VAN ITALLIE, T. B. (1965). *Amer. J. Gastroent.*, **43**, 549.

IBER, F. L., HARDOON, E. & SANGREE, M. H. (1963). *Clin. Res.*, **11**, 185.

JARNUM, S. & JENSEN, H. (1966). *Scand. J. Gastroent.*, **1**, 306.

JEFFRIES, G. H., CHAPMAN, A. & SLEISENGER, M. H. (1964). *New Engl. J. Med.*, **270**, 761.

JOHNSTON, J. M. (1968). "Handbook of Physiology," Sect. 6, 1353, Amer. Physiol Soc., Washington, D.C.

KAYDEN, H. J., SENIOR, J. R. & MATTSON, F. H. (1967). *J. Clin. Invest.*, **46**, 1695.

KELLER, P. J. (1968). "Handbook of Physiology," Sect. 6, 2605, Amer. Physiol. Soc., Washington, D.C.

McGILL, D. B. & NEWCOMER, A. D. (1967). *Gastroenterology*, **53**, 371.

NEWCOMER, A. D. & McGILL, D. B. (1966). *Gastroenterology*, **51**, 481.

PITKANEN, E. & SVINHUFVUD, U. (1965). *Ann. Med., Exptl. Biol. Fernia* (Helsinki), **43**, 250.

PLOTKIN, G. R. & ISSELBACHER, K. J. (1964). *New Engl. J. Med.*, **271**, 1033.

SCHNEIDER, A. J., KINTNER, W. B. & STIRLING, C. E. (1966). *New Engl. J. Med.*, **274**, 305.

SEMENZA, G. (1968). "Handbook of Physiology," Sect. 6, 2543, Amer. Physiol. Soc., Washington, D.C.

SENIOR, J. R. (1964). *J. Lipid. Res.*, **5**, 495.

STEWART, J. S., POLLACK, D. J., HOFFBRAND, A. V., MOLLIN, D. L. & BOOTH, C. C. (1967). *Quart. J. Med.*, **36**, 425.

TAYLOR, W. H. (1968). "Handbook of Physiology," Sect. 6, 2567, Amer. Physiol. Soc., Washington, D.C.

VAN DE KAMER, J. H., BOKKEL HUINICK, H. T. & WEYERS, H. A. (1949). *J. biol. Chem.*, **177**, 347.

VAN DEST, B. W., FORDTRAN, J. S., MORAWSKI, S. G. & WILSON, J. D. (1968). *J. Clin. Invest.*, **47**, 1314.

WEIJERS, H. A., VAN DE KAMER, J. H., DICKE, W. K. & IJSSELING, J. (1961). *Acta Pediatrica Scand.*, **50**, 55.

WESER, E. & SLEISENGER, M. H. (1967). *J. Clin. Invest.*, **46**, 499.

WHITBY, L. G. & LANG, D. (1960). *J. Clin. Invest.*, **39**, 854.

WINITZ, M., GRAFF, J., GALLAGHER, N., NORKIN, A. & SEEDMAN, D. A. (1965). *Nature*, **205**, 741.

WISEMAN, G. (1968). "Handbook of Physiology," Sect. 6, 1277, Amer. Physiol. Soc., Washington, D.C.

WORMSLEY, K. G. (1963). *Gut*, **4**, 261.

WYNGAARDEN, J. B., SEGAL, S. & FOLEY, J. B. (1957). *J. Clin. Invest.*, **36**, 1395.

III. ABNORMALITIES OF BILE SALT METABOLISM

The bile acids of man are C24 carboxylic acids containing the steroid nucleus. They are derived from 5 β-cholanoic acid (cholanic acid) by substitutions in positions 3, 7 and 12 of the nucleus (Sobotka, 1937, 1938; Fieser & Fieser, 1949, 1959; Haslewood, 1967).

These compounds (III–VI, Fig. 19.6) containing a carboxyl group at C24 are called bile acids or free or unconjugated bile acids. In this form they occur only in traces in normal blood and bile, and indeed only infrequently in pathological conditions. When released from the liver cell into the bile, the bile acids are conjugated with the amino acids glycine or taurine by a peptide link at C24 to form the bile salts; the term "salts" implies the conjugation rather than whether the resulting acid compound is present as an undissociated acid or as an anion. The fact that either glycine or taurine can be combined with each of the bile acids means that a rather large number of individual compounds is possible; all six of the conjugates containing the common human bile acids, cholic acid, chenodeoxycholic acid and deoxycholic acid are normally found in blood and bile.

The importance of the distinction between the free bile acids and the corresponding conjugated bile salts lies in the great difference in their chemical properties. The former are typical organic acids of molecular weight about 400, insoluble in water and aqueous acids, soluble in alkaline solution and in certain organic solvents, from which they may be crystallized, sometimes with difficulty. On the other hand, the conjugated bile salts are very freely soluble in water. The resulting solutions, even if dilute, have conspicuous properties as detergents, forming stable emulsions with oils and fats, and being powerful haemolytic agents. Examination of models indicates that the molecules, as in synthetic detergents, have a hydrocarbon portion clearly separated from the hydrophilic polar groups concentrated on one side of the molecule (Haslewood, 1967).

Primary and Secondary Bile Acids

Normal human bile contains conjugates of cholic acid and chenodeoxycholic acid as its major constituents (Wootton & Wiggins, 1953; Isaksson, 1953). These compounds are made by

the liver cells and secreted into the hepatic bile, they are therefore called primary bile acids. After passage into the gut, a proportion of bile salt is altered by the chemical action of the intestinal bacteria, the most important changes being de-conjugation and conversion of cholic acid to deoxycholic acid by removal of the hydroxyl group at C7.

The deoxycholic acid so formed constitutes the

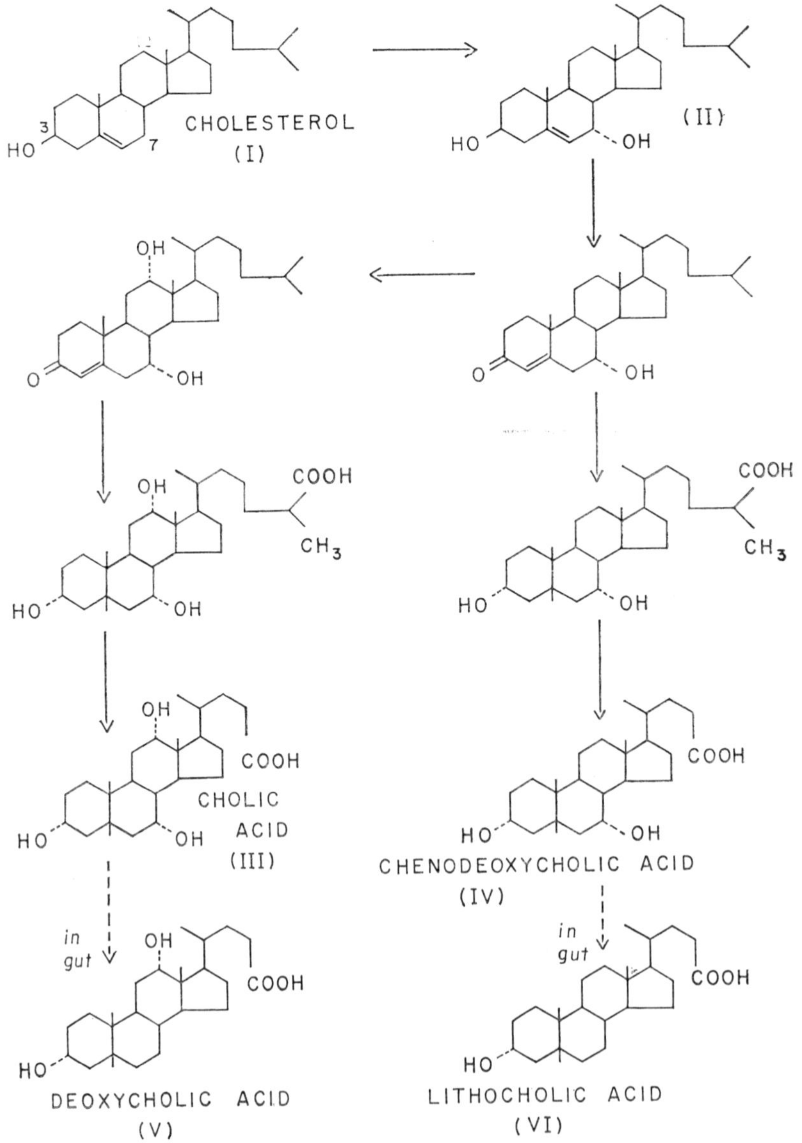

FIG. 19.6. Biosynthetic pathways from cholesterol to the bile acids. Certain of the intermediate stages have been omitted.

most important secondary bile acid; together with unchanged primary bile acids, it is reabsorbed in the ileum (Bergstrom, Lundh & Hofmann, 1963) by an active transport mechanism (Lack & Weiner, 1961) and transported in the portal blood back to the liver as a component of the entero-hepatic circulation (see Josephson, 1943). Con-jugated again with a fresh molecule of amino acid, the deoxycholic acid is excreted into the bile.

In the new-born infant (Encrantz & Sjovall, 1959) and in the patient with a complete bile fistula (Hellstrom & Sjovall, 1961; Carey & Williams, 1963) this contact between primary bile acid and intestinal bacteria does not occur, con-sequently there is an absence of deoxycholic acid in the bile. Analogous changes in the composition of the bile salts are found when the bile of "germ-free" animals is compared with that of the normal animal.

Biosynthesis of the Primary Bile Acids

The primary bile acids are made in the liver from cholesterol by a series of enzymic conver-sions (for details see Haslewood, 1967). An abbre-viated scheme is shown in Fig. 19.6 (omitting several intermediates and possible minor path-ways) and indicates how chenodeoxycholic acid (IV) results when reduction at C3 precedes 12α-hydroxylation, while cholic acid (III) is the product of the reactions occurring in the reverse order.

In the gut, apart from deconjugation, the principal bacterial action appears to be the pro-duction of deoxycholic acid (V) from cholic acid. No doubt the trace of lithocholic acid (VI) also found in human bile originates from a similar action on chenodeoxycholic acid (Bergstrom, 1962; Norman & Short, 1962).

The Enterohepatic Circulation

It is possible to determine the turnover of bile acids in the human by an isotope technique. An isotopically-labelled bile acid is administered and bile samples collected at intervals for several days. Analysis of the bile and determination of the specific activity of the contained bile acids enables the size of the bile acid pool and the rate of production of each acid to be calculated. This procedure has been done for cholic acid (Lind-stedt, 1962) and chenodeoxycholic acid (Daniels-son, Eneroth, Hellstrom, Lindstedt & Sjovall, 1963). Myant (1969) has deduced the correspond-ing pool size for deoxycholic acid from the observed concentration in duodenal juice. The results indicate that both cholic and chenodeoxy-cholic acid are produced at a rate of 0·2–0·4 g./day;

(0·4–1 mMole/day); the pool sizes are in the range of 0·5–2·5 g. (1–5 mMole) and the half-life of the compounds 2 to 6 days. The pool size of deoxycholic acid is about 0·7 g. (1·4 mMole).

Not all of the bile salt reaching the intestine is reabsorbed, either as an unchanged compound or after bacterial action. A proportion is lost into the large intestine and is excreted after further bacterial action which converts the acids into a variety of end-products (Eneroth, Gordon, Ryhage & Sjovall, 1966; Eneroth, Gordon & Sjovall, 1966).

Since in the steady state the daily production of bile acid must equal the loss in the faeces, a check on the daily production rate can be made by faecal analysis. Kinsell (1968) lists a number of estimates; although for technical reasons there is a wide spread of results, in general the figures are in reasonable agreement, indicating a daily production of about 0·5–1 g./day (1–2 mMole/day).

Serum Bile Acids

Carey (1958) and MacIntyre & Wootton (1960), in reviewing the reported levels of bile acids in blood, pointed out how variable were the results. Evidently, up to that time, many of the published methods were so inaccurate that the results were almost meaningless. Since then, technical methods for separating and estimating steroids have been developed, and procedures based on several different principles such as differential spectro-photometry (Carey, 1958), fluorimetry (Osborn, Wootton, da Silva & Sherlock, 1959; Panveli-walla, Lewis, Wootton & Tabaqchali, 1969) or gas-liquid chromatography (Sandberg, Sjovall, Sjovall & Turner, 1965) have been found to give closely similar results. The more recent methods are further able to distinguish free and conjugated acids and the proportions of the latter conjugated with glycine and taurine. In the normal fasting person the total serum bile acids lie in the range 0–2·5 μg/ml. (0–5 μM). Free bile acids were not detected in blood by Panveliwalla et al. (1969), who found that the amounts of cholic and cheno-deoxycholic acid compounds were roughly equal and in the range of 0–1 μg/ml. (0–2 μM). In this respect, their results are substantially in agreement with those of Carey (1958) and Sandberg et al. (1965). The latter authors also described concen-trations of deoxycholic acid conjugates which were appreciable, although less than those of the primary bile acids. It is therefore evident that the liver clearance of secondary bile acids is normally effective.

The relative proportions of taurine and glycine

conjugates are normally rather variable; glycine/taurine ratio usually being in the range of 1·1–6.

Bile Acids in Liver Disease

The metabolism of the bile acids undergoes important changes in cases of established liver disease. All authors agree that the blood level of total bile salts rises in cases of jaundice. In most of the modern reports, the values in obstructive jaundice or biliary cirrhosis were found to be in the range of 5–200 μg/ml. (10–400 μM); in cases of cirrhosis, levels about half as high were found.

There is a change in the composition as well as the amount of circulating bile salts. Carey (1958) reported that in biliary obstruction, the cholic acid concentration rose as well as the concentration of the dihydroxy bile acids, so that the normal proportions were preserved. In contrast, liver cell damage resulted in a disproportional increase in the dihydroxy bile acids, so reducing the dihydroxy/trihydroxy ratio to less than one. Carey regarded this as an important prognostic sign. His results were generally confirmed by others (Rudman & Kendall, 1957; Osborn et al., 1959) except that the latter authors were unable to attach much prognostic importance to the figures obtained. It seems that the increase in the dihydroxy acid proportion can be explained as an interference with the action of the 12α-hydroxylase necessary for the synthesis of cholic acid (in the diseased liver, there are considerable alterations in liver cell enzymes; Schersten, 1967) and also possibly as a decrease in the liver clearance of secondary bile acids.

A distressing symptom which is frequently experienced by patients with biliary obstruction is intractable pruritus. It has been attributed to the action of retained bile salts in the skin, although the mechanism by which an increased bile salt concentration results in itching is by no means apparent. In support of this theory are the facts that:

(a) an increased skin concentration has been demonstrated in obstructive jaundice (Schoenfield, Sjovall & Penman, 1967),

(b) serum bile acids are increased in patients with pruritus and jaundice (Carey, 1958; Brule & Cottet, 1942) and

(c) lowering of serum bile acids following surgical action (Varco, 1947) or administration of anion-exchange resin (Carey & Williams, 1961) is often accompanied by relief of the pruritus.

However it is evident that other factors must also be involved, since the pruritus is also relieved by steroid administration (Sherlock, 1958) and the correspondence between mean total bile acid value and itching is by no means exact (Osborn et al., 1959).

Another clinical observation of great antiquity relating to obstructive jaundice is that the urine of such patients may have a very low surface tension—the basis of the Hay's test using flowers of sulphur. It has been generally believed that bile salts are the surface tension lowering agent, but the evidence for this assumption is lacking and it cannot stand up to quantitative examination. The most recent work available (Gregg, 1967) suggests that only about 20 mg. of bile salt were excreted daily in the urine of his patient with stricture of the common bile duct and secondary biliary cirrhosis, and many previous attempts to isolate bile salts from suitable urine specimens have failed.

The Bile Acids and Cholesterol

In the biosynthesis of the bile acids (Fig. 19.6), the first reaction which converts cholesterol (I) into hydroxycholesterol (II) appears to be rate-limiting (Bergstrom, 1959). The enzyme responsible in mammalian liver is a 7α-hydroxylase and uses molecular oxygen. The reaction rate, i.e. the enzyme activity, is governed by a feed-back mechanism, in which the rate of bile acid formation is controlled by the amount of bile salts absorbed from the intestine. In animals, drainage of the bile results in an increase in the rate of production (Thompson & Vars, 1954) which can be reversed by infusing bile salts into the duodenum (Bergstrom & Danielsson, 1958). Boyd (1969) has shown that the enzyme activity increases about seven to ten times normal under these conditions while Moutafis, Myant & Tabaqchali (1968) found bile acid production to be increased five-fold in two patients with ileal resections which interfered with intestinal absorption.

Bile itself is of course the major vehicle for the excretion of excess cholesterol and malfunction of this excretory pathway may be responsible for the formation of gallstones. Cholesterol alone is quite insoluble in water but solutions of conjugated bile salts can dissolve appreciable quantities (Neiderhiser & Roth, 1968). It is now thought that most if not all of the cholesterol in bile is carried in micelles which contain also lecithin and bile salts (Juniper, 1965; Neiderhiser, Roth & Webster, 1966). At a constant water composition of 90%, corresponding to bile, the amount of cholesterol which can be held in micellar solution without crystallizing depends in a complicated manner on the relative proportions of lecithin and bile salts. The relationship can be expressed as phase diagrams with triangular co-ordinates

(Hofmann & Small, 1967); in general terms, cholesterol will tend to separate if there is insufficient bile salts and too much lecithin for the cholesterol content. The quantitative results of bile analyses can be plotted on the diagram; when this is done, the points for bile of patients with normal biliary tracts fall inside the micellar area, while those corresponding to lithogenic biles fall outside, indicating the likelihood of cholesterol crystallization.

In an experimental animal, gallstones may be produced by altering the proportions of these constituents, for example by feeding cholestyramine or cholesterol (see Freston & Bouchier, 1968). The significance of this work to human gall-bladder disease has yet to be determined.

Bile Salts and the Gut

The absorption of fat by the jejunum (Borgstrom, Dahlquist, Lundh & Sjovall, 1957) is associated with micellar formation (see p. 689) and requires the presence of sufficient quantities of conjugated bile salts (Hofmann, 1965). Unused bile salts are normally reabsorbed almost completely in the ileum. Derangements of this mechanism are now thought to be the principal, if not the only, cause of the steatorrhoea which frequently follows bacterial colonization of the upper intestine or the loss of ileal absorptive power.

The stagnant loop syndrome results from conditions leading to stagnation of the contents of the small intestine, such as diverticulosis of the jejunum or after surgical procedures resulting in a blind loop of intestine. The upper intestine normally possesses a transient bacterial population. When stasis occurs, a permanent population similar to that found in the lower intestine is established (Shiner & Drassar, 1969). The microorganisms interfere with vitamin B_{12} absorption and increase the urinary indican excretion by breakdown of tryptophan (Tabaqchali, Okubadejo, Neale & Booth, 1966). Another result of bacterial action is a fall in the concentration of conjugated bile salts in the fasting jejunal juice from a normal value of 5–10 mM to the range 1–5 mM (Tabaqchali, Hatzioannou & Booth, 1968). The level of taurine conjugates is lowered more than that of the glycine conjugates, and the dihydroxy-acid conjugates more than the cholic conjugates. Free bile acids, which are normally absent in the jejunum, can be found in high concentration (Donaldson, 1965; Tabaqchali & Booth, 1966). Serum bile acids reflect this aberration (Fig. 19.7). The values found are strikingly

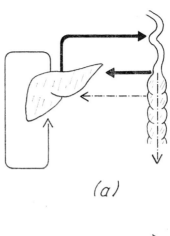

(a)

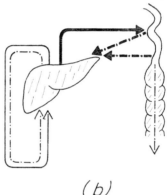

(b)

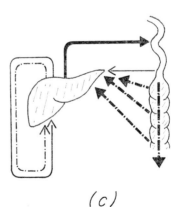

(c)

FIG. 19.7. The enterohepatic circulation of the bile salts. (*a*) in the normal subject, (*b*) in the stagnant loop syndrome, and (*c*) after ileal resection. Conjugated bile salts are indicated by solid arrows, free bile acids by dotted arrows. An indication of the quantitative importance of a pathway is given by the thickness of the line.

high (13–52 μM), almost entirely due to the presence of free bile acids and there is often a complete absence of taurine conjugates (Lewis, Panveliwalla, Tabaqchali & Wootton, 1969). Proof that the abnormality is indeed the result of bacterial action is provided by the return towards a normal pattern after the administration of appropriate antibiotics (Tabaqchali & Booth, 1966; Rosenburg, Hardison & Bull, 1967).

The presence of large amounts of free deoxycholic acid in the abnormal gut contents, and the discovery that this compound interfered with esterification of fatty acids (Dawson & Isselbacher, 1960) has led to the suggestion that there may be a direct toxic action on the jejunal mucosa (Rosenberg *et al.*, 1967). Tabaqchali *et al.* (1968) have shown that the mucosa is normal in these cases and have produced other arguments against the toxic action theory; moreover the measured bile salt concentration is less in some cases at least than the critical micellar concentration (Hofmann & Small, 1967) so that on the

present evidence, the condition would appear to be a straightforward bile salt depletion.

A somewhat similar biochemical condition is found in patients with extensive ileal disease or after massive ileal resections (Fig. 19.7). In such patients, excessive faecal losses of bile salts occur as shown by the administration of labelled conjugates. (Playout, Lack & Weiner, 1965; Austad, Luck & Tyor, 1967). The half-life of the bile salt pool in this condition is shorter than normal (Hofmann & Grundy, 1965; Van Deest, Fordtran, Morawski & Wilson, 1968) and the small bowel total bile salts are reduced, usually to the 1–5 mM range (McLeod & Wiggins, 1968). Taurine conjugates seem to be particularly affected. The blood levels show a picture similar to that of the blind loop syndrome, with high free bile acid concentrations and a reduction in taurine conjugates (Lewis *et al.*, 1969), a picture which is now thought to be sufficiently specific to make the estimation of blood levels worth consideration as a diagnostic investigation.

References

AUSTAD, W. I., LUCK, L. & TYOR, M. P. (1967). *Gastroenterology*, **52**, 638.

BERGSTROM, S. (1959). In "Hormones and Atherosclerosis," p. 31, Academic Press, New York.

BERGSTROM, S. (1962). *Fed. proc.*, **21**, 28.

BERGSTROM, S. & DANIELSSON, H. (1958). *Acta physiol. Scand.*, **43**, 1.

BERGSTROM, S., LUNDH, G. & HOFMANN, A. (1963). *Gastroenterology*, **45**, 229.

BORGSTROM, B., DAHLQUIST, A., LUNDH, G. & SJOVALL, J. (1957). *J. Clin. Invest.*, **36**, 1521.

BOYD, G. S. (1969). Paper read at a meeting of the Steroid Biochemistry Group of the Biochemical Society, 14th April, 1969.

BRULE, M. & COTTET, J. (1942). *Presse. Med.*, **50**, 369.

CAREY, J. B. (1958). *J. Clin. Invest.*, **37**, 1494.

CAREY, J. B. & WILLIAMS, G. (1961). *J. Am. Med. Assoc.* **176**, 432.

CAREY, J. B., & WILLIAMS, G. (1963). *J. Clin. Invest.*, **42**, 450.

DANIELSSON, H., ENEROTH, P., HELLSTROM, K., Lindstedt, S. & Sjovall, J. (1963). *J. biol. Chem.*, **7**, 2299.

DAWSON, A. M. & ISSELBACHER, K. J. (1960). *J. Clin. Invest.*, **39**, 730.

DONALDSON, R. M. (1965). *J. Clin. Invest.*, **44**, 1815.

ENCRANTZ, J. C. & SJOVALL, J. (1959). *Clin. Chim. Acta*, **4**, 793.

ENEROTH, P., GORDON, B., RYHAGE, R. & SJOVALL, J. (1966). *J. Lipid Res.*, **7**, 511.

ENEROTH, P., GORDON, B., SJOVALL, J. (1966). *J. Lipid Res.*, **7**, 524.

FIESER, L. F. & FIESER, M. (1949). "Natural Products Related to Phenanthrene," 3rd Ed. New York: Reinhold.

FIESER, L. F. & FIESER, M. (1959). "Steroids," New York: Reinhold.

FRESTON, J. W. & BOUCHIER, I. A. D. (1968). *Gut*, **9**, 2.

GREGG, J. A. (1967). *Nature* (Lond.), **214**, 29.

HASLEWOOD, G. A. D. (1967). "Bile Salts," London: Methuen.

HELLSTROM, K. & SJOVALL, J. (1961). *Acta physiol. Scand.*, **51**, 218.

HOFMANN, A. F. (1965). *Gastroenterology*, **48**, 484.

HOFMANN, A. F. & GRUNDY, S. M. (1965). *Clin. Res.*, **13**, 254.

HOFMANN, A. F. & SMALL, D. M. (1967). In "Annual Review of Medicine," p. 333.

ISAKSSON, B. (1953). *Acta Soc. Med. Upsala*, **59**, 307.

JOSEPHSON, B. (1943). *Physiol. Rev.*, **21**, 463.

JUNIPER, K. (1965). *Amer. J. Med.*, **39**, 98.

KINSELL, L. W. (1968). *Prog. Bioch. Pharm.*, **4**, 59.

LACK, L. & WEINER, I. M. (1961). *Am. J. Physiol.*, **200**, 313.

LEWIS, B., PANVELIWALLA, D., TABAQCHALI, S. & WOOTTON, I. D. P. (1969). *Lancet*, **1**, 219.

LINDSTEDT, S. (1962). *Clin. Chem. Acta*, **7**, 1.

MACINTYRE, I. & WOOTTON, I. D. P. (1960). *Ann. Rev. Biochem.*, **29**, 635.

McLEOD, G. M. & WIGGINS, H. S. (1968). *Lancet*, **1**, 873.

MOUTAFIS, C. D., MYANT, N. B. & TABAQCHALI, S. (1968). *Clin. Sc.*, **35**, 537.

MYANT, N. B. (1969). *Recenti. Prog. Med.*, in press.

NEIDERHISER, D. H. & ROTH, H. P. (1968). *Proc. Soc. Exp. Biol. Med.*, **128**, 221.

NEIDERHISER, D. H., ROTH, H. P. & WEBSTER, L. T. (1966). *J. Lab. Clin. Med.*, **68**, 90.

NORMAN, A. & SHORT, M. S. (1962). *Proc. Soc. Exp. Biol.* (N.Y.), **110**, 552.

OSBORN, E. C., WOOTTON, I. D. P., DA SILVA, L. C. & SHERLOCK, S. (1959). *Lancet*, **2**, 1049.

PANVELIWALLA, D., LEWIS, B., WOOTTON, I. D. P. & TABAQCHALI, S. (1969). *J. Clin. Path.*, in press.

PLAYOUST, M. R., LACK, L. & WEINER, I. M. (1965). *Am. J. Physiol.*, **208**, 363.

ROSENBERG, I. H., HARDISON, W. G. & BULL, D. M. (1967). *New Eng. J. Med.*, **276**, 1391.

RUDMAN, D. & KENDALL, F. E. (1957). *J. Clin. Invest.*, **36**, 530.

SANDBERG, D. H., SJOVALL, J., SJOVALL, K. & TURNER, D. A. (1965). *J. Lipid Res.*, **6**, 182.

SHERLOCK, S. P. V. (1958). "Diseases of the Liver and Biliary System." Oxford: Blackwell.

SHINER, M. & DRASSAR, B. S. (1969). *Gut*, in press.

SCHERSTEN, T. (1967). *Acta Chir. Scand.*, suppl. 373.

SCHOENFIELD, L. J., SJOVALL, J. & PENMAN, E. (1967). *Nature* (Lond.), **213**, 93.

SOBOTKA, H. (1937). "Physiological Chemistry of the Bile." London: Baillière, Tindall & Cox.

SOBOTKA, H. (1938). "Chemistry of the Steroids." London: Baillière, Tindall & Cox.

TABAQCHALI, S. & BOOTH, C. C. (1966). *Lancet*, **2**, 12.

TABAQCHALI, S., HATZIOANNOU, J. & BOOTH, C. C. (1968). *Lancet*, **2**, 12.

TABAQCHALI, S., OKUBADEJO, D. A., NEALE, G. & BOOTH, C. C. (1966). *Proc. Roy. Soc. Med.*, **59**, 1244.

THOMPSON, J. C. & VARS, H. M. (1954). *Am. J. Physiol.*, **179**, 405.

VAN DEEST, B. W., FORDTRAN, J. S., MORAWSKI, S. G. & WILSON, J. D. (1968). *J. Clin. Invest.*, **47**, 1314.

VARCO, R. L. (1947). *J. Lab. Clin. Med.*, **21**, 43.

WOOTTON, I. D. P. & WIGGINS, H. S. (1953). *Biochem. J.*, **55**, 292.

Chapter 20

THE PANCREAS

by

Henry T. Howat

Manchester Royal Infirmary

CHEMICAL PHYSIOLOGY

The acinar cells, the "centro-acinar" cells and the duct epithelium of the pancreas produce the exocrine secretion. It is convenient in our present state of knowledge to consider the external secretion of the pancreas as an admixture of two juices —one inorganic, the other organic—which are excreted into the duodenum in varying proportions according to prevailing physiological stimuli. The inorganic component, a watery fluid containing salts, and made alkaline by a high concentration of bicarbonate, is secreted in response to secretin which is released from the duodenal mucosa on contact with acid chyme. The alkaline, aqueous juice from the pancreas, together with bile, dilutes and neutralizes the hydrochloric acid as it is received by the duodenum from the stomach (Wormsley & Mahoney, 1967; Banks, Dyck, Dreiling & Janowitz, 1967), and hence exerts a self-regulatory control on the flow of pancreatic juice as the rising pH diminishes the release of secretin. The organic component, the enzyme juice, secreted by a dual nervous and hormonal mechanism, contains the enzymes necessary for the further digestion of carbohydrate, protein and fat in the lumen of the small intestine. Though the release of the hormone pancreozymin from the duodenal mucosa by digestive products, of which peptones and amino acids are most active (Wang & Grossman, 1951), is the principal physiological stimulus of enzyme flow (Harper, 1959), the vagus nerve has long been known to mediate in enzyme release. The possible neurohormonal interrelationships which exist when the pancreas responds to a meal are as yet unresolved (Harper, Blair & Scratcherd, 1962). The acinar cell elaborates the main digestive enzymes of the pancreas, but this highly specialized cell does not produce the bulk of the water or bicarbonate. The source of these inorganic constituents is uncertain, but Grossman & Ivy (1946), Wang, Grossman & Ivy (1948), and Grossman, Wang & Wang (1951) have suggested that the production of water and bicarbonate is a function of the cells of the intralobular ducts and "centro-acinar" cells. Becker (1962) reported that Manzke (1959) has demonstrated by histochemical methods that carbonic anhydrase, enzymically concerned in bicarbonate formation, is selectively concentrated in the duct epithelium, but is virtually absent from the acinar cells of at least three animal species, the rat, the mouse and the guinea-pig.

In addition to the dominant intestinal phase of pancreatic exocrine secretion, the pancreas, like the stomach, responds to cephalic and gastric phases of stimulation. Sham feeding markedly increases enzyme output both in dog and man (Preshaw, Cooke & Grossman, 1966; Sarles, Bauer & Prezlin, 1965); in the dog at least part of the response is mediated by the vagal release of gastrin from the pyloric antrum. In man the pancreatic response to a sham meal is established within 2–4 min., somewhat earlier than the gastric response to cephalic stimulation which suggests that a direct vagal effect predominates (Sarles, Dani, Prezlin, Souville & Figarella, 1968). Distension of both body and antrum of the stomach produces an increase in volume and enzyme output of pancreatic juice both in animals and man (White, Hayama & Magee, 1960; White & Magee, 1963; Blair, Brown, Harper & Scratcherd, 1966). Vagotomy abolishes the response to distension of the body, which is presumably mediated by vagal-vagal reflexes of the type described by Harper, Kidd & Scratcherd (1959) in cats, but the response to antral distension may at least partly be due to a hormonal effect, since extracts of antral mucosa (Blair, Clark, Harper,

Lake & Scratcherd, 1961; Blair *et al.*, 1966) and pure gastrin (Gregory & Tracy, 1964) increase the output of enzyme (a pancreozymin–like effect) from the pancreas.

STRUCTURE AND FUNCTION OF THE PEPTIDE HORMONES OF THE ALIMENTARY TRACT

Gastrin

Synthesis has followed determination of the amino acid sequence of several of the peptide hormones of the alimentary tract. The structure of the gastrin polypeptides of different species has been elucidated since the first synthesis of hog gastrin (Anderson, Barton, Gregory, Hardy, Kenner, MacLeod, Preston, Sheppard & Morley, 1964; Gregory, Hardy, Jones, Kenner & Sheppard, 1964; Bentley, Kenner & Sheppard, 1966). In all species gastrin is a heptadecapeptide amide, the N-terminal residue is pyroglutamyl and the C-terminal residue is phenylalanine amide. The C-terminal tetrapeptide sequence, Try-Met-Asp-Phe(NH$_2$), common to all gastrins, is an essential requirement for the physiological actions of gastrin (Morley, Tracy & Gregory, 1965). In man as in the pig, two gastrins are known; the peptides H II and G II only differ from human gastrin I (H1) and hog gastrin I (G1) in possessing a sulphate group bound in ester form to the tyrosyl residue. In human gastrins leucine replaces methionine which occupies position 5 of the molecule of hog gastrin.

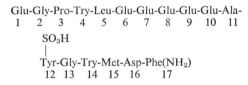

FIG. 20.1. Human Gastrin II (the N-terminal Glu is in the pyro form).

In addition to stimulating acid and pepsin secretion from the stomach and gastro-intestinal tone and motility (Gregory & Tracy, 1964; Gregory, 1967) gastrin possesses a slight secretin and a powerful pancreozymin-like effect but no cholecystokinetic activity. Tracy & Gregory (1964) considered that the whole range of biological activities displayed by the parent gastrin molecule is possessed by the C-terminal tetrapeptide sequence. Substitution of the amino acid residues of the tetrapeptide reduces its acid-stimulating power; enzyme production by the pancreas is virtually lost (Beswick, Howat & Morris, 1968).

Cholecystokinin-pancreozymin

It came as some surprise when Mutt & Jorpes (1967) announced that cholecystokinin-pancreozymin is built up of 33 amino acid units in which the amino acid sequence of the C-terminal tetrapeptide is identical to that of gastrin (Fig. 20.2). Jorpes & Mutt (1966) consider that cholecystokinin and pancreozymin cannot be separated; indeed that they are probably identical chemically.

$$SO_3H$$
$$|$$
Asp-Tyr-Met-Gly-Try-Met-Asp-Phe(NH$_2$)

Fig. 20.2. C-terminal octapeptide of cholecystokinin-pancreozymin.

Antibodies to the gastrin molecule have been evoked in rabbits by immunization with synthetic human gastrin 1 conjugated to bovine serum albumin, and a sensitive immunoassay method developed (McGuigan, 1968a). Immunological cross reactivity has been established between the C-terminal tetrapeptide amide of gastrin and cholecystokinin (McGuigan, 1968b). Gastrin has been identified by immunofluorescent techniques in interspersed differentiated epithelial cells of the antral mucosa of both pig and man (McGuigan, 1968c).

Caerulein

Methanol extracts of the skin of an Australian frog, *Hyla caerulea*, contain an active principle, caerulein, which has a hypotensive effect, and a powerful stimulant action on certain extravascular smooth muscles and on gastric and pancreatic secretions (Anastasi, Erspamer & Endean, 1967; Erspamer, Bertaccini, De Caro, Endean & Impicciatore, 1967). Caerulein-like polypeptides are also recovered from other Australian and South American amphibians. In these the physiological action of caerulein is not known. Anastasi, Erspamer & Endean (1967, 1968) have isolated caerulein in pure form, and Bernardi, Bosisio, De Castiglione & Goffredo, (1967) have confirmed the proposed structure. Caerulein bears a close resemblance to gastrin II (Fig. 20.3).

$$SO_3H$$
$$|$$
Glu-Gln-Asp-Tyr-Thr-Gly-Try-Met-Asp-Phe(NH$_2$)

Fig. 20.3. Caerulein (the N-terminal Glu is in the pyro form).

The decapeptide is much more potent on a weight basis than gastrin in stimulating acid secretion by the stomach, than cholecystokinin in contracting the gall bladder, or than pancreozymin in increasing enzyme output of the pancreas. Sulphation of the tyrosinyl residue is of decisive importance in determining the pharmacological activity of caerulein. The parent molecule is 10 to over 100 times more active than desulphated caerulein; on desulphation cholecystokinetic activity is virtually lost (Beswick & Howat, unpublished).

Secretin

Secretin is a polypeptide composed of 27 amino acids and 11 different amino acids. Cystine, methionine, tyrosine, tryptophan, proline, isoleucine and lysine are not represented. The features of the structure of secretin are its strongly basic nature and its similarity to glucagon (Fig. 20.4). Jorpes (1968) has suggested that as secretin is a strongly basic peptide of low molecular weight, it is at neutral reaction electrostatically bound to ionized carboxyl groups of the cell proteins, not easily extracted by water or saline. When hydrochloric acid enters the duodenum the negative charge of the cell proteins is reduced; possibly they acquire a positive electric charge. Secretin, set free as a hydrochloride in a highly ionized state, freely enters into the blood by diffusion. The similarity in structure of secretin to glucagon is of considerable interest in view of the suggestion that secretin acts as an insulin-releasing factor (Dupré, 1964; Dupré, Rojas, White, Ungar & Beck, 1966). Glucagon in both cats and dogs inhibits secretin-stimulated pancreatic secretion in contrast to its stimulatory effect on the flow of hepatic bile (Walker & Necheles, 1956; Dyck, Hoexter, Rudick & Janowitz, 1968).

Secretin

His-Ser-Asp-Gly-Thr-Phe-Thr-Ser-Glu-Leu-Ser-Arg-
Leu-Arg-Asp-Ser-Ala-Arg-Leu-Gln-Arg-Leu-Leu-
Gln-Gly-Leu-Val(NH$_2$)

Glucagon

His-Ser-Gln-Gly-Thr-Phe-Thr-Ser-Asp-Tyr-Ser-Lys-
Tyr-Leu-Asp-Ser-Arg-Arg-Ala-Gln-Asp-Phe-Val-
Gln-Try-Leu-Met-Asn-Thr

Fig. 20.4. Structures of Secretin and Glucagon.

Pure synthetic hog secretin and pure natural hog secretin have the same spectrum of actions and are equal in potency on a weight basis. Secretin stimulates the flow and bicarbonate output from the pancreas, stimulates the flow and bicarbonate output of bile, stimulates Brunner's glands and inhibits gastric motility and the acid secretion of the gastrin-stimulated stomach (Vayne, Stening, Brooks & Grossman, 1968; Grossman, 1968). Indeed Johnson & Grossman (1968) conclude that secretin is the inhibitory hormone or chalone (enterogastrone) released on contact of acid in the duodenum.

It has long been known that pancreatic juice contains the active kinin forming the enzyme kallikrein and an active kininase. Kinins play a role in the functional vasodilatation of glandular tissues. Hilton & Jones (1968) have recently shown that in the cat the juice obtained in response to a first dose of secretin has a high kinin-forming activity, and that the concentration falls off considerably in response to successive doses of secretin, a "wash-out" effect. Acetylcholine and pancreozymin in contrast greatly increase kinin-forming activity. Among the tissues in which primary prostaglandins have been demonstrated is the pancreas (Bergström, 1967).

ELECTRON MICROSCOPY

The introduction of refined techniques of electron microscopy, by which high resolution has been achieved in ultra-thin slices, has largely replaced histochemical methods in the study of the acinar cell. Compared with the acinar cells the cells of the intercalary ducts and "centro-acinar" cells are relatively structureless, and are characterized by a paucity of membranous material according to Ekholm & Edlund (1959), who studied the ultrastructure of the human exocrine cells of the pancreas in three fasting patients who for various reasons were subjected to laparotomy. The scarcity of a-cytomembranes (endoplasmic reticulum) in ductule cells provides supporting evidence that they are not concerned with active protein synthesis; on the other hand the presence of microvilli on the apical surface of these cells indicates either a secretory or absorptive function.

The ultrastructure of the cytoplasmic elements of the acinar cell in man (Ekholm & Edlund, 1959; Gadrat & Ribet, 1962) is similar in detail to that of the mouse (Sjöstrand & Hanzon, 1954a; Weiss, 1953), of the guinea-pig (Palade, 1956a,b; Palade & Siekevitz, 1956), and of the cat (Hermodsson, 1965); indeed it resembles strikingly on electron microscopy other cells, which, like the peptic cell of the stomach, are actively engaged in protein synthesis. The cytoplasm contains the rounded zymogen granules which, orientated towards the ductules, predominate apically, and is rich in membranes most numerous in the basal zone. These paired cytomembranes enclose the endoplasmic reticulum, and bear on the outer surface small adherent granules, about 150 Å in diameter, which, variously named microsomal particles or ribosomes, are largely aggregations of ribonucleoproteins. These roughly granular a-cytomembranes, the characteristic feature of cells engaged in protein synthesis, contrast with the less numerous agranular, smooth γ-cytomembranes found in the region of the Golgi apparatus. Current knowledge of the ultrastructure of the acinar cell has been reviewed by Sjöstrand (1962) and Hermodsson (1965), who have given an account of the molecular structure of its membranous components in various stages of secretory activity of the pancreas.

COMBINED CHEMICAL AND CYTOLOGICAL STUDIES

Siekevitz & Palade (1958a,b,c) have made combined cytological and chemical investigations on acinar cell fractions of the guinea-pig at various stages of digestion. In fasting guinea-pigs the trypsin-activatable proteases taken as a group (TAPase) and ribonuclease (RNase) are concentrated to the greatest extent in the zymogen granule fractions, a finding which fits the hypothesis, long proposed, that the zymogen granule is a temporary intracellular depot for digestive enzymes or enzyme precursors. The bulk of the remainder is present in the microsomal fractions; but when the guinea-pig is fed after a fast, within an hour the TAPase and RNase activity of the microsomal fraction increase markedly, at a time when the cavities of the endoplasmic reticulum contain numerous intracisternal granules and when the content of the microsomal vesicles increases in density (Siekevitz & Palade, 1958b).

After fractionating the microsomes in such a way as to dissolve the membranous vesicles but not the granules, they obtained a concentrate of granules in which the concentration of TAPase and RNase activity rose to levels similar to those in purified zymogen fractions. From the same microsomal preparations they also isolated ribonucleoprotein particles, presumably detached from the microsomal membranes as a result of the deoxycholate treatment, and found that these particles also possessed significant amounts of TAPase and RNase activity. To explain these findings Siekevitz & Palade postulated that the post-prandial increase in enzymic activity is due to the synthesis of new enzymes by the microsomes (a view first suggested by Weiss (1953) to explain his electron photomicrographs), and assumed that these enzymes are temporarily segregated into the intracisternal granules which thus appear as precursors of the mature zymogen granules of the cell. They brought forward as evidence to support these views the results of a further study (Siekevitz & Palade, 1958c), in which they followed the variations in and intracellular migration of the amount and concentration of radioactivity in the proteins of various cell fractions and subfractions for a period after labelling the proteins *in vivo* with DL-leucine-1-^{14}C. This paper confirmed the rapidity with which radioactive amino acids are incorporated into the proteins of the pancreas (Hansson, 1959) and the rapid turnover of proteins by the pancreas. When the same methods are applied to the synthesis of specific enzymes, it has been demonstrated that bovine trypsinogen and chymotrypsinogen (Keller, Cohen & Neurath, 1959, 1961) and murine ribonuclease (Morris & Dickman, 1960) are also synthesized at very high rates.

Caro (1961) traced the passage of pancreatic proteins labelled with leucine-^{3}H through the acinar cell. After some 15–20 min. some 70% of the radioautographic grains were localized in the large vacuoles of the Golgi region. Palade, Siekevitz & Caro (1962), Siekevitz & Palade (1960) and Redman, Siekevitz & Palade (1966) identified four stages of synthesis, intracellular transport and storage: a first stage of synthesis on ribosomes attached to rough endoplasmic reticulum; immediate transfer into the cisternae of the rough endoplasmic reticulum; subsequent transport into central condensing vacuoles of the Golgi zone (Caro & Palade, 1964), the area in which Sjöstrand & Hanzon (1954b) and Sjöstrand (1962) observed "precursor granules" and considered that the Golgi apparatus may be responsible for the formation of the membranes which enclose the zymogen granules; the zymogen granules represent the fourth stage, prior to discharge into the lumen, where they are dissolved at the pH of pancreatic juice.

Hokin & Hokin (1958) studied the incorporation of ^{32}P into phospholipids, which takes place during cholinergic stimulation and in response to pancreozymin. The greatest increase was in the turnover of phosphoinositide; other phosphatides were less markedly involved. The greatest phospholipid turnover was in the microsomal fraction. These events did not occur in response to secretin, and in the case of cholinergic drugs (though not pancreozymin) were inhibited by atropine.

Radioautographic studies have shown that phosphatidylinositol is evenly incorporated into rough and smooth membranes. The kinetics of incorporation did not support the hypothesis that smooth and rough membranes may be derived one from the other (Hokin & Huebner, 1967). Hokin has recapitulated the evidence which has led him to argue that increased synthesis of phosphatidylinositol in response to acetylcholine and pancreozymin is therefore concerned with the formation of new intracellular membranes (Hokin, 1967).

It is not known if the mechanism proposed by Palade's group is obligatory or whether it represents the state of affairs while the gland is actively secreting as well as during the storage period. Nor is it conclusively proved that the non-proteolytic enzymes, amylase and lipase, are also or always transported in this way, since amylase and lipase are recovered proportionately less in the zymogen fraction and more in the microsomal and final supernatant fractions (Van Lancker & Holtzer, 1959; Hansson, 1959). This may be due to leaching out of enzyme during the handling process. An alternative pathway may be the release of enzyme from the ribonucleoprotein particles into the cell sap, from which they are carried across the smooth-surfaced membranes of the zymogen vacuoles, which are probably derived from the Golgi membranes (Hokin, 1967). This is unlikely. Jamieson & Palade (1967) recently pulse-labelled guinea-pig slices with radioactive leucine, incubated in "chase" medium for variable times and separated by differentiated and gradient centrifugation into individual fractions of zymogen granules, total microsomes (the peripheral elements of the Golgi complex), rough microsomes (the rough-surfaced endoplasmic reticulum) and supernatant fluid. The kinetics of the synthesis and intracellular transport of enzyme in this system provide direct evidence that the secretory proteins are transported from the cisternae of the rough-surfaced endoplasmic reticulum via the small vesicles of the Golgi complex to condensing vacuoles. The low and relatively constant radioactivity of proteins in the supernatant fluid supports the view that synthesized zymogen proteins are transported entirely within a membrane system and not through the matrix of the cytoplasm.

The native proteins of the pancreatic cell are protected from the proteolytic action of these enzymes, which are stored and transported across the cell in the zymogen granules to be discharged into pancreatic ducts (Siekevitz & Palade, 1958b), where they disintegrate in the alkaline pancreatic juice. But the enzymes of the zymogen granules are proteins also sensitive to attack by proteolytic agents. A second protective mechanism exists since trypsin, chymotrypsin and the carboxypeptidases are synthesized and stored as inactive precursors, the zymogens, trypsinogen, chymotrypsinogen and the procarboxypeptidases. Trypsinogen is activated to trypsin by enteropeptidase (enterokinase) on reaching the duodenum, and chymotrypsinogen and the procarboxypeptidases are activated rapidly in the presence of free trypsin. A third line of defence exists since a trypsin inhibitor has been found in both pancreatic extracts and pancreatic juice. A trypsin inhibitor is also present in blood serum.

THE PANCREATIC PROTEINS

During the past decade much information has been gained on the enzyme content of the pancreas and pancreatic juice. Keller, Cohen & Neurath (1958) and Keller & Cohen (1961) showed that the chromatographic profile of the proteolytic enzymes of bovine pancreatic juice is similar to the relative proportions found in pancreatic tissue, in zymogen granules and in microsomal subfractions. Greene, Hirs & Palade (1963) extended these observations to amylase and lipase, and Marchis-Mouren (1959, 1965), and Marchis-Mouren, Charles, Ben Abdeljlil & Desnuelle (1961) demonstrated well marked amylase and ipase peaks in both dog and pig pancreatic juice on chromatography successively on diethylaminoethyl cellulose (DEAE) and carboxymethyl cellulose (CM). Specimens of human pancreatic juice are usually obtained by drainage of the pancreatic duct after surgical operation and in circumstances which are not usually physiological. According to Keller & Allen (1967) pancreatic juice in man has been reported to contain amylase, lipase, cholesterol esterase, phospholipase and phosphatase, as well as chymotrypsinogen, trypsinogen and a trypsin inhibitor. Extracts of human pancreas have been reported to contain in addition ribonuclease and elastase. Several enzymes have been isolated in purified form from extracts of human pancreas, notably crystalline amylase, two forms of ribonuclease and trypsin. Keller & Allen (1967) have separated the proteins of human pancreatic juice at pH 6·5 into anionic and cationic fractions. The cationic proteins include amylase, lipase, RNase and a pancreatic trypsin inhibitor; the anionic proteins include chymotrypsinogen, procarboxypeptidases A and B, and two components showing tryptic activity. They separated the cationic proteins on polyacrylamide gel and identified the bands by histochemical methods.

Zones containing amylase, lipase, RNase and pancreatic trypsin inhibitor were localized. The level of the inhibitor was such that 1 ml. of pancreatic juice containing 4 mg. of protein inhibited about 0·08 mg. of bovine trypsin. The inhibitor is a small, basic protein, soluble in 2·5 % trichloroacetic acid. It differs from the Kunitz bovine inhibitor in its slower migration rate in polyacrylamide gel at pH 4·1 and in its kinetic properties.

The hydrolytic activities of trypsin and the other pancreatic peptidases are most conveniently determined by following the reaction toward synthetic substrates with a Radiometer pH stat. Desnuelle (1961) has reviewed the properties and kinetics of pancreatic lipase, and emphasizes that lipase acts exclusively on emulsified esters. Hence the choice of substrate to measure the activity of lipase is of some importance; the substrate according to Desnuelle should be an emulsion of long-chain triglycerides, such as that on which lipase acts physiologically in the duodenum. Barrowman & Borgström (1968) have separated lipase (glycerol ester hydrolase) of rat pancreatic juice from a larger molecular weight enzyme (carboxylic ester hydrolase) by gel filtration and ion-exchange chromatography, and studied the specificity of the two enzymes for a series of substrates proposed for assay of lipase. Methods employing emulsified long chain triglycerides are still the most specific for the assay of pancreatic lipase. Dispersions of the chromogenic β-naphthyl laurate and oleate, and p-nitrophenyl laurate, are split principally by lipase: however the addition of bile salt, even in low concentrations to the incubation systems, alters the specificity of these substrates in favour of the esterase. Human pancreatic a-amylase has been obtained in a pure crystalline state (Meyer, Fischer, Bernfeld & Duckert, 1948). It acts on the unbranched polysaccharide of starch, amylose, by the hydrolytic splitting of a-1,4-glucosidic linkages. A rapid primary action yields dextrins of relatively low molecular weight, reducing markedly the viscosity of the substrate and altering the iodine colour, which ranges from violet to purple to brown according to chain length. The dextrins are further degraded to polysaccharides of smaller molecular weight which no longer stain with iodine; then, in a second much slower reaction, a mixture of maltose and maltotriose is formed; eventually maltotriose is split slowly, the end products of exhaustive action being 13 % glucose and 87 % maltose. The action of a-amylase on the branched polysaccharide amylopectin is analogous, here the a-1,4-glucosidic linkages are split in a random manner to yield a final degradation product in which the proportions of glucose and maltose differ. The presence of Cl^- ions is necessary for the activity of human α-amylase. The human pancreas seems to contain an antagonistic system of an amylase inhibitor and activator. The removal of the first, and at a later stage of purification the second, produces alternating increases and decreases of activity, a phenomenon always observed in the purification of human pancreatic amylase (Bernfield, 1951).

INORGANIC CONSTITUENTS

Apart from its protein content the characteristic chemical feature of pancreatic juice is its alkalinity due to a high concentration of bicarbonate. Bicarbonate and chloride concentrations vary inversely; the sum of the two anions expressed in milliequivalents is constant and approximates the total base of blood plasma (Thomas, 1950). The small amount of phosphate present is rather less than in blood plasma. The concentrations of the cations sodium and potassium are also equivalent to that of blood plasma, though the calcium concentration is somewhat lower. Dreiling & Janowitz (1956) have confirmed the observations made by Lagerlöf (1942) in man that bicarbonate and chloride vary inversely; at low rates of secretion, the chloride is high, at high rates of secretion bicarbonate is high. Little is known of the mechanisms by which bicarbonate enters pancreatic juice. Presumably it can come either from the blood plasma or from CO_2 derived from cellular metabolism or both. There is a hyperbolic relationship between concentration of bicarbonate and volume of pancreatic juice (Dreiling & Janowitz, 1959), and a linear relationship between output of bicarbonate and volume of juice in patients whose gall bladders have been removed (Lagerlöf, Rudewald & Perman, 1960). Dissociation of the relationship between HCO_3^- and volume can be brought about by acetazolamide, an inhibitor of carbonic anhydrase, which diminishes the total fluid and output of bicarbonate in response to secretin. The maximum bicarbonate concentration, however, remains high at low rates of secretion. In most patients with chronic pancreatitis and after ACTH there is a low maximal bicarbonate concentration, when compared with normal subjects at equivalent rates of flow. Dreiling & Janowitz (1959) did not consider that these data are compatible with the older admixture hypotheses—that the pancreas elaborates a solution of HCO_3^- isotonic with plasma, to which varying amounts of electrolytes, mainly Cl^-, are added from other sources (ulti-

mately the interstitial fluid), the final composition of the fluid depending on the varying proportions of the various fluids added. In its place they have proposed a new exchange hypothesis. In this case a primary secretion of isotonic HCO_3^- is modified by an interchange of HCO_3^- for Cl^- derived from interstitial fluid as the fluid passes down the intercalary ductules. At the highest rates of secretion there is the least time for exchange, at the lowest rates the greatest time for exchange. Acetazolamide would in this case have a double action, inhibition of the amount secreted into the duct system of the pancreas and interference with HCO_3^-/Cl^- exchange mechanism (Dreiling & Janowitz, 1959). Implicit in this statement is the suggestion of an active reabsorption of HCO_3^- and not a simple passive transfer of HCO_3^- and Cl^- between the ductules and interstitial fluid. In chronic pancreatitis and after ACTH a structural or functional modification of the ductules is thought to account for the shift in the bicarbonate flow relationships. In a cat secreting pancreatic juice of low enzyme content at a maximal rate of flow in response to a continuous infusion of secretion, an injection of pancreozymin increases the enzyme content of the juice for about 5 min. During the period of increased enzyme output there is a slight increase in the flow, a decrease in bicarbonate concentration and an increase in chloride concentration (Case, Harper & Scratcherd, 1969). Presumably the source of the chloride ion in this instance is the acinar cell.

When Ribet, Pascal & Sannou (1967) estimated the maximal bicarbonate secretory capacity in man by continuous infusion of secretin intravenously, they noted that while the volume of duodenal contents continued to rise as the dose of secretin was raised, bicarbonate concentration fell and chloride concentration rose. Similar findings were reported in man by Wormsley (1968a). Henrickson (1968) did not find this anomaly when synthetic secretin was given. Since in duodenal contents the admixture of unknown quantities of bile and intestinal juice might be a source of error, Ribet, Pascal, Vaysse & Bouchard (1968) repeated the experiments in dogs in which the pancreatic duct was cannulated and confirmed the dissociation of anions at high flow rates. No dissociation was obtained when the pancreas was stimulated by duodenal acidification (Pascal, Vaysse, Augier & Ribet, 1968). Although the exchange hypothesis can account for the secretory pattern at low and moderate rates, the dissociation at high secretory rates in response to secretin is best explained as a result of the pharmacological action of secretin in accordance with a two-component hypothesis, water and chloride being produced from an unknown source by large (pharmacological) doses of secretin.

PANCREATIC INSUFFICIENCY

When a large part of the pancreas has been destroyed or the major pancreatic duct blocked, exocrine secretory insufficiency may manifest itself by the appearance of excessive fat and organic nitrogenous substances in the stools. Such evidence of digestive impairment consequent on acinar dysfunction is a relatively late manifestation of chronic pancreatitis and cancer of the pancreas. In individual patients with comparable pancreatic destruction considerable variations in functional disability are found. Even complete obstruction of the major pancreatic and common bile ducts by cancer of the head of the pancreas with pancreatic achylia may not lead to obvious steatorrhoea.

Deficient exocrine aqueous secretion rarely causes manifest symptoms, though the lack of this factor may contribute to the development of peptic ulcer encountered in some patients with pancreatic achylia. It is only when the external secretion is diverted from the alimentary tract, as may occur when an external fistula of the main pancreatic duct is present, that the loss of fluid and electrolytes, principally bicarbonate, from the body may lead to dehydration and a metabolic acidosis which is troublesome to control.

The absorption of iron in physiological doses is increased in pancreatic insufficiency due to chronic pancreatitis (Davis & Badenoch, 1962). This is not due to the lowered pH in the duodenum as a result of deficient excretion of bicarbonate by the pancreas since absorption can be reduced by the addition of a freeze dried extract of whole pancreas (Viokase) to the test dose of iron. The active factor in pancreas appears to be water-soluble and heat labile. It is also present in pancreatic juice (Davis & Biggs, 1965, 1967). Anaemia is not a prominent feature of cancer of the pancreas until invading tumour ulcerates into the stomach or duodenum.

INVESTIGATION OF PANCREATIC DYSFUNCTION

In clinical practice pancreatic dysfunction can be assessed:

(a) indirectly—from evidence of impaired digestion and absorption of food,

(b) by the presence of an increased concentra-

tion of pancreatic enzymes in body fluids, either in the resting state or after stimulation of the pancreas (evocative tests),

(c) by assessing the incorporation of radioactive amino acids into the proteins of the acinar cells of the pancreas,

(d) by estimating pancreatic secretory capacity directly from the amount and character of the duodenal contents, obtained by intubation after stimulating the pancreas to secrete,

(e) from coincidental evidence of endocrine pancreatic dysfunction.

Impaired digestion and absorption of food

Neither balance test procedures, in which fat and nitrogen are measured, nor tolerance test procedures provide an early index of pancreatic dysfunction; nor as a rule do they distinguish between faulty digestion due to pancreatic dysfunction and faulty absorption due to dysfunction of the small bowel. If steatorrhoea is demonstrated this distinction is most conveniently made by a glucose tolerance test, the values of which are frequently elevated in pancreatic disease and depressed in small intestinal disease (Gaddie, Thomas, Smith & French, 1957). Fat balance studies are most useful in pancreatic disease in evaluating how much and how often pancreatin should be given in substitution therapy to the individual patient. Estimation of the total daily excretion of fat in the stool by the method of van de Kamer, Huinink & Weyers (1949) has not yet been displaced by other more sensitive methods. The technique is designed to measure fatty acids with a chain length greater than 14 carbon atoms; medium chain fatty acids are not recovered quantitatively with this method (Saunders, 1967; Braddock, Fleishner & Barbero, 1968).

Starch tolerance test

Althausen & Uyeyama (1954) compared blood glucose levels following the administration of 100 g. of Lintner's soluble starch and 100 g. of glucose. A smaller increase of blood sugar values after the starch than after the glucose they deemed characteristic of pancreatic insufficiency. Sun & Shay (1961) have evaluated this test in 101 patients with no pancreatic disease and 43 patients with pancreatic disease, and confirmed the normal values defined by the original authors. In their hands a positive starch tolerance test proved a reliable indication of pancreatic disease; on the other hand a negative test did not rule out pancreatic disease. Althausen & Uyeyama (1961) have commented on criticism of the method, and stress the importance of meticulously preparing the starch, since there is no doubt that many patients find the starch test meal unpalatable and in some cases more distressing than duodenal intubation. These workers considered the starch tolerance test to be as sensitive as the secretin test, and to be especially reliable in patients with diffuse cancer of the pancreas; it was positive in two-thirds of their patients with chronic pancreatitis, especially in those with more advanced disease. The use of amylose in place of starch, while more palatable, does not increase diagnostic accuracy (O'Loughlin & Howat, unpublished).

Amylase

Amylase is the term applied to hydrolytic enzymes which digest starch. Human pancreatic amylase is an α-amylase which has been obtained in the crystalline pure state. Many methods of determining amylase activity have been developed, the most important of which measure either a decrease in viscosity or a change of iodine colour or an increase of reducing power. The dextrinizing and saccharogenic activities are now most commonly measured. Amylose is used as an alternative substrate to starch in clinical practice (Street & Close, 1956). Since the activity of amylase depends on the nature of the substrate, and may change in the presence of protein, by increase of pH and even by dilution, the use of the term "amylase unit", though convenient, is strictly inaccurate. The large variety of methods for determining the amount of reducing substance liberated creates variable results. These factors make comparison of data from different laboratories difficult.

Serum amylase

Though the saccharogenic and iodometric methods of estimating amylase in serum do not give closely parallel results (Heinkel, 1961), from the practical point of view a pathological rise is manifested by both methods, either of which can be used to establish a clinical diagnosis.

In addition to the pancreas and salivary glands, the liver, Fallopian tubes (Green, 1957) and possibly striated muscle and even fat depots may be sources of serum amylase. The serum amylase is relatively constant for an individual in good health (Elman, Arneson & Graham, 1929; Sullivan & Knight, 1960). A rise follows acute pancreatitis or pancreatic duct obstruction so long as sufficient functioning acinar tissue remains. Though a raised serum amylase cannot be taken as pathognomonic evidence of pancreatitis, the highest values are usually seen in acute pancreatitis. In some cases the rise is evanescent or

negligible. Rises are seen in mumps and infective parotitis, in gall stones especially when sited in the common bile duct or neck of the gall bladder, in perforated peptic ulcer, small gut obstruction and peritonitis (Burnett & Ness, 1955). In practice care must be taken in assessing the significance of a raised amylase in serum taken in the 24 hr. following morphine, codeine and even pethidine, all of which cause spasm of the sphincter of Oddi. Low values are occasionally obtained in liver disease and in pancreatic destruction.

Following pioneer work by Delcourt & Delcourt (1953) many attempts have been made to separate and identify, in both normal and pathological sera, amylases arising from different sources, in particular the salivary and pancreatic amylases. McGeachin & Lewis (1959) and Dreiling, Janowitz & Josephberg (1963), using paper electrophoresis and an iodometric marker, found that the greater part of "amylase" in normal sera was associated with the albumin fraction, though in acute pancreatitis the peak of amylase was associated with γ-globulin. In normal serum the sum of the iso-amylases present in the various fractions exceeded the amylase content of the whole normal serum but not in acute pancreatitis, a discrepancy which they suggested was due to an amylase inhibitor present in normal serum but not in the serum of patients with acute pancreatitis. When a saccharogenic technique replaced the iodometric method, it became apparent that this anomaly was not due to amylase inhibitor but could be best explained as an artefact resulting from decolorization of the starch iodine indicator by albumin (Wilding, 1963, 1965; Delcourt, Delcourt & Wettendorff, 1964; Searcy, Ujihira, Hayashi & Berk, 1964). Recent work has confirmed the findings of Baker & Pellegrino (1954) who showed that on paper electrophoresis amylase is associated with γ-globulin (Ujihira, Searcy, Berk & Hayashi, 1965; Berk, 1967). This is true also of cellulose column chromatography (Berk, 1967), though on agar gel electrophoresis two peaks of amylase are present, one in normal serum attributed to hepatic amylase, a second in the serum of patients with acute pancreatitis which is similar in position to pancreatic and salivary amylase (Joseph, Olivero & Ressler, 1966). Berk (1967) detected two distinct peaks by polyacrylamide gel electrophoresis, the slower of which corresponded to pancreatic amylase, the faster to parotid gland amylase. The study of isoamylases on Sephadex G-100 and G-75 is further complicated by a specific absorption of amylase on the polysaccharide framework of the dextran gels which leads to retardation on the column (Wilding,

1963; Gelotte, 1964). No such interaction is observed on sephadex G-25.

In certain circumstances amylase in human serum may form a macromolecular complex, possibly with a protein, the size of which precludes its excretion by the urine (Wilding, Cooke & Nicholson, 1964; Berk, Kizu, Wilding & Searcy, 1967). The macroamylase has been shown by electrophoretic studies on polyacrylamide gel not to be the same in all cases. Since these patients with macroamylaseaemia have persistently raised serum amylase with normal or low urinary values, a simultaneous serum amylase and urinary amylase is recommended as a simple screening procedure prior to chromatography. Levitt, Goetzl & Cooperband (1968) believe that there are two types of macroamylaseaemia. They have encountered two elderly female patients with chronic diarrhoea and malabsorption due to steatorrhoea associated with subtotal villous atrophy on intestinal biopsy. The serum amylase activity was very high and was practically all associated with a molecule approximately 11S in size. Normal amylase, and the amylase present in serum in acute pancreatitis, has a sedimentation coefficient of approximately 4·5S. In three other patients with no clinical evidence of malabsorption the serum amylase values were less high and the macroamylase was approximately 7S in size.

Urinary amylase

Amylase is cleared from the blood by the kidney. McGeachin & Hargan (1956) have studied the renal clearance of amylase in normal man. Mean clearance values were 2·08 ± 0·10 ml./min. (range 1·0–3·25) in man and significantly less in women. Amylase clearance remained constant with moderate diuresis and increasing serum amylase concentration. More recently Blainey & Northam (1967) determined the renal clearance of amylase in nine normal subjects and 106 patients who had renal disease of varying severity, from the amyloclastic activity of serum and 4-hr. urine samples. Amylase clearance, at all degrees of renal function is directly related to creatinine clearance (mean 3%, range 2 to 6%). There seems therefore no advantage in determining urinary amylase over the much simpler assay of serum amylase concentration (Levitt, 1968). In a single patient with acute pancreatitis the amylase clearance rate maintained a constant relationship to glomerular filtration rate over a wide range of serum amylase levels. In renal insufficiency the serum amylase level rises in proportion to the fall of amylase clearance, but seldom exceeded twice the upper limit of normal.

In the absence of renal insufficiency, Saxon, Hinckley, Vogel & Zieve (1957) found the excretion rate of amylase in the urine was always abnormal when the serum concentration was abnormal; as a rule the urinary values were more abnormal. In acute pancreatitis the urinary values may remain abnormal for 7–10 days longer than the serum values which is difficult to explain unless there is an alteration of amylase clearance to creatinine clearance in acute pancreatitis (Levitt, 1968). Many workers in estimating urinary amylase have used 24-hr. or at least 6-hr. collections. Saxon et al. (1957), however, found that a 24-hr. specimen gave no more accurate results than a 1-hr. specimen. To minimize collection difficulties they advised a single 2-hr. collection expressing the results in units excreted/hr., as did Gambill & Mason (1964). In acute oliguric failure much higher levels of serum amylase, in excess of twice the upper limit of normal, are occasionally encountered. In some at least of these a terminal pancreatitis may be present. Meroney, Lawson, Rubini & Carbone (1956) found that plasma amylase concentration may be raised in acute renal insufficiency without evidence of associated pancreatitis. In their cases haemodialysis did not consistently reduce elevated amylase levels. When the raised serum amylase does not conform to the clinical picture Sachar & Weinhaus (1956) have suggested that it is important to check that renal clearance for amylase is normal by ensuring that the amount of amylase excreted in the urine in one hour exceeds the amount in 100 ml. of serum.

The urinary zymograms of *a*-amylase fall into two groups, a slower pancreatic group and a faster salivary group (Aw, 1966). Aw, Hobbs & Wootton (1967) observed that the ratio of pancreatic isoamylases in urine to absolute values of urinary amylase in 40 controls range from 0·9–3·4. This ratio was lower than 0·9 in seven of eight patients who had established chronic pancreatitis.

Amylase in peritoneal and pleural fluid

Zollinger, Keith & Ellison (1954) and Keith, Zollinger & McCleery (1950) thought examination of peritoneal fluid and assessment of its amylase content might contribute to the diagnosis of acute pancreatitis some 3–4 days after the onset of illness, when serum amylase values might have returned to normal. Values exceeding 300 Somogyi units were considered to support a diagnosis of acute pancreatitis. Amerson, Howard & Vowles (1958), however, did not find that the amylase content of the peritoneal fluid provided a reliable means of distinguishing between acute pancreatitis and acute perforation. In 17 of 26 patients with acute perforation the peritoneal fluid amylase exceeded 200 Somogyi units and in three patients it exceeded 1,500 units.

Amylase may be present in pleural fluid associated with acute pancreatitis.

Serum lipase

During the course of pancreatic disease, serum lipase varies with serum amylase. Though the two do not run wholly parallel, elevation of one is invariably associated with elevation of the other (Berk, 1967). As with amylase, high values may be found in perforated ulcer, intestinal obstruction and peritonitis not associated with pancreatic disease. As with amylase too, opiates may cause a rise, and abnormal values are not infrequently seen in gall stones, less commonly in subacute hepatitis and cirrhosis of the liver, and rarely in metastatic carcinoma of the liver.

Desnuelle (1961) has summarized the work done in his laboratory in Marseilles on lipase, and has discussed again the kinetics of the lipase reaction (Desnuelle, Reboud & Ben Abdeljlil, 1962), when he re-emphasized that pancreatic lipase acts exclusively on emulsified esters, preferably emulsified long-chain triglycerides, since lipase acts at the interface of emulsified globules and is inactive in aqueous solution. In clinical practice most workers use some modification of the Loerenhart technique described by Cherry & Crandall (1932), in which the substrate is emulsified olive oil. Burton, Hammond, Harper, Howat, Scott & Varley (1960b) were unable to estimate changes in the esterase content of serum in patients with pancreatitis when tributyrin was used as substrate according to the method of Goldstein & Roe (1943) and Goldstein, Epstein & Roe (1948), though Lagerlöf (1945) has used tributyrin as a substrate to measure "lipase" after activation with calcium oleate. Serum lipase is somewhat more specific than serum amylase. Despite improvements in technique, and in reducing incubation time in recent years (Ticktin, Trujillo, Evans & Roe, 1965), sufficient experience has not yet been gained in all clinical situations to permit an appraisal of these modifications.

Trypsin

It is not yet possible to measure trypsin in serum. Nardi (1958) used the substrate benzoyl-l-arginine amide hydrochloride and found increased amounts of ammonia released after incubating sera from patients with pancreatic disease. It is doubtful, however, whether the method can be validly applied to measure trypsin in sera, since this synthetic substrate is not specific for trypsin and may be hydrolyzed by plasmin and perhaps other proteases present in serum. Though some reports claim that anti-tryptic activity is reduced in severe acute pancreatitis, no direct proof is available that trypsin is released in pancreatic necrosis. Neither has the role played by the release of kinins been convincingly demonstrated. Some six double blind studies have now been published which show that aprotinin (Trasylol), when compared with an inert placebo, has no favourable effect on the pain, clinical course or mortality of acute pancreatitis (Nardi, 1963; Skyring, Singer & Tornya, 1965; Almgren, Edlund, Norback & Gelin, 1966; Trapnell, Talbot & Capper, 1967; Baden, Jordal, Lund & Zachariae, 1967; Edlund, 1968). The prophylactic value of aprotinin is difficult to evaluate since the incidence of post-operative pancreatitis is low and difficult to predict. Controlled evidence suggests that aprotinin does not prevent the development of post-operative acute pancreatitis (Baden, Jordal, Lund & Zachariae, 1967; Skinner, Corson & Nardi, 1968).

Assays of faecal trypsin and chymotrypsin may be of value in establishing a diagnosis of primary atresia of the pancreas and fibrocystic disease of the pancreas (mucoviscidosis) in children. Chymotrypsin and trypsin concentration in stools have been used to demonstrate severe pancreatic insufficiency in adults (Haverback, Dyce, Gutentag & Montgomery, 1963), but low faecal levels may sometimes be found, as in coeliac disease, when duodenal trypsin levels are normal (MacGowan & Wells, 1962).

Other enzymes circulating in blood serum although not specific for pancreatic disease, are sometimes found to be increased in pancreatitis or cancer of the pancreas. Elevated values of serum alkaline phosphatase, serum leucine aminopeptidase and the serum transaminases usually can be attributed to extrahepatic biliary obstruction, or the intrahepatic biliary obstruction of metastatic deposits.

Tests suggesting acute pancreatic necrosis

Kowlessar & McEvoy (1956) found a marked and sustained rise in serum deoxyribonuclease I activity in patients with true necrosis of the pancreas, but only a temporary minimal elevation in acute pancreatic oedema. An increased DNase activity persists for one to three weeks in severe pancreatitis (Roos, 1966). It is claimed to be not only of prognostic value, but also of diagnostic value after values of amylase have returned to normal. Electrolyte disturbances are a feature of the more severe forms of acute haemorrhagic pancreatic necrosis. The most specific of these is depletion of serum Ca from the 3rd to 11th days, since the fatty acid released by lipolysis in the upper abdomen combines with Ca to deplete the amount readily available circulating in the blood (Edmondson & Fields, 1942; Edmondson & Berne, 1944). It is only after several days that the serum concentration of calcium returns to normal. Edmondson, Berne, Homann & Wertman (1952) believe that this fall of serum Ca can be used as a prognostic index of the severity of the process. Mazumdar (1961) has reported methaemalbuminaemia in a fatal case of acute pancreatic necrosis. Methaemalbumin has been demonstrated both spectroscopically and electrophoretically in the blood of six patients with acute haemorrhagic pancreatitis, five of whom died; but none was found in six patients with the milder form of acute pancreatic oedema. Since haptoglobin persisted in the serum, Northam, Rowe & Winstone (1962) considered that the methaemalbuminaemia is not due to intravascular haemolysis, but arises when haematin or methaemalbumin, released after pancreatic digestion of the gross haemorrhagic effusion in the peritoneal cavity, are absorbed into the circulation. Methaemalbuminaemia is encountered in other acute abdominal emergencies associated with bleeding, such as ectopic pregnancy and bowel infarction (Bank, Barbezat, Marks & Silber, 1968).

Evocative tests

The rise in serum amylase and lipase values, which is such a feature of acute pancreatitis and relapsing acute pancreatitis, is less common and less striking in the more chronic forms of pancreatic disease, relapsing chronic pancreatitis, chronic pancreatitis and cancer of the pancreas. Popper & Nicheles (1943) showed experimentally in dogs, whose pancreas was maximally stimulated by secretin and a parasympathomimetic drug such as mecholyl, that the serum lipase rose in those animals in which the pancreas was normal; but no rise was obtained when the acinar tissue had previously atrophied or been destroyed. When, however, a submaximal stimulus, secretin alone, was given, no rise in serum lipase was found in normal dogs, though a rise could be obtained when the pancreatic duct had been recently tied (Popper, Olson & Necheles, 1943). Evocative serum studies have developed along two main lines which correspond to these experimental findings.

A maximal stimulus has been given (frequently combined with morphine to contract the sphincter of Oddi) in order to elicit a rise in enzymes in the blood from the normal pancreas, but in the absence of active functioning acini no appreciable or a negligible rise would result. The object is to demonstrate normal acinar function. Under the conditions of this morphine-secretin test about 30% of normal individuals showed no appreciable rise (Myhre, Nesbitt & Hurly, 1949), a proportion too high to justify the use of this *obstructive–evocative test* in clinical practice.

In the alternative method, a submaximal stimulus of the pancreas is chosen which leads to no appreciable rise in serum enzymes when the gland is normal but when the outflow of pancreatic juice is obstructed a significant rise is obtained. Such a rise is only found when acinar function is still retained. These conditions exist in the early stages of cancer of the head of the pancreas, or ampullary cancer at the onset of jaundice, and in chronic pancreatitis when considerable acinar function remains. When, however, increasing duct obstruction leads to impairment of pancreatic flow or acinar destruction and atrophy accompany the later stages of chronic pancreatic disease, then a significant rise in serum enzymes is less often seen.

Burton and his colleagues (1956, 1960b), who used secretin followed by pancreozymin as the stimulus, found that this *simple evocative test* was more frequently positive when the outflow from the pancreas, assessed from the volume of the duodenal contents, was normal than when it was reduced. Reduction in the volume of pancreatic secretion was associated with greater impairment of glucose tolerance, which further supports the idea that it is in the more moderate, rather than in the more extreme degrees of pancreatic impairment, that the simple evocative test in man is likely to be positive. These workers found indications of pancreatic disease in their combined groups of chronic pancreatitis, and cancer of the pancreas in 86% of patients, when they used an oral glucose test in conjunction with the simple evocative test of acinar function (Table 20.1). They based their results on absolute values and not on the increase proportional to the pre-stimulation value. From what has been said about isoamylases of serum of differing origins, it seems to be good practice to continue to do so until accurate estimations of serum amylase of pancreatic origin can be made. Serum lipase was considered to be a more sensitive index of chronic pancreatic disease than serum amylase in both the fasting control specimens and in the post-evocative values. Kirshen, Gambill & Mason (1965) preferred urinary amylase to serum amylase values in a similar evocative test.

TABLE 20.1

Simple evocative test (secretin-pancreozymin)

	Cancer of pancreas	Chronic pancreatitis	Total
Total . .	55 cases	49 cases	104
Positive simple evocative test	20	23	46
Impaired G.T.T. . .	29	23	52
Positive combined tests .	47	43	90 (86%)

The evocative test is not a specific test of pancreatic disease and false positive evocative tests quite often are encountered particularly in hepatic and biliary tract disease, and in other conditions affecting the upper abdomen. None the less, Howat (1962) has re-emphasized that the simple evocative test has considerable clinical value, in that it may focus attention on the pancreas at an earlier stage of the lesion when confirmation of a pancreatic lesion is otherwise difficult. It is most valuable in the first ten days of obstructive jaundice due to ampullary cancer, before pancreatic function deteriorates. Sun & Shay (1957) and Shay, Sun, Chey & O'Leary (1961) have also confirmed the value of a simple evocative test, and have used this test in association with either the starch tolerance test or ^{131}I-labelled triolein excretion in the stools, since both of these tests of digestive function become positive as acinar function progressively decreases. However, other more precise and informative methods of demonstrating impaired acinar function such as the examination of duodenal contents following secretin and pancreozymin have been developed.

Pancreatic scanning

Pancreatic scanning provides a visual record of the pancreas as well as a test of pancreatic function. Following intravenous injection, ^{75}Se-selenomethionine is incorporated into enzymic proteins of the acinar cells of the pancreas, and the gamma emission recorded by external scintillation scanning, either as a colourscan or a photoscan. The liver also accepts ^{75}Se-methionine and at the time of scanning radioactivity is frequently recorded in duodenal mucosa. Visualization of the normal pancreas is adequate in 75 to 85% of cases. Failure to visualize the normal pancreas may be due to an overlying enlarged liver. In interpreting a pancreatic scan it is useful to have a prior liver scan using [99]Tc Technetium sulphur colloid for comparison. In a few patients in whom pancreatic function is apparently normal the pancreas may not be adequately seen, so it is difficult to attribute non-visualization to a pathological process, though it is known that in active acute pancreatitis, in chronic pancreatitis and some cases of cancer of the pancreas uptake is diffusely reduced. Greater diagnostic reliance can be placed on pancreatic displacements and on localized filling defects indicative of pancreatic neoplasm. A scan may provide important, occasionally the sole, corroborative evidence of a lesion of the body or tail of the pancreas. "Cold spots" due to tumours of a size greater than 2 to 3 cm. may be detected under ideal conditions. Insulin contains no methionine, so insulinomas may present as "cold spots". Enhanced uptake by non β-cell tumours of Zollinger-Ellison type has been reported (Brown, Sircus, Smith, Donaldson, Dymock, Falconer & Small, 1968). Scanning is used as a screening test of pancreatic function in the sense that an unequivocally normal pancreatic scan is strong evidence that the gland is normal (Melmed, Agnew & Bouchier, 1968).

Although the isotope tends during the later excretion phases to be concentrated in the central or periductal areas of the pancreas, so far no method permits adequate visualization of the ducts of the pancreas. Attempts have been made by computer techniques to assess pancreatic function quantitatively and to separate the liver scan from the pancreatic scan by subtraction techniques, but so far these have met with little success. At present pancreatic scans are best interpreted by comparing the photoscan with the observer's appreciation of the normal.

Pancreatic secretory capacity

The composition of the pancreatic juice reaching the duodenum provides the only direct method of estimating pancreatic secretory capacity in man. The method is not entirely satisfactory since the duodenal contents are a mixture of fluids derived from the biliary tract, small intestine and pancreas. In health, fasting duodenal contents obtained free from contamination by gastric contents show wide variations, though the bicarbonate concentration tends to be low and the enzyme concentration high. The fasting duodenal contents from even quite severely damaged pancreatic glands may also show high enzyme concentration after a period of fasting, so some means of stimulating the pancreas to secrete is used. As stimulants, different workers have given food and food products, olive oil, skimmed milk, hydrochloric acid and ether, either into the stomach or duodenum. The classical technique is the quantitative aspiration of duodenal contents over a period of 60–80 min. after stimulating the gland with a single submaximal dose of secretin intravenously, as devised by Ågren & Lagerlöf (1936) and Lagerlöf (1942). Dreiling (1955), who has extensive experience of this method, has described the technique of the secretin test. The duodenal contents collected in response to secretin contain a variable amount of bile, since secretin is a choleretic agent as well as a stimulant of the aqueous pancreatic juice (Grossman, Janowitz, Ralston & Kim, 1949). When the gall bladder is normal, however, frequently the amount of bile present in the 2nd or 3rd 10-min. fraction following a *single* intravenous injection of secretin disappears (Ågren & Lagerlöf, 1937; Dreiling & Lipsay, 1951), and virtually pure pancreatic juice is obtained. At this time the concentration of bicarbonate is maximal, and this figure is taken as an index of pancreatic function. In addition to the volume recovered, the bilirubin and enzyme concentration have been measured. Lagerlöf (1942) gave quantitative values for volume, bicarbonate and enzyme output in response to a standard dose of secretin, and Dreiling (1955) gave the normal limits in a larger series of cases. Dreiling (1951, 1953) has observed that in cancer of the pancreas the characteristic feature is a ductal obstruction which leads to a reduced volume of duodenal contents, but a normal concentration of bicarbonate in response to secretin, while in chronic pancreatitis with consequent acinar destruction a normal volume associated with a diminished maximal bicarbonate concentration is typically found. Obstruction of the common bile duct in cancer of the head of the pancreas tends to accentuate this distinction.

After cholecystectomy, and when gall bladder function is diminished or absent, an increased volume of duodenal contents is obtained in response to an injection of secretin. This also is found in cirrhosis of the liver. The greatest volumes, however, are encountered in haemochromatosis when an increase of three or four times may be obtained in response to a standard single injection of secretin. If the maximal bicarbonate response to secretin is taken as an index of pancreatic function, in many of these cases a significantly low value is obtained when compared with normal. However, in these cases the total output of bicarbonate usually falls within normal limits. Burton and his colleagues (1960a) prefer to minimize the effects of a variable admixture of bile and intestinal juice on duodenal aspiration by assessing the total output of bicarbonate and enzyme produced over a period in response to the stimulus.

Many authors have not been impressed by the value of estimating the pancreatic enzymes in response to secretin. This in part is due to the inaccuracies inherent in estimating enzyme activity, which are greater than the errors in estimating bicarbonate. Burton, Evans, Harper, Howat, Oleesky, Scott & Varley (1960a), Marks & Tompsett (1958) and Sun & Shay (1960) have given the specific enzyme stimulant pancreozymin intravenously in the course of the secretin test. Burton *et al.* (1960a) considered a reduced enzyme output in the post-pancreozymin fractions of the secretin-pancreozymin test to be a more sensitive index of impaired pancreatic function than a diminished bicarbonate output in post-secretin samples, a finding which they found was somewhat more significant in cancer of the pancreas than in chronic pancreatitis.

The secretin-pancreozymin test permits a direct quantitative assessment of pancreatic excretory function, both of the aqueous bicarbonate juice and enzyme juice. After a mild attack of acute pancreatitis normal function is rapidly restored, but should this be delayed the likelihood of permanent structural damage, the basis of chronic pancreatitis becomes more likely. Occasionally in active mild pancreatitis increased values may be obtained (Table 20.2). Impaired tests are always found in patients with pancreatic steatorrhoea. Recently Howat (1963, 1968a,b) has reiterated that while a reduced maximal bicarbonate concentration and reduced bicarbonate output following a standard sub-maximal dose of secretin is the characteristic response in chronic pancreatitis and relapsing chronic pancreatitis as opposed to post-acute pancreatitis and relapsing acute pancreatitis, in duct obstruction, either due to stricture or stone or cancer blocking the pancreatic duct, a diminished volume results. The secretin-pancreozymin test interpreted in the clinical context is therefore not only an important diagnostic tool but provides a reliable guide to the treatment and prognosis of the individual patient.

TABLE 20.2

Secretin-pancreozymin test (Howat, 1968a)

| | | Decreased values in duodenal contents | | | |
| | | Post-secretin | | Post-pancreozymin | |
	Cases	Volume	Max. HCO_3^-	HCO_3^- output	Amylase output
Acute pancreatitis .	40	2(4)*	6	7(7)*	3(1)*
Chronic pancreatitis .	30	17	27	28	24
Cancer of the pancreas	34	21	23	26(1)*	28

*The figures in parentheses refer to significantly increased values sometimes obtained in acute phases of pancreatitis.

Burton and his colleagues (1960c), whose extracts of pancreozymin contain cholecystokinin which contracts the gall bladder, estimated the bile content of their fractions following this stimulus and devised a new semi-quantitative test of gall bladder function which correlated well with the results of oral cholecystography and seemed to be superior to secretin test of biliary function. This cholecystokinin test, as do all other tests which involve biliary pigment assessment, depends on the preservation of normal liver function. It proves to be of the greatest value in elucidating the causes of obstructive jaundice, prior to operation, (Table 20.3), and in confirming impaired function in a gall bladder which had not outlined on oral cholecystography (Howat, 1965). Cytological studies of the duodenal contents may provide confirmatory evidence of the presence of cancer in about half the cases of pancreatic cancer at the time of testing, although tetracycline fluorescence is less helpful in duodenal contents that contain bile (Burton & Cunliffe, 1966).

Continuous infusions of larger doses of secretin have been given to elicit "maximal" bicarbonate output by the pancreas analogous to maximal acid production by the stomach (Hartley, Gambill & Summerskill, 1965; Sarles, Bauer & Preslin, 1965; Banwell, Northam & Cooke, 1967). Wormsley (1968) has shown the validity of this method of assessing pancreatic function, but it is doubtful if the method adds information commensurate with the added cost and discomfort to the patient. Should synthetic secretin become freely available in clinical practice, it is possible that maximal stimulation of the pancreas will become more widely used in selected cases.

Dissociation of the enzymes of the pancreas has been shown to take place in animals in response to changes of dietary intake (adaptation). In man however, reports of dissociation of excreted enzymes have been most likely due to the inaccurate techniques and methods used to demonstrate enzyme activity. However, Sarles, Bauer & Prezlin (1965) found a pronounced fall off in the

TABLE 20.3

Obstructive Jaundice—67 cases (Howat, 1968a)

| | | Cholecystokinin test | | | Secretin-pancreozymin test | |
| | | Bilirubin index | | | | |
	No.	>100	<100	0	Normal	Abnormal
Gall-stones . . .	19	0	17	2	15	4
Cancer of biliary tract .	10	0	0	10	10	0
Cancer of ampulla of Vater	6	2	2	1	1	4
Cancer of head of pancreas	23	1	3	1	2	21
Other causes . . .	9					

output of lipase after 5 to 7 hours' continuous stimulation by secretin in man, though amylase, trypsin and chymotrypsin activity did not diminish. It is difficult to explain these results which so far do not seem to have been confirmed by other workers.

Lundh (1962), following the work of Borgström, Dahlquist, Lundh & Sjövall (1957) on intestinal absorption in man and of Lundh (1958) on intestinal absorption after gastric resections, has reintroduced a test meal as the pancreatic stimulus. The meal, composed of dried milk with vegetable oil to which dextrose is added to give a final composition of 6% fat, 5% protein and 15% carbohydrate, includes polyethyleneglycol as a reference substance to calculate the amount of absorption of the constituents of the meal. Samples are collected at intervals of 10 min. in the 1st hr. and 30 min. for a 2nd hr. by means of a fine polyvinyl tube lying in the duodenum or upper jejunum. The concentration of trypsin is determined using benzoyl-l-arginine-ethyl ester as the specific substrate. In normal subjects during the first 20–30 min. there is an initial peak of trypsin concentration followed by a fall and a slower secondary rise. Since the initial peak is only encountered in the first meal of the day after a period of fasting (Lundh & Borgström, 1962), it may represent a washing-out of preformed enzyme by a secretin mechanism, but since it is shortly followed by or accompanies a peak in bile pigment concentration it may represent a combined secretin-pancreozymin mechanism. Low concentrations of trypsin are found in chronic pancreatitis, pancreatic insufficiency and cancer of the pancreas, and the authors concluded that it is a simple and reliable method of evaluating pancreatic exocrine function. This test is of particular value in the investigation of advanced pancreatic disease when steatorrhoea is present (Cook, Lennard-Jones, Sherif & Wiggins, 1967). Hartley, Gambill, Engstrom & Summerskill (1966) and Zieve, Mulford & McHale (1966) found that the secretin-pancreozymin test gives greater discrimination than the Lundh test meal in the diagnosis of pancreatic disease.

Evidence of endocrine pancreatic dysfunction

Transient glycosuria and hyperglycaemia during the course of an acute abdominal emergency frequently suggest the possibility of acute pancreatitis. The disturbance is often mild, and as the patient recovers carbohydrate tolerance returns to normal, though occasionally permanent diabetes persists after recovery from a severe acute haemorrhagic pancreatitis. The chance finding of glycosuria in a patient with obscure upper abdominal symptoms may draw attention to a cancer of the pancreas or chronic relapsing pancreatitis. As these lesions progress there is a tendency for carbohydrate tolerance to become progressively impaired. Burton and his colleagues (1960c) have used the oral glucose tolerance test in conjunction with a simple evocative test in the diagnosis of pancreatic lesions. As yet there is no evidence that a glucose tolerance test after steroids or a tolbutamide tolerance test is superior in this context to a simple 50 g. glucose tolerance test.

AN APPRAISAL OF PANCREATIC FUNCTION TESTS (Howat, 1962, 1968)

Elevated serum amylase and lipase or urinary amylase, though not specific tests, are, when taken in conjunction with the clinical features, of great assistance in arriving at the often overlooked diagnosis of acute pancreatitis. The clinician may seek to use studies of pancreatic function to establish proof that a previous attack of abdominal pain may have been caused by pancreatitis. After an interval, evidence in support of this may not be readily obtained, since in the absence of complications, complete restitution of function accompanies the restitution of structure that takes place after acute pancreatitis. Even in severe necrosis, when surgery has eradicated the complications, a return to normal, albeit with some scarring, results. It is therefore important, during attacks of pain in the upper abdomen, to obtain serum for enzyme estimations and to repeat these even during a remission from pain. Minor elevations above the normal for the individual may still prove to be significant, although similar rises may accompany biliary tract disease. The most common cause of relapsing acute pancreatitis is the presence of gall-stones, removal of which terminates the attacks. Indeed, many patients are relieved of relapsing acute pancreatitis by surgery without the surgeon suspecting that pancreatitis has ever been present. During early relapsing chronic pancreatitis and in the early stages of cancer of the pancreas and cancer of the ampulla of Vater, serial enzyme studies are again helpful, and the simple evocative test, in which the enzymes are measured in serum in response to secretin and pancreozymin, and pancreatic scanning can be used as screening measures to uncover evidence of pancreatic disease; more severe pancreatic damage may be revealed when a glucose tolerance test or one of the tests of digestive capacity of the pancreas is added. The simple evocative test can, however, be performed at the same time as the secretin-pancreozymin test in which the duodenal contents are aspirated; this combination of tests provides the most valuable and complete appraisal of pancreatic function, and at the same time possesses the additional advantage of assessing gall bladder function.

The secretin-pancreozymin test is a sensitive test of pancreatic dysfunction in both chronic pancreatitis and cancer of the pancreas. The characteristic feature of chronic pancreatitis is a diminished maximal bicarbonate concentration and output of bicarbonate following secretin. The finding of pancreatic insufficiency distinguishes relapsing chronic pancreatitis from relapsing acute pancreatitis, the course and treatment of which are different. A reduced enzyme output in the post-pancreozymin samples provides a more sensitive index of pancreatic dysfunction in cancer of the pancreas than in chronic pancreatitis. But the secretin-pancreozymin test provides additional information; if the volume of the duodenal contents is also diminished, there is *prima facie* evidence of duct obstruction, due to stone, stricture or cancer. From the clinical assessment of the patient it is not usually difficult to determine which of these is present. A low volume may be the only finding to suggest a simple stricture or solitary stone obstructing the main pancreatic duct which is amenable to surgery. The secretin-pancreozymin test provides decisive information on the integrity of both pancreatic and biliary systems, essential to the management of the patient with pancreatic disease, which cannot be obtained in any other way short of operation.

References

ÅGREN, G. & LAGERLÖF, H. O. (1936). *Acta med. scand.*, **90**, 1.

ÅGREN, G. & LAGERLÖF, H. O. (1937). *Acta med. scand.*, **92**, 359.

ALMGREN, K. G., EDLUND, Y., NORBACK, B. & GELIN, L. E. (1966). *XXI Congr. int. de Chir. Philadelphia.* Sept. 1965, p. 356.

ALTHAUSEN, T. L. & UYEYAMA, K. (1954). *Ann. intern. Med.*, **41**, 563.

ALTHAUSEN, T. L. & UYEYAMA, K. (1961). *Gastroenterology*, **40**, 470.

AMERSON, R. J., HOWARD, J. M. & VOWLES, K. D. J. (1958). *Ann. Surg.*, **147**, 245.

ANASTASI, A., ERSPAMER, V. & ENDEAN, R. (1967). *Experientia*, **23**, 699.

ANASTASI, A., ERSPAMER, V. & ENDEAN, R. (1968). *Arch. Biochem. Biophys.*, **125**, 57.

ANDERSON, J. C., BARTON, M. A., GREGORY, R. M., HARDY, P. M., KENNER, G. W., MACLEOD, J. K., PRESTON, J., SHEPPARD, R. C. & MORLEY, J. S. (1964). *Nature*, **204**, 933.

AW, S. E. (1966). *Nature*, **209**, 298.

AW, S. E., HOBBS, J. R. & WOOTTON, I. D. P. (1967). *Gut*, **8**, 402.

BADEN, H., JORDAL, K., LUND, F. & ZACHARIAE, F. (1967). *Acta chir. scand. Suppl.*, **378**, 97.

BAKER. R. W. & PELLEGRINO, C. (1954). *Scand. J. clin. Lab. Invest.*, **6**, 94.

BANK, S., BARBEZAT, G. O., MARKS, I. N. & SILBER, W. (1968). *Brit. Med. J.*, **2**, 86.

BANKS, P. A., DYCK, W. P., DREILING, D. A. & JANOWITZ, H. D. (1967). *Gastroenterology*, **53**, 575.

BANWELL, J. G., NORTHAM, B. E. & COOKE, W. T. (1967). *Gut*, **8**, 50.

BARROWMAN, J. A. & BORGSTRÖM, B. (1968). *Gastroenterology*, **55**, 601.

BECKER, V. (1962). "The exocrine Pancreas", Ciba Foundation Symposium, p. 56. London, J. & A. Churchill Ltd.

BENTLEY, P. H., KENNER, G. W. & SHEPPARD, R. C. (1966). *Nature*, **209**, 583.

BERK, J. E. (1967). *J. Amer. med. Assoc.*, **199**, 98.

BERK, J. E., KIZU, H., WILDING, P. & SEARCY, R. L. (1967). *New. Eng. J. Med.*, **277**, 941.

BERGSTRÖM, S. (1967). *Science*, **157**, 382.

BERNARDI, L., BOSISIO, G., DE CASTIGLIONE, R. & GOFFREDO, O. (1967). *Experientia*, **23**, 700.

BERNFIELD, P. (1951). *Adv. Enzymol.*, **12**, 379.

BESWICK, F. B., HOWAT, H. T. & MORRIS, A. I. (1968). *J. Physiol.*, **197**, 71P.

BLAINEY, J. D. & NORTHAM, B. E. (1967). *Clin. Sci.*, **32**, 377.

BLAIR, E. L., BROWN, J. C., HARPER, A. A. & SCRATCHERD, T. (1966). *J. Physiol.*, **184**, 812.

BLAIR, E. L., CLARK, D. C., HARPER, A. A., LAKE, H. J. & SCRATCHERD, T. (1961). *J. Physiol.*, **157**, 17 P.

BORGSTRÖM, B., DAHLQUIST, A., LUNDH, G. & SJÖVALL, J. (1957). *J. clin. Invest.*, **36**, 1521.

BRADDOCK, L. I., FLEISHER, D. R. & BARBERO, G. J. (1968). *Gastroenterology*, **55**, 165.

BROWN, P. W., SIRCUS, W., SMITH, A. N., DONALDSON, A. A., DYMOCK, I. W., FALCONER, C. W. A. & SMALL, W. P. (1968). *Lancet*, **1**, 160.

BURNETT, W. & NESS, T. D. (1955). *Brit. med. J.*, **2**, 770.

BURTON, P. A. & CUNLIFFE, W. J. (1966). *Lancet*, **1**, 1002.

BURTON, P., EVANS, D. G., HARPER, A. A., HOWAT, H. T., OLEESKY, S., SCOTT, J. E. & VARLEY, H. (1960a). *Gut*, **1**, 111.

BURTON, P., HAMMOND, E. M., HARPER, A. A., HOWAT, H. T., OLEESKY, S. & VARLEY, H. (1956). *Gastroenterologia* (Basel), **86**, 463.

BURTON, P., HAMMOND, E. M., HARPER, A. A., HOWAT, H. T., SCOTT, J. E. & VARLEY, H. (1960b). *Gut*, **1**, 125.

BURTON, P., HARPER, A. A., HOWAT, H. T., SCOTT, J. E. & VARLEY, H. (1960c). *Gut*, **1**, 193.

CARO, L. G. (1961). *J. biophys. biochem. Cytol.*, **10**, 37.

CARO, L. G. & PALADE, G. E. (1964). *J. cell. Biol.*, **20**, 473.

CASE, R. M., HARPER, A. A. & SCRATCHERD, T. (1969). *J. Physiol.*, **201**, 335.

CHERRY, J. A. & CRANDALL, L. A. (1932). *Amer. J. Physiol.*, **100**, 266.

COOK, H. B., LENNARD-JONES, J. E., SHERIF, S. M. & WIGGINS, H. S. (1967). *Gut*, **8**, 408.

DAVIS, A. E. & BADENOCH, J. (1962). *Lancet*, **2**, 6.

DAVIS, A. E. & BIGGS, J. C. (1965). *Gut*, **6**, 140.

DAVIS, A. E. & BIGGS, J. C. (1967). *Amer. J. dig. Dis.*, n.s., **12**, 293.

DELCOURT, A. & DELCOURT, R. (1953). *C. R. Soc. Biol.*, **147**, 1104.

DELCOURT, A., DELCOURT, R. & WETTENDORFF, P. (1964). *C. R. Soc. Biol.*, **158**, 656.

DESNUELLE, P. (1961). *Adv. Enzymol.*, **23**, 129.

DESNUELLE, P., REBOUD, J. P., & BEN ABDELJLIL, A. (1962). "The Exocrine Pancreas", Ciba Foundation Symposium, p. 90. London, J. & A. Churchill, Ltd.

DREILING, D. A. (1951). *Gastroenterology*, **18**, 184.

DREILING, D. A. (1953). *Gastroenterology*, **24**, 540.

DREILING, D. A. (1955). *J. Mt. Sinai Hosp.*, **21**, 363.

DREILING, D. A. & JANOWITZ, H. D. (1956). *Amer. J. Med.*, **21**, 98.

DREILING, D. A. & JANOWITZ, H. D. (1959). *Amer. J. dig. Dis.*, n.s., **4**, 137.

DREILING, D. A., JANOWITZ, H. D. & JOSEPHBERG, L. J. (1963). *Ann. intern. Med.*, **58**, 235.

DREILING, D. A. & LIPSAY, JOAN J. (1951). *Gastroenterology*, **17**, 242.

DUPRÉ, J. (1964). *Lancet*, **2**, 673.

DUPRÉ, J., ROJAS, L., WHITE, J. J., UNGAR, R. H. & BECK, J. C. (1966). *Diabetes*, **15**, 555.

DYCK, W. P., HOEXTER, B., RUDICK, J. & JANOWITZ, H. D. (1968). *Clin. Res.*, **16(2)**, 283.

EDLUND, Y. (1968). Third meeting European Pancreatic Club, Prague. To be published.

EDMONDSON, H. A. & BERNE, C. J. (1944). *Surg. Gynec. Obstet.*, **79**, 240.

EDMONDSON, H. A., BERNE, C. J., HOMANN, R. E. & WERTMAN, M. (1952). *Amer. J. Med.*, **12**, 34.

EDMONDSON, H. A. & FIELDS, I. A. (1942). *Arch. intern. Med.*, **69**, 177.

EKHOLM, R. & EDLUND, Y. (1959). *J. Ultrastruct. Res.*, **2**, 453.

ELMAN, R., ARNESON, N. & GRAHAM, E. A. (1929). *Arch. Surg. Chicago*, **19**, 943.

ERSPAMER, V., BERTACCINI, G., DE CARO, G., ENDEAN, R. & IMPICCIATORE, M. (1967). *Experientia*, **23**, 702.

GADDIE, R., THOMAS, G., SMITH, N. & FRENCH, J. M. (1957). *Quart. J. Med.*, n.s. **26**, 121.

GADRAT, J. & RIBET, A. (1962). *Path. et Biol.*, **10**, 61.

GAMBILL, E. E. & MASON, H. L. (1964). *J. lab. clin. Med.*, **63**, 173.

GELOTTE, B. (1964). *Acta Chem. scand.*, **18**, 1283.

GOLDSTEIN, N. P., EPSTEIN, J. H. & ROE, J. H. (1948). *J. lab. clin. Med.*, **33**, 1047.

GOLDSTEIN, N. P. & ROE, J. H. (1943). *J. lab. clin. Med.*, **28**, 1368.

GREEN, C. L. (1957). *Amer. J. Obstet. Gynec.*, **73**, 402.

GREENE, L. J., HIRS, C. H. W. & PALADE, G. E. (1963). *J. biol. Chem.*, **238**, 2054.

GREGORY, R. A. (1967). p. 827. Handbook of Physiology. Section 6. Alimentary Canal. Vol. 2. Publ. Amer. Physiol. Soc. Washington. D.C.

GREGORY, H., HARDY, P. M., JONES, D. S., KENNER, G. W. & SHEPPARD, R. C. (1964). *Nature*, **204**, 931.

GREGORY, R. A. & TRACY, H. J. (1964). *Gut*, **5**, 103 & 107.

GROSSMAN, M. I. (1968) Third Meeting European Pancreatic Club. Prague. To be published.

GROSSMAN, M. I. & IVY, A. C. (1946). *Proc. Soc. exp. Biol. N.Y.*, **63**, 62.

GROSSMAN, M. I., JANOWITZ, H. D., RALSON, H. & KIM, K. S. (1949). *Gastroenterology*, **12**, 133.

GROSSMAN, M. I., WANG, C. C. & WANG, K. J. (1951). *Proc. Soc. exp. Biol. N.Y.*, **78**, 310.

HANSSON, E. (1959). *Acta physiol. scand.*, **46**, Suppl. 161.

HARPER, A. A. (1959). *Gastroenterology*, **36**, 386.

HARPER, A. A., BLAIR, E. L. & SCRATCHERD, T. (1962). The Exocrine Pancreas. Ciba Foundation Symposium. p. 168.

HARPER, A. A., KIDD, C. & SCRATCHERD, T. (1959). *J. Physiol.*, **148**, 417.

HARTLEY, R. C., GAMBILL, E. E., ENGSTROM, G. W. & SUMMERSKILL, W. H. J. (1966). *Amer. J. dig. Dis.* n.s., **11**, 27.

HARTLEY, R. C., GAMBILL, E. E. & SUMMERSKILL, W. H. J. (1965). *Gastroenterology*, **48**, 312.

HAVERBACK, B. J., DYCE, B. J., GUTENTAG, P. J. & MONTGOMERY, D. W. (1963). *Gastroenterology*, **44**, 588.

HEINKEL, K. (1961). *Bibl. gastroent.*, **4**, 120.

HENRICKSON, F. W. (1968). Third meeting European Pancreatic Club. Prague. To be published.

HERMODSSON, L. H. (1965). The ultrastructure of exocrine pancreas cells as related to secretory activity. Uppsala. Almquist & Wiksells.

HILTON, S. M. & JONES, M. (1968). *J. Physiol.* **195**, 521.

HOKIN, L. E. (1967). p. 935. Handbook of Physiology. Section 6. Vol. 2. *Amer. Physiol. Soc.* Washington. D.C.

HOKIN, L. E. & HOKIN, M. R. (1958). *J. biol. Chem.*, **233**, 805.

HOKIN, L. E. & HUEBNER, I. (1967). *J. cell. Biol.*, **33**, 521.

HOWAT, H. T. (1962). *Gastroenterology*, **42**, 72.

HOWAT, H. T. (1963). *Practitioner*, **191**, 42.

HOWAT, H. T. (1965). p. 249. In "The Biliary System". Ed. W. Taylor. Oxford. Blackwell.

HOWAT, H. T. (1968a). *J. Roy. Coll. Phycns. Lond.*, **3**, 85.

HOWAT, H. T. (1968b). *Postgrad. med. J.*, **44**, 76.

JAMIESON, J. D. & PALADE, G. E. (1967). *J. cell. Biol.*, **34**, 377 & 597.

JOHNSON, L. R. & GROSSMAN, M. I. (1968). *Amer. J. Physiol.*, **215**, 885.

JORPES, J. E. (1968). *Gastroenterology*, **55**, 157.

JORPES, E. & MUTT, V. (1966). *Acta physiol. scand.*, **66**, 196.

JOSEPH, R. M., OLIVERO, E. & RESSLER, N. (1966). *Gastroenterology*, **51**, 377.

KAMER, J. H. VAN DE, HUININK, H. & WEYERS, H. A. (1949). *J. biol. Chem.*, **177**, 345.

KEITH, L. M., ZOLLINGER, R. M. & MCCLEERY, R. S. (1950). *Arch. Surg. Chicago*, **61**, 930.

KELLER, P. J. & ALLEN, B. J. (1967). *J. biol. Chem.*, **242**, 281.

KELLER, P. J. & COHEN, E. (1961). *J. biol. Chem.*, **236**, 1407.

KELLER, P. J., COHEN, E. & NEURATH, H. (1958). *J. biol. Chem.*, **233**, 344.

KELLER, P. J., COHEN, E. & NEURATH, H. (1959). *J. biol. Chem.*, **234**, 311.

KELLER, P. J., COHEN, E. & NEURATH, H. (1961). *J. biol. Chem.*, **236**, 1404.

KIRSHEN, R., GAMBILL, E. E. & MASON, H. L. (1965). *Gastroenterology*, **48**, 579.

KOWLESSAR, O. D. & MCEVOY, R. K. (1956). *J. clin. Invest.*, **35**, 1325.

LAGERLÖF, H. O. (1942). *Acta med. scand.*, Suppl. 128.

LAGERLÖF, H. O. (1945). *Acta med. scand.*, **120**, 407.

LAGERLÖF, H. O., RUDEWALD, M. B. & PERMAN, G. (1960). *Acta med. scand.*, **168**, 269.

LANCKER, J. L. VAN & HOLTZER, R. L. (1959). *J. biol. Chem.*, **234**, 2359.

LEVITT, M. (1968). *Gastroenterology*, **54**, 128.

LEVITT, M. D., GOETZL, E. J. & COOPERBAND, S. R. (1968). *Lancet*, **1**, 340.

LUNDH, G. (1958). *Acta chir. scand.*, Suppl. 231.

LUNDH, G. (1962). *Gastroenterology*, **42**, 275.

LUNDH, G. & BORGSTRÖM, B. (1962). The Exocrine Pancreas. Ciba Foundation Symposium, p. 259. London, J. & A. Churchill, Ltd.

MCGEACHIN, R. L. & HARGAN, LILA A. (1956). *J. appl. Physiol.*, **9**, 129.

MCGEACHIN, R. L. & LEWIS, J. P. (1959). *J. biol. Chem.*, **234**, 795.

MCGOWAN, G. K. & WELLS, M. R. (1962). *J. clin. Path.*, **15**, 62.

MCGUIGAN, J. E. (1968a). *Gastroenterology*, **54**, 1005.

MCGUIGAN, J. E. (1968b). *Gastroenterology*, **54**, 1012.

MCGUIGAN, J. E. (1968c). *Gastroenterology*, **55**, 315.

MANZKE, E. (1959). Quoted by Becker, V. (1962).

MARCHIS-MOUREN, G. (1959). Quoted by Desnuelle, P. (1961).

MARCHIS-MOUREN, G. (1965). *Bull. Soc. Biol.*, **47**, 2207.

MARCHIS-MOUREN, G., CHARLES, M., BEN ABDELJLIL, A. & DESNUELLE, P. (1961). *Biochem. Biophys. Acta*, **50**, 186.

MARKS, I. N. & TOMPSETT, S. L. (1958). *Quart. J. Med.* n.s., **27**, 431.

MAZUMDAR, P. M. H. (1961). *Brit. med. J.*, **2**, 1617.

MELMED, R. N., AGNEW, J. E. & BOUCHIER, I. A. D. (1968). *Quart. J. Med.*, n.s., **37**, 607.

MERONEY, W. H., LAWSON, N. L., RUBINI, M. E. & CARBONE, J. (1956). *New Engl. J. Med.*, **255**, 315.

MEYER, K. H., FISCHER, E. H., BERNFIELD, P. & DUCKERT, F. (1948). *Arch. Biochem.*, **18**, 203.

MORLEY, J. S., TRACY, H. J. & GREGORY, R. A. (1965). *Nature*, **207**, 1356.

MORRIS, A. J. & DICKMAN, S. R. (1960). *J. biol. Chem.*, **235**, 1404.

MUTT, V. & JORPES, E. (1967). *Biochem. biophys. res. Comm.*, **26**, 392.

MYHRE, J., NESBITT, S. & HURLY, J. T. (1949). *Gastroenterology*, **13**, 127.

NARDI, G. L. (1958). *J. lab. clin. Med.*, **52**, 66.

NARDI, G. L. (1963). *New Eng. J. Med.*, **268**, 1065.

NORTHAM, B. E., ROWE, D. S. & WINSTONE, N. E. (1962). *Brit. med. J.*, **1**, 260.

PALADE, G. E. (1956a). *J. biophys. biochem. Cytol.*, **2**, suppl. 85.

PALADE, G. E. (1956b). *J. biophys. biochem. Cytol.*, **2**, 417.

PALADE, G. E. & SIEKEVITZ, P. (1956). *J. biophys. biochem. Cytol.*, **2**, 671.

PALADE, G. E., SIEKEVITZ, P. & CARO, L. G. (1962). The Exocrine Pancreas. Ciba Foundation Symposium. p. 23.

PASCAL, J-P., VAYSSE, N., AUGIER, D. & RIBET, A. (1968). *Scand. J. Gastroent.*, **3**, 444.

POPPER, H. L. & NECHELES, H. (1943). *Gastroenterology*, **1**, 490.

POPPER, H. L., OLSON, W. H. & NECHELES, H. (1943). *Surg. Gynec. Obstet.*, **77**, 471.

PRESHAW, P. M., COOKE, A. R. & GROSSMAN, M. I. (1966). *Amer. J. Physiol.*, **210**, 629.

REDMAN, C. M., SIEKEVITZ, P. & PALADE, G. E. (1966). *J. biol. Chem.*, **241**, 1150.

RIBET, A., PASCAL, J-P. & SANNOU, N. (1967). *Arch. Mal. App. dig.*, **56**, 677.

RIBET, A., PASCAL, J-P., VAYSSE, N. & BOUCHARD, J. P. (1968). *Scand. J. Gastroent.*, **3**, 401.

ROOS, K. (1966). First Meeting of European Pancreatic Club, London. *Gut.*, **7**, 301.

SACHAR, L. A. & WEINHAUS, R. (1956). *Arch. Surg. Chicago*, **73**, 305.

SARLES, H., BAUER, J-B. & PREZLIN, G. (1965). *Arch. Mal. App. dig.*, **54**, 177.

SARLES, H., DANI, R., PREZLIN, G., SOUVILLE, C. & FIGARELLA, C. (1968). *Gut*, **9**, 214.

SAUNDERS, D. R. (1967). *Gastroenterology*, **52**, 135.

SAXON, E. J., HINKLEY, W. C., VOGEL, W. C. & ZIEVE, L. (1957). *Arch. intern. Med.*, **99**, 607.

SEARCY, R. L., UJIHIRA, I., HAYASHI, S. & BERK, J. E. (1964). *Clin. Chim. Acta*, **9**, 505.

SHAY, H., SUN, D. C. H., CHEY, W. Y. & O'LEARY, D. (1961). *Amer. J. dig. Dis.*, n.s., **6**, 142.

SIEKEVITZ, P. & PALADE, G. E. (1958a). *J. biophys. biochem. Cytol.*, **4**, 203.

SIEKEVITZ, P. & PALADE, G. E. (1958b). *J. biophys. biochem. Cytol.*, **4**, 309.

SIEKEVITZ, P. & PALADE, G. E. (1958c). *J. biophys. biochem. Cytol.*, **4**, 557.

SIEKEVITZ, P. & PALADE, G. E. (1960). *J. biophys. biochem. Cytol.*, **7**, 619.

SJÖSTRAND, F. S. (1962). The Exocrine Pancreas. Ciba Foundation Symposium, p. 1. London, J. & A. Churchill, Ltd.

SJÖSTRAND, F. S. & HANZON, V. (1954a) *Exp. Cell Res.*, **7**, 393.

SJÖSTRAND, F. S. & HANZON, V. (1954b). *Exp. Cell Res.*, **7**, 415.

SKINNER, D. B., CORSON, J. G. & NARDI, G. L. (1968). *J. Amer. med. Assoc.*, **204**, 945.

SKYRING, A. P., SINGER, A. & TORNYA, P. (1965). *Brit. Med. J.*, **2**, 627.

STREET, H. V. & CLOSE, J. R. (1956). *Clin. Chim. Acta*, **1**, 256.

SULLIVAN, J. F. & KNIGHT, W. A. (1960). *Amer. J. dig. Dis.*, n.s., **5**, 246.

SUN, D. C. H. & SHAY, H. (1957). *Gastroenterology*, **32**, 212.

SUN, D. C. H. & SHAY, H. (1960). *Gastroenterology*, **38**, 570.

SUN, D. C. H. & SHAY, H. (1961). *Gastroenterology*, **40**, 379.

THOMAS, J. E. (1950). The external secretion of the pancreas. Springfield, Ill., Charles C. Thomas.

TICKTIN, H. E., TRUJILLO, N. P., EVANS, P. F. & ROE, J. H. (1965). *Gastroenterology*, **48**, 12.

TRACY, H. J. & GREGORY, R. A. (1964). *Nature*, **204**, 935.

TRAPNELL, J. E., TALBOT, C. H. & CAPPER, W. M. (1967). *Amer. J. dig. Dis.*, **12**, 409.

UJIHIRA, I., SEARCY, R. L., BERK, J. E. & HAYASHI, S. (1965). *Clin. Chem.*, **11**, 97.

VAYNE, M., STENING, G. F., BROOKS, F. P. & GROSSMAN, M. I. (1968). *Gastroenterology*, **55**, 260.

WANG, C. C. & GROSSMAN, M. I. (1951). *Amer. J. Physiol.*, **164**, 527.

WANG, C. C., GROSSMAN, M. I. & IVY, A. C. (1948). *Amer. J. Physiol.*, **154**, 358.

WALKER, L. & NECHELES, H. (1956). *Amer. J. Physiol.*, **187**, 638.

WEISS, J. M. (1953). *J. exp. Med.*, **98**, 607.

WHITE, T. T., HAYAMA, T. & MAGEE, D. F. (1960). *Gastroenterology*, **39**, 615.

WHITE, T. T. & MAGEE, D. F. (1963). *Gastroenterology*, **45**, 698.

WILDING, P. (1963). *Clin. Chim. Acta*, **8**, 918.

WILDING, P. (1965). *Clin. Chim. Acta*, **12**, 97.

WILDING, P., COOKE, W. T. & NICHOLSON, G. L. (1964). *Ann. intern. Med.*, **60**, 1053.

WORMSLEY, K. G. (1968). *Gastroenterology*, **54**, 197.

WORMSLEY, K. G. & MAHONEY, M. P. (1967). *Lancet*, **1**, 657.

ZIEVE, L., MULFORD, B. & McHALE, A. (1966). *Amer. J. dig. Dis.*, n.s., **11**, 685.

ZOLLINGER, R. M., KEITH, L. M. & ELLISON, E. H. (1954). *New. Engl. J. Med.*, **251**, 497.

Chapter 21

CONNECTIVE TISSUE DISORDERS

by

E. G. L. Bywaters and L. E. Glynn
Rheumatism Research Unit, Canadian Red Cross
Memorial Hospital, Taplow, Bucks.

THE CHEMISTRY OF NORMAL CONNECTIVE TISSUE

THE connective tissues of the body are all composed of the same four morphological components, namely cells, vessels, fibres and so-called "ground substance". The latter substance constitutes the medium in which the other three components are embedded and is itself a material of immense complexity. The proportions of these four constituents, however, vary greatly between the different types of connective tissue, for example, fibres predominating in tendon, cells in adipose tissue and ground substance in areolar tissue. The composition of connective tissue, therefore, varies widely between tissues of different type, and the first step in any chemical study of this tissue is the separation of its components for individual analysis. Compara-

tively little attention has been directed towards the chemistry of the cells or vessels, but the years since the last war have witnessed a prodigious effort to elucidate the chemical and physical structure of the fibres and their supporting matrix.

Collagen and Reticulin

Excluding nerve fibres, three types of fibre, collagen, reticulin and elastin, are histologically distinguishable in connective tissue and more recently cellulose has been reported (Hall & Saxl, 1961). Collagen fibres occur in wavy bundles; the individual fibres, about 2 μ thick, are composed of fibrils of 0·1 μ in thickness and separable from each other by teasing (Gross & Schmitt, 1948).

Much of the recent work has been done on bovine skin collagen, but the detailed amino acid composition of a large and diverse variety of collagens is now available and fully reviewed by Eastoe (1967). Collagen is a fibrous protein with a characteristic X-ray diffraction pattern, is insoluble in cold water but readily soluble on boiling to form gelatin. This entails an irreversible change with loss of its fibrous structure. Although gelatin is readily attacked by most proteolytic enzymes such as trypsin, papain and pepsin, native mammalian collagen is only attacked by the last. Heat, urea and other denaturing agents, however, greatly increase the susceptibility to proteolysis, and collagen so treated is readily acted upon by trypsin and papain (Neuman & Tytell, 1950; Axelrod & Martin, 1953). Sherry, Troll & Rosenblum (1954) have shown that native collagen is digestible by several enzymes to which it has always been regarded as resistant, provided the pH is sufficiently low, 2-4·5 for papain or ficin, 1·5 for animal cathepsins and leucocyte extracts. The amino acid composition has been worked out in great detail, and of the 421 amino acid residues in the molecule 419 have been identified (Bowes & Kenten, 1948). Apart from elastin, and possibly cryoglobulin (Mandema, van der Schaaf & Huisman, 1955), collagen is the only protein of mammalian origin to contain hydroxyproline. This is present to the extent of 14%, and its estimation in the hydrolysate of the material extracted on autoclaving forms the basis of the most widely used method of determining the collagen content of a tissue (Neuman & Logan, 1950). Of the other amino acids, tryptophan and cystine are absent, methionine is present to less than 1%, whilst proline 15%, glycine 26% and glutamic acid 11% form the bulk of the remaining residues. Hydroxylysine, although only present to 1·3% is, like hydroxyproline, found almost exclusively in collagen. Perhaps more informative than the composition expressed as a percentage of the total weight is composition expressed as the number of residues of each amino acid per 1000 residues (Ruben et al., 1963). This shows that glycine constitutes one-third of all the residues, proline plus hydroxyproline about one-quarter, and alanine about one-ninth. The elucidation of the complete primary sequence of the amino acids has not yet been achieved but the present position has been well summarized by Hannig & Nordwig (1967): (1) the primary structure is discontinuous with regions composed mainly of neutral amino acids (i.e. apolar regions) and others in which the polar amino acids are concentrated; (2) the non-polar regions are particularly rich in sequences -Gly-Pro-R where R can be either Hypro, Ala, Gly, Glu, Arg, Asp,

Phe, Thr or Ser. These amino acid triplets make up 33–35% of the whole primary structure. It is here, too, that clostridial collagenase exerts its specific action hydrolysing the bond between R and glycine in the sequence P - R - ↓ G - P where P is either proline or hydroxyproline, G is glycine or sometimes alanine, and R any other amino acid; (3) the non-polar regions correspond to the light bands seen on electron microscopy and are, as just stated, the sites of collagenase attack.

No free amino or imino groups were detected by Bowes & Moss (1951), using Sanger's fluorodinitrobenzene method, from which they conclude that the molecule is extremely large, with a molecular weight greater than 1,500,000, or that it has a cyclic structure or that the end-groups are not free but linked to a polysaccharide. A small number of end-groups, however, mostly aspartic acid, were found in collagen modified by heat or alkali treatment (Bowes & Moss, 1954). Gustavson (1955), from a comparative study of various collagens from fish and mammals, concludes that their stability is due to H-bonding between the OH groups of hydroxyproline and adjacent CO.NH groups. This relationship, however, is not substantiated by Watson's figures (Watson, 1958) for the composition of the collagen-like protein in earthworm cuticle, nor by those of Piez & Gross (1960) on fish collagens, who found a correlation between the shrinkage temperature (Ts) and total imino acid content as well as with hydroxyproline. They therefore concluded that the Ts of these fish collagens is not determined by H bonds to the OH group, but to the stability imparted to the molecule by the restriction of rotation associated with each imino acid, proline or hydroxyproline, in the peptide chain.

X-ray diffraction studies and electron microscopy have led to remarkable advances in our knowledge of the structure of the collagen molecule, and the manner in which the molecules are built up into fibres. It is now generally agreed by the investigators in this field that the collagen molecule consists of three peptide chains, each in the form of a helix, twisted together into a coiled coil, the whole arrangement being stabilized by intramolecular H bonding between CO and NH groups of the constituent amino acids (Ramachandran & Kartha, 1954; Rich & Crick, 1955).

The three-chain structure of collagen deduced from the X-ray studies has been fully confirmed by the isolation of the individual chains by Piez and his collaborators (Piez, Weiss & Lewis, 1960). Using heat-denatured acid-soluble collagen they were able by chromatography on carboxy-methyl cellulose to separate two fractions designated α and β, the former with about one-third the molecular weight of the intact collagen molecule, namely 100,000 compared to 300,000. The molecular weight of the β fraction was about twice that of the α component and is now known to consist of two α chains covalently linked. The relative proportions of α and β chains obtained depend upon the origin of the parent material and the degree to which the chains are covalently linked. In most of the soluble forms of collagen such interchain linkage is relatively small in amount and the bulk of the material obtained on thermal denaturation is in the α form. Piez, Lewis, Martin & Gross (1961) showed that there were at least two different forms of α chain, α_1 and α_2 differing in their amino acid composition and these could form β components β_{11} and β_{12}, in which the subscripts indicate the constituent α chains.

The nature of the bonds present in β chains binding the two α chains together has now been established. It was evident from the amino acid requirements for the formation of a triple helix that only part of the molecule could exist in this form. Other parts must necessarily be non-helical, and these being more accessible are more susceptible to proteolytic enzymes such as chymotrypsin and pepsin. These, presumably non-helical, enzyme-susceptible areas are referred to as the telopeptides. Since removal of these peptides results in an increase in the α at the expense of the β chains it may be concluded that the interchain cross-links are confined to these telopeptides. Confirmation has come from the study of the fragment cleaved from the chains by cyanogen bromide. As shown by Gross & Witkop (1962) this is highly specific for peptide bonds involving methionine. At the point of cleavage this yields a C-terminal homoserine lactone, and a new N-terminal amino acid is formed. By comparing the peptides so released from α_1, α_2 and β_{12} chains Bornstein & Piez (1966) found that a small peptide present in the α chains was missing from the β chains, but a new double chain peptide was present, thus indicating the site of the interchain cross-link. The significant peptides in the α chains were: one of 15 residues in α_1, and 14 residues in α_2, in both of which lysine occupied position 5. In some samples, however, this lysine residue was replaced by an aldehyde derivative, namely the δ-semi-aldehyde of α-amino-adipic acid and this, apparently by an aldol type condensation, forms a covalent link to its neighbouring chain. The blocking of these aldehydes by lathyrogenic agents like β amino-propionitrile may well account for the abnormalities of collagen maturation which are such a striking feature of osteolathyrism.

At present only three types of bond are generally accepted as participating in the structure of collagen, the covalent peptide bond, the hydrogen bond, and electrovalent bonds between free amino and free carboxyl groups. Insolubility of collagen in saturated LiBr which dissolves H-bonded structures suggests, however, the presence of some other strong bond, possibly an ester linkage. This agrees with the observation of Grassman (cit. Crawhall & Elliott, 1955) that reduction of procollagen by lithium borohydride releases amino alcohols on subsequent hydrolysis, since reduction of free carboxyl groups occurs only when they are previously esterified.

Soluble collagens. Although collagen is regarded as an insoluble protein it has long been known that a small proportion of rat tail tendon, for example, will go into solution in dilute acetic acid (Nageotte, 1927). Recently, more elaborate fractionations have been attempted, using various buffer solutions as solvent, in an attempt to identify the metabolic precursors of the mature insoluble fraction. Thus, Neuberger and his collaborators (Harkness, Marks, Muir & Neuberger, 1954) have separated the proteins of young rabbit skin into four fractions, an "alkali-soluble fraction" soluble in phosphate buffer at pH 9, an "acid-soluble fraction" by extracting the phosphate-insoluble residue with a citrate buffer at pH 3·8, insoluble collagen which is obtained as gelatin by autoclaving the residue from the two previous extractions, and finally the residue remaining undissolved after autoclaving. A fraction similar to the acid-soluble fraction of Neuberger had previously been obtained by Orekhovich (1950) from fresh calf skin. Since more of this fraction was obtainable from young animals than old, Orekhovich regarded it as a precursor of ordinary collagen and therefore called it procollagen. Studies of the turnover rate of collagen and its various soluble fractions, utilizing for this purpose glycine labelled with ^{14}C in the alpha position, have shown, however, that this view is probably incorrect. The radioactivity of these various fractions of skin collagen, obtained from rabbits at regular intervals after the administration of the labelled amino acid, indicates that the insoluble fraction is remarkably stable with an extremely low rate of turnover, but that the changes in radioactivity of the alkali-soluble fraction are compatible with its being a true precursor of all the other collagen fractions (Harkness *et al.*, 1954). By comparison the radioactivity of the acid-soluble fraction increased and decreased very slowly, thus suggesting that it is not a necessary intermediate in the formation of all skin collagen.

The composition of these various skin fractions is of interest for the light it throws on the maturation process from soluble to insoluble collagen. Both Bowes and Neuberger and their collaborators (Bowes, Elliott & Moss, 1953; Harkness *et al.*, 1954) have found that the soluble fractions are significantly richer in hydroxyproline and poorer in tyrosine. These fractions are also poorer in hexosamine. Bowes has therefore suggested that the maturation process is brought about by the action of a tyrosine-rich, hydroxyproline-poor substance—probably a mucopolysaccharide or mucoprotein. Neuberger, however, prefers to regard this tyrosine-rich material as a contaminant difficult to remove but not chemically linked with collagen in the living tissue.

The two soluble fractions of collagen, unlike gelatin, retain their submicroscopic structure which is readily revealed by electron microscopy of the appropriate precipitate. Nageotte, as long ago as 1927, recognized that collagen dissolved in weak acetic acid could be reprecipitated in fibrous form. Gross, Highberger & Schmitt (1952), in a study of the factors involved in the fibrogenesis of collagen *in vitro*, were impressed by the ability of serum acid glycoproteins at 10^{-9} molar concentration to precipitate the acid-soluble collagen as fibres with the 640 Å spacing typical of the native protein. This action of the glycoprotein, however, was by no means specific; thrombin, papain and adrenocorticotropic hormone all shared this property. It soon became apparent, however, that weak acetic acid solutions of collagen contain all the ingredients necessary for formation of typical collagen fibrils, and these can be precipitated as such merely by treatment with sodium chloride of appropriate ionic strength (1% NaCl, pH 6–7). Analysis of fibres precipitated in this way still showed the presence of hexosamine (Gross *et al.*, 1952). The possible role of heparin in *in vivo* fibrogenesis is still being studied. Gross and his colleagues, using solutions of collagen derived from the swim bladder of the carp, found that heparin was unable to precipitate fibres with the 640 Å spacing. Morrione (1952), however, using collagen from the dura mater of new-born babies, found typical collagen fibrils in the precipitate obtained on the addition of heparin in dilutions of up to one in 80,000. In

view of the widespread distribution of mast cells in connective tissues this is of great theoretical interest.

A small amount of polysaccharide appears to be firmly bound to collagen and resists extraction by 0·2 N-KOH for many weeks (Consden, Glynn & Stainier, 1953). Its function is as yet far from clear, but it could be either an integral part of the molecule or a cementing substance between them, or some larger aggregate such as the tactoids described by Banfield (1952). Further information on the problem of the maturation of collagen has been obtained by the studies of Gross on the thermal precipitation of neutral salt-soluble collagen. This form of collagen obtained by extraction of connective tissue at 4° C (Jackson & Fessler, 1955) is precipitated in fibrous form by warming to 37° C, but redissolves on cooling. Gross (1958), however, has shown that the degree of re-solution is a function of the time the material is kept insoluble at 37° C. Thus, whereas the precipitation at 37° C is completely reversible if cooling is undertaken immediately, after 48 hr. at 37° C only 10% goes into solution again on cooling. Since it is improbable that non-collagen components play a role in this phenomenon, Gross suggests that time allows the associated molecules to find their most stable and sterically matched fit, thus permitting the establishment of more cross-linking H bonds.

From the vast amount of work on solubilization of collagen, well summarized by Piez (1967), it can be concluded that the collagen molecule is a rod-shaped rigid structure 3000 Å long and 15 Å in diameter, with a molecular weight of 300,000. It is formed from three chains, two α_1 and one α_2, in helical formation held together as a super helix by hydrogen bonds supplemented by various covalent bonds of which the aldehyde cross-link of Bornstein & Piez (1966) is the best established. For a full discussion of the possible cross-linkages, both intra- and intermolecular, see the review by Harding (1965). This molecular unit from which all collagen is built has been termed tropocollagen. It is soluble below pH 5 at ionic strengths from 0 to 0·15; but around neutrality most collagens remain soluble at higher ionic strengths than 0·15. The solubility is, however, highly temperature-dependent as already discussed.

Soluble collagen can be readily precipitated in fibrous form by variations of temperature, ionic strength and the presence of specific precipitating agents. At least three varieties of fibre have been recognized by electron microscopy of these precipitates (Gross *et al.*, 1954), namely the native type with a repeat period of 640 Å, fibrous long spacing (FLS) with a centro-symmetric period of 2800 Å and segment long spacing (SLS) also with a period of 2800 Å but showing distinct polarization by which the two ends, A and B, could be distinguished.

The various sub-bands which can be recognized with the electron microscope can be interpreted as evidence that the tropocollagen molecule has a length which is non-integral with respect to the conspicuous D period, namely 4·4 D, and that the arrangement of the molecules to form protofibrils is accomplished by a staggering of the molecules by one D period with reference to its neighbours. This results in the native fibril in an overlap zone of 0·4 D and a "hole" zone of 0·6 D in every period of 640 Å. The various sub-bands within each 640 Å period are also explicable on the basis of a regular alternation of structure along the individual α chains. That these consist of linear peptides joined end to end by non-peptide, possibly ester linkages has already been suggested by the work of Gallop (1964) on the fragmentation of the chains by hydroxylamine. Molecular weight determination of the fractions so obtained suggests that the α_1 chain consists of five such sub-units and the α_2 of seven (Hodge, Petruska & Bailey, 1965). Gallop (1967), however, interprets his findings as evidence for six sub-units per chain.

In the absence of any convincing evidence in favour of any other factors as responsible for the thermal and metabolic stability of collagen it would appear that this stability is mainly attributable to the intrinsic structure of collagen as stabilized by its H bonding (Courts, 1960; Brown, Consden & Glynn, 1958). The influence of H bond breakers upon the thermal stability, enzyme susceptibility and *in vivo* absorbability (Glynn, 1957–8) strongly confirms this conclusion.

In the absence of any mammalian enzymes capable of breaking down collagen within the physiological pH range of the connective tissues it has been difficult to account for the readiness with which it is undoubtedly removed in various physiological and pathological conditions. At least two collagenases, however, have been recently demonstrated in vertebrate tissues, the first by Gross and his colleagues (Kang, Nagai, Piez & Gross, 1966) in the tail of the metamorphosing frog tadpole, and the second in a variety of mammalian tissues including bone and synovial membrane from rheumatoid joints (Evanson *et al.*, 1968). Both these enzymes are active at pH 7 and yield fragments capable of further digestion by other enzymes in the tissue fluids.

Reticulin. The question of the relationship of the polysaccharide to the protein fibre is of special interest in considering the nature of reticulin fibres. These are distinguished histologically from collagen fibres by their more delicate structure, their branching and tendency to form networks and by their being impregnated by various silver techniques, staining black therewith in contrast to collagen fibres which stain brown or pink. Under the electron microscope the fibres are indistinguishable from those of collagen, but occur in membranes composed of a network of fibrils 100-600 Å thick lying in an amorphous matrix. The fibrils, like those of collagen, go into solution on boiling, but the matrix remains undissolved (Kramer & Little, 1953). No differences have been detected between the X-ray diffraction patterns of collagen and reticulin.

The matrix of reticulin gives a positive reaction with the Hotchkiss-McMannus periodic acid-Schiff stain, and is undoubtedly rich in polysaccharide material. Since the fibres themselves are closely related chemically to collagen (Bowes & Kenten, 1949), it is suggested that the differences in their histological reactions, especially to silver impregnation, are attributable to a quantitative and possibly qualitative difference in the relationship of the fibres to the interfibrillar matrix (Glynn & Loewi, 1952; Tomlin, 1953). This is supported by Brewer's observation on differences in birefringence between collagen and reticulin (Brewer, 1957). He found that, whereas the form birefringence of both types of fibre and the intrinsic birefringence of collagen are positive, the intrinsic birefringence of reticulin is negative, suggesting the presence on the reticulin fibre of a material oriented at right angles to the fibre axis. The excess of polysaccharide in reticulin (Kramer & Little, 1953) could perhaps account for its greater resistance to solution on boiling in water. Bowes (1953) has suggested that the failure of such solutions to gel on cooling might result from the breakdown of the collagen of reticulin by the excessive boiling required to bring it into solution. The quantitative difference between the polysaccharide content of collagen and reticulin has been confirmed by Glegg, Eidinger & Leblond (1953). On hydrolysis, both types of tissue yielded glucose, galactose, mannose and fucose, but a rough quantitative comparison showed that reticulin contained at least five times as much of these sugars as did collagen.

A more recent analysis of reticulin isolated from renal glomeruli (Kefalides & Winzler, 1966) has confirmed its essential similarity to collagen with higher content of carbohydrate, but revealed a considerably greater amount of hydroxylysine.

Snellman (1963), on the basis of his studies of reticulin from skin and spleen, has suggested that guanosine triphosphate is also intimately associated with the tropocollagen of reticulin.

Elastin

Of the three types of fibre peculiar to connective tissue, elastin is the least understood. Under the light microscope elastin fibres appear straight and sometimes branched, and differ both from collagen and reticulin in staining reactions (Maximow & Bloom, 1944). Elastin is highly resistant to boiling water or formic acid and remains in the undissolved residue after autoclaving. Apart from collagen, it is the only protein in mammalian tissues to contain significant quantities of hydroxyproline, i.e. 2·0% (Bowes & Kenten, 1949). The predominant amino acids are glycine, leucine, valine and proline. Tryptophan, tyrosine, lysine, histidine and the sulphur-containing amino acids are either absent or present in quantities less than 1%. Elastase, an enzyme capable of dissolving elastin, has been obtained from beef pancreas (Balo & Banga, 1950) and shown to consist of two components, a mucopolysaccharidase and a protease (Hall, Reed & Tunbridge, 1952). Its action on elastin is essentially that of a protease. This has been clearly shown by Thomas & Partridge (1960) in an extensive study of a large variety of enzymes reported to possess elastolytic properties. Without exception these enzymes such as papain, ficin, bromelin and elastase itself are potent proteases with a wide range of peptide specificity, their elastolytic and proteolytic activity running closely parallel. The failure of such enzymes as trypsin, chymotrypsin and pepsin to attack elastin is attributed by Thomas & Partridge either to their restricted peptide-bond specificity, or inability to penetrate the cross-linked structure.

By the sequential action of several proteases followed by amino acid carboxypeptidases, Partridge, Elsden & Thomas (1963) isolated the regions of the elastin network containing the cross-linking regions of the constituent peptide chains. From these they were then able to isolate and characterize two new amino acids, desmosine and isodesmosine, each consisting as shown of a central pyridine nucleus with four side chains each terminating in an α amino acid, and thus capable of incorporation into four peptide chains. Different samples of elastin contain 1·4 to 2·8 of these cross-linking molecules per 1000 residues. The elasticity of elastin therefore is probably related to that of rubber in which long linear molecules are cross-linked at wide intervals to

I-Desmosine

II-Isodesmosine

form a single network. Because of its open structure elastin is susceptible to the action of a wide range of proteolytic enzymes, but only those capable of acting on a variety of peptide bands. Those like trypsin and chymotrypsin with restricted activity are almost without effect because of the very low content of the appropriate polar amino acids.

Ground Substance

The density with which the fibres are packed in different forms of connective tissue varies enormously from tendon at one extreme to the loose subcutaneous areolar tissue at the other. The material between the fibres is termed the ground substance and its composition and function differ widely in different sites, e.g. bone, cartilage and fascia. This ground substance is a gel, mostly composed of water, and intervenes everywhere between the blood and lymph vessels on the one hand and the metabolizing cells on the other. It is in fact the physical expression of the "milieu interne", and plays a major role in transport, storage and exchange of water and electrolytes. In view of its undoubted physiological and pathological importance, its comparative neglect by investigators until quite recently is surprising. In the light of present knowledge it is best regarded as a gel which owes its gel structure to the proteins and polysaccharides in solution. The gel-like nature of this substance in the dermal connective tissue has been particularly well illustrated by McMaster & Parsons (1950).

The identity of the materials constituting the ground substance is being currently studied in many centres, and much progress has been made since Meyer & Palmer (1934) first isolated hyaluronic acid. Chain & Duthie in 1939 showed that hyaluronic acid was a substrate for the spreading factor isolated from testes by Duran-Reynals (1928). Chondroitin sulphuric acid has also been shown to be a substrate for this testicular enzyme, and the presence of both these polysaccharides in dermal connective tissue has been confirmed (Pearce & Watson, 1949; Meyer & Chaffee, 1941).

The systemic effect of diseases such as rheumatic fever and rheumatoid arthritis upon the connective tissue ground substance was revealed by the studies of Bywaters, Holborow & Keech (1951). They found a considerable delay in these diseases in the reconstitution time of the dermal barrier to the spread of an indicator such as haemoglobin, following an intradermal injection of hyaluronidase. These findings have recently been confirmed and extended by Laskin, Engel, Joseph & Pollak (1961), using an electrometric method for serial measurements of displaced Donnan potentials in the dermis.

The polysaccharides now identified in various connective tissues are, excluding the blood group substances, at least eight in number. They are mostly acidic in character owing to the presence of uronic acid, sulphuric acid or both. The non-sulphated acid polysaccharides are hyaluronic acid and chondroitin. The sulphated polysaccharides are chondroitin sulphates A, B and C, keratosulphate (Meyer, Linker, Davidson & Weissmann, 1953) and heparitin, a sugar related to heparin but of a lower degree of sulphation (Linker, Hoffmann, Sampson & Meyer, 1958). Chondroitin sulphates A, B and C are polymers built up of a repeating unit consisting of a uronic acid in a β 1:3 linkage with a sulphated N-acetylgalactosamine. In chondroitin sulphate A and C the uronic acid is glycuronic acid, in the B variety it is iduronic acid. The sulphate radical is attached to C_4 in chondroitin sulphates A and B and to C_6 in chondroitin sulphate C. The hexosaminidic linkage in all three sugars has the β 1:4 configuration. Keratosulphate is composed of equimolar proportions of galactose, N-acetylglucosamine and sulphate, but little is known of how these are related in the intact molecule. The relative amounts of these polysaccharides vary considerably in different types of connective tissue and at different stages of maturation and ageing. In general there is a tendency for hyaluronic acid to decrease with age and for the sulphated polysaccharides to increase (Loewi & Meyer, 1958). Remarkable quantitative changes are found in various diseases, e.g. gargoylism.

The synthesis of the various polysaccharides has undergone a remarkable clarification since the discovery by Leloir and his colleagues (Caputto, Leloir, Cardine & Paladine, 1950) of the role of the nucleoside diphosphate derivatives of the sugars in hexose and polysaccharide metabolism. These nucleosides, or activated sugars so called, are capable in the presence of appropriate enzymes of undergoing a variety of transformations involving epimerization, oxidation or reduction so that all the known polysaccharides of the connective tissues are capable of synthesis from glucose. Similarly the synthesis of the sulphated sugars is mediated via activated sulphate in the form of adenosine 3-phosphate-5-phosphato sulphate (Hilz & Lipmann, 1955) usually referred to as PAPS.

It is now clear that the various polysaccharides do not exist in the connective tissues as free compounds but are covalently linked to protein. Such protein polysaccharides have been most extensively studied in cartilage (Pal & Schubert, 1965) from which many different fractions have been isolated differing mainly in the proportion of protein to polysaccharide. The protein is non-collagenous, with glycine constituting only some 10% of the residues, and hydroxyproline absent. The present concept of the structure of these compounds envisages a central protein core to which the polysaccharide chains are attached at intervals along the peptide chain. Since even the most highly purified preparations contain both chondroitin sulphate and keratan sulphate it is probable that both polysaccharides are present on individual protein molecules. This of course is essentially similar to the currently held view concerning the structure of the water-soluble blood group substances in the body secretions (Morgan & Watkins, 1956).

The linkage area between the polysaccharide and the protein has received especial study by Roden and his colleagues (Gregory, Laurent & Roden, 1964; Roden & Smith, 1966). For chondroitin-4-sulphate they have clearly shown that the linkage is via the hydroxyl group of serine by means of the following sequence: glycuronic acid (1–3)-N-acetyl galactosamine sulphate (1–4) glycuronic acid (1–3) galactose (1–3) galactose (1–4) xylose-O-serine. An identical link has been found between heparin and protein, but the protein linkage of keratan sulphate is probably even more complex (Bray, Lieberman & Meyer, 1967).

Cartilage

Cartilage precedes bone in both phylo- and ontogenesis: it determines the form of bone and, because it covers the "business end", its function also. Thus its biochemical abnormalities have importance for students of growth, locomotion, congenital and acquired deformities, and old age. Its basic composition has only in recent years been fully studied (Eichelberger, Akeson & Roma, 1958). Water comprises 75–80%, becoming less with age. Electrolytes show certain differences from other tissues both in the intra- and in the extracellular phase; the latter preponderates and comprises collagen fibres, polysaccharide protein complex and ultrafiltrate. Associated with its avascularity, metabolism of cartilage in the adult is mainly glycolytic (Bywaters, 1937; Hills, 1940) like that of non-nucleated erythrocytes, although in the young there is relatively more oxidative phosphorylation (Rosenthal et al., 1941; Whitehead, 1960). Although at birth the polysaccharide consists mainly of chondroitin sulphate A, it is almost entirely replaced in early adult life by chondroitin sulphate C and kerato-sulphate in a ratio of 2·5:1 (Kaplan & Meyer, 1959); sialic acid is also reported to be present (Anderson, 1962). No genetically determined retention of chondroitin sulphate A, akin to that of foetal haemoglobin, has yet been described, but in gargoylism (Hurler's syndrome), chondroitin sulphate B is present up to 12% in cartilage, as well as chondroitin sulphates A and C. Storage occurs in various organs together with heparitin sulphate, and it is excreted in large amounts in the urine (Dorfman & Lorinez, 1957; Meyer et al., 1958).

Chondroitin sulphate exists in cartilage as a chondromucoprotein, bound covalently to a protein first isolated by Shatton & Schubert in 1954, and found to be rich in tyrosine (Partridge & Davis, 1958). Protein constitutes about one-third of the complex. The softening and collapse of cartilage produced in rabbits injected with crude extracts containing papain (Thomas, 1956) is due to rupture of the protein-chondroitin bond, with subsequent loss of polysaccharide from the cartilage and its appearance in serum and urine (Tsaltas, 1958). In young rabbits deformities appear, due to involvement of epiphyseal cartilage (Hulth & Westerborn, 1959). Resynthesis occurs rapidly unless hydrocortisone or similar steroid is given (McCluskey & Thomas, 1959). Similar effects are seen in hypervitaminosis

A (Thomas et al., 1960) and with plasmin in vitro (Lack & Rogers, 1958) and in vivo (Lack, 1959). The latter process may play some part in the local removal of cartilage in areas of inflammation, and in the formation of fibrinoid. Still not understood is the rare condition of atrophic polychondritis, where, sometimes in association with a rheumatoid type of arthritis and sometimes without, inflammatory infiltration and removal of cartilage occurs in ears, eyes, nose, bronchi and joints (Gordon et al., 1948; Bean et al., 1958). One case has shown a positive Rose-Waaler test (Davies & Kelsall, 1961). The condition seems responsive to steroid (Pearson et al., 1960).

The commonest and indeed "universal" disease of cartilage is the osteoarthrosis of advancing years, where the cartilage of the bone ends becomes thinned, frayed and worn away down to the underlying bone. This process is associated with loss of polysaccharide relative to collagen (Matthews, 1952; Loewi, 1953). Similar changes occur with age in the nucleus pulposus of the intervertebral disc (Happey, Wiseman & Naylor, 1961). While "wear and tear" accounts for some part of this process, there is great individual variation, partly genetically determined (Stecher & Hersh, 1944). It seems possible that metabolic factors may play some part, since the Silberbergs found (1950) that a high-fat diet accelerated the appearance of such changes in mice. Other than progeria, which is ill-understood, the only metabolic abnormality producing generalized osteoarthritic change is ochronosis, due to absence of homogentisic acid oxidase. The pigmented polymer localizes in cartilage and makes it brittle leading to early degenerative changes (O'Brien, Banfield & Sokoloff, 1961).

The problem of Ca deposition in connective tissue is discussed under calcinosis, but it should perhaps be mentioned here that abnormal Ca deposition in cartilage occurs not only in ochronosis, in hypervitaminosis D and in hyperparathyroidism, but also as a hereditary disease, chondrocalcinosis (Rubens-Duval et al., 1961). Its mechanism is unknown.

RHEUMATOID ARTHRITIS

Introduction

Rheumatoid arthritis is a crippling disease of unknown aetiology affecting primarily the synovial membrane of joints, bursae and tendon sheaths. Earlier work suggesting a significant hereditary factor in its pathogenesis has been seriously challenged by the studies of Bunim et al. (1964) on the incidence of the disease in various

Red Indian tribes. To avoid selection bias the only satisfactory method of studying the problem is by surveys of whole populations, not just comparing the incidence in relatives of affected and non-affected individuals. Such studies reveal little if any evidence of heredity on the incidence of either the disease or its associated serological manifestations (v.i.).

No evidence for any specific endocrine or biochemical abnormality has emerged, despite various claims (never confirmed) ranging from abnormalities of erythrocyte K to blood serotonin concentration, or various amino acid or muco-polysaccharide excretion rates or of noradrena-line:adrenaline ratios in urine.

The primary changes in rheumatoid arthritis seem to occur in the connective tissues of certain moving parts; these changes have been characterized morphologically, but not yet biochemically, although some information is beginning to emerge about the rheumatoid nodule, a zone of necrosis, surrounded by proliferating histiocytes and other inflammatory cells, which not infrequently occurs in the neighbourhood of tendons, bursae and over bony prominences. This will be discussed first. Next will be considered what are probably secondary phenomena, reflections of this primary change, occurring in the blood serum and in the synovial fluid. Finally, the specificity of these biochemical changes will be discussed.

Biochemical and Biophysical Changes in Rheumatoid Nodules and Synovium

The necrotic material in the centre of a rheumatoid nodule bears some resemblance to fibrin (and hence has been called "fibrinoid" material). Fawns & Landells (1954), using fresh tissue cut on the freezing microtome and examined by phase contrast and polarized light as well as by conventional fixation and staining procedures, have re-emphasized the two distinct parts of this material, a fibrillar portion resembling collagen in all respects except that it is argyrophil, and a granular portion refractile but not birefringent and not argyrophil, staining occasionally dark blue like fibrin with Mallory's phosphotungstic acid-haematoxylin and staining deeply with the periodic acid-Schiff procedure like a polysaccharide. Unlike the fibrillar component, these granules are digested by trypsin but not by collagenase. They give a strong reaction for tyrosine with Millon's reagent. Ziff and his co-workers (Bien & Ziff, 1951; Kantor, Sokoloff, Smith & Ziff, 1951; Ziff, Kantor, Bien & Smith, 1953) found that by conventional staining criteria 80% of fibrinoid material from such rheumatoid

nodules was extractable by 0·1 N-NaOH or crystalline trypsin, but was not extracted by collagenase, borate buffer at pH 7·8, testicular hyaluronidase or streptokinase-activated plasmin. Trypsinized or alkali-extracted tissue showed empty spaces in areas previously occupied by fibrinoid; strands of intact collagen fibres previously obscured became visible. The extracts contained negligible amounts of hydroxyproline. All the hydroxyproline of the nodule is adequately accounted for by the collagen and elastin extractable therefrom (Bien & Ziff, 1951). Unfortunately, no figures are given for the total amount of material extracted or of its nitrogen content. Further evidence comes from X-ray diffraction studies of such nodules in which Kellgren and others (Kellgren, Ball, Astbury, Reed & Beighton, 1951) have shown the absence of the typical collagen pattern and recognizable X-ray evidence of true fibrin in the necrotic centre. Electron microscopic studies have shown that this centre is characterized by amorphous material rather than by collagen fibres.

In the somewhat similar but less orientated nodules of rheumatic fever, Consden, Glynn & Stanier (1953) have noted the presence of increased amounts of tyrosine-rich material and poly-saccharide, the latter composed predominantly of galactose and glucosamine. Fibrin has been shown to be present in the nodules of rheumatic fever and rheumatoid arthritis by immuno-fluorescent methods (Gitlin, Craig & Janeway, 1957), as well as γ-globulin (Vasquez & Dixon, 1957). A useful review is that by Movat (1957).

The recent discovery of a collagenase produced by rheumatoid synovium in tissue culture may well indicate the means of collagen destruction in this disease (Evanson, Jeffrey & Krane, 1968). It is inactivated by serum so that intimate contact between the enzyme-producing cells and the substrate is probably necessary as is seen for example with pannus and the underlying cartilage.

Collagen in rheumatoid arthritis. There is little evidence of any abnormality in the primary or tertiary structure of collagen in rheumatoid arthritis. Steven (1966), however, has shown that the collagen obtained from affected synovia is more susceptible than normal collagen to proteolytic enzymes such as pronase. It is also lacking an alkali-resistant cross-link, so that on boiling alkali-treated collagen from rheumatoid tissue 80–90% goes into solution whereas the comparably treated normal collagen is only solubilized to about 30% (Steven, 1966). Whether this deficiency of cross-linkage is due to faulty synthesis or partial disruption resulting from the inflammatory process remains to be determined. In view of the role of a copper-containing enzyme in the oxidation of lysine which is apparently a step in the formation of the cross-link of collagen described by Bornstein & Piez (1966), it is interesting that about 50% of patients with rheumatoid arthritis excrete in their urine an excess of a copper-binding ligand (Gerber, 1966). In a series of 215 non-rheumatoid patients comparable levels of the ligand were found in only 5%.

Changes in Synovial Fluid and Blood

If rheumatoid inflammation occurs in one joint only, and particularly if this is a small joint, changes in synovial fluid occur, but the circulating blood shows no detectable change. We deduce, therefore, that these primary changes in rheumatoid synovial connective tissue and lining membrane modify first the character of the synovial fluid and secondly, if the change is sufficiently intense and widespread, the blood. A possible exception (see later) is the globulin responsible for the Rose-Waaler test.

Synovial fluid. With the increased permeability of the capillaries in the inflamed synovial membrane, the synovial fluid is increased in amount, the total protein concentration increases, and the proportion of proteins of larger molecular weight (globulins) begins to rise towards that in the blood (Svartz & Olhagen, 1948; Perlmann, Ropes, Kaufman & Bauer, 1954). At the same time, perhaps because of the increased flow of plasma filtrate into the joint, the amount of hyaluronic acid-protein complex in the fluid increases in total quantity, but its concentration falls. The character of the precipitate brought about by acetic acid in the presence of protein changes. The decrease depends usually on the degree and chronicity of change in the synovial membrane. The glucose content falls by a variable amount from its usual level which is equal to that in the blood. These changes are fully detailed in the monograph by Ropes & Bauer (1952). Cortisone acetate and, to a more marked degree, hydrocortisone reverse these changes (Dixon & Bywaters, 1953), perhaps by decreasing capillary permeability, when either injected locally or when given systemically in adequate doses. Enzymes such as aminotripeptidase appear in the fluid, as in any inflammatory effusion (Ziff, Simson, Scull, Smith, Shatton & Mainland, 1955).

The hyaluronate isolated from synovial fluid by filtration through a millipore filter (Ogston & Stanier, 1950) has a limiting viscosity number, lower than that of the hyaluronate obtained from normal joints (Sundblad, 1965), clear evidence of a reduction in molecular weight. It is not, however, clear whether this is the result of degradation or faulty synthesis.

Of especial interest in view of the widely held view that the joint changes are the result of a local immunological reaction is the low level of complement in the synovial fluid compared with that in blood taken at the same time (Perkin & Zvaifler, 1964). The observation that the γ-globulin in the fluid may exceed the concentration in the plasma has also been attributed to a local immune response leading to synthesis of γ-globulin by plasma cells in the synovial membrane itself. This synthetic capacity of the rheumatoid synovial membrane has indeed been established *in vitro* by Smiley, Jacks & Ziff (1968).

Changes in the blood. The acute phase changes in the blood of rheumatoid arthritis patients— fibrinogen increase, mucoprotein increase—are non-specific and occur in any inflammatory condition. They were reviewed in the previous edition of this book (pp. 819-823).

Other substances characterizing the serum of patients with rheumatoid arthritis depend for their recognition as yet on biological rather than biochemical properties. These may be listed briefly thus:

(1) *Serum complement* is said to be increased in rheumatoid arthritis (Wedgewood & Janeway, 1953).

(2) *Non-specific hyaluronidase inhibitor* (Faber & Iverson, 1952), thought to be a heparin-like material (Glick & Sulven, 1951).

(3) A *factor producing necrosis* in the isolated skin of guinea-pigs (Boake & Lovell, 1954; Lovell, Pryce & Boake, 1954).

(4) *C-reactive protein*, an α_1-globulin reacting with the somatic C substance of pneumococci, which is increased in the serum and in effusions of many inflammatory conditions including rheumatoid arthritis (Hill, 1951). This substance as well as mucoprotein is independent of the γ-globulin response to antigenic stimulation since it occurs in patients with agammaglobulin-aemia (Good, 1954).

(5) *The Rose-Waaler test.* The ability of rheumatoid sera to potentiate the agglutination of various particles has been known for many years, but it was only with the discovery of the Rose-Waaler reaction that its significance became appreciated. It is now known that this property of rheumatoid sera is due to the presence of a fast moving γ-globulin, with sedimentation

coefficient of 19s that is capable of reacting in certain circumstances with the slower moving γ-globulin with a sedimentation coefficient of 7s. The reaction between these two globulins has many of the features of an antigen–antibody reaction, the 7s globulin playing the role of antigen. Further support for this view comes from the observation that the factor is not confined to the γ M fraction but that the other fractions such as the IgA and IgC may also participate, thus bringing the factor into line with other antibodies (Adachi et al., 1969).

The use as a histochemical reagent of heat-aggregated 7s γ-globulin conjugated with fluorescein has revealed the presence of the rheumatoid factor in plasma cells in various parts of the body, especially in the synovial membrane and in the lymph nodes, as well as free within the germinal centres. The ultracentrifugal studies of Franklin and his collaborators (1957) have shown that in serum, and presumably also in vivo, the rheumatoid factor exists loosely combined with several molecules of 7s γ-globulin, the complex possessing a sedimentation coefficient of 22s. The 19s molecule is itself composed of 7s units, apparently held together by S–S bonds, since it is readily dissociated into these units by reagents such as mercaptoethanol.

There is still some difference of opinion as to whether the rheumatoid factor (i.e. the 19s rheumatoid γ-globulin) can react with native human 7s globulin, or whether the latter must first undergo some change in configuration so as to expose the appropriate reactant groups. The weight of evidence certainly favours the latter (Aho, 1961). It is presumably a change of this sort that is undergone by the molecules of 7s γ-globulin when adsorbed on to particles of latex or bentonite, or when tanned on to red cells, that enables these various preparations to be used for the detection of the rheumatoid factor; and similarly when the 7s globulin is bound to its carrier by immune forces as in the original test with sheep cells coated with rabbit amboceptor.

The lack of specificity with regard to the origin of the 7s γ-globulin with which the rheumatoid factor can react was at first regarded as evidence against the immune nature of the reaction. Further work, however, has clearly shown that these apparently non-specific cross reactions are in no way different from the cross reactivity shown by classical antibodies to serum proteins. It is moreover the cross reactivity that is the specific feature of the rheumatoid factor. Thus, in several diseases, e.g. syphilis, sarcoidosis and viral hepatitis, positive tests for rheumatoid factor may be obtained if the reactant 7s globulin is of human origin, but they are almost invariably negative when tests using rabbit globulin, e.g. the sensitized sheep cell test, are employed.

Such evidence as is at present available is against the participation of the rheumatoid factor in pathogenesis, although there is a good positive correlation between its presence and the development of subcutaneous nodules and complications such as arteritis. If, as is now almost unanimously agreed, the factor is an auto-antibody against the patient's own modified γ-globulin, this emphasizes rather the role of immunological reactivity in the development of the disease, without the factor itself necessarily participating in the actual formation of lesions. The appearance of virtually indistinguishable rheumatoid lesions in subjects with agammaglobulinaemia supports this interpretation. Other antibody-like substances, more commonly found in systemic lupus, also occur, but less frequently, in the sera of rheumatoid arthritics.

Many cases of chronic inflammatory arthritis do not possess the rheumatoid factor, e.g. ankylosing spondylitis, psoriatic arthritis, Reiter's syndrome and the arthritis associated with ulcerative colitis or agammaglobulinaemia; and in some cases of rheumatoid arthritis and Still's disease it can only be detected by the highly sensitive inhibition test (Ziff et al., 1956). Furthermore, population surveys have revealed its presence in some individuals who have no sign of arthritis. Despite these discrepancies it is proving invaluable in genetic and epidemiological studies.

Specificity of Serological Changes

With the exception of the last, none of the above changes is in any way specific, being given, for the most part, not only by serum from closely related conditions like rheumatic fever, etc., but also from such chronic diseases with tissue destruction as chronic bacterial infections, myocardial infarction, etc. They are thus comparable with the changes in iron-binding capacity, serum iron and serum copper levels seen in rheumatoid arthritis and other inflammatory diseases (Brendstrup, 1953). Some of these changes are useful in differentiating certain related conditions: thus colloidal gold flocculation is seen in 79% of cases with rheumatoid arthritis, but much less commonly in ankylosing spondylitis, 24% according to Hart, Robinson, Allchin & Maclagan (1949), and in rheumatic fever only if there is coexistent heart failure.

Nor are the changes in the synovial fluid in any way specific; similar alterations in protein and sugar content are seen in any inflammatory condition, as also are the alterations in viscosity and synovial mucin precipitability.

Abnormalities in the metabolism of several amino acids have been revealed by a study of their excreted metabolites. The best established of these is that involving tryptophan which reveals itself as an excessive excretion of 3-hydroxy-anthranilic acid (McMillan, 1960; Bett, 1962) and of kynurenine (Bett, 1962), a further degradation product of tryptophan. The excessive excretion of kynurenine by rheumatoid subjects is especially well revealed by a loading dose of L-tryptophan and the increase can be prevented by intra-muscular or oral pyridoxine. There is no other evidence of pyridoxine deficiency in these patients and the nature of the metabolic fault is still obscure. The abnormal kynurenine excretion also falls as disease activity declines.

The production of taurine from cystine requires pyridoxine so that any deficiency of this vitamin would be expected to lead to a fall in the output of taurine. The observation of Rylance (1969), however, showed the reverse: the urinary excretion of taurine was significantly greater in rheumatoid subjects than in controls and tended towards normal in patients on aspirin. The basis of the disturbance is unknown but is probably attributable to excessive cell destruction.

An abnormality in tyrosine metabolism is suggested by the observation of McCormick, Robinson, Smith & Day (1962) that p-hydroxy-phenyllactic acid was detectable in 40% of rheumatoid patients but in only 1·8% of normal subjects. It was unaffected by supplements of ascorbic acid.

Several reports have appeared in recent years of a folate deficiency in rheumatoid arthritis as shown by reduction in plasma level (Gough, McCarthy, Read, Mollin & Walters, 1964; Deller, Urban, Ibbotson, Horwood, Milazzo & Robson, 1966). Nevertheless the deficiency of folate in the red cells is much less pronounced, implying a greater efficiency of folate utilization in these patients, a conclusion confirmed by the rarity of megaloblastic changes despite the low folate levels in plasma and red cells (Omer & Mowat, 1968). The known masking effect of iron deficiency on the megaloblastic changes of folate deficiency (Herbert, 1965) may well be operating here.

The folate deficiency associated with rheumatoid arthritis does not appear to result from nutritional deficiency or impaired absorption. It

is presumably the result of increased metabolic demand or deviation but where or how is quite unknown. The increased cellular activity of the affected tissue seems a likely site for increased metabolic demand but the lack of correlation of the deficiency with the duration or severity of the disease makes this unlikely.

In summary, therefore, although the biochemical approach to the problem of rheumatoid arthritis promises to be fruitful, no great headway has yet been made in the study of tissue lesions; the changes in blood and synovial fluid demonstrated so far are secondary and non-specific, with the exception of the appearance of the substance giving the Rose-Waaler test.

GOUT AND URATE ACCUMULATION

Introduction

Although urate was first crystallized from the serum by Garrod in 1848, only in the last few years has the problem of gout clearly crystallized from its previous amorphous state. Gout is a "crystallosis". We have now considerable information about various mechanisms of the urate accumulation which always precedes overt gout, about the final common mechanism which produces the actual attack and about the disposal of urate, as well as, in addition, efficient and adequate management both of the acute attack and of the symptomless hyperuricaemia which accompanies it. These advances have come about at an increasingly rapid rate, proceeding logically from the pioneer discoveries of Scheele (1776), of Wollaston (1797), Garrod (1848) and Fischer (1895) (reviewed historically by Copeman, 1964) to the newer work of the last 20 years.

Mechanisms of the Acute Attack

The acute inflammation of the gouty attack is due to the local formation of urate crystals, monosodium urate monohydrate (Howell et al., 1963); a similar syndrome can be reproduced artificially by the injection of crystals of sodium urate of a certain size (Seegmiller et al., 1962) or of cortisone crystals (Faires & McCarty, 1962), and is seen naturally in the syndrome called "pseudogout" due to the precipitation of calcium pyrophosphate crystals. Such urate crystals are ingested by polymorphonuclear leucocytes and can be found both free in synovial fluid and intracellularly in synovial cells: they need to be differentiated from calcium pyrophosphate monohydrate crystals (causing "pseudogout") by their shape and their strong negative birefringence (technique, Oster & Pollister, 1955). However, typical calcium pyrophosphate crystals may be

E. G. L. BYWATERS AND L. E. GLYNN

found occasionally in synovial fluid from classical gout (Currey & Sweetenham, 1965). Chemotaxis and phagocytosis with release of kinins from polymorphonuclear leucocytes by activation of Hageman factor (Kellermeyer & Breckenridge, 1965) and decrease in pH due to lactate accumulation are associated with the progressive build-up of the inflammation. Why urate crystals should precipitate in bursae, tendons, synovial membrane and cartilage is uncertain. Deposition in the superficial layers of articular cartilage (Sokoloff, 1957) suggests diffusion from the synovial fluid, where levels are usually similar to those of serum (Ropes & Bauer, 1953). In certain instances with crystals, a higher fluid/serum ratio may be found (Reeves, 1965).

Since the metabolism of adult cartilage is predominantly glycolytic (Bywaters, 1937) the resultant lactic acid accumulation and decreased pH would favour crystallization as perhaps would also "steric exclusion" (Laurent, 1964).

Tissue levels of lactate depend also on blood levels and will thus fluctuate considerably in relation to fasting, exercise, alcohol ingestion, etc. It seems quite possible that the occasional attack of gout that occurs with serum urate within a normal range on uricosuric therapy may be due to fluctuating levels of urate and "solubility-factors" in the neighbourhood of dissolving gouty tophi. What is certain is that serum and tissue content must be of a level such that supersaturation is present and precipitation can occur where local modifying factors are propitious. This critical level is very variable: thus, the acute gouty attack may occur with levels only just above normal limits and yet often fails to occur in uraemia with serum levels up to 40 mg./100 ml., well above the theoretical levels quoted (6–8 mg./100 ml.). Supersaturation studies, mostly in connection with uric acid stone formation in urine (Fried & Vermeulen, 1964), involve both true supersaturation and the protective effect of colloid and complexing-ions. Further work is needed in this sphere with plasma and other tissue fluids, where normally the urate content is that of a protein-free plasma filtrate. The exception is cerebrospinal fluid—about one-tenth of serum levels (Rosenbloom et al., 1967), due to absence of xanthine oxidase, the resultant oxypurines being actively secreted from CSF to blood by the choroid plexus (Berlin, 1969).

Serum Urate and Methods for its Determination

While urate crystal detection in tissues or body fluids is the only laboratory criterion for gout,

serum urate levels are most useful in its diagnosis, taken in conjunction with clinical history and provided the patient is not taking salicylate or other drugs influencing serum levels (Table 21.1). Both salicylate and various other drug effects depend on dosage, since both renal secretion and renal absorption of water are decreased and the net effect depends therefore on drug concentration.

TABLE 21.1

Drugs that produce decreased serum levels

High dosage salicylate
Chlorothixene (taractan)
Benzofurane, etc.
Bishydroxycoumarol
Benemid
Sulfinpyrazone
Urelim

Drugs that produce increased serum levels

Low dosage salicylate
Pyrazinamide
Nicotinic acid (ref. *Brit. med. J.*, 1964, **ii**, 1181)
Chlorothiazide, etc.
Guanethidine
Quinethazone
Mecamylamine (Dollery et al., 1960)
Pempidine (Fry & Barlow, 1962)

No effect

Methyldopa (Daley & Evans, 1962)
Mefenamic, flufenamic acid (Latham et al., 1966)
Indomethacine (Emmerson, 1967)
Ethacrynic acid
Frusemide (Lasix) (Humphreys, 1966)

(It must be remembered that many proprietary preparations include salicylate along with other drugs.)

There are, however, a great deal many more people with raised serum urate levels than with gout; 2% of hyperuricaemic males develop gout per year as against an annual incidence in the total population of 0.1% (O'Sullivan, 1968).

Much argument has been engendered because of the continuing use of unsatisfactory methods for the estimation of uric acid, utilizing the classical phosphotungstic acid colour reaction after protein precipitation. It has long been known that the reduction of tungstic acid by uric acid to give a blue colour, first noticed by Frabot in 1904 and utilized in the classical blood methods of Folin (1933, 1934) and Benedict & Behre (1931), is given by many reducing substances other than uric acid. However, some uric acid may be lost in the protein precipitate and a factor appears in the tungstate filtrate which inhibits to some extent the colour development (Bulger & Johns, 1941), leading some to prefer ferricyanide reduction methods (Brøckner-Mortensen, 1937; Bulger & Johns, 1941; Silverman & Gubernick, 1947). Effects of non-uric acid chromogens account for 10–15% of the uric acid level (Block & Geib, 1947), although Bulger & Johns (1941) assert that in gout with a high serum uric acid level, the total non-uric acid chromogen is not increased. These non-uric acid chromogens behave similarly to uric acid in many ways and their excretion is accelerated by uricosuric drugs (Wolfson, Huddlestun & Levine, 1947; Wolfson, Levine & Tinsley, 1947; Robinson & Block, 1946). The erythrocytes contain a higher and more variable proportion of chromogen than does plasma. Serum or plasma is therefore to be preferred for the estimation (Jacobson, 1938). Tophi are said to contain sodium monourate only (Brandenberger & Schinz, 1950), *without* non-uric acid chromogen (Wolfson, Huddlestun & Levine, 1947). The only completely satisfactory method is that using ultraviolet spectrophotometry (introduced by Kalckar & Shafran, 1947) following uricase digestion (introduced by Blauch & Koch, 1938). (For modern techniques, see Liddle, Seegmiller & Laster, 1959.) For ordinary clinical purposes, modifications of the older colorimetric methods are relatively satisfactory and simpler. (For comparison of these modifications, see Hendry *et al.*, 1959.) Normal serum values are below 6·5 mg./100 ml. for men and 6·0 mg. for women using the direct Benedict & Behre (1931) method (Stecher *et al.*, 1949); below 6·0 mg. and 5·5 mg. respectively using the indirect method of Folin (Smyth *et al.*, 1948*a*, *b*) or below 7·5 mg./100 ml. for men by the enzymic spectrophotometric method (Wyngaarden, 1960). It is essential that a laboratory should establish normal values for the method it uses: most now use one of the colorimetric methods adapted to the (Technicon) autoanalyser. Even this shows a great deal of variation from laboratory to laboratory (Bywaters & Holloway, 1964; O'Sullivan, 1968), but such variability is less than with non-automated methods. It is not necessary for routine purposes to estimate true urate levels with and without uricase since Healy has shown (*cit.* Decker, 1968) with an automated colorimetric method that the correction for non-urate chromogen was small in normals (less than 0·1 mg./100 ml.) and in gout (less than 0·2 mg./100 ml.), being large only in chronic uraemia. Hypoxanthine and xanthine are measured by enzymic conversion to urate (Chalmers & Watts, 1968).

Purine Metabolism in Health

Serum urate falls from a mean neonatal figure of 5·6 mg./100 ml. (Marks *et al.*, 1968) to a low level between 10 days and 2 years of age, rising gradually thereafter (Castello *et al.*, 1968) until the puberty spurt, to a higher level in boys than in girls. The mean serum urate concentration in females very rarely reaches that of the male even after the menopause (O'Sullivan, 1968) for reasons possibly to do with the differential nucleoprotein turnover of spermatazoa and ova, but still far from clear.

Whereas in most mammals, purines are broken down through urate to allantoin, man and the primates lack uricase. Some have seen in this a possible reason for primate supremacy (Orowan, 1955). The stimulating effects of such methyl purines as caffeine and the well-known gouty tendency of historically outstanding persons have combined with the more recently ascertained association of aggression, drive, executive ability or achievement in business, factory (Dunn *et al.*, 1963), military (Stetten & Hearon, 1959), school (Kasl *et al.*, 1966) or university personnel to reinforce this belief. However, an alternative possibility is that serum uric acid levels might be the result of "achievement" etc. and all that goes with it (Montoye *et al.*, 1967). Differences in mean urate levels between populations may be in part genetically determined, but environmental factors such as diet may also play a part. It is interesting to note that while relatives of high serum uric acid probands had a high mean serum uric acid, the same was true also of these probands' spouses (Popert & Hewitt, 1962). The indirect effects of dietary peculiarities on enzyme induction (Rowe & Wyngaarden, 1966), on renal handling as in fasting, due to β-hydroxybutyrate competition (Scott, McCallum & Holloway, 1964; Goldfinger *et al.*, 1965; McLachlan & Rodnan, 1967) and in alcoholism, due to lactate (Lieber, 1965) or on feedback inhibition, are probably more important than the direct contribution of the digested fragments to the synthetic pool. The higher liver xanthine oxidase in gout may possibly be attributable to this (Carcassi *et al.*, 1969).

The normal adult body pool of 1·2 g. (0·9–1·6) is maintained by urinary and intestinal excretion of urate and oxypurines, on the one hand, and by synthesis of purines from simple components on the other (Fig. 21.1). The turnover rate (determined isotopically) is 0·5–1·1 g./day, mean

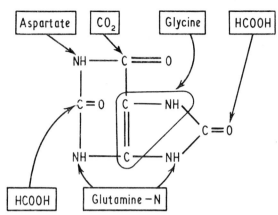

FIG. 21.1.   Uric acid and its component precursors.

0·7 g./day. Only 50–70% of the purine synthesized appears in the urine, the rest being broken down in the gut by bacterial action.

The purine nucleus forms the basis of cellular

activity and proliferation and indeed of life itself. It is built up by a sequence of steps from the first committed reaction—that of phosphoribosyl pyrophosphate with glutamine. The pathway thereafter leads (Fig. 21.2) to inosinic acid, from which on the one hand purine is built up into nucleoprotein and through which, on the other, nucleoproteins are broken down to oxypurines and uric acid. As in all enzymically determined sequences there is feedback inhibition, the most important of which is probably that governing the first committed step.

In health, feedback mechanisms ensure an equilibrium adequate for demand—but we know little yet about the details. Most of our knowledge has come about through the investigation of disease. Through study of the Lesch-Nyhan syndrome (*q.v.*), for instance, American investigators have shewn us that what has been called the "salvage pathway" whereby hypoxanthine and guanine are reconverted back to inosinic acid through the agency of hypoxanthine-guanine

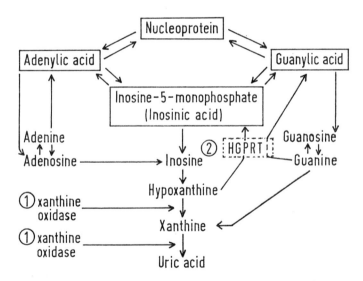

PATHWAYS OF PURINE BREAKDOWN (modified from Wyngaarden and Seegmiller)

Note sites of enzyme action :-

① Xanthine oxidase, blocked by allopurinol

② Hypoxanthine-guanine phosphoribosyl transferase
    absent in Lesch-Nyhan syndrome

FIG. 21.2. Pathways of purine breakdown (modified from Wyngaarden and Seegmiller). (Reproduced from "Gout and other Metabolic Disorders" in "Textbook of the Rheumatic Diseases" (4th Edition) ed. Copeman, W. S. C., Livingstone, Edinburgh, 1969.)

phosphoribosyl (HGPR) transferase and thereby made available again to synthetic build-up, is of considerable importance. Much of this remains to be worked out: we know something, however, of the excretory mechanisms.

Urinary uric acid accounts for the major part of purine excretion in man. About one-third of the total output is excreted in the faeces as the bacterial breakdown products—mainly ammonia —of intestinally secreted urate. Urinary urate is derived mainly from tubular secretion, an active process, inhibited by pyrazinamide, but, due no doubt to the convoluted processes of evolution, this definitive act is preceded by a prologue, whereby urate filtration through the glomerular basement membrane, 100% according to direct measurements, is then completely reversed by almost 100% reabsorption in the proximal convoluted tubule—a process affected to a certain extent by competition for transport mechanisms by penicillin, benemid, etc.

It has always been difficult to differentiate these diverse renal mechanisms, and, apart from direct glomerular puncture, most of our information has come from the action of drugs and the use of the stop-flow method on the final urinary excretion. A more basic controversy is still unsettled—concerning urate-binding. Despite claims to the contrary (Alvsaker, 1965), most people believe that urate is not bound to protein in any way relevant to passage through glomerular or capillary membranes. Alvsaker's recent claims have been denied by Sheikh & Møller (1968). They conclude, using equilibrium dialysis, ultra-filtration and gel filtration methods, that binding of urate to albumin (5% at 20° C and 37° C) is small and therefore will have only negligible physiological implications.

Mechanisms of Urate Accumulation in Disease

There are three possible mechanisms of abnormal urate accumulation:

(i) Decreased destruction;
(ii) Decreased excretion;
(iii) Increased formation.
These are not mutually exclusive.

(i) *Decreased destruction* plays no part in urate accumulation or gout. Intestinal secretion (and the consequent bacterial breakdown) is greater, not less, in people with raised serum uric acid levels (Sorensen, 1965). The resultant ammonia is excreted partly in the faeces and partly in the urine.

(ii) *Decreased excretion.* Overt renal disease with nitrogen retention and hyperuricaemia seldom causes gout, but occasionally cases may be seen when gout can undoubtedly be ascribed to the hyperuricaemia induced by primary renal disease, e.g. in renal artery stenosis (Page & Kimmelstiel, 1966) or traumatic ischaemia (Mertz & Schindera, 1968). Richet *et al.* (1965), record 17 such cases including polycystic disease, membranous nephritis, amyloidosis, preceding gout by 10–20 years. The rarity of such cases is accounted for probably by the compensatory tubular mechanisms which come into play in ordinary renal disease (McPhaul, 1968).

On the other hand, decreased urate clearance of some degree is seen in a high proportion of cases of gouty patients, that is, in people who have long-standing hyperuricaemia and often without nitrogen retention. Such impairment is only very rarely associated with tophaceous deposits of urate in the kidney; and similarly only very rarely do we see the acute oliguria of uric acid crystal blockage, usually in rashly treated secondary gout due to reticulosis or polycythaemia. The hyperuricaemia and gout associated with hypercalcaemia is seen most commonly in hyperparathyroidism (Bywaters *et al.*, 1963), but may perhaps occur also with the hypercalcaemia of sarcoidosis (Scott, Dixon & Bywaters, 1964). It is probably due to renal tubular damage associated with calcium deposition, as many have shown nephrocalcinosis.

Other types of disease associated with decreased clearance include myxoedema (Ryckewaert *et al.*, 1967; Scott, 1966) and lactic acidosis, either familial (Sussman *et al.*, 1968) or isolated (Isomaki & Kreus, 1968).

Perhaps the most interesting forms of renal hyperuricaemia are those associated with hypertension and with plumbism, the former because it is common and the latter because it is nowadays rare.

Hypertension was associated with hyperuricaemia in 47% of 217 cases (Cannon *et al.*, 1966), but this cluster includes also hypertriglyceridaemia (Feldman & Wallace, 1964), hypercholesterolaemia (Harris-Jones, 1957), atherosclerosis (Gertler *et al.*, 1951), and in hyperlipidaemia (types 3, 4 and 5 with respectively hyperdysbetalipoproteinaemia, hyperprebeta- and mixed hyperlipidaemia) (Fredrickson *et al.*, 1967). Breckenridge (1966), studying cases at the Royal Postgraduate Medical School, found that 27% of untreated hypertensives had serum urate concentrations above 7·0 mg./100 ml. (males) or 6 mg./100 ml. (females). In such cases, turnover-rate was found to be normal (Arnott *et al.*, unpublished), although the pool of miscible uric acid was increased, as might be expected. Thus hyperuricaemia in these cases could be ascribed to renal secretory tubular defect, perhaps part of the same lesion that produced the hypertension.

Another type of hyperuricaemia is that leading to "Saturnine gout" due to plumbism, and also probably produced by renal tubular defect ("Bleiniere"). Saturnine gout as in Garrod's day (1870) is seen in painters (Ludwig, 1957) and others industrially exposed, and, in this day of the amateur, in those who make cider (Walls, 1969) and wine (Gounelle *et al.*, 1967) using lead glazed vessels, in distillers of "moonshine" whisky who use lead-patched accumulators (Morgan *et al.*, 1966), in burners of lead batteries (Ehrlich & Chokatos, 1966) and in children who eat the peeling lead paint of Queensland verandahs (Emmerson, 1963).

Thus, summarizing, there seems to be a specific tubular defect in renal hyperuricaemia not entailing nitrogen retention but presumably interfering with the active secretion of urate and perhaps of neutral amino acids (Kaplan *et al.*, 1969), and it is this segmental function that is affected by pyrazinamide (Petty & Dalrymple, 1964). Finally, there appears to be defective urate excretion in most over-producers (*q.v.*).

(iii) *Increased urate formation.* Over-production of urate is the most important mechanism in most patients with gout, and is due either (*a*) to increased nucleoprotein turnover (formerly called "secondary" gout) or (*b*) to aberrations of the metabolic pathway. An indication of increased production is given by a 24-hourly urinary excretion of more than 600 mg.; a more accurate measure is given by the incorporation of isotopically labelled precursor (such as glycine).

(*a*) *Increased nucleoprotein turnover* leading to hyperuricaemia is seen predominantly in myelo-proliferative disease, first and foremost poly-cythaemia vera, and sometimes secondary polycythaemia, in myeloid leukaemia and less frequently lymphocytic leukaemia, lymphosarcoma, occasionally in megaloblastic anaemia, sickle cell anaemia and oesteogenesis imperfecta. In these conditions there is both an increased formation and an increased breakdown of nucleoprotein. The body pool of urate is increased in one-third of these patients, serum urate is increased and daily urinary excretion usually exceeds 600 mg. There is also an increased incorporation of isotope label with urate, but, as in health, this occurs between the 10th and 14th day rather than in the first week, as occurs in "primary gout".

That is, purine is being metabolized through the normal pathways but at an excessive rate.

Increased nucleoprotein turnover seems a likely cause of the hyperuricaemia of psoriasis since there is a direct correlation between the extent of skin involvement and the serum uric acid level (Eisen & Seegmiller, 1961); 36% of patients with psoriatic arthritis have a raised serum uric acid level (Beveridge & Lawson, 1967).

(*b*) *Over-production of urate due to aberrations of the metabolic pathway.* So-called "primary" gout is usually due to over-production of urate, not as in the preceding category from increased nucleoprotein formation and breakdown along normal channels, but via "shunt" pathways: if these patients are given isotope-labelled glycine, the peak of labelled urinary urate occurs early, during the first few days rather than as in normals during the second week. However, several different mechanisms may be distinguished, and without doubt more remain to be discovered and characterized; the most dramatic and well known is that displayed in the Lesch-Nyhan syndrome, very well covered at the Vermont meeting of October 1967 (Proceedings edited by Bland, 1968). Others briefly mentionable include partial qualitative HGPRT deficiency (Kelley *et al.*, 1967*a*, *b*) and simulating syndromes —phenocopies without HGPRT deficiency (Nyhan *et al.*, 1969), mongolism (Down's syndrome) (Fuller *et al.*, 1962; Kaufman & O'Brien, 1967), glycogen storage disease of several types (*q.v.*) and hereditary fructose intolerance (Perheentupa & Raivio, 1967; Howell, 1968).

The *Lesch-Nyhan syndrome* was first described in 1963 (Lesch & Nyhan, 1963). The full syndrome comprises mental retardation, choreoathetosis, spastic cerebral palsy, self-mutilation and aggressive behaviour associated with hyperuricaemia and perhaps later tophaceous gout. It occurs in young boys and is inherited as an X-linked recessive character. There is excessive urate synthesis, about twenty times normal, with greatly increased urinary excretion. Seegmiller and his colleagues (1967) have shown that skin fibroblasts and erythrocytes in this sex-linked disorder lack the enzyme hypoxanthine–guanine phosphoribosyl transferase (HGPRTse). No activity is measurable in brain or liver. In normal circumstances this enzyme converts hypoxanthine and guanine in the presence of phosphoribosyl pyrophosphate (PRPP) (which contributes its ribose-5-phosphate) back to their respective mononucleotides, inosinic (IMP) and guanylic acid GMP): it also converts xanthine to xanthylic acid (XMP). This "re-utilization" is performed for adenine by a separate enzyme (APRTse) which has been found deficient in another family without, however, urate abnormalities (Kelley *et al.*, 1968); in the Lesch-Nyhan children the latter enzyme is not only present but increased and changed in regard to its heat-stability.

Thus, in normal man nucleic acid synthesis can proceed directly from the first step in purine synthesis (glutamine + PRPP) through inosinic acid (IMP), or alternatively it can derive through HGPRTse and APTse from the free purine bases guanine and adenine—the so-called "salvage" route. How such enzyme deficiency produces the accelerated urate synthesis of the Lesch-Nyhan syndrome continues to be a subject of much discussion and experiment: decreased feedback inhibition at the first committed stage and rate-limiting step of purine synthesis (PRPP + glutamine mediated by PRPP amido-transferase) might be produced by decrease in guanylic acid; the availability of PRPP would also be increased (discussed fully by Kelley, 1968) and this has been shown to be increased in Lesch-Nyhan fibroblast cell cultures (Rosenbloom, 1968) which have, as expected, increased purine synthesis and lack HGPRTse. (Azathioprine does not inhibit purine synthesis in these patients since they lack the enzyme necessary to convert it to the nucleotide responsible for its pseudo-feedback inhibition of PRPP amido-transferase.)

Mosaicism in female heterozygotes, postulated by Seegmiller *et al.* has been confirmed (Migeon *et al.*, 1968), providing the third example of the Lyon hypothesis. The relationship of biochemical changes to neurological dysfunction remains an exciting field for research. As Bland has pointed out, "the possibility that we might identify biochemical mechanisms mediating aggressive human behaviour is of great importance in human affairs" (1968), but the self-mutilation produced in the rat by the equivalent in man of 80 cups of coffee/day has not so far provided a very meaningful answer. Nor has early detection (at 94 hours after birth (Marks *et al.*, 1968)) and prompt treatment of these children with allopurinol, with satisfactory fall in serum urate levels, provided any protection against the development of mental retardation, spasticity and self-mutilation.

Study of this fascinating mutation is complicated (perhaps ultimately made easier) by the existence of phenocopies, e.g. a patient with retarded development, mental retardation, unusual autistic behaviour with extreme hyperuricaemia and over-production of urate, but normal levels of HGPRTase. On allopurinol the total purine excretion fell as in normals, as did the ratio of hypoxanthine to xanthine, unlike the full L–N syndrome. On the other hand, adenine PRTase was increased (Nyhan *et al.*, 1969). Hooft *et al.* (1968), has recorded a girl of 3 years with mental retardation, choreoathetosis and self-mutilation with normal serum uric acid levels, heavy isotope incorporation but maximal at the fifth day (not at 12 as in Lesch-Nyhan syndrome) and slightly increased urate excretion.

Partial deficiency of this important enzyme has been shown to occur in adult gouty over-producers of urate (Kelley *et al.*, 1967*a*, *b*). A personal case recorded by Bluestone (1968) (and included by Kelley *et al.*, in their comprehensive review, 1969) showed mental impairment and epilepsy; allopurinol has helped his gout, reduced his tophi and enabled him to hold down a job.

Urine uric acid/creatinine ratio, normally 0·5 in adults (1·5 in first week of life), is increased to 3·2 in Lesch-Nyhan syndrome, 1·0 in adult partial deficiency, up to 0·75 in secondary gout and up to 0·53 in ordinary gout (Kaufman *et al.*, 1968). The definitive enzyme method measures the incorporation of ^{14}C-labelled hypoxanthine or guanine into inosinic or guanylic acid by red cells or fibroblasts (Berman *et al.*, 1968; Kelley *et al.*, 1967*a*, *b*).

A quite different metabolic fault associated with over-production of urate is *glycogen storage disease*. This has been classified into a number of different types depending on the particular enzyme defect (*q.v.*). Type I (lacking glucose-6-phosphatase) is associated with hyperuricaemia (Alepa *et al.*, 1967; Fine & Strauss, 1967) and gout (von Hoyningen-Huene, 1966), only partly explained by competition with urate excretion by lactate and keto acids at the renal tubular level. Increased synthesis has been shown by Kelley *et al.* (1968), and by Jakovic & Sorensen (1967). Another type of glycogen storage disease associated with absence of liver phosphorylase and increased lactate levels (Type VI) is also associated with hyperuricaemia (Brombacher *et al.*, 1964). Howell has suggested that deficiency of glucose-6-phosphatase blocking the conversion of glycogen to glucose might lead to increased conversion of glucose-6-phosphate to PRPP (reviewed by Howell, 1968), but this would not apply to Type VI with hyperuricaemia.

New methods for the control of gout and hyperuricaemia have also been modelled on analogue blockade—e.g. allopurinol, an analogue of hypoxanthine effectively blocking the conversion of hypoxanthine and xanthine to uric acid by xanthine oxidase (Scott, 1966 (ed.)). Perhaps the most exciting aspect of the entire field is the relationship to learning and intellectual and mental development: elucidation of mechanisms in these rather esoteric cases might be of universal value.

VARIETIES OF TISSUE CALCIFICATION

The deposition of calcium salts in the tissues of the body is of several kinds:

(i) *Preceding and associated with normal bone formation* (developmental).

(ii) *Senescent calcification*, seen in costal cartilage of healthy people often at comparatively early ages and due not to any alteration of serum levels but to local cartilage changes (*q.v.*).

(iii) *Dystrophic calcification*, seen in scar tissue, degenerating fibroids, tuberculous glands, walled-off abscesses, atherosclerotic plaques, following fat necrosis (e.g. in acute pancreatitis) muscle necrosis in myocardial infarction or crush syndrome, in paraplegia or poliomyelitis, in the intervertebral discs in alkaptonuria, and in the blood vessels and ligaments in the heredo-familial vascular and articular calcification described by Sharp (1954). The serum levels and metabolism of phosphorus and calcium are not deranged in these patients, and the deposition depends upon a local anomaly.

In a wide survey of autopsy and biopsy material or pathological tissue calcification, 96% of specimens showed apatite (Gatter & McCarty, 1967), all except the pineal gland, carbonate apatite, and four examples of Whitlockite (β Ca_3 $(PO_4)_2$ or β calcium orthophosphate.)

(iv) *Metastatic calcification*, seen in conditions such as hyperparathyroidism, hypoparathyroidism, pseudo-hypoparathyroidism, hyperphosphataemia due to renal disease, sarcoidosis, hypervitaminosis D, excessive intake of milk and alkaline powders, and generalized affections of bone (as from myelomatosis, leukaemia, sarcoidosis, Paget's disease, osteomyelitis or metastatic carcinoma). In this group there are abnormalities of calcium and phosphate levels in the blood plasma and tissue fluid, and a Ca $\times$ P product usually greater than 40 associated with the deposition of calcium in the lungs, kidney, cornea, arteries, stomach, pulmonary vein and left atrium; this distribution is dependent (Wells, 1915) on local alkalinity and a low CO_2 tension due to excretion of acid, and was not seen for instance by Egoville (1938) in the stomach of a patient without free acid secretion.

(v) *Oxalosis.* This is a rare condition where calcium oxalate is deposited in the media of arteries, in bone marrow and other organs, particularly the kidneys where it may make up to 10·3% of the wet weight of the kidney (Chon & Donohue, 1952), leading to progressive renal failure. There is usually no deposition in joints (Scowen, Stansfeld & Watts, 1959), although gout-like arthropathy has been recorded (McLaurin *et al.*, 1961). It probably represents the late stage of primary hyperoxaluria, a familial genetically determined enzyme defect resulting in an over-production of oxalate from glyoxylate (Scowen, Crawhall & Watts, 1958), perhaps abated by carbimide treatment (Solomons, Goodman & Riley, 1967).

(vi) *Chondrocalcinosis or pseudogout.* Chondrocalcinosis articularis diffusus (Losada *et al.*, 1957; Ravault, Lejeune & Maitrepierre, 1959) or "pseudogout" (McCarty, Kohn & Faires, 1962) is a condition where calcium pyrophosphate dihydrate ($Ca_2P_2O_7.2H_2O$) is deposited symmetrically throughout the body in articular cartilage and fibrocartilage, and often in the synovial membrane of joints and tendon sheaths. Clinically it is characterized by recurrent attacks of joint pain and inflammation, usually in the knees but involving sometimes elbows, hips, wrists, ankles and shoulders.

The attacks are acutely painful, transient and recurrent, often being mistaken for true gout, showing local swelling, heat, redness and tenderness. One or more joints may be involved, and like gout, a chronic lesion may follow repeated attacks. Radiologically, calcification is seen in hyaline, and more characteristically in fibrocartilage—e.g. in the triangular ligament of the wrist, and the menisci of the knee. Similar cartilage calcification is seen in Wilson's disease (Boudin, Pepin & Hubault, 1963) and in haemochromatosis (Hamilton *et al.*, 1968), where attacks of pseudogout may occur, also without hypercalcaemia. Similar deposits in cartilage, fibro- and hyaline, are seen radiologically in hypercalcaemic states of which the most important is hyperparathyroidism (Bywaters, Dixon & Scott, 1963). Not only is the distribution similar but the crystals appear also to be calcium pyrophosphate. Other deposits may occur in hypercalcaemic states which need differentiation from "pseudogout". Patients with sarcoidosis may also have calcific deposits with pseudogout attacks (Solomon & Channick, 1960; Cabot Case Record, 1961), and such deposits may persist long after the transient hypercalcaemia has subsided, as in a patient we have followed for many years, briefly referred to by Scott (1966).

The diagnosis is confirmed by aspiration of

synovial fluid in which crystals of calcium pyrophosphate may be found free or within leucocytes, easily recognized in polarized light. They must be distinguished from the sodium urate crystals of gout, and this distinction is achieved not only by their shape but more reliably by determination of the sign of bire-fringence (Currey, 1968) or as a research procedure by X-ray diffraction.

The biochemical mechanism of calcium pyro-phosphate crystal precipitation and why it should preponderantly occur in cartilage are not known. Its occurrence in families (Zitnan & Sit'aj, 1963) supports a genetic mechanism, but no enzyme defect has yet been discovered. It seems possible that local pyrophosphatase might be lacking or inhibited. Like so many other metabolic anomalies, the end result may be produced by several different mechanisms and the calcification seen in overt hypercalcaemia due most frequently to hyperparathyroidism obviously has a more direct mechanism.

(vii) *Other types of para-articular calcium salt deposition* include that of calcium hydrogen phosphate dihydrate ($CaHPO_4 2H_2O$), crystals with strong positive birefringence showing radiologically in the menisci of the knee joint as punctate deposits of small size (McCarty *et al.*, 1966) and also of apatite (McCarty & Gatter, 1966). The latter is associated with recurrent acute inflammatory episodes in the neighbourhood of joints and in bursae or as solitary deposits in the menisci of the knees (McCarty *et al.*, 1966). In addition, Currey *et al.* (1966) have tentatively identified some crystals in the knee joint as those of calcium oxalate with strong positive birefringence. Calcific polytendinitis (Cohen & Bywaters, 1969) or peritendinitis calcanea (Bossi, 1954) may present with acute episodes resembling gout and are thought to be due to hydroxy-apatite deposition (Thompson *et al.*, 1968).

(viii) *Calcinosis.* This is a deposition of Ca salts in the connective tissue of skin, panniculus and fasciae, usually without demonstrable alteration in serum levels of calcium, phosphate or alkaline phosphatase, or in metabolism apart from tissue retention. It has usually been regarded as a disease *sui generis*, although some regard it as only a manifestation of tissue injury in certain collagen diseases, e.g. dermatomyositis and scleroderma (Wheeler, Curtis, Cawley, Grekin & Zheutlin, 1952). However, the majority of patients with scleroderma or dermatomyositis fail to develop calcification, even in some cases after massive dosage of vitamin D (Cornbleet &

Struck, 1937). Conversely, many patients with calcinosis fail to give a history of or show signs consistent with dermatomyositis or scleroderma. Radiological examination in the early stage of connective tissue inflammation may fail to show calcification (Rothstein & Welt, 1936 (Case 2); Rudolph, 1934). We have examined biopsy material from a boy who later developed calcinosis universalis and found little abnormality except muscle atrophy, collagen fibre increase and collections of monocytes and plasma cells. We conclude that in certain people a local or generalized inflammatory or degenerative lesion of connective tissue, resembling clinically derma-tomyositis or scleroderma, leads to the deposition of calcium salts in connective tissue locally or generally.

These deposits have been frequently analysed (see reviews and references listed by Wheeler *et al.*, 1952). The most reliable analyses indicate that this type of pathological calcium deposit is similar chemically to normal bone salt, an apatite approximating to dahlite with a formula of $2Ca_3(PO_4)_2.CaCO_3$ (see detailed discussion by Armstrong, 1950). This is not surprising since both bone salt and calcinotic deposits must be in equilibrium with the homeostatically maintained tissue fluid. This gives a theoretical Ca/P ratio of 2·2/1, agreeing well with Bauer, Marble & Bennett's (1931) figure of 2·16 and Brooks' (1934) ratio of 2·15, both from calcinotic nodules. Most authors give 80% $Ca_3(PO_4)_2$, 15 to 22% $CaCO_3$, e.g. Piersall (1933), Bolam (1935). The residual Ca/P ratio of those two analyses (i.e. total Ca *minus* carbonate Ca) reaches 1·87 and 1·88 and for Bolam (1935) 1·78, compared with a theoretical ratio of 1·94 for dahlite and a value for bone ranging between 1·88 and 2·01 (Kramer & Shear, 1928). Other analyses are more variable (Turpin, Brun & Guillamin, 1934; Comroe, Chamberlin & Sunderman, 1939). Water is a variable fraction, from 50 to 67%, with traces of Mg and Fe, 13 and 80 mg./100 g. respectively (Turpin *et al.* 1934) and minimal amounts of uric acid (4 mg./100 g.), cholesterol (415 mg./100 g.), and fatty acids (1% dry weight) according to Bauer *et al.* (1931). X-ray diffraction studies showed an apatite pattern (Pedersen, 1943; Zellweger, 1948; Cornbleet, Reed & Reed, 1949) as is seen also in aortic calcification. Material from one of our cases of dermatomyositis with calcinosis has shown 15 mg. Ca per 100 mg. wet weight (Loewi & Dorling, 1964) and has been identified by X-ray diffraction as apatite (Cochrane & Davies, 1965) as has material from *calcinosis cutis* (Paegle, 1966).

While blood levels of Ca, P or phosphatase are usually normal in calcinosis, occasionally high levels are reported from reliable sources (e.g. Brooks, 1934, whose patient showed 12·1–13·7 mg. Ca/100 ml., 5·2–7·7 mg./100 ml. inorganic P and 0·3–0·4 Kay units alkaline phosphatase/100 ml.). We have two boys aet. 12 and 14 under observation with a plasma alkaline phosphatase ranging up to 25 and 28 King-Armstrong units per 100 ml. respectively, not explicable in terms of liver or bone disease and with no abnormality other than calcinosis. The upper level of normal at this age would be 15 K.A. units/100 ml. Pedersen (1943) has described a case with raised blood uric acid in the absence of azotaemia. Azotaemia usually indicates metastatic rather then dystrophic calcification.

Metabolic balances are usually normal (e.g. Friedlander, 1930; and references in Atkinson & Weber, 1938; Wheeler et al. 1952), but may show Ca and P retention even on low Ca intake (Bauer et al., 1931; Brooks, 1934) due presumably to deposition in the soft tissues. A negative balance has occasionally been seen (e.g. by Turpin et al. 1934), but this need occasion no surprise, since it is well recognized that these Ca deposits often disappear rapidly with or without specific treatment, cf. Craig & Lyall (1931) in 6 weeks; Brooks (1934), Briggs & Illingworth (1952) in 6 weeks; Swanson, Forster & Iob (1933) in 5 weeks; Sheldon (1938), although Sheldon's case may have been one of hypervitaminosis D. We conclude, therefore, that in dystrophic calcification and in calcinosis universalis the important abnormality is a local one, in the calcifying tissue itself.

(ix) *Tumoral calcinosis.* These large often rapidly growing deposits, usually over buttocks, trochanters or other bony areas (McClatchie & Bremner, 1969) have been described in sibs (Duret, 1899, cit. Lafferty, Reynolds & Pearson, 1965). The chalky masses (12 G.% of calcium) consist of almost pure tribasic calcium phosphate $Ca_3(PO_4)_2$ (Lafferty et al., 1965) which showed a daily net accretion of 200 mg./day but an exchange of 5 G./day calcium. These authors, using isotope incorporation, found calcium metabolism normal, and alkaline phosphatase normal, but noted, as have others, a high serum phosphorus, attributed by Wilber and Statopolsky (1968) to an inherited reduction in tubular response to the phosphaturic action of parathyroid hormone. There is obviously, however, a local factor which determines where and in what tissue the calcium is deposited.

The Local Factor

We know little as yet of the processes by which Ca salts are deposited in some tissues under normal conditions, e.g. to form bones. As McLean (1952) has remarked, "What is it that keeps everything else from being calcified?" Our knowledge of pathological calcification is even less complete, but many of the steps may prove to be of a similar character. In general, while the formation of Ca soaps as a result of fat breakdown may occur as an initial step, for instance, in acute pancreatitis, and while phosphate liberation from necrotic muscle in the "crush syndrome" may cause immediate precipitation of calcium phosphate, these are initial steps only and occur only under unusual conditions. Ultimately, and in all long-standing calcification, Ca salts of varying composition are deposited in a certain kind of matrix which may be normal epiphyseal cartilage, ageing rib cartilage or connective tissue which contains not only several varieties of chondroitin sulphate (Meyer & Rapport, 1951) but also other polysaccharides. What is the abnormality of the matrix in calcinosis which determines the local formation of such precipitates? Histologically there may be fibrosis, some mild round cell infiltration with a few giant cells and fibroblast proliferation surrounding the Ca deposits. Muscle is normal apart from some atrophy: connective tissue only is affected, usually that of subcutaneous tissue and fasciae, occasionally of the fat lobules surrounding individual fat cells (Bolam, 1935; Bauer et al., 1931). Occasionally a "hyaline degeneration" of connective tissue has been noted, but its significance is not clear (Jaddasohn, 1910; Versé, 1912), and we ourselves have also noted apparent calcification of individual fibres in fixed tissue sections as one of the initial changes. These fibres stain weakly with the periodic acid-Schiff method until after decalcification with versene when they stain more strongly; they resemble elastic fibres.

Chondroitin sulphuric acid may be important in normal and pathological calcification since it binds calcium (in the absence of serum, Howard, 1953). Cartilage probably acts somewhat like an ion-exchange resin, absorbing Ca ions up to the point where deposition as phosphate occurs, then taking up more (Eichelberger & Roma, 1954; Sobel & Burger, 1954). Its milliequivalent capacity to take up Na, Ca or Ba is proportional to its sulphate content (Boyd & Neuman, 1951). Calcification of cartilage in vitro is prevented by previous exposure to protamine (Sobel, 1952) and to a metachromatic dye such as toluidine blue, both of which are known to combine with chondroitin sulphate. These basic dyes, however, unlike alizarin, permit cartilage to remove Ca and phosphate from solution (Miller, Waldman & McLean, 1952). In support of this is the observation by Levine, Rubin, Follis & Howard (1949) that amorphous material from a calcinotic nodule stains metachromatically and gives a positive periodic-Schiff reaction, as also do the crystals. After decalcification the crystal sites also stain metachromatically. This still fails to indicate why some connective tissues containing polysaccharide calcify and others do not. As in bone, the collagen fibres of cartilage may act as crystal inducers, and, once crystal seeding has occurred, body levels of Ca and P are adequate to maintain apatite formation. Solomons & Neuman (1960) suggest that the ϵ-amino group of collagen is the inducing site; and that an inhibitor normally exists, perhaps organic phosphate, normally hydrolysed locally by phosphatase in the process of Ca deposition and bone formation. It is known that collagen fibres reconstituted in phosphate buffer undergo rapid calcification *in vivo* (Mergenhagen *et al.*, 1960). In costal cartilage which calcifies with age, the ageing process is associated with a decrease in relative quantity and in polymerization (judged by viscosity and periodate consumption) of chondroitin sulphate (Loewi, 1953). This is shown histochemically by decreased metachromasia and increased periodic-Schiff staining.

In chondrocalcinosis, pyrophosphate accumulation in cartilage may be due to local lack of pyrophosphatase. This (as alkaline phosphatase) is thought to destroy pyrophosphate which itself is an inhibitor of Ca salt precipitation (Fleish and Neuman, 1961) perhaps by absorption on to existing hydroxy-apatite crystals. However, in hypophosphatasia with greatly decreased alkaline phosphatase and increased renal excretion of pyrophosphate (Russell, 1965) although bone is defective, there is no cartilage calcification.

Treatment

From the gross overall biochemical viewpoint, patients with calcinosis have too much Ca. Depletion measures have improved a few patients, but many fail to gain relief and progression occurs. Rarely, spontaneous recovery is seen, but in some of such recorded cases there is the possibility of confusion with hypervitaminosis D. The use of "sequestrene" (ethylenediamine tetra-acetate) in the form of the trisodium salt by mouth will remove Ca from the gut (Rubin, 1953), but this is of little practical use. Intravenous EDTA given over a three-week period has produced functional and radiological improvement in calcinosis universalis (Davies & Moe, 1959). Longer established but perhaps less effective methods include a low Ca diet and the giving by mouth of disodium hydrogen phosphate in a dosage of 4 g. with each meal (Craig & Lyall, 1931). Ca deposits in sarcoidosis disappear with steroid therapy. Corticotropin has been followed by improvement in some cases of calcinosis (Briggs & Illingworth, 1952), but usually is disappointing (Silva, Ponde & Lichtenberg, 1953; Scott & DeLilly, 1954). It has been observed to increase the Ca output in the bile (Burnett & Flink, 1954).

AMYLOIDOSIS

In view of the recent publication (Mandema *et al.*, 1968) of the proceedings of a symposium on amyloid disease covering all aspects, including biochemical, this topic is not included in the present book.

References

The Chemistry of Normal Connective Tissue
ANDERSON, A. J. (1962). *Biochem. J.*, **82**, 372.
AXELROD, A. E. & MARTIN, C. J. (1953). *Proc. Soc exp. Biol., N.Y.*, **83**, 463.
BALO, J. & BANGA, I. (1950). *Biochem. J.*, **46**, 384.
BANFIELD, W. G. (1952). *Proc. Soc. exp. Biol., N.Y.*, **81**, 658.
BEAN, W. B., DREVETS, C. C. & CHAPMAN, J. S. (1958). *Medicine*, **54**, 353.
BORNSTEIN, P. & PIEZ, K. A. (1966). *Biochemistry*, **5**, 3803.
BOWES, J. H. (1953). In "Nature and Structure of Collagen", p. 49. Ed. Randall, J. T. Discussion. London, Butterworth.

BOWES, J. H., ELLIOTT, R. G. & MOSS, J. A. (1953). In "Nature and Structure of Collagen", p. 199. Ed. Randall, J. T. London, Butterworth.
BOWES, J. H. & KENTEN, R. H. (1948). *Biochem. J.*, **43**, 358.
BOWES, J. H. & KENTEN, R. H. (1949). *Biochem. J.*, **45**, 281.
BOWES, J. H. & MOSS, J. A. (1951). *Nature (Lond.)*, **168**, 514.
BOWES, J. H. & MOSS, J. A. (1954). *Biochem. J.*, **55**, 735.
BRAY, B. A., LIEBERMAN, R. & MEYER, K. (1967). *J. biol. Chem.*, **242**, 3373.
BREWER, D. B. (1957). *J. Path. Bact.*, **74**, 371.

BROWN, P. C., CONSDEN, R. & GLYNN, L. E. (1958). *Ann. rheum. Dis.*, **17**, 196.

BYWATERS, E. G. L. (1937). *J. Path. Bact.*, **44**, 247.

BYWATERS, E. G. L., HOLBOROW, E. J. & KEECH, M. K. (1951). *Brit. med. J.*, **2**, 1178.

CAPUTTO, R., LELOIR, L. F., CARDINI, C. E. & PALADINI, A. C. (1950). *J. biol. Chem.*, **184**, 333.

CHAIN, E. & DUTHIE, E. S. (1939). *Nature (Lond.)*, **144**, 977.

CONSDEN, R., GLYNN, L. E. & STANIER, W. M. (1953). *Biochem. J.*, **55**, 248.

COURTS, A. (1960). *Biochem. J.*, **74**, 238.

DAVIES, H. R. & KELSALL, A. R. (1961). *Ann. rheum. Dis.*, **20**, 189.

DORFMAN, A. & LORINCZ, A. E. (1957). *Proc. nat. Acad. Sci.*, **43**, 443.

DURAN-REYNALS, F. (1928). *C.R. Soc. Biol., Paris*, **99**, 6.

EASTOE, J. E. (1967). In "Treatise on Collagen". Vol. 1; p. 1. Ed. Ramachandran G. N., Academic Press, New York.

EICHELBERGER, L., AKESON, W. H. & ROMA, M. (1958). *J. Bone Jt. Surg.*, **40-A**, 142.

EVANSON, J. M., JEFFREY, J. J. & KRANE, S. M. (1968). *J. clin. Invest.*, **47**, 2639.

GALLOP, P. M. (1964). *Biophys. J.*, **4**, 79.

GLEGG, R. E., EIDINGER, D. & LEBLOND, C. P. (1953). *Science*, **118**, 614.

GLYNN, L. E. (1957–8). Lectures on the Scientific Basis of Medicine. University of London. London, Vol. 7, p. 359.

GLYNN, L. E. & LOEWI, G. (1952). *J. Path. Bact.*, **64**, 329.

GORDON, E. J., PERLMAN, A. W. & SCHECHTER, N. (1948). *J. Bone Jt. Surg.*, **30-A**, 944.

GRASSMAN, quoted by CRAWHALL, J. C. & ELLIOTT, D. F. (1955). *Nature (Lond.)*, **175**, 299.

GREGORY, J. D., LAURENT, T. C. & RODEN, L. (1964). *J. biol. Chem.*, **239**, 3312.

GROSS, E., HIGHBERGER, J. H. & SCHMITT, F. O. (1954). *Proc. nat. Acad. Sci., USA*, **40**, 679.

GROSS, E. & WITKOP, B. (1962). *J. biol. Chem.*, **237**, 1856.

GROSS, J. (1958). *J. exp. Med.*, **108**, 215.

GROSS, J., HIGHBERGER, J. H. & SCHMITT, F. O. (1952). *Proc. Soc. exp. Biol., N.Y.*, **80**, 462.

GROSS, J. & SCHMITT, F. O. (1948). *J. exp. Med.*, **88**, 555.

GUSTAVSON, K. H. (1955). *Nature (Lond.)*, **175**, 70.

HALL, D. A., REED, R. & TUNBRIDGE, R. E. (1952). *Nature (Lond.)*, **170**, 264.

HALL, D. A. & SAXL, H. (1961). *Proc. roy. Soc. B.*, **155**, 202.

HANNIG, K. & NORDWIG, A. (1967). In "Treatise on Collagen". Vol. 1; p. 73. Ed. Ramachandran, G. N.: Academic Press, New York.

HAPPEY, F., WISEMAN, A. & NAYLOR, A. (1961). *Nature (Lond.)*, **192**, 868.

HARDING, J. J. (1965). *Adv. Protein Chem.*, **20**, 109.

HARKNESS, R. D., MARKO, A. M., MUIR, H. M. & NEUBERGER, A. (1954). *Biochem. J.*, **56**, 558.

HILLS, G. M. (1940). *Biochem. J.*, **34**, 1070.

HILZ, H. & LIPMANN, F. (1955). *Proc. nat. Acad. Sci., Wash.*, **41**, 880.

HODGE, A. J., PETRUSKA, J. A. & BAILEY, A. J. (1965). In "Structure and function of connective and skeletal tissues". Ed. Fitton-Jackson, S., Harkness, R. D., Partridge, S. M. & Tristram, G. R. Butterworths, London.

HULTH, A. & WESTERBORN, O. (1959). *J. Bone Jt. Surg.*, **41-B**, 836.

JACKSON, D. S. & FESSLER, J. H. (1955). *Nature (Lond.)*, **176**, 69.

KANG, A. H., NAGAI, Y., PIEZ, K. A. & GROSS, J. (1966). *Biochemistry*, **5**, 509.

KAPLAN, D. & MEYER, K. (1959). *Nature (Lond.)*, **183**, 1267.

KEFALIDES, N. A. & WINZLER, R. J. (1966). *Biochemistry*, **5**, 702.

KRAMER, H. & LITTLE, K. (1953). In "Nature and Structure of Collagen", p. 33. Ed. Randall, J. T. London, Butterworth.

LACK, C. H. (1959). *J. Bone Jt. Surg.*, **41-B**, 384.

LACK, C. H. & ROGERS, H. J. (1958). *Nature (Lond.)*, **182**, 948.

LASKIN, D. M., ENGEL, M. B., JOSEPH, N. R. & POLLAK, V. E. (1961), *J. Clin. Invest.*, **40**, 2153.

LINKER, A., HOFFMANN, P., SAMPSON, P. & MEYER, K. (1958). *Biochim. biophys. acta*, **29**, 443.

LOEWI, G. (1953). *J. Path. Bact.*, **65**, 381.

LOEWI, G. & MEYER, K. (1958). *Biochim. biophys. acta*, **27**, 453.

McCLUSKEY, R. T. & THOMAS, L. (1959). *Amer. J. Path*, **35**, 819.

McMASTER, P. D. & PARSONS, R. J. (1950). *Ann. New York Acad. Sci.*, **52**, 992.

MANDEMA, E., VAN DER SCHAAF, P. C. & HUISMAN, T. H. J. (1955). *J. Lab. clin. Med.*, **45**, 261.

MATTHEWS, B. F. (1952). *Brit. med. J.*, **2**, 1295.

MAXIMOW, A. A. & BLOOM, W. (1944). "A Textbook of Histology", p. 55. 4th Ed. Philadelphia, Saunders.

MEYER, K. & CHAFFEE, E. (1941). *J. biol. Chem.*, **138**, 491.

MEYER, K., GRUNBACH, M. M., LINKER, A. & HOFFMAN, P. (1958). *Proc. Soc. exp. Biol., N.Y.*, **97**, 275.

MEYER, K., LINKER, A., DAVIDSON, E. A. & WEISSMANN, B. (1953). *J. biol. Chem.*, **205**, 611.

MEYER, K. & PALMER, J. W. (1934). *J. biol. Chem.*, **107**, 629.

MORGAN, W. T. J. & WATKINS, W. M. (1956). *Nature (Lond.)*, **177**, 521.

MORRIONE, T. G. (1952). *J. exp. Med.*, **96**, 107.

NAGEOTTE, J. (1927). *C.R. Soc. Biol., Paris*, **96**, 172, 464 & 828.

NEUMAN, R. E. & LOGAN, M. A. (1950). *J. biol. Chem.*, **186**, 549.

NEUMAN, R. E. & TYTELL, A. A. (1950). *Proc. Soc. exp. Biol., N.Y.*, **73**, 409.

O'BRIEN, W. M., BANFIELD, W. G. & SOKOLOFF, L. (1961). *Arth. & Rheumat.*, **4**, 137.

OREKHOVICH, K. D. (1950). *C.R. Acad. Sci. U.R.S.S.*, **71**, 521.

PAL, S. & SCHUBERT, M. (1965). *J. biol. Chem.*, **240**, 3245.

PARTRIDGE, S. M. & DAVIS, H. F. (1958). *Biochem. J.*, **68**, 298.

PARTRIDGE, S. M., ELSDEN, D. F. & THOMAS, J. (1963). *Nature (Lond.)*, **197**, 1297, and **200**, 651.

PEARCE, R. H. & WATSON, E. M. (1949). *Canad. J. Res., E.*, **27**, 43.

PEARSON, C. M., KLINE, H. M. & NEWCOMER, V. D. (1960). *New Engl. J. Med.*, **263**, 51.

PIEZ, K. A. & GROSS, J. (1960), *J. biol. Chem.*, **235**, 995.

PIEZ, K. A., WEISS, E. & LEWIS, M. S. (1960). *J. biol. Chem.*, **235**, 995.

PIEZ, K. A., LEWIS, M. S., MARTIN, G. R. & GROSS, J. (1961). *Biochim. biophys. Acta.*, **53**, 596.

PIEZ, K. A. (1967). In "Treatise on Collagen". Vol. 1; p. 207. Ed. Ramachandran, G. N.: Academic Press, NewYork.

RAMACHANDRAN, G. N. & KARTHA, G. (1954). *Nature (Lond.)*, **172**, 269.

RICH, A. & CRICK, F. H. (1955). *Nature (Lond.)*, **176**, 915.

RODEN, L. & SMITH, R. (1966). *J. biol. Chem.*, **241**, 5949.

ROSENTHAL, O., BOWIE, M. A. & WAGONER, G. (1941). *J. cell. comp. Physiol.*, **17**, 221.

RUBENS-DUVAL, A., VILLIAUMEY, J. & LUBERTZKI, D. (1961). *Rev. Rhumat.*, **28**, 423.

RUBIN, A. L., PFAHL, D., SPEAKMAN, P. T., DAVISON, P. F. & SCHMITT, F. O. (1963). *Science*, **139**, 37.

SHATTON, J. & SCHUBERT, M. (1954), *J. biol. Chem.*, **211**, 565.

SHERRY, S., TROLL, W. & ROSENBLUM, E. D. (1954). *Proc. Soc. exp. Biol., N.Y.*, **87**, 125.

SILBERBERG, R. & SILBERBERG, M. (1950). *Amer. J. Path.*, **26**, 113.

SNELLMAN, O. (1963). *Acta. chem. scand.*, **17**, 1057.

STECHER, R. M. & HERSH, A. H. (1944). *J. clin. Invest.*, **23**, 699.

THOMAS, J. & PARTRIDGE, S. M. (1960). *Biochem. J.*, **74**, 600.

THOMAS, L. (1956). *J. exp. Med.*, **104**, 245.

THOMAS, L., MCCLUSKEY, R. T., POTTER, J. L. & WEISSMANN, G. (1960). *J. exp. Med.*, **111**, 705.

TOMLIN, S. G. (1953). *Nature (Lond.)*, **171**, 302.

TSALTAS, T. T. (1958). *J. exp. Med.*, **108**, 507.

WATSON, M. R. (1958). *Biochem. J.*, **68**, 416.

WHITEHEAD, R. G. (1960). *J. Bone Jt. Surg.*, **42**-B, 155.

Rheumatoid Arthritis

ADACHI, M., ATSUMI, T., SAITO, N., NAKAMURA, M. & HORIUCHI, Y. (1969). *Int. Arch. All.* **35**, 77.

AHO, K. (1961). *Ann. Med. exp. Biol. Fenn.*, **39**, Suppl. 7.

BETT, I. M. (1962). *Ann. rheum. Dis.*, **21**, 63.

BIEN, E. J. & ZIFF, M. (1951). *Proc. Soc. exp. Biol., N.Y.*, **78**, 327.

BOAKE, W. C. & LOVELL, R. R. H. (1954). *Brit. J. exp. Path.*, **35**, 350.

BRENDSTRUP, P. (1953). *Acta med. scand.*, **146**, 384.

BUNIM, J. J., BURCH, T. A. & O'BRIEN, W. M. (1964). *Bull. rheum. Dis.*, **15**, 349.

CONSDEN, R., GLYNN, L. E. & STAINER, W. M. (1953). *Biochem. J.*, **55**, 248.

DELLER, D. J., URBAN, E., IBBOTSON, R. N., HORWOOD, J., MILAZZO, S. & ROBSON, H. N. (1966), *Brit. med. J.*, **1**, 765.

DIXON, A. ST. J. & BYWATERS, E. G. L. (1953). *Clin. Sci.*, **12**, 15.

EVANSON, J. M., JEFFREY, J. J. & KRANE, S. M. (1968). *J. clin. Invest.*, **47**, 2639.

FABER, V. & IVERSON, M. (1952). *Acta med. scand.*, **143**, 436.

FAWNS, H. T. & LANDELLS, J. W. (1954). *Ann. rheum. Dis.*, **13**, 28.

FRANKLIN, E. C., HOLMAN, H. R., MÜLLER-EBERHARD, H. J. & KUNKEL, H. G. (1957). *J. exp. Med.*, **105**, 425.

GERBER, D. A. (1966). *Arthr. Rheum.*, **IX**, 795.

GITLIN, D., CRAIG, J. M. & JANEWAY, C. A. (1957). *Amer. J. Path.*, **33**, 55.

GLICK, D. & SYLVEN, B. (1951). *Science*, **113**, 388.

GOOD, R. A. (1954). *J. Lab. clin. Med.*, **44**, 803.

GOUGH, K. R., MCCARTHY, C., READ, A. E., MOLLIN, D. L. & WALTERS, A. H. (1964). *Brit. med. J.*, **1**, 212.

HART, F. D., ROBINSON, K. C., ALLCHIN, F. M. & MACLAGAN, N. F. (1949). *Quart. J. Med.*, **18**, 217.

HERBERT, V. (1965). *Ann. Rev. Med.*, **16**, 359.

HILL, A. G. S. (1951). *Lancet*, **2**, 807.

KANTOR, T., SOKOLOFF, L., SMITH, A. & ZIFF, M. (1951). *Ann. rheum. Dis.*, **10**, 471.

KELLGREN, J. H., BALL, J., ASTBURY, W. T., REED, R. & BEIGHTON, E. (1951). *Nature*, **168**, 493.

LOVELL, R. R. H., PRYCE, D. M. & BOAKE, W. C. (1954). *Brit. J. exp. Path.*, **35**, 345.

MCCORMICK, J. N., ROBINSON, R., SMITH, P. & DAY, J. (1962). *Ann. rheum. Dis.*, **21**, 79.

MCMILLAN, M. (1960). *J. clin. Path.*, **13**, 140.

MEHL, J. W., GOLDEN, F. & WINZLER, R. J. (1949). *Proc. Soc. exp. Biol. N.Y.*, **72**, 110.

MOVAT, H. Z. (1957). *Amer. J. med. Sci.*, **236**, 373.

OGSTON, A. G. & Stanier, J. E. (1950). *Biochem. J.*, **46**, 364.

OMER, A. & MOWAT, A. G. (1968). *Ann. rheum. Dis.*, **28**, 24.

PERKIN, T. J., Jr. & ZVAIFLER, N. J. (1964). *J. clin. Invest.*, **43**, 1372.

PERLMANN, G. E., ROPES, M. W., KAUFMAN, D. & BAUER, W. (1954). *J. clin. Invest.*, **33**, 319.

ROPES, M. W. & BAUER, W. (1952). "Synovial Fluid Changes in Joint Disease". Cambridge, Mass., Commonwealth Fund. Harvard Univ. Press.

RYLANE, R. J. (1969). *Ann. rheum. Dis.*, **28**, 41.

SMILEY, J. D., SACHS, C. & ZIFF, M. (1968). *J. clin. Invest.*, **47**, 624.

STEVEN, F. S. (1966). *Ann. rheum. Dis.*, **25**, 563.

SUNDBLAD, L. (1965). In "The amino sugars". Ed. Balazs, E. A., Jeanloz, R. W. Academic Press, New York. p. 230.

SVARTZ, N. & OLHAGEN, B. (1948). *Acta med. scand.*, **130**, Suppl. 206, **456.**

VAZQUEZ, J. J. & DIXON, F. J. (1957). *Lab. Invest.*, **6**, 205.

WEDGEWOOD, R. J. P. & JANEWAY, C. A. (1953). *Pediatrics*, **11**, 569.

ZIFF, M., BROWN, P., LOSPALLUTO, J., BADIN, J. & McEWEN, C. (1956). *Amer. J. Med.*, **20**, 500.

ZIFF, M., KANTOR, T., BIEN, E. & SMITH, A. (1953). *J. clin. Invest.*, **32**, 1253.

ZIFF, M., SIMPSON, J., SCULL, E., SMITH, A., SHATTON, J. & MAINLAND, D. (1955). *J. clin. Invest.*, **34**, 27.

Gout and Urate Accumulation

ALEPA, F. P., HOWELL, R. R., KLINENBERG, J. R. & SEEGMILLER, J. E. (1967). *Amer. J. Med.*, **42**, 58.

ALVSAKER, J. O. (1965). *Scand. J. clin. Invest.*, **17**, 1, 9. 467 & 476.

ARNOTT, R., GLASS, H., HOLLOWAY, V. & SCOTT, J. T. (1966). (Unpublished.)

BENEDICT, S. R. & BEHRE, J. A. (1931). *J. biol. Chem.*, **92**, 161.

BERLIN, R. D. (1969). *Science*, **163**, 1194.

BERMAN, P. H., BALIS, M. E. & DANKIS, J. (1968). *J. Lab. clin. Med.*, **71**, 247.

BEVERIDGE, G. W. & LAWSON, A. A. (1967). *Scot. med. J.*, **12**, 21.

BLAND, J. H. (1968). *Fed. Proc.*, **27**, 1021.

BLAUCH, M. B. & KOCH, F. C. (1938). *Proc. Soc. exp. Biol.*, *N.Y.*, **38**, 638.

BLOCK, W. D. & GEIB, N. C. (1947). *J. biol. Chem.*, **168**, 747.

BLUESTONE, R. (1968). *Proc. roy. Soc. Med.*, **61**, 1119.

BRANDENBERGER, E. & SCHINZ, H. R. (1950). *Experientia*, **6**, 188.

BRØCKNER- MORTENSEN, K. (1937). *Acta med. scand.*, Suppl. 84.

BROMBACHER, P. J., CREVELD, S. VAN, DAMME, J. P., HUIJING, F. & PLOEM, J. E. (1964). *Acta med. scand.*, **176**, 269.

BRECKENRIDGE, A. (1966). *Lancet*, **1**, 15.

BULGER, H. A. & JOHNS, H. E. (1941). *J. biol. Chem.*, **140**, 427.

BYWATERS, E. G. L. (1937). *J. Path. Bact.*, **44**, 247.

BYWATERS, E. G. L., DIXON, A. ST. J. & SCOTT, J. T. (1963). *Ann. rheum. Dis.*, **22**, 171.

BYWATERS, E. G. L. & HOLLOWAY, V. P. (1964). *Ann. rheum. Dis.*, **23**, 236.

CANNON, P. J., STASON, W. B. & DEMARTINI, F. E. (1966). *New Eng. J. Med.*, **275**, 457.

CARCASSI, A., MARCOLONGO, R., MARINELLO, E., RIARIO-SFORZA, G. & BOGGIANO, C. (1969). *Arth. Rheum.*, **12**, 17.

CASTELLO, D., MORELLI, M. T., ROSMINO, G. C. & BALLARIO, R. (1968). *Minerva Pediat.*, **20**, 151.

CHALMERS, R. A. & WATTS, R. W. (1968). *Analyst*, **93**, 354.

COPEMAN, W. S. C. (1964). "A Short History of the Gout and the Rheumatic Diseases". California University Press.

CURREY, H. L. F. & SWEETENHAM, K. V. (1965). *Brit. med. J.*, **2**, 481.

DALEY, D. & EVANS, B. (1962). *Brit. med. J.*, **2**, 156.

DECKER, J. (1968). "Population Studies of the Rheumatic Diseases". Proc. 3rd Internat. Symposium, New York, June 5–10 1966. Eds. Bennet, P. H. & Wood, P. H. N. Excerpta Medica Foundation, p. 382.

DOLLERY, C. T., DUNCAN, H. & SCHUMER, B. (1960). *Brit. med. J.*, **2**, 832.

DUNN, J. P., BROOKS, G. W., MAUSNER, J., RODNAN, G. P. & COBB, S. (1963). *J.A.M.A.*, **185**, 431.

(Editorial) (1964). *Brit. med. J.*, **2**, 1181.

EHRLICH, J. & CHOKATOS, J. (1966). *Arch. int. Med.*, **118**, 572.

EISEN, A. Z. & SEEGMILLER, J. E. (1961). *J. clin. Invest.*, **40**, 1486.

EMMERSON, B. T. (1963). *Aust. Ann. Med.*, **12**, 310.

EMMERSON, B. T. (1967). *Brit. med. J.*, **2**, 272.

FAIRES, J. S. & McCARTY, D. P. (1962). *Arth. Rheum.*, **5**, 295.

FELDMAN, E. B. & WALLACE, S. L. (1964). *Circulation*, **29**, 508.

FINE, R. N. & STRAUSS, J. (1967). *Amer. J. Dis. Childh.*, **112**, 572.

FOLIN, O. (1933). *J. biol. Chem.*, **101**, 111.

FOLIN, O. (1934). *J. biol. Chem.*, **106**, 311.

FRABOT, C. (1904). *Ann. chim. Anal.*, **9**, 371.

FREDRICKSON, D. S., LEVY, R. & LEES, R. S. (1967). *New Eng. J. Med.*, **276**, 215.

FRIED, F. A. & VERMEULEN, C. W. (1964). *Invest. Urol.*, **2**, 131.

FRY, L. & BARLOW, K. A. (1962). *Brit. med. J.*, **1**, 920.

FULLER, R. W., LUCE, M. W. & MERTZ, E. T. (1962). *Science*, **137**, 868.

GARROD, A. B. (1848). *Med. Chir. Trans.*, **31**, 83.

GARROD, A. B. (1870). *Lancet*, **2**, 781.

GERTLER, M. M., GARN, S. M. & LEVINE, S. A. (1951). *Ann. int. Med.*, **34**, 1421.

GOLDFINGER, S., KLINENBERG, J. R. & SEEGMILLER, J. E. (1965). *New Eng. J. Med.*, **272**, 351.

GOUNELLE, M., BOUDENE, C., CHOLLEY, A. *et al.* (1967). *Bull. Soc. Med. Hop. Paris.*, **118**, 1041.

HARRIS JONES, J. N. (1957). *Lancet*, **1**, 857.

HENDRY, P. I. A., WHITE, K. H. & STRANGER, I. J. (1959). *Med. J. Aust.*, **2**, 956.

HOOFT, C., VAN NEVEL, C. & DE SCHAEPDRYVER, A. F. (1968). *Arch. Dis. Childh.*, **43**, 734.

HOWELL, R. R. (1968). *Fed. Proc.*, **27**, 1078.

HOWELL, R. R. (1968). *Fed. Proc.*, **27**, 1082.

HOWELL, R. R., EANES, E. D. & SEEGMILLER, J. E. (1963). *Arth. Rheum.*, **6**, 97.

HUMPHREYS, D. M. (1966). *Brit. med. J.*, **1**, 1024.

ISOMAKI, H. & KREUS, K.-E. (1968). *Acta med. scand.*, **184**, 293.

JACOBSON, B. M. (1938). *Ann. intern. Med.*, **11**, 1277.

JAKOVIC, S. & SORENSEN, L. B. (1967). *Arth. Rheum.*, **10**, 129.

KALCKAR, H. M. & SHAFRAN, M. (1947). *J. biol. Chem.*, **167**, 429.

KAPLAN, D., DIAMOND, H., WALLACE, S. L. & HALBERSTAM, D. (1969). *Ann. rheum. Dis.*, **28**, 180.

KASL, S. V., BROOKS, G. W. & COBB, S. (1966). *J.A.M.A.*, **198**, 713.

KAUFMAN, J. M. & O'BRIEN, W. M. (1967). *New Eng. J. Med.*, **276**, 953.

KAUFMAN, J. M. GREENE, M. L. & SEEGMILLER, J. E. (1968), *J. Pediat.*, **73**, 583.

KELLERYMEYER, R. W. & BRECKENRIDGE, R. T. (1965). *J. Lab. clin. Med.*, **65**, 307.

KELLEY, W. N. (1968). *Fed. Proc.*, **27**, 1047.

KELLEY, W. N., ROSENBLOOM, F. M., HENDERSON, J. F. & SEEGMILLER, J. E. (1967a). *J. clin. Invest.*, **46, 1078**.

KELLEY, W. N., ROSENBLOOM, F. M., HENDERSON, J. F. et al. (1967b). *Proc. nat. Acad. Sci. USA*, **57**, 1735.

KELLEY, W. N., LEVY, R. I., ROSENBLOOM, F. M., HENDERSON, J. F. & SEEGMILLER, J. E. (1968). *J. clin. Invest.*, **47**, 2281.

KELLEY, W. N. & SEEGMILLER, J. E. (1968). *J. Pediat.*, **72**, 488.

KELLEY, W. N., GREENE, M. L., ROSENBLOOM, F. M., HENDERSON, J. F. & SEEGMILLER, J. E. (1969). *Ann. int. Med.*, **70**, 155.

LATHAM, B., RADCLIFF, F. & ROBINSON, R. G. (1966). *Amer. phys. Med.*, **8**, 242.

LAURENT, T. C. (1964). *Nature*, **202**, 1334.

LESCH, M. & Nyhan, W. L. (1963). *J. Pediat.*, **63**, 729.

LIDDLE, L., SEEGMILLER, J. E. & LASTER, L. (1959). *J. Lab. clin. Med.*, **54**, 903.

LIEBER, C. S. (1965). *Arth. Rheum.*, **8**, 786.

LUDWIG, G. D. (1957). *Arch. int. Med.*, **100**, 802.

MacLACHLAN, M. J. & RODNAN, G. P. (1967). *Amer. J. Med.*, **42**, 38.

McPAUL, J. J. (1968). *Metabolism*, **17**, 430.

MARKS, J. F., BAUM, J., KEELE, D. K. et al. (1968). *Pediatrics*, **42**, 357.

MARKS, J. F., KAY, J., BAUM, J. & CURRY, L. (1968). *J. Pediat.*, **73**, 609.

MERTZ, D. P. & SCHINDERA, F. (1968). *Ger. med. Monthly*, **13**, 414.

MIGEON, B. R., DER KALOUSTIAN, V. M., NYHAN, W. L. et al. (1968). *Science*, **160**, 425.

MONTOYE, H. J., FAULKNER, J A., DODGE, H. J., MIKKELSEN, W. M., WILLIS, P. W. & BLOCK, W. D. (1967). *Ann. int. Med.*, **66**, 838.

MORGAN, J. M., HARTLEY, M. W. & MILLER, R. E. (1966). *Arch. int. Med.*, **118**, 17.

NYHAN, W. L., JAMES, J. A., TEBERG, A. J., SWEETMAN, L. & NELSON, L. G. (1969). *J. Pediat*, **74**, 20.

OROWAN, E. (1955). *Nature*, **175**, 683.

OSTER, G. (1955). "Physical Techniques in Biological Research", Vol. 1. Eds. Oster, G. & Pollister, A. W. New York, Academic Press Inc., p. 439.

O'SULLIVAN, J. B. (1968). "Population Studies of the Rheumatic Diseases". Proc. 3rd Internat. Symposium, New York, June 5–10 1966. Eds. Bennet, P. H. & Wood, P. H. N. Excerpta Medica Foundation, p. 377.

PAGE, L. B. & KIMMELSTIEL, P. (1966). *New Eng. J. Med.*, **274**, 1374.

PERHEENTUPA, J. & RAIVIO, K. (1967). *Lancet*, **2**, 528.

PETTY, T. L. & DALRYMPLE, G. V. (1964). *Ann. int. Med.*, **60**, 898.

POPERT, A. J. & HEWITT, J. V. (1962). *Ann. rheum. Dis.*, **21**, 154.

REEVES, B. (1965). *Ann. rheum. Dis.*, **24**, 569.

RICHET, G., MIGNON, F. & ARDAILLOU, R. (1965). *Presse Med.*, **73**, 633.

ROPES, M. W., & BAUER, W. (1953). "Synovial fluid changes in Joint Disease". Cambridge, Mass., Harvard University Press.

ROSEMBLOOM, F. M. (1968). *Fed. Proc.*, **27**, 1063.

ROSENBLOOM, F. M., KELLEY, W. N., MILLER, J., HENDERSON, J. F. & SEEGMILLER, J. E. (1967). *J.A.M.A.*, **202**, 175.

ROWE, P. B. & WYNGAARDEN, J. B. (1966). *J. biol. Chem.*, **241**, 5571.

RYCKEWAERT, A., MASSE, C., JURMAND, S. H. et al. (1967). *Sem. Hop. Paris.*, **43**, 3059.

SCOTT, J. T. (1966). *Proc. roy. Soc. Med.*, **59**, 310.

SCOTT, J. T. (1966). Ed. Symposium on Allopurinol. *Ann. rheum. Dis.*, **25**, No. 6 (Suppl.).

SCOTT, J. T., DIXON, A. St. J. & BYWATERS, E. G. L. (1964). *Brit. med. J.*, **1**, 1070.

SCOTT, J. T., McCALLUM, F. M. & HOLLOWAY, V. P. (1964). *Clin. Sci.*, **27**, 209.

SEEGMILLER, J. E., HOWELL, R. R. & MALAWISTA, S. E. (1962). *J.A.M.A.*, **180**, 469.

SEEGMILLER, J. E., ROSENBLOOM, F. M., & KELLEY, W. N. (1967). *Science*, **155**, 1682.

SHEIKH, M. I. & MOLLER, J. V. (1968). *Biochem. biophys. Acta*, **158**, 456.

SILVERMAN, H. & GUBERNICK, I. (1947). *J. biol. Chem.*, **167**, 363.

SMYTH, C. J., COTTERMAN, C. W. & FREYBERG, R. H. (1948a). *J. clin. Invest.*, **27**, 749.

SMYTH, C. J., STECHER, R. M. & WOLFSON, W. Q. (1948b). *Science*, **108**, 514.

SOKOLOFF, L. (1957). *Metabolism*, **6**, 230.

SORENSEN, L. B. (1965). *Arth. Rheum.*, **8**, 694.

STECHER, R. M., HERSH, A. H. & SOLOMON, W. M. (1949). *Ann. intern. Med.*, **31**, 595.

STETTEN, D. W. & HEARON, J. Z. (1959). *Science*, **129**, 1737.

SUSSMAN, K. E., ALFREY, A., KIRSCH, W., ZWEIG, P. & MESSNER, F. (1968). *J. Lab. clin. Med.*, **72**, 1022.

VON HOYNINGEN-HUENE, C. B. J. (1966). *Arch. int. Med.*, **118**, 471.

WALLS, A. D. F. (1969). *Brit. med. J.*, **1**, 98.

WOLFSON, W. Q., HUDDLESTUN, B. & LEVINE, R. (1947). *J. clin. Invest.*, **26**, 995.

WOLFSON, W. Q., LEVINE, R. & TINSLEY, M. (1947). *J. clin. Invest.*, **26**, 991.

WOLLASTON (1797). *Phil. Trans.*, **87**, 386.

WYNGAARDEN, J. B. (1960). *Arth. Rheum.*, **3**, 414.

Varieties of Tissue Calcification

ARMSTRONG, W. D. (1950). Transactions of the 2nd Conference on Metabolic Interrelationships, 1950. Josiah Macy Jr. Foundation, p. 11.

ATKINSON, F. R. B. & WEBER, F. P. (1938). *Brit. J. Derm. Syph.*, **50**, 267.

BAUER, W., MARBLE, A. & BENNETT, G. A. (1931). *Amer. J. med. Sci.*, **182**, 237.

BOLAM, M. (1935). *Brit. J. Derm. Syph.*, **47**, 340.

BOSSI, R. (1954). *Br. J. Radiol.*, **27**, 692.

BOUDIN, G., PEPIN, B. & HUBAULT, A. (1963). *Bull. Soc. med. Hop. Paris*, **114**, 617.

BOYD, E. S. & NEUMAN, W. F. (1951). *J. biol. Chem.*, **193**, 243.

BRIGGS, J. N. & ILLINGWORTH, R. S. (1952). *Lancet*, **2**, 800.

BROOKS, W. D. W. (1934). *Quart. J. Med.*, **3**, n.s., 293.

BURNETT, W. & FLINK, E. B. (1954). *J. Lab. clin. Med.*, **44**, 777.

BYWATERS, E. G. L., DIXON, A. ST. J. & SCOTT, J. T. (1963). *Ann. rheum. Dis.*, **22**, 171.

Cabot Case Record (1961). *New Eng. J. Med.*, **265**, 135.

CHON, L. T. & DONOHUE, W. L. (1952). *Pediatrics*, **10**, 660.

COCHRANE, W. & DAVIES, D. V. (1965). *Ann. rheum. Dis.*, **24**, 147.

COHEN, LORD, & BYWATERS, E. G. L. (1969). In: "Textbook of the Rheumatic Diseases", Edn. 4. Ed. Copeman, W. S. C. Livingstone, p. 428.

COMROE, B. I., CHAMBERLIN, G. W. & SUNDERMAN, F. W. (1939). *Amer. J. Roentgenol.*, **41**, 749.

CORNBLEET, T., REED, C. I. & REED, B. P. (1949). *J. invest. Derm.*, **13**, 171.

CORNBLEET, T. & STRUCK, H. C. (1937). *Arch. Derm. Syph.*, *Chicago*, **35**, 188.

CRAIG, J. & LYALL, A. (1931). *Brit. J. Chld. Dis.*, **28**, 29.

CURREY, H. L. F. (1968). *Proc. R. Soc. Med.*, **61**, 969.

CURREY, H. L. F., KEY, J. J., MASON, R. M. & SWETTENHAM, K. V. (1966). *Ann. rheum. Dis.*, **25**, 295.

DAVIES, H. & MOE, P. J. (1959). *Pediatrics*, **24**, 780.

DURET, M. H. (1899). *Bull. Soc. anat. Paris*, **74**, 225. (Cited Lafferty, F. W. *et al.* (1965). *Amer. J. Med.*, **38**, 105.)

EGOVILLE, J. W. (1938). *Arch. Path.*, **26**, 1047.

EICHELBERGER, L. & ROMA, M. (1954). *Amer. J. Physiol.*, **178**, 296.

FLEISH, H. & NEUMAN, W. F. (1961). *Amer. J. Phys.*, **200**, 1296.

FRIEDLANDER, J. (1930). *Dtsch. Arch. klin. Med.*. **166**, 107.

GATTER, R. A. & McCARTY, D. J. (1967). *Arch. Path.*, **84**, 346.

HAMILTON, E., WILLIAMS, R., BARLOW, K. A. & SMITH, P. M. (1968). *Quarterly J. Med.*, **37**, 171.

HOWARD, J. E. (1954). Transactions of the 5th Conference on Metabolic Interrelationships, 1953. Josiah Macy Jr. Foundation, p. 127.

JADDASOHN, J. (1910). *Arch. Derm. Syph.*, *Wien*, **100**, 317.

KRAMER, B. & SHEAR, M. J. (1928). *J. biol. Chem.*, **79**, 121.

LAFFERTY, F. W., REYNOLDS, E. S. & PEARSON, O. H. (1965). *Amer. J. Med.*, **38**, 105.

LEVINE, M. D., RUBIN, P. S., FOLLIS, R. M. & HOWARD, J. E. (1949). Transactions of the 1st Conference on Metabolic Interrelationships, 1949. Josiah Macy Jr. Foundation, p. 41.

LOEWI, G. (1953). *J. Path. Bact.*, **65**, 381.

LOEWI, G. & DORLING, J. (1964). *Ann. rheum. Dis.*, **23**, 272.

LOSADA, M. L., COX, F. L., RODRIQUEZ, J. V., ROUBAN, E. T. & SILVA, L. R. (1957). *Ann. rheum. Dis.*, **16**, 454.

McCARTY, D. J., KOHN, N. N. & FAIRES, J. S. (1962), *Ann. int. Med.*, **56**, 711.

McCARTHY, D. J., HOGAN, J. M., GATTER, R. A. & GROSSMAN, M. (1966). *J. Bone Jt. Surg.*, **48-A**, 309.

McCARTHY, D. J. & GATTER, R. A. (1966). *Arth. Rheum.*, **9**, 804.

McCLATCHIE, S. & BREMNER, D. (1969). *Brit. med. J.*, **1**, 153.

McLAURIN, A. W., BEISEL, W. R., McCORMICK, G. J. & SCALETTAR, R. (1961). *Ann. int. Med.*, **55**, 70.

MERGENHAGEN, S. E., MARTIN, G. R., RIZZO, A. A., WRIGHT, D. N. & SCOTT, D. B. (1960). *Biochim. Biophys Acta*, **43**, 563.

MEYER, K. & RAPPORT, M. M. (1951). *Science*, **113**, 596.

MILLER, Z. B., WALDMAN, J. & McLEAN, F. C. (1952). *J. exp. Med.*, **95**, 497.

PAEGLE, R. D. (1966). *Arch. Path.*, **82**, 474.

PEDERSEN, J. (1943). *Acta med. scand.*, **113**, 373.

PIERSALL, C. E. (1933). *Radiology*, **20**, 164.

RAVAULT, P. P., LEJEUNE, E. & MAITREPIERRE, J. (1959). *Rev. Lyon. Med.*, **8**, 1095.

ROTHSTEIN, J. L. & WELT, S. (1936). *Amer. J. Dis. Child.*, **52**, 368.

RUBIN, M. (1954). Transactions of the 5th Conference on Metabolic Interrelationships. Josiah Macy Jr. Foundation, 1953, p. 355.

RUDOLPH, C. C. (1934). *J. Pediat.*, **4**, 342.

RUSSELL, R. G. (1965). *Lancet*, **2**, 461.

SCOTT, J. T. (1966). *Proc. R. Soc. Med.*, **59**, 310.

SCOTT, R. B. & DeLILLY, M. R. (1954). *Amer. J. Dis. Child.*, **87**, 55.

SCOWEN, E. F., CRAWHALL, J. C. & WATTS, R. W. E. (1958). *Lancet*, **2**, 300.

SCOWEN, E. F., STANSFELD, A. G. & WATTS, R. W. E. (1959). *J. Path. Bact.*, **77**, 195.

SHARP, J. (1954). *Ann. rheum. Dis.*, **13**, 15.

SHELDON, J. H. (1938). *Proc. R. Soc. Med.*, **31**, 1119.

SILVA, F., PONDE, A. DE A. & LICHTENBERG, F. (1953). *Arch. Derm. Syph.*, *Chicago*, **68**, 588.

SOBEL, A. E. (1952). Transactions of the 4th Conference on Metabolic Interrelationships, 1952. Josiah Macy Jr. Foundation, p. 113.

SOBEL, A. E. & BURGER, M. (1954). *Proc. Soc. exp. Biol.*, *N.Y.*, **87**, 7.

SOLOMON, R. B. & CHANNICK, B. J. (1960). *Ann. int. Med.*, **53**, 1232.

SOLOMONS, C. C., GOODMAN, S. & RILEY, C. M. (1967). *New Eng. J. Med.*, **276**, 207.

SOLOMONS, C. C. & NEUMAN, W. F. (1960). *J. biol. Chem.*, **235**, 2502.

SWANSON, W. W., FORSTER, W. G. & IOB, L. V. (1933). *Amer. J. Dis. Child.*, **45,** 590.

THOMPSON, G. R., MING TING, Y., RIGGS, G. A., FENN, H. ELLEN & DENNING, R. M. (1968). *J.A.M.A.*, **203,** 464.

TURPIN, R., BRUN, C. & GUILLAMIN, C. O. (1934). *Pr. med.*, **11,** 1561.

VERSÉ, M. (1912). *Beitr. path. Anat.*, **53,** 212.

WELLS, H. G. (1915). *Arch. intern. Med.*, **15,** 74.

WHEELER, C. E., CURTIS, A. C., CAWLEY, E. P., GREKIN, R. H. & ZHEUTLIN, B. (1952). *Ann. intern. Med.*, **36,** 1050.

WILBER, J. F. & STATOPOLSKY, E. (1968). *Ann. int. Med.*, **68,** 1044.

ZELLWEGER, H. (1948). *Helv. paediat., Acta,* **3,** 287.

ZITNAN, D. & SIT'AJ, S. (1963). *Ann. rheum. Dis.*, **22,** 142.

Amyloidosis

MANDEMA, E., RUINEN, L., SCHOLTEN, J. H. & COHEN, A. S. (1968). "Amyloidosis", Excerpta Medica Foundation, Amsterdam.

Chapter 22

DISORDERS OF BONE AND CALCIUM METABOLISM

by

Russell Fraser and Iain MacIntyre
Royal Postgraduate Medical School, London

GENERAL

THOUGH bone contains only 44% water, its solid constituents maintain an active equilibrium with their counterparts in the extracellular fluid. Thus not only can bone diseases (e.g. bone tumours) lead to abnormalities in the composition of plasma and so of urine, but also abnormalities in the composition of extracellular fluid (e.g. uraemia) may cause secondary disorders in bone.

The solid matter of bone is made up of a few cells and an intercellular substance compounded of three main constituents; two of these together comprise the intercellular matrix or osteoid tissue, i.e. the collagen fibres bound together by the mucopolysaccharide cement substance; the third constituent, the mineral, is found as crystals mainly of calcium and phosphate assembled along the collagen fibres, and comprises two-thirds of the dry weight.

The Structure of Bone

The entire surface of bone is covered with a curtain of cells controlling exchange from the bone. Three main types of cells are found in bone: (1) enclosed osteocytes which maintain the structure, (2) osteoblasts, found on the growing surfaces which control new bone formation, and (3) osteoclasts, giant cells occurring at the sites of resorption, in which process they are intimately involved. The proportions of these cells vary in response to certain general stimuli; thus, osteoblasts increase with more rapid matrix formation as in rickets or healing fractures, and osteoclasts multiply with increased resorption as in hyperparathyroidism with bone disease.

The intercellular tissue of bone differs from that of other tissues mainly as a result of its property of calcifiability in the presence of normal extracellular fluid. By special techniques, un-decalcified bone sections can be cut showing a dense collagen web, in relation to which lie the bone crystals, canaliculi and spaces for the cells (Figs. 22.1 and 22.2). When thin shavings of bone are decalcified in ethylenediamine tetra-acetic acid at pH 7 and then agitated in water, the collagen fibres are exposed and can be seen with the electron microscope (Fig. 22.3). When the bone shavings are treated with hyaluronidase to dissolve instead the cement matrix, the bone crystals remain and are seen clinging to the collagen fibres.

There are two main types of bone: (1) cortical bone, mainly in the diaphyses of long bones, and comprised of interlocked Haversian systems in which each unit is an osteon controlled by a central osteocyte; and (2) trabecular bone or spongiosa, mostly in the axial skeleton and ends of long bones, whose surrounding endosteo-membrane contains its controlling osteocytes. The latter or trabecular bone is the most active metabolically and it responds to mechanical and hormonal stimuli.

Bone Growth and Replacement

Growth of bone can occur either from connective tissue (membranous bone formation) or from some types of cartilage (endochondral bone formation). Since there are more stages in endo-chondral bone formation, disorders of bone formation show more characteristic histology at the metaphysis or costochondral junctions. In addition, throughout the whole life of all bones there is a steady replacement continuing *in situ*, new bone formation by osteoblasts occurring on some bone surfaces, and on others resorption by osteoclasts. This steady replacement of bone involves new matrix as well as new crystals and is additional to the dynamic ion-exchange established between the bone crystals and the body fluid. It should be remembered that the deposition of radioactive tracer isotopes will illustrate a summation of these processes, not simply a picture of new bone formation. The rate of this steady replacement by new bone tissue varies in different parts of the skeleton, with disease, and steadily declines with age (Fig. 22.4).

In all these sites, this laying down of bone requires first the formation of the characteristic bone matrix or osteoid, and then its calcification; its removal requires the dissolution of both the osteoid and the crystals. Both the formation of osteoid and the conferring on it of the property of calcifiability are under the control of osteoblasts. Despite much study, the chemical mechanisms involved in the formation and resorption of bone are ill-understood (*see below*).

Resorption is a random process whose control is ill-understood—one factor is mineral homeostasis. Initially the resorption cavity extends as a tunnel and after some months the function of the site changes to bone formation and concentric laminae of new bone are laid down. Koelliker (1873) described the important role of the osteoclast in this process, and its importance in the reconstruction of bone during growth as well as in the adult's constant bone replacement. Bone resorption occurs in the sites where osteoclasts are seen and its rate varies with their abundance. The general rate of bone resorption rises with increase in parathyroid activity and in acidosis,

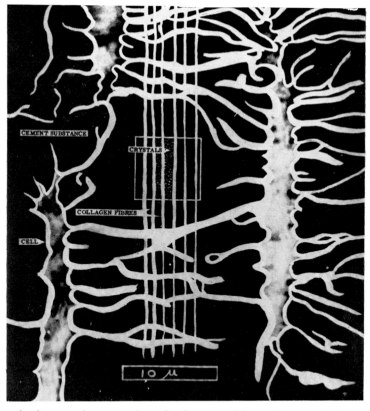

Fig. 22.1. Schematic electron microscope view of a fragment of bone (after autoclaving to remove organic component) retouched to show canaliculi and collagen fibres. The collagen fibres have been represented diagrammatically in the extracellular matrix space by white vertical lines. Magnification about 4000 ×. From Robinson, R. A. (1952). *J. Bone Joint Surg.*, **34**-A, 389.

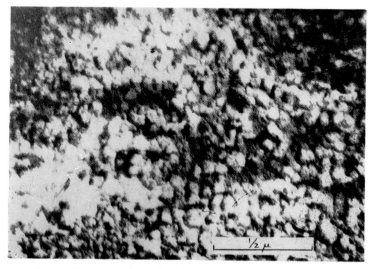

Fig. 22.2. Electron micrograph of a section of undecalcified, osmic-acid fixed, and *n*-butyl-methacrylate-embedded human rib cortex; shadowed. Note plaques of crystals. Magnification about 61,300 ×. From Robinson, R. A. & Watson, M. L. (1952). *Anat. Rec.*, **114**, 402.

[To face p. 752.

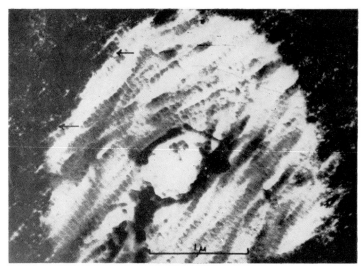

FIG. 22.3. Electron micrograph of a section of ethylenediamine-tetra-acetate—partly-decalcified, osmic-acid-fixed bone, embedded as in Fig. 22.2. The crystals apparently lie mainly at the doublet-bands of the collagen fibres. Magnification about 32,300 ×. From Robinson, R. A. & Watson, M. L. *Anat. Rec.*, **114**, 409.

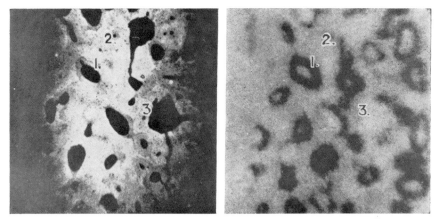

FIG. 22.4. Section of femur from dog given ^{32}P 3 days previously, (*a*) left, microradiograph, (*b*) right, auto-radiograph. Note that the ^{32}P uptake is high in (1) a young Haversian system, is low in (2) an old Haversian system, and is zero in (3) bone tissue surrounding a resorption cavity. Magnification about 27 ×. From Engfeldt, B., Engström, A. & Zetterström, R. (1952). *Biochimica et Biophysica Acta*, **8**, 375.

and decreases in alkalosis and in response to calcitonin. Whether the general level of activity is mediated by humoral control of the decalcification, with osteoclasts then proliferating for the dissolution of the protein matrix (Jaffé, 1933), or by humoral control of osteoclast activity remains unsettled. Hancox (1949) concluded that there is no direct evidence that osteoclasts erode bone. A local factor is involved in bone resorption; during growth the metaphysis is singled out for reconstruction in a process including considerable osteoclastic resorption followed by appositional bone formation. Possibly both chelating mechanisms and hyaluronidase-like or proteolytic enzymes may be involved. The mechanism must simultaneously depolymerize mucopolysaccharides, digest collagen, and hold calcium and phosphate in solution.

Bone Matrix and Collagen

The bone matrix is primarily collagen which is apparently similar to the collagen elsewhere in the body. The amino acids glycine and hydroxyproline (HP) each comprise about one-third of its weight. Essentially all the HP in the body is in collagen or its degradation products, of which none is resynthesized into collagen, so that the level of circulating HP should index the rate of collagen turnover, to which bone appears to make the main contribution. The basic molecular unit of collagen is tropocollagen, a rod-like macro-molecule of length about 3000 Å, 14 Å diameter, molecular weight 300,000 and composed of three helically coiled polypeptide chains. The chains are held together intramolecularly by linkages involving especially the glycines and HPs, while similar intermolecular linkages bond these units together into the fibres of insoluble or mature collagen. Its synthesis starts intracellularly with the ribosomes forming protocollagen, i.e. polypeptide chains containing proline and lysine; and when these still-intracellular chains reach a sufficient length, an hydroxylating enzyme converts these constituent amino acids to HP and hydroxylysine, and so the chains are converted to tropocollagen units which are then extruded extracellularly as fibres. At first these fibres are "soluble collagen" (i.e. can be extracted with saline), but they mature to "insoluble collagen" by progressively developing additional intramolecular and intermolecular cross linkages. These fibres show on electron microscopy a banded periodicity of 640 Å, dependent probably on the tropocollagen molecular units being arranged in a staggered array in the fibrils. Less is known of the catabolism of collagen; a probably specific collagenase first transforms insoluble to soluble collagen and then to smaller peptides, which are then removed mainly as soluble peptide units, though in part as free amino acids.

Bone Crystals and Ion-exchange

With the electron microscope (Fig. 22.3), the bone crystals have been seen best after autoclaving or glycerol-ashing to dissolve the matrix (Robinson, 1952); trabecular crystals with long axes (3–400 Å) in the direction of the collagen fibres, nearly as wide, and 25–50 Å thick (Robinson, 1952). The crystals of both bone and teeth resemble the larger ones of synthetic basic calcium phosphate (hydroxyapatite; $3 Ca_3(PO_4)_2 . Ca(OH)_2$). Normal bone salt is a compound mainly of calcium, phosphate, hydroxyl ions and water, which has a calcium/phosphate (Ca/P) molar ratio of 1·5 and which gives the X-ray diffraction pattern of the hydroxyapatite lattice —i.e. a lattice structure common to a series of solid basic calcium phosphates whose molar Ca/P can vary from 1·3 to 2·0. The crystals also contain carbonate and citrate and a mixture of small amounts of other ions, especially Na^+, Mg^{++}, K^+, Cl^- and F^-. The crystals are best regarded as a slightly impure basic calcium phosphate in which carbonate is incorporated. The Ca/P molar ratio of hydroxyapatite is 1·66, while that of bone is 1·5, implying that bone is more highly hydrated and less alkaline, with some Ca exchanged from H_3O^+. To explain this variability without change of the lattice, it is suggested that these crystals can allow both surface adsorption and some internal substitution with the lattice remaining intact.

The surfaces can absorb water, CO_2, Na^+, citrate, proteinate and trace minerals. The rapid initial but slow final equilibrium found with isotopes suggests that ions can also be exchanged into the bone crystals (Falkenheim, Neuman & Hodge, 1947). This slower exchange into the crystals, called isomorphic substitution, can occur only up to a certain extent and does not involve any other change in the crystal.

It is envisaged that the free crystal surfaces adsorb a surface hydration shell, which is in rapid equilibrium with the surrounding medium and so via the osteocytes with the extracellular fluid; and with which the interior ions of the crystal establish a slow but measurable equilibrium. Many crystals lie on the surface with some unshared sides, and on these is formed the hydration shell. When powdered bone is freed of its organic matter, by autoclaving or glycerol-ashing, the total area of crystal surfaces can be estimated by CO_2 adsorption or isotope exchange. Such estimates range from 64 to 200 m²/g. bone ash, which correspond to over 100 acres for a 70 kg. man. Even if only a small proportion of these surfaces is available in the presence of organic matrix, there must be several acres over which a few litres of fluid circulate (Neuman & Neuman, 1953).

Thus, bone resembles in some respects an ion-exchange column, with its hydration shell in equilibrium with the surrounding fluid medium, to which its crystal composition, as noted, slowly adjusts up to a definite though limited extent. But bone exchanges both cations and anions; the exchangeable ions are linked principally by electrostatic forces, and the exchange is pH-dependent as well as being a function of mass. Isotope studies, even *in vitro* with dead bone, have shown the rapidity with which these exchanges can occur, for example with ^{32}P, ^{45}Ca and with Ur, Sr, Na, etc. (Hodge, Gavett & Thomas, 1946; Singer & Armstrong, 1951; Lacroix, 1952; Zetterström, 1952). There is evidence that in bone the CO_2 is mostly surface-adsorbed rather than incorporated as ionic HCO_3^-. Displacement of two Ca ions can occur either for four ions of Na or H_3O^+ or for two ions of Sr or Pb, or for one of Ur, though not for K or Ba, and the surface anions exchange with HCO_3^-, OH^-, $PO_4^{\equiv}$, and citrate. Thus, some foreign ions can exchange with the hydration layer of the bone crystals. Because of some ill-understood specific affinity of the organic matrix of bone, deposition can also occur in it of other foreign ions whose nuclear forces will not permit ion-exchange; such as mostly the rare earths, Americium, Ba, Yt, Az, Ce, Ga (Dudley & Maddox, 1949; Dudley, Maddox & La Rue, 1949). These foreign ions which deposit in bone also frequently hydrolyse in the body to form a colloid, which fraction is then deposited in the reticulo–endothelial system (Schubert, 1951; Brucer, Andrews & Bruner, 1953).

The extent to which the organic matrix modifies the ion-exchange is not known; the crystals are intimately mixed with the matrix, and all exchanging ions must permeate through it. Ashing powdered bone greatly accelerates its rate of ion-exchange. Further, exchanges with newly deposited bone mineral (e.g. at the metaphysis) are much more rapid than with that of older bone, either *in vitro* (Neuman & Mulryan, 1950; Amprino, 1952; Carlsson, 1952; Lacroix, 1952) or *in vivo* (Hodge *et al.*, 1946; Engfeldt, Engström & Zetterström, 1952), and these differences are diminished by low-temperature ashing. Rachitic skeletons fix a larger percentage of isotope-like growing bones (Copp, Hamilton, Jones, Thompson & Cramer, 1951; Carlsson, 1952), and as any skeleton matures a smaller fraction of water, CO_2, Na and other mineral remains in equilibrium with the body fluids. This decline with age is partly due to the poorer circulation and the decreasing water content of the ageing bones.

Samples of dead-bone powder (human or calf), equilibrate with solutions of Ca and P, over the pH range 6·6–7·8, and have been found to yield a relatively constant solubility product,

$$[Ca^{++}]^3 \times [PO_4^{\equiv}]^2 = 4\cdot1 \times 10^{-27},$$

whether equilibrium is approached from super-saturation or under-saturation. On this basis normal human extracellular fluid ($[Ca^{++}]$ = 6 mg./100 ml. and $[P]$ = 3 mg./100 ml.) implies an equilibrium with bone at pH 6·8 which is similar to the intracellular pH (MacGregor & Nordin, 1960). These authors suggest that the bone crystals may be maintained at this pH presumably by cellular activity.

Bone Calcification

Both humoral and local factors are involved in the calcification of bone. The composition of body fluids may limit calcification, as in rickets, or cause excessive bone resorption as in renal failure. It has been difficult to define bone solubility in simple physico-chemical terms, such as a solubility product, and it must be remembered that the *in vivo* conditions also include the cells and organic matrix round the crystals. Rachitic cartilage has been used to measure the adequacy of the humoral factors. Fig. 22.6 shows that parathyroid extract increases the calcifying qualities of serum, and Fig. 22.5 shows an attempt to define the limits of biological solubility for varying pH and P concentrations with constant Ca concentration. Thus for bone at a pH near 6·8, a simple product of Ca × P only approximately indexes calcifiability with varying P concentrations, while a tendency to acidosis is unfavourable as also is uraemia (*vide infra*).

However, local factors, some inhibiting and some facilitating, are probably the major ones which initiate calcification in bone. Since collagen from various sources will calcify in a metastable solution of Ca and P, some local factors must prevent calcification in most sites. The main known factors in this inhibition are the covering of the collagen by fully polymerized mucopolysaccharide ground substance, and the pyrophosphate found in all body fluids as well as in

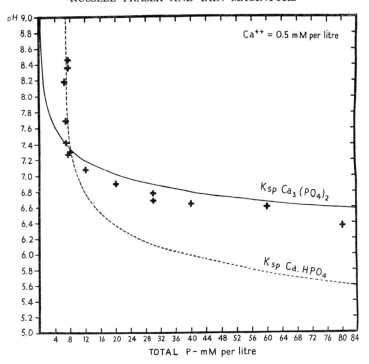

FIG. 22.5. The "limits of biological solubility". The minimal concentrations for calcification in rachite cartilage exposed to inorganic solutions *in vitro*. With constant total Ca concentration (0.5 m-mol./l.), at various pH levels, the minimal total phosphate (P) causing calcification was determined and plotted (+). Lines have been drawn representing solubility products of $CaHPO_4$ (from $pK_{sp} = 5.47$; Shear & Kramer, 1928), and $Ca_3(PO_4)_2$ (from $pK_{sp} = 23.1$; Logan & Taylor, 1937). Note that above pH 7.3 calcification follows the solubility product of $CaHPO_4$, and below pH 7.3 that of $Ca_3(PO_4)_2$. (From F. C. McLean, "Metabolic aspects of convalescence" (1946). Transactions of the 14th Macy Conference, p. 33.)

bone where it is approximately 5% of the phosphorus. Pyrophosphate can inhibit the precipitation of calcium and phosphorus from metastable solutions (Fleisch & Bisaz, 1964), and also inhibit the dissolution of hydroxyapatite crystals. It may also keep the calcium and phosphorus in urine from forming crystals. Howard and his associates have isolated a small polypeptide from human urine which has similar effects, but is 500 times more potent than pyrophosphate in inhibiting the calcification of ricketic cartilage; as it also circulates in plasma it may be even more important than the pyrophosphate but its source is not known.

Bone formation is initiated over an area by the osteoblasts elaborating an extracellular collagen matrix, osteoid, which within a further 4 to 8 days they modify to become calcifiable. At the bone-forming surfaces the edge of the osteoid adjoin-ing the bone can be identified by special stains as a calcification front (Bordier, Matrajt, Hioco, Hepner, Thompson & Booth, 1968). In rickets, such a calcification front does not develop in the osteoid which instead goes on thickening excessively. The changes which the osteoblasts effect in this region to permit crystal nucleation probably include, (1) a local excess of alkaline phosphatase (which is also a pyrophosphatase, and so removes the pyrophosphate inhibition), (2) depolymerization of the acidic mucopoly-saccharide and so exposure of the collagen along with consequentially increasing local concentrations of Ca ions. Then the initial step is phosphorylation of sites on the native collagen fibrils which as they are laid down in bone probably provide the template which initiates calcification (Glimcher, 1959). The initial mineral phase in bone may be an amorphous Ca phosphate which

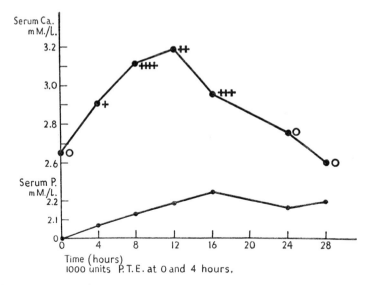

F<small>IG</small>. 22.6. The "limits of biological solubility", tested on serum from dog after administration of parathyroid extract (PE). The animal was given 1000 units of PE at 0 hr. and again at 4 hr. Serum withdrawn at 0, 24 and 28 hr. produced no calcification of rachitic cartilage *in vitro*; serum withdrawn at 4, 8, 12 and 16 hr. produced +, + + + +, + + and + + + calcification respectively. (From F. C. McLean, "Metabolic aspects of convalescence" (1946). Transactions of the 14th Macy Conference, p. 34.)

is recrystallized with time to true hydroxy-apatite (Glimcher, 1968). It seems that the highly specific stereochemical configuration of mature-type collagen fibrils can initiate heterogeneous nucleation of apatite crystals from a metastable Ca–P solution. Experiments adding metastable Ca–P solutions to various reconstituted and native collagens have found that this occurs only with native-type fibrils (640 Å axial repeat representing one type of aggregation state of the tropocollagen macromolecules); evidently the specificity lies in the manner of packing the collagen macromolecules, for reconstituting native-type fibrils, and demineralized bone collagens resulted in the loss of this property of nucleation catalysis. Apparently the constituent ions of the apatite lattice in solutions interact with appropriately matched and spaced side-chain groups of the native collagen fibril; much of the bonding is apparently of phosphate. Microscopic studies have regularly shown the first crystals as small seeds in rhythmic sites along the fibrils.

Active osteoblasts, or cartilage cells in calcifying cartilage, are characterized by the presence in them of alkaline phosphate, glycogen, and phosphorylase (Robison, McLeod & Rosenheim, 1930; Gutman & Gutman, 1941; Roche, 1947,

1950). These all disappear from the scorbutic animal's cells along with its loss of ability both to form osteoid and to calcify it into bone; and reappear when ascorbic acid administration restores these abilities (Sebrell & Harris, 1954). Sobel (1950) has shown that the local calcification mechanism may be reversibly inactivated, e.g. by shaking bone slices for 2 hrs. in a Ca solution to which has been added a second ion which he regards as a competitor (Be, Cu, Mg, Sr, Na or I). After similar subsequent shaking of them in the solution of $CaCl_2$ without any added competing ions, the slices are again calcifiable. It has been well shown that phosphatase is invariably present at the site of calcification in bone, cartilage and teeth and that it appears with the development of ossification centres.

RELATED METABOLISM

The normal human adult skeleton contains about 1200 g. Ca, 530 g. P, 11 g. Mg (see Table 22.1). There is little knowledge as yet of the importance of Mg in bones, where 58% of the body's Mg is found. Since the skeleton contains 99% of the body's Ca and 87% of its P, we shall be much concerned with the biochemistry of these elements. The other main site of the body's

P is muscle (10%), where it occurs in an N/P ratio by weight of 14·7; P occurs in the bones in a Ca/P ratio by weight of 2·2. These ratios are useful in considering metabolic data; for, when the body's P balance is changing and account has been taken of associated changes in Ca and N balance, and in plasma levels, it is possible to apportion the factors involved in the P balance by the use of these ratios (Albright & Reifenstein, 1948).

TABLE 22.1

Composition of human adult skeleton

(after Shohl, 1939)

	Total (g.)	Total weight of skeleton (%)	Skeletal fraction of total body content (%)
Water	5100	44·0	10
Ca	1150	9·5	99·7
P	530	4·6	87·6
Na	18·7	0·16	28·6
Mg	11	—	58·9

Plasma Levels

Plasma calcium. There is practically no Ca in the blood corpuscles. Plasma Ca occurs in two main forms: that bound to protein and the ultra-filtrable fraction. The content of the CSF and other extracellular fluids is similar to the ultra-filtrable fraction, but CSF in particular is probably a secretion whose Ca content usually, though not always, reflects plasma ultrafiltrate (Herbert, 1933; Howard, 1954). It has been claimed that discordance between these is characteristic of parathyroid disorders, but many doubt this. The normal level of total serum Ca is 4·9—5·5mEq/l.

The first successful method for estimating serum Ca was that of Kramer & Tisdall (1921), in which Ca was directly precipitated from blood serum by addition of ammonium oxalate. The precipitate was thrice washed with dilute ammonia and finally titrated with $KMnO_4$ after dissolution in acid. This method was modified by Tisdall in 1923, who preferred to wash the precipitate only twice, and modified again in 1925 by Clark & Collip, who considered the most accurate results were obtained by washing the oxalate precipitate with only one portion of dilute ammonia. These latter authors emphasized that the method depended entirely upon compensation of errors for its accuracy. MacIntyre (1955) found by using radioactive isotopes that the concomitant precipitation of Mg oxalate compensated to a varying degree for the losses of Ca oxalate in the washings which together amounted to 5 to 10% of the total in the Tisdall (1923) procedure. Results by the Tisdall procedure, then, are probably lower than the true values for serum Ca by something like 3 to 4%. The higher results obtained with the Clark & Collip procedure (1925) approach more closely to the true values. The chelating methods for serum Ca (Lehmann, 1953; Baron & Bell, 1959) in which the Ca of the serum is titrated with ethylene–diamine tetra-acetate yield results which are in general agreement with those by the Kramer–Tisdall procedure (1921). The most recent chelating methods are probably more precise than the oxalate precipitation procedures. The flame photometer, now universally used for

TABLE 22.2

Biochemical findings in bone disease

(N = normal; L = low; H = high; Sl = slightly)

	Alkaline Phosphatase (K.A. units/100 ml.)	Phosphorus (mg./100 ml.)	Calcium (mg./100 ml.)
Normal	(N3–13)	N ($2\frac{1}{2}$–$4\frac{1}{2}$)	N (9–11)
Rickets & osteomalacia	N or H (25–40)	L ($\frac{1}{2}$–$2\frac{1}{2}$)	N (or L)
Hypophosphatasia	L (0–7)	N	N-H ($9\frac{1}{2}$–18)
Hypoparathyroidism	N	H ($4\frac{1}{2}$–10)	L (5–7)
Hyperparathyroidism	N or H (20–200)	L ($\frac{1}{2}$–$2\frac{1}{2}$) (or N)	H (11–20)
Osteitis deformans	H (20–200)	N	N
Metastatic carcinoma	N-H (10–50)	N or L	N (or H)
Osteogenic sarcoma	H (10–40)	N	N
Multiple myeloma	N	N or L	N-H (10+)
Fractures	Sl H (10–20)	N	N

the estimation of Na and K in biological material, is coming into widespread use for the rapid and more accurate determination of serum Ca. MacIntyre (1957) indicates that flame photometric results are a little higher than those yielded by the titrimetric procedures; 95% of healthy subjects have serum Ca values in the range 4·9–5·5 mEq./l. (MacIntyre, 1962); a similar normal range has been obtained by Gordan (1961) and Ikkos (1961).

Circulating Levels of Phosphorus and Phosphatase

Inorganic phosphate. The normal plasma phosphate (P) level is 2·5–4·5 mg./100 ml., varying within this range according to intake and also in a diurnal rhythm. It is about 1–2 mg./100 ml. higher in children and acromegalics. It is nearly all ultrafiltrable (Handler & Cohn, 1951; Hogben & Bollman, 1951; Hopkins, Howard & Eisenberg, 1952). It has been found that plasma P is partly protein-bound and only 85% free (Loken, Havel, Gordan & Whittington, 1960). Similar levels tend to be found in other fluids, though CSF, which is a secretion, is lower. Though starvation, or other conditions involving acidosis, withdraws Ca and P from the bones and tissues, the circulating levels are little altered. The P level fluctuates in the normal range according to intake and falls in P-depleted states, e.g. in recovery from cell dehydration such as after diabetic acidosis. It falls after insulin or glucose administration when glucose moves intracellularly. Otherwise, the serum P level reflects mainly renal homeostasis, parathyroid function or a deficiency in vitamin D. The rise in uraemia tends to lower serum Ca. The fall in hyperparathyroidism and the rise in hypoparathyroidism is associated with opposite changes in serum Ca. Deficiency of vitamin D is generally associated with some fall in serum P as well as in serum Ca; the Ca × P product generally falls. In contrast to hyperparathyroidism, in vitamin D excess or in other bone decalcifying disease the serum P (and phosphatase) remains normal, while serum Ca may rise. Artificial raising of serum Ca by Ca infusions, or by large oral doses of soluble Ca salts, raises serum P 1–2 mg./100 ml., due partly but not entirely to parathyroid suppression.

Plasma alkaline phosphatase. It was shown by Martland & Robison (1926) that the blood plasma contains a phosphatase similar to that of the bone. Its optimum activity is at an alkaline pH, and it is activated by Mg ions. Many tissues contain alkaline phosphatase; osteoblasts of bone, liver, small intestine, kidney and placenta are particularly rich sources. The enzymes from these tissues can be distinguished from each other by kinetic measurements and substrate specificity, response to inhibitors, electrophoretic mobility and resistance to denaturation by heat, urea or acid pH. In the normal adult, the circulating alkaline phosphatase appears to be largely of liver type according to the above criteria, with a small, genetically-determined contribution from the intestine in some individuals. There may also be a component of bone phosphatase. In physiological or pathological conditions in which there is enhanced osteoblastic activity, e.g. during normal growth, or in Paget's disease, hyperparathyroidism, osteogenic sarcoma, etc., the plasma alkaline phosphatase is increased and takes on the characteristics of the bone enzyme.

Methods for the estimation of plasma or serum alkaline phosphatase activity involve the hydrolysis of an orthophosphate ester by the enzyme at alkaline pH, and subsequent estimation of either the inorganic phosphate or the non-phosphate residue released by cleavage of the substrate. Many substrates have been used in this estimation. Choice of substrate is usually made so as to allow the non-P part of the molecule to be determined easily and sensitively by a second reaction (e.g. the phenol released from phenylphosphate), or so that the non-P residue is coloured without further chemical treatment (e.g. the *p*-nitrophenol derived from *p*-nitrophenyl phosphate is yellow in alkaline solution). These two substrates, together with *a*-glycerophosphate (inorganic P is measured following hydrolysis of this substrate), are those most commonly used in clinical estimations of alkaline phosphatase. Many modifications of phosphatase methods have been described, with a consequent proliferation of units in which plasma phosphatase activity may be reported. The three units in most general use are: King–Armstrong units (substrate, phenyl phosphate), Bodansky units (*a*-glycerophosphate) and Bessey–Lowry units (*p*-nitrophenyl phosphate). These units are usually reported per 100 ml. of plasma or serum. A given preparation of alkaline phosphatase hydrolyses these three substrates at different rates; furthermore, alkaline phosphatases from different tissues act on a range of substrates to give distinct patterns of relative activity, and this is especially true of intestinal and placental phosphatases compared with those from other tissues. Comparisons of results obtained by different methods of assay are therefore difficult, since plasma or serum contains a mixture of phosphatases from several sources. Adoption of

International Units of enzyme activity (i.e micromoles of substrate hydrolysed per minute) will reduce the confusion of phosphatase units to some extent, but it must be remembered that these are not absolute units, and that the nature of the substrate, temperature, pH and other conditions must still be specified.

An indication of the relative magnitudes of several phosphatase units can be seen in Table 22.3.

TABLE 22.3

Plasma alkaline phosphatases by several methods

(Units per 100 ml. plasma, normal ranges, units according to different authors' definitions)

Kay (1930)	0·1–0·2
Jenner & Kay (1932)	3–13
King & Armstrong (1934)	3–13
Bodansky (1933)	1·5–5
Shinowara, Jones & Reinhart (1942)	2·8–8·6
Huggins & Talalay (1945)	3–15

TABLE 22.4

Normal plasma alkaline phosphatase
(King–Armstrong units)

Healthy laboratory workers and others:

American (*Reiner*, 1953)	4·0–10·0
British (*King & Wootton*, 1956)	(3·3) 4·5–9·5 (12·9)
Canadian (*King & Armstrong*, 1934)	3·0–13·0
Danish (*Buch & Buch*, 1939)	4·4–13·2
Swedish (*Arner & Swedin*, 1949)	2·0–8·0
German civilians (*Stern*, 1948):	
35 men	4·0 ± 2·0
33 women	3·0 ± 2·1
71 children	12·5 (5–28)
Pregnant women, British (*Young* et al., 1946):	
First 24 weeks (261 cases)	4·3 ± 2·0
32 weeks–term (220 cases)	10·5 ± 3·0
Post-partum (1 week)	10·4 ± 3·5
Post-partum (6 months)	7·6 ± 2·5
Infants 0–3 yr., British (*Gray & Carter*, 1949):	
Normals (56)	17 (11–20)
Clinical rickets (64)	25–40 (− 76)
Early rickets	35

Normal values of alkaline phosphatase. The normal range for alkaline phosphatase in serum has been repeatedly determined, and a range of

3–13 King–Armstrong units/100 ml. is generally accepted for adults (Table 22.4). Considerably higher levels are found in growing children, reaching levels of about 25 K.A.U./100 ml. The phosphatase level is correlated with the extent of bone growth and declines to adult values after puberty. A small difference in serum phosphatase levels between men and women has been noted (Dent & Harper, 1962), and there is evidence of a slight rise in later life. A slight or moderate increase in serum alkaline phosphatase usually occurs during the last trimester of pregnancy, due to the entry of placental phosphatase into the maternal circulation.

Plasma alkaline phosphatase in bone disease. The phosphatase level in these diseases is correlated with the extent of osteoblastic activity. Highest values are observed in Paget's disease, in which the raised alkaline phosphatase level is usually the only chemical abnormality of the serum, and in osteogenic sarcoma. In Paget's disease constant phosphatase levels may be maintained for several years, an increase indicating an extension of the disease. Phosphatase levels in hyperparathyroidism may range between normal and high values, depending on the degree of bone involvement, and similar considerations apply in rickets and osteomalacia.

Secondary cancerous deposits in bone which stimulate osteoblastic activity (e.g. from prostatic or breast cancers) cause a raised alkaline phosphatase activity. In these patients a differential analysis of the alkaline phosphatase into bone and liver components may be helpful in determining whether metastases in liver or bone are present. In the case of bone metastases which are of an osteolytic rather than an osteoblastic type, serum acid phosphatase may be raised, alkaline phosphatase remaining normal. Diseases of bone which raise serum Ca such as sarcoidosis or multiple myelomatosis do not usually raise the serum alkaline phosphatase activity. Low serum alkaline phosphatase levels (0–3 K.A.U./100 ml.) are characteristic of the congenital abnormality of hypophosphatasia, in which calcification is deficient.

Calcium

Absorption. Compared with other common metals, such as K and Na, the speed of absorption of Ca is slow, and the amount that can be absorbed per day is limited, even under optimal conditions. However, this limitation is only important either during recovery from bone depletion or in pregnancy and lactation; in which last state the needs for Ca are so high that balance of Ca is almost impossible with any diet. Although tracer amounts of ^{45}Ca placed in the upper intestine equilibrate with the blood almost as rapidly as after intravenous injection, more than tracer amounts cannot move so fast (Rubin, 1954). A single large oral dose of 2 g. of Ca as a soluble salt such as the gluconate will raise the plasma Ca temporarily to a peak of $+1\cdot5$ mg./ 100 ml. at 2 hr. associated with increased urinary loss (Shohl, 1939).

Ca is absorbed mainly in the duodenum and the upper small intestine by mucosal cells containing a specific carrier protein whose production is dependent on the supply of vitamin D (Wasserman & Taylor, 1968). The amount secreted into or absorbed from the large intestine is negligible (Nicolaysen, 1934). Absorption by this specific mechanism is accelerated by parathormone and other hormonal regulators. The proportion of Ca absorbed may be increased to a much smaller extent by raising the ratio of Ca/P in the diet, the acidity of the upper intestine, or by giving extra Ca as a soluble organic salt, e.g. lactate or gluconate (Schmidt & Greenberg, 1935; Shohl, 1939; Nicolaysen, Eeg-Larsen & Malm, 1953). If a systemic acidosis is induced, this has an opposite effect on the retention of Ca by the body (Shohl, 1939), and so the effects of changes in the acid-base balance in the diet may be complex. If the Ca is given as CaCl$_2$, the most soluble salt, this also produces a systemic acidosis and so involves mixed effects. Faulty absorption of fat, i.e. steatorrhoea, is always associated with decreased Ca absorption; though up to 0·5 g./day may be found in the faeces as soaps (Nicolaysen et al., 1953), this loss probably depends mainly on the associated vitamin D deficiency.

Ca absorption may be assessed either in an acute test (a medium oral load with tracers, or a large oral load alone) or in a balance procedure. The latter assesses net absorption, or true absorption less the endogenous faecal loss which may itself be abnormal. Net absorption must be assessed in relation to the dietary Ca (see Tables 22.5 and 22.6 and Fig. 22.7.) While it is fairly steadily about 33% of dietary Ca, it will be adapted with urinary excretion to achieve balance, provided the dietary Ca is above the minimum Ca requirements. The Ca secreted into the gut and the endogenous faecal Ca loss are measurable by intravenous tracers as discussed on p. 764. In balance procedures it is usual to assess endogenous Ca metabolism on low Ca intake (100–150 mg./day), or on the assessed "home" intake in order to avoid adaptation; and to assess net absorption either on "home" intake or on a standard medium (1 g./day) or high (2+ g./day) Ca intake (see Table 22.5).

An adaptation of the efficiency of the absorption of Ca for low levels of intake can apparently occur, but its mechanism is not clear. It is particularly well shown with young rats, and is even more efficient when they have increased vitamin D intake (Nicolaysen & Jansen, 1939). Some humans are better absorbers of Ca than

Ca INTAKE & NET ABSORPTION

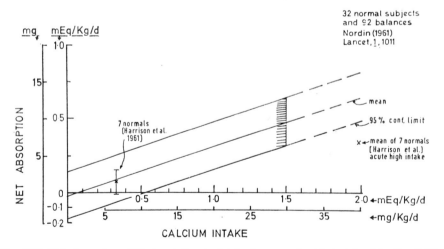

FIG. 22.7. Net absorption of Ca in relation to intake for normal subjects (after Nordin, 1961).

TABLE 22.5

Sample balance data on moderate calcium diets

(Clinically important values are italicized)

Diagnosis[1]	Concurrent treatment (if any)	Ca in mg./24 hr.				Source
		Intake	Urine	Faeces	Balance	
1 a. Normal (adult)	—	500	180	340	− 20	McCance (1954)
1 b. Normal (children: mean)	—	920	74	666	+ 180	Macy (1942)
2 a. Simple osteomalacia (Oriental)	(hospital diet probably corrected deficit)	1470	*3*	1147	+ *320*	Liu et al. (1940)
2 b. Simple osteomalacia (steatorrhoea)	—	1400	44	1614	− 258	Fraser (unpublished)
3 a. Vit. D-resistant rickets ♂ 4½ yr.	—	760	40	640	+ 80	Albright, Butler & Bloomberg (1937)
		1430	60	1260	+ 110	Albright, Butler & Bloomberg (1937)
3 b. Vit. D-resistant osteomalacia	—	1500	75	1075	+ 350	Fraser (unpublished)
4 a. Vit. D-resistant rickets ♂ 6 yr. (Fanconi syndrome)	—	793	65	654	+ 74	Bickel et al. (1952) (Bld. urea = 23 mg./100 ml.)
4 b. Vit. D-resistant ♂ 16 yr.	—	3000	*520*	1350	+ *1130*	Salassa et al. (1954)
5. Uraemic osteodystrophy "renal rickets"	—	1054	69	*1173*	− *188*	Bickel et al. (1952) (Bld. urea = 144 mg./100 ml.)
6. Osteoporosis (post menopausal)	—	780	*340*	580	− *140*	Albright & Reifenstein (1948)
7. Thyrotoxicosis	—	780	*420*	936	− *576*	Fraser (unpublished)
8 a. Hypoparathyroidism	—	1200	60	1220	− 80	Albright & Reifenstein (1948)
8 b. Hypoparathyroidism on therapy	Vit. D$_2$ (10 mg./d.)	1200	60	140	+ 1000	Albright & Reifenstein (1948)
9. Primary hyperparathyroidism	—	1100	*465*	265	+ *370*	Albright & Reifenstein (1948)
10 a. Sarcoidosis (hypercalcaemia)	—	960	140	500	+ 320	Anderson et al. (1954)
10 b. Sarcoidosis (hypercalcaemia)	Cortisone (100 mg./d.)	960	140	860	− 40	Anderson et al. (1954)

[1] Cases quoted are adults unless stated otherwise.

TABLE 22.6

Sample balance data on low calcium diet

(Clinically important values are italicized)

Diagnosis	Concurrent treatment (if any)	Ca in mg./24 hr.				Source
		Intake	Urine	Faeces	Balance	
1. Normal adult (mean)	—	110	60	200	− 150	Bauer et al. (1929)
2. Hypoparathyroidism	—	100	*23*	83	− 6	Albright & Reifenstein (1948)
3. Primary hyperparathyroidism	—	216	*600*	134	− 518	Fraser (unpublished) (178449)
4. Polycystic fibrous dysplasia	—	90	100	220	− 230	Albright, Butler, Hampton & Smith (1937)
5. Hypercalcaemic sarcoid	—	190	*210*	80	− 100	Anderson et al. (1954)
6. Idiopathic hypercalcuria	—	150 / 350	*240* / *360*	53 / 90	− 143 / − 100	Albright et al. (1953)
7. Thyrotoxicosis	—	145	*158*	204	− 217	Fraser (unpublished)
8. Hypercalcaemia with breast carcinoma secondaries	Stilboestrol (15 mg./day)	135	*670*	not estimated	− 535+	Kennedy et al. (1953)
9. Uraemic osteodystrophy	—	210	90	*380*	− 260	Albright, Drake & Sulkowitch (1937)
10 a. Osteomalacia (simple)	—	100	*30*	150	− 80	Liu et al. (1940)
10 b. Osteomalacia (due to steatorrhoea)	—	100	*10*	190	− 100	Bennett et al. (1932)
11. Vit. D-resistant osteomalacia	—	150	*120*	110	− 80	Fraser (unpublished)
12. Treated osteomalacia due to renal tubular acidosis	Vit. D$_2$ (1–2 mg./day) + Na lactate (300 m-equiv./day)	73	*160*	55	− 142	Albright et al. (1946)

others, though whether this is in part dependent on vitamin D supply is not clear (McCance, 1954). Though adaptive changes in absorptive efficiency have not been shown in humans on short term studies, Malm (1958) has studied adaptation over 2–8 months in 26 men taking diets of 400–900 mg. Ca/day and found that 23 of them could adapt with varying speed. Further, either selective adaptation in the race or individual adaptation of absorption must have occurred to explain the efficient absorption shown for Ceylonese children (Nicholls & Nimalasuriya, 1939) and a Peruvian prison (Hegsted, Moscoso & Collazos, 1952) where balances were achieved on intakes of Ca below 400 mg./day. Various studies have been made of Ca balance to try to determine the smallest intake which does not involve a negative balance; this "Ca requirement" appears to vary among individuals from 3–15 mg./kg./day (Nordin & Smith, 1965). Defective net absorption of Ca is a feature of malabsorption, relative or absolute vitamin D deficiency, i.e. of either simple or D-resistant osteomalacia (Stanbury, Lumb & Nicholson, 1960), and excessive Ca absorption is found in idiopathic hypercalcuria, and in hypercalcaemic sarcoid in which an associated vitamin D hypersensitivity has also been shown.

Acute absorption tests assess true absorption. Nordin and his colleagues (Peacock, Knowles & Nordin, 1968) have proposed a test of acute Ca deprivation followed by a load suitable for assessing hypercalcuria for its dependence on hyperabsorption. After overnight fasting, their normals had urinary excretions of 0.08 ± 0.02 mg./100 ml. G.F.R. In hypercalcuric subjects, corresponding basal fasting values were found only after 16 hr. fasting. After an oral Ca load (100 mg. Ca citrate/kg. as suspension, following an overnight fast) the normal subjects excreted over the next 8 hr. 40–180 mg. urinary Ca, while hyperabsorbing hypercalcurics excreted 190–300 mg. during a similar 8-hr. period. Tracer Ca absorption tests are usually performed by giving to fasting subjects 5–10 μC ^{47}Ca or 1 μC ^{45}Ca with some 5–20 m-Eq. carrier as a soluble Ca salt, and usually measuring the plasma at 2 hr. when the normal peak occurs (0.8 to 2.0%/litre). Alternatively the 0–24 hour urine specific activity, or 6-day faecal or whole body Ca may be measured; or more complex double tracer tests can use the second dose given intravenously to correct for Ca cleared from the plasma. Nordin, Young, Oxby & Bulusu (1968) have suggested a procedure for using a single tracer absorption test with plasma samples

at 1 and 2 hr. from which they derive a possibly adequate correction for clearance of the absorbed Ca from plasma. Such acute absorption tests show increased true absorption in hyperparathyroidism, vitamin D overdosage or hypersensitivity as in sarcoid, and idiopathic hypercalcuria with or without renal stones; and decreased absorption in renal disease, and corticosteroid overdosage but only in some cases of malabsorption.

Urinary excretion of calcium. Plasma Ca is probably about 50% filtrable by the glomerulus (the ultrafiltrable fraction). Under all circumstances a large proportion of the filtered Ca is reabsorbed by the tubules; normally about 99%, giving an average ultrafiltrable Ca clearance of about 0.4 ml./min.

Probably because of the technical difficulties involved in plasma ultrafiltration, there have not been many studies of the renal handling of Ca. Neuman & Chen (1954) report observations in the dog on the ratio of ultrafiltrable Ca clearance to the G.F.R., measured by endogenous creatinine (the Ca to creatinine clearance ratio, Ca/Cr CR). Like similarly excreted substances, the Ca/Cr CR also rises steadily with rising serum Ca levels. Further study is needed of the factors which influence this clearance. It is probably influenced by serum P level [probably a rise of P lowers both serum and urinary Ca (Howard, 1954)], PAH or diodrast excretion (which increases it considerably) and parathormone.

Urinary Ca excretion on a range of known intakes in studies of 606 normal individuals of varying age and size has been analysed by Knapp (1947). She showed that the urinary excretion correlated more closely with the non-obese weight than with the intake or age. After allowing for body weight, she found only slight changes in urinary excretion in relation to intake with diets up to 10 mg./kg./24 hr. (Fig. 22.8). The range is quite wide suggesting that, even after allowing for size, endogenous factors are the main determinants of urinary Ca. Pyrah & Raper (1955) also find the range of normal urinary Ca extends up to 350 mg./24 hr. Long-term studies by Nicolaysen et al. (1953) on 30 normal men on intakes planned to be constant at either 900 mg. or 450 mg. showed each individual's excretion to fluctuate $\pm 20\%$ about his mean level, while these ranged from the group mean by -50 to $+100\%$. To distinguish renal hypercalcuria from that dependent on hyperabsorption, the urinary Ca excretion can be measured on low Ca intake (under 200 mg./day); to which most of the equilibration is completed after 1 to 2 days; on

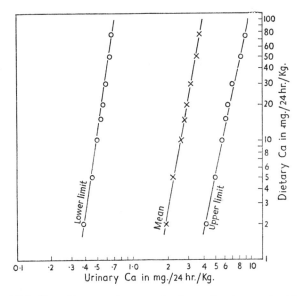

FIG. 22.8. The wide normal range of urinary Ca of normal subjects
in relation to dietary Ca. (Redrawn from Knapp (1947).)

this intake normal urinary Ca is 50–150 mg./day
or at least under 200 mg./day (Nordin & Smith,
1965). As noted earlier, a Ca deprivation test
can do this by withdrawing Ca foods for 24 hr.

Urinary Ca excretion may be raised by increasing the dietary acid intake or its Ca/P ratio,
by ingesting such salts as those of Ca and Mg or
large vitamin D doses, and by skeletal immobilization (Shohl, 1939), but especially by
hyperparathyroidism, by bone-invasive disease,
hyperthyroidism and acromegaly and by idiopathic hypercalcuria. It is lowered in nephrosis
(Emerson & Beckman, 1945; Jones, Peters,
Morgan, Coles & Mallick, 1967), uraemia,
hypoparathyroidism, by chronic thiazide diuretics
to immobilized or other subjects (Rose, 1966),
alkalosis and in vitamin D deficiency, though not
always in vitamin D resistant rickets. Sweat losses
of Ca are probably small (Eisenberg & Gordan,
1961).

Calcium tracers. The body's avidity for Ca has
been assessed by Ca tolerance tests* when these
give sufficient Ca for the "excess Ca" to be
measurable (e.g. 15 mg. Ca/kg. over 4 hr).
However, without disturbing the body's Ca
equilibrium, indices of the body's transfer of Ca
can be obtained from the use of Ca tracers.
Four tracers are readily available, ^{45}Ca (half-life

* These tests also measure the phosphaturia
response to hypercalcaemia.

164 days, beta emitter), ^{47}Ca (half-life 4·7 days,
γ emitter), ^{85}Sr (65 days, γ emitter), or stable ^{88}Sr
which can be measured in a flame photometer
(Fraser, Harrison & Ibbertson, 1960). Sr appears
to be deposited in the bones by the same process
as Ca, entering the bone crystals and exchanging
equivalently for Ca. While the intestine discrimi-
nates greatly against orally administered Sr
(Spencer, Li, Samachson & Laszlo, 1960),
variations in its absorption parallel those of Ca
(Wasserman, Comar & Papadopoulou, 1957),
but faecal losses of intravenously injected tracer
Ca or Sr are not widely divergent (Dow &
Stanbury, 1960; Spencer et al., 1960). Renal
clearance of Sr is three to five times that of Ca
(Harrison, Raymond & Tretheway, 1955).
Double tracer experiments with ^{45}Ca and ^{85}Sr
gave similar pool sizes and disappearance
constants in man (Dow & Stanbury, 1960). The
same autoradiographic pattern is seen in bone
(Engfeldt, Bjornerstedt, Clemedson & Engström,
1954), though minor differences in release from
bone have been noted (Talmage, Elliott, Davis
& Enders, 1957a; Talmage, Schooley & Comar,
1957b; Likins, Posner, Kunde & Craven, 1959).
Such findings are important for the problem of
radio-toxicity of ^{90}Sr.

The tracer is usually given intravenously at
0 hr. and its disposal indexed from the plasma
or urine measurements of specific activity, often
supplemented by faecal, skeletal or whole body

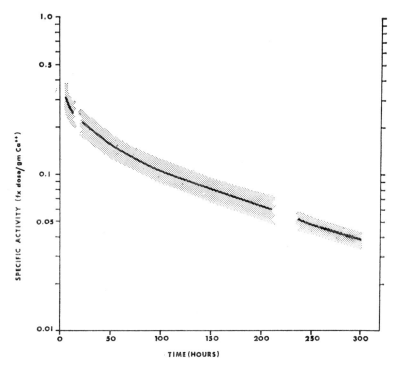

Fig. 22.9. ^{47}Ca or ^{45}Ca tracer tests: values from normal subjects for plasma and for urine Ca specific activity (uncorrected) for first 5 days after i.v. dose (mean $\pm$ standard deviation for each time interval shown). (From Heaney & Skillman, 1964.)

measurements. Since urine and faecal losses can be deducted, appropriate analysis of the disappearance curve can derive indices of the body's or the skeleton's avidity for Ca, including possibly a less valid index of bone resorption. The measured faecal loss can index endogenous faecal loss (Heaney & Skillman, 1964), while oral doses can measure true absorption rather than the net absorption measured on balances.

Skeletal measurements. Fig. 22.9 shows the tracer measurements obtained in normals after a single intravenous dose of ^{47}Ca, and Fig. 22.10 similar data obtained with stable ^{88}Sr as tracer. Fig. 22.11 shows the good correlation between skeletal avidity indexed by this Sr tracer test and that measured by "Ca excess" in a Ca tolerance test, as is also found if Sr is infused and excess Ca + Sr is used in the calculation (Mazzuoli, Biagi & Coen, 1961). Both such tests have revealed increased skeletal avidity, for example in osteomalacia (Fraser *et al.*, 1960).

Such tracer data when corrected for urine and faecal losses reflect the summation of the disposal of Ca over various mostly bony sites. This bone disposal involves two main processes, deposition into new bone and a two-way ion-exchange, to which gradually becomes added some contribution from bone resorption as the resorption sites become labelled from ion-exchange. However, as abnormalities in bone deposition are likely to involve corresponding changes in ion-exchange, tracer disposal rates usually index but over-estimate new bone formation—except when bone is qualitatively changed as in osteomalacia when matrix is over-produced but not properly calcified.

Analysis of these data can be of varying complexity, but these tracers suggest three main Ca pools, (1) a rapidly exchangeable pool, the measurable exchangeable Ca space (V_{CaE}) which includes the ECF Ca, most soft tissue Ca, and that on all accessible bone surfaces, (2) a slowly exchanging deeper bone pool, and (3) a still deeper pool practically inaccessible until resorption invades it. The simplest type of analysis as in Fig. 22.10 measures the transfer from the first to the deeper pools as if it were a simple one-way transfer—the "apparent accretion rate" (Kb or

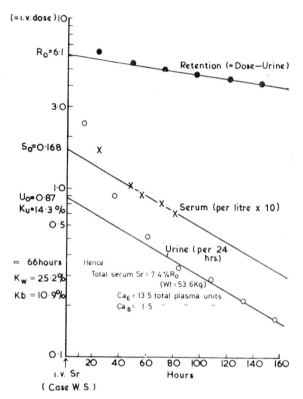

FIG. 22.10. Sample strontium (Sr) test result: the calculation of exchangeable Ca space (V_{CaE} or Ca_E) and daily deposited Ca (V_{CaB} or Ca_B). (From Fraser, Harrison & Ibbertson, 1960, *Quart. J. Med.*, **29**, 85.)

A). Plots of the plasma or urine specific activity measurements (Fig. 22.9) generally show three main phases—an initial rapid fall over the first 2 to 3 days as the Ca mixes through the rapidly exchangeable pool (the exchangeable space C_{CaE}), the second an approximately exponential decay over 2 to 6 days, whose slope probably reflects the rate of transfer from this pool or the apparent accretion or deposition rate (Kb or A); and, after these phases, which are shorter in younger or growing bone, comes the third or slower disappearance slope which often starts at a recognizable break when Ca turnover is rapid, is less nearly exponential, and whose lessened slope reflects tracer returning from deep bone partly by resorption and partly by ion exchange.

Simple indices of the apparent skeletal disposal rate (e.g. 24 hr. Ca space) reflect skeletal avidity for Ca, or after 24 hr. the exchangeable Ca plus apparent accretion rate (see Fig. 22.12). Slightly more analysis as in Fig. 22.10 measures separately the exchangeable Ca space and the apparent bone accretion rate as if the latter were a simple one-way loss into a deeper pool; from the starting level and the slope of the exponential fall, both corrected for urine and faecal losses. Anderson and his colleagues (Anderson, Osborn, Tomlinson & Walls, 1964; Anderson, Tomlinson, Osborn & Wise, 1967*b*) have shown that the same three disappearance phases of the curve may better fit a power function, on a log–log plot. Other analyses based on the two compartment models with two-way exchange derive a lower accretion rate possibly involving less exchange. In normals, the exchangeable Ca is 3–7 g. or under 1% of the skeleton, while the apparent bone deposition rate is 0·3–0·5 g./day or 10% of the skeleton per year; but tetracycline methods suggest that true bone formation may be only about one-fifth of this.

Among hypercalcaemic conditions, hyperparathyroidism and vitamin D poisoning have high accretion rates (Fraser *et al.*, 1960; Eisenberg & Gordan, 1961), except in very mild degrees. High

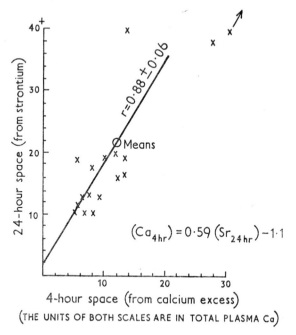

FIG. 22.11. Seventeen combined Ca and Sr infusions: the correlation of 24 hr. Sr space and 4 hr. Ca space. The Ca "space" in litres of plasma = the total body retention of the infusion divided by the excess Ca found at the same sime per litre of plasma. The serum excess = the Ca concentration at 4 hr. after starting the infusion *minus* the Ca concentration before infusion. (From Fraser *et al.*, 1960, *Quart. J. Med.*, **29**, 85.)

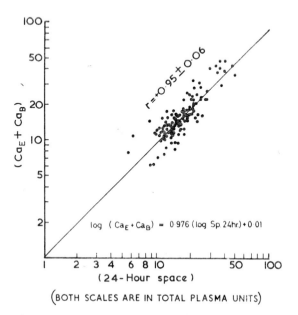

FIG. 22.12. The correlation between (Ca$_E$ and Ca$_B$) and 24 hr. Sr space in 128 Sr tests. (From Fraser *et al.* 1960, *Quart. J. Med.*, **29**, 85.)

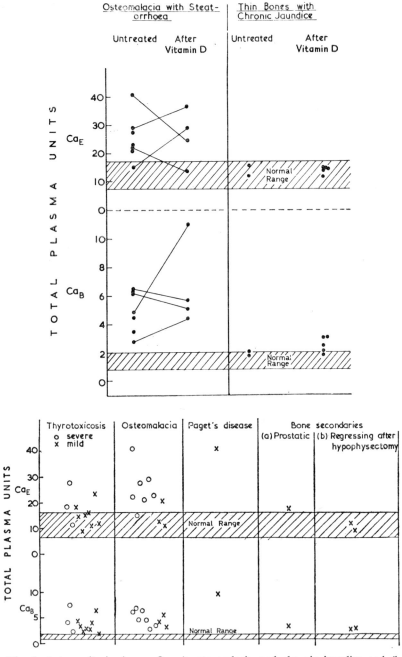

Fig. 22.13. The Sr test results in (upper figure) osteomalacia and chronic jaundice and (lower figure) "hypermetabolic" bone disease without hypercalcaemia. (From Fraser *et al.*, 1960, *Quart. J. Med.*, **29**, 85.)

accretion rates are also found in normo-calcaemic Paget's disease, sclerosing bone secondaries, in osteomalacia, hyperparathyroidism and acromegaly (Fig. 22.13). Exceptionally severe deficiency osteomalacia has shown a small pool and decreased accretion (Harris, Hoffenberg & Black, 1965). Most local bone lesions have an increased local uptake of Ca tracer probably due to reactive new bone formation (Corey, Kenny, Greenberg, Pazianos, Pearson & Laughlin, 1961; Gynning, Langeland, Lindberg & Waldeskog, 1961), the only exception so far being myeloma.

Other measurements. Single intravenous or preferably double tracer methods can enable measurement of endogenous faecal Ca loss. Endogenous faecal Ca ranges 130 ± 50 mg./day and rises with increased dietary Ca; from a total intestinal Ca secretion of 194 ± 73 mg./day (Heaney & Skillman, 1964). Secreted Ca varies little with metabolic state, though there is an increased loss in some malabsorption states, probably from gut surface losses (Joplin, Melvin, Hepner, Neale & Bordier, 1969).

Phosphate

Absorption. Except in herbivora, primary P deficiency is unknown; this "aphosphorosis" is relievable by P salts and clinically resembles rickets (Shohl, 1939). Excluding phytate, most dietary P is well absorbed unless there is an abnormal intestinal excess of some poorly absorbed heavy metal, which has been administered as a salt, such as Al, Be, Fe, etc., or an excess of Ca. In these circumstances insoluble phosphates are formed in the gut, and if the quantities are sufficient, low-P rickets may be produced. Oral doses of soluble inorganic phosphates are rapidly absorbed, temporarily raising serum P levels, and nearly all being rapidly excreted in the urine. Normally, whatever the intake, faecal excretion is small and ranges 20 to 40% of it.

Urinary excretion. Normally a large proportion (about 90 to 95%) of filtered P is reabsorbed, and this proportion is increased when the blood level falls, with a threshold normally occurring at approximately 2 mg./100 ml. In the absence of P deficiency due to recent acute loss such as in the recovery from diabetic acidosis, and of any considerable change in bone status (e.g. the starting of treatment for rickets, etc.), the urinary excretion normally reflects the intestinal absorption of P, via its influence on serum P levels, and so is usually a high percentage of the intake (60 to 80%).

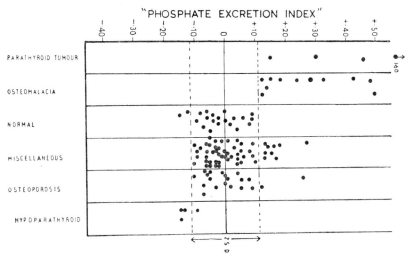

FIG. 22.14. "Urinary phosphate excretion index" in parathyroid disorders and in certain metabolic bone diseases.

$$\text{Urinary PE index} = \frac{C_P}{C_{Cr}} - \frac{\text{serum P (mg./100 ml.)}}{20} + 0.05$$

$\left(\dfrac{C_P}{C_{Cr}} = \text{ratio of phosphate clearance to that of creatinine.}\right)$

Note: (1) high values in primary hyperparathyroidism and in secondary hyperparathyroidism of osteomalacia, and in a few miscellaneous and osteoporotic cases; (2) low values in hypoparathyroidism. (From Nordin & Fraser (1956).)

Whether the excretion is normal is probably best assessed from its relation to the blood level. Normal urinary P excretion with low or relatively low levels in the plasma will occur when renal glomerular function is normal but tubular reabsorption is lowered—notably with hyperparathyroidism, but also in Cushing's syndrome, after cortisone injections (Roberts & Pitts, 1953), and so presumably with various stress states, or with certain primary renal tubular defects. Low excretions relative to the blood level (usually shown by high blood levels with normal urinary excretions) occur in hypoparathyroidism as well as with general renal failure.

Nordin & Fraser (1956) have evolved a formula for assessing the urinary excretion of P in the light of serum P and total renal function (GFR), the urinary phosphate excretion index:

$$C_p/C_{cr} - \frac{\text{ser P (mg.)}}{20} + 0 \cdot 05 = 0 \pm 0 \cdot 12;$$

where C_p/C_{cr} = the ratio of the clearance of P to that of creatinine and serum P (mg.) = serum P in mg./100 ml. Using the data assembled by Milne, Stanbury & Thompson (1952) and their own, they found that this could distinguish normal cases from either hypoparathyroidism or primary and secondary hyperparathyroidism. The index would also be raised in glycosuria, cortisone treatment, vitamin D intoxication, renal tubular defects, etc. It should, however, be a reliable means of excluding the suspicion of hyperparathyroidism (see Fig. 22.14). Several other types of index of P excretion are also used (Thomas, Connor & Morgan, 1958; Gordan, 1962), many of which do not make allowance for serum P. It is now clear that an additional factor needing attention in the excretion indices is the dietary P, for a high P intake tends to increase phosphaturia and a low P intake to reduce it (Fraser, 1960; Gordan, 1962). It is recommended, therefore, that when testing for suspected hyperparathyroidism, the patient be on a diet of low P, best achieved by adding 120 ml. Al(OH)$_3$ gel and 2·5 g. Ca/day; while a high P diet is best for suspected hypoparathyroidism. Hyperparathyroid patients will have a higher P excretion index at any P intake than do the normals, provided both groups have been on the same P intake (Gordan, 1962). If special precision is desired, the theoretical renal P threshold may be measured by giving an intravenous infusion of buffered Na phosphate over 180 min. and deriving a regression line of urinary P on plasma P (Hyde, Vaughan, Jones, McSwiney & Prunty, 1960); normally the threshold is over 2·0 mg./100 ml.

and it is lowered in hyperparathyroidism and other conditions causing phosphaturia.

Supplements of phosphate. Inorganic phosphate has been given intravenously or orally not only to treat hypercalcaemia, due either to malignancy or to inoperable hyperparathyroidism, but also to treat phosphate-diabetes or vitamin D resistant "osteomalacia" (Nagent de Deuxchaisnes & Krane, 1965, 1967; Smith & Dick, 1968c); its possible use has also been explored in recurrent renal stone formers (Bernstein & Newton, 1966) as well as in osteoporosis. A neutral mixture of P salts is used to give ½–1 g. P t.d.s. (or the equivalent daily dose intravenously during 6 to 8 hr.)

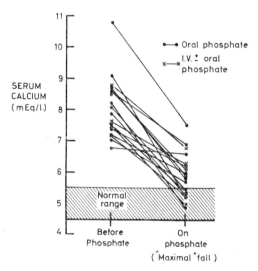

EXTENT OF "MAXIMAL" FALL IN SERUM CALCIUM

(18 courses in 13 patients)

FIG. 22.15. Treatment of hypercalcaemia by oral or i.v. phosphate supplements: extent of maximal fall in serum Ca seen over 18 courses in 13 patients by first to fifth day (From Thalassinos & Joplin, 1968.)

There is no doubt about its effective relief of malignant hypercalcaemia (Goldsmith & Ingbar, 1966; Kahil, Orman, Gyorkey & Brown, 1967; Massry, Mueller, Silverman & Kleeman, 1968; Thalassinos & Joplin, 1968), for which it is probably the most efficacious emergency treatment (Fig. 22.15), being more rapid and more universally effective than corticosteroids without necessitating intravenous administration as does EDTA or sulphate. It is essentially an emergency measure which enables effective treatment of the primary disease, but it can remain effective in courses lasting weeks (Thalassinos & Joplin, 1968). Its chronic administration is also effective in restoring the serum Ca and P to normal in hyperparathyroidism (Albright & Reifenstein, 1948; Dent, 1967), and also in promoting the healing of phosphate-diabetes osteomalacia and so minimizing the hazards of vitamin D intoxication in managing this disease. Such supplements are effective mainly by their action on bone, for in malignant hypercalcaemia it lowers urinary Ca (Herbert, Lemann, Petersen & Lennon, 1966); serum P is little altered a few hours after the infusion, and metastatic calcification is probably not increased, as judged from post mortem evidence (Thalassinos & Joplin, 1968). Following such supplements given to thyroparathyroidectomized animals, Pechet, Bobadilla, Carroll & Hesse (1967) found isotopic and histological evidence of increased bone formation. In phosphate-diabetes osteomalacia it causes acutely an increased hydroxyprolinuria, a rising alkaline phosphatase and other evidence of bone healing and correction of the osteomalacia (Smith & Dick, 1968c). It is also said to enhance the action of calcitonin in reducing bone resorption (Hirsch, 1968).

Magnesium

Magnesium (Mg) is present in all living tissues and is essential for life. Our knowledge of Mg metabolism has grown in recent years, but we still know relatively little of the role of Mg in normal metabolism and even less of its part in disease.

Evolutionary aspects. The enzymes activated by Mg may be summarized as follows:

1. Alkaline phosphatases and pyrophosphatases are all activated by Mg and inhibited by beryllium. Enzymes transferring phosphates from ATP or to ADP are also activated.

2. Mg ions are necessary whenever thiamine pyrophosphate is required as a co-factor.

3. Enolase requires the presence of Mg in high concentration.

4. Some peptidases, such as leucine aminopeptidase, require Mg.

The dependence of so many vital reactions on Mg and the abundance of Mg in the body is to be expected from the fact that Mg was one of the major cations present in the pre-Cambrian seas in which life first evolved. Anaerobic glycolysis was one of the most primitive energy-yielding processes to evolve; hence its occurrence in both the yeast cell and the muscle cell and the importance of Mg for most of the reactions. The importance of Mg as an enzyme activator and the occurrence of the element in tissues are both legacies of the common marine origin of life.

Physiology. Mg is the fourth most abundant cation in the body. The contents of Ca, sodium and potassium are 60,000, 5500 and 3000 m-equiv., respectively. The total body content of Mg is 2000 m-equiv. Half of the total body Mg is present in bone and the remainder is mainly inside body cells. Although only a very small proportion (about 1%) of the total body Mg is in the extracellular fluid, the plasma concentration is maintained within the limits of 1·5 to 1·8 m-equiv./l.

Absorption and excretion. A normal diet contains about 20 m-equiv. Mg/day. Of this, two-thirds is unabsorbed and excreted in the faeces. The remainder is absorbed and excreted in the urine. Although it has been reported that Mg absorption is enhanced by vitamin D, this vitamin does not play a dominant role as it does for Ca. It seems that Mg is handled by the kidney and the gut by a transport system which has some factors in common with Ca.

Magnesium homeostasis. Several hormones have been shown to influence the handling of Mg. These include aldosterone, vasopressin and parathyroid hormone. Of these it seems that only parathyroid hormone is normally concerned with Mg regulation. There is now evidence that the level of plasma Mg affects the secretion rate of parathyroid hormone. An increased level of plasma Mg produces inhibition, and low levels an enhancement. Parathyroid hormone diminishes Mg excretion in the urine and enhances Mg absorption from the gut. The effect of parathyroid hormone on the skeleton is of less importance for Mg than it is for Ca since the proportion of Mg in bone is very small. We do not understand how the body regulates both Mg and Ca if they both depend on parathyroid hormone. The interrelation of Mg with calcitonin remains to be determined.

Magnesium deficiency. Experimental Mg deficiency has been thoroughly studied in the rat. Hypercalcaemia is usually produced and this is thought to be due to stimulation of the production of parathyroid hormone. Mg deficiency also occurs in man in the following situations:

1. *The malabsorption syndrome.* Hypomagnesaemia of some degree occurs in about one-quarter of cases of this syndrome. It may be severe enough to merit specific treatment in as many as 10%. As would be expected, the cause is abnormal Mg losses in faeces.

2. *Parathyroid disease.* The plasma Mg falls

after removal of a parathyroid tumour. A post-operative fall in plasma Mg almost always occurs, but is much more marked in cases with severe bone disease and in cases in which hypo-magnesaemia was present preoperatively. The latter abnormality occurs when preoperative vomiting has been marked or when hyper-magnesiuria has been prominent. Increased loss of Mg in the urine is presumably due to the effect of the increased tubular load of a divalent cation due to hypercalcaemia. This outweighs the effect of parathyroid hormone in increasing tubular absorption.

3. *Chronic alcoholism.* The occurrence and symptomatology of hypomagnesaemia in chronic alcoholism have been described. It seems likely that Mg deficiency is due to increased urinary loss in the face of diminished intake. The reason for the urinary loss is not clear.

4. Prolonged or severe loss of body fluids (e.g. vomiting, diarrhoea).

5. Diuretic therapy, especially thiazide di-uretics in large doses.

6. Hypercalcaemia from any cause.

7. Renal tubular acidosis.

8. Tubular necrosis in the recovery phase.

9. Portal cirrhosis.

10. Primary aldosteronism.

In these situations plasma Ca is more often reduced than increased.

Symptomatology of Magnesium Deficiency

Three points may be made about the clinical picture:

1. Tetany, in the sense of painful peripheral muscle cramps, is not a feature of pure Mg deficiency. Since hypocalcaemia often co-exists with hypomagnesaemia, classic tetany is quite often seen, but disappears when electrolyte abnormalities other than hypomagnesaemia are relieved. It is considered that hypomagnesaemia alone may cause classic tetany. However, this is probably unusual because we have not noted this to occur in a large clinical experience.

2. There are signs and symptoms which are of non-specific nature but which can be ascribed to Mg deficiency when they are promptly relieved by therapy. Thus, muscular weakness, vertigo, mental changes (especially extreme irritability and aggressiveness), tremors and non-specific electroencephalographic and electrocardiographic changes may occur in various combinations. These may be sufficiently characteristic to allow clinical diagnosis, but usually the picture is as non-specific as in most cases of potassium deficiency.

3. The cardinal feature of most cases of Mg deficiency is a tendency to potentially fatal seizures.

Diagnosis and Treatment

Diagnosis requires the easy availability of reliable serum Mg estimations and awareness of the clinical situations in which Mg deficiency may occur. Severe and persistent hypomagnesaemia is worth treating because fatal seizures may occur and because it seems likely that renal damage may be induced. In the presence of very low initial levels (0·8 m-equiv./l. or less), treatment should begin with intravenous administration of magnesium chloride: 2 m-equiv./kg. may safely be given intravenously over 4 hr. In less severe cases, repletion may be accomplished gradually by administration of 0·25 to 0·5 m-equiv./kg./day until the plasma Mg is normal. In severe malabsorption, larger amounts may be necessary, even up to 4 m-equiv./kg./day in divided doses.

It may be useful to give Mg supplementation routinely after removal of a parathyroid adenoma. This should certainly be done when there has been severe preoperative vomiting or when bone disease is marked. When plasma Mg analyses are readily available, supplementation may be reserved for those cases of parathyroid tumour in which hypomagnesaemia has been demonstrated.

Urinary Hydroxyproline

The circulating levels of hydroxyproline (HP) are generally indexed from urinary excretion rates, for there is good evidence that these mirror plasma levels (Prockop & Kivirikko, 1967), and the method is reasonably sensitive and specific (Kivirikko, Laitinen & Prockop, 1967). Of total urinary HP only 5% is free HP, for much of the free amino acid is metabolized to urea and CO_2; the peptide HP similarly derived from the degradation of collagen, accounts for the majority of the total HP measurable after hydrolysis (Kivirikko *et al.*, 1967). The threshold for HP peptides is so low that the rate of renal clearance approximates the GFR (Prockop & Kivirikko, 1967). The relatively unique fate and source of HP enable its measurements to index collagen turnover, to which bone collagen probably contributes more than half. Since gelatin-free diets contribute little to urinary HP, and proline is only hydroxylated after its incorporation into the polypeptide protocollagen or whose synthesis it is not re-utilized, practically all the body's HP is derived from the catabolism of collagen.

Clearly several different types of alterations in collagen metabolism could alter the rate of urinary excretion, as well as increases or decreases in the overall collagen turnover; nevertheless its excretion rate seems often to reflect the latter. As indicated in Fig. 22.16 changes in the urinary HP excretion rate may arise also from variations in the proportions of soluble and insoluble collagen, since isotope studies have shown that soluble collagen is more rapidly metabolized to HP. The normal adult values (i.e. over 21 years) are 15–43 mg./24 hr. or 9–24 mg./24 hr./m².

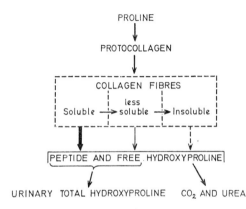

FIG. 22.16. Scheme of metabolism of hydroxyproline (after Prockop & Kivirikko, 1967).

For younger growing children the values are 3 or 4 times this range per unit surface area, perhaps partly because of a higher proportion of soluble collagen. The urinary excretion of HP is increased with over-secretion of growth hormone, thyroxine or parathyroid hormone, and tends to be decreased in the opposite disorders, though a decrease is less easily defined in adults. It is also increased in other conditions which involve lysis of bone, generalized catabolism and rickets or osteomalacia (Laitinen, 1967), in which appropriate treatment with vitamin D (Smith & Dick, 1968b) or phosphate (Smith & Dick, 1968c) increases it further. The increase in rickets may reflect the increased osteoblastic activity, possibly less maturation of collagen in the wide osteoid seams, and probably also the usually associated secondary hyperparathyroidism (Anderson, Bannister, Parsons & Tomlinson, 1967a). It is

reduced in scurvy and increased in lathyrism and in some patients with Marfan's syndrome, probably because of defective conversion of soluble to insoluble collagen. Urinary HP is usually normal in "collagen diseases".

METABOLIC REGULATORS AFFECTING BONE

Control Mechanisms

Skeletal homeostasis. Although the skeleton is being constantly remodelled, in normal adults this occurs without net change in total skeletal mass. Yet, when young adults are suddenly immobilized with paralytic poliomyelitis, there occurs a dramatic skeletal loss and hypercalcuria, which suggests that a major factor maintaining skeletal replacement is the constant stimulation by mechanical stresses. Indeed a mechanism for this stimulation has been suggested by Becker, Bassett & Bachman (1964) who recorded from an excised dead or living bone and found that a potential difference was induced between the end and the midshaft when a bending stress was imposed. Presumably basic cellular activities provide basic rates of bone formation and resorption, which are adapted in response to both this stimulation and the others ensuring Ca–P homeostasis.

Calcium–phosphate homeostasis. There appears to be no special hormonal mechanism which regulates plasma P, although several hormones, especially parathyroid hormone, are known to increase renal P clearance. There is little evidence however that changes in plasma P have a direct influence on parathyroid hormone secretion rate. It is perhaps not surprising therefore that the plasma P is less precisely controlled than is plasma Ca which is under detailed hormonal control. The three main regulators of Ca metabolism in man are parathyroid hormone, calcitonin and vitamin D. The actions of calcitonin and vitamin D are discussed in detail elsewhere. In this section we shall summarize their influence on Ca homeostasis.

In young animals, such as the rat, the main influence on plasma Ca is the turnover rate of bone. Here, the most important factor in plasma Ca regulation is the osteoclastic resorption of bone under the influence of parathyroid hormone. The effects of parathyroid hormone on the gut and kidney are far less significant than its effect on bone in this case. This is also true in generalized Paget's disease in adult man in which the turnover rate of bone may be twenty times greater than normal. However, the situation is different in normal adults. In this case the action of parathyroid hormone on the gut and kidney is more important than its effect on osteoclastic resorption of bone. This is because the changes in Ca flow into and out of extracellular fluid, produced by changes in gut and renal function, are much greater than those produced by changes in bone resorption.

Calcitonin is normally present in adult plasma and appears to play a role in regulating bone resorption. It has relatively little effect on plasma Ca in adults, although it may be important in plasma Ca regulation in babies and young children.

Vitamin D

Vitamin D, or exposure to the sun so that the vitamin is synthesized from precursors in skin, is essential for normal health. Vitamin D is stored in the liver, but only in relatively small amounts. Two forms of vitamin D are known, vitamin D_2 (calciferol) and vitamin D_3 (cholecalciferol).

Vitamin D_2 is produced by irradiation of ergosterol; vitamin D_3 from irradiation of 7-dehydrocholesterol. This latter is the normal process in man, in whom ergosterol is not absorbed. The structures of these vitamins are shown in Fig. 22.17. The requirement of vitamin D for most infants is less than 400 units daily. However, although adequate for children with fair skins, this may be inadequate for dark-skinned children in northern latitudes. In Europe and the U.S.A. many foods are fortified with calciferol, but this procedure has sometimes produced poisoning of children by excessive intake of the vitamin. For this reason new official standards have recently been proposed which minimize this risk by limiting the content of vitamin D in national dried milk, cod liver oil and infant cereals.

Action of vitamin D. Very recently, DeLuca (1968) has shown that vitamin D is converted to an active form (25-hydroxycholecalciferol). It seems possible that this is the substance which is responsible for most of the effects of vitamin D in man, and that some revision of our present hypothesis may prove necessary. For example, it is possible that some cases of resistance to vitamin D may result from failure to convert the vitamin to a metabolically active form. Vitamin D has three sites of action:

1. *Intestine.* Vitamin D is essential for Ca absorption. However, the precise mechanism involved is completely unknown, although recently Wasserman, (1968) has suggested that

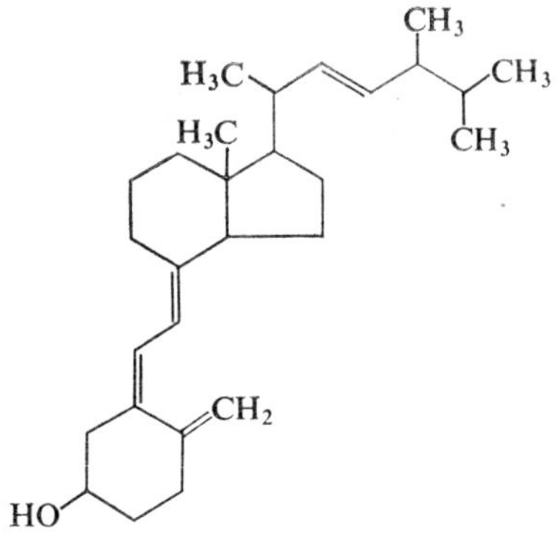

VITAMIN D_2
ergocalciferol

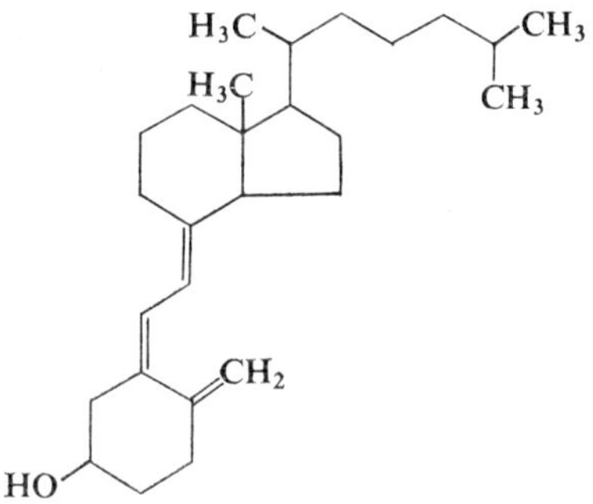

VITAMIN D_3
cholecalciferol

25-hydroxycholecalciferol

FIG. 22.17. Structural formulae of vitamin D_2 and vitamin D_3.

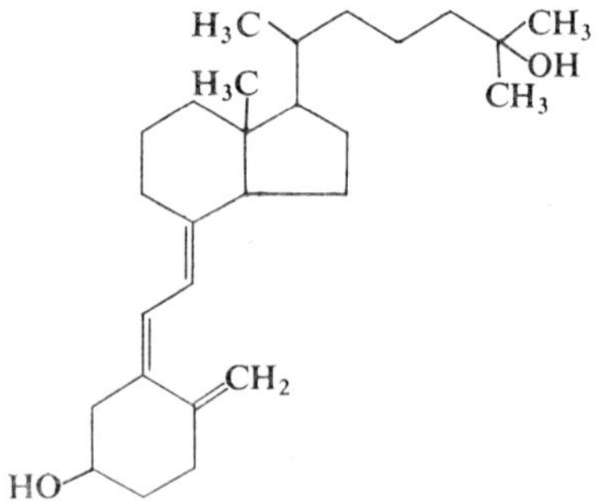

the administration of vitamin D to rachitic animals results in the synthesis of a Ca-binding protein in the intestinal mucosa. This protein is thought to be essential for Ca absorption. However, much more work is required. There is no doubt however that an outstanding defect in man in vitamin D deficiency is a failure to absorb dietary Ca.

2. *Bone.* Although it has been claimed that rickets is entirely secondary to the failure to absorb Ca from the gut, there seems little doubt that vitamin D also has a direct action on bone. This action is a complex one, but it appears both to aid mineralization of collagen and, in addition, to increase bone resorption. The latter effect is most easily seen with large doses, but may occur to a small extent even with physiological amounts of the vitamin.

3. *Kidney.* Vitamin D in large doses increases renal excretion of P, mimicking the action of parathyroid hormone. However, this effect, although predominant in parathyroidectomized animals, is not seen in intact animals. Indeed, in animals with increased secretion of parathyroid hormone, vitamin D diminishes urinary P excretion.

Relationship with parathyroid hormone. Vitamin D appears to be necessary for the action of parathyroid hormone on bone in the rat. Although the evidence is quite strong, not all investigators are agreed. In man there is no conclusive evidence that vitamin D deficiency alone prevents the action of parathyroid hormone. Other factors appear to be involved. For example, Mg and vitamin D may both be co-factors required for the action of parathyroid hormone so that only when both are deficient is the action of parathyroid hormone on bone insufficient.

Parathyroid Hormone

Historical aspects. The parathyroid glands were discovered by Owen (1862) during a post-mortem dissection of an Indian rhinocerus, but it was Sandström (1880) who gave the first complete description. Erdheim (1906) suggested the relationship of parathyroids to Ca metabolism and bone disease when he showed that in para-thyroidectomized rats defects occurred in the skeleton and enamel of the teeth. From these animal observations and further studies in patients, he concluded correctly that the para-thyroids secreted a hormone involved with bone Ca, and that the parathyroid function was dependent upon serum Ca levels. It was then observed that the tetanic convulsions of para-thyroidectomized animals could be prevented by the administration of Ca salts, showing that they were not due to a circulating toxin as was then thought. That a low plasma Ca stimulated parathyroid hormone was suggested by Marine (1914); Schlagenhaufer (1916) and Maresch (1916) made the further suggestion that the para-

thyroid hormone might produce abnormal levels of plasma Ca in disease. This led Mandl (1925) to the first clinical diagnosis of a parathyroid adenoma successfully treated by surgery.

Chemistry. Bovine parathyroid hormone has been obtained in a highly purified state and shown to consist of a single chain of 83 amino acids. A partial structure of the molecule has been proposed by Potts, Keutmann, Niall, Deftos, Brewer & Aurbach (1967), and they have recently suggested that a portion of the molecule consisting of 20 amino acids near the amino terminus may contain most of the biological activity. Their earlier views that the carboxyl end of the molecule was more important for biological activity have now been modified. Further progress in the field requires a knowledge of the complete structure of parathyroid hormone and confirma-tion of this structure by synthesis. The situation is very unsatisfactory at the moment. Although active extracts were prepared by Collip (1925), there is still no International Standard available for parathyroid hormone. This has serious consequences in research. For example, estimates of potency of extracts in different laboratories cannot be compared and differences of an order of magnitude are to be expected. An agreed unit based on a solid standard is required.

Action. Parathyroid hormone has at least three sites of action:

1. *Bone.* The hormone acts directly on osteo-clasts to increase activity and rate of bone resorption. This action requires vitamin D and perhaps Mg.

2. *Renal.* Parathyroid hormone produces a marked increase in P excretion and a fall in the excretion of Ca and Mg. Parathyroid hormone retains its renal action even in vitamin D deficiency.

3. Parathyroid hormone increases absorption of Ca and Mg from the intestinal tract. This action may also require vitamin D, although this has not been fully studied.

The secretion of parathyroid hormone is controlled by alterations in plasma Ca. This was first studied by Patt & Luckhardt (1942), although their evidence was poor; Copp & Davidson (1961) produced much better evidence from perfusion studies in dogs. But Sherwood, Potts, Care, Mayer & Aurbach (1966) were the first to demonstrate by immunoassay that by raising or lowering plasma Ca the plasma levels of para-thyroid hormone were lowered or raised, respec-tively. This work has been amply confirmed. However, Richelle & Care (1967) have shown that

Mg also influences secretion of parathyroid hormone as suggested by MacIntyre, Boss & Troughton (1963). This suggests that parathyroid hormone controls Mg as well as Ca, although alterations in parathyroid hormone excretion probably have less effect on Mg than on Ca.

The earlier controversy on whether the Ca-raising effect of parathyroid hormone depended on an action on bone (McLean & Urist, 1968) or was secondary to the presence of plasma P has now been resolved. The level of plasma P is certainly very important in changing plasma Ca levels, perhaps more important than the level of osteoclastic resorption in adult man. Nevertheless, parathyroid hormone acts directly on bone as proposed by McLean & Urist (1968) and this action may be dominant under certain circumstances.

Calcitonin

Existence. Copp, Cameron, Cheney, Davidson & Henze (1962) in Vancouver tested current hypotheses of Ca regulation by perfusing thyroparathyroid glands in dogs. They found that their results could only be explained by postulating the existence of a new Ca-lowering hormone which they called calcitonin. Kumar, Foster & MacIntyre (1963) soon confirmed their work and went on to show that the thyroid rather than the parathyroid, as claimed by Copp and colleagues, was the source of the hormone (Foster, Baghdiantz, Kumar, Slack, Soliman & MacIntyre, 1964). These workers also concluded that the activity of crude rat thyroid extracts in lowering plasma Ca (first shown by Hirsch, Gauthier & Munson, 1963) was due to their calcitonin content.

Chemistry. Porcine calcitonin is a single chain polypeptide consisting of 32 amino acids with a 1–7 disulphide bridge at the amino terminus and prolinamide at the carboxyl terminus. Human calcitonin is very different in structure. Although it also consists of a single chain of 32 amino acids and has prolinamide at the carboxyl terminus and retains the disulphide bridge, there are 18 substitutions in the sequence as compared to the porcine hormone. In addition, an active dimer of the human hormone has been shown to exist.

These large differences in structure between hormones of closely related species are unusual in protein hormones. The significance of the differences is not understood, but deductions about the action of human calcitonin from experiments with porcine material may have to be treated with caution until they are confirmed.

Secreting cells. It is now known that the cells which secrete calcitonin (C-cells), although present mainly in the thyroid in lower mammals, largely make up a special endocrine gland in birds and reptiles. This gland is known as the ultimobranchial body, and its function has been a mystery until recently. The situation in man may differ from that in lower mammals. In man, C-cells are found in parathyroid and thymus as well as in the thyroid gland. This is not unexpected on embryological grounds since the C-cells are found in the primitive pharynx in the ultimobranchial region below the third and fourth pouches. The C-cells therefore make up a separate endocrine system whose distribution differs in different species.

Action. When porcine or human calcitonin is injected intravenously in young rats there is a rapid fall in plasma Ca and P. This is due to inhibition of osteoclastic resorption of bone. Porcine calcitonin also has an effect on the kidney. An increased excretion of P has been demonstrated in the rat and increased excretion of P, Ca, Mg and sodium has been shown in man. The effect of the human hormone on renal function has not yet been studied.

Function of Calcitonin in Man

Although porcine calcitonin is effective in lowering plasma Ca in man in certain diseased states, porcine calcitonin produces little effect on plasma Ca in normal adults when given by single intravenous injection. This probably means that osteoclastic resorption of bone is less important in Ca homeostasis in adults, and that the gut and kidney play a greater part than has been recognized. In diseases in which bone turnover is greatly increased, such as Paget's disease, porcine calcitonin produces a dramatic fall in plasma Ca.

Calcitonin is however present in normal adult plasma and increases in concentration after Ca infusion. This means that it must modify the action of parathyroid hormone on bone and it presumably plays a role in preventing excessive bone resorption. Whether this role is important physiologically remains to be determined.

Significance of Calcitonin in Disease

The plasma levels of calcitonin have yet to be studied in metabolic bone disease and it is possible that calcitonin is responsible for some disorders of Ca homeostasis and bone. It has been suggested that calcitonin may play a role in osteopetrosis and in pseudohypoparathyroidism. The latter seems unlikely but in both cases detailed studies will have to be made. However, there is no doubt that plasma calcitonin levels are markedly increased in medullary carcinoma of the thyroid. This disease may represent a cancer of the C-cells and it is not surprising that high plasma levels are found. The tumours are extremely rich in calcitonin and it was from this source that the human hormone was first isolated. The very high plasma levels which may be found in this disease are useful for diagnosis and may result in detection of metastases or recurrences before they are evident clinically. The high plasma levels are not usually associated with disorders of Ca homeostasis. Several possibilities have to be considered to explain this apparent anomaly. The most likely is that even marked inhibition of osteoclastic bone resorption does not produce hypocalcaemia in the adult since this is not a major factor in maintenance of normal plasma Ca levels. However, there are several other possibilities which have to be considered: increased production of parathyroid hormone in compensation; circulation of the hormone in an inactive form; and insensitivity of the skeleton to the hormone.

Therapeutic Use of Calcitonin

Hopes have been expressed that calcitonin might prove useful in the management of osteoporosis. This remains a possibility which will require to be investigated by careful trials. It is also possible that calcitonin may be effective in treating hypercalcaemia when this is due to increased bone resorption. It might also be useful in treating the bone disease of inoperable parathyroid adenoma.

BONE DISEASES

Parathyroid Disorders

Metabolic bone disease is likely to be generalized, though possibly with its brunt more on certain skeletal areas. Local or patchy bone disease, however, may become very widespread, and may also cause metabolic effects. Generalized undue thinning of bone (caused metabolically) may be due to osteomalacia (defective calcification), osteoporosis or bone atrophy, or osteitis fibrosa (excessive bone destruction). The radiologist can sometimes help with the recognition of certain signs characteristic of one or other of these generalized bone diseases, Looser's zones, or Milkman fractures in osteomalacia, periosteal erosions on the fingers and sometimes cystic changes in osteitis fibrosa, or predominant involvement of the spine with sparing of the lamina dura in osteoporosis; but these features are not always present. The main biochemical tests used to distinguish between these types of causes are: the serum concentrations of Ca, P and phosphatase (see Table 22.2), the urinary Ca excretion on low Ca diets or on ordinary diets (see Tables 22.5 and 22.6), the faecal Ca excretion on standard diets of moderate or high Ca (1 or 2 g. Ca/day), and also infusion tests and acute absorption tests. Immunoassay of parathormone and calcitonin and other hormones should be available shortly to supplement such diagnostic procedures (Editorial, 1968).

In certain diseases which affect the bone, secondary hyperparathyroidism is apt to occur as a part of the body's reaction to the disease, and will then add its own manifestations to those due to the primary disease. This occurs notably in chronic uraemia, where it is one of the factors causing uraemic osteodystrophy, and in rickets or osteomalacia. Factors tending to lower circulating ionized Ca levels initiate the response and so the lowering is minimized by the parathyroid's response. In uraemia both the rising serum P and also unidentified "anti-calcification" factors in serum impair the availability of Ca ions. Injections of P cause parathyroid hyperplasia (Albright & Reifenstein, 1948); and enlarged parathyroids have been found in uraemia (Pappenheimer & Wilens, 1935; Snapper, 1949; Magnus & Scott, 1936), and in osteomalacia (Erdheim, 1907; Wilder, Higgins & Sheard, 1935; Liu, Chu, Su, Yu & Cheng, 1940); in one example of the former the total parathyroid weight was 11 g. (Albright & Reifenstein, 1948). The associated radiological finding of subperiosteal osteodystrophy (Teall, 1928; Dent & Hodson, 1954) suggests that these parathyroids are also active.

Hypoparathyroidism

Hypoparathyroidism does not cause bone disease, but rather latent or manifest tetany, at times epileptic fits, atrophic skin and nails, monilia infections, cataracts and metastatic calcification in the soft tissues, conjunctiva and cornea and brain tissue, especially the basal ganglia. Its metabolic signs are low Ca and high P with normal alkaline phosphatase in the serum, with low urinary Ca and also low urinary P for such a high serum P level. Both ionized and protein-bound Ca are low. Especially in children, a proportion of such cases also have steatorrhoea (Williams & Wood, 1959). Lowered parathyroid reserve may be revealed by an EDTA test (Jones & Fourman, 1963a, b; Michie, Stowers, Frazer & Gunn, 1965) revealing inefficient restoration of a lowered Ca. "Hypo-parathyroidism," subclinical apart from such tests, is said to cause neurasthenic and nervous symptoms (Fourman & Royer, 1968); among thyroidectomy cases, postoperative tetany or low serum Ca is reported in $\frac{1}{2}$ to 6%, but defective EDTA tests in 25%. Idiopathic hypopara-thyroidism (Bronsky, Kushner, Dubin & Snapper, 1958) is the other common type; which is some-times associated with Addison's disease and/or other endocrine deficiencies, with corresponding circulating antibodies. Replacement treatment is by oral calciferol at about 2–5 mg./day or dihydrotachysterol (AT10), though replacement is imperfect tending to hypercalcuria when attaining sufficient lowering of serum P.

Pseudohypoparathyroidism

Pseudohypoparathyroidism (Albright & Reifenstein, 1948) is a familial disorder causing an identical syndrome, including Ca gout, which is associated with a typical body build and shape of hands and face—notably short fourth and fifth metacarpals ("brachymetacarpal dwarfs"), as are also seen in Turner's syndrome. Lee, Tashjian, Streeto & Frantz (1968) have produced strong evidence that the primary defect is unresponsive to parathormone as originally postulated. Immunoassayable parathormone was raised in the peripheral veins and normal in parathyroid tissue; while in response to infused parathormone, no rise in urinary cyclic AMP was seen, as found in normals. While calcitonin was high in the thyroid tissue, total thyroidectomy did not ameliorate the hypocalcaemia. In some milder cases (pseudo-pseudohypoparathyroidism) the blood chemistry is normal despite the skeletal abnormalities; and in others there is abnormal blood chemistry along with radiological signs of hyperparathyroidism in the bones—presumably due to residual responsiveness remaining in the bones (Kolb & Steinbach, 1962).

Primary Hyperparathyroidism

Primary hyperparathyroidism may be mani-fested as bone disease, but more often as kidney stones or nephrocalcinosis (Albright & Reifen-stein, 1948; Cook & Keating, 1945), hypertension or vague ill health. The bone disease is osteitis fibrosa (see Figs. 22.18 and 22.19) or excessive bone destruction often associated with bone pains, and in severe cases bone cysts due either to osteo-clastic tumours (Albright & Reifenstein, 1948; Snapper, 1949) or cysts from haemorrhages. Primary hyperparathyroidism may also present as arthritis in which pseudo-gout with chondro-

calcinosis may be a feature (Melvin, Joplin & Fraser, 1966). Severe cases may get acute attacks of nausea and vomiting due to hypercalcaemic crises (when the Ca rises to about 17 mg./100 ml.), which can progress to uraemia and death prob-ably from the renal and cardiac effects of the hypercalcaemia. Probably only severe cases get evident bone disease, but an increased Ca tracer turnover is an almost universal feature, as also increased osteolysis discernible in bone biopsies specially studied. The pathological basis is usually an adenoma which is not infrequently multiple (Woolner, Keating & Black, 1952; Norris, 1946), and rarely there may be generalized apparently primary hyperplasia either with a characteristic "Wasserhelle" cell hypertrophy (Castleman & Cope, 1951), or with chief cell nodular hyperplasia. An interesting unexplained association is that hyperparathyroidism may occur with multiple endocrine adenomas, espe-cially of the pituitary and pancreatic islet cells (Underdahl, Woolner & Black, 1953). The basis is very rarely carcinoma (Albright & Reifenstein, 1948; Young & Emerson, 1949).

Typical biochemical findings are needed to confirm the diagnosis, for bone X-ray and routine histology may be normal (see Fig. 22.18). Unless renal complications have supervened, the serum Ca is high, and the serum P low or normal with phosphaturia. The diagnosis may be difficult to establish if complicating renal disease has developed, for the serum P then tends to rise into the normal range and phosphaturia is a feature of all severe uraemias; very rarely with severe uraemia, even the serum Ca may be normal (Snapper, 1949). Such frankly uraemic cases can closely simulate tertiary hyperpara-thyroidism (see below) whose treatment how-ever is similar. There are other causes of hyper-calcaemia and hypercalcuria, usually with normal P, when hyperparathyroidism is unlikely; hypervitaminosis D, various other bone-invasive diseases such as myeloma and other tumours of bone, cast-immobilized fractures and sarcoid, as well as some malignant tumours without bone invasion (see below). In any hypercalcaemia, these usually need excluding, and plasma alkaline phosphatase will often help. If this is raised, with a high serum Ca and a low serum P, hyper-parathyroidism is likely; if it is not raised, and there is also radiological thinning of bone, hyperparathyroidism is most unlikely, whatever the blood urea. But hyperparathyroidism without evident bone disease may have a normal serum alkaline phosphatase, and in such cases other malignancies and invasive bone disease must be

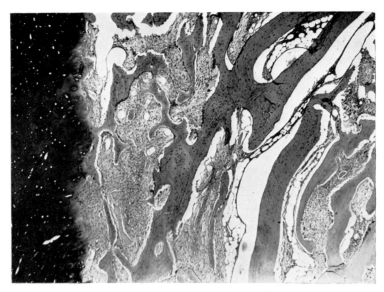

FIG. 22.18. Iliac crest bone biopsy. Primary hyperparathyroidism with bone disease. *Note*. (1) many osteoclasts eroding the edges of trabeculae; (2) fibrous invasion of marrow (osteitis fibrosa). Decalcified section, 30 ×.

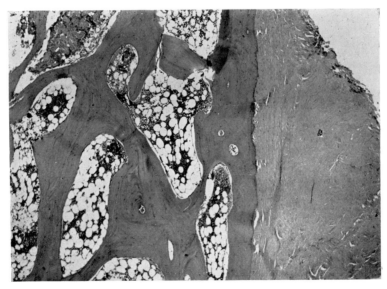

FIG. 22.19. Iliac crest bone biopsy. Primary hyperparathyroidism without bone disease. *Note*. Normal trabeculae and marrow in the spaces. Decalcified section, 30 ×.

[*To face p. 778.*

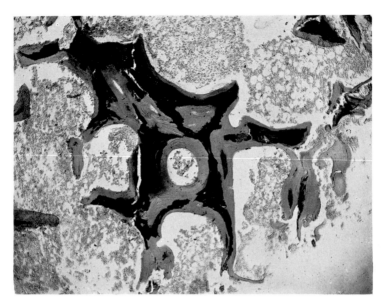

FIG. 22.20. Iliac crest bone biopsy. Osteomalacia. Note dark-stained calcium only in centre of wide trabeculae—surrounded by wide uncalcified osteoid seams. Undecalcified section, von Kossa Stain, 30 ×.

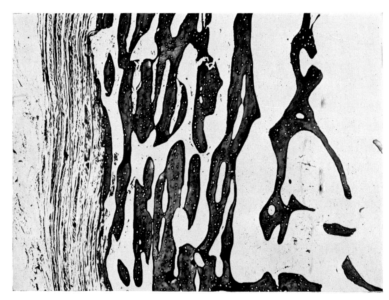

FIG. 22.21. Iliac crest bone biopsy. Osteoporosis. Note thin, but otherwise normal trabeculae (cf. above or normal bone in Fig. 22.19); their calcification seemed to be normal on an undecalcified section, 30 ×.

carefully excluded. Rarely some of these other causes of hypercalcaemia may give the typical serum Ca and P levels of uncomplicated primary hyperparathyroidism, so that they should always be considered before diagnosing hyperparathyroidism. Hypercalcuria with hypophosphataemia but normocalcaemia occurs in induced acidosis (Shohl, 1939), and in idiopathic hypercalcuria (Albright, Hennemann, Benedict & Forbes, 1953). With these last findings, but no acidosis, serial blood samples should be taken to be sure that hypercalcaemia indicative of hyperparathyroidism has not been missed. With definite hypercalcaemia of doubtful basis, finding a raised bone accretion rate by a tracer test can clinch its cause as hyperparathyroidism (Fraser *et al.*, 1960); and in doubtfully low serum P, a phosphaturia test may confirm (Nordin & Fraser, 1960; Fraser, 1960). The cortisone test is also helpful in such doubtful cases—hyperparathyroid hypercalcaemia practically never suppressing during the test, while many but not all of the others do (Dent, 1956). Immunoassays of parathormone and calcitonin are almost available to help clarify many such diagnostic problems (Editorial, 1968). But identical syndromes can arise when extra-osseous malignancies produce parathormone, similarly immuno-assayable (see below).

The only treatment is operative; location of the tumour is by no means easy, for it may be found over a wide area in the neck and mediastrinum. Postoperatively the bones become avid for Ca, and care is needed temporarily to avoid tetany which can be severe and even fatal (Ca injections and oral calciferol). Significant bone repair will occur within months, but complete restoration may not be complete for years. Mg deficiency may be a postoperative problem after parathyroidectomy in cases with bone disease (Hanna, North, MacIntyre & Fraser, 1961).

Secondary and Tertiary Hyperparathyroidism

Disorders tending to lower serum Ca cause compensatory increase of parathormone secretion and so tend to restore serum Ca at the cost of some lowering of the serum P; such compensatory hyperplasia, or secondary hyperparathyroidism, is seen especially in conditions causing uraemia or rickets and osteomalacia. When such secondary hyperparathyroidism becomes sustained over many years of increasing severity, it can become autonomous probably from adenomas developing within the hyperplastic parathyroid—tertiary

hyperparathyroidism, which can be difficult to distinguish from primary hyperparathyroidism severe enough to cause uraemia. Several instances initiated from uraemia have been published and some from steatorrhoea with osteomalacia (Davies, Dent & Watson, 1968).

Rickets or Osteomalacia

Rickets or osteomalacia is characterized by defective calcification of bone, often shows excessive amounts of matrix and is associated usually with low Ca absorption, low serum levels of Ca and/or P along with a high level of alkaline phosphatase. Rickets, the disease seen in the young, differs from osteomalacia only in its having epiphyseal manifestations. There are two main types:

1. *Simple or deficiency osteomalacia*, associated with a vitamin D deficiency due to dietary or absorption defect (Bassett, Keutman, Hyde, van Alstine & Russ, 1939), which is correctable by ordinary standard vitamin D dosage (1–10,000 i.u./day) provided this is injected when there is absorption defect.
2. *Vitamin D-resistant osteomalacia*, due to various causes other than vitamin D deficiency, which responds only to high vitamin D dosage (upwards from 50,000 i.u./day) or other treatments. The main features, i.e. the bone pathology and the basic abnormalities of serum biochemistry, are common to both these types and will be discussed in connection with the former type.

Simple or Deficiency Osteomalacia

This can be produced in rats if deficiency of either Ca or P (Shohl, 1939) is added to a vitamin D deficiency. In man, this last deficiency alone suffices to cause simple osteomalacia; though a deficiency of dietary Ca may sometimes contribute to the bone disease in oriental and tropical dietaries which, mainly cereals and vegetables, may provide under 250 mg. Ca/day (Snapper, 1949). In Western countries, except in wartime or among infants, simple osteomalacia is likely to depend not upon deficient diet or sunlight exposure, but rather on defective absorption of vitamin D, e.g. on steatorrhoea. Rickets used to be extremely frequent; for example, it was found in 95% of post mortems on infants (4–18 months) in Dresden in 1901–05. Hunger osteopathy (osteomalacia) was seen in Germany after the first World War, and in France and the Netherlands after the second (Justin-Besancon,

1942; de Gennes & Mahoudean, 1943; Pompen, La Chapelle, Groen & Mercx, 1946). In steatorrhoea or chronic jaundice (Snapper, 1949), the osteomalacia may be overt; but it is often subclinical (Atkinson, Nordin & Sherlock, 1956). It is also an important post-gastrectomy complication in elderly subjects when the additional factors of poor diet and confinement to home often contribute (Thompson, Neale, Watts & Booth, 1966b; Chalmers, Conacher, Gardner & Scott, 1967).

The defective calcification is evident both in endochondral bone formation (causing a typical histopathology in the cartilage-bone transition in such areas as the epiphyseal cartilage-metaphysis junction) and also in the steady replacement of all bone, causing thickened osteoid seams of uncalcified matrix best seen on the trabeculae. Bone biopsy is an important method of confirming the diagnosis, which however can be unreliable without undecalcified sections. Wide osteoid seams are then a characteristic finding, and a more striking characteristic is the *loss of the calcification front*, the special staining area normally seen at the junction between calcified bone and osteoid (Bordier et al., 1968) (see Fig. 22.20). The bones in osteomalacia become soft rather than brittle, and show symmetrical partial cracks at stress points, the Looser's zones or Milkman's fractures seen on X-ray, which occur only in osteomalacia. Osteomalacia may be associated with protein, Ca and other malnutrition, e.g. in hunger osteopathy or steatorrhoea, and then may be complicated by osteoporosis; this may lessen but should not remove these histological signs of osteomalacia. Other systemic effects are to be seen in rickets and osteomalacia, sometimes tetany due to low serum Ca, but more often irritability and weakness, and a myopathy (Smith & Stern, 1967; Thomas, 1967) due to the cellular effects of the electrolyte disorder. In rickets, with its epiphyseal involvement, there is always retardation of growth and widening of the epiphyses; in children, widening and radiolucency of the metaphysis are the earliest signs. As already noted, secondary hyperparathyroidism is a feature of rickets, which accelerates the thinning of bone (Salvesen & Böe, 1953) and is probably secondary to the lowering of serum Ca.

The biochemical signs of osteomalacia are (i) lowered serum Ca or P (particularly the latter), usually but not always sufficient to give a Ca × P product below 30 mg./100 ml., (ii) a raised serum alkaline phosphatase, except sometimes with minimal lesions, gross malnutrition, uraemia, or

confinement to bed (Gray & Carter, 1949), (iii) metabolic data (see Table 22.5) on a moderate Ca intake ($\frac{1}{2}$–1 g./day) showing a low urinary Ca below 50–150 mg. (the normal range of a low Ca diet), and a low net Ca absorption. Excluding the low urinary Ca, all the above features are found in all types of osteomalacia. Confirmation that the osteomalacia is simple can be obtained by demonstrating the response (increased Ca absorption) after a standard vitamin D dosage (see Table 22.6). In the minimal grades, the serum changes may not be discernibly abnormal, probably because of secondary hyperparathyroidism, but the urinary Ca is usually, though not always, lowered (Snapper, 1949). The demonstration of an excessive retention of an intravenous Ca dose may be an even more sensitive index of minimal osteomalacia (Nordin & Fraser, 1956). In untreated rickets and osteomalacia the urinary HP tends to be high, and when appropriate therapy is given, an effective bone healing response is reflected in an immediate sharp rise in urinary HP, not seen when vitamin D or inorganic P is given to normals, presumably due to increased collagen turnover with the healing in the bone (Smith & Dick, 1968a, b; Anderson, Bannister, Parson & Tomlinson, 1967a). With simple osteomalacia this response is seen to vitamin D (Smith & Dick, 1968b), and with D-resistant osteomalacia to P therapy (Smith & Dick, 1968c). Tritium-vitamin D absorption tests show vitamin D absorption decreased in the osteomalacia of steatorrhoea and gastrectomy; and assays of serum vitamin D show low levels in these cases but normal levels in D-resistant hypophosphataemic osteomalacia (Thompson et al., 1966b).

It is not clear why in some patients osteomalacia is associated with lowering mainly of the serum Ca, and in others with lowering mainly of the serum P. Lowering of serum Ca, at times to tetany levels, is probably more likely when greater severity or duration has more severely depleted the bone Ca store or the body's vitamin D (Harris et al., 1965), and when for some reason there has been less secondary hyperparathyroidism. Rarely the tetany of steatorrhoea is associated with blood levels indicative of and probably due to hypoparathyroidism (Salvesen & Böe, 1953), and then large parathyroid-replacement doses of vitamin D will be needed to correct the disorder. Mild healing, often with temporary tetany, is caused in osteomalacia by starvation or other acidosis, or on giving citrate (Shohl, 1939), probably as these measures raise either the circulating levels of serum P and ionized Ca.

Vitamin D-resistant Osteomalacia

Typical osteomalacia may often be the presenting clinical disorder in this group of conditions arising from causes other than vitamin D deficiency—probably mostly from renal tubular defects or leaks which lower the body's circulating levels of Ca or P, and so the Ca × P product. As a group, excepting some rare uraemic osteodystrophies, they generally show the following differences from simple osteomalacia:

1. No evident cause for vitamin D deficiency.

2. Urinary Ca often normal even on a low Ca diet.

3. Effective treatment needs either unphysiologically high vitamin D dosage (1–40 mg./day) (to cause excessive Ca absorption) or therapy other than vitamin D, which restores a strongly positive Ca balance and the serum levels of Ca, P and phosphatase, while healing the bone radiologically and histologically (Salassa, Power, Ulrich & Hayles, 1954).

4. On renal function tests there is in most instances evidence of abnormal tubular function with normal glomerular function. These cases, as indeed most cases of osteomalacia, show an excessive urinary P loss for their serum P level, whose basis may be either a renal leak (Dent, 1952) or secondary hyperparathyroidism or both.

These conditions may be grouped as follows:

Renal tubular acidosis. The main sign of this is the lowered plasma bicarbonate and pH with raised Cl. On renal testing the ammonia production under acid load is defective (Wrong & Davies, 1959), and there may also be proteinuria, some fixation of the urinary specific gravity and a tendency for K loss, but none of the other tubular defects characteristic of the Fanconi syndrome. Treatment is effected by giving sufficient $NaHCO_3$ or Shohl's Na citrate–citric acid solution to correct the acidosis; initiation of treatment may be accelerated with 50–100,000 i.u. vitamin D, but this is not needed to maintain the cure.

Fanconi's syndrome. This is a familial disorder which may be evident from infancy or only become manifest in adult life; one type of the infantile form is associated with and possibly due to cystinosis. There is generally a slighter degree of acidosis in this condition, evidenced by lowered serum bicarbonate and pH (Milne, Stanbury & Thompson, 1952); but ammonia production by the kidney is usually normal. One or more of the following characteristic associated disorders is always found—glycosuria, amino-aciduria, ketonuria, fixation of urinary specific gravity, defective water diuresis or a tendency to K loss (Dent, 1952; Bickel *et al.*, 1952). Abnormal urinary amino acids can be shown by chromatography and the total excretion of them is excessive, i.e. over 1 to 2% of the total nitrogen (Stowers & Dent, 1947). A specific proximal renal tubular defect has been described (Clay, Darmady & Hawkins, 1953). An allied familial disorder has been described by Lowe, Terry & MacLachan (1952).

Vitamin D-resistant Rickets

This resembles Fanconi's syndrome in having a familial incidence, and both infantile and adult forms (Dent, 1956); it may be the minimal form. No disorder, other than those described above as characteristic of vitamin D-resistant osteomalacia, can be demonstrated; thus the condition may depend on a urinary leak of either Ca or P or both, though the possibility of a primary disorder of bone calcification has not been excluded. Appropriate treatment is oral P supplemented with vitamin D (Wilson, York, Jaworski & Yendt, 1965; Nagent de Deuxchaines & Krane, 1967; Smith & Dick, 1968c).

Hypervitaminosis D. At well above the therapeutic dose range toxic effects may be produced; probably in man from chronic administration of at least 150,000 i.u./day (Freeman, Rhoads & Yeager, 1956; Kaufman, Beck & Wiseman, 1947). Biochemical abnormalities appear in the sub-toxic dosage range—raised serum Ca with or without some rise in the serum P and decreased faecal Ca (Crimm & Strayer, 1934). As the toxic range is entered, evidence of bone destruction dominates and is accompanied by hypercalcuria; serum Ca and P levels still show the same abnormalities, though rarely the serum P may be lowered (Albright & Reifenstein, 1948). The mechanism of the excessive bone destruction is not clear. Serum citrate is always high, the bone phosphatase is much decreased (Baumgartner, King & Page, 1929) and the bone shows wide osteoid seams which will calcify *in vitro* in normal serum (Follis, 1954). Associated with the excessive bone destruction, metastatic calcification develops in the sites common to other causes of excessive calcification, the most important being the kidney; ultimately uraemia supervenes, which may be lethal. The toxicity may become manifest clinically either because of uraemia or because of toxic symptoms associated with hypercalcaemia—anorexia and malaise, possibly vomiting or diarrhoea, and polyuria. Apart from stopping the vitamin D the important treatment is cortisone and saline infusion to promote diuresis.

Hypervitaminosis A. This is a rare but interesting cause of skeletal thinning with fracture and haemorrhages, general malaise, growth failure and skin lesions (Moore & Wang, 1945; Rodahl, 1950; Nieman & Klein Obbink, 1954). Acute toxicity is doubtful, but chronic toxicity is well established experimentally. The bones become thin in association with signs of cellular hyperactivity (Wolbach, 1946), usually attributed to excessive bone destruction (Barnicot, 1950) but also to defective bone formation (Irving, 1949). The effects have been studied *in vitro* (Fell & Mellanby, 1952). Parts of the syndrome may arise from a secondary deficiency of other vitamins. Excess carotene or carotenaemia has never produced this syndrome. The syndrome has been reported mostly in infants (Knudson & Rothman, 1953), but also in adults occasionally (Sulzberger & Lazar, 1951; Frey & Shoch, 1952). The minimal chronic toxic dose in man is probably 600,000 i.u./day and about one-sixth of this for children.

Idiopathic hypercalcaemia in infants. This syndrome, virtually unknown in America, was relatively common in Great Britain in varying severity. The clinical and biochemical features strongly resemble those of hypervitaminosis D, especially the high Ca retention, and the beneficial effects of low-Ca diets and of cortisone (Bonham Carter, Dent, Fowler & Harper, 1955; Morgan, Mitchell, Stowers & Thomson, 1956; Stapleton, MacDonald & Lightwood, 1956). This disorder may be due to over-dosage of, or hypersensitivity to, vitamin D (and hence the supplements of vitamin D in various prepared food products have now been reduced).

Osteoporosis

This, the commonest metabolic bone disease, is characterized by a diffuse thinning of the bones, due to diminution in the total amount of bony tissue, i.e. bone atrophy with fewer and thinner trabeculae, without evidence of any qualitative defect in the residual bone (see Fig. 22.21). This is probably the end result of various metabolic disorders affecting the skeleton. The disease is commonly first brought to notice by fractures, for in bone atrophy the breaking stress of bone increases much more quickly than the ash content (Bell, Dunbar, Beck & Gibb, 1967). In early cases the thinning is predominantly in the spine and pelvis, but even in advanced cases the lamina dura around teeth is uninvolved.

Though the condition is common, and an important cause of fractures in the elderly, its cause remains obscure. A useful clinical classification is into (*a*) the "common" or "typical" form found in post-menopausal or senile subjects, (*b*) the "secondary" type where it is one feature of a wider syndrome such as Cushing's syndrome, thyrotoxicosis, hyperparathyroidism, and malabsorption or post-gastrectomy, and (*c*) the "atypical" forms found in various conditions such as disuse atrophy, prolonged Ca deficiency, gross malnutrition as in anorexia nervosa, a post-pregnancy type and the "idiopathic" form seen in young adults and children (Berglund & Lindquist, 1960; Dent & Friedman, 1965). A rarer recently recognized form has been seen in patients and rats given heavy and prolonged heparin therapy—possibly from excessive osteolysis from enzymes released from bone cells (Griffith, Nichols, Asher & Flanagan, 1965). Experimental osteoporosis has been induced by feeding low Ca diets to rats (Harrison & Fraser, 1960), or cats (Scott, Greaves & Scott, 1961) and is characterized by greatly enhanced resorption which is minimized by parathyroidectomy, like the osteoporosis of disuse.

The basic abnormalities in common or typical, i.e. post-menopausal and senile, osteoporosis still await adequate elucidation. At the time of diagnosis, most subjects show a normal range of bone formation, as first shown by the Ca isotope studies (Fraser *et al.*, 1960; Eisenberg & Gordan, 1961) and since confirmed by semi-quantitative microradiographic studies (Jowsey, Kelly, Riggs, Biano, Scholz & Gershon-Cohen, 1965) though estimates by biopsy after tetracycline-labelling have suggested decreased bone formation (Villanuela, Frost, Ilnicki, Frame, Smith & Arnstein, 1966). Evidence is accumulating that in association with this normal rate of bone formation, resorption is increased as assessed both by two-pool Ca tracer analysis (Whedon, 1968) and by analysis of bone biopsies. During the development of the bone atrophy a considerable negative Ca balance must have built up, possibly very slowly; but at diagnosis urinary and faecal Ca excretion, including the endogenous faecal loss, are generally normal, as also is urinary HP excretion. Thus disproportionate osteolysis without the usual compensatory bone formation has evidently developed; but why has the skeletal homeostasis been inadequate?

Popular surveys show an increasing incidence in older decades both of fractures and of decreased radiological bone density (Meema, 1966; Meema & Meema, 1967). Possibly because the more rapid bone turnover in younger subjects may make them more resistant to the causes of osteoporosis, there is a steady skeletal loss with age, at least in the surveyed Atlantic populations. From routine hospital post-mortems Caldwell & Collins (1961) found a steady thinning of vertebral bone with age, e.g. from 72 mg. Ca/ml. bone at ages 26–65 years to 60 mg. Ca/ml. at ages 76–85 in males and from 70 to 59 mg. Ca/ml. in females for the same ages. Meema (1966) and Meema & Meema (1967) find that thinning of metacarpal cortices falls with age more rapidly after middle age, especially in women and noticeably after their artificial or natural menopause. Decreased mechanical stress may be another factor, at least in some subjects. When paralysis develops and imposes severe immobilization, isotope and other studies have shown that this causes considerably increased blood flow and accelerated resorption without adequate compensatory increase of bone formation (Heaney, 1962, 1968). How often in the apparently uncomplicated cases an abnormal previous Ca metabolism has contributed is hard to say—whether low dietary Ca, or hypercalcuria, or a poor adaptation of their Ca absorption to these factors (Nordin, 1961; Whedon, 1968), sometimes arising from partial vitamin D deficiency, sometimes from minor steatorrhoea or other gastro-intestinal disorders affecting Ca or other absorption. Nordin (1961) has found that typical osteoporotics do not lower their urinary Ca on low Ca diets as readily as normals, and that they tend to be on a lower Ca intake. A low Ca diet with normal vitamin D supplies has produced osteoporosis and not osteomalacia in animals (Crawford, Gribetz, Diner, Hurst & Castleman, 1957; Harrison & Fraser, 1960). Harrison, Fraser & Mullan (1961) found that about 70% of these typical osteoporotics, when given a high Ca intake increase their net Ca absorption, and they diminish their bone resorption; but this response is apt to be temporary (Whedon, 1968). While an inherited defect in bone collagen formation and remodelling, osteogenesis imperfecta, causes a similar abnormality, no evidence of an analagous defect has been found in the common form.

Oestrogens and androgens, whose deficiency may contribute to the hypogonadal and postmenopausal incidence, have been found to lower urinary Ca loss and not to alter the accretion rate of Ca (Eisenberg, 1960) but to decrease its resorption by bone. Hormonal factors are involved in the incidence of several types of secondary osteoporosis. Thyrotoxicosis is associated with hypercalcuria, increased bone resorption, bone turnover of Ca and urinary

HP, and so when severe or in elderly subjects causes osteoporosis. Cortisol excess is associated with decreased Ca absorption, increased bone resorption and impaired collagen formation as well as decreased bone formation in the severer degrees. Growth hormone is an important stimulus to periosteal bone growth, and increases the bone turnover of Ca and HP (Laitinen, 1967); so that osteoporosis is a feature of hypopituitarism. Though often stated so, it is not found in acromegaly—where the frequent kyphosis probably arises from lax ligaments, while X-rays show excessive periosteal bone which recedes after treatment; and its nearly universal hypercalcuria is usually reversible on correction of the acromegaly, while it is associated with hypercalcaemia in 25%, in about half of which cases it is reversible on correction of the acromegaly while the others require parathyroidectomy (Nadarajah, Hartog, Redfern, Thalassinos, Wright, Joplin & Fraser, 1968). Other rarer causes of osteoporosis include—hyperparathyroidism with minimal bone disease, xanthomatosis, vitamin A excess, and vitamin C deficiency.

Administration of fluorine has increased the Ca retention (Rich, Ensinck & Fellows, 1961; Bernstein & Cohen, 1967) and probably impairs osteolysis, but its dosage (10–60 mg./day) and place in therapy are still empirical. Calcitonin also awaits assessment of its place in therapy (Foster, Doyle, Bordier, Matrajt & Tun-Chot, 1967). Oestrogen and androgen treatment (Henneman, Carroll & Albright, 1956) may prevent new fractures, as may administration of Ca, but restoration of normal bone density remains a problem (Fraser, 1962; Doyle, Gutteridge, Joplin & Fraser, 1967).

Uraemic Osteodystrophy

Renal disease is associated with bone disease (i.e. renal osteodystrophy) in at least three circumstances:

1. That described here where the bone disease is secondary to chronic renal failure, i.e. that involving glomerular failure and due to diffuse renal disease.

2. Vitamin D-resistant osteomalacia or rickets secondary to renal tubular defect, already described on p. 781.

3. Primary hyperparathyroidism which has caused renal disease and perhaps also renal failure.

A bone disease secondary to chronic renal failure is probably best described as uraemic osteodystrophy because it has varying bone manifestations of obscure pathogenesis, while the signs of chronic renal glomerular failure are its only associated signs; possibly it always develops when renal failure is sufficiently chronic. It has been described as "renal rickets", "renal osteitis fibrosa," or "renal secondary hyperparathyroidism," but its manifestations are often mixed.

The bone abnormalities of chronic renal failure are often sub-clinical and recognized only by X-ray or post-mortem; but they may cause bone softening and consequent deformities, epiphyseal enlargement, and bone pain. Bone thinning is a feature of most types. They occur especially in children whose more rapid bone growth is more liable to disclose it, but they also occur in adults. They are thus often associated with congenital renal lesions. The features of the renal failure are usually dominant, but sometimes the bone disorder may bring the patient to the doctor. There are always evident signs of renal failure, i.e. general malaise, involving often anaemia and pigmented skin, and always proteinuria and the blood biochemistry of renal failure, as well as impairment of general and bone growth. Hypertension and retinitis are often but not always absent (Snapper, 1949; Follis, 1950).

Several types of bone lesion are seen, the different types often being present in the same patient:

1. Manifestations probably of the general growth retardation, i.e. delayed epiphyseal closure, usually with widening of the epiphyseal line on X-ray, and general atrophy of the bone (Claireaux, 1953; Snapper, 1949).

2. Osteomalacia or rickets in a minor or more rarely in a major degree (Follis, 1950).

3. Subperiosteal erosions especially at the metaphyses, probably due to secondary hyperparathyroidism (Dent & Hodson, 1954).

4. Severe osteitis fibrosa, though rarely to the degree of cyst formation, showing histologically excessive bone destruction with irregular eroded edges on bone trabeculae, excessive osteoclasts, and fibrosis extending into the marrow (see Fig. 22.18) (Gilmour, 1947; Rule & Grollman, 1947; Albright & Reifenstein, 1948; Follis, 1950).

5. Osteosclerosis, or excessive density of bone apt to be seen particularly in vertebrae, skull and subperiosteally in the shafts of limb bones, and showing histologically as irregularly thick bone (Claireaux, 1953; Crawford, Dent, Lucas & Martin, 1954; Bell & Garner, 1966).

All except type 5 are associated with thinning of bone. It is perhaps commonest to see a mixture of types 2, 3 and 4, with type 2 or 4 dominant (Parsons, 1927; Ginzler & Jaffé, 1941; Gilmour, 1947). Often the earlier developments show only types 1 and 2 while the more chronic show predominantly type 4 with some features of type 5. Though this osteosclerosis may occur with primary hyperparathyroidism which has caused uraemia, it is especially characteristic of uraemic osteodystrophy. In the more chronic lesions, there is frequently extensive associated metastatic calcification (in its typical sites except that there is rarely much in the kidneys), which tends to be more pronounced than with correspondingly severe bone disease from primary hyperparathyroidism (Mulligan, 1947). Most cases of uraemic osteodystrophy have associated hyperparathyroidism, which is usually secondary or merely compensatory, and is revealed by subperiosteal erosions or the more severe features of osteitis fibrosa. This hyperparathyroidism may be recognized as autonomous or tertiary, when severe bone disease does not seem relievable by vitamin D without raising the serum Ca or increasing the metastatic calcification, when otherwise the serum Ca becomes raised spontaneously and the metastatic calcification prominent, or when persistent hypercalcaemia is revealed after dialysis has eliminated the uraemia.

Management of uraemic osteodystrophy is becoming increasingly important now that renal failure is treated by dialysis or transplant. A large proportion of patients frequently dialysed seem to develop signs of metabolic bone disease or hypercalcaemia as the uraemia is controlled (Wing, 1968). During dialysis Ca balance may alter unless the dialysis fluid closely approximates the concentration of plasma unfiltrable Ca—too high levels tending to cause nausea, and too low possibly leading to features of continuing hyperparathyroidism with metastatic calcification (Pendras & Erikson, 1966). Wing (1968) offers evidence that the optimal concentration for Ca is 6.0 ± 0.2 m-equiv./l. provided any raised serum P is reduced with oral aluminium hydroxide to minimize the metastatic calcification.

The mechanism of production of the osteodystrophy in renal failure remains obscure. There is probably a general toxic interference with bone as with other growth. Uraemic serum ultrafiltrate will not calcify rachitic cartilage as does normal serum (Yendt, Connor & Howard, 1955), and gut sacs from uraemics show impaired Ca transfer (Kessner & Epstein, 1965). The acidosis is probably not an important factor, but the main cause seems to be antagonism to vitamin D (Stanbury et al., 1960; Stanbury & Lumb, 1966;

Dent, Harper & Philpot, 1961), along with varying secondary or tertiary hyperparathyroidism. The urinary Ca is strikingly low, as also in non-uraemic nephrosis (Emerson & Beckman, 1945; Jones et al., 1967) and gut absorption of Ca low; oral alkalies diminish the Ca loss (Litzow, Lemann & Lennon, 1967; Clarkson, Warren McDonald & Wardener, 1967); but aluminium hydroxide, while increasing the already high faecal P, does not increase Ca absorption (Fletcher, Jones & Morgan, 1963). The serum unionized ultrafiltrable Ca is raised (Walser, 1962; Walser, Robinson & Duckett, 1963). With the mainly osteomalacic bone disorder total serum Ca tends to be low, but normal with the predominantly hyperparathyroid bone disease (Stanbury & Lumb, 1966). When the parathyroid response is sufficient to overcome the vitamin D-resistance it apparently involves osteitis fibrosa. After the GFR fall under 24% the serum P tends to rise (Goldman & Bassett, 1954) and then metastatic calcification to show. The osteosclerosis is a later development after a period with other lesions, and it may depend on excessive calcitonin response. The earlier stages of uraemic osteodystrophy are treatable with carefully adjusted, often large doses of Vitamin D, perhaps aided by oral alkalies or Ca. The vitamin D dose needed will fall after the bone disease is corrected or when the uraemia is corrected. When vitamin D treatment is ineffective on the bone, or metastatic calcification a problem, tertiary hyperparathyroidism is suspect; and total parathyroidectomy followed by vitamin D replacement therapy can be very effective for both the bone disease and the metastatic calcification (Felts, Whitley, Anderson, Carpenter & Bradshaw, 1965; Wilson et al., 1965; Stanbury & Lumb, 1966).

Biochemical abnormalities will always be found in the blood of these patients; most consistently those of uraemia, blood urea usually over 100 mg./100 ml. (very occasionally 50–100 mg./100 ml.), frequently anaemia, generally acidosis with low bicarbonate, usually (almost always) raised P (Snapper, 1949), and a slightly or occasionally considerably lowered serum Ca. Uraemic osteodystrophy can generally be distinguished from hyperparathyroidism associated with secondary renal failure by the latter showing raised serum and urine Ca, and nephrocalcinosis sufficient to show on X-ray, or at least one of these three. Vitamin D-resistant osteomalacia due to renal tubular disease is distinguishable by its showing low serum P, and none of the features of uraemia.

Miscellaneous
Osteopetrosis

This rare disease presents either in infancy in a severe and ultimately fatal form, or in a milder adolescent form. The former is inherited as an autosomal recessive. The basic defect in resorption and remodelling causes the bone to become dense with clubbed metaphyses and narrowed marrow spaces and nerve foraminae. There is associated hyperabsorption of Ca with a low urinary excretion and on bone biopsy no osteoclasts. The chronic benign form causes shortness and a tendency to fractures. Serum biochemistry is normal except for a raised acid phosphatase, and an unresponsiveness to the stimuli for osteolysis, such as parathormone and vitamin D, and a tendency to hypocalcaemia on a low Ca diet (Fraser, Kooh, Chan & Cherian, 1968).

Extraosseous Malignancy Causing Hypercalcaemia

Syndromes mimicking the biochemical and other abnormalities of hyperparathyroidism are being increasingly recognized as due to malignant tumours without bone involvement, from various organs especially kidney, bladder and lung. Several of these have been shown to be hyperparathyroid from the tumour producing polypeptides cross-reacting with parathormone, while others may produce an osteolytic sterol (Gordan, Cantino, Erhardt, Hansen & Lubich, 1966).

Invasive Bone Disease

Various diseases which can invade the bone on a widespread scale may produce secondary metabolic effects and a syndrome which can simulate those of primary metabolic bone disease. This may occur especially with osteolytic secondary malignancy spreading to bone, marrow neoplasia such as myeloma, sarcoidosis and occasionally primary bone diseases such as Paget's disease or sarcoma. This syndrome arises from widespread osteolysis. Immobilization is especially apt to exacerbate this syndrome, as it decreases normal bone deposition so important to these patients with their excessive bone resorption. In some instances where bone secondaries have been treated with oestrogens or androgens an exacerbation or development of this hypercalcaemic syndrome has followed—usually either in those tumours proving unresponsive to the endocrine treatment, or when the institution of the treatment has coincided with increased immobilization (Kennedy, Tibbets, Nathanson & Aub, 1953).

Radiologically there may be no signs of

patchiness in the bone thinning to give a clue. Hypercalcuria with normal plasma levels of Ca, P and phosphatase is the earliest metabolic feature. Measurement of the hypercalcuria associated with bone secondaries offers a method of assessing the effectiveness of the hormone or other treatment of the tumour (Pearson, West, Hollander & Treves, 1954). There may also be hypercalcaemia and in severe cases this may rise to levels producing the hypercalcaemic syndrome, with vomiting and secondary renal impairment and uraemia. Metabolically this syndrome resembles vitamin D intoxication. In invasive bone disease without hypercalcaemia, in which there is good reactive bone repair, the phosphatase may be raised. When there is also hypercalcaemia, the condition is often distinguishable from hyperparathyroidism by the normal plasma P and phosphatase. But when the hypercalcaemia is complicated by renal impairment, the evidence of the primary bone disease process may be needed to exclude hyperparathyroidism, whose hypophosphataemia can then be masked by uraemia. Occasionally more chronic bone invasive disease leads to osteosclerosis—when the reaction to the invasion predominates over its osteolytic effects, e.g. the bony sclerosis which may develop in myelofibrosis, or locally around prostatic secondaries.

Multiple Myeloma

Bone invasion without obvious cause is not infrequently due to this condition (Adams, Alling & Lawrence, 1949). Radiologically there may be merely diffuse bony radiolucency. In about two-thirds of these cases there is hypercalcuria and in about half, hypercalcaemia (Gutman, Tyson & Gutman, 1936). When there is renal involvement there may be Ca metastases. Plasmacytomas mostly arise first in the marrow, soon spreading into the bone, and are generally in multiple sites when first recognized. Their especial sites are the skull, vertebrae and pelvis. There is generally an associated anaemia and renal involvement is frequent, with protein urea and/or renal failure.

The disease is generally associated with abnormal serum and urinary proteins. Serum electrophoresis (Rundles, Cooper & Willett, 1951) usually shows an abnormal protein travelling as a sharp band with γ-globulin or between it and the B-globulin.

Boeck's Sarcoidosis

This granuloma occasionally produces "punched out" osteolytic lesions in bone, especially in the hands, but then generally without evidence suggesting disordered bone metabolism. But occasionally, in other cases usually without these radiological lesions, this disorder leads to hypercalcaemia, hypercalcuria and at times nephrocalcinosis, in association usually with renal failure and possibly also renal involvement with sarcoid (Longcope & Freiman, 1952). These latter cases may show generalized skeletal decalcification. In this type of case the presenting symptoms are often those of hypercalcaemia or renal failure and the condition may simulate hyperparathyroidism rather closely— the absence of hypophosphataemia having less diagnostic help since there is nearly always associated renal failure. The hypercalcaemic state resembles that of vitamin D intoxication in having an associated low faecal Ca, and in the hypercalcaemia being partly reducible by a low Ca diet (Hennemann, Carroll & Dempsey, 1954; Anderson, Dent, Harper & Philpot, 1954). These metabolic features respond dramatically to cortisone or ACTH treatment, which also shrinks the granulomas of this condition (Klatskin & Gordon, 1953; Anderson et al., 1954). Sarcoid patients have been found to be abnormally sensitive to the hypercalcaemic action of vitamin D (Scadding, 1950). Various explanations have been offered for these hypercalcaemic effects of sarcoid, but it is probably due to excessive absorption of Ca from the gut due to this unexplained hypersensitivity to vitamin D.

Paget's Disease

This is a patchy disease of bone which frequently becomes relatively widespread. Urinary Ca loss on low intakes may be excessive, but serum Ca and P are usually normal except with patients immobilized with fractures. There is often an associated tendency to vascular calcification. It was originally thought to be an inflammatory disease because of the increased vascularization which it shows, but its basis is obscure. It is associated with bone destruction of a type which apparently provokes reactive bone formation to an extent almost suggesting neoplasia. Histologically, early lesions show predominantly an excess of osteoclasts destroying normal bone, surrounded by osteofibrosis extending into the marrow. Most lesions also show a concurrent extensive irregular replacement by bone of a bizarre texture, with a mosaic of cement lines instead of normal Haversian systems; and the bone becomes widened and its trabecular system coarser, so giving the resulting "spongy hypertrophy".

The disease is relatively common and is said

to affect 3% after the age of 40 (Schmorl, 1949). The common sites are the spine, the pelvis and the skull. The early purely osteolytic lesion may be seen in the skull, osteoporosis circumscripta cranii. Reflecting probably the associated active bone replacement, there is always associated increased plasma alkaline phosphatase, except in very occasional "burnt-out" cases. Dramatic acute changes in Ca metabolism have been produced with calcitonin including relief of bone pain (Bijovet, van der Sluys Veer & Jansen, 1968) and with mitramycin.

Mammary Carcinoma and Bone Secondaries

In the blood plasma of patients with carcinoma of the breast (female and male) there is an increase in the concentration of the glycolytic and phosphatase enzymes. These return to, and remain within, normal limits on successful treatment, e.g. through suppression of pituitary activity by implantation in the pituitary of radio-active yttrium (Jegatheesan & Joplin, 1960; Joplin & Jegatheesan, 1962). High levels of total acid phosphatase are usually indicative of meta-stases in the skeleton. Campbell & King (1962) found increased plasma levels of both acid and alkaline phosphatase in breast cancer patients with osteoblastic and with osteolytic metastases, with the acid phosphatase relatively more raised in the latter. This recalls the common finding of a raised acid, as well as alkaline, plasma phos-phatase in Paget's disease (King & Jegatheesan, 1959). In mammary cancer, patients without bone secondaries had normal levels of both phosphatases.

Osteogenesis Imperfecta

A congenital mesenchymal defect resembling osteoporosis.

Hypophosphatasia

A "rickets with deficiency of alkaline phos-phatase activity" starting generally in children and also more rarely in adults is a disorder characterized by defective bone calcification and associated with low levels of alkaline phosphatase activity in bone and serum. Ca tracers show a normal exchangeable pool and a reduced bone deposition rate unlike rickets, but correlating with the histological signs of reduced osteo-blastic activity (Eisenberg & Pimstone, 1967). The alkaline phosphatase activity of the tissues of kidneys and other organs as well as that of the bones, leucocytes and blood plasma, is either not measurable or is extremely low (Scaglione & Lucey, 1956; Curranino, Neuhauser, Reyersbach

& Sobel, 1957; MacDonald & Shanks, 1957), and its absence or near absence seems in some way to be related to the presence of ethanolamine phosphate in the urine of these patients (McCance, Morrison & Dent, 1955; Fraser, 1957; Cusworth, 1958), for the alkaline phosphatase activity may fluctuate along with inverse changes in the ethanolamine phosphate (Eisenberg & Pimstone, 1967). Balance measurements show a tendency to lose more Ca in urine than faeces, but other-wise a normal balance. Serum Ca and P and phosphaturia measurements are normal. The condition has been recognized in adults (Fraser, 1957; Owen & Peskin, 1958; Eisenberg & Primstone, 1967). Beisel, Austen, Rosen & Herndon (1960) diagnosed hypophosphatasia in a 36-year-old male who suffered an incomplete femoral fracture after minimal trauma. Predni-sone, oestrogen and steroid therapy were in-effective, but there was gradual healing oɪ the fractures during two prolonged metabolic balance studies when both Ca and P were retained.

Hyperphosphatasia

Chronic osteopathy with extremely high serum alkaline phosphatase (and somewhat raised acid phosphatase), but with Ca, P and other bio-chemical constituents at normal levels, has been described by Marshall (1962); other cases by Swoboda (1958) and Caffey (1961). The whole skeleton was involved, and there was massive new bone formation with bowing of the legs and obstruction of the upper air passages.

Polycystic Fibrous Dysplasia

In this condition localized areas of osteitis fibrosa occur in the skeleton, without, however, generalized decalcification or any other indication of generalized bone metabolic disorder. This skeletal abnormality is associated with brown skin spots and at times other endocrine disorders —notably precocious puberty in females. Its importance is its possible confusion with hyper-parathyroidism—indeed Albright believes that some of von Recklinghausen's original cases, because of the distribution of their lesions, were due to this disorder. The tendency for a regional distribution in the skin and bone lesions suggests either a neurological or an embryological explanation (Albright & Reifenstein, 1948).

The skeletal lesions may progress during child-hood and adolescence; thereafter there is usually stabilization or progressive sclerosis. The affected areas of the skeleton show by X-ray, either widening with thinned cortex and apparent cyst formation, or in the older lesions increased density, and often cause pathological fractures. Plasma alkaline phosphatase is raised with extensive lesions, but there are no other biochemical abnormalities.

Neurofibromatosis

As well as pigmented skin spots, bone lesions also occur in this condition, most commonly kyphoscoliosis, either due to neurofibromas extending into bone, or to an associated vitamin D-resistant osteomalacia which may co-exist (Swan, 1954).

Fluorosis and Fluoride Metabolism

Fluorine (F, atomic number 9; atomic weight 19·00) is the first member of the halogen series of the elements which form Group VIIB of the Periodic Table (Mendeleeff's classification). The relative insolubility of CaF_2 compared with that of the Ca salts of Cl, Br and I is one of the striking differences between F and the other halogens.

Despite the low solubility of CaF_2, the absorption of F^- from the alimentary tract is remarkably effective; when ingested in solution as either NaF or CaF_2 little F^- is present in the faeces of human beings (Machle, Scott & Largent, 1942; Machle & Largent, 1943). About 50% of the F^- absorbed from the gut following the ingestion of salts by healthy human subjects is excreted in the urine, the remainder being retained almost exclusively by the skeleton (Carlson, Singer & Armstrong, 1960). The latter authors found that 4 hr. after the ingestion of radioactive ^{18}F the soft tissues showed only very low activity; the renal clearance of F^- in the two adults studied was greater than that of Cl^-, and increased with urine flow. F^- clearance was always less than creatinine clearance; tubular reabsorption of F^- from the glomerular filtrate was about 55%.

The concentration of F in whole blood in humans is approximately 280 μg./100 ml. (Krebs, 1950), 70% being present in the plasma (Carlson, Singer & Armstrong, 1960). When drinking water is F^- free, the concentration of F in the urine is 0·3–0·5 p.p.m. (0·3–0·5 mg./l.) (Cockburn, 1961); the excretion by the kidney increases with oral intake. Largent & Heyroth (1949) found a normal level of 0·5–1·3 p.p.m. and 2·0–15·0 p.p.m. in persons imbibing F, while Siddiqui (1955) estimated an average of 2·75 p.p.m. in fluorotic patients and 3·4 p.p.m. in a case who had removed to an area with no detectable F in the drinking water. Tooth enamel normally contains 10–34 mg. of F/100 g.

of dried material, while the concentration in dentine is 24–76 mg./100 g. On a high F diet, the F content of the enamel is increased (Eastoe, 1961).

The F content of bone increases with the level of intake; in a group of persons whose drinking water had contained 0·1–0·4 p.p.m. of F for periods of from 20–30 years the bone F increased linearly with intake from 40–400 mg./100 g. of dry fat-free bone (Zipkin, 1960). This author found no histological abnormalities in bone related to F^- ingestion when the F concentration was as high as 564 mg./100 g. The deposition of F in the skeleton results when the concentration in the body fluids is as low as 100 μg./100 ml. (Neuman & Neuman, 1958). Neuman, Neuman, Main, O'Leary & Smith (1950) consider that at such levels the principal reaction in bone involves the exchange of F^- ions for OH^- groups, and that the exchange is not limited to the surface of the bones.

The increased incidence of osteoporosis among some residents has been attributed to the low F content (less than 0·1 p.p.m.) of the drinking water in the area surveyed (Leone, Stevenson, Besse, Hawes & Dawber, 1960); by contrast increased bone density occurred in individuals examined in another district in which the drinking water contained as much as 8 p.p.m. of F (Leone, 1960). An improvement in Ca balance, resulting from a marked decrease in the urinary excretion of the element, was demonstrated in a case of osteoporosis who had been treated with 60 mg. of NaF/day for several months (Rich & Ensinck, 1961).

The addition of 1·0 p.p.m. of F to the drinking water has been claimed to prevent dental caries (Ast, Finn & McCaffrey, 1950; for review see Stones, 1954). The results of surveys reported by Arnold (1960) demonstrate the beneficial effects of F^- in reducing the occurrence of dental caries in children. On the other hand, the condition of "mottled teeth" (Black & McKay, 1916) was claimed by Churchill (1931) to be due to an excess of F (2–13 p.p.m.) in the water. In a district where the water contained 4–5 p.p.m. of F, Ainsworth (1933) and Bowes & Murray (1936) found that 90% of the children had "mottled teeth". Grey and chalk-white patches seen on the teeth are the first evidence of chronic F poisoning.

A more serious condition is that of osteosclerosis, which results from industrial exposure to excessive amounts of F. This was first observed by Møller & Gudjonsson (1932) in Denmark, and was given the name "fluorosis". An investiga-

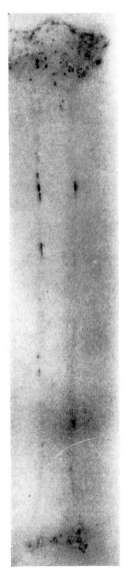

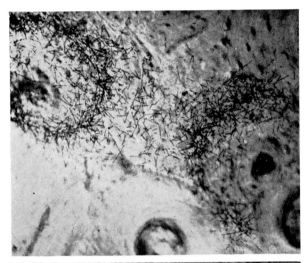

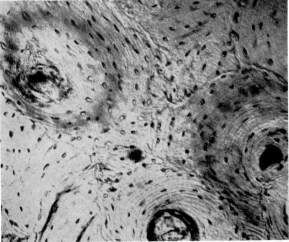

FIG. 22.22. Autoradiograph of section of human tibia from patient who died of radium poisoning.

Note irregular areas of deposition which is mostly at the end of the bone.

FIG. 22.23. Autoradiograph and photomicrograph of a section of cortical bone of humeral shaft of same patient as Fig. 22.22.

Note alpha tracks indicating radium only in some lamellae of some Haversian systems. About 175 ×. (Both illustrations are reproduced from W. B. Looney & L. A. Woodruff (1953). *Arch. Path.*, **56,** 1.)

[*To face p.* 788.

tion by the Medical Research Council (1949) in Scotland found a similar occurrence of fluorosis amongst the livestock feeding on grass near the factory of an aluminium industry where F^- was contained in the fumes from the smelting process. In the bones of both humans and animals an increased density was observed, there was formation of osteophytes, with varying calcification of ligaments, tendons and interosseous fasciae. Although the bony changes are most marked in the vertebrae, all parts of the skeleton may be affected. When severe, the condition of fluorosis may be marked by backache, stiffness and difficulty of movement. Siddiqui (1955) described calcification of the ligaments, with marked involvement of the cervical spine, in Indians living in villages whose well water contained 5–13 p.p.m. of F. Many of the cases had marked projections from the tibiae, bowing of the shaft and exostoses of the skull. Pigmented patches and pitting of the teeth were common.

The most reliable methods for F^- estimation involve (1) ashing the tissue or fluid; (2) isolation of F by distillation (Willard & Winter, 1933); and (3) colorimetric estimation of F^-. The colorimetric estimation is based on the bleaching action of the F^- ion on coloured metal-dye complexes, e.g. zirconyl-eriochrome cyanine R read at 568 mμ (Singer & Armstrong, 1959).

Radium Poisoning
and the allied hazards of Fission Products)

Many of the elements normally foreign to the body tend, when introduced into the circulation in soluble form, to be stored in the bones much as in an ion-exchange column. In the first few days there is some concurrent urinary excretion and removal by the reticulo-endothelial system and liver with subsequent faecal excretion, but thereafter the retention is almost exclusively in the bones, and its loss from them is very slow. Though this limits the acute toxicity, it not only handicaps the elimination of chronic intoxication (e.g. of lead), but also may lead to local toxic effects (e.g. fluorosis, see above). One special and now important type of such local toxicity is the radiation effect from absorbed foreign ions which are radioactive. The uranium fission products now constitute perhaps the main potential hazard for poisoning with such foreign bone-seeking elements (Hamilton, 1947). And so the knowledge now available about chronic radium and mesothorium poisoning in the human has acquired an enhanced importance; for in animals these behave very like the fission products.

Before this selective deposition in bone can occur, a soluble form has to reach the circulation; and fortunately many of the fission products are insoluble and not absorbed, whether inhaled or swallowed (Hamilton, 1947). After injection some of these elements (e.g. gallium; Brucer et al., 1953) may partly precipitate in colloidal form, which fraction is then removed by the liver, so diminishing the proportion deposited in bone. Inhaled insoluble radium does not penetrate beyond the respiratory tract, though it leaves its serious chronic effects there (Aub, Evans, Hemplemann & Martland, 1952). The bone deposition of the soluble salts occurs in two main patterns: (1) that of those Type 1 elements whose ionic characteristics permit entry into the bone salt, first by surface ionic exchange and subsequently by gradual incorporation into new bone as it is laid down (^{226}Ra, and notably Sr among the fission products); and (2) that of those Type 2 elements with ionic features which do not permit this entry into bone salt, but which nevertheless have a special affinity for bone matrix (most of the rare earths of the lanthanide and actinide series; which include barium, plutonium, other fission products and mesothorium). These depositions are patchy, probably in relation to the blood supply, and the rate of growth and of metabolism, i.e. mostly at epiphyses, in trabeculae particularly those of the proximal bones, and least in compact bone where they are scattered sparsely on the younger Haversian systems (see Figs. 22.22 and 22.23). With ^{226}Ra some sites receive none, and the variation in concentration among the sites of bone deposition varies about tenfold (Norris, 1946). Type 1 elements will deposit on the crystals deep to the normal thin osteoid seams; but Type 2 elements will be surface deposits in this osteoid, i.e. nearer the marrow and to the bone cells. Perhaps for these reasons Type 2 elements more readily produce marrow damage and osteogenic and fibroblastic tumours.

Dial painters of the pre-1930 era received mixtures of ^{226}Ra (a Type 1 element) and of mesothorium (a Type 2 element) and so had more severe toxic effects than later groups of patients (Aub et al., 1952). Patients were also injected between 1910 and 1930 with pure radium (^{226}Ra) and have been followed up carefully. The early asymptomatic radiological signs, seen 10–20 years later, are small scattered nodules of radiolucency, to which are added later patches of increased density, and in more severe cases patches of necrosis and occasional sarcomas (Looney, Hasterlik, Brues & Skinmont, 1955). At 20 years

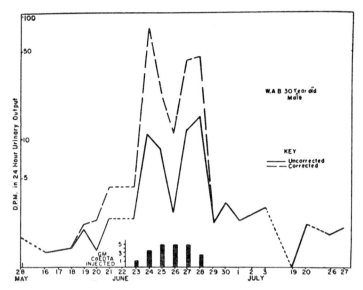

FIG. 22.24. The urinary excretion of plutonium by man following the intravenous administration of calcium ethylenediamine tetra-acetate. (From Rubin, M. (1954). Fifth Macy Conference on Metabolic Inter-relations, 1953, p. 352. New York, Josiah Macy Foundation.)

after the injections, about 70% of the radon being produced in them is exhaled; this can be measured and also the rest of the radon retained in the body can be estimated by γ-counting of the body. From these two measurements the total body content of radium, and also its duration in the body, can be calculated (Norris, Speckman & Gustavson, 1955).

The normally slow removal of these deposited elements can be enhanced if chelating agents are given soon after the poisoning (Fig. 22.24); but when as much as one week's new bone has been subsequently deposited, chelating agents cause little preferential removal of the poison. Several attempts have been made to deliver therapeutic radiation to bone tumours by injection of similar bone-seeking radioisotopes, but the specific concentration in the tumour sites has been poor.

References

ADAMS, W. S., ALLING, E. L. & LAWRENCE, J. S. (1949). Amer. J. Med., 6, 141.

AINSWORTH, N. J. (1933). Brit. dent. J., 55, 233.

ALBRIGHT, F. A., BURNETT, C. H., PARSON, W., REIFENSTEIN, E. L. & ROOS, A. (1946). Medicine, 25, 399.

ALBRIGHT, F. A., BUTLER, A. M. & BLOOMBERG, E. (1937). Amer. J. dis. Childh., 54, 529.

ALBRIGHT, F. A., BUTLER, A. M., HAMPTON, A. D. & SMITH, P. (1937). N. Eng. J. Med., 216, 727.

ALBRIGHT, F. A., DRAKE, T. G. & SULKOWITCH, W. H. (1937). Bull. Johns Hopk. Hosp., 60, 377.

ALBRIGHT, F. A., HENNEMANN, P. H., BENEDICT, P. H. & FORBES, A. P. (1953). Proc. Roy. Soc. Med., 46, 1077.

ALBRIGHT, F. A. & REIFENSTEIN, E. C. (1948). "The Parathyroid Gland and Metabolic Bone Disease". Baltimore, Williams & Wilkins.

AMPRINO, R. (1952). Experientia, 8, 380.

ANDERSON, J., BANNISTER, D. W., PARSONS, V. & TOMLINSON, R. W. S. (1967a). Cal. Tiss. Res., 1, 183.

ANDERSON, J., DENT, C. E., HARPER, C. & PHILPOT, G. R. (1954). Lancet, 2, 720.

ANDERSON, J., OSBORN, S. B., TOMLINSON, R. W. S. & WALL, M. (1964). Quart. J. Med., 33, 421.

ANDERSON, J., TOMLINSON, R. W. S., OSBORN, S. B. & WISE, M. E. (1967b). Lancet, 1, 930.

ARNER, O. & SWEDIN, B. (1949). Acta chir scand., 97, 135.

ARNOLD, F. A. (1960). Arch. industr. Hlth., 21, 308.

AST, D. B., FINN, S. B. & McCAFFREY, I. (1950). Amer. J. publ. Hlth., 40, 716.

ATKINSON, M., NORDIN, B. E. C. & SHERLOCK, S. (1956). Quart. J. Med., 25, 299.

AUB, J. C., EVANS, R. D., HEMPLEMANN, L. H. & MARTLAND, H. S. (1952). Medicine, 31, 221.

BARON, D. N. & BELL, J. L. (1959). J. clin. Path., 12, 143.

BARNICOT, N. A. (1950). J. Anat., Lond., 84, 374.

BASSETT, S. H., KEUTMANN, E. H., HYDE, H. V. Z., VAN ALSTINE, H. E. & RUSS, E. (1939). J. clin. Invest., 18, 101, 121.

BAUER, W., ALBRIGHT, F. A. & AUB, J. C. (1929). *J. clin. Invest.*, **7**, 75.

BAUMGARTNER, L., KING, E. J. & PAGE, I. H. (1929). *Biochim. Z.*, **213**, 170.

BECKER, R. D., BASSETT, C. A. & BACHMAN, C. H. (1964). *In* "Bone Biodynamics", p. 209. Ed. Frost H. M., Boston, Little Brown & Co.

BEISEL, W. R., AUSTEN, K. R., ROSEN, H. & HERNDON, E. G. JR. (1960). *Amer. J. Med.*, **29**, 369.

BELL, G. H., DUNBAR, O., BECK, J. S. & GIBB, A. (1967). *Cal. Tiss. Res.*, **1**, 75.

BELL, J. & GARNER, A. (1966). *J. Path. Bact.*, **91**, 563.

BENNETT, T. I., HUNTER, D. & VAUGHAN, J. M. (1932). *Quart. J. Med.*, **1**, 603.

BERGLUND, G. & LINDQUIST, B. (1960). *Clin. Orthop.*, **17**, 259.

BERNSTEIN, D. S. & COHEN, P. (1967). *J. clin. Endocr.*, **27**, 197.

BERNSTEIN, D. S. & NEWTON, R. (1966). *Lancet*, **2**, 1105.

BICKEL, H., BARR, H. S., ASTLEY, R., DOUGLAS, A. A., FINCH, E., HARRIS, H., HARVEY, C. G., HICKMANS, E. M., PHILPOTT, M. G., SMALLWOOD, W. C., SMELLIE, S. M. & TEALL, C. G. (1952). *Acta pediat., Stockh., Supple.*, **90**.

BIJVOET, O. L. M., VAN DER SLUYS VEER, J. & JANSEN, A. P. (1968). *Lancet*, **1**, 876.

BLACK, G. V. & McKAY, F. S. (1916). *Dent. Cosmos.*, **58**, 132.

BODANSKY, A. (1933). *J. biol. Chem.*, **101**, 93.

BONHAM CARTER, R. E., DENT, C. E., FOWLER, D. I. & HARPER, C. M. (1955). *Arch. Dis. Childh.*, **30**, 399.

BORDIER, PH., MATRAJT, H., HIOCO, D., HEPNER, G. W., THOMPSON, G. R. & BOOTH, C. C. (1968). *Lancet*, **1**, 437.

BOWES, J. H. & MURRAY, M. M. (1936). *Brit. dent. J.*, **60**, 556.

BRONSKY, D., KUSHNER, D. S., DUBIN, A. & SNAPPER, I. (1958). *Medicine (Balt·)*, **37**, 317.

BRUCER, M., ANDREWS, G. A. & BRUNER, H. D. (1953). *Radiology*, **61**, 534.

BUCH, I. & BUCH, H. (1939). *Acta med. scand.*, **101**, 211.

CAFFEY, J. (1961). "Pediatric X-ray Diagnosis". 4th Ed., p. 1044. Chicago.

CALDWELL, R. A. & COLLINS, D. H. (1961). *J. Bone Jt. Surg. (Brit.)*, **43-B**, 346.

CAMPBELL, D. M. & KING, E. J. (1962). *Biochem. J.*, **81**, 23P.

CARLSON, C. H., SINGER, L. & ARMSTRONG, W. D. (1960). *Proc. soc. exp. Biol. Med.*, **104**, 235.

CARLSSON, A. (1952). *Acta physiol. scand.*, **26**, 200, 212.

CASTLEMAN, B. & COPE, O. (1951). *Bull. Hosp. Jt. Dis.*, **12**, 368.

CHALMERS, J., CONACHER, W. D. H., GARDNER, D. L. & SCOTT, P. J. (1967). *J. Bone Jt. Surg.*, **49-B**, 403.

CHURCHILL, H. V. (1931). *J. industr. Engng. Chem.*, **23**, 996.

CLAIREAUX, A. E. (1953). *J. Path. Bact.*, **65**, 291.

CLARK, E. P. & COLLIP, J. B. (1925). *J. biol. Chem.*, **63**, 461.

CLARKSON, E. M., WARREN, R. L., McDONALD, S. J. & WARDENER, H. E. DE (1967). *Clin. Sci.*, **32**, 11.

CLAY, R. D., DARMADY, E. M. & HAWKINS, M. (1953). *J. Path. Bact.*, **65**, 551.

COCKBURN, B. F. (1961). *In* "Biochemist's Handbook", ed. Long, C. p. 919. London, D. van Nostrand Co. Ltd.

COLLIP, J. B. (1925). *J. biol. Chem.* **63**, 395.

COOK, E. N. & KEATING, F. R. (1945). *J. Urol.*, **54**, 525.

COPP, D. H., CAMERON, E. C., CHENEY, B. A., DAVIDSON, A. G. F. & HENZE, K. G. (1962). *Endocrinology*, **70**, 638.

COPP, D. H., HAMILTON, J. G., JONES, D. C., THOMPSON, D. M. & CRAMER, C. (1951). Trans. IIIrd Conf. Metabolic Interrelations, 1951. New York, Josiah Macy Junior Foundation, 226.

COPP, H. & DAVIDSON, A. G. F. (1961). *Proc. Soc. exp. Biol. (N.Y.)*, **107**, 342.

COREY, K. R., KENNY, P., GREENBERG, E., PAZIANOS, A., PEARSON, O. H. & LAUGHLIN, J. S. (1961). *Amer. J. Roentgenol.*, **85**, 955.

CRAWFORD, J. D., GRIBETZ, D., DINER, W. C., HURST, P. & CASTLEMAN, B. (1957). *Endocrinology*, **61**, 59.

CRAWFORD, T., DENT, C. E., LUCAS, P. & MARTIN, N. H. (1954). *Lancet*, **2**, 981.

CRIMM, P. D. & STRAYER, J. W. (1934). *Amer. J. Med. Sci.*, **187**, 557.

CURRANINO, G., NEUHAUSER, E., REYERSBACH, G. C. & SOBEL, E. (1957). *Amer. J. Roentgenol.*, **78**, 392.

CUSWORTH, D. C. (1958). *Biochem. J.*, **68**, 262.

DAVIES, D. R., DENT, C. E. & WATSON, L. (1968). *Brit. med. J.*, **3**, 395.

DELUCA, H. F. (1968). Personal communication.

DENT, C. E. (1952). *J. Bone Jt. Surg.*, **34-B**, 266.

DENT, C. E. (1956). *Brit. med. J.*, **1**, 230.

DENT, C. E. (1967). *Lancet*, **2**, 613.

DENT, C. E. & FRIEDMAN, M. (1965). *Quart. J. Med.*, **34**, 177.

DENT, C. E. & HARPER, C. M. (1962). *Lancet*, **1**, 559.

DENT, C. E., HARPER, C. M. & PHILPOT, G. R. (1961). *Quart. J. Med.*, **30**, 1.

DENT, C. E. & HODSON, C. J. (1954). *Brit. J. Radiol.*, **27**, 605.

DOW, E. C. & STANBURY, J. B. (1960). *J. clin. Invest.*, **39**, 885.

DOYLE, F. H. (1961). *Brit. J. Radiol.*, **34**, 698.

DOYLE, F. H., GUTTERIDGE, G. H., JOPLIN, G. F. & FRASER, R. (1967). *Brit. J. Radiol.*, **40**, 241.

DUDLEY, H. C. & MADDOX, G. C. (1949). *J. Pharmacol.*, **96**, 224.

DUDLEY, H. C., MADDOX, G. E. & LA RUE, H. C. (1949). *J. Pharmacol.*, **96**, 135.

EASTOE, F. (1961). *In* "Biochemists Handbook". Ed. Long, C., p. 772. London, D. van Nostrand Co. Inc.

Editorial. (1968). *New Eng. J. Med.*, **279**, 1230.

EISENBERG, E. (1960). *In* "Biological Activities of Steroids in Relation to Cancer". Eds. Pincus, G. & Vollmer, E. P. New York, Academic Press.

EISENBERG, E. & GORDAN, G. S. (1961). *J. clin. Invest.*, **40**, 1809.

EISENBERG, E. & PIMSTONE, B. (1967). *Clin. Orthop.*, **52**, 199.

EMERSON, K. & BECKMAN, W. W. (1945). *J. clin. Invest.*, **24**, 564.

ENGFELDT, B., BJORNERSTEDT, R., CLEMEDSON, C.-J. & ENGSTRÖM, A. (1954). *Acta orthop. scand.*, **24**, 161.

ENGFELDT, B., ENGSTRÖM, A. & ZETTERSTRÖM, R. (1952). *Biochim. Biophys. Acta*, **8**, 375.

ERDHEIM, J. (1906). *Mitt. Grenzgeb. Med. Chir.*, **16**, 632.

ERDHEIM, J. (1907). Sitzungsber, d. K. Akad. Wissensch. Wein, 2a. *Math.-Naturw.*, **116**, 811.

FALKENHEIM, M., NEUMAN, W. F. & HODGE, H. C. (1947). *J. biol. Chem.*, **169**, 713.

FELL, H. B. & MELLANBY, E. (1952). *J. Physiol.*, **116**, 320.

FELTS, J. H., WHITLEY, J. E., ANDERSON, D. E., CARPENTER, H. M. & BRADSHAW, H. H. (1965). *Ann. intern. Med.*, **62**, 1272.

FLEISCH, H. & BISAZ, S. (1964). *Experimentia*, **20**, 276.

FLETCHER, R. F., JONES, J. H. & MORGAN, D. B. (1963). *Quart. J. Med.*, **32**, 321.

FOLLIS, R. H. (1950). *Bull. Johns Hopk. Hosp.*, **87**, 593.

FOLLIS, R. H. (1954). Trans. 5th Conference on Metabolic Interrelations. New York, Josiah Macy Junior Foundation, 228.

FOSTER, G. V., BAGHDIANTZ, A., KUMAR, M. A., SLACK, E., SOLIMAN, H. A. & MACINTYRE, I. (1964). *Nature (Lond.)*, **202**, 1303.

FOSTER, G. V., DOYLE, F. H., BORDIER, PH., MATRAJT, H. & TUN-CHOT, S. (1967). *Amer. J. Med.*, **43**, 691.

FOURMAN, P. & ROYER, P. (1968). *In* "Calcium Metabolism and the Bone". 2nd Ed. Oxford, Blackwells.

FRASER, D. (1957). *Amer. J. Med.*, **22**, 730.

FRASER, D., KOOH, S. W., CHAN, A. W. & CHERIAN, A. G. (1968). *Calc. Tiss. Res.*, **2**, Supple., 52.

FRASER, R. (1960). *Proc. 1st Int. Congr. Endocr.*, Copenhagen, p. 113.

FRASER, R. (1962). *J. Bone Jt. Surg.*, **44-B**, 485.

FRASER, R., HARRISON, M. & IBBERTSON, K. (1960). *Quart. J. Med.*, **29**, 85.

FREEMAN, S., RHOADS, P. S. & YEAGER, L. B. (1956). *J.A.M.A.*, **130**, 197.

FREY, R. & SHOCH, A. (1952). *Dermatologica*, **194**, 80.

DE GENNES, L. & MAHOUDEAU, C. (1943). *Bull. Soc. Med. Hop., Paris*, **59**, 408.

GILMOUR, J. R. (1947). *In* "The Parathyroid Glands and Skeleton in Renal Disease". p. 157. London, Oxford University Press.

GINZLER, A. N. & JAFFÉ, H. L. (1941). *Amer. J. Path.*, **17**, 293.

GLIMCHER, M. J. (1959). *Rev. Mod. Phys.*, **31**, 359.

GLIMCHER, M. J. (1968). Proc. VIth Int. Europ. Symp. Calc. Tiss., Lund, 1968. *Calc. Tiss. Res.*, 2 supple., p. 1.

GOLDMAN, R. & BASSETT, S. H. (1954). *J. clin. Endocr.*, **14**, 278.

GOLDSMITH, R. S. & INGBAR, S. H. (1966). *New Eng. J. Med.*, **274**, 1.

GORDAN, G. S. (1961). *Texas State J. Med.*, **57**, 578.

GORDAN, G. S. (1962). *Rec. Prog. Horm. Res.*, **18**, 297.

GORDAN, G. S., CANTINO, T. J., ERHARDT, L., HANSEN, J. & LUBICH, W. (1966). *Science*, **151**, 1226.

GRAY, J. D. & CARTER, F. S. (1949). *Arch. dis. Childh.*, **24**, 189.

GRIFFITH, G. C., NICHOLS, G., ASHER, J. & FLANAGAN, B. (1965). *J.A.M.A.*, **193**, 91.

GUTMAN, A. B. & GUTMAN, E. B. (1941). *Proc. Soc. exp. Biol., N.Y.*, **48**, 687.

GUTMAN, A. B., TYSON, T. L. & GUTMAN, E. B. (1936). *Arch. intern. Med.*, **57**, 379.

GYNNING, J., LANGELAND, P., LINDBERG, S. & WALDESKOG, B. (1961). *Acta radiol. (Stockh.)*, **55**, 119.

HAMILTON, J. G. (1947). *Radiology*, **49**, 325.

HANCOX, N. M. (1949). *Biol. Rev.*, **24**, 448.

HANDLER, P. & COHN, D. V. (1951). *Amer. J. Physiol.*, **164**, 646.

HANNA, S., NORTH, K. A. K., MACINTYRE, I. & FRASER, R. (1961). *Brit. med. J.*, **2**, 1253.

HARRIS, F., HOFFENBERG, R. & BLACK, E. (1965). *Metabolism*, **14**, 1101.

HARRISON, M. & FRASER, R. (1960). *J. Endocr.*, **21**, 191, 197, 207.

HARRISON, M., FRASER, R. & MULLAN, B. (1961). *Lancet*, **1**, 1015.

HARRISON, G. E., RAYMOND, W. H. A. & TRETHEWAY, H. C. (1955). *Clin. Sci.*, **14**, 681.

HEANEY, R. P. (1962). *Amer. J. Med.*, **33**, 188.

HEANEY, R. P. (1968). *In* "Clinical Endocrinology II". Eds. Astwood, E. B. & Cassidy, C. E. p. 349. New York, Grune & Stratton.

HEANEY, R. P. & SKILLMAN, T. G. (1964). *J. Lab. Clin. Med.*, **64**, 29.

HEGSTEAD, D. M., MOSCOSO, I. & COLLAZOS, C. C. (1952). *J. Nutrit.*, **46**, 181.

HENNEMAN, P. H., CARROLL, E. L. & ALBRIGHT, F. (1956). *Ann. N.Y. Acad. Sci.*, **64**, 343.

HENNEMANN, P. H., CARROLL, E. L. & DEMPSEY, E. F. (1954). *J. clin. Invest.*, **33**, 941.

HERBERT, F. K. (1933). *Biochem. J.*, **27**, 1978.

HERBERT, L. A., LEMANN, J. Jr., PETERSEN, J. R. & LENNON, E. J. (1966). *J. clin. Invest.*, **45**, 1886.

HIRSCH, P. E. (1968). *Proc. Symp. Thyrocalcitoninin, London 1967*, p. 11. London, Heinemann.

HIRSCH, P. F., GAUTHIER, G. F. & MUNSON, P. L. (1963). *Endocrinology*, **73**, 244.

HODGE, H. C., GAVETT, E. & THOMAS, I. (1946). *J. biol. Chem.*, **163**, 1.

HOGBEN, O. A. M. & BOLLMANN, J. L. (1951). *Amer. J. Physiol.*, **164**, 670.

HOPKINS, T., HOWARDS, J. E. & EISENBERG, H. (1952). *Bull. Johns Hopk. Hosp.*, **91**, 1.

HOWARD, J. E. (1954). Trans. 5th Conference Metabolic Interrelations, 1953. New York, Josiah Macy Junior Foundation.

HUGGINS, C. B. & TALALAY, P. (1945). *J. biol. Chem.*, **159**, 279.

HYDE, R. D., VAUGHAN JONES, R., MCSWINEY, R. R. & PRUNTY, F. T. G. (1960). *Lancet*, **1**, 250.

IKKOS, D. (1961). Personal communication.

IRVING, J. G. (1949). *J. Physiol.*, **108**, 92.

JAFFÉ, H. L. (1933). *Arch. Path.*, **16**, 63, 236.

JEGATHEESAN, K. A. & JOPLIN, G. F. (1960). *Proc. Roy. Soc. Med.*, **53**, 197.

JENNER, H. D. & KAY, H. D. (1932). *Brit. J. exp. Path.*, **13**, 22.

JONES, J. H., PETERS, D. K., MORGAN, D. B., COLES, G. A. & MALLICK, N. P. (1967). *Quart. J. Med.*, **36**, 301.

JONES, K. H. & FOURMAN, P. (1963a). *Lancet*, **2**, 119.

JONES, K. H. & FOURMAN, P. (1963b). *Lancet*, **2**, 121.

JOPLIN, G. F. & JEGATHEESAN, K. A. (1962). *Brit. med. J.*, **1**, 827.

JOPLIN, G. F., MELVIN, K. E. W., HEPNER, G. W., NEALE, G. & BORDIER, PH. (1969). (In preparation.)

JOWSEY, J. (1966). *Amer. J. Med.*, **40**, 485.

JOWSEY, J., KELLY, P. J., RIGGS, J. L., BIANCO, A. J., SCHOLZ, D. A. & GERSHON-COHEN, J. (1965). *J. Bone Jt. Surg.*, **47-A**, 785.

JUSTIN-BESANCON, L. (1942). *Bull. Soc. Méd. Hôp., Paris*, **58**, 328.

KAHIL, M., ORMAN, B., GYORKEY, F. & BROWN, H. (1967). *J.A.M.A.*, **201**, 721.

KAUFMAN, P., BECK, R. D. & WISEMAN, R. D. (1947). *J.A.M.A.*, **134**, 688.

KAY, H. D. (1930). *J. biol. Chem.*, **89**, 235, 249.

KENNEDY, B. J., TIBBETS, D. M., NATHANSON, I. T. & AUB, J. C. (1953). *Cancer Res.*, **13**, 445.

KESSNER, D. M. & EPSTEIN, F. H. (1965). *Amer. J. Physiol.*, **209**, 141.

KING, E. J. & ARMSTRONG, A. R. (1934). *Canad. med. Ass.*, **31**, 376.

KING, E. J. & JEGATHEESAN, K. A. (1959). *J. clin. Path.*, **12**, 85.

KING, E. J. & WOOTTON, I. D. P. (1956). Microanalysis in Medical Biochemistry. 3rd Ed. London, J. & A. Churchill.

KIVIRIKKO, K. I., LAITINEN, O. & PROCKOP, D. J. (1967). *Anal. Biochem.*, **19**, 249.

KLATSKIN, G. & GORDON, M. (1953). *Amer. J. Med.*, **15**, 484.

KNAPP, E. L. (1947). *J. clin. Invest.*, **26**, 182.

KNUDSON, A. G. & ROTHMAN, P. E. (1953). *Amer. J. Dis. Childh.*, **85**, 316.

KOELLIKER, A. (1873). Die normale Resorption. Leipzig, F. W. Voegl.

KOLB, F. O. & STEINBACH, H. L. (1962). *J. clin. Endocr.*, **22**, 59.

KRAMER, B. & TISDALL, F. F. (1921). *J. biol. Chem.*, **41**, 339.

KREBS, H. A. (1950). *Ann. Rev. Biochem.*, **19**, 410.

KUMAR, M. A., FOSTER, G. V. & MACINTYRE, I. (1963). *Lancet*, **2**, 480.

LACROIX, P. (1952). *Experientia*, **8**, 426.

LAITINEN, O. (1967). *Acta endocr. supple.*, **120**, 1.

LARGENT, E. J. & HEYROTH, F. F. (1949). *J. industr. Hyg.*, **31**, 134.

LEE, J. B., TASHJIAN, A. H., STREETO, J. M. & FRANTZ, A. G. (1968). *New Eng. J. Med.*, **279**, 1179.

LEHMANN, J. (1953). *Scand. J. clin. Lab. Invest.*, **5**, 203.

LEONE, N. C. (1960). *Arch. industr. Hlth.*, **21**, 324.

LEONE, N. C., STEVENSON, C. A., BESSE, B., HAWES, L. E. & DAWBER, T. R. (1960). *Arch. industr. Hlth.*, **21**, 326.

LIKINS, R. C., POSNER, A. S., KUNDE, M. L. & CRAVEN, D. L. (1959). *Arch. Biochem.*, **83**, 472.

LITZOW, J. R., LEMANN, J. & LENNON, E. (1967). *J. clin. Invest.*, **46**, 280.

LIU, S. H., CHU, H. I., SU, C. C., YU, T. F. & CHENG, T. Y. (1940). *J. clin. Invest.*, **19**, 327.

LOKEN, H. F., HAVEL, R. J., GORDAN, G. S. & WHITTINGTON, S. L. (1960). *J. biol. Chem.*, **235**, 3645.

LONGCOPE, W. & FREIMAN, D. G. (1952). *Medicine*, **31**, 1.

LOONEY, W. B., HASTERLIK, R. J., BRUES, A. M. & SKINMONT, E. (1955). *Amer. J. Roentgenol.*, **73**, 1006.

LOONEY, W. B. & WOODRUFF, L. A. (1953). *Arch. Path.*, **56**, 1.

LOWE, C. U., TERRY, M. & MACLACHAN, E. A. (1952). *Amer. J. Dis. Childh.*, **83**, 164.

McCANCE, R. A. (1954). Trans. 5th Conference Metabolic Interrelations, 1953. New York, Josiah Macy Junior Foundation, 166.

McCANCE, R. A., MORRISON, A. B. & DENT, C. E. (1955). *Lancet*, **1**, 131.

MACDONALD, A. M. & SHANKS, A. (1957). *Arch. Dis. Childh.*, **32**, 304.

MACGREGOR, J. & NORDIN, B. E. C. (1960). *J. biol. Chem.*, **235**, 1215.

MACHLE, W. & LARGENT, E. J. (1943). *J. industr. Hyg. Toxicol.*, **25**, 112.

MACHLE, W., SCOTT, E. W. & LARGENT, E. J. (1942). *J. Industr. Hyg. Toxicol.*, **24**, 199.

MACINTYRE, I. (1955). *Rev. Trav. chim. Pays-Bas.*, **74**, 498.

MACINTYRE, I. (1957). *Biochem. J.*, **67**, 164.

MACINTYRE, I. (1962). *Advances in Clinical Chemistry*, **4**, 1.

MACINTYRE, I., BOSS, S. & TROUGHTON, V. A. (1963). *Nature (Lond.)*, **198**, 1058.

MACY, I. G. (1942). Nutrition and Chemical Growth in Childhood. Vol. 1, p. 161, Springfield, Thomas.

McLEAN, F. C. (1946). *Trans. 14th Macy Conference.* p. 33, 34.

McLEAN, F. C. & URIST, M. R. (1968). Bone: fundamentals of the physiology of skeletal tissue. 3rd Ed. Chicago and London, University of Chicago Press.

MAGNUS, H. A. & SCOTT, R. B. (1936). *J. Path. Bact.*, **42**, 665.

MALM, O. J. (1958). *Scand. J. Clin. Lab. Invest.*, 10 supple., 36.

MANDL, F. (1925). *Wien. Klin. Wschr.*, **38**, 1343.

MARESCH, R. (1916). *Frankft. Z. Path.*, **19**, 159.

MARINE, D. (1914). *Proc. Soc. exp. Biol. (N.Y.)*, **11**, 117.

MARSHALL, W. C. (1962). *Proc. Roy. Soc. Med.*, **55**, 238.

MARTLAND, M. & ROBISON, R. (1926). *Biochem. J.*, **29**, 847.

MASSRY, S. G., MUELLER, S., SILVERMAN, A. G. & KLEEMAN, C. R. (1968). *Clin. Res.*, **16**, 128.

MAZZUOLI, G., BIAGI, E. & COEN, G. (1961). *Arch. Med., Scand.*, **170**, 21.

MEDICAL RESEARCH COUNCIL MEMORANDUM. Industrial Fluorosis (1949). No. 22. London, H.M.S.O.

MEEMA, H. E. (1966). *J. Bone Jt. Surg.*, **48-A**, 1138.

MEEMA, H. E. & MEEMA, S. (1967). *Canad. Med. Ass. J.*, **96**, 132.

MELVIN, K. E. W., JOPLIN, G. F. & FRASER, T. R. (1966). *Proc. Roy. Soc. Med.*, **59**, 595.

MICHIE, W., STOWERS, J. M., FRAZER, S. C. & GUNN, A. (1965). *Brit. J. Surg.*, **52**, 503.

MILNE, M. D., STANBURY, S. N. & THOMPSON, A. E. (1952). *Quart. J. Med.*, **21**, 61.

MØLLER, P. F. & GUDJONSSON, S. V. (1932). *Acta radiol. stockh.*, **13**, 269.

MOORE, T. & WANG, Y. L. (1945). *Biochem. J.*, **39**, 222.

MORGAN, H. G., MITCHELL, R. C., STOWERS, J. M. & THOMSON, J. (1956). *Lancet*, **1**, 925.

MULLIGAN, R. M. (1947). *Arch. Pathol.*, **43**, 177.

NADARAJAH, A., HARTOG, M., REDFERN, B., THALASSINOS, N., WRIGHT, A. D., JOPLIN, G. F. & FRASER, R. (1968). *Brit. med. J.*, **4**, 797.

NAGANT DE DEUXCHAISNES, C. & KRANE, S. M. (1965). *J. clin. Invest.*, **44**, 1078.

NAGANT DE DEUXCHAISNES, C. & KRANE, S. M. (1967). *Amer. J. Med.*, **43**, 508.

NEUMAN, W. F. & CHEN, P. S. (1954). Trans. 5th Conf. Metabolic Interrelations, 1953. New York, Josiah Macy Junior Foundation, 130.

NEUMAN, W. F. & MULRYAN, B. J. (1950). *J. biol. Chem.*, **185**, 705.

NEUMAN, W. F. & NEUMAN, M. W. (1953). *Chem. Rev.*, **53**, 1.

NEUMAN, W. F. & NEUMAN, M. W. (1958). *In* "The Chemical Dynamics of Bone Mineral". p. 97. University of Chicago Press.

NEUMAN, W. F., NEUMAN, M. W., MAIN, E. R., O'LEARY, J. & SMITH, F. J. (1950). *J. biol. Chem.*, **187**, 655.

NICHOLLS, L. & NIMALASURIYA, A. (1939). *J. Nutrit.*, **18**, 563.

NICOLAYSEN, R. (1934). *Skand. Arch. Physiol.* 69 suppl.

NICOLAYSEN, R., EEG-LARSEN, N. & MALM, O. J. (1953). *Physiol. Rev.*, **33**, 424.

NICOLAYSEN, R. & JANSEN, J. (1939). *Acta paediat., stockh.*, **23**, 405.

NIEMAN, C. & KLEIN OBBINK, H. J. (1954). *Vitam. & Horm.*, **12**, p. 69. New York, Academic Press Inc.

NORDIN, B. E. C. (1961). *Lancet*, **1**, 1011.

NORDIN, B. E. C. & FRASER, R. (1956). Ciba Foundation Symposium on Bone Structure and Metabolism. London, Churchill.

NORDIN, B. E. C. & FRASER, R. (1960). *Lancet*, **1**, 947.

NORDIN, B. E. C. & SMITH, D. A. (1965). *In* "Diagnostic Procedures in Disorders of Calcium Metabolism". London, Churchill.

NORDIN, B. E. C., YOUNG, M. M., OXBY, C. & BULUSU, L. (1968). *Clin. Sci.*, **35**, 177.

NORRIS, E. H. (1946). *Arch. Path.*, **42**, 261.

NORRIS, W. P., SPECKMAN, T. W. & GUSTAVSON, P. F. (1955). *Amer. J. Roentgenol.*, **73**, 785.

OWEN, J. A. Jr. & PESKIN, H. (1958). *Clin. Res.*, **6**, 249.

OWEN, R. (1862). *Trans. Zool. Soc. Lond.*, **4**, 31.

PAPPENHEIMER, A. M. & WILENS, S. L. (1935). *Amer. J. Path.*, **11**, 73.

PARSONS, L. G. (1927). *Arch. Dis. Childh.*, **2**, 1.

PATT, H. M. & LUCKHARDT, A. B. (1942). *Endocrinology*, **31**, 384.

PEACOCK, M., KNOWLES, F. & NORDIN, B. E. C. (1958). *Brit. med. J.*, **2**, 729.

PEARSON, O. H., WEST, C. D., HOLLANDER, V. P. & TREVES, N. E. (1954). *J.A.M.A.*, **154**, 234.

PECHET, M. M., BOBADILLA, E., CARROLL, E. L. & HESSE, R. H. (1967). *Amer. J. Med.*, **43**, 696.

PENDRAS, J. P. & ERICKSON, R. V. (1966). *Ann. intern. Med.*, **64**, 293.

POMPEN, A. W. M., LA CHAPELLE, E. H., GROEN, J. & MERCX, A. P. M. (1946). *Acta brev. neerl. Physiol.*, **14**, 26.

POTTS, J. T. Jr., KEUTMANN, H. T., NIALL, H., DEFTOS, L. J., BREWER, H. B. Jr. & AURBACH, G. D. (1967). *In* "Parathyroid Hormone and Thyrocalcitonin (Calcitonin)". Proc. IIIrd Parathyroid Conference. Eds. Talmage, R. V. & Belanger, L. F. Excerpta Medica Foundation

PROCKOP, D. J. & KIVIRIKKO, K. I. (1967). *Ann. intern. Med.*, **66**, 1243.

PYRAH, L. N. & RAPER, F. P. (1955). *Brit. J. Urol.*, **27**, 333.

REINER, M. (1953). Standard Methods of Clinical Pathology. New York, Academic Press.

RICH, C. & ENSINCK, J. (1961). *Nature, (Lond.)*, **191**, 184.

RICH, C., ENSINCK, J. & FELLOWS, H. (1961). *J. clin. Endocr.*, **21**, 611.

RICHELLE, L. & CARE, A. D. (1967). Unpublished observations.

ROBERTS, K. E. & PITTS, R. F. (1953). *Endocrinology*, **52**, 324.

ROBINSON, R. A. (1952). *J. Bone Jt. Surg.*, **34-A**, 389.

ROBINSON, R. A. & WATSON, M. L. (1952). *Anat. Rec.*, **114**, 409.

ROBISON, R., MacLEOD, M. & ROSENHEIM, A. H. (1930). *Biochem. J.*, **24**, 1927.

ROCHE, J. (1947). *Ann. Nutrit., Paris*, **1**, 3.

ROCHE, J. (1950). "The Enzymes: Chemistry and Mechanism of Action". Eds. Sumnmer, J. B. & Myrback, K., Vol. 1, pt. 1. New York, Academic Press.

RODAHL, K. (1950). *Skr. norsk. Polar-instituut., No. 95, Oslo,* Hypervitaminosis A.

ROSE, G. A. (1966). *Brit. J. Surg.,* **53,** 769.

RUBIN, M. (1954). Trans. 5th Conference Metabolic Interrelations, 1953. New York, Josiah Macy Junior Foundation, 163, 344, and 352.

RULE, C. & GROLLMAN, A. (1947). *Ann. intern. Med.,* **20,** 63.

RUNDLES, R. W., COOPER, G. R. & WILLETT, R. W. (1951). *J. clin. Invest.,* **30,** 1125.

SALASSA, R. M., POWER, M. H., ULRICH, J. A. & HAYLES, A. B. (1954). *Proc. Mayo Clin.,* **29,** 214.

SALVESEN, H. A. & BÖE, J. (1953). *Acta med. scand.,* **146,** 290.

SANDSTRÖM, I. (1880). *Upsala Läk.-Fören. Förh.,* **15,** 441.

SCADDING, J. G. (1950). *Brit. med. J.,* **1,** 745.

SCAGLIONE, P. R. & LUCEY, J. F. (1956). *Amer. J. Dis. Childh.,* **92,** 493.

SCHLAGENHAUFER, (1916). *Munch. med. Wschr.,* **63,** 56.

SCHMIDT, C. L. A. & GREENBERG, D. M. (1935). *Physiol. Rev.,* **15,** 297.

SCHMORL, G. (1949). *Ergebn. inn. Med., Kinderheilk.,* **4,** 402.

SCHUBERT, J. (1951). *Nucleonics,* **2,** 13, 66, 59.

SCOTT, P. P., GREAVES, J. P. & SCOTT, M. G. (1961). *Brit. J. Nutr.,* **15,** 35.

SEBRELL, W. H. & HARRIS, R. S. (1954). "The Vitamins". Vol. 2. New York, Academic Press.

SHERWOOD, L. M., POTTS, J. T. Jr., CARE, A. D., MAYER, G. P. & AURBACH, G. D. (1966). *Nature (Lond.),* **209,** 52.

SHINOWARA, G. Y., JONES, L. M. & REINHART, H. L. (1942). *J. biol. Chem.,* **142,** 921.

SHOHL, A. T. (1939). "Mineral Metabolism". New York, Reinhold Publishing Corporation.

SIDDIQUI, A. H. (1955). *Brit. med. J.,* **1,** 1408.

SINGER, L. & ARMSTRONG, W. D. (1951). *Proc. Soc. exp. Biol., N.Y.,* **76,** 229.

SINGER, L. & ARMSTRONG, W. D. (1959). *Anal. Chem.,* **31,** 105.

SMITH, R. & DICK, M. (1968a). *Clin. Sci.,* **35,** 575.

SMITH, R. & DICK, M. (1968b). *Lancet,* **1,** 279.

SMITH, R. & DICK, M. (1968c). *Clin. Sci.,* **34,** 43.

SMITH, R. & STERN, G. (1967). *Brain,* **90,** 593.

SNAPPER, I. (1949). "Medical Clinics on Bone Disease". 2nd Ed. New York, Interscience Publications.

SOBEL, A. E. (1950). Trans 2nd Conference on Metabolic Interrelations, 1950. New York, Josiah Macy Junior Foundation.

SPENCER, H., LI, M., SAMACHSON, J. & LASZLO, D. (1960). *Metabolism,* **9,** 916.

STANBURY, S. W. (1960). *In* "Recent Advances in Renal Disease". Ed. Milne, M. D. p. 181. London, Pitman Medical Publishing Co.

STANBURY, S. W. & LUMB, G. A. (1966). *Quart. J. Med.,* **35,** 1.

STANBURY, S. W., LUMB, G. A. & NICHOLSON, W. F. (1960). *Lancet,* **1,** 793.

STAPLETON, T., MACDONALD, W. B. & LIGHTWOOD, R. (1956). *Lancet,* **1,** 932.

STERN, M. I. (1948). *Brit. J. Nutrit.,* **1,** 182.

STONES, H. H. (1954). *Brit. dent. J.,* **96,** 173.

STOWERS, J. M. & DENT, C. E. (1947). *Quart. J. Med.,* **16,** 275.

SULZBERGER, M. B. & LAZAR, M. P. (1951). *J.A.M.A.,* **146,** 788.

SWAN, G. F. (1954). *Brit. J. Radiol.,* **27,** 623.

SWOBODA, W. (1958). *Helvt. paediat. acta.,* **13,** 292.

TALMAGE, R. V., ELLIOTT, J. R., DAVIS, R. & ENDERS, A. C. (1957a). *Fed. Proc.,* **16,** 127.

TALMAGE, R. V., SCHOOLEY, J. C. & COMAR, C. L. (1957b). *Proc. Soc. exp. Biol. N.Y.,* **95,** 413.

TEALL, C. G. (1928). *Brit. J. Radiol.,* **21,** 25.

THALASSINOS, M. & JOPLIN, G. F. (1968). *Brit. med. J.,* **4,** 14.

THOMAS, P. K. (1967). *Postgrad. Med. J.,* **43,** 103.

THOMAS, W. C. Jr., CONNOR, T. B. & MORGAN, H. G. (1958). *J. Lab. Clin. Med.,* **52,** 11.

THOMPSON, G. R., LEWIS, B. & BOOTH, C. C. (1966a). *J. clin. Invest.,* **45,** 94.

THOMPSON, G. R., NEALE, G., WATTS, J. W. & BOOTH, C. C. (1966b). *Lancet,* **1,** 623.

TISDALL, F. F. (1923). *J. biol. Chem.,* **56,** 439.

UNDERDAHL, L. O., WOOLNER, L. B. & BLACK, B. M. (1953). *J. clin. Endocr.,* **13,** 20.

VILLANUELA, A., FROST, H., ILNICKI, L., FRAME, B., SMITH, R. & ARNSTEIN, R. (1966). *J. Lab. clin. Med.,* **68,** 599.

WALSER, M. (1962). *J. clin. Invest.,* **41,** 1454.

WALSER, M., ROBINSON, B. H. B. & DUCKETT, J. M. (1963). *J. clin. Invest.,* **42,** 456.

WASSERMAN, R. M. (1968). Personal communication.

WASSERMAN, R. M., COMAR, C. L. & PAPADOPOULOU, D. (1957). *Science,* **126,** 1180.

WASSERMAN, R. M. & TAYLOR, A. N. (1968). *J. Biol. Chem.,* **243,** 3978 and 3987.

WHEDON, G. D. (1968). *In* "Clinical Endocrinology". Eds. Astwood, E. B. & Cassidy, C. E., p. 349. New York, Grune & Stratton.

WILDER, R. M., HIGGINS, G. M. & SHEARD, C. (1935). *Ann. intern. Med.,* **7,** 1059.

WILLARD, H. H. & WINTER, O. B. (1933). *Industr. Engng. Chem. Anal. Ed.,* **5,** 7.

WILLIAMS, E. & WOOD, C. (1959). *Arch. Dis. Childh.,* **34,** 302.

WILSON, D. R., YORK, S. E., JAWORSKI, Z. F. & YENDT, E. R. (1965). *Medicine,* **44,** 99.

WING, A. J. (1968). *Brit. med. J.,* **4,** 145.

WOLBACH, S. B. (1946). *Proc. Inst. Med., Chicago,* **16,** 118.

WOOLNER, L. B., KEATING, F. R. & BLACK, B. M. (1952). *Cancer,* **5,** 1069.

WRONG, O. & DAVIES, H. E. F. (1959). *Quart. J. Med.*, **28**, 259.

YENDT, E. R., CONNOR, T. B. & HOWARD, J. E. (1955). *Bull. Johns Hopk. Hosp.*, **96**, 1.

YOUNG, J. H. & EMERSON, K. (1949). *Ann. intern. Med.*, **30**, 823.

YOUNG, J., KING, E. J., WOOD, E. & WOOTTON, I. D. P. (1946). *J. Obstet. Gynaec. Brit. Emp.*, **53**, 251.

ZETTERSTRÖM, R. (1952). *Biochem. Biophys. Acta.*, **8**, 283.

ZIPKIN, I. (1960). *Arch. industr. Hlth.*, **21**, 329.

Chapter 23

DISORDERS OF THE REPRODUCTIVE ORGANS

by

P. M. F. BISHOP and I. F. SOMMERVILLE

Guy's Hospital and the Institute of Obstetrics and Gynaecology, London

CLINICAL ASPECTS

METHODS OF HORMONE ASSAY

THE object in this chapter is to review the endocrine disorders of the male and female gonads with particular reference to the information concerning these disorders which has been and in future may be more frequently obtained by studies of the estimation or assay of steroid hormones and gonadotropins. In order to do this we have thought it desirable to give an account of the clinical aspects of intersexual states, precocious puberty and sexual precocity, and endocrine tumours of the testis and ovary, and to record the findings up-to-date of levels of 17-ketosteroids, oestrogens, pregnanediol and gonadotropins in these disorders. Little information is at present available concerning blood levels of these hormones.

We have divided the chapter into two parts, the first clinical and the second dealing with the laboratory aspects of the subject. The introduction of laboratory details into the clinical section would, in our opinion, distract the attention of the reader, whereas the critical review of existing laboratory methods gains force by being uninterrupted by a discussion of the pathology, clinical picture and methods of treatment of the various disorders. Many of the conditions we discuss occur rarely and in many cases there has been an unfortunate lack of co-operation between the clinician and the laboratory. This is seldom the fault of the laboratory worker, but if he can make himself more familiar with the clinical aspects of the condition he is investigating he may enlighten the clinician and encourage him to submit more of his interesting cases to laboratory analysis.

CLINICAL ASPECTS

by P. M. F. BISHOP

INTERSEXUALITY

True Hermaphroditism

This is a rare condition of which about 150 cases have been reported (Overzieher, 1961). The gonads consist of a testis on one side and an ovary on the other, or of a testis (or ovary) on one side and an ovotestis on the other, or of bilateral testes and ovaries or ovotestes. There is usually a palpable gonad and this is nearly always a testis although ovotestes may be found in an inguinal hernia. Nevertheless ovarian tissue is rarely found outside the abdomen although five cases of bilateral scrotal ovotestes are mentioned by Ferrier (1965) as occurring in sibs in two different families. The external genitalia vary considerably in appearance, but hypospadias, partial or complete failure of labioscrotal fusion, cryptorchidism and an inguinal hernia should make one suspect the diagnosis. Bodily configuration varies from almost normal male to almost normal female, but three-quarters of the reported cases have been reared as males, though 80% develop "gynaecomastia" at puberty and 50% menstruate (a uterus is present, in fact, in practically every case). Indeed ovulation has been demonstrated in over 25%, though spermatogenesis is exceedingly rare (Federman, 1967). According to Guinet (1965) more than 80% are chromatin-positive and most true hermaphrodites have a 46/XX karyotype indistinguishable from that of a normal female. It is generally agreed, however, that testicular elements can develop only in the presence of a Y-chromosome. There are many possible explanations of the absence of a Y-chromosome in cases of true hermaphroditism. The chromosomal pattern may, in fact, be a mosaic, of which the Y-containing sex chromosome pattern has not been discovered. It may in fact exist only in the gonads. Or else one of the X-chromosomes may carry a testis-determining gene of a Y-chromosome, so that the sex chromosome pattern should be represented as 46/XXY. Finally, true hermaphroditism may be due to double fertilization of an egg by two sperms one containing an X-chromosome and the other a Y-chromosome giving rise to an XX/XY-chromosome.

In a case described by Zachariae (1955) only one gonad (a testis) had been identified when nuclear sexing was studied. The pattern was chromatin-positive, and it was therefore clear that the other gonad contained ovarian tissue and that the case was one of true hermaphroditism.

Hormone studies have not shown a characteristic pattern that might be useful in identifying the condition. It would seem, therefore, that hormone studies are of little value in the diagnosis of true hermaphroditism, nor do they seem to bear any relation to the degree of activity of the gonads as indicated by histological studies. In fact, the only way to diagnose true hermaphroditism is to submit both gonads to biopsy.

Male Pseudohermaphroditism

"Pseudohermaphroditism" indicates that the remaining structures of the reproductive tract do not entirely correspond with the sex of the gonads. Thus "male pseudohermaphroditism" suggests that the gonads are testes, but that certain elements of the reproductive tract are female.

All these individuals have normal male sex chromosome patterns (46/XY) and in all cases there is a strong possibility that careful enquiry will reveal other members of the family with similar abnormalities. This is especially emphasized in cases of testicular feminization in which the ratio of females to unaffected males to affected males is 2:1:1 so that the patients with testicular feminization comprise about half the males at risk. Transmission is through the mother and the genetic abnormality may be a sex-linked recessive trait, manifest in the male or a sex-limited autosomal dominant. In some families the "carrier" mothers are, of course, fertile and normally developed women but may have scanty sexual and body hair or a delayed menarche.

Many theories have been put forward to account for the feminization or incomplete masculinization which is the characteristic feature of this condition, but the current theory is that there is a variable lack of sensitivity not only of the reproductive tract but of the tissues that normally display male secondary sex characters. Many hormonal studies have now been carried out on these patients, and in some cases before and after gonadectomy, and although the results are by no means consistent they do not suggest that the condition is due to abnormally high levels of oestrogen production or abnormally low levels of androgen production.

"Masculine" and "indifferent" types of male pseudohermaphroditism. In the masculine type the individual in every way resembles a normal male, though the presence of a uterus and Fallopian tubes may be discovered by chance. The indifferent

type consists of those cases where it may be difficult to identify the sex of the infant at birth, for the phallus may resemble a large clitoris, or a small penis at the base of which the urethra opens, and the scrotum may be bifid and lead into a vagina. The vagina, on the other hand, may enter the posterior urethra or consist of a non-patent cord leading from the uterus to the posterior urethra. The testes may be suspended from the broad ligaments or may be found at any point on the pathway of descent into the scrotum. The bodily habitus is usually male though gynaeco-mastia may develop during adolescence.

"Testicular femization." "Feminine" type of male pseudohermaphroditism. This is a condition in which the individual appears to be a normal female on superficial observation. Sometimes the build is eunuchoid and the girl is tall and thin. In other cases the breasts are overdeveloped, though the nipples may be somewhat immature. Usually axillary and pubic hair is absent, though there may be a few hairs on the vulva. The labia are poorly developed, especially the labia minora. The clitoris is normal or small. The vagina ends blindly, but is usually long enough to permit satisfactory intercourse. The internal genitalia are absent or rudimentary. The gonads may be situated intra-abdominally at the site of normal ovaries, or they may be in the inguinal canals, or in the labia majora. They are testicles and consist of seminiferous tubules usually with no sign of germinal epithelium and there may be a marked increase of interstitial cells. These testicles, especially if they are intra-abdominal, show a greater tendency to become malignant than the undescended testicle of the otherwise normal male and on this account most authorities recommend castration. Federman (1967) states that 25% of the reported cases of testicular feminization that had reached the age of 30 without being castrated had a malignant testicular tumour, usually described as a "germinoma".

Earlier (Hauser, 1961) it was supposed that the urinary levels of oestrogen were higher than in normal males, though lower than in normal females, and that the level generally drops to zero after castration indicating that the testicles are the sole source of the oestrogen, though even as early as 1953 Morris had found urinary 17-oxosteroid and oestrogen excretion to be within the ranges for normal men. Griffiths, Grant & Whyte (1963) were the first to report an *in vitro* study on a testis in this condition and showed that it could form androstenedione and testosterone but not oestrogen. Jeffcoate, Brooks & Prunty (1968) have studied the androgen and oestrogen

secretion in two patients with testicular feminization. Male levels of testosterone secretion were indicated by measurement of the urinary production rates of testosterone *in vivo*, the testosterone levels in peripheral and testicular venous plasma and the synthesis of testosterone from ^{14}C-progesterone *in vitro*. Secretion of oestrogen was low, as judged by low oestrogen production rates and the failure to detect oestrogen in the testicular vein plasma or to synthesize oestrogen *in vitro*. Chorionic gonadotropin administration greatly increased the secretion of testosterone and of oestrogen. This suggests that the testis is secreting oestrogens in a normal male fashion.

Perhaps the most striking feature of this syndrome is the absence of pubic and axillary hair in the majority of cases. The absence of "sexual" hair growth in the presence of normal 17-oxosteroid figures intrigued Wilkins (1965) who demonstrated the presence of pubic hair follicles by biopsy; he believed therefore that the follicles lacked sensitivity to normal female levels of androgen and were thus "superfeminine" in their resistance to androgen. The picture of hairless women with feminized testicles is the key to the aetiology of male pseudohermaphroditism which presents a spectrum of syndromes from the almost normal male, with perhaps a mild degree of hypospadias or an undescended testicle, to the almost normal phenotypic female who has no sexual or body hair and whose gonads are in fact testicles, a spectrum which reveals the degree of variability of the lack of sensitivity of the tissues to androgen.

Gonadal Dysgenesis

Turner (1938) described the syndrome of primary amenorrhoea, short stature, cubitus valgus and webbing of the neck. Sharpey-Schafer (1941) thought that the fundamental lesion was a defect of the ovaries and Varney, Kenyon & Koch (1942), and Albright, Smith & Fraser (1942) confirmed this suggestion by finding elevated urinary gonadotropin values. The condition was now referred to as "ovarian agenesis", the sub-group in which there was webbing of the neck being known as "Turner's syndrome". In 1954 it was found that many of these patients were chromatin-negative (Polani, Hunter & Lennox; Wilkins, Grumbach & Van Wyk). Later it was suggested that the association of red-green colour blindness, which seldom occurs in women, with the chromatin-negative pattern in ovarian agenesis, was compatible with an XO-chromosome anomaly (Polani, Lessof & Bishop, 1956) or even mosaicism (Danon & Sachs, 1957) in some cases.

The introduction of the technique of chromosome analysis has confirmed both these suggestions (Ford, Jones, Polani, Almeida & Briggs, 1959; Ford, 1961). The condition has been renamed "gonadal dysgenesis". The fundamental chromosomal lesion is that there is something wrong with the second X-chromosome. It is completely absent in all the cells giving rise to the classical 45/XO Turner's syndrome. Or else there is a structural modification, such as the formation of an isochromosome for the long arm of the X, so that the chromosome consists of two long arms instead of a long and a short arm, with consequent loss of important genic material normally carried on the short arm. Or there may be deletion of a portion of the second X-chromosome, or there may be mosaicism, so that only some cells contain sex chromosomes that suffer from one or other of these anomalies. The commonest group of chromatin-negative gonadal dysgenesis is XO and this group consists of cases of classical Turner's syndrome. Less common chromatin-negative cases are mosaics such as XO/XX, XO/XY or XO/XYY. All these have one stem line possessing only one X-chromosome and this enables them to be chromatin-negative. If, on the other hand, the stem line of the cells represented in the culture studied contained the XX pattern the individual would be chromatin positive. The chief chromatin-positive mosaic patterns are XO/XX, XO/XXX and XO/XX/XXX (Bishop, 1964). These cases tend to have less characteristic Turner's stigmata clinically, and more signs of feminization, such as occasional menstrual periods.

The gonad is a rudimentary structure lying in the broad ligament; after the normal age of puberty, secondary female sexual development fails to take place so that the mammary glands and the external genitalia remain infantile, pubic and axillary hair is scanty or absent, and menstruation does not occur. The condition is associated with a variety of congenital anomalies, such as cubitus valgus, "shield" chest, Madelung's deformity of the wrist, shortening of the fourth or fifth metacarpals or both, oesteoporosis, pigmented naevi, malformation of the auricles (of the ear), renal anomalies, congenital lymphoedema of the legs, feet and hands, coarctation of the aorta and red-green colour blindness (Bishop, Lessof & Polani, 1960a). There is a significantly increased incidence of diabetes mellitus and many of the patients have significant titres of antibodies to thyroglobulin and some had Hashimoto's thyroiditis (Engel & Forbes, 1965).

Urinary gonadotropin levels are always elevated and the output of 17-oxosteroids is lower than the normal female average in about half the cases (Bishop et al., 1960a).

"Pure" gonadal dysgenesis. The three cardinal features of Turner's syndrome are short stature, lack of gonadal tissue, and congenital anomalies. The group of cases labelled "pure" gonadal dysgenesis is so called because the patients are not short—indeed, they may be tall and eunuchoid in habitus—and have no congenital anomalies. In fact the only cardinal feature they exhibit is gonadal dysgenesis, their gonads being represented by fibrous streaks. They present as cases of primary amenorrhoea with lack of secondary sex characteristics and they may be chromatin-positive. They show a great tendency to develop malignant gonadal tumours, such as dysgerminomas or gonadoblastomas. It is prudent therefore to visualize the gonads (or gonadal streaks) in all cases of suspected "pure" gonadal dysgenesis. Urinary gonadotropin titres of course are high in these cases.

"Mixed" gonadal dysgenesis. There have been many reports (e.g. Meyer (1925), Baer (1927), Pich (1937), del Castillo, de la Balze & Argonz (1947), Gordan et al. (1955), Grumbach, Ducharme & Moloshok (1955) and Greenblatt et al. (1956)) of cases of ovarian dysgenesis or agenesis showing clinical signs of masculinization due to presence in the rudimentary ovaries of cells of medullary origin, and in 1964 Sohval proposed the term "mixed" gonadal dysgenesis to describe these cases and in 1967 Federman reviewed 37 published cases plus five seen by him at the Massachusetts General Hospital. Either there is no gonad on one side, or else it is represented by a streak and in one case by a tumour. The gonad on the other side was either a testis or a tumour. The tumours have been described as seminomas, dysgerminomas, gonadomas and gonadoblastomas and should certainly be removed as should the tumours found in cases of pure gonadal dysgenesis. All the patients had a uterus and one or more Fallopian tubes, but some also had a vas. On the whole the internal genitalia favoured the female, but in over half the cases the external genitalia were considered ambiguous. Twenty-six were raised as females and 10 as males. In the remaining six information was not available. Somatic stigmata of Turner's syndrome were present in 13 cases, but specifically stated to be absent in 16 and not mentioned in 13. Five of the patients raised as females showed breast development at puberty and they all had a gonadal tumour. None of the patients raised as males developed gynaecomastia. Five patients presented with an inguinal hernia which on operation revealed an uterus and

tube. This syndrome has been called *hernia uteri inguinale in the male*. These patients are always considered to be normal males, though the contralateral testis may be undescended. Some of these patients have actually been found to be fertile. Clearly there is considerable overlap clinically between this condition and the masculine or indifferent type of male pseudohermaphroditism, true hermaphroditism and Turner's syndrome. The true hermaphrodite has a testis plus ovary. Turner's syndrome is associated with bilateral streaks, the male pseudohermaphrodite has a testis plus a testis, whereas mixed gonadal dysgenesis consists of a testis plus a streak. With regard to the cytogenetics of the condition, the essential features are mosaicism, of which one stem is XO, similar to Turner's syndrome with bilateral "streaks", and the other, or one of the other stems, contains a Y-chromosome. For instance, nine out of 24 patients who underwent chromosomal analysis had the mosaic pattern XO/XY.

Male "Turner's syndrome". Webbing of the neck as well as some of the congenital anomalies just mentioned, associated with testicular abnormalities, such as cryptorchidism, have been so far reported in 15 cases in the literature (Polani, 1961).

Female Pseudohermaphroditism

This condition is the result of congenital adrenal hyperplasia occurring between the third month (by which time the genital ducts have differentiated) and the fifth month of foetal life (when the urogenital sinus has completed its differentiation). Thus, the Fallopian tubes, uterus and upper vagina are normally developed, the urogenital sinus persists and the lower part of the vagina opens into it just before it appears on the surface as the urethral meatus. Posterior to this opening a shallow vulvar groove covered with mucous membrane masks the normal position of the vaginal orifice. The labia minora are either absent or rudimentary; the labia majora are hypertrophied and may be fused to resemble a scrotum; the phallus is considerably hypertrophied and anchored by chordee. Congenital adrenal hyperplasia is due to a defect in the enzymatic biosynthesis of cortisol from progesterone. This consists of hydroxylation of the progesterone molecule at the 11-, 17- and 21-carbon atoms.

The commonest enzyme deficiency is of 21-hydroxylase which therefore impairs the synthesis of cortisol but not of the C_{19} steroids which do not possess the ethyl side chain attached to the 17-carbon atom. The lack of cortisol releases the

Progesterone

Cortisol

pituitary from the normal restraining action on the output of corticotropin, which is therefore secreted in abundance and leads to excessive production of androgens.

This would account for the intense virilization which is the characteristic feature of the syndrome, leading to hirsutism, lack of mammary development, a muscular physique and amenorrhoea. The child grows rapidly, but there is early closure of the epiphyses and by the time of adolescence the girl is shorter than her contemporaries and her arms and legs are very short in comparison with her trunk. In male infants with congenital adrenal hyperplasia, the excessive androgenic influence becomes apparent at about the age of 3 years as a form of sexual precocity known as *macrogenitosomia precox* with marked masculinization and enlargement of the penis, growth of sexual and body hair, abnormal muscularity and rapid statural growth followed by stunting due to early closure of the epiphyses. Though the penis is large, the testes are small and atrophied owing to the inhibitory action of the adrenal androgens on the output of gonadotropin.

Administration of cortisone or one of its analogues, by mouth, restores the normal cycle of biosynthesis to some extent. The cortisone checks the output of corticotropin, and thus suppresses the excessive production of androgen with a marked fall in the output of 17-oxosteroids. At the same time it supplies adequate amounts of glucocorticoid to prevent the onset of Addisonian crises. By curbing the excessive production of corticotropin pituitary gonadotropins are at last released and in the female normal ovarian function is established, leading to regular menstruation, breast development and the adoption of a more female habitus. These women can of course now conceive and go through pregnancy with the birth of a normal child.

These cases can be distinguished from other cases of pseudohermaphroditism by the high urinary 17-oxosteroid levels which are dramatically lowered by administration of cortisone. There is also an increased output of pregnanetriol which is a specifically diagnostic observation. In the more severe cases there is a marked tendency to salt loss. This is partly because the cortisol precursors cause a diuresis of Na^+ and Cl^-, and partly because the 21-hydroxylase deficiency leads to inadequate production of aldosterone to combat the excessive excretion of salt by the renal tubules. If the salt-losers are infants the predominant urinary metabolite is 11-ketopregnanetriol, whereas older children characteristically excrete pregnanetriol (Bergstrand, Birke & Plantin, 1959). Whereas classical cases show marked signs of virilization at birth and progressive masculinization during infancy and childhood, there are cases in which the enzyme defect gives rise to less marked changes. For instance cases have been reported in which virilization did not become manifest until some time after birth (Green et al., 1950) or in which despite marked virilization regular ovulatory cycles occurred and pregnancy was achieved (Southren, Saito, Laufer & Soffer, 1961). Bahner & Schwarz (1961) describe the case of a man with macrogenitosomia precox with normal, rather than atrophied, testes who was the father of two children. They postulate that atrophy of the testes is due to excessive production of oestrogen by the adrenal, and that the over-production of androgen without oestrogen may lead to true precocious puberty rather than sexual precocity. Dominguez (1961) made in vitro studies of bilateral testicular tumours removed from a boy with congenital adrenal hyperplasia, and found that they synthesized large quantities of 17α-hydroxyprogesterone indicating a low degree of activity of 21-hydroxylase and side-chain-splitting activity. Schoen, di Raimondo & Dominguez (1961), who give a clinical account of this case, suggest that the development of testicular tumours in such cases is a potential danger and that they possess the biosynthetic activity of abnormal adrenal tissue. They emphasize that corticoid therapy from an early age is essential to suppress the excessive output of corticotropin and thus prevent the testicular tumour development. Wilkins (1965) was convinced that in cases in which the testes are enlarged this is due to hyperplasia of aberrant adrenal cells. Under cortisone therapy these testes have been reported to shrink and the 17-oxosteroid output can be completely suppressed by cortisone therapy.

There is a group of cases of congenital adrenal hyperplasia associated with hypertension. The enzyme defect in these cases is not lack of 21-hydroxylase but probably complete absence of 11β-hydroxylase. This leads to accumulation of deoxycorticosterone (DOC) as a precursor of cortisol, which accounts for the raised blood pressure. The biosynthetic block produced by the absence of 11-hydroxylase gives rise to 17α-hydroxy-11-deoxycorticosterone (Compound S) of which the urinary metabolite is tetrahydro-S. Bongiovanni (1961) has described another enzyme defect giving rise to congenital adrenal hyperplasia, namely deficiency of the 3β-dehydrogenase. This is the enzyme that converts pregnenolone ($Δ^5$-pregnen 3β01-20-one) to progesterone ($Δ^4$-pregnen-3,20-dione). Three infants were involved and they all died.

Pregnenolone   Progesterone

Further, there are the two infants reported by Prader & Siebenmann (1958) suffering from congenital lipoid hyperplasia of the adrenals and four other cases recorded in the literature. Three were males with testes and chromatin-negative nuclear sex, and three were females with ovaries and a chromatin-positive pattern. All had female external genitalia and bilateral adrenal hyperplasia due to accumulation of lipids and cholesterol. Here the enzymic block is in one of the first steps in adrenocortical biosynthesis, namely the conversion of cholesterol to pregnenolone. The female external genitalia in the male cases are probably accounted for by inability to produce foetal testosterone, which is necessary for differentiation of the male reproductive tract. Other cases of lipoid adrenal hyperplasia have also been reported, for instance O'Doherty (1964).

Finally, a form has been described by Bongiovanni (1966) due to lack of 17-hydroxylase. This was discovered in an adult female with hypertension and no secondary sexual development.

The urinary output of 17-oxosteroids and oestrogens was virtually nil.

Female pseudohermaphroditism of non-adrenal origin. Cases of female pseudohermaphroditism of non-adrenal origin are comparatively rare. Brentnall (1945) reported a case in which the mother developed an arrhenoblastoma during the pregnancy, and Javert & Finn (1941) describe two other mothers with arrhenoblastomas who had miscarriages, the foetuses showing signs of female pseudohermaphroditism. A few cases have been reported in which no apparent masculinizing influence was derived from the mother (Wilkins, 1965; Papadatos & Klein, 1954). More recently there have been numerous reports of non-adrenal female pseudohermaphroditism occurring in infants of mothers treated with androgens or progestogens with androgenic properties during pregnancy for threatened abortion or a history of repeated miscarriages. The extent of the masculinization depends not only on the androgenic potency of the compounds and the dosage and length of time during which they were administered, but also on the stage in pregnancy when they were given. Enlargement of the clitoris is a universal finding, but it may be accompanied by partial or complete fusion of the labioscrotal folds, if treatment is begun before the thirteenth week, or persistence of the urogenital sinus with the vagina opening into the posterior urethra. One case has been described (Moncrieff, 1958) with absence of the vagina. In contrast to the cases of congenital adrenal hyperplasia no further masculinization takes place after birth, and the urinary 17-oxosteroid levels are within the normal range and no abnormal metabolites, such as pregnanetriol, are found in the urine. Apart from androgens, such as methyltestosterone and methylandrostenediol, ethisterone, norethisterone and norethynodrel have been responsible for foetal masculinization. Indeed Grumbach, Ducharme & Moloshok (1959) point out that norethisterone is comparable in its androgenic activity to methyltestosterone. That progesterone itself can induce foetal masculinization has not been established, though Hayles & Nolan (1958) report one case in which the mother was given a total of 30 mg. This, however, is a very small dose. In three other cases (Grumbach *et al.*, 1959) other hormone preparations were also administered (methyltestosterone in one instance and large doses of stilboestrol in the other two). Wilkins (1965) collected records of 100 cases of non-adrenal female pseudohermaphroditism. In 32 cases the mother, during her pregnancy, had been treated with ethisterone: 36 mothers had received nor-

ethisterone, one norethynodrel, 15 a recognized androgen, two progesterone, four stilboestrol and 10 had received no hormonal therapy. The four cases in which the mother had been given stilboestrol were reported by Bongiovanni *et al.* (1959), and they suggest that there may be temporary foetal or maternal adrenocortical hyperplasia under the influence of large doses of stilboestrol in selected cases. These effects must be rare, for Bongiovanni and his colleagues point out that at the Joslin Clinic 950 diabetic pregnant women have been treated with female sex hormones. Seven hundred were given large doses of stilboestrol throughout pregnancy. No case of abnormal development of the genitalia of the offspring was noted. Indeed there is probably great individual variation in sensitivity of the foetus, as exemplified by the case reported by Vandekerckhove (1954) of a woman with carcinoma of the breast who received a total of 6·85 g. of methylandrostenediol throughout her pregnancy, and gave birth to a normal female infant.

DISORDERS OF THE TESTIS

Precocious Puberty

It is valuable to distinguish "precocious puberty" from "sexual precocity". In the former condition all the features of normal puberty are present, but they have developed prematurely, that is, before the age of 10. Sexual precocity indicates that as the result of excessive production of androgen at an abnormally early age some or all of the stigmata of adolescence or the adult state develop before the age of 10, with the exception of testicular growth and spermatogenesis. Indeed, the circulation of excessive androgen tends to produce testicular atrophy.

Precocious puberty may be either "constitutional" or due to neurogenic lesions affecting the hypothalamic sex centre. It is very rare in boys and the combined experience of Seckel (1946), Jolly (1955) Thamdrup (1961) and Wilkins (1965) has brought to light only 180 cases. One hundred and seventeen were of the "*constitutional*" or "*idiopathic*" type. The "*constitutional*" type (in which no organic cause or lesion can be found) is almost certainly genetically determined, and has a strong tendency to occur in males of certain families often in more than one generation. In the case of boys, signs of precocious development tend to occur very early, in contrast to what happens in girls. Usually these children develop a strong sexual urge, which may lead to an embarrassing social situation. The 17-oxosteroid output may be slightly increased as compared with the normal figure for the boy's chronological age, but it is not abnormally high as it would be if the condition were one of sexual precocity due to adrenocortical overactivity. Urinary gonadotropins may be demonstrated which they would not be in cases of sexual precocity. Finally, should it be possible to obtain consent to perform a testicular biopsy, mature spermatogenesis will be revealed.

Precocious puberty due to *neurogenic causes* occurred in the Seckel-Jolly-Thamdrup-Wilkins series in 65 cases, namely in roughly one-third of the total, and therefore, in the absence of obvious abnormal neurological signs, a ventriculogram should be examined before it is assumed that the case is constitutional in origin. The lesion is usually a pineal tumour or a hypothalamic disorder, such as a hamartoma. Both in the pineal and hypothalamic lesions and indeed in many or most of the cases of constitutional precocious puberty the normal mechanism of inhibition of gonadotropin-releasing factor from the hypothalamus is interrupted. In some cases there are accompanying signs of a neurological lesion, such as internal hydrocephalus, diabetes insipidus, somnolence, obesity, temperature disturbances or cranial nerve palsies. The hormonal pattern is the same as in constitutional precocious puberty, namely, demonstrable output of gonadotropin and slightly raised 17-ketosteroid levels. The testes are of adult size and spermatogenesis is present.

Sexual Precocity

Sexual precocity in boys is as rare as precocious puberty. It was caused by *congenital adrenal hyperplasia* (macrogenitosomia precox) in 53 cases of the Seckel-Jolly-Thamdrup-Wilkins series. There is thought to be a special tendency for the cases of male congenital adrenal hyperplasia to develop adrenal crises, but this may be because the cases often remain undiagnosed, and therefore untreated until the age of 3 or more when precocious puberty begins to be evident. Addisonian crises occurring before this time may be labelled "infantile convulsions" and may be fatal because corticosteroid therapy has not been instituted. The high output of urinary 17-oxosteroids is significantly suppressed by dexamethasone, or further considerably raised by the ACTH-stimulation test. This distinguishes these cases from those caused by a postnatal *adrenocortcal tumour*, of which there were 16 in the Seckel-Jolly-Thamdrup-Wilkins series. If the adrenal overactivity commences after birth but during the first decade, it is nearly always due to a tumour,

usually malignant, and not to hyperplasia. Clinically, it may be difficult to distinguish the condition from macrogenitosomia precox, but in the case of a tumour, the precocity develops rapidly with a very high output of 17-oxosteroids. A history of precocity or female pseudohermaphroditism in siblings is suggestive of congenital adrenal hyperplasia, and there may be a history of "convulsions" or other episodes indicating Addisonian crises. Malignant adrenocortical tumours are "autonomous" of corticotropin control. Though these tumours are malignant the prognosis depends on whether they are still encapsulated at operation. If there has been no local spread or distant metastases the prognosis is good.

Sexual precocity may also be caused by an *interstitial cell tumour* of the testicle. This is extremely rare; Bishop, Van Meurs, Willcox & Arnold (1960*b*) collected 25 cases from the literature, and added one of their own. Wilkins (1965) brings the total of published cases up to 33. Further cases have been since reported but the total up to date is probably not more than 50. The age of onset is generally between 3 and 6 years. The tumour is usually palpable and the diagnosis therefore easy, but this has not been so in two cases reported in our series, in which exploration of the adrenal was undertaken. The tumour is usually benign and if it is the prognosis is good. The 17-oxosteroid level was recorded in 15 of the 33 cases referred to by Wilkins, and ranged between 2·9 and 550 mg./24 hr. Only in three were the pre-operative values within normal limits for the patient's age; in the rest they were significantly or grossly raised. This is somewhat surprising because it has been the impression that gonadal androgens are, biologically, strikingly active, but contribute only modestly to the total 17-oxosteriod excretion, wheras the opposite is true of adrenal androgens. It is true that in some of the cases that showed high levels of urinary 17-oxosteroid excretion the interval between the onset of signs of androgenic overactivity and the ititial estimation of 17-oxosteroids was relatively great, suggesting that the production of androgens by the tumour progressively increased. Nevertheless, one might suspect that in the cases where the 17-oxosteroid level was greatly raised the tumour consisted of adrenal-rest cells rather than of testicular Leydig cells. One of the supposedly characteristic features of Leydig cells, as opposed to cells of adrenocortical origin, is the presence of crystalloids of Reinke. Unfortunately, the presence or absence of these structures has not been clearly established in the histological reports of any of the cases showing high values. The case of Savard *et al.* was very fully investigated by fractionation of the individual 17-oxosteroids and also by incubation of tissue slices of the tumour with labelled testosterone, progesterone, cholesterol and acetate. The pre-operative fractionation studies showed that androsterone and aetiocholanolone were the two metabolites present in highest concentration, and that they appeared in approximately equal amounts, indicating that testosterone and androstenedione were the principal virilizing hormones which are normally derived from testicular tissue. Nevertheless, the identification of certain 11β-hydroxy-steroids indicated the presence of the enzyme 11β-hydroxylase, which is normally found only in adrenal tissue. In addition, histological examination of the tumour cells clearly revealed crystalloids of Reinke, and the authors therefore question the tissue specificity of both the crystalloids of Reinke and the capacity to elaborate 11β-hydroxy-steroids. A case is reported by Engel, Lanmar, Scully & Villee (1966) in which the histological diagnosis strongly suggested an interstitial tumour of the testis and not an adrenal-rest tumour, although no crystalloids of Reinke were detected. The preoperative 17-oxosteroid level was 7·5 to 13 mg./24 hr. and fell to 3 mg. within 2 days of the operation (Normal value for a 4-year-old boy, which he was, being < 1 mg./24 hr.). The tumour was incubated with acetate-1-^{14}C and the labelled steroids identified not only indicated the presence of 11β-hydroxylase but the presence of cortisol. Indeed another case has been described by Besch, Watson, Barry, Hanwi, Mostow & Gwinup (1963) in which cortisol was formed from progesterone secreted by a patient with unilateral testicular tumour with clinical signs of Cushing's syndrome. Pure interstitial cell tumours are therefore difficult to distinguish from adrenal-rest cell tumours despite the urinary 17-oxosteroid levels.

Interstitial cell tumours in adults. These are rather more frequent in adults than in children (Dalgaard & Hesselberg, 1957), but they often produce no endocrine manifestations. When they do the picture is one of feminization rather than excessive virilization and gynaecomastia is the commonest manifestation, sometimes associated with aspermia, impotence and loss of libido. The output of 17-oxosteroids may be considerably raised. Ward, Krantz, Mendeloff & Haltiwanger (1960) found levels up to 1860 mg./24 hr. in one case associated with gynaecomastia, and also very high output of urinary oestrogens. According to Dalgaard & Hesselberg about 10% are malignant.

Other Testicular Tumours

Though the histogenesis and site of origin (testis or adrenal cortex) of interstitial cell tumours is by no means clear, the classification and nomenclature of other testicular tumours is controversial and hormonal studies have not up to now helped very much in the diagnosis, indications for treatment and the prognosis. There are Sertoli cell tumours, the rarest of all testicular tumours, seminomas and teratomas, the commonest, comprising roughly 90% of all testicular tumours. Most of the teratomas, which occur predominantly in younger men, between the ages of 20 and 30, and comprise about 40% of all testicular tumours, are considered to be more malignant and radio-resistant than the seminomas, which comprise about 50% and develop later in life. With the object of indicating the degree of malignancy of the teratomas some sort of classification has been proposed—indeed at least two classifications—one British (the Testicular Tumour Panel and Registry, Collins & Pugh, 1964) and one American (Friedman & Moore, 1964, and Dixon & Moore, 1952). The Testicular Tumour Panel and Registry have tried to classify the teratomas roughly according to the malignancy from "Teratoma Differentiated" (TD) through "Malignant Teratoma Intermediate A and B" (M.T.I.A. or M.T.I.B.) to "Malignant Teratoma Anaplastic" (M.T.A.). As a subdivision of the latter there is "Malignant Teratoma Trophoblastic" (M.T.T.).

As far as the endocrine aspects of these tumours are concerned we can consider Sertoli cell tumours, seminomas, teratomas and especially trophoblastic teratomas. *Sertoli cell tumours* occur comparatively frequently in dogs and usually produce signs of feminization. The Testicular Tumour Panel and Registry (Collins & Symington, 1964) have only six on their books and the London Hospital series (Hope-Stone, Blandy & Dayan, 1963) only one. The first one to be reported in a human being instead of a dog was Teilum's case (1958). These tumours are benign and usually cause feminization such as gynaecomastia, loss of libido and impotence. It was consequently thought that the Sertoli cells secreted oestrogen but it is more probable that any oestrogen produced by the testis is due to conversion of androstenedione produced by the Leydig cells to oestrone. The commonest testicular tumour, the *seminoma*, is the least malignant and 80% of the patients who undergo an orchidectomy and subsequent radiotherapy on account of this tumour survive five years and then die subsequently of some other cause. It used to be said that in some cases of seminoma there was abnormally high urinary output of follicle-stimulating gonadotropin (F.S.H.) where in teratomas and especially chorionepitheliomas human chorionic gonadotropin (H.C.G.) was excreted in large amounts. Unfortunately these estimations of urinary gonadotropin do not seem to be very helpful in classification or in prognosis. The origin and nature of the gonadotropic activity is unknown. The Friedman test for pregnancy was positive in 40 out of 121 patients with testicular tumours (Moon & Hullinghorst, 1948). Dixon & Moore (1952) recorded a positive Aschheim-Zondek test in 20 out of 24 patients with seminoma and in 154 out of 251 cases with various types of teratoma. These positive tests are due chiefly to the presence of H.C.G. in the urine. Though the presence of gonadotropins in the urine does not specify the degree of malignancy of the tumour, its persistence following orchidectomy indicates the presence of metastases. Urinary 17-oxosteroids and oestrogens in patients with seminomas and teratomas show no consistent abnormalities. (I am indebted to a great extent for this information to the excellent review article by Dayan, 1966.)

Testicular Deficiency

The most convenient and practical classification of testicular deficiency is that suggested by Heller & Nelson (1948). This primarily divides testicular deficiency into two main groups, depending on whether there are signs of eunuchoidism or not. The former group is then subdivided according to whether the lesion is primarily testicular (hypergonadotropic) or primarily hypophyseal (hypogonadotropic). None of the methods of classification is perfect and each can be criticized on one ground or another, but the Heller-Nelson classification still seems the best and will be adopted here.

Testicular deficiency with eunuchoidism. (a) *Hypogonadotropic eunuchoidism.* The bodily habitus is tall and eunuchoid, and secondary sex characters are poorly developed. The testicles are small and biopsy shows a histological picture similar to that of the normal prepubertal testis, namely small tubules containing a few spermatogonia and undifferentiated Sertoli cells; no Leydig cells are present. Because of the absence of Leydig cells the plasma testosterone levels are significantly lowered. Gonadotropins cannot be demonstrated in the urine, and indeed the condition is one of indefinitely delayed puberty. Recently, treatment of this condition with human menopausal gonadotropin ("Pergonal") has been given experimental trials and is said to be effective

in about one-third of the cases. This preparation contains a high concentration of F.S.H. which stimulates the maturation of spermatozoa. Strictly speaking this treatment is indicated only in cases of *germinal cell arrest* associated with low titres of urinary gonadotropins.

In a small number of cases belonging to this group there was evidence of the development of the germinal epithelium, either up to the primary spermatocyte stage or even to the extent of full maturation with production of spermatozoa. This relatively rare sub-group is referred to as *"fertile eunuchs"*. Could they achieve sexual potency they might become fathers.

Hypogonadotropic eunuchoidism must be differentiated from pituitary infantilism, adult pituitary failure and delayed puberty. In cases of *pituitary infantilism* there is evidence of lack of other pituitary influences than the gonadotropic. For instance, the "infantilism" or "dwarfism" indicates failure of somatotropic hormone production, and there is often an associated hypothyroidism as shown by low BMR values. In this condition there is usually a very low output of urinary 17-oxosteroids, possibly indicating both gonadal and adrenocortical failure, whereas in hypogonadotropic eunuchoidism the 17-oxosteroid value is usually in the low normal range. The bone age is usually extremely retarded and indeed the epiphyses of the long bones may never unite. *Adult pituitary failure* due, for instance, to a craniopharyngioma or chromophobe adenoma usually diagnosed by the X-ray appearances of the pituitary fossa or by suprasellar calcification, may be distinguished from hypogonadotropic eunuchoidism when the former supervenes in adult life after normal physical development has already taken place. There will then be gradual failure of gonadal function associated possibly with secondary hypothyroidism and adrenocortical deficiency. Finally, *delayed puberty* is difficult to differentiate from hypogonadotropic eunuchoidism, which indeed is a condition of indefinitely delayed puberty. Administration of a therapeutic trial of injections of chorionic gonadotropin—our dosage regime is 1500 I.U. three times a week for 6 weeks, and possibly for another 6 weeks—initiates puberty which then proceeds spontaneously in cases of delayed puberty, but in cases of hypogonadotropic eunuchoidism the condition relapses when the treatment is abandoned. Delayed puberty is a common occurrence; hypogonadotropic eunuchoidism is extremely rare.

(b) *Hypergonadotropic eunuchoidism.* This condition may be separated into two main groups depending on whether testicular failure occurs during infancy or childhood, or whether it develops during puberty.

(i) *Prepubertal testicular failure* is a term which is convenient to use for patients one sees at about the age of 16 or 18 who have not yet achieved secondary sexual maturity. On examination no testicular tissue can be palpated though one may be able to distinguish tissue that might be epididymal or vas deferens. The testis has apparently disappeared, and it is seldom possible to determine why this has happened. These cases present as primary testicular deficiency with complete lack of secondary sexual characters. Their urinary gonadotropins are high and their 17-oxosteroids (or urinary or plasma testosterone levels) are low. They are obviously sterile and require replacement therapy with androgens.

(ii) *Klinefelter's syndrome (Seminiferous tubule dysgenesis)*. This syndrome, first described by Klinefelter *et al.* (1942) as consisting of gynaecomastia, small testes showing hyalinization of the tubules and apparently normal Leydig cells, aspermia and raised urinary gonadotropin output, is now known to be due to a chromosomal anomaly in which chromatin-positive nuclear sexing is commonly associated with an XXY-chromosomal pattern. The cytogenetics of this condition have become more complicated in recent years and cases in which three or even four X-chromosomes are present have been recorded. The more X-chromosomes that are present the greater the tendency to mental deficiency. The karyotype XXYY has recently been recognized. Two Y-chromosomes are frequently associated with tall stature and violently aggressive criminal behaviour. Cases of Klinefelter's syndrome have been described with no chromosomal abnormality. They have a less pronounced gonadal defect. The individual develops normally until the pubertal age. The testicles then remain small and firm, and microscopically show hyalinization of the seminiferous tubules with complete absence of germinal epithelium and only occasional presence of Sertoli cells. Relatively few seminiferous tubules are to be found, and there is evidence of their atresia in the presence of "ghost" tubules. The interstitial tissue is in fact hyperplastic, and may be seen in clumps or islands. Some of the patients show signs of androgenic deficiency, such as eunuchoid proportions with increased span length as compared with height, and increased lower measurements as compared with upper measurement, scanty pubic and axillary hair and defective beard growth. Some develop gynaecomastia, though these individuals are often rather virile in relation to the rest of their secondary sex characters. After the age of normal puberty the urinary gonadotropin levels are elevated, and the urinary 17-oxosteroid output is low normal or actually subnormal. The plasma testosterone levels are significantly diminished (Federman, 1967) and there is a lack of response to exogenous administration of chorionic gonadotropin.

Testicular deficiency without eunuchoidism. This constitutes a far commoner group of cases consisting mainly of men who until they submitted themselves to investigations in connection with infertility were unaware that they were suffering from aspermia or oligospermia. Physically there is no sign of androgenic failure. On the other hand, testicular biopsy reveals pathological changes in the seminiferous tubules and germinal epithelium (except in those cases in which the aspermia is due to bilateral congenital absence or blockage of a portion of the deferent ducts, and the seminiferous tubules and their contents are therefore histologically normal). The pathological changes consist of germinal cell aplasia; or arrest of maturation of the germinal epithelium at the primary spermatocyte stage; or disorderly arrangement of germinal elements which normally follow each other in an orderly sequence of maturation until the fully developed spermatozoa reach the centre of the lumen of the seminiferous tubule; or peritubular fibrosis which deprives the tubule of its blood supply and thus leads to degeneration and gradual disappearance of the elements of the germinal epithelium, so that Sertoli cells only are left to be identified in the hyalinized tubule.

Gynaecomastia

The general consensus of opinion is that gynaecomastia results either from the circulation of excessive oestrogen or else from a lowered androgen/oestrogen ratio. The oestrogen/17-oxosteroid urinary excretion ratio was studied in a group of Bantu subjects suffering from gynaecomastia, and compared with a group of normal Bantu controls. A possibly significant increase was found in the gynaecomastia series (Bloomberg *et al.*, 1958). Gregoris (1957) estimated urinary oestrogen and 17-oxosteroid output in patients with severe liver disease, some of whom were suffering from gynaecomastia. The oestrogen output was not increased in the gynaecomastia group, but the 17-oxosteroid output was diminished. Exogenous administration of oestrogen certainly produces gynaecomastia. In some individuals the mammary tissue is excessively sensitive to normal oestrogen levels. For instance, about 80% of boys at puberty develop gynaecomastia; in the majority this consists merely of slight tenderness and swelling of the nipple or the transient development of a hard subareolar plaque; in a few instances, however, the degree of gynaecomastia causes the youth embarrassment, and furthermore the mammary swelling fails to regress and may therefore require plastic surgery. There are a number of circumstances in which the occurrence of gynaecomastia is difficult to explain. It has, for instance, very occasionally been reported following the administration of certain drugs such as digitalis and strophanthin, or in association with debilitating diseases such as thyrotoxicosis, sprue and severe diabetes. It has been a prominent feature of the results of improved nutrition in repatriated prisoners-of-war. Furthermore, there are many cases occurring in adult men for which no cause can be found. There is, however, considerable evidence that in a number of conditions the gynaecomastia is due to oestrogen secreted by the Leydig cells of the testis. For instance, gynaecomastia has been found in connection with interstitial cell tumours of the testis in 3 out of 26 prepubertal cases (Bishop *et al.*, 1960*a*) and in six adult cases (Hermann *et al.*, 1958). Maddock *et al.* (1952) describe patients in whom the sole remaining testicular structure was clumps of Leydig cells, and found the urinary oestrogen excretion to be higher than in castrates. Furthermore, following administration of chorionic gonadotropin to seven normal men, they found a striking increase in oestrogen excretion, and testicular biopsy revealed hyperplasia and signs of increased secretory changes in the Leydig cells accompanied by signs of tubular damage. It is not uncommon to find that administration of HCG in the treatment of undescended testicle or retarded development leads to the appearance of gynaecomastia, which has also been reported in connection with chorionepithelioma, seminoma and teratoma of the testis, all of which tumours may produce chorionic gonadotropin. Hall (1959) examined material obtained by testicular biopsy in over 50 cases of gynaecomastia attending the Department of Endocrinology at Guy's Hospital, and found the predominant histological feature to be clumping and hyperplasia of the Leydig cells. In certain conditions associated with gynaecomastia it is clear that the adrenal cortex is the source of the oestrogen production. It seems possible, in fact, that the production of oestrogen may, in certain circumstances, be transferred from the testicle to the adrenal cortex. Gynaecomastia is also found in some cases of prepubertal testicular failure. In these cases the testis obviously cannot produce the hormone which causes the

gynaecomastia, and if it is admitted that this is oestrogen it presumably comes from the adrenal cortex. Details are given by Wallach *et al.* (1957) of 34 cases of adrenocortical carcinoma associated with gynaecomastia. The production of biologically active oestrogens by these tumours is clearly established. In Wallach *et al.*'s case equilenin, a weak oestrogen present in the urine of pregnant mares, was isolated from the tumour, this being the first occasion on which it has been demonstrated in the human subject. There was an elevated urinary excretion of oestrogen with normal 17-oxosteroid levels.

DISORDERS OF THE OVARY

Precocious Puberty

Wheras "*constitutional*" precocious puberty is as rare an occurrence in boys as is precocious puberty due to neurogenic causes, in girls it accounts for between 80 and 90% of the cases, and although the differential diagnosis should be carefully considered the child should not be lightly submitted to radical investigative procedures (such as laparotomy to exclude a granulosa cell tumour). In boys there is a strong hereditary disposition, whereas in girls the condition is usually sporadic. Once the menarche is established it is likely that the menstrual cycles will be ovulatory, and the demonstration of the typical biphasic temperature pattern (relatively low before ovulation and relatively high after ovulation), or the finding of pregnanediol in the urine during the second half of the cycle, will certainly differentiate the condition from sexual precocity. These children may therefore conceive, though Jolly (1955) does not consider precocious sexual interest to be at all common in the girls, as it undoubtedly is in the boys belonging to this group. Nevertheless, Wilkins (1965) points out that 70 of 310 girls with precocious puberty became pregnant before the age of 14, and that 18 pregnancies occurred between the ages of 5 and 10. Because of the production of oestrogen at an early age the girls grow conspicuously tall, but the epiphyses unite prematurely and in adult life the individuals tend to be short and stocky. Urinary gonadotropins can be demonstrated in normal adult levels and the 17-oxosteroid output is high for the child's age. Wilkins (1965) applied the terms *premature thelarche* and *pubarche* to the conditions in which there is precocious development of the breast and of the pubic and axillary hair respectively. In the cases of premature thelarche of which Wilkins quotes 56 as against 102 cases of idiopathic female sexual precocity the breast development is the only premature feature, and it is probable that the mammary tissue is excessively sensitive and is stimulated to growth by the normal prepubertal concentrations of circulating oestrogen. The breast enlargement becomes evident at between 1 and 3 years of age. On the other hand, in some cases of premature pubarche the bone age is from one to four years in advance of the chronological age, and Thamdrup (1955) has found a slightly increased excretion of 17-oxosteroids and reducing corticoids in most of the cases of his series of 17 patients, which indicates premature activation of adrenal androgens, as Silverman et al. (1952) suggested. Seven of the 29 patients of the series of Silverman et al. (1952) were mentally retarded, but this was thought to be a coincidence. However, all the children in Thamdrup's series were mentally retarded and 12 suffered from a severe cerebral disorder. One girl died at the age of 4½ years and microscopical examination of the hypothalamic region revealed atrophic ganglion cells. It seems possible, therefore, that premature pubarche may be of *neurological* origin and due to a disturbance of the cerebral regulation of adrenal androgen production via the pituitary. In the majority of cases, however, the condition is presumably due to increased sensitivity of the sexual hair follicles to normal prepubertal levels of androgen. *Polyostotic fibrous dysplasia* was first described by Albright et al. (1937), and consists of a syndrome in which there are scattered bone lesions, often unilateral, areas of pigmentation of the skin and premature puberty. The bone lesion consists of osteitis fibrosa, though in certain places the bone may show increased density, and Thannhauser (1944) has suggested that there may be overgrowth of bone at the base of the skull causing pressure on the hypothalamus. Urinary gonadotropins have been absent or low in the cases in which they have been estimated. It is curious that polyostotic fibrous dysplasia is almost entirely confined to girls, although Falconer, Cope & Robb-Smith (1942) described a case in a boy and Jolly (1955) mentions two other cases, and more recently Benedict (1966) has reported a fourth case, whereas precocious puberty associated with pineal tumours nearly always occurs in boys.

Endocrine Tumours of the Ovary

The majority of ovarian tumours are "silent" and do not betray their presence by producing clinical evidence of disturbance of ovarian function. Endocrine tumours of the ovary may be feminizing or masculinizing. Feminizing tumours are the only cause of sexual precocity in girls.

Masculinizing tumours have never been described as occurring before puberty, so that heterosexual precocity, that is, prepubertal virilism, is never due to ovarian causes. Between the menarche and the menopause feminizing tumours most characteristically give rise to the menstrual pattern of metropathia haemorrhagica, which consists of episodes of prolonged bleeding varying in amount from a trickle to a flooding, and alternating with non-bleeding phases of variable duration. After the menopause feminizing tumours produce post-menopausal bleeding as the most prominent sign. Masculinizing tumours may develop at any time after puberty or the menopause.

Sexual precocity due to feminizing ovarian tumours. Uterine bleeding is usually the first clinical sign, and often precedes breast development. This is in contrast to cases of precocious puberty in which mammary development and incipient pubic hair growth antedate the first menstrual period. There may be either single episodes of bleeding or else the irregular bleeding pattern characteristic of metropathia haemorrhagica. In less than half the cases bleeding is fairly regular, and resembles the non-ovulatory cycles which so often characterize the first few months of normal menstrual life. In some cases bleeding occurs for the first time after removal of the tumour—"oestrogen withdrawal" bleeding. Later the breasts and external genitalia begin to show adolescent changes and the feminine bodily contours appear. According to Wilkins (1965) a palpable abdominal tumour was present in most cases by the time that signs of sexual development became evident. The contralateral ovary remains infantile. Owing to the increased osteoblastic activity which oestrogen induces, the long bones increase in size and the child becomes taller than other children of her own age, though there is little advancement of the bone age.

Removal of the tumour leads to regression of signs of precocity much more frequently than in the case of interstitial cell tumour of the testicle, especially if the child is operated upon as early as possible, for after the age of eight regression is unlikely to take place. Treatment in a child should be conservative and is usually confined to removal of the affected ovary and tube. At this age the growth, if it is a granulosa cell tumour, is nearly always unilateral and the prognosis is good even though there may be histological evidence of low-grade malignancy.

Though granulosa cell tumours are the most frequent cause of female sexual precocity, they nevertheless occur very rarely in children. Thompson et al. (1967) reviewed 53 ovarian tumours occurring in children, at the Mayo Clinic since 1905. Only five were "functioning" tumours and all of these were granulosa-cell tumours. No hormone studies had been undertaken pre-operatively, but one case in which there was a recurrence showed no excess of urinary oestrogen. Wilkins (1965) quotes 31 identified cases and 30 in which the type was not identified in the series reported by Seckle, plus one each in Jolly and Thamdrup's series and two in Wilkins' own series. Feminizing neoplasms other than granulosa cell tumours have been reported as leading to sexual precocity. In Seckel's series there were six tera-tomas and four chorionepitheliomas. Seckel & Plotz (1955) collected four cases of luteoma from the literature and added one of their own. Granulosa-theca cell tumours have also been described for instance by Tweedie (1958) (two cases) and such cases may fall into the category that Seckel described as "type not identified". Another granulosa-theca cell tumour was repor-ted by Scarpa et al. (1959). Very few hormone studies have been undertaken in these cases up to date. In the four cases of chorionepithelioma collected from the literature by Seckel (1946), which developed between the ages of 6 and 8 and were exceedingly malignant, chorionic gona-dotropin was demonstrated in the tumour in one case and in the urine in the remaining cases. Bruk et al. (1960) believe that theirs is the first report of quantitative biochemical oestrogen estimation in granulosa-cell tumours causing sexual precocity. They found the total urinary oestrogen levels to be not so high as in normal adult females at mid-cycle, whereas in other cases reported the oestro-gen levels have been assayed biologically and have been found much higher than in normal adults. This suggests that active oestrogens other than oestradiol, oestrone and oestriol, may be pro-duced by granulosa cell tumours. They also found elevated levels of urinary gonadotropin ("F.S.H.") which suggests that these tumours are not auto-nomous, but are under some degree of pituitary control. Marsh et al. (1962) report a case of granulosa cell tumour occurring in a 26-month-old girl with sexual maturation and elevated urinary oestrogens. In vitro studies of the tumour tissue showed a high capacity of conversion of ^{14}C-testosterone to radioactive oestrogen.

Feminizing Ovarian Tumours in Adults

Though these tumours must be considered unusual even in adult life, they occur more commonly than they do in children. Pratt (1937) collected 200 cases from the literature, and since that date there have been other series reported,

such as those of Henderson in 1942 (30 cases), Hodgson, Dockerty & Mussey (1945) (62 tu-mours), Haines & Jackson (1950) and Matthew (1955). Of the 40 cases of Haines & Jackson's series 60% occurred between the ages of 40 and 60, whereas the majority (24) of the 43 cases collected by Matthew (1955) over a period of 17 years (from the Gynaecological Department of Edinburgh University) developed over the age of 50 with the greatest incidence in the seventh decade.

Menstrual disturbance is the commonest and usually the only clinical symptom. Periods of amenorrhoea may occur in the premenopausal group, and may alternate with episodes of pro-longed and heavy bleeding. On the other hand there may be no interruption of normal menstrual rhythm, and in any case in a premenopausal woman menstrual irregularity alone could hardly lead to the suspicion of the presence of a femini-zing tumour, even if the endometrium showed cystic glandular hyperplasia. Post-menopausal bleeding, however, is more likely to give rise to suspicion, although Fahmy (1933) found that a granulosa cell tumour was present in only three out of 937 patients complaining of postmeno-pausal bleeding. Behrens (1959) collected records of 264 post-menopausal patients with ovarian tumours. The endometrium showed proliferation in 78. Of these only 28 had granulosa-cell or theca-cell tumours that might be expected to pro-duce oestrogen which would stimulate endometrial proliferation.

The tumour itself may vary in size from a minute lesion discovered accidentally to a growth weigh-ing 15·5 kg. (Pratt, 1950). It is therefore not always palpable on bimanual examination, though in the majority of cases it is, and in Haines & Jackson's series abdominal pain and swelling due to the tumour were prominent features. The uterus, on the other hand, is almost always enlarged, sometimes considerably, owing to the influence of the oestrogen produced by the tumour. The clinical features are mainly due to oestrogen production by the tumour, whether this be a true granulosa-cell tumour, a thecoma or a granulosa-thecoma.

Very few hormonal studies have been under-taken that have so far reached the literature. Paschkis et al. (1958) suggest a classification according to the hormones produced by the tumour, as follows: granulosa-theca cell, oestro-gen with suppression of gonadotropins; thecoma, oestrogen in large amounts; luteinized granulosa-theca cell (luteoma), oestrogen and progesterone; and chorionepithelioma, chorionic gonadotropin with secondary production of oestrogen and progesterone.

Masculinizing Tumours of the Ovary

Until the seventh week of intra-uterine life the gonad cannot be regarded as an endocrine organ, and the cortex and medulla contain primitive cells which are capable of differentiating later into ovarian and testicular structures respectively. It is possible, however, that certain of these primitive cells may remain dormant during the stages of normal embryonic development and may, very rarely, differentiate at some time during post-natal life. This is believed to be the explanation of the origin of testicular seminomas. The homo-logue of this tumour, which the French refer to as a seminoma of the ovary, is the *dysgerminoma*, a relatively uncommon tumour which is generally supposed to produce no hormones, and develops chiefly in adolescent girls and young women, the "carcinoma puellarum". Hughesdon (1966) dis-agrees with the commonly held opinion that these tumours develop from the "indifferent" cells of the early gonad and his studies lead him confi-dently to believe that the tumours arise from female germ cells, namely oocytes.

At a later stage of embryonic development, when gonadal differentiation commences, sex cords derived from the gonadal mesenchyme make their appearance, and if the gonad is to become a testis they are canalized to form the seminiferous tubules. If, on the other hand, the gonad develops into an ovary a second wave of differentiation is superimposed upon the testicular scaffolding, though remnants of the original testicular struc-ture may persist and give rise to a tumour in later life.

Such a tumour is known as an *arrhenoblastoma*, and three types are described, depending on the degree of differentiation of the testicular struc-tures. The most highly differentiated, the so-called testicular adenoma of Pick, contains tubules, a rete testis and islands of Leydig cells. It is rare and seldom produces endocrine manifestations. At the other extreme there is the equally rare and highly undifferentiated growth which closely resembles a sarcoma and almost always gives rise to virilism. The intermediate group, which includes most of the cases of arrhenoblastoma, is represented by a tumour that consists of a mass of dense fibrous tissue resembling a fibrosarcoma in which is embedded tubules, sex cords and Leydig cells. If it has grown to a reasonable size this tumour gives rise to virilism.

These tumours are rare and only few of them have fallen into the hands of steroid chemists

capable of studying them expertly. The charac-teristic feature of most of them is that when they display androgenic features they are intensely virilizing though the urinary 17-oxosteroid output is within the normal range or only slightly raised. This is in favour of their being of gonadal origin rather than developing from cells that are funda-mentally adrenocortical. Stimulation studies with ACTH and chorionic gonadotropin and suppres-sion tests with dexamethasone and oestrogen have not as yet solved the problem, nor have fractiona-tion studies designed to determine whether the principal androgens produced are derived from gonadal tissue or from adrenocortical cells. Crystalloids of Reinke, thought to be characteris-tic of testicular Leydig cells, have been sought for and sometimes found, but there is no absolute agreement among the experts as to their exact origin. In the last edition of this book an attempt was made to report the whole literature to date in great detail, but it made confusing reading. Since then there have been few important reviews that have clarified either the classification or the histo-genesis of masculinizing tumours of the ovary. The purely pathological nomenclature of these tumours—whether they are arrhenoblastomas, masculinovoblastomas, lipoid-cell virilizing tu-mours, or even hypernephromas of the ovary—is not of primary concern in the present context and until some agreement is reached as to the signifi-cance of the biochemical evidence it seems merely confusing to present the details of the few and conflicting reports that have so far been received. Hughesdon's chapter in Modern Trends in Gynaecology (1966) though primarily concerned with histogenesis rather than biochemistry, perhaps summarizes the position concerning one type of potentially androgenic tumour. He points out that over 100 "lipoid cell tumours" have now been reported, a minority of which behave like adrenal tumours, having a high 17-oxosteroid excretion level and responding to stimulation with ACTH but not with chorionic gonadotropin. He believes however that this reflects the native ability of neoplastic ovarian tissue to produce any derivative of intermediate mesoderm rather than the tumours originating in pre-formed adreno-cortical tissue.

THE POLYCYSTIC OVARY SYNDROME

(Stein-Leventhal Syndrome)

The classical features of this condition are bilateral ovarian enlargement, amenorrhoea, infertility, hirsutism, obesity and vague abdominal pain (Stein & Leventhal, 1935). Unfortunately the classical features by no means invariably occur in any individual case, and diagnosis therefore may be difficult. For instance infertility, which is the commonest complaint (in those cases in which it could be a complaint) occurred in only 75% of 296 cases reported in the literature (Goldzieher & Green, 1962). No other of the classical symptoms was present in more than 50% of the cases. For example, although amenorrhoea is the classical menstrual pattern and occurred in 47% of 350 cases, regular periods occurred in 16% of 253 cases, and 61 biphasic basal temperature patterns were recorded in 13% of 77 cases, whereas corpora lutea were found at operation in 19% of 322 cases. It therefore becomes necessary wherever possible to visualize the ovaries by culdoscopy or other means. Classically the ovaries are enlarged and in Goldzieher & Green's series submitted to operation they were in 25 out of 29 cases.

On macroscopic examination not only are the ovaries usually obviously enlarged but they appear firm, smooth, flattened, sclerotic and bluish white ("oyster" ovaries). This is due to thickening of the tunica albuginea and is almost invariable. On cutting into them they appear to be polycycstic, though no large follicular cysts are found, and the cortex is thick and fibrotic. On microscopical examination numerous microcystic follicles are encountered, many of them surrounded by hyperplastic theca interna cells, though there is no frank luteinization of the theca.

Hormone estimations have now been performed in a considerable number of cases, and the results have been reviewed by Goldzieher & Green (1962) and by Shearman (1966). The steroidal deviations of the Stein-Leventhal syndrome have led to the postulation of many hypotheses. It seems to be universally agreed that the polycystic ovary produces excessive quantities of androgen perhaps due to the increased number of active follicles engaged in steroidogenesis (Kase, 1964), perhaps due to enzyme defects such as impairment of 19-hydroxylase, preventing androstenedione conversion to oestradiol, or to lack of the aromatizing enzyme preventing the aromatization in ring A which is characteristic of oestrogens. Short & London (1961) extracted androstenedione from cyst fluid but could find no oestrone or oestradiol in it. Giorgi (1963) confirmed the presence of androstenedione but did find oestradiol in the cyst fluid. Despite the relatively inefficient oestrogen synthesis as compared with the excessive amounts of androgen produced, the Stein-Leventhal ovary is quite capable of secreting amounts of oestrogen similar to those found in the follicular phase of the normal cycle.

There is also evidence for increased and disturbed adrenocortical steroidogenesis with increased production of dehydroepiandrosterone and urinary excretion of pregnanetriolone, which might suggest a slight impairment of 21-hydroxylase formation, such as one gets in congenital adrenal hyperplasia leading to increased androgen formation and diminished synthesis of cortisol.

The restoration of normal ovulatory cycles by wedge-resection or by administration of clomiphene suggests that the ovarian and adrenal abnormalities may be due to deranged activity of the pituitary or hypothalamus. At the moment these postulations are hard to explore because of the methodological difficulties in regard to gonadotropin assay and especially of FSH isolation and quantitative measurement. Identification of the hypothalamic gonadotropin (L.H.)-releasing factor is still unsatisfactory.

Certainly the results of wedge-resection of the ovaries are remarkably satisfactory. Stein (1966) reported conception in 82% of 83 women submitted to bilateral wedge resection. This is the experience of other authors. Unfortunately, however, regression of hirsutism occurs relatively seldom. It may be supposed that fairly radical wedge-resection would produce these satisfactory results simply by removing the excessive luteinized thecal cells, thus allowing the remaining ovarian structures to respond normally to pituitary gonadotropic influences. It has been found, however, that even when the ovaries are merely bisected and the two halves sewn together, back-to-back, equally satisfactory results are achieved. This is in favour of the mechanical theory that the thickened capsule prevents ovulation.

References

ALBRIGHT, F., SMITH, P. H. & FRASER, R. (1942). *Amer. J. med. Sci.*, **204**, 625.
ALBRIGHT, F., BUTLER, A. M., HAMPTON, A. O. & SMITH, P. (1937). *New England. J. Med.*, **216**, 727.
BAER, W. (1927). *Arch. Gynäk.*, **51**, 3241.
BAHNER, F. & SCHWARZ, G. (1961). *Acta endocr. Kbh.*, **38**, 236.

BEHRENS, H. (1959). *Arch. Gynäk.*, **193**, 270.
BENEDICT, P. H. (1966). *Amer. J. Dis. Child.*, **111**, 426.
BERGSTRAND, C. G., BIRKE, G. & PLANTIN, L.-O. (1959). *Acta endocr. Kbh.*, **30**, 500.
BESCH, P. K., WATSON, D. J., BARRY, R. D., HAMWI, G. L., MOSTOW, J. & GWINUP, G. (1963). *Steroids*, **1**, 644.

BISHOP, P. M. F. (1964). *Brit. med. J.*, **1**, 1255.

BISHOP, P. M. F., LESSOF, M. H. & POLANI, P. E. (1960a). *Mem. Soc. Endocrinol.*, **7**, 162.

BISHOP, P. M. F., VAN MEURS, D. P., WILLCOX, D. R. C. & ARNOLD, D. (1960b). *Brit. Med. J.*, **1**, 238.

BLOOMBERG, B. M., MILLER, K., KEELEY, K. J. & HIGGINSON, J. (1958). *S. Afr, J. med. Sci.*, **23**, 83.

BONGIOVANNI, A. M. (1961). *J. clin. Endocrin.*, **21**, 860.

BONGIOVANNI, A. M. (1966). Exc. Med.—2nd Intern. Congr. on Hormonal Steroids. Milan. p. 8.

BONGIOVANNI, A. M., EBERLEIN, W. R., SMITH, J. D. & McPADDEN, A. J. (1959). *J. clin. Endocrin.*, **19**, 1608.

BRENTNALL, C. P. (1945). *J. Obst. Gynaec. Brit. Emp.*, **52**, 235.

BRUK, I., DANCASTER, C. P. & JACKSON, W. P. U. (1960). *Brit. Med. J.*, **2**, 26.

DEL CASTILLO, E. B., DE LA BALZE, F. A. & ARGONZ, J. (1947). *J. clin. Endocrin.*, **7**, 385.

COLLINS, D. H. & PUGH, R. C. B. (1964). *Brit. J. Urol.*, **36**, Suppl. 1.

COLLINS, D. H. & SYMINGTON, T. (1964). *Brit. J. Urol.* **36**, Suppl. 2.

DALGAARD, J. B. & HESSELBERG, F. (1957). *Act. path. microbiol. Scandinav.*, **41**, 219.

DANON, M. & SACHS, L. (1957). *Lancet*, **2**, 20.

DAYAN, A. (1966). "Hospital Medicine", p. 126.

DIXON, F. J. & MOORE, R. A. (1952). "A.F.I.P. Atlas of Tumour Pathology". **8**, 31b and 32. Washington, D.C.

DOMINGUEZ, O. V. (1961). *J. clin. Endocrin.*, **21**, 663.

ENGEL, E. & FORBES, A. P. (1965). *Medicine*, **44**, 135.

ENGEL, L. L., LANMAN, GERTRUDE, SCULLY, R. E. & VILLEE, DOROTHY B. (1966). *J. clin. Endocrin.*, **26**, 381.

FAHMY, E. C. (1933). *J. Obstet. Gynaec. Brit. Emp.*, **40**, 506.

FALCONER, M. A., COPE, C. L. & ROBB-SMITH, A. H. T. (1942). *Quart. J. Med.*, n.s., **11**, 121.

FEDERMAN, D. D. (1967). "Abnormal Sexual Development". London, W. B. Saunders.

FERRIER, P. E. (1965). *Lancet*, **1**, 1401.

FORD, C. E. (1961). "Human Chromosomal Anomalies". (Eds. Smith, D. R. & Davidson, W. M.), p. 23. London, Staples.

FORD, C. E., JONES, K. W., POLANI, P. E., ALMEIDA, J. C. DE & BRIGGS, J. H. (1959). *Lancet*, **1**, 711.

FRIEDMANN, N. B. & MOORE, R. A. (1946). *Milit. Surg.*, **99**, 573.

GIORGI, E. P. (1963). *J. Endocrin.*, **27**, 225.

GOLDZIEHER, J. W. & GREEN, J. A. (1962). *J. clin. Endocrin.*, **22**, 325.

GORDAN, G. S., OVERSTREET, E. W., TRAUT, H. F. & WINCH, G. A. (1955). *J. clin. Endocrin.*, **15**, 1.

GREEN, O. C., MIGEON, C. J. & WILKINS, L. (1960). *J. clin. Endocrin.*, **20**, 929.

GREENBLATT, R. B., CARMONA, N. & HIGDON, L. (1956). *J. clin. Endocrin.*, **16**, 235.

GREGORIS, L. (1957). *Act. med. Patavina*, **17**, 277.

GRIFFITHS, K., GRANT, J. K. & WHYTE, W. G. (1963). *J. clin. Endocrin.*, **23**, 1044.

GRUMBACH, M. M., DUCHARME, J. R. & MOLOSHOK, R. E. (1959). *J. clin. Endocrin.*, **19**, 1369.

GUINET, P. (1965). *Minerva pediatrica*, **17**, 611.

HAINES, M. & JACKSON, I. (1950). *J. Obstet. Gynaec. Brit. Emp.*, **57**, 737.

HALL, P. F. (1959). "Gynaecomastia". New South Wales, Australian Med. Publish. Co.

HAUSER, C. A. (1961). "Die Intersexualität". (Ed. Overzieher, C.), p. 261. Stuttgart, Thieme.

HAYLES, A. B. & NOLAN, R. B. (1958). *Proc. Mayo. Clin.*, **33**, 197.

HELLER, C. G. & NELSON, W. O. (1948). *J. clin. Endocrin.*, **8**, 345.

HENDERSON, D. N. (1942). *Amer. J. Obstet.*, **43**, 194.

HERMANN, W. L., BUCKNER, F. & BASKIN, A. (1958). *J. clin. Endocrin.*, **18**, 834.

HODGSON, J. E., DOCKERTY, M. B. & MUSSEY, R. D. (1945). *Surg. Gynec. Obstet.*, **81**, 631.

HOPE-STONE, H. F., BLANDY, J. P. & DAYAN, A. D. (1963). *Brit. med. J.*, **1**, 984.

HUGHESDON, P. E. (1966). *Obst. and Gynec. Survey*, **21**, 245.

JAVERT, C. T. & FINN, W. F. (1951). *Cancer*, **4**, 60.

JEFFCOATE, S. L., BROOKS, R. V. & PRUNTY, F. T. G. (1968). *Brit. med. J.*, **1**, 208.

JOLLY, H. R. (1955). "Sexual Precocity". Springfield, Ill., Thomas.

KASE, N. (1964). *Amer. J. Obst. and Gynec.*, **90**, 1268.

KLINEFELTER, H. F., REIFENSTEIN, E. C. & ALBRIGHT, F. (1942). *J. clin. Endocrin.*, **2**, 615.

MADDOCK, W. O., EPSTEIN, M. & NELSON, W. O. (1952). *Ann. N.Y. Acad. Sci.*, **55**, 657.

MARSH, J. M., SAVARD, K., BAGGETT, B., VAN-WYK, J. J. & TALBERT, L. M. (1962). *J. clin. Endocrin.*, **22**, 1196.

MATTHEW, G. D. (1955). *Proc. Roy. Soc. Med.*, **48**, 724.

MEYER, R. (1925). *Virchows Arch.*, **255**, 33.

MONCRIEFF, A. (1958). *Brit. med. J.*, **2**, 267.

MOON, H. D. & HOLLINGHORST, R. L. (1948). *Amer. J. Path.*, **24**, 1067.

MORRIS, J. M. (1953). *Amer. J. Obstet. Gynec.*, **65**, 1192.

O'DOHERTY, N. J. (1964). *Guy's Hosp. Rep.*, **113**, 368.

OVERZIEHER, C. (1961). "Die Intersexualität". (Ed. Overzieher, C.), p. 188. Stuttgart, Verlag.

PAPADATOS, C. & KLEIN, R. (1954). *J. Pediat.*, **45**, 662.

PASCHKIS, K. E., RAKOFF, A. E. & CANTAROW, A. (1958). "Clinical Endocrinology". London, Cassell.

PICH, G. (1937). *Beitr. path. Anat.*, **98**, 218.

POLANI, P. E. (1961). *Brit. med. Bull.*, **17**, 200.

POLANI, P. E., HUNTER, W. F. & LENNOX, B. (1954). *Lancet*, **2**, 120.

POLANI, P. E., LESSOF, M. H. & BISHOP, P. M. F. (1956). *Lancet*, **2**, 118.

PRADER, A. & SIEBENMANN, R. E. (1958). "Symposium on Nuclear Sex". (Eds. Smith D. R. & Davidson, W. M.) London, Heinemann.

PRATT, F. B. (1937). *J. Obstet. Gynaec. Brit. Emp.*, **44**, 880.

PRATT, J. P. (1950). "Modern Trends in Obstetrics and Gynaecology". (Ed. Bowes, K.), p. 534. First Series, London, Butterworth.

SCARPA, J. B., BEHERAN, H., RAICES, A. A. & BUR, G. E. (1959). *Amer. J. Obstet.*, **78**, 821.

SCHOEN, E. J., DI RAIMONDO, V. & DOMINGUEZ, O. V. (1961). *J. clin. Endocrin.*, **21**, 578.

SECKEL, H. P. G. (1946). *Med. Clin. N. Amer.*, **30**, 183.

SECKEL, H. P. G. & PLOTZ, E. J. (1955). *Ztschr. Kinderhlk.*, **76**, 593.

SHARPEY-SCHAFER, E. P. (1941). *Lancet*, **2**, 559.

SHEARMAN, R. P. (1966). *Obstet. and Gynec. Survey*, **21**, 1.

SHORT, R. V. & LONDON, D. R. (1961). *Brit. med. J.*, **1**, 1724.

SILVERMAN, S. H., MIGEON, C., ROSEMBERG, E. & WILKINS, L. (1952). *Pediatrics*, **10**, 426.

SOHVAL, A. R. (1964). *Amer. J. Med.*, **36**, 281.

SOUTHREN, A. L., SAITO, A., LAUFER, A. & SOFFER, L. J. (1961). *J. clin. Endocrin.*, **21**, 675.

STEIN, I. F. (1966). In "Ovulation". (Ed. Greenblatt, R. G.) p. 150. Lippincott.

STEIN, I. F. & LEVENTHAL, J. L. (1935). *Amer. J. Obst. and Gynec.*, **29**, 181.

TEILUM, G. (1958). *Cancer*, **11**, 769.

THAMDRUP, E. (1955). *Acta Endocr. Kbh.*, **18**, 564.

THAMDRUP, E. (1961). "Precocious Sexual Development". Springfield, Ill., Thomas.

THANNHAUSER, S. J. (1944). *Medicine*, **23**, 105.

THOMSPON, J. P., DOCKERTY, M. B., SYMMONDS, R. E. & HAYLES, A. B. (1967). *Amer. J. Obst. and Gynec.*, **97**, 1059.

TURNER, H. H. (1938). *Endocrinology*, **23**, 566.

TWEEDIE, F. J. (1958). *Amer. J. Obstet.*, **75**, 964.

VANDEKERCKHOVE, D. (1954). *Ann. Endocrin.*, **15**, 513.

VARNEY, R. F., KENYON, A. T. & KOCH, F. C. (1942). *J. clin. Endocrin.*, **2**, 137.

WALLACH, S., BROWN, H., ENGLERT, E. & EIK-NES, K. (1957). *J. clin. Endocrin.*, **17**, 945.

WARD, J. A., KRANTZ, S., MENDELOFF, J. & HALTIWANGER, E. (1960). *J. clin. Endocrin.*, **20**, 1622.

WILKINS, L. (1965). "The Diagnosis and Treatment of Endocrine Disorders in Childhood and Adolescence". 3rd Ed., Springfield, Ill., Thomas.

WILKINS, L., GRUMBACH, M. M. & VAN WYK, J. J. (1954). *J. clin. Endocrin.*, **14**, 1270.

ZACHARIAE, F. (1955). *Acta Endocr. Kbh.*, **20**, 331.

METHODS OF HORMONE ASSAY

by IAN F. SOMMERVILLE

IN the preceding sections, the results of the assay of the gonadotropic and gonadal hormones have been cited in connection with disorders of reproductive function. The following comments are intended to aid in assessing the usefulness and limitations of methods of assay in the light of recent advances in technique. It will be appreciated that this aspect of endocrinology is in a phase of rapid development and, although many methods of assay constitute imperfect and indirect indices of endogenous hormone secretion, the application of new and powerful physico-chemical procedures for microanalysis is making an increasing contribution to our knowledge of reproductive physiology and pathology.

There is no ideal method of assay, only a method which may be ideal for the purpose of the investigator. Thus, in a study of steroid metabolism it may be essential to use a chemical technique of the highest degree of specificity for the quantitative determination of a single steroid compound, whereas it may be unwise to single out one of the metabolites of an ovarian hormone when attempting to deduce the level of endogenous secretion. Much must be learned about the intermediary metabolism of the steroid hormones before one can distinguish between an absolute deficiency of production of a hormone and a relative deficiency due to its deflection into abnormal metabolic pathways, and before one can assess the hormonal environment of the target cells or the importance of variations in tissue responsivity. A high degree of sensitivity, accuracy, precision and specificity is essential for the determination of the relatively low concentrations of steroids in systemic blood and tissue or for labour-saving micro-methods for urinary analysis. In the past, attempts to improve the analytical procedures were frequently open to the criticism that this was effected by progressive elaboration rather than innovation. During the past five years this situation has been completely changed by two major advances—the development of techniques for the quantitative determination of steroids by thin-layer and gas-liquid chromatography and the use of radioimmunoassay for the determination of human pituitary gonadotropins.

BIO-ASSAY OF PITUITARY GONADOTROPIN

In this section, comment will be confined to work upon the purification and bio-assay of two of the three gonadotropic factors which are believed to be secreted by the human pituitary—the follicle-stimulating hormone (FSH) and the luteinizing or interstitial cell-stimulating hormone (LH or ICSH). The third gonadotropin, prolactin (which is probably identical with luteotropin, LTH), will not be discussed.

Preparation of gonadotropin from human pituitaries. Highly active preparations with follicle-stimulating activity have been prepared from the pituitary glands of sheep (Li, Simpson & Evans, 1949; Woods & Simpson, 1960) and pigs (Steelman & Segaloff, 1959), but clinical trials with these animal preparations yielded inconclusive results. Subsequently, the purification of FSH from human pituitaries was reported (Li, 1958; Gemzell, Diczfalusy & Tillinger, 1958; Steelman, Segaloff & Andersen, 1959). The material prepared by Gemzell and his co-workers precipitated with $(NH_4)_2SO_4$ at saturations between 55% and 75% and the fraction precipitating at 55% saturation was found to possess mainly luteinizing activity (LH). Thus it appeared to be possible to obtain from human pituitaries at least partially purified fractions which exhibit either FSH or LH activities. More recently, chromatography on DEAE-cellulose has been employed by most workers for the purification of FSH, followed by gel filtration on Sephadex-G (Roos & Gemzell, 1964; Parlow, Condliffe, Reichert & Wilhelmi, 1965). Furthermore, although very highly purified FSH preparations are unstable, material suitable for administration to patients can be obtained from human glands in a relatively high state of purity and with adequate potency (Crooke, Butt, Palmer, Morris, Edwards & Anson, 1963; Butt, 1967). A satisfactory procedure for the preparation of LH from human pituitaries has been described by Hartree, Butt & Kirkham, (1964); human LH is more stable than FSH.

Preparation of pituitary gonadotropin from human urine. In the past, kaolin absorption was employed for the purification of urinary gonadotropin of pituitary origin (Scott, 1940; Dekanski, 1949) and a product designated HMG24 prepared by Dekanski by kaolin adsorption and acetone precipitation was selected as the International Reference Preparation (1st IRP-HMG: *Bull. World Health Org.*, 1960). On the other hand, more active material was prepared by adsorption on cabunite by Johnsen (1955) and by ion-exchange chromatography (Bourrillon, Got & Marcy, 1960; Albert, Derner, Stellmacher, Lieferman & Barnum, 1961). Finally, a new standard prepared by the kaolin technique and purified by chromatography on permutit (Donini, Puzzuoli & Montezemolo, 1964) was selected as the 2nd IRP-HMG.

Bio-assay in human plasma. Although it is over 30 years since gonadrotropic activity was demonstrated in the serum of ovariectomized women (Fluhman, 1929), it was many years before the purification of plasma pituitary gonadotropin was studied in detail (Antoniades, Pennel, McArthur, Ingersoll, Ulfelder & Oncley, 1957). This was achieved by purification of human plasma with ethanol and zinc salts with controlled ionic strength, and protein concentration. Apostolakis (1960) described a method for the estimation of plasma gonadotropin in post-menopausal women, and in other non-pregnant individuals in whom the plasma concentration is relatively high. In 1964, McArthur, Antoniades, Larson, Pennell, Ingersoll & Ulfelder demonstrated the presence of both FSH and LH in the plasma of post-menopausal women. The former was assayed by the rat ovary augmentation test and the latter in terms of the weight increase of the ventral prostate of the hypophysectomized rat.

Bio-assay in human urine. Of the numerous methods employed for the extraction of "total urinary gonadotropin" of pituitary origin (urinary HPG), kaolin adsorption and tannic acid precipitation have been most widely employed (Albert, 1955; Johnsen, 1958; Loraine & Brown, 1956). The mixture of FSH and LH is then assayed by the effect upon the uterine weight of immature mice as described by Klinefelter, Albright & Griswold (1943) in terms of the second IRP-HMG. Alternatively, the increase in the rat ovarian weight may be used (Albert, 1959) but this appears to be a less sensitive method.

Attempts to determine FSH or predominantly FSH activity by bio-assay are of especial interest because of the difficulties in achieving satisfactory determination by the new technique of radioimmunoassay (see below). The ovarian augmentation assay is useful for this purpose and depends upon the increase in the ovarian weight of immature rats (Steelman & Pohley, 1953) or mice (Brown, 1955) when this effect is potentiated by the administration of human chorionic gonadotropin (HCG). The mouse augmentation test is more sensitive. Igarashi & McCann (1964) used the mouse uterine weight as the end-point in an augmentation test (with lower doses of HCG) and obtained a further increase in sensitivity. As discussed in the following section, LH can be readily determined by radioimmunoassay but it may still be of interest to employ bio-assay by one of the laborious methods depending upon the weight increase of the ventral prostate in hypophysectomized rats (Greep, Van Dyke and Chow,

1942; McArthur, 1952) or the ovarian ascorbic acid depletion test (OAAD) of Parlow (1961). The latter technique has the disadvantage that, in its present form it is not applicable to urinary extracts.

With regard to variations in the urinary excretion of HPG during the menstrual cycle or of predominantly FSH or LH activities, results are conflicting but certain points of agreement have emerged. A mid-cycle peak in the excretion of HPG has been observed in a proportion of cycles (Brown, Klopper & Loraine, 1958; Johnsen, 1959); there is a peak in LH excretion at mid-cycle or associated with the occurrence of ovulation (McArthur, 1952; Loraine & Brown, 1956; Fukushema, Stevens, Gannt & Vorys 1964); FSH is excreted in lower amounts in the luteal phase but evidence is very conflicting about the occurrence of peaks. In a recent study of 23 healthy young women, Rocca & Albert (1967) carried out daily assays of urinary FSH and found an increase for the first few days of the cycle, maintenance of this for the remainder of the follicular phase and for the early luteal phase followed by a decrease until the end of the cycle. There was considerable variation between individual subjects but FSH excretion was similar in consecutive cycles of the same subjects.

IMMUNOASSAY AND RADIOIMMUNO-ASSAY OF GONADOTROPINS

Since 1960, immunological methods have been widely employed for the determination of human chorionic gonadotropin—using haemagglutination inhibition (Wide & Gemzell, 1960) or complement fixation (Brody & Carlström, 1961); inert particles such as latex may be used as a substitute for red blood cells (Goss & Taymor, 1962). Using either approach, attempts have been made to develop procedures for the estimation of FSH and LH and the cross reaction between anti-HCG and human LH has been used for the immunological assay of urinary LH by the haemagglutination technique (Wide, Roos & Gemzell, 1961; Butt, Crooke & Cunningham, 1961) or using latex particles (Rizkallah, Taymor, Park, & Batt, 1965). With regard to FSH, preliminary results indicate that the complement-fixation technique may be applicable and haemagglutination inhibition has also been investigated but it is probable that radioimmunoassay techniques will be more efficient. A sensitive and rapid radioimmunoassay for LH (or HCG) in human blood or urine has been reported by Wilde, Orr & Bagshawe (1967) using a double antibody precipitation technique, similar to that employed for insulin (Hales & Randle, 1963). The HCG is iodinated with ^{125}I by the technique previously used for the preparation of iodinated growth hormone (Greenwood, Hunter and Glover, 1963) although the latter used ^{131}I and ^{131}I-HCG has also been used for the radioimmunoassay of LH (or HCG) by Franchimont (1966). Recently, Faiman & Ryan (1967) and Saxena, Demura, Gandy & Peterson (1967) have described techniques for the radioimmunoassay of FSH. While it is evident that further work is indicated upon FSH determination in biological fluids by this approach, the advent of radioimmunoassay of LH is a major advance and has the advantage that a large number of assays can conveniently be performed simultaneously and the result obtained within 24 hours of receiving the specimen. It will be evident, however, that immunological methods do not necessarily equate with potency nor can this important point readily be elucidated by comparison of the results of immunoassay with those of bio-assay. Further advances in our knowledge of the chemistry of the gonadotropins must be made before the study of the gonadotropins can pass into the phase of biochemical investigation.

ASSAY OF OESTROGENS

Since the early observations of Allen & Doisy (1923) upon the induction of vaginal cornification in ovariectomized mice, bio-assay of the urinary oestrogens has been widely studied (Emmens, 1950) and Szego & Roberts (1946) used bio-assay to investigate the protein-bound oestrogen in blood. Unfortunately, however, the Allen-Doisy technique and its modifications are too laborious for routine clinical use, although it would be premature to consider that they have been entirely replaced by current chemical techniques. At the present state of knowledge, it is important to confirm that the small amounts of urinary oestrogens chemically determined are indeed oestrogenic in nature. This must be borne in mind when evaluating attempts to remove extra-ovarian oestrogens by such procedures as total adrenalectomy, involving the application of chemical techniques to urinary extracts which may contain only a few micrograms of the supposed oestrogen. Furthermore, it may be unwise to limit attention to the clinical significance of only the three principal urinary oestrogens.

These oestrogens are readily estimated by the Kober colour reaction, the pink colour produced when a steroid oestrogen is heated with a mixture of phenol and sulphuric acid, the mixture cooled, diluted with water and reheated (Kober, 1931; Brown, 1952). But in men and post-menopausal women the oestrogen output is so low that the proportion of non-oestrogen chromogens is overwhelming, and the Kober colour due to the oestrogens is masked. In the past, considerable work has been devoted to attempts to eliminate interference by other chromogens or to correct for such interference in the final reaction (Jayle, Crepy & Judas, 1943; Stevenson & Marrian, 1947). Jayle & Crepy (1950) eliminated pigments by the introduction of hydrolysis with phosphotungstic acid. In addition, numerous attempts have been made to separate the oestrogens one from another. Mather (1942) separated oestriol from oestrone and oestradiol-17β by distribution between benzene and sodium carbonate; Stimmel (1946) employed adsorption chromatography on alumina, and Engel, Slaunwhite, Carter & Nathanson (1950) carried out a systematic investigation of the separation of oestrogens by counter-current distribution. This technique has the advantage that each compound is characterized by a physical constant.

More sensitive than the Kober colour is the fluorescence which develops when phenolic steroids are treated with strong sulphuric acid. This phenomenon has been studied extensively by Bates & Cohen (1950). Alternatively, Finkelstein, Hestrin & Koch (1947) used phosphoric acid, and Garst, Nye, Maron & Friedgood (1950) described a fluorescent reaction between oestrogens and phthalic anhydride. Braunsberg, Stern & Swyer (1955) preceded fluorimetric assay by partition chromatography on celite. A modified Kober reaction has been introduced by Ittrich (1958). This involves selective extraction of the colour complex by p-nitrophenol in chloroform, and results in an increase in sensitivity with a decrease in interference by non-specific chromogens.

The choice of the ideal method for the hydrolysis of the urinary oestrogens from their conjugation as glucuronides or sulphates is still far from settled. It might be hoped that the less pigmented extracts which result from enzymic hydrolysis would contain less interfering substances. On the other hand, Bauld (1955) suggested that the substances which interfere with the Kober reaction may not be pigments present originally in the urine, but may arise from colourless precursors which become pigmented on contact with alkali.

An important advance in the efficacy of chemical techniques for the determination of urinary oestrogens resulted from the co-operative studies of Brown (1955a) and Bauld (1955), and the final method evolved by Brown has been widely adopted. The method incorporates a phase-change purification step involving methylation of the phenolic fraction; the methylated oestrogens are then further purified and separated from one another by chromatography on alumina columns, and are estimated by a modification of the Kober reaction. Interfering colours are corrected for by the spectrophotometric method of Allen (1950). This procedure permits the separation and quantitative determination of 2–4 μg. of each of the three oestrogens per 24-hr. urine specimen. In using the method particular care is required in the standardization of the alumina.

The advent of this technique, and its application to the normal menstrual cycle (Brown, 1955b), provided an accurate picture of the cyclical changes in the urinary excretion of the three steroids. There is an "ovulation peak" followed by a sudden fall in the excretion of all three compounds (oestriol lags about 24 hr. behind the others). There then occurs a rise to a second peak, the "luteal maximum", at about the 21st day of the cycle, and finally a fall towards menstruation. In a study of 10 cycles from eight healthy women, Brown obtained the following values: Ovulation peak: oestriol (0–15 μg./24-hr.); oestrone 11–31 μg./24-hr.); oestradiol-17β (4–14 μg./24-hr.). Luteal maximum: oestriol (8–72 μg./24-hr.); oestrone (10–23 μg./24-hr.) and oestradiol-17β (4–10 μg./24-hr.). Extending this study, Brown (1956) carried out a unique series of analyses of the urinary oestrogen excretion of a woman from before the beginning of a normal pregnancy, up to delivery, and then during the puerperium, lactation and the re-establishment of menstruation. A saponification step introduced by Bauld (1956) was subsequently incorporated in the method of Brown (Brown, Bulbrook & Greenwood, 1957). In the author's laboratory this modified Brown method is used for all assays in non-pregnant subjects. For studies in pregnancy, the determination is confined to urinary oestriol, and the method modified accordingly. Since interference may result from the administration of such laxatives as senna, cascara and phenolphthalein, it is necessary to stop laxatives or replace with liquid paraffin and to allow time for clearance of phenolphthalein before collection of specimens for assay. In patients receiving the tranquillizer, Equanil, spuriously high urinary oestriol values are obtained unless the saponification step is used.

By use of the Girard reaction and partition

chromatography of the oestrogens in each of the Girard fractions, Givner, Bauld & Vagi (1960) have developed a method for the quantitative determination in human urine of 2-methoxy-oestrone, oestrone, Ring D α-ketolic oestrogens, oestradiol-17β, 16-epioestriol and oestriol. This is a lengthy procedure, but should yield important information upon the excretion of this more complete series of urinary oestrogens. Gas-liquid chromatography has also been used for determination of some of these compounds (Wotiz & Chattoraj, 1964) and gas-liquid chromatography preceded by gel filtration and purification has been used for the analysis of a wide spectrum of oestrogens in human bile and urine (Adlercreutz, Salokangas & Luukkainen, 1967). These workers stress the importance of achieving adequate specificity and are obtaining evidence for identity by combined gas-chromatography and mass spectrometry (Luukainen & Adlercreutz, 1967).

Methods have been developed for the chemical determination of oestrogens in blood and tissues. Thus, a modification of the Brown method has been applied to the determination of oestrogens in placental tissue (Diczfalusy & Lindquist, 1956) and foetal blood (Diczfalusy & Magnusson, 1958). This technique suffers from the relatively low sensitivity of the Kober reaction and H_2SO_4 fluorescence has been employed by Preedy & Aitken (1961). This procedure involves partition chromatography on a celite column and is suitable for assays in foetal or maternal plasma in late pregnancy.

The measurement of oestrogens in the peripheral venous blood of non-pregnant women has been a difficult task, due to the extremely low concentrations in a sample of reasonable volume. Considerable progress has been made, however, with the development of more sensitive methods of detection. These procedures utilize microfluorometry (Ichii, Forchielli, Pearloff & Dorfman, 1963; Roy, Harkness & Kerr, 1965), double isotope derivative formation (Svendsen, 1960; Svendsen & Sorensen, 1964; Slaunwhite & Neely, 1963), and gas-liquid chromatography with electron-capture detection (Wotiz, Charransol & Smith, 1967; Attal, Hemdeles & Eik-Nes, 1967; Exley & Chamberlain, 1967). Ichii et al. (1963) have reported that the mean value for both free oestrone and oestradiol-17β in the plasma of healthy premenopausal women is 0·03 μg./100 ml. Roy et al. (1965) have measured the total (free and conjugated) oestrone, oestradiol-17β and oestriol in the peripheral blood of women during the menstrual cycle. Their mean values for the follicular and ovulatory phases—

expressed as μg./100 ml. are as follows: oestrone: 0·020 and 0·070; oestradiol: 0·013 and 0·028; oestriol: 0·025 and 0·037. The sensitive isotopic method described by Svendsen (1960) and modified in a subsequent report (Svendsen & Sorensen, 1964), involves the formation of isotopically labelled pipsyl esters. The results indicate that the plasma concentration of free oestrone and oestradiol during the menstrual cycle are in the order of 0·03–0·10 μg./100 ml. plasma, with the highest values occurring in the middle third of the cycle. Gas-liquid chromatography has been employed with electron-capture detection to measure total plasma oestrone, oestradiol and oestriol as the heptafluorobutyrate derivatives (Wotiz et al., 1967). The mean values for oestrone, oestradiol, and oestriol in non-pregnant women were 0·24, 0·17 and 0·23 μg./100 ml. respectively. Attal et al. (1967) reported free oestrone values to be 0·018–0·125 μg./100 ml. in plasma of women with normal ovulatory cycles. These results were obtained by the use of 3-methyl-17-pentafluorophenylhydrazone, for gas chromatographic measurement with an electron capture detector. The technical difficulties involved in the analyses of plasma oestrogens are emphasized in a recent review (O'Donnell & Preedy, 1967), but it is probable that these will be overcome in view of the now rapid advancement in the development of ultra-sensitive and specific techniques for the determination of low concentrations of steroids in biological fluids

It must be emphasized that the clinical value, whether as a guide to diagnosis, therapy or prognosis, of the assay of oestrogens in urine or blood is largely untested. It may be strictly limited, and a test of the functional capacity of the ovary, similar to that employed in studying adrenocortical function, may be more informative than the mere measurement of the urinary excretion of oestrogens of endogenous origin.

ASSAY OF PROGESTERONE AND PREGNANEDIOL

Until 1954, attempts to assess the level of endogenous secretion of the hormone of the corpus luteum depended either upon the biological assay of the concentration of progestogenic activity in the blood, or upon such indirect evidence as could be obtained by the chemical estimation of pregnanediol or other progesterone metabolites in the urine. The former approach was complicated by difficulties in the histological interpretation of the results of such sensitive methods as that of Hooker & Forbes (1947), and by the fact that there was considerable discrepancy between the values obtained by different methods (Hoffman & v. Lam, 1941; Forbes, 1951). Furthermore, the observation of high values by bio-assay, and repeated failure even to detect the hormone by chemical means in peripheral human blood (Haskins, 1950; Butt, Morris, Morris & Williams, 1951; Wiswell & Samuels, 1951) raised the question, which is still pertinent, as to the importance of other progestogenic hormones and the status of progesterone as the principal progestogen in human physiology. The latter approach suffers from the fact that urinary pregnanediol (there are several closely related pregnanediols in human urine) may arise from precursors other than progesterone and that, since the urinary level is the end-result of a rather complex metabolism, deduction of hormone secretion from metabolite excretion may not be possible in physiological and pathological states.

It was encouraging, therefore, when progesterone was isolated from the human placenta (Salkanick, Noall, Zarrow & Samuels, 1952) and was detected in the ovarian vein of the ewe and the sow (Edgar, 1953). Finally, the hormone was identified in human peripheral venous blood collected after the 6th month of pregnancy (Zander, 1954; Zander & Simmer, 1954). This was achieved by the repeated purification by paper chromatography of pooled extracts of blood, and the application of colour reactions and ultraviolet and infra-red spectroscopy. The concentration of the hormone in umbilical venous blood is considerably higher than that of the peripheral venous blood of the mother (Zander & von Münstermann, 1954; Sommerville, 1957; Aitken, Preedy, Eton & Short, 1958), and the progesterone concentration in placental tissue has been estimated at different stages of pregnancy (Zander & von Münstermann, 1956). With regard to other progestogens, it should be noted that two closely related compounds, both exhibiting progestational activity, have been isolated from human follicles, corpora lutea and placentae (Zander, Forbes, von Münstermann & Neher, 1958). These are 20α- and 20β-hydroxy-pregn-4-en-3-one. The 20α epimer has been identified in human pregnancy plasma (Short, 1960).

The first spectrophotometric methods for the determination of plasma progesterone involved spectrophotometry of the Δ^4-3-ketone at 240 mμ, (Zander & Simmer, 1954; Short, 1958). Subsequently, derivatives were formed—for example, the dinitrophenylhydrazone (Hinsberg, Pelzer & Seuken, 1956); the isonicotinic acid hydrazone (Sommerville & Deshpande, 1958) and the

thiosemicarbazone (Sommerville, Pickett, Collins & Denyer, 1963). These techniques were satisfactory for the study of peripheral blood levels in the second and third trimesters of pregnancy (in the range 5–30 μg./100 ml. plasma) but did not possess adequate sensitivity for studies in nonpregnant women. Fluorescence techniques were also investigated but were liable to overestimation.

Subsequent methods have involved either the preparation of isotopically labelled derivatives or gas-liquid chromatography (GLC). Thus sodium (^{3}H)—borohydride was used by Woolever & Goldfein (1963) and a double isotope derivative technique with progesterone-4-^{14}C and ^{35}S-thiosemicarbazide was described by Riondel, Tait, Tait, Gut & Little (1965). The latter method is very sensitive and has a high degree of accuracy but the labour involved has precluded its application on a large scale.

The use of isotopic and gas-chromatographic methods for the determination of plasma progesterone in the non-pregnant has been the subject of a recent review (van der Molen & Aakvaag, 1967) and three techniques appear to possess adequate sensitivity—the isotope derivative method of Riondel et al. (1965); the reduction of progesterone to 20β-hydroxypregn-4-en-3-one with formation of the chloroacetate for electron capture detection as described by **van der Molen & Groen** (1965) and a relatively simple method in which thin-layer chromatography is followed by GLC using a flame ionization detector and automatic electronic integration (Wyman & Sommerville, 1966, 1968). These two gas chromatographic techniques incorporate a labelled internal standard and calculation of the result in terms of a second non-labelled standard which is added before GLC.

As an alternative to correction in terms of two internal standards, overall correction for the recovery of the labelled standard was effected by combustion of the effluent gas and proportional counting (Collins & Sommerville, 1964; Sommerville & Collins, 1965) but this technique requires further development for determination of the hormone in the follicular phase of the menstrual cycle.

It may be concluded that valid determination of plasma progesterone can now be performed over the range of concentrations observed in the menstrual cycle.

Plasma pregnanediol was estimated after infusion of progesterone (Sommerville, 1952) and subsequently in a combined determination of the hormone and metabolite (Sommerville &

Deshpande, 1958). This method was adequate for the study of peripheral blood levels in pregnancy and of foetal blood (Deshpande & Sommerville, 1958; Deshpande, Turner & Sommerville, 1960). Evidence for the identity of the steroid (5β-pregnane-$3a$, $20a$-diol) was obtained by infra-red spectroscopy (Oertel & Eik-Nes, 1960) and this compound, its 3β-isomer and 5β-pregnane-$3a$-ol-20-one have been identified after intravenous administration of progesterone-4-^{14}C (Thijssen & Zander, 1966). For the determination of plasma pregnanediol in the non-pregnant woman, a gas-liquid chromatographic method has been developed and preliminary results were reported (Sheerin & Sommerville, 1968). It is probable that useful information will be derived from the serial analysis of plasma progesterone and pregnanediol in women with ovarian dysfunction.

Urinary pregnanediol is excreted throughout the menstrual cycle in amounts which are vast compared with the concentration of most steroids in peripheral venous blood. For example, in the follicular phase of the cycle a plasma progesterone concentration of $0 \cdot 05$ μg./100 ml. ($0 \cdot 005$ μg./10 ml. plasma analysed) may be accompanied by a urinary pregnanediol excretion of 1 mg./24-hour (50 μg. in the 1/20th of the 24 hr. specimen analysed). For this reason, valid results have been obtained by methods which do not involve the use of isotopes either as internal standards or for derivative formation. Similarly, although gas-chromatographic methods have been evolved (e.g. Wotiz, 1963) it is customary to use the established method of Klopper, Michie & Brown (1955) which involves adsorption chromatography, before and after acetylation, and colorimetry. During an ovulatory cycle there is a rise in urinary pregnanediol excretion from $0 \cdot 5$–$1 \cdot 0$ mg./24 hr. in the follicular phase to 2–8 mg./24 hr. in the luteal phase. As emphasized by Borth & de Watteville (1952) daily determinations throughout the cycle reflect the function of the corpus luteum but, in practice, the clinical indications for urinary pregnanediol assay are quite limited; when required, serial analyses are essential—for example to assess the effect of agents for the suppression or stimulation of ovarian function.

ASSAY OF URINARY PREGNANETRIOL, PREGNANETRIOL-11-ONE AND Δ^5-PREGNENETRIOL

It has long been known that pregnanetriol is excreted in large amounts in the urine of patients with adrenocortical hyperfunction (Butler & Marrian, 1937; Mason & Kepler, 1945), and the assay is of clinical value in assessing the efficacy of corticoid therapy in congenital adrenal hyperplasia. More recently it has been demonstrated that a cyclic change in urinary pregnanetriol excretion occurs during the menstrual cycle (Pickett, Kyriakides, Stern & Sommerville, 1959; Fotherby, 1960; Pickett & Sommerville, 1962). There are several closely related methods for the determination of urinary pregnanetriol (Stern, 1957; Bongiovanni & Eberlein, 1958; Fotherby & Love, 1960), and additional evidence for the identity of the final product of the Stern method has been obtained (Pickett & Kellie, 1962).

There is increasing interest in the determination of pregnanetriol-11-one (pregnane-$3a$, $17a$, $20a$-triol-11-one), Δ^5-pregnenetriol (Δ^5-pregnene-3β, $17a$, $20a$-triol) and related steroids. A thorough investigation of the urinary excretion of these steroids has been conducted by Cox (1959, 1960) and Wilson, Lipsett & Ryan (1961). Pregnanetriol-11-one has not been detected in the urine of healthy subjects, but is present in the urine of patients with adrenal hyperplasia (Finkelstein, von Euw & Reichstein, 1953). Recently Cox & Shearman (1961) reported the presence of pregnanetriol-11-one and of abnormally high amounts of Δ^5-pregnenetriol in the urine of patients with the Stein-Leventhal syndrome. Stern & Barwell (1963) have described a method for the determination of Δ^5-pregnenetriol and have applied the method to two groups of patients—one group designated as examples of the Stein-Leventhal syndrome on clinical grounds; the other not so designated but exhibiting one or more of the features of the syndrome. In 65% of the first group, the urinary excretion was more than $0 \cdot 2$ mg./24 hr. whereas in 94% of the second group it was below this level.

By far the most widely employed method for the estimation of the total neutral 17-oxosteroids (17-KS) is based upon the characteristic colour which develops when a methylene ketone reacts with m-dinitrobenzene in alkaline solution (Zimmermann, 1935; Callow, Callow & Emmens, 1938; Holtorff & Koch, 1940). It should be emphasized that the reaction is liable to interference not only by non-ketonic contaminants but by steroid ketones with ketonic groups at positions other than C-17, and that these colorimetric difficulties are only partly met by the use of correction factors based upon the light absorption of the reaction mixture at different wavelengths. In Great Britain, the Medical Research Council (1951) suggested the adoption of a standard procedure (based upon that of Robbie & Gibson,

1943), not so much with the idea that this is superior to other modifications of the method of Callow *et al.* (1938), but so that results obtained by different laboratories will be more comparable. The clinical significance of the estimation of the total 17-KS will not be discussed further. It is illustrated in the preceding sections, and its general application has been comprehensively reviewed (Mason & Engstrom, 1950). In the majority of healthy men and women, the urinary excretion of total neutral 17-KS is in the range 12–18 mg./24 hr. and 6–12 mg./24 hr. respectively, but values in the range of 6–20 mg./24 hr. have been reported in apparently healthy individuals of either sex. In old age the urinary excretion may be as low as 20% of these values.

Partial or complete fractionation of this group of steroids is informative. Separation of ketones from non-ketones with consequent purification of the former is effected by the use of Girard T reagent (Girard & Sandulesco, 1936), and the micro-Girard fractionation of Talbot, Berman, MacLachlan & Wolfe (1941) is convenient for this purpose. A further separation depends upon the fact that steroid compounds with a hydroxyl group at C-3 in a position *cis* to the methyl group at C-10 usually form insoluble digitonides. These digitonin-precipitable steroids are designated β-hydroxy-17-KS, and non-precipitable compounds are designated α-hydroxy-17-KS. Dehydro*epi*androsterone and *epi*androsterone are β-hydroxycompounds, whereas androsterone and its C-5 stereoisomer, aetiocholanolone, are α-hydroxy-17-KS. Many attempts have been made to effect separation of individual 17-KS, notably the pioneer work of Dingemanse, Huis in't Veld & de Laat (1946) and Dobriner, Lieberman & Rhoads (1948). An important technical advance was the introduction of gradient elution chromatography (Lakshmanan & Lieberman, 1954). In this technique an eluting solvent of gradually increasing polarity is applied to an adsorption column, and separations are improved by sharpening of the individual zones on the chromatogram. In the method of Kellie & Wade (1955), a micro-modification of the Zimmermann reaction is applied and the colours are analysed by spectrophotometry. However, although fractionation of the neutral 17-KS has been useful in the study of adrenocortical function, the application of this technique to the study of androgens in women has been of limited value. As indicated above, the urinary excretion of neutral 17-KS in healthy men and women may fall in the same range. In this range also fall the values obtained in the majority of patients with idiopathic hirsutism,

the Stein-Leventhal syndrome, and most ovarian tumours—for example, arrhenoblastoma—although the mean excretion in healthy women is lower than that of hirsute women or men. Accordingly, the determination of neutral 17-KS in individual patients gives little information about ovarian androgen production, although this simple test should be applied to specimens from all hirsute women in order to assess adrenocortical function (in addition to the determination of the 17-hydroxycorticosteroids). As the neutral 17-KS are mainly derived from non-androgenic or weakly androgenic precursors (notably dehydroepiandrosterone) a significant rise in the secretion rate of the principal androgen —testosterone—may not be reflected by a detectable increase in the urinary excretion of androsterone, aetiocholanolone or total neutral 17-KS. For this reason the determination of testosterone is much more informative.

ASSAY OF TESTERONE AND EPITESTOSTERONE

Determination of the blood production rate of testosterone in terms of the metabolic clearance rate and the mean plasma concentration in systemic blood, indicates that the production rate of the androgen is more than twenty-fold higher in men than in women, and it may be deduced— with certain reservations—that the secretion rate of testosterone is more than fifty times higher in men (Horton & Tait, 1966; Tait & Horton, 1966). This direct approach to the study of androgen secretion cannot be used for routine work due to the complexity of the technique and the inadvisability of administering isotopically labelled steroids to pre-menopausal women, but very valuable information can be gained by determination of testosterone in the peripheral venous blood or of testosterone glucuronide in the urine.

The main technical problem associated with the determination of plasma testosterone arises from the low concentrations of the hormone in the peripheral venous blood of women. In 1961, a method was reported by Finkelstein, Forchielli & Dorfman, based on the fact that testosterone can be enzymically converted to oestradiol-17β and oestrone (Ryan, 1959) and the latter compounds estimated by fluorimetry. Application of this method revealed a mean plasma testosterone concentration of 0·56 μg./100 ml. in men (range 0·10–0·98 μg.) and a mean of 0·12 μg./100 ml. in women (range 0·02–0·26 μg.) (Forchielli, Sorcini, Nightingale, Brust & Dorfman, 1963). Subsequently, this method has been widely applied to the study of hirsutism and virilism and observation of high plasma concentrations in a large proportion of patients (Conti, 1967). The method is sufficiently sensitive to detect 1 μg./100 ml.; it is rather time-consuming for general use. As in the case of plasma progesterone determination, more recent techniques have involved either double isotope dilution or gas-liquid chromatography. With regard to the former type of method the technique of choice would be either that of Riondel Tait, Gut, Tait, Joachim & Little (1963) which involves formation of the ^{35}S-thiosemicarbazone, or the technique described by Burger, Kent & Kellie (1964) which involves formation of the tritiated acetate of testosterone-4-^{14}C, and is a modification of the method of Hudson, Coghlan, Dulmanis, Winton & Ekkel (1963). Application of these techniques gave similar results for plasma testosterone in men, but the values in women obtained by the method of Riondel et al. (1963) were lower than those obtained by the other methods (0·06 ± 0·03 μg./100 ml.). Using the technique of Riondel et al. (1963) and subtracting for a nonspecific blank, the mean value for plasma testosterone in healthy women was found to be 0·03 μg./100 ml. (Lobotsky, Wyss, Segre & Lloyd, 1964). The double isotope methods are extremely laborious, and subsequent work has been mainly concerned with attempts to devise accurate and specific methods for determination by thin-layer and gas-liquid chromatography. A significant advance was the introduction of electron capture detection for this purpose (Brownie, van der Molen, Nishizawa & Eik-Nes, 1964). By this technique the mean plasma concentration in men was 0·42 ± 0·6, and in women 0·06 ± 0·03 μg./100 ml. The method of Brownie et al. was applied to the study of larger groups of healthy human subjects by van der Molen, Groen & Peterse (1966); the mean concentration in men was 0·68 μg./100 ml. (0·34–1·49) and in 46 women there was a mean of 0·052 μg./100 ml. However, in 14 individuals the concentration fell below the lower limit of detection (0·02 μg./100 ml.) so that the true mean range was considered to be between 0·036 and 0·052 μg./100 ml. In the method of Brownie et al. (1964) the monochloroacetate is used as electron capturing derivative whereas the heptafluorobutyrate gives a larger detector response with an increase in sensitivity. Procedures have already been outlined involving the use of this derivative (Exley, 1966) and a method has been developed in the author's laboratory involving thin-layer chromatography, a modified reaction for the formation of testosterone mono-heptafluorobutyrate, an electron capture detector

with ^{63}Ni as the radioactive source, and automatic electronic digital integration. This procedure has recently been evaluated in detail with calculation of the total random theoretical error and practical errors, and it is concluded that valid determinations can be performed throughout the range of plasma concentrations of healthy women and men. In 41 healthy males there was a mean of 528 ± 261 nanograms/100 ml. plasma, and in 20 healthy females the mean was 40 ± 14 ng./100 ml. (Collins, Sisterson, Koullapis, Mansfield & Sommerville, 1968).

Testosterone is present in urine as the glucuronide and was first isolated from this source by Schubert and Wehrberger (1960). It should be noted that urinary testosterone glucuronide is not only derived from the testosterone which has been secreted into the circulation but that the conjugate may be formed in the liver without the passage of free testosterone of hepatic origin into the blood stream. For this reason urinary testosterone determination is not a direct index of testosterone production but as there is no significant difference between the ratio of the testosterone blood production rates of men as compared to women and the mean urinary testosterone excretion in either sex this factor does not detract from the use of the urinary assay in practice. Since 1960 numerous techniques have been described and these will not be discussed in detail. The 17α-epimer of testosterone —epitestosterone—is also present in urine (Korenman, Wilson & Lipsett, 1964; Brooks & Giuliani, 1964) but convincing evidence for the presence of this steroid in blood has not yet been presented. In the earlier procedures the two epimers were measured as one product (Camacho & Migeon, 1963; Vermeulen & Verplancke, 1963; Futterweit, McNiven, Guerra-Garcia, Gilbree, Drosdowsky, Siegal, Soffer, Rosenthal & Dorfman, 1964), and there was some overlap between the lower limit of excretion in men and the upper limit in women. Subsequently, the epimers were separated by gas-liquid chromatography (Brooks, 1964; Sparagana, 1965; da Nicola, Dorfman & Forchielli, 1966). However, these techniques were applied to a relatively small number of specimens with conflicting results. Thus, similar values for urinary testosterone and epitestosterone were reported for four healthy men (Brooks, 1964); the excretion of epitestosterone was reported to be lower than that of testosterone in nine men (Sparagana, 1965), whereas similar values for the epimers were reported for a further 12 men (da Nicola, Dorfman & Forchielli, 1966). Furthermore, the latter observed very high concentrations of epitestosterone in hirsute women. Using a method developed in the author's laboratory (Sommerville, 1965, Sommerville et al., 1968a, b) the following results were reported by Ingiulla, Forleo, Galli & Severi (1968): a mean of 5·5 µg./ 24 hr. for testosterone and of 6·9 µg for the epimer in 12 pre-menopausal women; means of 78 µg. and 49 µg. in five young men. In a study of 26 hirsute women, the same authors reported elevated values, but the excretion of epitestosterone was not of the order reported by da Nocola et al. Although further work upon epitestosterone is indicated, it is encouraging to note that there is considerable agreement as to the range of excretion of the testosterone glucuroniside. Thus, using a technique for testosterone only, Vermeulen (1966) reported a mean excretion of 7·0 µg. testosterone/24 hr. in 12 healthy

women (2·9–12·1) and for 50 men the mean was 124·2 µg./24 hr. (30–351·8 µg.). In this study there was a 20 : 1 ratio between the results in men aged 25–45 years and those of pre-menopausal women, i.e. a similar ratio to that reported for blood production rates, as indicated above. The simultaneous determination of testosterone in blood and urine should be of interest. With regard to the analysis of random samples, it should be emphasized that major changes in the day to day excretion of the androgen may occur in hirsute women, as indicated by a preliminary report (Sommerville et al., 1968). This report also confirms the finding of Ingiulla et al. (1968) that, whereas urinary testosterone excretion is relatively constant throughout the normal menstrual cycle, there is a cyclical change in epitestosterone excretion—with a significant rise in the luteal phase.

References

ADLERCREUTZ, H., SALOKANGAS, A. & LUUKKAINEN, T. (1967). Mem. Soc. Endocrinol., 16, 89.
AITKEN, E. H., PREEDY, J. R. K., ETON, B. & SHORT, R. V. (1958). Lancet, 2, 1096.
ALBERT, A. (1955). Proc. Mayo. Clin., 30, 552.
ALBERT, A. (1959). Fertil. Steril., 10, 60.
ALBERT, A., DERNER, L., STELLMACHER, V., LIEFERMAN, J. & BARNUM, J. (1961). J. Clin. Endocrin., 21, 1261.
ALLEN, E. & DOISY, E. A. (1923). J. Amer. med. Ass., 81, 819.
ALLEN, W. M. (1950). J. clin. Endocrin., 10, 71.
ANTONIADES, H. N., PENNEL, R. B., McARTHUR, J. W., INGERSOLL, F. M., ULFELDER, H. & ONCLEY, J. L. (1957). J. biol. Chem., 228, 863.
APOSTOLAKIS, M. (1960). J. Endocrin., 19, 377.
ATTAL, J., HEMDELES, S. M. & EIK-NES, K. B. (1967). Anal. Biochem., 20, 394.
BATES, R. W. & COHEN, H. (1950). Endocrinology, 47, 166, 182.
BAULD, W. S. (1955). Mem. Soc. Endocrin., 3, 11.
BAULD, W. S. (1956). Biochem. J., 63, 488.
BONGIOVANNI, A. M. & EBERLEIN, W. R. (1958). Analyt. Chem., 30, 388.
BORTH, R. & WATTEVILLE, H. DE (1952). Vitam. and Horm., 10, 141.
BOURRILLON, R., GOT, R. & MARCY, R. (1960). Acta endocr. Kbh., 35, 225.
BRAUNSBERG, H., STERN, M. I. & SWYER, G. I. M. (1955). Mem. Soc. Endocrin., 3, 41.
BRODY, S. & CARLSTRÖM, G. (1961). Nature (Lond.), 189, 841.
BROOKS, R. V. (1964). Steroids, 4, 117.
BROOKS, R. V. & GIULIANI, G. (1964). Steroids, 4, 101.
BROWN, J. B. (1952). J. Endocrin., 8, 196.
BROWN, J. B. (1955a) Biochem. J., 60, 85.
BROWN, J. B. (1955b). Lancet, 1, 320.
BROWN, J. B. (1956). Lancet, 1, 704.

BROWN, J. B., BULBROOK, R. D. & GREENWOOD, F. C. (1957). J. Endocrin., 16, 49.
BROWN, J. B., KLOPPER, A. & LORAINE, J. A. (1958). J. Endocrinol., 17, 401.
BROWN, P. S. (1955). J. Endocrin., 13, 59.
BROWNIE, A. C., MOLEN, H. J. VAN DER, NISHIZAWA, E. E. & EIK-NES, K. B. (1964). J. clin. Endocr. Metab., 24, 1091.
BULL. World Health Org. (1960). 22, 563.
BURGER, H. G., KENT, J. R. & KELLIE, A. E. (1964). J. clin. Endocr. Metab., 24, 432.
BUTLER, G. C. & MARRIAN, G. F. (1937). J. biol. Chem., 119, 565.
BUTT, W. R. (1967). "Hormone Chemistry", London, D. van Nostrand.
BUTT, W. R., CROOKE, A. C. & CUNNINGHAM, F. J. (1961). Proc. Roy. Soc. Med., 64, 647.
BUTT, W. R., MORRIS, P., MORRIS, C. J. O. R. & WILLIAMS, D. C. (1951). Biochem. J., 49, 434.
CALLOW, N. H., CALLOW, R. K. & EMMENS, C. W. (1938). Biochem. J., 32, 1312.
CAMACHO, M. & MIGEON, C. J. (1963). J. Clin. Endocr. Metab., 23, 301.
COLLINS, W. P., SISTERSON, J. M., KOULLAPIS, E. N., MANSFIELD, M. D. & SOMMERVILLE, I. F. (1968). J. Chromatog., 37, 33.
COLLINS, W. P. & SOMMERVILLE, I. F. (1964). Nature (Lond.), 203, 836.
CONTI, C. (1967). "Endocrine functions of the Ovary", Ed. Jayle, M. J. p. 491. Oxford, Pergamon Press.
COX, R. I. (1959). J. biol. Chem., 234, 1693.
COX, R. I. (1960). Acta endocr. Kbh., 33, 477.
COX, R. I. & SHEARMAN, R. P. (1961). J. clin. Endocrin., 21, 586.
CROOKE, A. C., BUTT, W. R., PALMER, R. F., MORRIS, R., EDWARDS, E. L. & ANSON, C. J. (1963). J. Obstet. Gynaec. Brit. Commonw., 70, 604.
DEKANSKI, J. (1949). British J. exp. Path., 30, 272.

DESHPANDE, G. N. & SOMMERVILLE, I. F. (1958). *Lancet*, **2**, 1046.

DESHPANDE, G. N., TURNER, A. K. & SOMMERVILLE, I. F. (1960). *J. Obstet. Gynaec. Brit. Emp.*, **67**, 954.

DICZFALUSY, E. & LINDQUIST, P. (1956). *Acta endocr. Khb.*, **22**, 203.

DICZFALUSY, E. & MAGNUSSON, A. M. (1958). *Acta endocr. Kbh.*, **28**, 169.

DINGEMANSE, E., HUIS IN'T VELD, L. G. & LAAT, B. M. DE (1946). *J. clin. Endocrin.*, **6**, 535.

DOBRINER, K., LIEBERMAN, S. & RHOADS, C. P. (1948). *J. biol. Chem.*, **172**, 241.

DONINI, P., PUZUOLI, D. & MONTEZEMOLO, R. (1964). *Acta endocr. Kbh.*, **45**, 156.

EDGAR, D. G. (1953). *Biochem. J.*, **54**, 50.

EMMENS, C. W. (1950). "Hormone Assay", p. 391. New York, Academic Press.

ENGEL, L. L., SLAUNWHITE, W. R., CARTER, P. & NATHANSON, I. T. (1950). *J. biol. Chem.*, **185**, 255.

EXLEY, D. (1966). "Androgens", **101**, 11. Excerpta Med. Int. Congr. Ser.

EXLEY, D. & CHAMBERLAIN, J. (1967). *Steroids*, **10**, 509.

FAIRMAN, C. & RYAN, R. J. (1967). *J. clin. Endocr. and Metab.*, **27**, 444.

FINKELSTEIN, M., EUW, J. VON & REICHSTEIN, T. (1953). *Helv. chim. Acta*, **36**, 1266.

FINKELSTEIN, M., FORCHIELLI, E. & DORFMAN, R. I. (1961). *J. clin. Endocrin.*, **21**, 98.

FINKELSTEIN, M., HESTRIN, S. & KOCH, W. (1947). *Proc. Soc. exp. Biol. N.Y.*, **64**, 64.

FLUHMANN, C. F. (1929). *J. Amer. med. Ass.*, **93**, 672.

FORBES, T. R. (1951). *Endocrinology*, **49**, 218.

FORCHIELLI, E., SORCINI, C., NIGHTINGALE, M., BRUST, N. & DORFMAN, R. I. (1963). *Analyt. Biochem.*, **5**, 416.

FOTHERBY, K. (1960). *Brit. med. J.*, **1**, 1545.

FOTHERBY, K. & LOVE, D. N. (1960). *J. Endocrin.*, **20**, 157.

FRANCHIMONT, P. (1966). *Ann. Endocr.*, **27**, 273.

FUKUSHIMA, M., STEVENS, V. G., GANNT, C. L. & VORYS, N. (1964). *J. Clin. Endocr. and Metab.*, **24**, 205.

FUTTERWEIT, W., MCNIVEN, M. L., GUERRA-GARCIA, R., GILBREE, N., DROSDOWSKY, M., SIEGEL, G. L., SOFFER, L. J., ROSENTHAL, I. M. & DORFMAN, R. I. (1964). *Steroids*, **4**, 137.

GARST, J. B., NYC, J. F., MARON, D. M. & FRIEDGOOD, H. B. (1950). *J. biol. Chem.*, **186**, 119.

GEMZELL, C. A., DICZFALUSY, E. & TILLINGER, K. G. (1958). *J. clin. Endocrin.*, **18**, 1333.

GIRARD, A. & SANDULESCO, G. (1936). *Helv. chim. Acta*, **19**, 1095.

GIVNER, M. L., BAULD, W. S. & VAGI, K. (1960). *Biochem. J.*, **77**, 406.

GOSS, D. A. & TAYMOR, M. L. (1962). *Endocrinol.*, **71**, 321.

GREENWOOD, F. C., HUNTER, W. M. & GLOVER, J. S. (1963). *Biochem. J.*, **89**, 114.

GREEP, R. O., VAN DYKE, H. B. & CHOW, B. F. (1942). *Endocrinol.*, **30**, 635.

HALES, C. N. & RANDLE, P. J. (1963). *Biochem. J.*, **88**, 137.

HARTREE, A. S., BUTT, W. R. & KIRKHAM, K. E. (1964). *J. Endocr.*, **29**, 61.

HASKINS, A. L. Jr. (1950). *Proc. Soc. exp. Biol., N.Y.*, **73**, 439.

HINSBERG, K., PELZER, H. & SEUKEN, A. (1956). *Biochem. Z.*, **328**, 117.

HOFFMANN, F. & V. LAM, L. (1941). *Zbl. Gynäk.*, **65**, 2014.

HOLTORFF, A. F. & KOCH, F. C. (1940). *J. biol. Chem.*, **135**, 377.

HOOKER, C. W. & FORBES, T. R. (1947). *Endocrinology*, **41**, 158.

HORTON, R. & TAIT, J. F. (1966). *Excerpta Med. Found. Int. Congr. Ser.*, **101**, 199.

HUDSON, B., COGHLAN, J., DULMANIS, A., WINTON, M. & EKKEL, I. (1963). *Aust. J. Exp. Biol. Med. Sci.*, **41**, 235.

ICHII, S., FORCHIELLI, E., PEARLOFF, W. H. & DORFMAN, R. I. (1963). *Anal. Biochem.*, **5**, 422.

IGARASHI, M. & MCCANN, S. M. (1964). *Endocrinol.*, **74**, 440.

INGIULLA, W., FORLEO, R. & GALLI, A. (1968) (in press). Research on Steroids, Vol. III, 259.

INGIULLA, W., FORLEO, R., GALLI, A. & SEVERI, S. (1968), "Gas Chromatogr. determ. of Hormonal Steroids", p. 183, Ed. Polvani. F., New York & London, Academic Press.

ITTRICH, G. (1958). *Hoppe-Seyles Z., physiol. Chem.*, **312**, 1.

JAYLE, M. F. & CREPY, O. (1950). *Bull. soc. chim. biol. Paris*, **32**, 1067.

JAYLE, M. F., CREPY, O. & JUDAS, O. (1943). *Bull. soc. chim. biol. Paris.*, **25**, 301.

JOHNSEN, S. G. (1955). *Acta endocr. Kbh.*, **20**, 101 and 106.

JOHNSEN, S. G. (1958). *Acta endocr. Kbh.*, **28**, 69.

JOHNSEN, S. G. (1959). *Acta endocr. Kbh.*, **31**, 209.

KELLIE, A. E. & WADE, A. P. (1955). *Biochem. J.*, **62**, 1P.

KLINEFELTER, H. F. Jr., ALBRIGHT, F. & GRISWOLD, G. C. (1943). *J. clin. Endocrin.*, **3**, 529.

KLOPPER, A., MICHIE, E. A. & BROWN, J. B. (1955). *J. Endocrin.*, **12**, 209.

KOBER, S. (1931). *Biochem. Z.*, **239**, 209.

KORENMAN, S. G., WILSON, H. & LIPSETT, M. B. (1964). *J. biol. Chem.*, **239**, 1004.

LAKSHMANAN, T. K. & LIEBERMAN, S. (1954). *Arch. Biochem.*, **53**, 258.

LI, C. H. (1958). *Proc. Soc. exp. Biol., N.Y.*, **98**, 839.

LI, C. H., SIMPSON, M. E. & EVANS, H. M. (1949). *Science*, **109**, 445.

LOBOTSKY, J., WYSS, H. I., SEGRE, E. J. & LLOYD, C. W. (1964). *J. Clin. Endocr. and Metab.*, **24**, 1261.

LORAINE, J. A. & BROWN, J. B. (1956). *J. Clin. Endocr. and Metab.*, **16**, 1180.

LUUKKAINEN, T. & ALDERCREUTZ, H. (1967). *Ann. Med. exp. Fenn.*, **45**, 264.

MCARTHUR, J. W. (1952). *Endocrinology*, **50**, 304.

McArthur, J. W., Antoniades, H. N., Larson, L. H., Pennell, R. B., Ingersoll, F. M. & Ulfelder, H. (1964). *J. Clin. Endocr.*, **24**, 425.

Mason, H. L. & Engstrom, W. W. (1950). *Physiol. Rev.*, **30**, 321.

Mason, H. L. & Kepler, E. J. (1945). *J. biol. Chem.*, **161**, 235.

Mather, A. (1942). *J. biol. Chem.*, **144**, 617.

Medical Research Council (1951). *Lancet*, **2**, 585.

Molen, H. van der & Aakwaag, A. (1967). "Hormones in Blood", Vol. II, p. 221, Ed., Grays C. H., & Bacharach A. L., London, Academic Press.

Molen, H. van der & Groen, D. (1965). *J. Clin. Endocr. and Metab.*, **25**, 1625.

Molen, H. van der, Groen, D. & Peterse, A. (1966). *Excerpta Med. Found. Int. Congr. Ser.*, **101**, 1.

Nicola, A. F. da, Dorfman, R. I. & Forchielli, E. (1966). *Steroids*, **7**, 351.

O'Donnell, V. J. & Preedy, J. R. K. (1967). "Hormones in Blood", Vol. II, p. 109, Ed., Gray C. H., & Bacharach A. L., London and New York, Academic Press.

Oertel, G. W. & Eik-Nes, K. B. (1960). *Arch. Biochem. Biophys.*, **86**, 144.

Parlow, A. F. (1961). "Human Pituitary Gonadotropins", p. 300, Ed. Albert A., Springfield, Illinois, C. C. Thomas.

Parlow, A. F., Condliffe, P. G., Reichert, L. E. & Wilhelmi, A. E. (1965). *Endocrinol.*, **76**, 27.

Pickett, M. T. & Kellie, A. E. (1962). *Acta endocr. Kbh.*, **41**, 129.

Pickett, M. T., Kyriakides, E. C., Stern, M. I. & Sommerville, I. F. (1959). *Lancet*, **2**, 829.

Pickett, M. T. & Sommerville, I. F. (1962). *Acta endocr. Kbh.*, **41**, 135.

Preddy, J. R. K. & Aitken, E. H. (1961). *J. biol. Chem.*, **236**, 1300.

Riondel, A., Tait, J. F., Gut, M., Tait, S. A. S., Joachim, E. & Little, B. (1963). *J. Clin. Endocr. and Metab.*, **23**, 620.

Riondel, A., Tait, J. F., Tait, S. A. S., Gut, M. & Little, B. (1965). *J. Clin. Endocr. and. Metab.*, **25**, 229.

Rizkallah, T., Taymor, M. L., Park, M. & Batt, R. V. (1965). *J. Clin. Endocr. and Metab.*, **25**, 943.

Robbie, W. A. & Gibson, R. B. (1943). *J. clin. Endocrin.*, **3**, 200.

Rocca, D. & Albert, A. (1967). *Mayo Clin. Proc.*, **42**, 536.

Roos, P. & Gemzell, C. A. (1964). *Biochim. Biophys. Acta*, **82**, 218.

Roy, E. J., Harkness, R. A. & Kerr, M. G. (1965). *J. Endocr.*, **31**, 177.

Ryan, K. J. (1959). *J. biol. Chem.*, **234**, 268.

Salhanick, H. A., Noall, M. W., Zarrow, M. X. & Samuels, L. T. (1952). *Science*, **115**, 708.

Saxena, R. B., Demura, H., Gandy, H. M. & Peterson, R. E. (1967). *J. Clin. Endocr. and Metab.*, **28**, 519.

Schubert, K. & Wehrberger, K. (1960). *Naturwissenschaften*, **47**, 281.

Scott, L. D. (1940). *Brit. J. exp. Path.*, **21**, 320.

Sheerin, B. M. & Sommerville, I. F. (1968) "Gas Chromatogr. Determ. of Hormonal Steroids", p. 278, Ed. Polvani, F. New York and London, Academic Press.

Short, R. V. (1958). *J. Endocrin.*, **16**, 415.

Short, R. V. (1960). *J. Endocrin.*, **20**, xv.

Slaunwhite, W. R. & Neely, L. (1963). *Anal. Biochem.*, **5**, 137.

Sommerville, I. F. (1952). *Proc. Roy. Soc. Med.*, **45**, 807.

Sommerville, I. F. (1957). *J. clin. Endocrin.*, **17**, 317.

Sommerville, I. F. (1965). "Gas Chromatography o Steroids in Biol. Fluids", p. 53, Ed. Lipsett, M. B. New York, Plenum Press.

Sommerville, I. F. & Collins, W. P. (1965). *Steroids*, Suppl. II, 22.

Sommerville, I. F., Collins, W. P. & Wyman, H. (1968) (in press). "Gas Chromatogr. Determ. of Hormonal Steroids", p. 85, Ed. Polvani, F., New York and London, Academic Press.

Sommerville, I. F. & Deshpande, G. N. (1958). *J. clin. Endocrin.*, **18**, 1223.

Sommerville, I. F., Fernandez, G. E., Marocchi, A. & Sharples, M. J. (1968b), Research on Steroids, Vol. III, 185.

Sommerville, I. F., Pickett, M. T., Collins, W. C. & Denyer, D. C. (1963). *Acta Endocr. Kbh.*, **43**, 101.

Sparagana, M. (1965). *Steroids*, **5**, 773.

Steelman, S. L. & Pohley, F. M. (1953). *Endocrinology*, **53**, 604.

Steelman, S. L. & Segaloff, A. (1959). *Rec. Prog. Horm. Research*, **15**, 115.

Steelman, S. L., Segaloff, A. & Andersen, R. N. (1959). *Proc. Soc. exp. Biol. N.Y.*, **101**, 452.

Stern, M. I. (1957). *J. Endocrin.*, **16**, 180.

Stern, M. I. & Barwell, J. O. H. (1963). *J. Endocrin.*, **27**, 87.

Stevenson, M. F. & Marrian, G. F. (1947). *Biochem. J.*, **41**, 507.

Stimmel, B. F. (1946). *J. biol. Chem.*, **162**, 99.

Svendsen, R. (1960). *Acta Endocrin.*, **35**, 161.

Svendsen, R. & Sorensen, B. (1964). *Acta Endocrin.*, **47**, 245.

Szego, C. M. & Roberts, S. (1946). *Proc. Soc. exp. Biol. N.Y.*, **61**, 161.

Tait, J. F. & Horton, R. (1966). "Steroid Dynamics", p. 396, Eds. Pincus, G., Nakaa, T., and Tait, J. F., New York and London, Academic Press.

Talbot, N. B., Berman, R. A., MacLachlan, E. A. & Wolfe, J. K. (1941). *J. clin. Endocrin.*, **1**, 668.

Thijssen, J. H. H. & Zander, J. (1966). *J. Acta Endocr. (Copenh.)*, **51**, 563.

Vermeulen, A. (1966). *Excerpta Med. Found. Int. Congr. Ser.*, **101**, 71.

Vermeulen, A. & Verplancke, J. C. M. (1963). *Steroids*, **2**, 453.

Wide, L. & Gemzell, C. A. (1960). *Acta endocr. Kbh.*, **35**, 261.

Wide, L., Roos, P. & Gemzell, C. A. (1961). *Acta Endocr.*, **37**, 445.

WILDE, C. E., ORR, A. H. & BAGSHAWE, K. D. (1967). *J. Endocr.*, **37**, 23.

WILSON, H., LIPSETT, M. R. & RYAN, D. W. (1961). *J. clin. Endocrin.*, **21**, 1304.

WISWELL, J. G. & SAMUELS, L. T. (1951). *Amer. J. med.*, **10**, 788.

WOODS, M. C. & SIMPSON, M. E. (1960). *Endocrinology*, **66**, 575.

WOOLEVER, C. A. & GOLDFEIN, A. (1963). *Int. J. appl. Radiat. Isotopes*, **14**, 163.

WOTIZ, H. H. (1963). *Biochim. Biophys. Acta*, **69**, 415.

WOTIZ, H. H., CHARRANSOL, G. & SMITH, I. N. (1967). *Steroids*, **10**, 127.

WOTIZ, H. H. & CHATTORAJ, S. C. (1964). *Analyt. Chem.*, **36**, 1466.

WYMAN, H. & SOMMERVILLE, I. F. (1966). *Excerpta Med. Found. Int. Congr. Ser.*, **111**, 200.

WYMAN, H. & SOMMERVILLE, I. F. (1968). *Steroids*, **12**, 63.

ZANDER, J. (1954). *Nature*, **174**, 406.

ZANDER, J., FORBES, T. R., MÜNSTERMANN, A. M. VON & NEHER, R. (1958). *J. clin. Endocrin.*, **18**, 337.

ZANDER, J. & MÜNSTERMANN, A. M. VON (1954). *Klin. Wschr.*, **32**, 894.

ZANDER, J. & MÜNSTERMANN, A. M. VON (1956). *Klin. Wschr.*, **34**, 494.

ZANDER, J. & SIMMER, H. (1954). *Klin. Wschr.*, **32**, 529.

ZIMMERMANN, W. (1935). *Z. physiol. Chem.*, **233**, 257.

Chapter 24

THE BIOCHEMISTRY OF NEOPLASTIC DISEASE

by

A. E. KELLIE

The Courtauld Institute of Biochemistry, The Middlesex Hospital Medical School, London, W.1

INTRODUCTION

UNLIKE many contributions to the present volume, this chapter does not deal with a metabolic lesion occurring in one anatomical system or organ, but with a fundamental aberration of growth which may arise in any growing tissue at any time. Cancerous growth is essentially a disease of multicellular organisms and in so far as growth, whether normal or neoplastic, is achieved by repeated cell division and cell enlargement, one approach to the study of the disease is the study of cell development and of the factors initiating and controlling it. Many readers, trained in the older disciplines, may question the justification of treating neoplastic disease as a biochemical disorder because of its complexity and because of our present ignorance of many aspects of cell division in higher animals, yet few would deny that ultimately the process must be capable of being expressed at cellular level in terms of cell biochemistry.

Any departure from normal cell division may not be immediately obvious, but once the abnormality is initiated it can perpetuate itself by transference in subsequent cell divisions until the so-called neoplastic tissue becomes a palpable mass. It is in this form that cancer is often encountered in the ward and the history of medicine suggests that at this stage attempts to reverse the process are rarely successful; in a broad sense, the efforts of the surgeon, physician and radiotherapist are concentrated on preventing the spread of the neoplasm by finding a selective means of destroying the abnormal growth without adversely affecting healthy cells and vital organs. Failure to control neoplastic growth at this advanced stage may be simply because, by the time the growth is manifest, the initial cellular event which began the abnormality may be remote and therefore irreversible.

THE CELL AT THE MICROSCOPIC LEVEL

Units of the Cell

Even at the level of the light microscope it is clear that the cell is not just a random collection of molecules in a transparent bag but a highly organized structure with physical compartments and subcellular particles. The higher resolution of the electron microscope reveals that the intricate organization extends to a fine structure approaching macromolecular dimensions (Bessis, 1960). In addition to the nucleus, the cytoplasm contains discrete bodies including the centrosome, mitochondria, smooth and rough endoplasmic reticulum, ribosomes, lysosomes, etc. Fairly recent developments in technique, notably in high speed centrifugation against a density gradient, have made it possible to separate these organelles from each other for individual study.

The *nucleus* has for many decades been regarded as the organizational centre of the cell. Under high power it is clearly separated from the cytoplasm by the nuclear membrane, but there is also microscopical evidence of a second membrane of cytoplasmic origin and a so-called perinuclear space between the two layers which may be in contact with the vacuolar space of the endoplasmic reticulum. In some regions these two layers are in contact with each other and the double layer is perforated by circular holes or "pores" which open and close and which may give access to the cytoplasm.

Within the *cytoplasm*, the *centrosome* (Golgi

bodies and centriole) frequently occupies a central position as befits the prominent role which this region of the cell plays in cell division. The *mitochondria*, 1–5 μ in length and shaped irregularly (like groundnuts) are surrounded by a double membrane 100–200 Å in thickness. This membrane projects into the interior of the mitochondria as a series of baffles, or *cristae*. These bodies contain protein and fat and are rich in the enzymes of the citric acid cycle; they are the sites of oxidative phosphorylation within the cell and as such they supply the energy for intermediate metabolism. The *endoplasmic reticulum* is a network of canaliculi or flattened vacuoles bounded by a membrane 50 Å thick. In some cells, these vacuoles may open to the cell surface or to the perinuclear space and they appear to form a vacuolar network varying in shape and length, which converts the cytoplasm into a sponge-like medium. In some areas the reticulum carries a large number of *ribosomes* (rough endoplasmic reticulum) which are attached to the cytoplasmic surface of the boundary membrane, and these bodies synthesize the specific proteins of the species. The protein appears to form in the lumina of the vacuolar spaces before transmission to other parts of the cell; this kind of reticulum is most prolific in cells which secrete large amounts of proteins and it may account for more than three-quarters of the cell space. Free ribosomes are found in the cytoplasm of some cells, but they are not necessarily functional in this form.

Cell Division

Cells can only be formed from other cells by the process of cell division. At the level of the light microscope, cell division (mitosis) is seen as a complex and organized procedure which may be observed in all growing tissues and which goes through the same fundamental stages of prophase, metaphase, anaphase, telophase and interphase, irrespective of the species or the site of growth. This is a basic process for all forms of life.

As might be expected, the nucleus plays a prominent part in preparing the cell for subdivision. One of the earliest and most significant events within the nucleus is the duplication of the chromosomes whereby two chromosome strands (chromatids) identical with that of the parent cell are produced. Duplication occurs during the late interphase but is incomplete as the chromatids remain attached to a central point of each chromosome, the centromere. The formation of the cell spindle and the organization of the centromeres with the attached chromatids at the equatorial plane of the spindle appears to be under the control of the centrosome. These changes occur during the metaphase which is terminated by the subdivision of the centromeres and the physical separation of the daughter cell chromosomes. Only when these processes are complete does division of the cytoplasm occur, followed by separation of the daughter cells.

When germ cells are being created the process of cell division takes a different form (meiosis). A parental cell (diploid state) undergoes two stages of cell division resulting in the formation of four germ cells with the modification that during the second division the chromosomes fuse and are reduced to half the normal number (haploid state). Subsequent fusion of male and female germ cells (gametes) restores the diploid state (zygote) and normal mitosis follows. In the late nineteenth century, geneticists noted that genes which controlled the inheritance of recognizable characteristics appeared to be physically associated with certain chromosomes at cell division. Genes which controlled recognizable traits, when present on the same chromosome, appeared to be inherited together; genes located on different chromosomes were frequently inherited in an independent manner. This pointer to the storage of genetic information in the genes resident on the chromosomes was widely recognized many years before its biochemical significance was understood.

Multicellular organisms arise by fusion of two haploid gametes and all cell growth results from the subsequent mitotic cell division of the diploid zygote. The changes whereby the unicellular zygote is converted into the metazoan adult are numerous and complex but are all fundamentally based on cell division. As growth to adult form is manifestly not a chance event, it is clear that the information which initiates and directs subsequent growth must be recorded in the single cell of the fertile ovum. Genetic information of similar complexity must be stored in the gamete which produces the next generation, and although proof is lacking, there are many indications that most, if not all somatic cells, have a record of the genetic complement of the species. Knowledge of the form in which this information is stored and of its transmission to daughter cells at division are clearly important aspects of the growth process.

Cell Growth

Microscopy throws little light on the mechanism of cell enlargement. In unicellular organisms enlargement of the cell reaches a point where cell division occurs and the identical daughter cells separate from each other and repeat the life history of the parent cell. The situation with

multicellular organisms is much more complex, and although growth does occur by repeated cell division, this alone cannot explain the complexity found in the adult form. Whereas the daughter cells of unicellular organisms are identical with the parent cell and with each other, this is not true of metazoan growth patterns. As growth proceeds through the embryological, foetal and juvenile stages there is a chronological change in the expression of the genetic message which differentiates the cells to carry out special functions and which organizes the formation of body organs.

THE CELL AT THE MOLECULAR LEVEL

Units of the Cell

A cell which reproduces two daughter cells, which in turn grow to maturity, must of necessity duplicate all cell constituents. At division, the contents of the parent cell may be shared so that each progeny contains all essential molecules, but growth requires that each shall increase in size and content. Because of the complexity of the process it is convenient to consider this problem in separate stages dividing the cell contents into the micro-molecules (Mol. Wt. $\ngtr$ 1000), responsible for energy requirements and intermediate metabolism, and the macro-molecules (Mol. Wt. 10^3–10^7) representing mainly the enzyme complement of the cell and its store of genetic information.

Micro-molecules as sources of energy, No viable cell can continue to exist without a source of energy. Animal cells which lack chloroplasts and therefore the ability to use solar energy directly, obtain the necessary energy by degrading more complex molecules in their food, releasing the stored energy of the covalent carbon to carbon bonds. The combustion is not accomplished directly by molecular oxygen but indirectly by the transfer of hydrogen along a chain of substrates and respiratory ferments. The release of energy is associated with this step-wise breakdown, being released at stages of the process, not as heat but as cellular energy stored in various forms as the so-called high energy bonds of phosphate esters. A most important store of this kind is achieved in the conversion of adenosine diphosphate to adenosine triphosphate which in turn supplies the energy for innumerable synthetic reactions within the cell. The salient features of this process, when glucose is the source of energy, may be followed in the steps of the Embden-Meyerhof transformation of glucose to pyruvic acid, and in the further oxidation of pyruvate to CO_2 and H_2O in the citric acid cycle (Baldwin, 1963; Mahler & Cordes, 1966). The stored energy is available for many kinds of work which must be performed within the cell, but undoubtedly, one of its principal functions is to promote the synthesis of both micro- and macro-molecules essential for cell growth.

Micro-molecules as sources of building units. Complex molecules of food not only supply the energy for cell growth but also the small carbon units which the cell must have in order to synthesize practically every molecule, irrespective of size, within the cell. A few molecules, e.g. the essential amino-acids and the vitamins, cannot be formed by some higher animals and these must be present in the diet; ancillary requirements of nitrogen, phosphorus, sulphur and other essential elements must also be obtained from extracellular sources. The pathways whereby cells are able to synthesize the essential structures required for life have been worked out in considerable detail and these are described in texts dealing with intermediary metabolism. Among the small units synthesized in this way are the building "bricks" of two important classes of macro-molecules, namely the amino-acids essential for protein formation and the sub-units of the nucleic acids, pentose sugars and the purine and pyrimidine bases.

Even in the presence of ample food supply and an adequate store of cellular energy, the cell is unable to break down complex food molecules without the catalytic effect of innumerable enzymes. These macro-molecules, which are predominantly protein in nature, catalyse each stage of the breakdown of energy-rich foodstuffs and each stage of the synthesis of the complex assembly of micro- and macro-molecules characteristic of the species. They play a predominant role in the cell for they are essential for the synthesis of all cell components including the proteins of which they are themselves composed. The type of enzymes synthesized controls the nature and behaviour of the cell.

The macro-molecules. The simplest macro-molecule of the animal cell is glycogen (Mol. Wt. ~ 1,000,000) which is formed enzymically from glucose units in the presence of uridine-5-triphosphate. It is a simple polymer which acts as a store of glucose and has no other functional role. Only four enzymes are necessary for the conversion of glucose into glycogen, an arrangement which requires little genetic information.

The structure of proteins. By comparison with glycogen, the proteins are macro-molecules of great complexity and specificity. Unlike the polysaccharides, they are not polymers of a single sub-

unit, but long chains of different amino-acids joined by repeated peptide bonds

$$—CO—CH—\underset{\underset{R_1}{|}}{NH}—CO—\underset{\underset{}{}}{CH}\overset{\overset{R_2}{|}}{}—NH—CO—\underset{\underset{R_3}{|}}{CH}—$$

In this linear form high molecular weights can be built up and as there are some 20 different amino-acids in animal protein the permutations of this primary structure are enormous; further increase in molecular complexity arises, as in insulin, from cross-linkage between adjacent strands. The three-dimensional structure of proteins imposed by specific binding and cross-linkage of the primary polypeptide chains endows each different protein with a unique but not necessarily stable form. The contours and crevices of the surface of the molecules are thought to provide the basis of the specificity of proteins, and of enzyme-substrate interrelationship. On the basis of stereochemical considerations, Pauling & Corey (1951) suggested that some long chain polypeptides may achieve stability by adopting a helical configuration and experimental support for this idea was provided by X-ray crystallographic studies carried out on myoglobin and haemoglobin (Kendrew, Dickerson, Strandberg, Hart, Davies, Phillips & Shore, 1960; Perrutz, 1962). The structure of several proteins and enzymes has been established showing some regions of the polypeptide chain in the form of an α-helix and others in unique folds stabilized by cross-linkage (Phillips, 1968). In the case of the enzyme lysozyme, which attacks bacterial cell walls, not only has the 3-dimensional structure of the enzyme been established but it has been shown that it is uniquely shaped to receive in a crevice of the molecule a hexose saccharide unit which is repeated as a polysaccharide structure in the bacterial cell wall. Proposals have been made for a possible mechanism of action of the enzyme at the molecular level (Blake, Mair, North, Phillips & Sarma, 1967).

All living cells are able to synthesize proteins and enzymes of many kinds, but the particular kind of protein which they do synthesize is dictated by the structure of a second important class of macro-molecules—the nucleic acids.

The structure of nucleic acids. The name nucleic acid is a misnomer which arose because the earliest sources of this class of compound were almost exclusively the nuclei of cells. It is now recognized that two distinct groups of nucleic acids exist; the deoxyribonucleic acids (DNA) and the ribonucleic acids (RNA). The DNA, which are almost entirely confined to the nuclei of mammalian cells,* are linear polymers of four different nucleotides (phosphate-deoxyribose-base). The polymeric link is formed between the phosphate residue and the deoxyribose unit of successive nucleotides forming a backbone structure in which the bases play no part

```
        /
  phosphate
        \
          deoxyribose—Base₁
        /
  phosphate
        \
          deoxyribose—Base₂
        /
  phosphate
        \
```

Linear polymers of very high molecular weight are formed in which the bases, adenine (A), guanine (G), thymine (T) and cytosine (C) stick out at right angles from the backbone, but whereas the backbone structure is very regular (—phosphate—deoxyribose—phosphate—deoxyribose—) the arrangement of the four bases is very irregular and provides the basis of the transfer of genetic information during cell division. It has been established that the stable DNA molecules of higher organisms exist as two polymeric chains twisting about each other as a regular double helix in which the purine (A & G) and pyrimidine (T & C) bases in opposite chains hydrogen-bond together to stabilize the macromolecule. The structure of one chain dictates that of the other as adenine will only bond with thymine (A—T) and guanine only with cytosine (G—C) (Fig. 24·1). The DNA molecule, therefore, resembles a very long twisted ladder in which the long elements are composed of alternating deoxyribose-phosphate units and the rungs of paired, complementary purine and pyrimidine bases. A consequence of this structure is that the ratios A:T and G:C in a DNA molecule must always be unity, whereas the ratio A+T: G+C in different DNA molecules varies widely.

Ribonucleic acids (RNA) are similar in structure to DNA in that they consist of linear polymers of four nucleotides, but they differ in two important respects. In the first place, the pentose sugar of these macromolecules is ribose, which differs from deoxyribose in having an additional hydroxyl group. The second distinctive feature of RNA molecules is that they contain the base uracil (U) in place of the closely related pyrimidine, thymine (T). These differences do not pre-

vent RNA molecules from forming a double helix with a single strand of DNA provided the convention that A pairs with U and G pairs with C is met, but RNA-DNA twin helices do not survive long in *in vivo* conditions. Whereas DNA molecules are very stable in the double helix form, RNA molecules usually exist and function as a single linear strand. The three-dimensional form of these structures is not known. In the growth process

Nucleotides

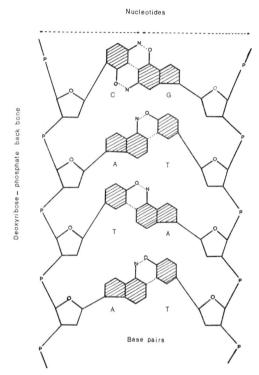

FIG. 24.1. Structure of a fragment of deoxyribonucleic acid molecule, showing deoxyribose-phosphate "backbone" and base-pairing of adenine (A)—guanine (G) and thymine (T)—cytosine (C)

of all cells three different types of RNA are encountered: ribosomal RNA (r-RNA), messenger RNA (m-RNA) and soluble or transport RNA (t-RNA); although all are synthesized in the nucleus in the presence of DNA they are usually found in the cytoplasm.

The Nature of the Genetic Material

Evidence of the identity of the genetic material, genes and chromosomes, with nucleic acid structures, is inferential but cumulative. In the case of simple virus particles, e.g. virus T4 which infects

---

* Traces of DNA have recently been found in mitochondria.

the bacterium *E. coli*, the invading parasite consists of a low molecular weight DNA double helix surrounded by a protective protein coat. When a cell is infected, *only the DNA strand enters the cell*, but once inside it uses the organized structures within the host cell to replicate the DNA material; the many reproduced strands not only code for the synthesis of the protective protein of the coat but they utilize the rough endoplasmic reticulum of the invaded cells for this synthesis. When the cell is destroyed and ruptured (lysed) it liberates many virus particles identical with the original virus. In more highly organized viable cells the genetic material is more complex: e.g. in *E. Coli*, approximately 100 genes out of a total of more than 1000 have been located on the circular DNA chromatin and recognized in terms of their contributions to the intermediary metabolism of the cell. With many approximations it has been calculated that the average gene is a linear polymer of 1000–1500 nucleotide pairs and as most bacteria must have several hundred, if not thousand, genes, the length and complexity of the DNA genetic strand must be very considerable.

The paramount role of the nucleus in directing the development of a cell in higher organisms is indicated by nuclear transplantation experiments in which nuclei from cells of a renal tumour of the frog were transplanted into de-nucleated frog oocytes, whereby growth of the synthetic cell was supported up to the tadpole stage (King & McKinnell, 1960; McKinnel, 1962). Similar experiments have also been carried out transplanting nuclei from normal cells of the intestinal epithelium into de-nucleated oocytes, sustaining growth to the adult, fertile toad (Gurdon, 1962; Gurdon & Uehlinger, 1966).

The Genetic Code

Undoubtedly one of the most important functions carried out by DNA is the direction of the synthesis of proteins and enzymes by the growing cell. DNA plays no direct part in this process, but nevertheless carries the necessary information concealed in its molecular structure. The deoxyribose-phosphate backbone is repetitive and can carry no specific information but it has been established that the instruction is recorded in the sequence of bases assembled on the linear DNA chain. The choice of nucleotide for any position is limited to the four alternatives which carry the bases A, G, C or T and hence, in a strand of "n" nucleotides, the possible permutations are 4^n. If one accepts as an approximation that a gene is composed of 1500 base pairs, the number of

permutations in this small DNA molecule reaches the enormous total of 4^{1500}, enough to permit an almost infinite variety of structural information.

Although DNA in the nucleus plays no direct part in protein synthesis, but transmits the necessary information to the ribosomes by relatively short lengths of specific m-RNA, it has been established that the order of bases in the DNA dictates the order of amino-acid selection at the remote site of protein synthesis. The DNA is read as a three-unit code; thus the sequence U—U—U in RNA codes for phenylalanine in the polypeptide chain, U—C—U codes for serine, G—U—U for valine and an RNA sequence of U—U—U—U—C—U—G—U—U will organize the synthesis of the tripeptide phenylalanine-serine-valine. In such a code the selection of four possible nucleotides for three adjacent positions is possible in $4^3(64)$ ways, more than sufficient to select the 20-odd amino-acids found in animal protein. In support of the hypothesis that the basic biochemical reactions of all cells are similar, it is of interest that the ribosomes of many types of cells interpret this basic code in precisely the same way.

Cell Division

For our present knowledge of the biochemistry of cell division we are greatly dependent on recent progress in the fields of virology and bacteriology; indeed, more is known about the reproduction of the bacterium *E. coli* than about any other cell division. Unfortunately we have little knowledge of the process of cell division in higher organisms and information available cannot be extended uncritically to multicellular organisms. According to contemporary belief, the basic biochemistry of cell growth and division is similar in all cells irrespective of whether they relate to the reproduction of a unicellular organism or to the growth of tissue in a higher animal. In the course of centuries of evolutionary change, it is not unlikely that many basic cellular processes have remained unchanged and indeed there is considerable experimental support for this belief. There is no evidence of the participation of a "vital force"; indeed there is great similarity in the intermediate metabolism of all cells and all the known biochemical reactions within cells obey the established laws of chemistry.

"Replication" of the chromosomal DNA. During the interphase stage of cell division the chromosomes duplicate themselves. The complementary structure of the twin DNA helix immediately suggests a means whereby the linear strands can be reproduced prior to cell division (Watson,

1965). Under suitable conditions, which include the presence of all four nucleotides found in DNA, a specific enzyme, deoxyribonucleic acid polymerase, and adenosine triphosphate, the twin strands of the DNA helix disengage and as they do so the exposed base pairs act as templates for the assembly of the corresponding nucleotides, according to the convention that an exposed adenine base will attract only a free thymine nucleotide and a guanine will anchor only a free cytosine nucleotide and vice versa (Fig. 24·2). As each

Cell Growth

After cell division, each daughter cell will have, in addition to the DNA record of information, a share of the components of the parent cell. Some of the compounds inherited will be fairly stable, but others will have a short biological life and will have to be replaced by further cell activity; it is almost certain that such activity will depend on the presence of many enzymes which themselves may have a limited life. The new cell must be able to adapt itself to changing internal and external

Parent DNA

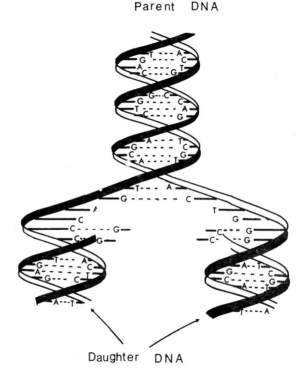

FIG. 24.2. Replication of chromosomal deoxyribonucleic acid; untwisting of parent DNA twin helix and formation of daughter helices by assembly of nucleotides by base pairing.

Daughter DNA

nucleotide in turn takes up its position on the template, the polymerase assembles the backbone of the new strands, linking adjacent units by means of a covalent ribose-phosphate bond. When this process is complete the positive strand "+" of the parent DNA has produced a new negative "−" strand, while the parent "−" strand has produced a new "+" strand, and the net result is the duplication of the entire DNA molecule. Experimental evidence suggests that the synthesis of the new strands proceeds in this way as the parent DNA untwines, and that the energy is supplied by the high energy bonds of adenosine triphosphate.

conditions and for this purpose requires a dynamic and therefore flexible system of development. Such a system would exist if cell components, especially enzymes, had a limited life but were continuously reproduced. This type of dynamic metabolism, which is thought to exist in all viable cells, lays great stress on the continuous formation of enzymes (proteins) within the cell.

"*Transcription*" *of DNA-dependent RNA.* Although DNA is confined to the nucleus of the cell, most protein synthesis occurs in the cytoplasm; "pulse-labelling" of amino-acids shows clearly that the newly formed polypeptide chain is associated with the cytoplasmic ribosomes which are rich in RNA. The RNA molecules can only be formed in the presence of DNA and are therefore formed in the nucleus and transported, with associated protein, from the nucleus to the endoplasmic reticulum. The formation of RNA ("transcription") resembles that of DNA (replication) in that both occur on an exposed DNA strand acting as an assembly template, but with the difference that in the formation of RNA, the pentose involved is ribose, and uracil mononucleotide (and not thymine) pairs with adenine. It is not known what factors determine whether an exposed DNA strand will act as a template for the replication of DNA or the transcription of RNA; both require the presence of a partially untwisted DNA helix although somewhat unexpectedly in the formation of RNA only one strand of the DNA is copied. Both processes require the presence of the correct nucleotide triphosphates and the correct polymerizing enzyme, DNA polymerase or RNA polymerase, to link up the assembled nucleotides; these enzymes are not interchangeable and the course of synthesis may be directed by the presence or absence of either enzyme.

The base ratios $A+U : G+C$ of synthesized RNA molecules are the same as those of the DNA strand $(A+T : G+C)$ on which they have been assembled but, unlike the DNA twin helix, the A:U and G:C ratios of the RNA molecule are not 1:1. This unexpected structure is possible because, as the RNA strand forms, it disengages from the template and, unlike DNA, does not form a twin helix. Whereas the replication of the DNA involves the entire molecule, the transcription of RNA is confined to relatively short lengths of the DNA template, and it is considered that coding of the template contains start and stop signals recognized by the RNA polymerase. Of the three different kinds of RNA produced in the nucleus, r-RNA codes for the synthesis of ribosomal protein within the nucleus; m-RNA codes for the formation of all other protein produced by the cytoplasmic ribosomes; t-RNA plays a special role in the assembly of amino-acids for incorporation in polypeptides. Clearly the molecular size of RNA is much less than that of DNA; a simple virus may have a DNA molecular weight of 1×10^8 corresponding to 50 genes with an average molecular weight of 2.5 million and each gene will code for several enzymes. Indeed, a group of enzymes within the cell responsible for sequential stages of the synthesis of a metabolite requiring several enzymic steps are often coded together in a linear section of the DNA; such a sequence is called an *operon*.

"*Translation" of RNA. Protein synthesis.* Protein synthesis in the cytoplasm never occurs in solution but always on the surface of a ribosome and always in the presence of m-RNA which carries the code for the sequence of amino-acids to be assembled. Under the electron microscope, ribosomes appear to consist of two subunits, the larger particle (50S) has a molecular weight of $\sim 1.8 \times 10^6$ and the smaller (30S) is about half this size. Both particles contain protein and RNA, and it has been established that the process of protein synthesis is initiated by the formation of a complex between m-RNA and the smaller unit. During the enlargement of the polypeptide chain there is a cycle of events which seems to involve the separation and recombination of the two subunits (Schlessinger, Mangiarotti & Apirion, 1967).

The amino-acids for assembly do not come directly into contact with the m-RNA at the ribosomal surface but are activated and prepared for assembly by combination with specific receptor molecules (t-RNA) which recognize the base sequence of the m-RNA code. These t-RNA molecules, which are specific for individual amino-acids, are coded for on the DNA as linear polynucleotides containing approximately 80 units; all t-RNA molecules begin with the nucleotide guanine (G, 5'-end) and all end with the nucleotide sequence C—C—A (3'-end) and union with the enzyme-activated amino-acid always occurs with the ribose of the terminal adenine nucleotide. Throughout most of their length these amino-acid–t-RNA complexes are base-paired so that they adopt a clover-leaf form in which the linear elements (stalks) form helical spirals, but in the vicinity of the U-bends (Fig. 24·3) three adjacent unpaired nucleotides (the anti-codon) are free to bind on to the 3-unit codon on the m-RNA; thus the leucine-t-RNA complex has an unpaired nucleotide sequence A—A—C which binds to an U—U—G base sequence on the m-RNA polynucleotide strand, and once in position a polypeptidase enzyme links the leucine to the growing polypeptide chain (Fig. 24·4). In this indirect manner the genetic message carried from generation to generation by the nuclear DNA directs the growth pattern of all cells by dictating the types of enzymes and proteins to be synthesized.

The nucleotide sequence of yeast alanine t-RNA (77 units), which is one of several which have been worked out in detail, has been shown to include nine unusual nucleotides (other than those containing A, G, C or U); several of the unusual bases differ from normal bases in that they are methylated at one or more positions, and it has been established that in some cases the methylation occurs after the nucleotide has been incor-

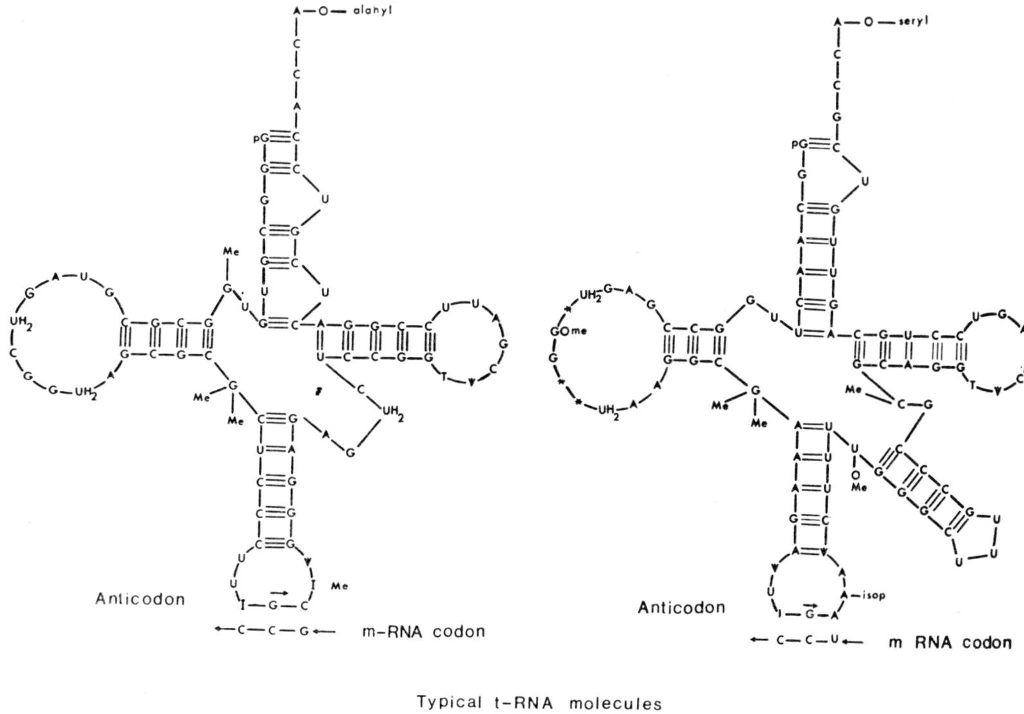

Typical t-RNA molecules

Fig. 24.3. Structure of typical transfer RNA (t-RNA) molecules.

porated in the t-RNA. These unusual bases are found in varying proportions in all t-RNA molecules so far analysed and their function is obscure, but one school of thought suggests that their presence near the anti-codon of t-RNA molecules may prevent base-pairing and thus expose the 3-unit code nucleotides. Recent analytical work has also revealed the presence of unusual bases in r-RNA; these include inosine, pseudo-uridine and dihydro-uracil as well as methylated derivatives of the common nucleosides. Methylation of these bases almost certainly occurs after the polymerization is complete and several specific DNA and RNA methylases have been described. It is noteworthy that a number of chemical carcinogens are able to methylate purine and pyrimidine bases of DNA and RNA molecules *in vivo*.

CELL GROWTH AND DEVELOPMENT

We have no precise knowledge of the factors which initiate the replication of the chromosomal DNA, a process which presages the formation of daughter cells. Thereafter, at the macromolecular level, growth can be seen as the integration of three basic processes, "replication" of DNA,

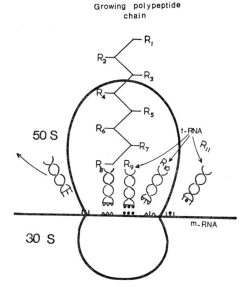

Fig. 24.4. Translation of messenger RNA (m-RNA) at ribosome. t-RNA represented symbolically in "twisted hairpin" form. R_1—R_{11}, etc., amino-acid residues.

27*

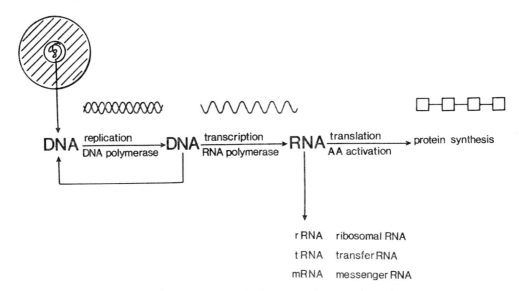

FIG. 24.5. Basic Dogma: Replication, transcription and translation.

"transcription" of DNA-dependent RNA and "translation" of the m-RNA into protein synthesis (Fig. 24.5). Provided each daughter cell has a replica of the parental DNA, a share of the enzyme complement of the parent cell and access to the same source of food supply, growth can continue in the new cells. When unicellular organisms are introduced into a nutrient solution there is an initial period (lag phase) pending the synthesis of essential metabolites, when reproduction and growth are restricted; this is followed by rapid reproduction (log phase) in which cell division and growth of successive generations proceed until either the food supplies are exhausted or it is no longer possible to maintain the composition of the environment because of accumulating by-products. At first sight, in this type of colony there is no control of growth; cells divide, the daughter cells are identical, they separate and each reproduces the life history of the parent cell.

Control of Growth in Unicellular Organisms

It is clear, however, even in "simple" unicellular organisms, that some control of the availability of genetic information is essential even if it is confined to the recognition of the type of food available or the sensing of accumulating by-products. It is considered that all of the genetic information is not continuously available but that selective mechanisms are present, according to the needs of the organism and the nature of the environment. Within newly formed cells some enzymes are required in much larger amounts than others; for example, as biosynthesis is impossible without energy, more priority must be given to the enzymes required for oxidative phosphorylation than to those responsible for the synthesis of stable catalytic co-factors. As the enzymes are proteins, these must represent a major proportion of new cell contents, and therefore the availability of amino-acids, purine and pyrimidine bases and pentose sugars must have high priority in the recently divided cell, although the requirement for some of these units may later decrease. The direction and control of protein synthesis is of paramount importance for it is this which ultimately decides the types of molecules produced by the cell. In unicellular organisms this control is exercised in a variety of ways, some coded for internally in the DNA chain and others dependent on external factors.

Operators, repressors and inducers. It has been previously indicated that where the synthesis of a cell molecule involves the consecutive action of a number of enzymes these are frequently coded for in an "operon", i.e. a length of DNA which is expressed by a single m-RNA carrier. In bacterial cells at least, the activity of many such operons is under regulation by repressor molecules, thought to be protein in nature, which are coded for by a DNA sequence in the neighbourhood of the operon. These repressor molecules indirectly control the availability of a portion of the genetic message; it was formerly thought that repressors might suppress the action of the operon by direct combination with the pertinent segment of the DNA, but this is now considered improbable. It has been shown that the functioning of an operon is directly controlled by an operator located in the DNA immediately adjacent to the operon; the nature of the operator is still uncertain, but it could be a start signal or a device for opening the twin DNA helices at the pertinent point.

Repressors may be present at all times but are not always functional, since if they were they would always suppress the functioning of the operon, but they can be influenced by small molecules which enter or accumulate in the cell. Molecules which inactivate the repressor and permit the synthesis of proteins or enzymes are the so-called inducers, whereas those which convert an inactive into an active repressor are called co-repressors. Such inducer and co-repressor compounds can markedly influence the type of protein synthesized by the cell; thus, the presence of the disaccharide lactose in the nutrient broth of bacteria may inactivate the repressor controlling the synthesis of β-galactosidase, an enzyme necessary for the hydrolysis of lactose. In an analogous manner the presence of excessive amounts of an individual amino-acid acting as a co-repressor may convert an inactive repressor into an active one, and thus suppress the synthesis of enzymes uniquely associated with the biosynthesis of the amino-acid in question.

It is not certain at which point the suppression of information occurs, for although the above account suggests that the transcription of DNA information is hindered in the nucleus other possibilities exist. The rate of synthesis of protein at the translational stage, m-RNA → protein, may be inhibited by interaction between the repressor and m-RNA in a manner which prevents the latter from becoming attached to the ribosomes. Alternatively, the repressor may only delay attachment so that the effective life of the m-RNA is reduced. In bacteria, the response to added inducers of co-repressors is very prompt, causing a fall in the amount of the corresponding m-RNA; this could be interpreted as support for the suppression of transcription but as the average life of m-RNA in bacterial cells at 37° is 1–6 min. the evidence does not exclude the possibility of increased destruction of m-RNA.

Code degeneracy, mis-sense and nonsense. The coding for the selection of amino-acids in the translation stage of growth (m-RNA → proteins) is not rigid, in the sense that many amino-acids are selected by more than one trinucleotide group (codon); thus phenylalanine is selected by t-RNA molecules carrying both sequences U—U—U and U—U—C, and serine by U—C—U and U—C—C. Because of this the code is said to be degenerate and although at present it appears that degeneracy involves the change of only one of the three codon nucleotides the universality of this arrangement has not yet been established. Errors in replication or transcription will produce an abnormal sequence of bases which results in the selection of wrong amino-acids (mis-sense); the replacement of one nucleotide for another could result in the normal protein being synthesized (because of degeneracy), but is more likely to result in the synthesis of a protein abnormal in the sense of one or two amino-acids (mis-sense). Such abnormal proteins may show some of the biological activity of the normal protein. Not all 64 codons, however, select amino-acids and there are clear indications of sequences, e.g. U—A—A and U—A—G (nonsense codons) which stop the reading of the m-RNA message and cause termination and detachment of the polypeptide chain. Thus it is clear that replacement of individual nucleotides in the sequence may cause either mis-sense or nonsense combinations, but because of degeneracy the former is more likely. The replacement of from one to three nucleotides in an m-RNA chain will result in the synthesis of a protein with an abnormal amino-acid, but the introduction of one or two additional nucleotides in a sequence will destroy all the coded intelligence which follows and will have far-reaching effects. Changes in DNA structure can arise by deletion, addition or by substitution of nucleotides; they may also be brought about by transformation of bases *in situ*.

Not only can the pattern of protein synthesis be influenced by variations in the biological lives of diverse m-RNAs, but there is evidence that where one m-RNA codes for several proteins, some end-products are produced in substantially greater amounts. This observation is interpreted as indicating that ribosomes may attach themselves at several points along the m-RNA and may be able to translate some parts of the message at greater speeds or more frequently than others. It does not necessarily follow that optimum synthesis would be achieved if enzymes responsible for sequential stages of a multistage process were produced in equal amounts.

Thus it has been possible to recognize some of the factors which control the release of genetic information in bacterial cells; among these are the operators, repressors, inducers and co-repressors which probably control the formation of m-RNA. In addition there is evidence of some control of the translational stage acting either by variation of the biological life of individual m-RNA or by control of the rate of translation.

Cell Growth in Multicellular Organisms

Too great emphasis cannot be placed on the recognition that our present knowledge of molecular change at the cell level is based, almost exclusively, on the reproduction and growth of unicellular organisms. As in the case of bacteria, we have scant knowledge of factors which cause the duplication of chromosomal DNA in the cells of multicellular organisms and we can only presume that at cell division a similar mechanism is used for the transfer of genetic information to daughter cells. There is experimental evidence that the "transcription" of DNA-dependent RNA and the "translation" of m-RNA in protein synthesis follows the conventional path in the cells of higher organisms (references, Harris, 1968).

It is feasible that the local development and organization of cell growth is mediated by hormonal mechanisms under genetic control. Embryonic organizers or inducers have been described but not characterized and there is some evidence that the signal for morphological change in the developing embryo is triggered off in some way by physical contact between separate parts of the embryo. There is more precise knowledge of tropic hormones secreted by the anterior pituitary lobe, e.g. somatotropin, which are essential for organ development and growth although the mechanism of action of these hormones on cells is unknown. Finally, it is recognized that the so-called hormone-dependent tissues in the body respond only to stimulus by specific molecules. Although it is clear that in each case the stimulus results in cell division and growth, the mechanism of action is unknown; it is probable that the hormonal secretion is itself under genetic control.

Cell Differentiation

Although it is reasonable to suppose that the basic biochemistry of all cells is the same, two simple but fundamentally important features of cell division in the multicellular organism distinguish this process from the analogous event in bacteria. In multicellular organisms the daughter cells are not necessarily identical and they do not separate. Not only is this true of the first division of the zygote, but it continues to be true, with cumulative effect, at each somatic cell division. At an early stage of embryological development, the timing varies from species to species, fundamental cell differentiation begins, and this presages the extensive morphological development

found in the adult form. If this change in behaviour at cell division is genetically controlled, and at present there appears to be no alternative possibility, then the source of the genetic information has new dimensions in time and location. It is clear that certain types of cellular differentiation are delayed until the appropriate stage of embryonic development has been reached. As might be expected, the DNA content of the mammalian cell is very much greater (at least a thousandfold) than that of the bacterial cell and we have at present little conception as to how the stepwise control of embryological and juvenile development is organized.

A differentiated cell not only retains the ability to divide but is also able to transfer to daughter cells and subsequent progeny some imprint of its modified character. The effect can only be understood, in terms of present knowledge, as a modification of the genetic message and as there is no cytological evidence of change in the chromosomes, some change in the availability of genetic information may be responsible. One hypothesis, based on the recognition of the action of repressors, suggests that a differentiated cell is one in which a very high proportion of the available information is suppressed, resulting in the activity of the cells being canalized into the production of a limited range of proteins. In support of this idea there is evidence that some of the m-RNA molecules of highly differentiated cells are metabolically stable and therefore have a relatively long active cell life. The cells of the liver which are responsible for the synthesis of plasma proteins lie in this category and so do the primitive red blood cells responsible for haemoglobin synthesis. It is probable that cells which secrete the main digestive enzymes are specialized in this way. In each of these tissues study of the rate of incorporation of radioactive bases necessary for RNA formation show that the re-formation of m-RNA in these cells is slow.

Control of Growth in Multicellular Organisms

Growth in normal cells. The limited amount of data available on the regulation of growth in the cells of multicellular organisms does not permit even primary conclusions to be drawn. It is widely accepted that in these cells, as in bacteria, the DNA of the chromosomes acts as a template on which RNA is synthesized, and that this RNA passes, in some way, to the polyribosomes of the cytoplasm where it, in turn, acts as a template for the assembly of proteins; but on the question of detail of the steps involved and of the regulation of the process, many opinions are held. Of the two main hypotheses at present advanced, the "genetic operator model" supposes that control of genetic expression is exercised by regulation of the "transcription" of DNA-dependent RNA within the nucleus. Regulation of "transcription" may be achieved either by controlling the number of genes active at any one time, presumably by some repressor mechanism, or by selective control of the rate of transcription of different operons.

The alternative hypothesis, the "cytoplasmic operator model", suggests that control is exercised in the cytoplasm by regulation of the "translation" stage. This concept lays considerable emphasis on the duration of the active cell life of diverse m-RNA, for there are many ways in which attachment of the messenger to the ribosome could be limited and active protein synthesis affected (references, see Harris, 1968). Among many mechanisms which have been advanced as areas of possible regulation, the earliest is that of control of disengagement of RNA from the DNA template. Alternative mechanisms suggest forms of control which operate during the transport of m-RNA from the nucleus to the polyribosomes, either during passage through the nuclear-cytoplasmic membrane or during transport across the cytoplasm. One specific suggestion is that the cell life of m-RNA is regulated as a balance between the protective effect of carrier ribosomal protein and the hydrolytic action of nucleases in the cytoplasm. There is also clearly the possibility of regulation of the rate of translation at the polyribosomes. These ideas are largely speculative and much experimental work remains to be done before useful conclusions can be drawn.

Just as we are ignorant of the factors which initiate and regulate cell growth in multicellular organisms, so we are ignorant of the mechanism whereby cell growth is terminated. Whereas a bacterial cell will divide, separate and grow indefinitely in the presence of ample nutrient supply, cells of multicellular organisms are self-limiting in their growth characteristics. These cells do not separate but adhere to form a contiguous mass of cells which builds up to form an organ; when the organ reaches adult size, growth automatically ceases. The mechanism whereby this limitation is imposed is uncertain, but there is evidence, based mainly on the behaviour of cells in tissue culture, that contact between neighbouring cells provides the signal to limit cell growth. This lack of information on cell growth, regulation and inhibition is disappointing and sets a limit, for the time being, on any attempt to interpret the loss of control which characterizes the cancer cell.

Growth in cancer cells. In many respects the growth characteristics of cancer cells resemble those of normal cells so closely that differentiation at the cell level is impossible. Unlike many infectious diseases, where it is possible to combat infection by exploiting the fact that the invading cell differs radically from that of the host, in neoplastic disease the abnormal cells are descended from normal tissue cells and are genetically closely related. The similarity is so great that it may be impossible to differentiate neoplastic cells from the normal cells from which they arise on biochemical or functional grounds; thus, cells produced in neoplasia of the adrenal cortex contain the same group of specialized steroidogenic enzymes and secrete the same biologically active hormones as do normal cortex cells. Many claims have been made of qualitative and quantitative differences between normal and neoplastic tissues but even if such differences could be substantiated there is no way of telling whether they are causes or effects, and, if effects, whether they represent primary or distant consequences of changed cell metabolism. One of the most difficult aspects of such comparisons is the problem of finding a comparable normal tissue.

Although an outstanding characteristic of cancer cells is the escape from homeostatic growth control, it is not always possible at an early stage to distinguish normal from cancer cells purely on the basis of rate of cell growth. Tumours arise most frequently in developing or replacement tissues in which growth itself is accelerated; moreover the rate of growth of tumour cells varies considerably from the slow growth of benign tumours to the rampant growth of invasive secondary deposits.

The most outstanding single difference is that irrespective of site of growth, cancer cells continue to divide and grow in locations where normal cells in a normal environment would not. It cannot be asserted that normal cells in the same environment as the cancer cells would remain normal, for to do so would be to exclude the possibility that an environmental factor might be responsible for the abnormal behaviour of the cancer cells. This is still a possibility, and reports continue to appear suggesting that tumour growth is influenced by environmental factors (Bulbrook, Hayward, Spicer & Thomas, 1962) but the weight of the experimental evidence at the present time is against it and very strongly suggests that the abnormality is inherent in the cancer cell. Indeed, both normal and neoplastic cells are found in close proximity in a common environment. The difference between these two types of cells lies not so much in the kind of cell produced as in the extent and form of growth; the normal cell grows in conformity with a recognizable pattern and when this pattern is complete, growth ceases. In contrast, cancer cells recognize no pattern of growth and no terminal form.

Reference has been made to "contact inhibition" between normal cells whereby they appear to recognize the proximity of each other and set a limit to cell growth. There is considerable specificity about this type of response as contiguous but unrelated cells show less tendency to adhere to each other. This has been demonstrated *in vitro* by using dilute trypsin concentrations to prepare free kidney and liver cells and by re-incubating the mixed cells in the absence of trypsin. Under these conditions normal kidney and liver cells aggregate together in separate masses. Free kidney cells incubated in a similar manner with free cells from a malignant skin carcinoma form a mixed aggregate (Watson, 1965). In this respect, cancer cells behave as though they were foreign to most normal tissues; neoplastic cells which remain at the site of origin acquire the ability to invade and disorganize normal tissue development because of their failure to recognize the presence of other normal cells. Many such cells do not remain attached to the primary tumour site, but are carried via the blood and lymphatic systems to new sites where they establish new malignant secondary deposits.

The fact that cells are highly differentiated affords no protection against the onset of neoplastic disease. Because of this, cancer may arise in almost any organ and assume so many forms that it must be regarded as a family of diseases related by the common characteristics of invasiveness and loss of control of cell division. In one respect there is common ground in the behaviour of cells modified by differentiation and those that have acquired neoplastic characteristics, namely the manner in which the new features of the cell are transmitted to daughter cells, and all subsequent progeny. Both of these forms of cell modification appear to be almost irreversible.

THE AETIOLOGY OF CANCER

According to a current hypothesis, the cancer cell originates from a typical somatic cell as a result of a faulty cell division which creates a permanent modification of the genetic record. While the main features of the typical cell are retained, including basic biochemistry and function, the mechanism of cell control is destroyed and with this goes the specific contact recognition of

the neighbourhood of other cells. It may be that these two properties are linked or inter-dependent, for escape from homeostatic control always appears to be associated with invasive tendencies. The modified cell growing autonomously is unable to fit in with the organized pattern of development of the species and eventually produces a palpable mass of contiguous cells.

This concept of the cancer cell lays emphasis on the inheritability of the genetic fault, and the little that we know about the mechanics of cell division points to the importance of the transfer of genetic information during replication of the DNA molecule. However much errors of transcription and translation may affect the development of individual cells, there is no recognized way in which these processes can modify the transmission of genetic information at cell division. It is because these basic facts are widely accepted that current theories of carcinogenesis are based on the assumption that some change in the transfer of DNA genetic structure is involved.

Three such possibilities have been considered, namely incomplete replication of the DNA code, complete replication of the code but with some inherited repressor action which denies the availability of the complete record, and finally the inheritance of the complete DNA code with additional extraneous genetic information. Perhaps combinations of these effects are involved, for the antigenic response of many tumour cells—that is, the reaction of other cells to the macromolecules present in the tumour—suggests that while new antigens, not present in normal cells, are formed (extraneous effect), a number of antibodies present in normal cells are lacking in the tumour (incomplete effect) Zilber, 1958; Heidelberger & Moldenhauer, 1956).

Chemical Carcinogenesis

A large number of pure chemical compounds can induce tumour formation in experimental animals. Not all of these compounds are structurally related but many have features in common and fall into main groups, including nitroso compounds, aromatic amines, polycyclic hydrocarbons and alkylating agents, etc. Perhaps it is not surprising that a biological event as complex as cell division should be sensitive to chemical reagents, but outside the above groups there is virtually no common structural feature and it is difficult to conceive how any common mechanism can explain their interference with the genetic record. It is also difficult to understand why randomly scattered cells become neoplastic while the majority of cells remain normal. In general tumours caused by topical administration, particularly by polycyclic hydrocarbons, arise at the site of application, but the majority of active compounds can also be administered subcutaneously or systemically to produce tumours at remote sites.

Although no common mechanism of action has been proposed, tentative hypotheses have been advanced to explain the action of certain groups of carcinogens. The theory of somatic mutation suggests that these compounds induce chemical modification of the DNA genetic record, either by anomalous base pairing during transcription or by preventing the entire record from being copied. By way of example, many active carcinogens are alkylating agents which are capable of alkylating or methylating purine and pyrimidine bases in nucleic acids under *in vivo* conditions, a modification which could induce permanent and far-reaching effects on cell behaviour. Another class of carcinogens includes compounds with two reactive sites on the molecule, e.g. 1,2-3,4-di-epoxybutane and bis-(2-chloroethyl)-methylamine, which are thought to act not by anomalous base-pairing but by joining opposite strands of the DNA molecule by covalent links, thus preventing the complete untwining of the double helix in replication (references, Brookes & Lawley, 1964).

An alternative theory of action implies faithful copying of all sections of the DNA molecule except those coding for repressor molecules, and particularly that portion of the record which controls cell division and growth. When this theory was originally advanced it was thought that repressor molecules were nucleic acids, but now that it is reasonably certain that many are protein in nature, the theory suggests that the carcinogen combines with and modifies the repressor protein in such a way that control over cell division is lost.

A satisfactory theory of carcinogenesis must also be capable of explaining the differences between the antigenic responses of tumours and those of normal cells. Many of the carcinogenic compounds possess considerable chemical reactivity and may react with molecules other than polynucleotides. The immunological theory of carcinogenesis suggests that chemical carcinogens not only modify the DNA record but also acting as haptens combine with protein to form new antigenic species. It is remotely possible that protein responsible for the repression of cell division reacts in this way and loses its ability to restrict growth, but lack of experimental support makes this hypothesis unattractive at present. Many of the tentative explanations cover some of the experimental facts, but none embraces all.

Suggestions have also been made that carcinogenesis is a two-stage process, involving an initiating agent such as urethane or benz[*a*]anthracene which establishes the neoplastic growth, and a promoter, e.g. croton oil, which stimulates abnormal cell growth when applied even after a long interval of time (Salaman, 1958).

Alkylating Agents

A high percentage of the known carcinogens, in spite of structural diversity, can act as biological alkylating agents; the collection includes epoxides, ethyleneimines, S- and N-mustard gas analogues, lactones, methanesulphonates, etc. Many of these compounds are mutagenic and several have been shown to methylate RNA- and DNA- bound purine and pyrimidine bases *in vivo* and *in vitro* (Lawley & Brookes, 1961; 1963). The principal site of attack is at the N-7 position of guanine and to a lesser extent at the N-3 position of adenine. Alkylation, and specifically methylation, at these positions may lead to anomalous base-pairing in the replication and transcription stages, the sequence G—C being paired as A—T and vice versa. Even if only small sections of the polynucleotide strand were affected in this way the consequences of the mis-sense in the cell could be quite marked.

Nor is this the only site where error could arise, for in an analogous way errors of translation may occur as a result of methylation of the same bases in t-RNA molecules whereby the 3-unit code for specific amino-acid selection may be altered. The significant part played by methylated bases in preventing base-pairing is clear from the cloverleaf arrangement of typical t-RNAs shown in Fig. 24·3. Adventitious methylation could conceivably disrupt these highly selective molecules and change the anti-codon sequence at the m-RNA codon site.

Nitroso Compounds

Many nitroso compounds such as dimethylnitrosamine, diazomethane, N-methyl-N-nitrosourethane, etc. are powerful carcinogens affecting a wide range of organs and species. The compounds produce acute and chronic lesions and their high potency is demonstrated by the fact that some tumours are induced by a single administration, indeed, in some cases the incidence of tumours appears to be delayed longer than the apparent metabolic life of the carcinogen. Within 3 hr. of the administration of a single dose of dimethylnitrosamine (50 mg./kg. body wt.), changes in the fine structure of rat liver cells have been observed, beginning characteristically with the disruption of ribonucleoprotein of the endoplasmic reticulum. The same compound also induces tumours in the kidney of the rat and by a variation of the route of administration tumours have been produced in the lung and in the epithelial lining of the oesophagus and bladder. The type and location of tumour formation varies widely with the compound administered, the dose, the route of administration and the experimental animal used. In rats, low doses of dimethylnitrosamine induce tumours in the liver during long-term experiments, whereas higher doses produce kidney tumours in a shorter period of time. This diverse effect of a single compound is believed to be due to the liver being unable to metabolize large doses so that some spill over into the excretory system occurs and the carcinogen gains access to the kidney which is more sensitive and produces fatal tumours more rapidly than the liver. The nitroso compounds, although chemically very active, are not metabolically very stable and are thought to break down in tissue to form diazoalkanes in the first instance; these unstable metabolites undergo further change with the formation of methylene or methyl carbonium ions, which act as powerful alkylating agents. Like many alkylating agents, the nitroso compounds are mutagenic but unlike most alkylating agents they induce tumours in a wide range of tissues. The nitroso group which is common to all compounds of the class is almost certainly the carcinogenic radical, while the remainder of the molecule, the "carrier", is believed to influence the degree of penetration of different tissues. This may be a reflection of the solubility or permeability of individual compounds.

A current view is that these compounds induce neoplastic change by alkylation of nucleotide bases *in situ*. Support for this concept has been provided by the administration of [^{14}C]dimethylnitrosamine to rats and by incubation of this compound with rat liver slices. Radioactivity was incorporated into liver and kidney DNA and RNA, mainly as 7-methylguanine and also into protein fractions as methylated histidines (Magee & Schoental, 1964). Metabolic studies of [7-^{14}C] methylguanine in rats have shown some incorporation of this compound into systems synthesizing nucleic acids, i.e. RNA in liver and DNA in the intestine and foetus (Craddock, Mattocks & Magee, 1968). It is interesting to note the effect which oxidative deamination of DNA bases by nitrous acid (HO . NO, c.f. nitrosamines → —N . NO) might have on the replication of the DNA strand. Adenine would be deaminated to hypoxanthine, which would pair with cytosine instead of thymine; cytosine deaminated to uracil would pair with adenine instead of guanine; and guanine deaminated to xanthine would continue to pair with cytosine. This simple change of —NH$_2$ groups to —OH groups, even if it affected only a few nucleotides, would have a marked effect on the genetic record. Thymine and uracil bases in RNA do not carry amino groups and would be unaffected.

Aromatic Amines

This group of carcinogens has special significance because some members of the group are important industrially and are known to be active in man. Compounds recognized as hazardous to humans include benzidine, *o*-tolidine, *o*-dianisidine, 1- and 2-naphthylamine, auramine, 4-aminobiphenyl, etc., and many other aromatic amines have been shown to be carcinogenic in experimental animals (Clayson, 1962). While it is prudent to regard all compounds of this class as potentially dangerous, the most active compounds appear to have at least two aromatic rings and the position *para* to the amino group either substituted or forming part of the aromatic ring system. Any satisfactory theory of action must be able to explain why some members of this class of compounds are apparently non-carcinogenic.

Tumours formed by these agents are frequently found in the excretory system, especially in the bladder and this observation has prompted the suggestion that metabolites of the administered compounds are responsible for tumour formation. One metabolic modification which has been considered is hydroxylation on the N-atom (N-hydroxylation); many aromatic amines, especially when administered as the acetamide derivatives, undergo N-hydroxylation and there is some evidence that these metabolites are more active than the administered compounds. Thus the potent carcinogen, 2-acetamidofluorene, which causes cancer of the bladder and liver of dogs, cancer of the ureters and bladder in rabbits, and tumours of many tissues in mice, is found as the glucuronide of N-hydroxy-2-acetamidofluorene in the urine of these animals (Miller, Wyatt, Miller & Hartmann, 1961). Many other carcinogens in this group, including 2-aminofluorene, 4-aminostilbene and 4-aminobiphenyl, are hydroxylated in this way and here too it has been shown that the N-hydroxyl derivatives are at least as active as the corresponding parent compounds. On the other hand, aniline and 2-naphthylamine are hydroxylated by rat liver but are not carcinogenic in this animal. Some *o*-hydroxyarylamines are carcinogenic and it has been alternatively suggested that *o*-hydroxylation may also produce carcinogenic metabolites (Clayson, 1953). No single explanation fits all compounds, and in this connection it has been reported (Miller & Miller, 1960) that rats can convert N-hydroxy-2-acetamidofluorene to 2-amino-1-fluorenol and that rabbit liver *in vitro* can change N-hydroxyarylacetamides to the corresponding *o*-acetamidophenols. This is some evidence that the two metabolites which have been cited as active agents are sometimes inter-convertible. It is noteworthy also that N-hydroxy derivatives of arylamines (I) have structural features, in common with hydroxyl

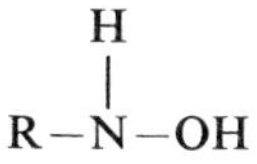

(I) 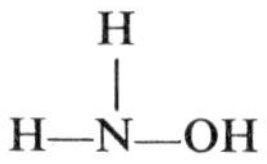 (II)

amine (II), a compound which reacts with the base cytosine, altering the molecule so that it no longer pairs with guanine.

The mechanisms of carcinogenesis proposed for aryl amines are still highly speculative. Suggestions that the parent compounds and their *o*-hydroxy derivatives form complexes with protein, with or without quininoid formation, do not appear to have very special significance. Similarly, evidence of interaction between *o*-hydroxy amines and nucleic acid *in vitro* offers no proof that this interaction occurs *in vivo* or that if it does, that it has any biological significance.

Polycyclic Hydrocarbons

Fusion of two or more benzenoid aromatic rings gives rise to a group of related compounds, the so-called polycyclic hydrocarbons, e.g. naphthalene, anthracene, phenanthrene, acridine, fluorene, etc. Not all the members of the group are carcinogenic, and although the earliest recognized chemical carcinogens are of this type, studies of chemical structure in relation to activity have been singularly barren. Several of the highly carcinogenic compounds are synthetic compounds which have not so far been found in nature, but at least two active compounds, benzo[*a*]pyrene and methylcholanthrene, have been found in natural products and are carcinogenic in man. The former compound has widespread distribution and has been found in coal tar, mineral oil, soot, cigarette tobacco tar, engine exhaust fumes and in the air of industrial towns (Harington, 1962).

It is not known whether these compounds are active directly or indirectly as metabolites, but as they frequently induce tumours at the site of administration the evidence favours the former mechanism; moreover, none of the known metabolites are carcinogenic. Because the group is large, and relatively few compounds have been subject to metabolic study, it is dangerous to generalize, but the most frequent form of metabolic attack, whether studied *in vivo*, or *in vitro* with microsomal preparations, appears to be the addition of the elements of hydrogen peroxide, across an aromatic double bond to form a glycol structure. This kind of addition reaction is often achieved biologically by the intermediate formation of epoxy compounds, many of which are carcinogenic, but in the case of polycyclic hydrocarbons no such epoxy compounds have been detected and the earliest recognized metabolic products are invariably no longer carcinogenic (references, see Boyland, 1964).

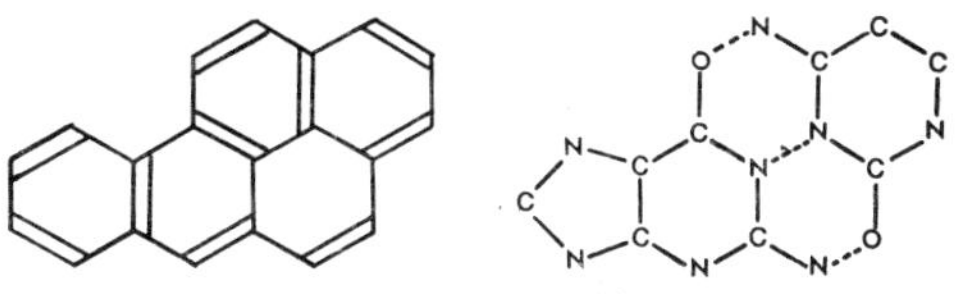

Benzo[*a*] pyrene   Guanine – Cytosine

Fig. 24.6. Superficial resemblance between the carcinogenic hydrocarbon benzo[*a*]pyrene and the base-paired structure between purine and pyrimidine nucleotides.

There is some evidence that polycyclic hydrocarbons can form complex molecules with purines and with DNA structures *in vitro*, but no *in vivo* experiments impart any physiological significance to these observations, nor has any attempt been made to correlate carcinogenic activity with polycyclic hydrocarbon-purine complex formation. Purely on theoretical grounds, Haddow (1961) commented on the superficial resemblance between the carcinogenic hydrocarbon benzo[*a*]pyrene and the base pair structure between guanine and cytosine (Fig. 24·6), suggesting that because interatomic distances were similar the intercalation of the polycyclic hydrocarbon between the twin helices of the DNA strands might occur.

CARCINOGENESIS BY VIRUS INFECTION

There is little doubt that some tumours arise as a result of virus infection of normal cells. At present the best documented examples are confined to species other than man, and perhaps the best-known are the Rous sarcoma virus (RSV) which causes tumours in chickens and the polyoma virus which infects the embryonic cells of many rodents. In addition, a related group of virus particles is almost certainly responsible for leukaemia in birds and mammals and possibly also in man. At the present time it is impossible to say what proportion of recognized tumours is caused by virus infection, as it is virtually impossible to locate and examine the primary interaction between virus particles and healthy cell *in vivo*. A more profitable approach is achieved by infection of somatic cells grown in tissue culture (Temin & Rubin, 1958; Vogt & Dulbecco, 1960).

Viruses exist only in parasitic association with living cells and they are dependent on the fine structure of the cells for their own reproduction. There is considerable variation in size and complexity, ranging from small bacteriophages, e.g. F2, Mol. Wt. 4×10^5, which are very dependent on host cell metabolism, to large and complex structures approaching the size of a small bacterium, e.g. smallpox virus, Mol. Wt. 4×10^9. All contain a central core of nucleotide genetic material surrounded by a protective coat. Unlike the cells which they infect, virus particles contain either DNA or RNA but not both. The viral polynucleotide may be single or double stranded but whatever the type, it normally exists in the form of a closed ring. The ring may be opened by artificial means but present evidence suggests that in this form the polynucleotide is not infective. The viral protective coat may be a single layer of small protein sub-units, as in polyoma, or a multi-layer protein coat incorporating lipid and polysaccharide structures.

Polyoma Virus

The polyoma virus has a circular double helix of DNA of low molecular weight which can code for not more than 10 protein molecules; it is spherical in shape and the infective core is surrounded by a geometrical arrangement of 72 identical protein sub-units. When the particle infects a cell the protein coat is jettisoned at the cell surface and only the DNA strand enters the cell, and subsequently the nucleus. Once in the nucleus, the virus may behave in one of two ways which may or may not be related; it is not possible to be sure on this point, since at this stage in each case the DNA strand becomes incorporated in the nucleus and is no longer recognizable. In the majority of infected cells the viral DNA plays a dominant role in directing the activity of the cell, supplanting the function of the cell genetic record and using the energy and metabolites stored in the cell to replicate its own DNA strands. These new strands code for the proteins characteristic of the virus and the synthesis is achieved on the endoplasmic reticulum of the cell. After an interval of time the cell is ruptured (lysed) and the newly formed virus particles are set free to infect other cells. In other cells, a relatively rare event may occur; after the incorporation of the viral DNA into the nucleus, the infected cell may not die but change radically and begin to divide and grow in a manner indistinguishable from a cancer cell. No infectious particles are produced by this type of cell and it is currently believed that within the tumour the polyoma DNA strand is integrated in some way with the host cell chromosome and that the combined genetic material dictates the behaviour of the new cell (Watson, 1965).

An analogy can be drawn between the behaviour of the viral DNA which infects a susceptible cell and some bacteriophages which invade so-called lysogenic bacteria. In the latter case the phage DNA is inserted into the host chromosome and to all intents behaves as part of it, being reproduced once at every cell division. There is experimental evidence which indicates that the incorporation of the phage DNA in the cell chromatin is achieved by the simultaneous breaking of host DNA and the viral circular strand, the broken ends rejoining to incorporate the linear phage DNA in the cell DNA strand. The phage DNA incorporated in the cell chromosome is called the prophage and it is extremely difficult to detect in this form; the only reliable evidence of its presence is when the prophage is rejected from the modified cell and begins to produce new virus particles by infecting other cells in the conventional way. No one has yet succeeded in recovering a virus particle from a polyoma-infected cell and the evidence of its presence is indirect, and is, in part, based on the immunological properties of the abnormal cell. Tumour cells produced by polyoma virus infection contain antigens which are absent from the healthy cell and which can be used to produce specific antibodies. These antibodies do not react with the normal cell or with the virus protein coat and the antigens which produce them seem to be coded for by a new sequence in the DNA strand (Sjögren, Hellström & Klein, 1961). It has been claimed that the antigens produced when the related virus SV.40 induces neoplastic changes in monkey cells are also present in infected cells reproducing the virus particle. A claim has also been made to have demonstrated the presence of integrated non-infective SV.40 virus in hamster tumours. A very small number of these cells, containing no detectable virus particles, inoculated into hamsters, produced tumours and, it is claimed, small amounts of virus (Sabin & Koch, 1963). It is assumed that the inoculum transferred viral genetic material in a non-infective state. Although such evidence is indirect and inconclusive, it provides a reasonable explanation why polyoma and related viruses induce tumours only in new-born or embryonic tissue (Stewart, Eddy & Borgese, 1958; Pietra, Spencer & Shubik, 1959). The ability to form antibodies is almost non-existent at the time of birth, so that the cells have practically no antibody resistance to infection and indeed any tumour virus present at this time may be accepted as homologous protein and may confer immunological tolerance towards subsequent virus infection (Billingham, Brent & Medawar, 1953). The ability of some host cells to survive infection by the virus is almost a necessity, since otherwise the host would die and the virus itself could not survive.

The smaller the virus particle, the less the genetic content of the DNA strand, the more dependent is the virus upon the endogenous sources of energy and metabolites in the host cell. Thus polyoma virus contains approximately 4800 base pairs and some single strand DNA viruses related to bacteriophage $\emptyset \times 174$ as few as 5000–6000 nucleotide units. This amount of genetic material is sufficient to code for not more than 1500–2000 amino-acid sequences, clearly insufficient to organize the synthesis of enzymes required for the formation of the micromolecules necessary for the formation of the DNA and protein of the new particles. One is forced to conclude either that the infective process is confined to actively dividing cells where the necessary micromolecules are already present or, if static cells are involved, that the virus must have some way of changing the cell metabolism and directing its synthetic activities into the required direction. It can be shown that the rate of DNA synthesis in virus T.2-infected cells is many times greater than that in non-infected cells.

Rous Chicken Sarcoma

The formation of tumours in chickens by Rous sarcoma virus is a more complex process. The Rous virus belongs to a group of so-called myxoviruses which vary considerably in size and are responsible for many diseases in animals and man, including mumps and influenza. Within the group, RSV is of medium size but is nevertheless many times greater than polyoma. The genetic material consists of a single-stranded RNA ring surrounded

by many protein subunits of different types and enclosed in a membrane composed of lipoprotein. Because of the presence of this lipid material in all members of the myxovirus group they are readily destroyed by lipid solvents such as ether and chloroform. The RNA strand of RSV contains about 30,000 nucleotides, more than sufficient to code for the protein sub-units of the coat, and it is probable that there are unidentified internal proteins which may or may not be active enzymes.

The reproduction of myxoviruses is unusual in that the host cell may be invaded simultaneously by several RNA strands, which are conventionally replicated in the nucleus and which use the cell polyribosomes to form proteins characteristic of the virus. However, the host cell is not lysed in the usual way, as the RNA strands associated with the newly formed proteins find their way to the cell surface and are budded off into the surrounding medium. This process does not necessarily cause cell death but changes the morphological form of the cell, so that in unrestricted cell growth and loss of contact inhibition it is indistinguishable from a malignant cancer cell.

Much of the early work with RSV was confused by failure to recognize that all RSV preparations were grossly contaminated by a related helper virus, Rous associated virus (RAV), which interferes with simple infection (Hanafusa, Hanafusa & Rubin, 1963). By means of modern tissue culture techniques it is possible to infect a susceptible chicken embryonic cell with a single RSV particle and under these circumstances some cells develop neoplastic properties but produce no new virus particles. The analogy between this stage and polyoma infection of mouse embryo cells is clear. Somewhat surprisingly, if the infection of the chick embryo tissue culture is carried out with a RSV preparation contaminated with RAV, cancer cell formation and virus production of RSV and RAV particles can go ahead simultaneously. The reason for these curious findings has been found in the demonstration that RSV is a defective virus unable to code for the synthesis of its own protective coat and only capable of being reproduced in the presence of a helper virus which supplies the protein layer. Experimental support for this theory has been provided by replacing the helper virus with a related virus (RIF) and demonstrating that the protein coat of the RSV particles is changed; in each case the coat is that of the helper virus (Watson, 1965). The helper viruses RAV and RIF will infect chicken cells, reproducing their type, but they do not induce neoplastic changes in the host cell.

The form adopted by the RSV RNA in infected

cells which are able to produce viral particles does not raise new problems, for although cellular RNA never acts as a template for the replication of RNA, a number of bacterial viruses are known which contain only single-stranded RNA ($+$) as a source of genetic information. These viruses on entering a host cell code for an enzyme not found in the healthy cell, which enables RNA replication to take place. The RNA twin helices then serve as templates for the synthesis of new single-stranded ($+$) RNA and new protein; as in the case of DNA-dependent RNA transcription, only the ($+$) RNA strand is formed.

The form adopted by the RSV in infected non-producing cells is much more difficult to ascertain, but is a problem, nevertheless, pertinent to the aetiology of cancer cells. If the viral RNA replicates itself in a non-producing cell as it does in a producing cell, then it is necessary to assume that at each mitotic cell division at least one particle enters each cell, for reversions from Rous sarcoma cells to normal cells have never been observed. Either so many replicates are present in the dividing cell that chance ensures the transfer of an infecting RNA molecule, or a mechanism exists for ensuring assembly of the infecting strands (RNA) at the axial plate as a normal cell chromosome. The alternative possibility is that the viral RNA is incorporated or transcribed as DNA into the host cell chromosome and is replicated as part of the host chromosome at each cell division. Such a mechanism would explain the inheritance of the neoplastic character by daughter cells but it creates a new precedent in that it supposes the transfer of genetic information in the direction of RNA to DNA to produce a mutation of the genetic record. No previous example of this reverse transfer of information (Fig. 24·5) is acknowledged but in support of the hypothesis is the claim that DNA isolated from RSV-infected cells contains nucleotide sequences complementary to those of the viral RNA. No such correspondence was found in DNA from non-infected cells.

DIFFICULTIES IN ESTABLISHING A UNITARY THEORY OF CARCINOGENESIS

The catalogue of carcinogenic chemicals already mentioned is by no means exhaustive, for many exogenous carcinogenic compounds are found in nature including the fungal toxins, e.g. aflatoxin and griseofulvin, the plant toxins, e.g. senecio alkaloids, insecticides, pharmaceuticals and even in simple metal-dextran preparations. There is little point in trying to discuss the mech-anism of action of such a heterogeneous collection of carcinogens in the light of the present inability to find a common mechanism of action at a cellular level for relatively simple chemical compounds. Even when it is possible, for example, to demonstrate the ability of an alkylating agent to modify a DNA strand, there is rarely sufficient experimental proof that it occurs *in vivo* at a cellular level and that the event is causally related to the subsequent appearance of a tumour.

A major barrier to progress, even in experimental carcinogenesis, is the remoteness in time and place between the carcinogenic stimulus and the neoplastic response. In an attempt to approach the cellular level, and to exclude as far as possible the complication of having, as *in vivo*, a mass of normal tissue, many studies are now carried out by somatic cell tissue culture. There is, however, some danger that experimental tumours maintained under these conditions may change in character from the original tumour line.

According to currently accepted ideas, the transfer of genetic information at cell division can only be expressed in terms of DNA structure and as long as the validity of this dogma is maintained, the vertical transmission of neoplastic growth characteristics in successive cell generations must imply some modification of DNA structure. Theories of chemical carcinogenesis usually suggest incomplete replication, due to repressor action or covalent linkage of DNA strands, or incorrect replication due to chemical interference with normal base pairing. In each case the daughter cell is a deficient cell, lacking some of the genetic information of a normal cell and possibly having some misinformation which interferes with the cell growth mechanism. In contrast, the virus theory of carcinogenesis implies the addition of genetic information to the host cell as provirus DNA incorporated into the host chromosomes; here again it is necessary to assume that modified information is responsible for the abnormal growth of infected non-producing cells. Either theory could explain the presence of new antigenic material in the neoplastic cell, but the virus theory, in its simplest form, does not explain the absence of some normal cell antigens.

According to supporters of the viral concept of carcinogenesis, chemical carcinogens either liberate or activate virus particles already in the susceptible cell.

ENDOGENOUS CARCINOGENS

In addition to the numerous exogenous compounds which can give rise to neoplastic growth,

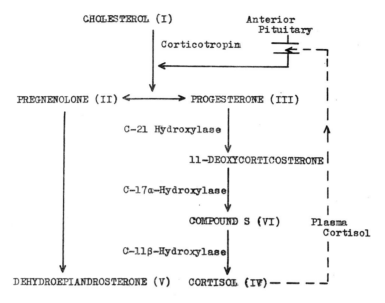

Fig. 24.7. Adrenogenital syndrome. Biogenesis of cortisol (IV) and dehydroepiandrosterone (V) with feed-back mechanism which inhibits the secretion of corticotropin.

Cholesterol (I); Pregnenolone (II); Progesterone (III); Compound S (VI).

there is reliable evidence that excessive amounts of some endogenous products can lead to hyperplasia, and occasionally to neoplasia. Many of the compounds which behave in this way are hormones, the secretion of which is controlled by homeostatic mechanisms. These compounds, e.g. thyroid factors, corticotropin and oestrogens, are responsible for growth and differentiation of endocrine glands or of hormone-dependent tissues, and it is the breakdown of the control mechanism which, somewhat infrequently, leads to overstimulation and hyperplasia. One of the best-understood examples of this type of abnormality has been recognized in adrenogenital syndrome.

Adrenogenital Syndrome

This relatively rare condition is characterized by adrenal hyperplasia and by the secretion of excessive amounts of androgenic steroids which in the foetus leads to pseudohermaphroditism, in the infant to precocious puberty and in the adult female to masculinization and hirsutism. Corticotropin secreted by the anterior lobe of the pituitary stimulates the growth and development of the adrenal cortex and as shown in Fig. 24·7 catalyses the conversion of cholesterol (I) to pregnenolone (II) and to progesterone (III). Within the cells of the cortex, pregnenolone is further metabolized by

independent routes to two products, one of which is cortisol (IV), a glucocorticoid, and the other dehydroepiandrosterone (V), an androgen precursor. The conversion of progesterone to cortisol involves the introduction of hydroxyl groups at positions C-11β, C-17α and C-21 of the steroid nucleus and the necessary steroid hydroxylases are present in normal adrenal tissue.

In recent literature, several cases of adrenal syndrome have been reported in which it has been possible to demonstrate the partial or complete inhibition of one or more of these hydroxylases essential for the biosynthesis of cortisol. Most frequently it is the activity of the enzyme responsible for the conversion of the penultimate metabolite (compound S, VI) to cortisol which is impaired, and this inhibition can be shown by the absence of normal cortisol metabolites from the urine and the presence of abnormal compound S metabolites (Mattox, Hayles, Salassa & Dion, 1964). As a net result of the biochemical lesion cortisol levels in peripheral plasma are subnormal. The neuro-hypophyseal region of the brain is sensitive to changing plasma cortisol levels; high concentrations suppress the secretion of the corticotropin by the anterior pituitary lobe and vice versa. Failure of adrenal hydroxylases leads, in this way, to excessive secretion of corticotropin, over-stimulation of the adrenal cortex and over-production of progesterone. Although the pregnenolone to cortisol metabolic route is inhibited, that leading to the formation of dehydroepiandrosterone is not, and this androgen precursor, produced in excessive amounts, causes masculinization. Provided neoplastic changes have not occurred, the clinical condition responds well to cortisol administration; abnormal metabolites disappear from the urine and, in the adult female, the symptoms of excessive androgen secretion slowly diminish. Further experimental evidence of the aetiology of this condition has been provided by the administration of metyrapone (2-methyl-1,2-di-3-pyridyl-1-propanone), a compound which selectively inhibits 11β-hydroxysteroid hydroxylase and which produces in experimental animals hyperplasia of the adrenal cortex and the other symptoms of adrenogenital syndrome (Dominguez & Samuels, 1963).

Hormone-dependent Tissues

That some advanced forms of neoplastic disease in humans are reversible is apparent from the seemingly genuine temporary remissions which have been obtained by the treatment of so-called hormone-dependent tumours with exogenous, antagonistic steroids. The effect is apparently confined to somatic tissues which, during normal growth, respond to hormone stimulation, e.g. the response of ovarian and breast tissue to oestrogens, but perhaps the best-documented cases relate to the treatment of carcinoma of the prostate with the potent oestrogen stilboestrol. Under this treatment it is reported that in a substantial percentage of cases there is relief of pain and objective evidence of the control of primary growth and the reduction in size of secondary deposits. The improvement is, however, only temporary and after an interval of time, which varies from case to case, growth in both primary and secondary deposits recommences. The tumour is then considered to be autonomous, i.e. no longer hormone-dependent (Huggins & Hodges, 1941).

The rationale of this therapy is that prostate cells, unlike most somatic tissues, respond to circulating androgen (testosterone) levels and although this is a normal physiological response, when neoplastic cells are present in the gland these, being genetically related, are also stimulated excessively to cell division and growth. At the present time it is considered that the administered oestrogen does not act directly on the prostate cells, although evidence on this point is not strong, but indirectly via the secretions of the anterior pituitary lobe. As in the case of corticotropin control, the hypothalamic region is sensitive to circulating oestrogen levels, high concentrations causing a reduction in the secretion of pituitary gonadotropins. In the male the interstitial cell stimulating hormone (LH) acts, in turn, on the Leydig cells of the testes which under normal conditions secrete testosterone. By this mechanism oestrogen administration is used to lower the level of circulating androgens and to exercise some control over neoplastic prostate growth. In a complementary but reverse way, androgen therapy (testosterone, methyltestosterone) is used to reduce circulating oestrogen levels in an attempt to exercise control over the growth of oestrogen-dependent breast tumours.

THE MOLECULAR BASIS OF HORMONE-DEPENDENCE

Recent experimental work has thrown considerable light on one aspect of hormone-dependent tissues. In a classical approach to this problem Jensen & Jacobson (1962) administered minute doses of high specific activity [6,7-³H]oestradiol (0.01–0.1 μg., 1–10 μC) to a group of immature female rats and studied the distribution of radioactivity in various tissues as a function of time. Radioactivity, expressed on a tissue weight basis, rose less rapidly in uterus, vagina and breast than in other somatic tissues, but the level subsequently reached was higher and this was maintained much longer than in other tissues. Although not more than 1 % of the dose accumulated in the uterus, the concentration of oestradiol in this organ (10^{-8}M) was greater than that in plasma (2×10^{-11}M) at any time indicating the presence of a selective absorption mechanism. Moreover, it was possible to demonstrate that the radioactivity in the uterus was due to unmetabolized oestradiol.

Similar tissue distribution experiments have been carried out with other oestrogenic and non-oestrogenic compounds. When [6,7-³H]oestrone was administered, the retention of radioacivity, though selective, was considerably lower than with [³H]oestradiol and examination of the radioactive material bound by the uterus showed considerable conversion of oestrone to oestradiol, suggesting that oestrone may only become active by metabolic conversion to oestradiol. Tissue distribution tests carried out with [6,7-³H]oestriol, which is a weaker oestrogen than oestradiol or oestrone, showed some binding of radioactivity by the uterus but radioactivity disappeared rapidly from the vascular compartment and the retention by the tissue was for a much shorter period than with oestradiol. Other compounds which are biologically active as oestrogens, including 17α-

methyloestradiol, 17α-ethynyloestradiol, and the non-steroid stilboestrol, showed a similar selective binding whereas testosterone, progesterone and 17α-oestradiol, a biologically inactive isomer of oestradiol, were not selectively retained (Jensen *et al.*, 1966). Puromycin and actinomycin D, which inhibit the synthesis of protein on the endoplasmic reticulum, do not interfere with the binding of oestradiol in this selective manner.

After the administration of [³H]oestradiol, autoradiography of uterine tissue sections shows radioactivity in both the endometrium (lamina propria) and the myometrium, with the concentration in the former being approximately twice that in the latter. Intracellular distribution showed radioactivity in both cytoplasm and nucleus but with some concentration at the cytoplasmic-nuclear membrane. Further insight into the distribution of radioactive oestrogen within the cell has been obtained by incubating homogenates prepared from the uteri of immature experimental animals, e.g. rats, rabbits and calves, with trace amounts of [6,7–³H]oestradiol. Under these *in vitro* conditions some radioactivity is bound to the homogenate which can then be analysed in terms of subcellular particles by high-speed centrifugation against a sucrose gradient. In this type of experiment the radioactivity is largely divided between the nuclear pellet and the cell supernatant fractions. Progress in studies of the nuclear-bound fraction has been disappointing but further analysis of the cell supernatant by gel-filtration and electrophoresis has shown the presence of two components with associated radioactivity; one particle, with a sedimentation constant of 9.5*S*, is apparently homogeneous and has the properties of specific oestrogen receptor, the other (3–6*S*) binds oestrogens, progesterone and testosterone in a much less specific manner (Toft, Shyamala & Gorski, 1967; Maurer & Chalkley, 1967). The 9.5*S* component has a molecular weight variously reported between 50,000–200,000 and is saturated with oestrogen at extremely low concentrations ($14 \times 10^{-7} \mu$M.) corresponding to a dissociation constant of 7×10^{-10}. Kinetic studies suggest that the oestrogen-binding sites are homogeneous, i.e. all of one kind, and on the assumption that they are uniformly distributed throughout the uterus, it has been calculated that this approximates to about 2500 sites per cell. The binding of [³H]oestradiol to the component is destroyed by proteolytic enzymes but not by deoxyribonuclease or by ribonuclease, enzymes which hydrolyse DNA and RNA respectively. The binding is heat-dependent, pH-dependent and is destroyed by agents which reduce —SH groups; in all these respects the 9.5*S* component behaves as though a substantial part of the molecule was protein in character. The binding occurs in the cold and does not require cellular organization or energy (Toft *et al.*, 1967).

Within half an hour of the administration of oestradiol *in vivo* to immature rats, it is possible to detect biochemical changes in uterine tissue *in vitro* which appear to be consequences of the binding of the hormone by the target organ (Hamilton, Teng & Means, 1968; Widnell, Hamilton & Tata, 1967). Early biochemical events include increased rate of synthesis of rapidly-labelled nuclear RNA and *de novo* synthesis of protein, events which might be interpreted as the initial steps leading to increased cellular proliferation. Excellent contemporary reviews of the work are available (Gorski, Noteboom & Nicolette, 1965; Korner, 1967; Hamilton, 1968).

These experimental results suggest that certain cells in the so-called hormone-dependent tissues of immature female animals remain dormant in the absence of oestrogenic stimulation. The cells contain specific receptor molecules which can bind very small amounts of biologically active oestrogenic compounds and that as a consequence there is new biochemical activity within these cells. It is not possible to associate this new cellular activity causally with the cell division and growth which characterize the recognized physiological response of the tissue to oestrogenic stimulation, but they are both consequences of the binding of oestrogens at the target organ, and they are conceivably related. The synthesis of DNA-dependent RNA and of protein are the kind of cell activity usually associated with cell growth. As it is possible to induce precocious development of secondary sexual characteristics in pre-adolescent animals, the receptor molecule may be present in the dependent tissue from an early stage of development.

A tentative hypothesis, advanced by Jacob & Monod (1961) to explain new cellular activity resulting from the appearance in the cell of new specific small molecules, is based on the assumption that the complete genetic record is present in virtually all cells, but that portions, and presumably substantial proportions, of the information are masked by repressor molecules. Specific molecules, e.g. oestradiol, gaining access to the nucleus combine with specific repressors and by so doing release additional genetic information which modifies cell behaviour. By analogy, the oestradiol or the protein-oestradiol complex must gain access to the nucleus and initiate cell division.

In this connection it is noteworthy that growth in the oestrogen-deficient uterus has been induced by treatment *in utero* with extracts of RNA prepared from uteri which had been stimulated *in vivo* by oestrogen (Segal, 1964; Segal, Davidson & Wada, 1965). In a related field Karlson (1963) has produced experimental support for the Jacob and Wood concept by showing that the steroid hormone, ecdysone, which brings about morphological changes in moulting insects, does so by stimulating RNA synthesis in the vicinity of the chromosomes.

The distribution of [^{3}H]oestradiol in cells of the uterine endometrium based on autoradiography is somewhat at variance with the results of high-speed centrifugation of endometrial homogenates; the former shows main concentration at the nuclear membrane whereas the latter suggests that a high proportion of the hormone is in the nucleus (Jensen, DeSombre & Jungblut, 1967). Jensen and his colleagues (Jensen, Suzuki, Kawashima, Stumpf, Jungblut & DeSombre, 1968) have examined the distribution of radioactive oestradiol in these cells at various time intervals after administration and have concluded that the supernatant receptor molecule (9.5S) behaves as a vehicle transporting oestradiol across the cytoplasm to the nucleus. Precisely what happens within the nucleus is uncertain, but there is some evidence that the 9.5S complex is transformed into a smaller (5S) oestradiol-containing particle.

A most significant aspect of the action of oestradiol on hormone-dependent tissue in relation to the study of neoplastic disease is that it appears to present a model system in which a specific and recognizable signal induces cell growth in dormant cells. Not only is there evidence that excessive administration of oestrogens to experimental animals induces tumours (Lacassagne, 1932) but it has been shown that oestrogen-dependent tumours can be induced in rats by the administration of dimethylbenzanthracene. Breast tumours produced in this way also appear to contain receptor molecules which specifically bind oestradiol (King, Gordon, Cowan & Inman, 1966).

The concept of receptor molecules which specifically bind hormones is not confined to oestrogens nor indeed to the steroid group. Homogenates of rat uteri also bind progesterone and testosterone on a receptor molecule which is clearly different from that which binds oestradiol (Toft, *et al.*, 1967) and the presence of a receptor molecule for testosterone derivatives in prostate tissue has also been reported (Anderson & Liao,

1968; Bruchovsky & Wilson, 1968). Recognized receptors for cortisol, aldosterone and thyroid factors have been described.

SUMMARY

In summary, it appears that cancer is an abnormal form of cell growth which can arise in almost any of the specialized tissues of the multicellular mammalian species. Because the affected cells retain their differentiated character, the abnormality presents itself in many forms and is best described as a family of diseases rather than a single entity. In contrast to the normal somatic cells from which they arise, neoplastic cells, although morphologically and functionally similar, appear to have lost the property of "contact inhibition" and they are no longer subject to the controls which limit cell division and growth in normal tissues. As a consequence of the defect, cancer cells are unable to fit into the normal pattern of organ formation but invade and disrupt local tissue at the site of origin; because of the loss of adhesive properties, cells may break away from the original cell mass and being carried in the blood and lymphatic systems to new sites, set up abnormal secondary growths.

It is significant that the abnormal growth characteristics of cancer cells are passed on to daughter cells formed by mitosis and the reversion to normal type cell at any subsequent generation appears to be a very rare if not an impossible event. In terms of what we know about cell division and the transfer of genetic information, the indirect evidence points strongly to the conclusion that the DNA structure of the cell chromosomes must in some way be modified. In human cancer, the onset of the first neoplastic change can rarely be traced and even in experimental cancer, which can be induced at will by a wide variety of agents, the response is often remote from the stimulus. The evidence available at the present time is insufficient to justify a unitary theory of carcinogenesis even though it is possible to imagine how some chemical carcinogens, some forms of virus infection or nuclear bombardment could alter the structure of the genetic material. The proof that some alkylating agents can methylate DNA, the demonstration that they do so *in vivo* does not necessarily establish this as the cause of the tumours which subsequently appear in a minority of exposed cells. The fault appears to be associated with the fidelity of the genetic record, and the lesion could quite easily have a biochemical basis. Whether or not we can establish the nature of this inherited defect depends, in part, upon whether or not we already understand that feature of cell division which is at fault. Any future work which adds to knowledge in the field of cell division and growth increases the chance of recognizing the basic cause.

References

ANDERSON, K. M. & LIAO, S. (1968). *Nature (Lond.),* **219,** 277.

BALDWIN, E. (1963). "Dynamic Aspects of Biochemistry". Cambridge Univ. Press, 4th Edit.

BESSIS, M. (1960). "The Ultrastructure of the Cell". Sandoz Monograph.

BILLINGHAM, R. E., BRENT, L. & MEDAWAR, P. B. (1953). *Nature (Lond.),* **172,** 603.

BLAKE, C. C. F., MAIR, G. A., NORTH, A. C. T., PHILLIPS, D. C. & SARMA, V. R. (1967). *Proc. Roy. Soc.* **B167,** 365.

BOYLAND, E. (1964). Polycyclic Hydrocarbons. *Brit. Med. Bull.,* **20,** 121.

BROOKES, P. & LAWLEY, P. D. (1964). Alkylating Agents. *Brit. Med. Bull.,* **20,** 91.

BRUCHOVSKY, N. & WILSON, J. D. (1968). *J. biol. Chem.,* **243,** 2012.

BULBROOK, R. D., HAYWARD, J. L., SPICER, C. C. & THOMAS, B. S. (1962). *Lancet,* **2,** 1238.

CLAYSON, D. B. (1953). *Brit. J. Cancer,* **7,** 460.

CLAYSON, D. B. (1962). Chemical Carcinogenesis. Churchill, London.

CRADDOCK, V. M., MATTOCKS, A. R. & MAGEE, P. N. (1968). *Biochem. J.,* **109,** 75.

DOMINGUEZ, O. V. & SAMUELS, L. T. (1963). *Endocrinology,* **73,** 304.

GURDON, J. B. (1962). *J. Embryol. exp. Morph.,* **10,** 622.

GURDON, J. B. & UEHLINGER, V. (1966). *Nature, (Lond.),* **210,** 1240.

GORSKI, J., NOTEBOOM, W. D. & NICOLETTE, J. A. (1965). *J. Cell. Comp. Physiol.* Suppl. 1, **166,** 91.

HADDOW, A. (1961). *Proc. Nat. Cancer Conf.,* **4,** 31.

HAMILTON, T. H. (1968). *Science,* **161,** 649.

HAMILTON, T. H., TENG, C-S. & MEANS, A. R. (1968). *Proc. Nat. Acad. Sci.,* **59,** 1265.

HANAFUSA, H., HANAFUSA, T. & RUBIN, H. (1963). *Proc. Nat. Acad. Sci. Wash.,* **49,** 572.

HARINGTON, J. S. (1962). *Nature, (Lond.),* **193,** 43.

HARRIS, H. (1968). "Nucleus and Cytoplasm". Clarendon Press, Oxford.

HEIDELBERGER, C. & MOLDENHAUER, M. G. (1956). *Cancer Res.,* **16,** 442.

HUGGINS, C. & HODGES, C. V. (1941). *Cancer Res.,* **1,** 293.

JACOB, F. & MONOD, J. (1961). *J. mol. Biol.,* **3,** 318.

JENSEN, E. V. & JACOBSON, H. I. (1962). *Recent Progr. Hormone Res.,* **18,** 387.

JENSEN, E. V., DESOMBRE, E. R. & JUNGBLUT, P. W. (1967). Oestrogen Receptors in Hormone-Responsive Tissues and Tumours, in "Endogenous Factors Influencing Host-Tumour Balance". Eds. Wissler, R. W., Dao, T. L. & Wood, S., Jr.: University of Chicago, p. 15.

JENSEN, E. V., JACOBSON, H. I., FLESHER, J. W., SAHA, N. N., GUPTA, G. N., SMITH, S., COLUCCI, V., SHIPLACOFF, D., NEUMANN, H. G., DESOMBRE, E. R. & JUNGBLUT, P. W. (1966). In "Steroid Dynamics". Eds. Nakao, T., Pincus, G. & Tait, J.: New York, Academic Press, p. 133.

JENSEN, E. V., SUZUKI, T., KAWASHIMA, T., STUMPF, W. E., JUNGBLUT, P. W. & DESOMBRE, E. R. (1968). *Proc. Nat. Acad. Sci.,* **59,** 632.

KARLSON, D. (1963). *Persp. biol. Med.* **6,** 203.

KENDREW, J. C., DICKERSON, R. E., STRANDBERG, B. E., HART, R. G., DAVIES, D. R., PHILLIPS, D. C. & SHORE, V. C. (1960). *Nature (Lond.),* **185,** 422.

KING, R. J. B., GORDON, J., COWAN, D. M. & INMAN, D. R. (1966). *J. Endocrin.,* **36,** 139.

KING, T. J. & MCKINNELL, R. G. (1960). "Cell Physiology and Neoplasia". University of Texas Press, p. 591.

KORNER, A. (1967). *Progr. Biophys. & Mol. Biol.,* **17,** 61.

LACASSAGNE, A. (1932). *Comptes Rendus,* **195,** 630.

LAWLEY, P. D. & BROOKES, P. (1961). *Nature (Lond.),* **192,** 1081.

LAWLEY, P. D. & BROOKES, P. (1963). *Biochem. J.,* **89,** 127.

MCKINNELL, R. G. (1962). *Am. Zool.,* **2,** 430.

MAGEE, P. N. & SCHOENTAL, R. (1964). *Brit. med. Bull.,* **20,** 102.

MAHLER, H. R. & CORDES, E. H. (1966). "Biological Chemistry". Harper and Row, London.

MATTOX, V. R., HAYLES, A. B., SALASSA, R. M. & DION, F. R. (1964). *J. clin. Endocrin. Metab.,* **24,** 517.

MAURER, H. R. & CHALKLEY, G. R. (1967). *J. mol. Biol.,* **27,** 431.

MILLER, E. C. & MILLER, J. A. (1960). *Biochim. biophys. Acta,* **40,** 380.

MILLER, J. A., WYATT, C. S., MILLER, E. C. & HARTMANN, H. A. (1961). *Cancer Res.,* **21,** 1465.

PAULING, L. & COREY, R. B. (1951). *Proc. Nat. Acad. Sci.,* **37,** 729.

PERRUTZ, M. F. (1962). "Proteins and Nucleic Acids: Structure and Function". Elsevier, Amsterdam.

PHILLIPS, D. C. (1968). Proc. of the Plenary Sessions, VII Internat. Congr. of Biochem., Tokyo, p. 63.

PIETRA, G., SPENCER, K. & SHUBIK, P. (1959). *Nature (Lond.),* **183,** 1689.

SABIN, A. B. & KOCH, M. A. (1963). *Proc. Nat. Acad. Sci. Wash.,* **49,** 304.

SALAMAN, M. H. (1958). *Brit. med. Bull.,* **14,** 116.

SCHLESSINGER, D., MANGIAROTTI, G. & APIRION, D. (1967). *Proc. nat. Acad. Sci.,* **58,** 1782.

SEGAL, S. J. (1964). *Anat. Rec.*, **148**, 334.

SEGAL, S. J., DAVIDSON, O. W. & WADA, K. (1965). *Proc. nat. Acad. Sci.*, **54**, 782.

SJÖGREN, H. O., HELLSTRÖM, I. & KLEIN, G. (1961). *Cancer Res.*, **21**, 329.

STEWART, S. E., EDDY, B. E. & BORGESE, N. (1958). *J. Nat. Cancer Inst.*, **20**, 1223.

TEMIN, H. M. & RUBIN, H. (1958). *Virology*, **6**, 669.

TOFT, D., SHYAMALA, G. & GORSKI, J. (1967). *Proc. nat. Acad. Sci.*, **57**, 1740.

VOGT, M. & DULBECCO, R. (1960). *Proc. nat. Acad. Sci. Wash.*, **46**, 365.

WATSON, J. D. (1965). "Molecular Biology of the Gene". Benjamin, New York.

WIDNELL, C. C., HAMILTON, T. H. & TATA, J. R. (1967). *J. cell. Biol.*, **32**, 766.

ZILBER, L. A. (1958). *Advanc. Cancer Res.*, **5**, 291.

INDEX

Anaemia, megaloblastic, folate deficiency, 195, 196
    following gastrectomy, 194
    in childhood, 195
    in sickle cell disease, 175
    of pregnancy, 196
  of chronic disorders, 161–163
  pernicious, 194, 459
    gastritis and, 547
  pyruvate-kinase deficiency, 167–168
  sideroblastic, 196–197
  spherocytosis in, 165
  urate increase in, 739
  vitamin B_{12} deficiency, 188–189
Anaesthesia, and the nervous system, 452–453
Andersen's disease. *See* Glycogenosis, type IV.
Androgens, action of, 315
  and thyroid gland, 429
  metabolism, 326–327
  secretion, muscles and, 510
  synthesis, pathways, 323
Angiokeratoma corporis diffusum, 629
Angiotensin, 244
  effect on aldosterone secretion, 269
  intra-renal role, 250–251
  measurement of, 244–246
  pharmacological properties, 244
  plasma levels in various clinical states, 246–250
  response of kidney to, in hypertension, 242
Angiotensinases, 244
Angiotensin-renin system, 242–244
Anion-exchange resins, 684
Antibodies, activity in urine, 531
  in auto-immune disease, 548
  synthesis, 529
  warm and cold, 546
Antibody combining site, 529–530
Anticonvulsant drugs causing anaemia, 196
Antidiuretic hormone, controlling urine flow, 263
  metabolism, in starvation, 22
Antigens, 524
  combination with antibody, 529
Antithyroid compounds, in thyrotoxicosis, 423
Appetite, 26, 27
Arginine, excretion, in cystinuria, 590, 592
Argininosuccinic aciduria, 580
Aromatic amines, as carcinogens, 842
Arrhenoblastoma, 811
Arteries, atheroma in, morphology, 636, 637
  fibrous plaque, 636, 637
  in atherosclerosis, 637
Arylsulphatase, 475
Ascites, in liver disease, 152
Atherosclerosis, 635–659
  aetiology, 637
  blood platelets in, 645–647
  diagnostic tests, 644–645
  dietary aspects, 648–653
  due to hyperlipaemia, 620
  hereditary aspects, 645
  hypercholesterolaemia and, 639–640
  lipid metabolism, 636, 637, 638, 639
  morphology, 635–637

Atherosclerosis, oestrogens and, 654
  plasma enzyme studies, 650–651
  plasma lipids in, 641–644
  preventive measures, 651
  thrombosis and, 647
  thrombotic theory, 638
  use of drugs, 653–656
Atromid, reducing plasma lipids, 654
Autoimmune disease, 543–549

BAL in porphyria, 226
Bacterial infection, causing hepatic necrosis, 145
  immunoglobulin levels in, 533
Bantu porphyria, 216, 226, 229
Basal metabolic rate, 396
  and body composition, 7
  in starvation, 21
Bassen-Kornzweig disease, 622
Bence Jones protein, metabolism, 540
  structure, 539
Benzopyrene, as carcinogen, 843
Benzothiadiazines, effect of insulin secretion, 43–44
Beri-beri, 458, 461
Beta thalassaemia major and minor, 177
Bicarbonate, and diffusion of ammonia, 678
  excretion, 271–272
  in colon, 668
  in pancreas, 667, 709
  in saliva, 665
Bicarbonate ions, in body fluids, 10
Bielschowsky disease, 627
Bile, 662, 666–667
  circulation of, 697, 699
Bile acids, 695
  and cholestrol metabolism, 648, 698–699
  in liver disease, 698
  in serum, 697–698
  primary and secondary, 696–697
Bile ducts, obstruction of, 137
Bile pigments, constitution of, 129–130
  metabolism, 129–133
  origin of, 129, 131
Bile salts, in intestine, 699–700
  metabolism, abnormalities of, 695–701
  relation to fat digestion, 689
Biliary cirrhosis, primary, 136, 617
  xanthomatous, lipid metabolism in, 617
Biliary obstruction, 698
Bilirubin, and kernicterus, 138
  change in liver, 130
  diazo reaction, 132
  early, 131–133
  metabolism, 129, 130
  over-production of, 134
Bladder, cancer of, 842
Blood, amino acids in, 555
    in Hartnup disease, 593
    in Wilson's disease, 599
  assay of oestrogens in, 818
  bile acids in, 697–698
  bioassay of gonadotropin in, 815

Progesterone, assay of, 818–820
  biosynthesis of, 310, 311, 312
  metabolism, 326
Prolinuria, 595
Propanolol, in hyperthyroidism, 424
Prostaglandins, 251
  atherosclerosis and, 649–650
  fatty acids as precursors, 649
Prostate, carcinoma, 302–303, 848
Protein, absorption, 694
  amounts in body, 2, 17
  contractile, in muscle, 491
  deficiency, causing acute yellow atrophy, 147
    causing liver necrosis, 146
  in liver in kwashiorkor, 29
  in muscle during atrophy, 498
  in nerve degeneration, 456
  in pancreas, 707, 708–709
  intake, effect on amino acid excretion, 555
  in tissue in phenylketonuria, 562
  iodo-, 385–388
  loss of in muscle, 30
  malabsorption, 694
  metabolism, action of cortisol, 313
    effect of glucagon on, 60–61
    effect of glucocorticoids, 57
    effect of insulin, 54, 55
    excretion of end products, 260–262
    in acute renal failure, 294
    in Addison's disease, 330–331
    in haemodialysis, 295
    in hyperthyroidism, 419
    in kwashiorkor, 28–30
    in nephrotic syndrome, 280–281
  monoclonal, pathological effects, 538, 542
  structure of in cell, 830
  synthesis in hyperthyroidism, 420
    in myxoedema, 412
  translation of, 834
Protein-calorie malnutrition, 27–31
  folate deficiency, 195–196
Protein-bound iodine, 397–398
  effect of certain drugs, 399
Protein flocculation tests, 139
Proteinuria, 276–278
  classification, 277
  in glomerulonephritis, 281
  in nephritis, 278
  in nephrotic syndrome, 279, 280–281
  non-selective, 281
  production of, 277
Protoporphyria, 216
  erythropoietic, aetiology, 226
  diagnosis, 229
Protoporphyrin, 217, 218, 219, 220
Protozoal infection, causing hepatic necrosis, 145
  immunoglobulin levels in, 533
Pruritis, in biliary obstruction, 698
  in liver disease, 151–152
Pseudogout, 734, 741
Pseudo-hermaphroditism, 344

Pseudohypoparathyroidism, 778
  calcitonin in, 776
Psychological factors, in obesity, 24
Pteroylglutamic acid, 182, 183
Puberty, delayed, 806
  precocious, 803–804, 808
Purgatives, addiction to, 675
Purine biosynthesis, 184
Purine metabolism, 736–738
Pyelonephritis, 285–286
Pyloric stenosis, 673
Pyridoxine deficiency, 197
Pyrimidine biosynthesis, 185
Pyrophosphate, in bone calcification, 755
Pyruvate, levels, in diabetes, 464
  in multiple sclerosis, 470
  in muscular activity, 470
  in periodic paralysis, 506
  in polyneuritis, 458, 460, 461
  in porphyria, 226
  in subacute combined degeneration of cord, 459
  metabolism in Fanconi syndrome, 597
Pyruvate-kinase deficiency, 167
Pyruvate tolerance test, 461

Radium poisoning, 789–790
Receptors, action of catecholamines on, 362, 366–367
Refsum's syndrome, 476, 618, 622
Renal artery lesions, causing uraemia, 290
Renal artery stenosis, 235, 248, 249
Renal blood flow, 257
Renal clearance tests, 256
Renal clearances, 256
Renal cortical necrosis, 290
Renal disease, associated with bone disease. See Uraemic osteodystrophy.
Renal failure, acute, 289–295
  treatment, 293–294
  chronic, 286–289
  urea in intestine in, 680
  use of ion-exchange resins, 683
Renal function, in multiple myelomatosis, 542
  in starvation, 22
  tests, 273–276
Renal glycosuria, 260, 297
Renal hypercalcuria, 763
Renal osteodystrophy, 297, 298
Renal transplantation, biochemical aspects, 288–289
Renal tubular acidosis, 297, 781
Renal tubular syndromes, 297–299
Renin, 242–243
  activity, in aldosteronism, 352
    in hyperaldosteronism, 348, 349, 351
    in pregnancy, 351
  and sodium excretion, 269
  inhibitor, 243
  intra-renal role, 250–251
  measurement of, 244–246
  plasma levels, in clinical states, 246–250
    in Conn's syndrome, 235
    normal, 247

PRINTED IN GREAT BRITAIN BY THE WHITEFRIARS PRESS LTD.
LONDON AND TONBRIDGE